图书在版编目(CIP)数据

黄帝内经:汉英对照/吴连胜、吴奇译.—北京:中国科学技术出版社,1997
ISBN 7-5046-2231-1

Ⅰ.黄… Ⅱ.吴… Ⅲ.黄帝内经-汉、英 Ⅳ.R221

中国版本图书馆 CIP 数据核字(97)第 06227 号

责任编辑:许 英 周跃庭
封面设计:麻仲学
正文设计:麻仲学
责任校对:梁艳红
Editor-in-charge by Xu Ying and Zhou Yaoting
Cover design by Jeffrey Z. X. Ma
Content design by Jeffrey Z. X. Ma
Proofread by Liang Yanhong

中国科学技术出版社出版
北京海淀区白石桥路 32 号 邮政编码:100081
新华书店北京发行所发行 各地新华书店经售
北京久恒文化科技公司照排
北京市艺辉胶印厂印刷
*
开本:787×1092 毫米 1/16 印张:53.25 字数:1336 千字
1997 年 12 月第 1 版 1997 年 12 月第 1 次印刷
印数:1—1500 册 定价:168.00 元

Yellow Empero's Canon of Internal Medicine

黄帝内经

(汉英对照)

Original Writer:(Tang Dynasty) Bing Wang
Englished by: Nelson Liansheng Wu, Andrew Qi Wu

原著:王 冰(唐)
英译:吴连胜 吴 奇

China Science & Technology Press
中国科学技术出版社
·北 京·

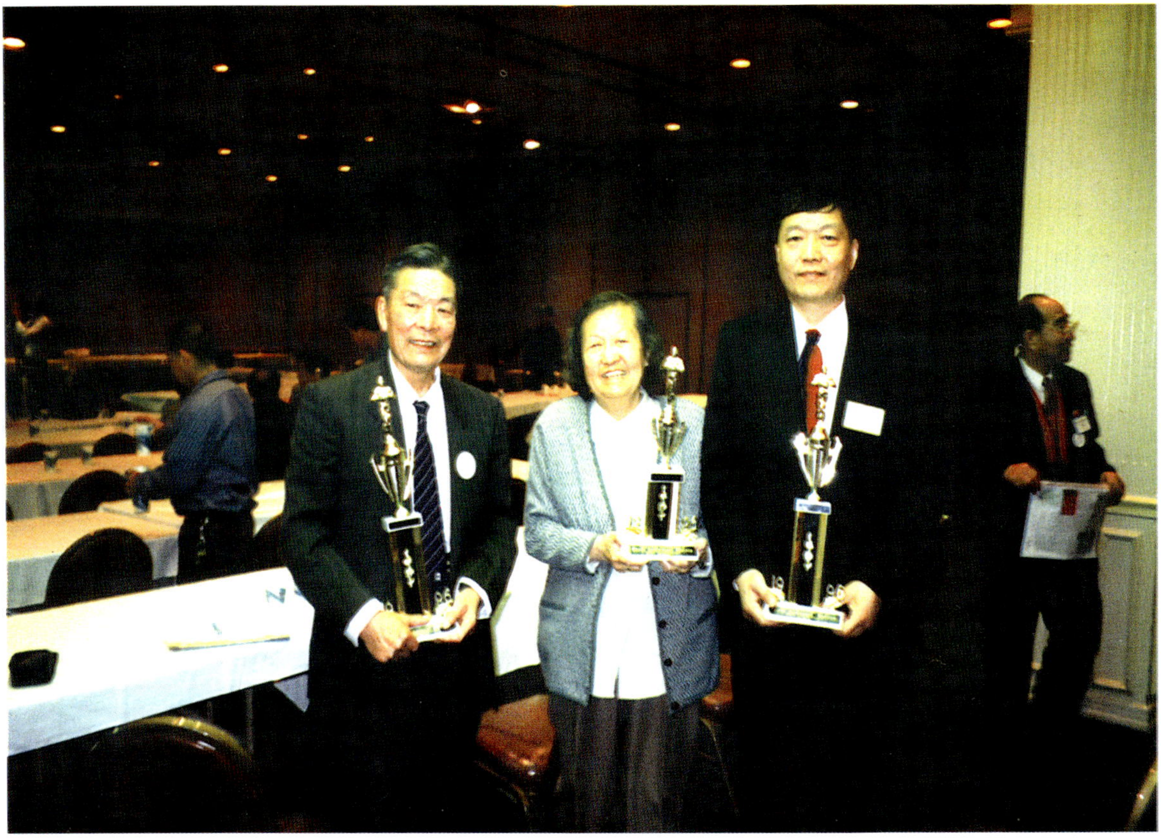

吴连胜（左）和他太太及儿子出席1996年在美国内华达州拉斯维加斯举行的第三届世界传统医学大会。

Mr. Nelson Liansheng Wu (left), his wife and son were in the Third Conference on the World Traditional Medicine at Las Vegas, Nevada, U.S.A., 1996.

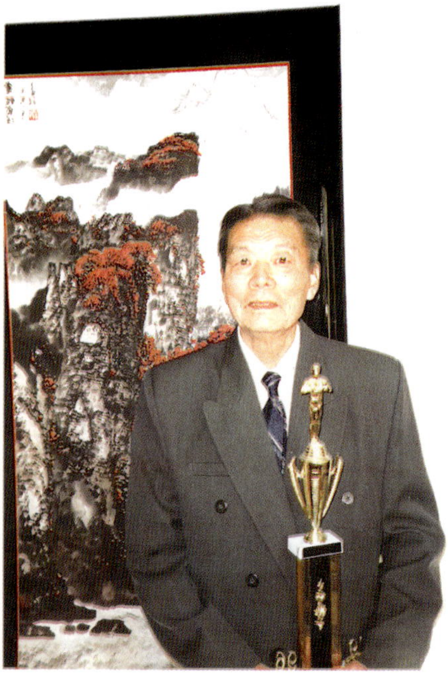

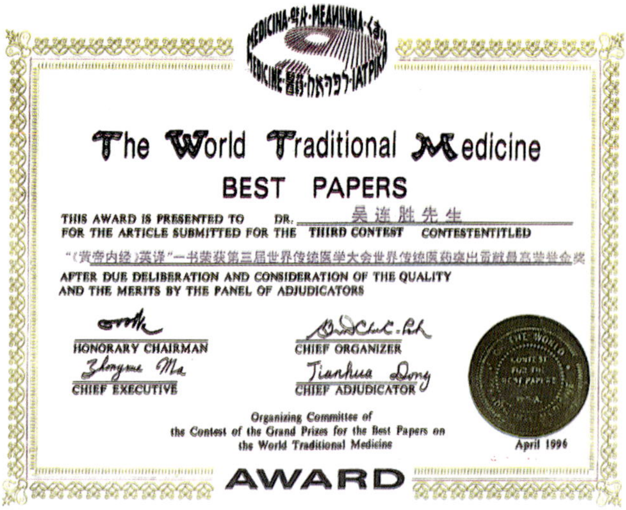

吴连胜先生所译《黄帝内经》一书，荣获第三届世界传统医学大会最高荣誉金奖。

Yellow Empero's Canon Internal Medicine, translated by Mr. Nelson Liansheng Wu, was awarded a gold medal of honor at the Third Conference on the World Traditional Medicine.

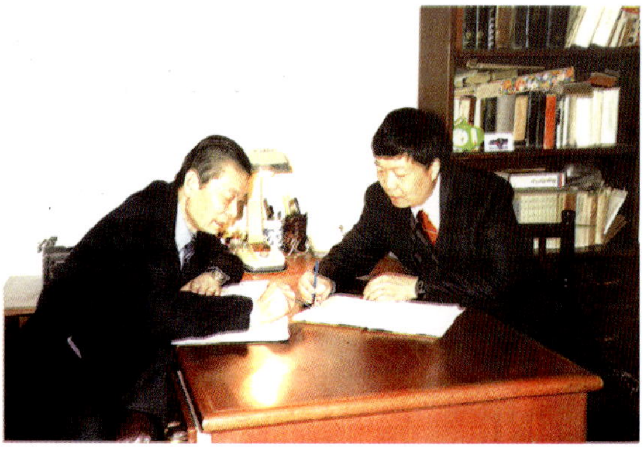

吴连胜先生和他的儿子吴奇医生在一起探讨中医理论。

Mr. Nelson Liansheng Wu and his son, Mr. Andrew Qi Wu are discussing the theories of traditional Chinese medicine.

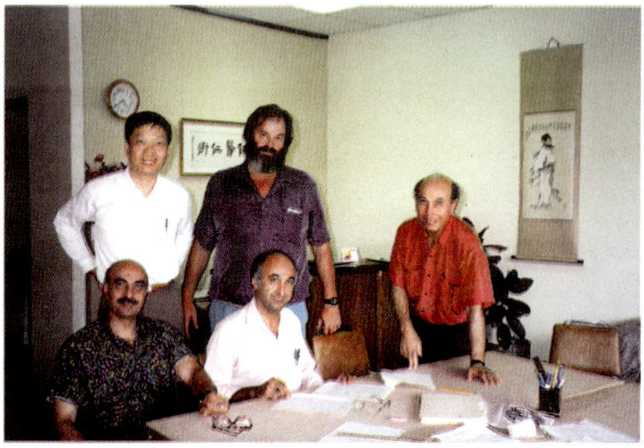

吴奇医生在美国他的中医诊所里，同他的学生们在一起。

Mr. Andrew Qi Wu and his students in his own clinic of traditional Chinese medicine in USA.

目　　录

Contents

素　　问

Su Wen

(Plain Questions)

评热病论篇第三十三
Chapter 33　Ping Re Bing Lun
　　　　　　(On Febrile Disease) ……………………………………………… (167)

逆调论篇第三十四
Chapter 34　Ni Tiao Lun
　　　　　　(On Maladjustments) …………………………………………… (171)

疟论篇第三十五
Chapter 35　Nüe Lun
　　　　　　(On Malaria) ……………………………………………………… (174)

刺疟篇第三十六
Chapter 36　Ci Nüe
　　　　　　(On Treating Malaria with Acupuncture) …………………… (182)

气厥论篇第三十七
Chapter 37　Qi Jue Lun
　　　　　　(The Diseases Due to the Intertransference of Cold and Heat Evils
　　　　　　Between Various Organs) …………………………………………… (186)

咳论篇第三十八
Chapter 38　Ke Lun
　　　　　　(On Cough) ……………………………………………………… (188)

举痛论篇第三十九
Chapter 39　Ju Tong Lun
　　　　　　(On the Pathology of Pain)
　　　　　　　…………………………………………………………………… (191)

腹中论篇第四十
Chapter 40　Fu Zhong Lun
　　　　　　(On Abdominal Diseases) ………………………………………… (196)

刺腰痛篇第四十一
Chapter 41　Ci Yao Tong
　　　　　　(The Pricking Therapy for Lumbago of Various Channels) ……… (200)

风论篇第四十二
Chapter 42　Feng Lun
　　　　　　(On Wind-evil) …………………………………………………… (204)

痹论篇第四十三
Chapter 43　Bi Lun
　　　　　　(On Bi-disease) …………………………………………………… (208)

痿论篇第四十四
Chapter 44　Wei Lun
　　　　　　(On Flaccidity) …………………………………………………… (213)

厥论篇第四十五
Chapter 45　Jue Lun

灵　枢
Ling Shu
(Spiritual Pivot)

序

王冰撰

夫释缚脱艰，全真导气，拯黎元于仁寿，济羸劣以获安者，非三圣道则不能致之矣。孔安国序《尚书》曰：伏羲、神农、黄帝之书，谓之三坟，言大道也。班固《汉书·艺文志》曰：《黄帝内经》十八卷，《素问》即其经之九卷也，兼《灵枢》九卷，乃其数焉。虽复年移代革，而授学犹存，惧非其人，而时有所隐，故第七一卷，师氏藏之，今之奉行，惟八卷尔。然而其文简，其意博，其理奥，其趣深，天地之象分，阴阳之候列，变化之由表，死生之兆彰，不谋而遐迩自同，勿约而幽明斯契，稽其言有徵，验之事不忒，诚可谓至道之宗，奉生之始矣。

Preface

Wang Bing

In releasing the bundages, overcoming of troubles, the preservation of one's natural state, the dredging of the breath, the rising of the great multitude to benevolence and long life, the guiding of the feeble and weak to attain tranquility, they can only be accomplished by using the methods of the three sages. The preface to《Book of History》(Shang Shu) by Kong An Guo said that the writings of Fu Xi, Shen Nong and the Yellow Emperor were called the "Three Mounds", and they were discussing the great way. In the treatise on the《Canons and Literature of History. Han Dynastry》, Ban Gu listed the Yellow Emperor's Canon of Internal Medicine in 18 rolls of which the "Plain Questions"(Su Wen) is 9 rolls and the "Spiritual Pivort"(Ling Shu) is 9 rolls, they made up the number of 18 rolls of the canon.

Although the years have changed and the age is different, yet the words have been held together and have been taught as a subject of study, so that, this book is still preserved. It was feared that the the wrong person might get the information, so, at times, some parts of it were hidden. And thus, the seventh roll was hidden by Master Shi, and the book "Plain Questions" we have now has only 8 rolls.

Be it as it may, yet its style is concise, its ideas are vast, its principles are recondite and its purpose is profound. With the help of it. The phenomena of heaven and earth are distinquished, the state of Yin and Yang are set forth, the causes of change are exhibited, and the symptoms of death or survival of the patient are made plain. It is not necessary to deliberate over these principles with others, they are unanimous far and near, and the implicitness is in perfect accord. If you examine the words in this document, you will find that they contain proof; if you test the facts, there will be no errors, thus, it can really be called the source of

the first principle and the beginning of preserving one's life.

假若天机迅发，妙识玄通，蒇谋虽属乎生知，标格亦资于诂训，未尝有行不由迳，出不由户者也。然刻意研精，探微索隐，或识契真要，则目牛无全，故动则有成，犹鬼神幽赞，而命世奇杰，时时间出焉。则周有秦公，魏有张公、华公，皆得斯妙道者也。咸日新其用，大济蒸人，华叶递荣，声实相副，盖教之著矣，亦天之假也。

Even if one has spontaneous natural talents, profound and wonderful knowledge, nevertheless he is still in need of texual and philological elucidations to put into exemplary form. One can not walk if there is no path, and one can not leave if there is no door.

Yet, if one concentrates his attention upon the research on the essence and traces the implicit and hidden sources of things, or knows truly the important features of this document, he will be able to know thoroughly the essentials like an expert chef, when slaughtering a cow, can see only the chinks of bones and muscles of the cow instead of seeing only the whole body of the cow, and he will be successful as if he had the mysterious assistance of the spirits and gods. In the past, many people were remarkable and were famous for a generation from time to time. Such as, in Zhou dynasty, there was his excellency Qin Yueren (about 220 B. C.), in Wei dynasty, there was his excellency Zhang Daoling (156 A. D.) and his excellency Hua Tuo (died 220 A. D.), all of them daily renewed their applications of the principles and greatly added the multitude of people, their brilliant foliage become florious, their reputation matched reality, which was, in all probability, achieved by their teaching and was also the bestowal of heaven.

冰弱龄慕道，夙好养生，幸遇真经，式为龟镜。而世本纰缪，篇目重叠，前后不伦，文义悬隔，施行不易，披会亦难，岁月既淹，袭以成弊。或一篇重出，而别立二名；或两论并吞，而都为一目，或问答未已，别树篇题；或脱简不书，而云世阙；重《合经》，而冠《针服》，并《方宜》而为《欬篇》，隔《虚实》而为《逆从》，合《经络》而为《论要》，节《皮部》为《经络》，退《至教》以《先针》，诸如此流，不可胜数。且将升岱岳，非迳奚为，欲诣扶桑，无舟莫适。乃精勤博访，而并有其人，历十二年，方臻理要，询谋得失，深遂夙心。时于先生郭子斋堂，受得等候师张公秘本，文字昭晰，义理环周，一以参详，群疑冰释。恐散于末学，绝彼师资，因而撰注，用传不朽，兼旧藏之卷，合八十一篇，二十四卷，勒成一部，冀乎究尾明首，寻注会经，开发童蒙，宣扬至理而已。

I, Wang Bing, admired the Way and always loved the care of one's health in my youth. Fortunately, I happened to come upon the Canon of the Yellow Emperor whose function was that of a mirror which can guide the treating. But the popular copies were disordered, there were duplications in the tables of contents, the first and the last parts of the book contradictory to each other, the words and their meaning were disparate, so that it was difficult to apply it in teaching and it was difficult to read and understand. These errors have been retained for years and they have been repeated so that they have produced corruptions of the text. Sometimes, one chapter appeared twice, and was given a different title. Sometimes, two discussions were combined, and one heading was given to both, Sometimes, when the answer to a question had not yet been completed, a title of a separate chapter was set up. Sometimes

the slips for writing had disappeared or were not written out, and the writer said, for example, "This age lacks such and such materials", The chapter of "On Channels" was repeated and titled as "The Needle". The "Proper Recipe" was absorbed to become the chapter of "The Cough". The chapter "Asthenia and Sthenia" was separated and named as "Adverseness and Agreeableness". The chapter "Channels and Collaterals" was titled as the "Important Discussion", and the "Part of Skin" simplified into "Channels and Collaterals". In this way, the supreme teaching was held back and the use of the needle was put in front. Matters of this sort were countless.

Any one who desires to ascend the Tai Yue (the Tai Mountain) can not succeed without a road; anyone who wishes to travel to Fu Sang (Japan) can not arrive there without a ship. So, I investigated diligently the original text and visited extensively the persons who could help me. After twelve years of study, now I finally understand the principles. I inquired into the right points and into the wrong points and the results satisfy my old desire.

I received the original secret, hidden edition of the foremost master, his excellency Zhang Zhongjing at the home of my teacher Guo Zi Zhai, The writing in this text is very clear, the principle and the reasoning of his texture are well-rounded; and by making use of it for purposes of interpretation, many doubtful points have disappeared like melted ice. As I am afraid his text may be lost in my hands and that, as a consequence, the teaching material will disappear, I wrote a commentary to it in order to perpetuate it eternally. I combined it with the text in my possession into one book of eighty-one chapters and twenty-four rolls. It is my intention to investigate the tail in order to understand the head, to investigate the commentaries in order to understand the classic, to develope the medical knowledge for the young men, and to spread widely the highest principles.

其中简脱文断，义不相接者，搜求经论所有，迁移以补其处，篇目坠缺，指事不明者，量其意趣，加字以昭其义。篇论吞并，义不相涉，阙漏名目者，区分事类，别目以冠篇首。君臣请问，礼仪乖失者，考校尊卑，增益以光其意。错简碎文，前后重叠者，详其指趣，削去繁杂，以存其要。辞理秘密，难粗论述者，别撰《玄珠》，以陈其道。凡所加字，皆朱书其文，使今古必分，字不杂糅，庶厥昭彰圣旨，敷畅玄言，有如列宿高悬，奎张不乱，深泉净滢，鳞介咸分，君臣无夭枉之期，夷夏有延龄之望，俾工徒勿误，学者惟明，至道流行，徽音累属，千载之后，方知大圣之慈惠无穷。时大唐宝应元年岁次壬寅序

Some paragraphs of this book in the original text are missing and its writing is interrupted, hence, the meaning of the different paragraphs cannot be combined. I tried to find the missing part for the classics and essays and transplanted them in order to fill the gaps. In this original edition some titles and topics have been lost, and there is no clarity in the explanations, thus, I guessed their meanings and clarified them by adding words. There is also some confusion in regard to different parts of chapters and their contents, in such cases of confusion, the contents of the successive sentences are not related to each other, and sometimes, there are titles missing; hence, I divided and arranged them according to classifications and gave them new titls.

The text consists of conversation of the emperor with his minister. Their conversations are not always in accordance with etiquette; in such cases, I added some words in order to shed light upon their exalted and humble position. There are also some wrong paragraphs and confused characters and some of which are overlapping; I attempted to determine their meaning and omitted those confused and overlapping parts in order to preserve the essential portions. The meaning of some words is very deeply hidden and it is difficult to explain them cursorily, hence, I am writing another book by the name of Xuan Zhu (Pearls of Mystery) to explain the meanings. All the words which were added by me are written in red, the purpose of which is to distinguish between the new and the old and to prevent confusion between the words.

All my efforts made with the purpose of clarifying the text to fulfil the loyal hopes and wishes of the Emperor and to bring out the profound words in such a way that they are like star suspended high in the sky where the Kui star cannot be confused with the Zhang star, and that they are like a deep well which is so clear that one can distinguishing fishes and turtles under the water. I also wish to prevent the Emperor and his subordinates from dying young and to give both the barbarrians and the Chinese the hope of prolonging their lives, and to clarify matters for the learners and to make the highest principle to prevail and to keep in continuous existence of it, so that after a thousand years, people will know that wisdom and kindness of the great sages were without limits.

This preface was written in the first year of Bao Ying of the great Tang dynasty (762 A.D.).

上古天真论篇第一

Chapte 1
Shanggu Tianzhen Lun
(On Human Preserving Health Energy in Ancient Times)

昔在黄帝，生而神灵，弱而能言，幼而徇齐，长而敦敏，成而登天。

Yellow Emperor of ancient time, was bright and clever when he was born, good at talking when he was a child, had a modest style of doing things and an upright character when he was young; in his youth, he was honest and possessed a strong ability of distinguishing what was right and what was wrong. He became an emperor when he grew up.

乃问于天师曰：余闻上古之人，春秋皆度百岁，而动作不衰；今时之人，年半百而动作皆衰者，时世异耶？人将失之耶？

Yellow Emperor asked the Taoist master Qibo, saying: "I am told the people in ancient times could all survive to more than one hundred years old, and they appeared to be quite healthy and strong in actions, but the people at present time are different, they are not so nimble in actions when they are only fifty, and what is the reason? Is it due to the change of spiritual principles or caused by the artificial behavior of men?"

岐伯对曰：上古之人，其知道者，法于阴阳，和于术数，食饮有〔《千金方》"有"下有"常"字〕节，起居有常〔《千金方》"常"下有"度"字〕，不妄作劳，故能形与神俱，而尽终其天年，度百岁乃去。今时之人不然也，以酒为浆，以妄为常，醉以入房，以欲竭其精，以耗散其真，不知持满，不时〔林校引别本"时"作"解"〕御神，务快其心，逆于生乐，起居无节，故半百而衰也。

Qibo answered: "Those who knew the way of keeping a good health in ancient times always kept in their behavior in daily life in accordance with the nature. They followed the principle of Yin and Yang and kept in conformity with the art of prophecy based on the interaction of Yin and Yang. They were able to modulate their daily life in harmony with the way of recuperating the essence and vital energy, thus they could master and practise the way of preserving a good health. Their behaviours in daily life were all kept in regular patterns such as their food and drink were of fixed quantity, their daily activities were all in regular times. They never overworked. In this way, they could maintain both in the body and in the spirit

substantiality, and were able to live to the old age of more than one hundred years.

But the people nowadays are quite different. They do not recuperate themselves according to the way of preserving a good health, but run in counter to it. They are addicted to drink without temperance, keep idling as an oldinary, indulge in sexual pleasures and use up their vital energy and ruin their health. They do not protect their primordial energies carefully as handling a utensil full of valuable things. They don't understand the importance of saving their energy but waste them rashly by doing what ever to their liking. They know not the joy of keeping a good health and have no regular pattern of their daily food, drink and activities. Therefore, they become decrepit when they are only fifty."

夫上古圣人之教下也〔"下也"二字误倒，应据《千金方》乙正，"下"字属下读〕，皆谓之〔《千金方》"谓"为"为"字〕，虚邪贼风，避之有时；恬惔虚无，真气从之，精神内守，病安从来。是以志闲而少欲，心安而不惧，形劳而不倦，气从以顺，各从其欲，皆得所愿。故美其食，任其服，乐其俗，高下不相慕，其民故曰〔王冰所据本"曰"作"自"〕朴。是以嗜欲不能劳其目，淫邪不能惑其心，愚智贤不肖不惧于物，故合于道，所以能年皆度百岁而动作不衰者，以其德全不危也。

"In anctent times people behaved according to the teaching of preserving health of the sages : All evil energies of various seasons are harmful to people, they attack the body when it is in general debility, and they should be defended anytime and everywhere. When one is completely free from wishes, ambitions and distracting thoughts, indifferent to fame and gain, the true energy will come in the wake of it. When one concentrates his spirit internally and keeps a sound mind, how can any illness occur?

"Therefore, those who are able to keep a leisured aspiration will not be afraid at the time when something terrible happens, those who have strong bodies will not feel fatigued after labour, and those who have a quiet spirit, their primordial energy will be moderate, their desires can be satisfied easily if only they are not insatiably greedy. It is precisely because of their having the above spiritual basis, they are able to adapt to any environment. They are not too particular about the quality and style of the costume, but feels at ease with local customs. They do not seek or admire the material comfortable life of others, so they are plain and honest.

"As they are having a quiet and stable state of mind, no desire can seduce their eyes, and no obscenity can entice their heart. Although the intelligence and moral character between different people are not the same, yet they can all attain the stage of giving no thought of personal gain or loss, and thus, they are all able to live according to the way of keeping a good health.

"The reason of those who can live more than one hundred years without being decrepit is that they can manage the way of keeping a good health thoroughly."

帝曰：人年老而无子者，材力尽邪？将天数然也。

Yellow Emperor asked: "People are unable to have any child when they are old, whether it is due to the exhaustion of their tendon's energy or it is the natural law of physiology?"

岐伯曰：女子七岁，肾气盛，齿更发长。二七而天癸至，任脉通，太冲〔《太平圣惠方》，并无“太”字〕脉盛，月事以时下，故有子。三七，肾气平均，故真牙生而长极。四七，筋骨坚，发长极，身体盛壮。五七，阳明脉衰，面始焦，发始堕。六七，三阳脉衰于上，面皆焦，发始白。七七，任脉虚，太冲脉衰少，天癸竭，地道不通，故形坏而无子也。

Qibo answered: "For a woman, her kidney energy becomes prosperous when she is seven, as kidney determines the condition of the bone, and teeth are the surplus of bone, her milk teeth fall off and the perminant teeth emerge when her kidney energy is prosperous; as hair is the extension of blood and the blood is transformed from the kidney essence, her hair will grow when the kidney is prosperous.

"Her Taingui (the substance necessary for the promotion of growth, developement and reproductive function of human body)appears at the age of fourteen(2×7). At this time, her Ren channel begins to put through, and her Chong channel becomes prosperous and her menstruation begins to appear. As all her physiological conditions being mature, she can be pregnant and bear a child.

"The growth of kidney energy reaches the normal status of an adult by the age of twenty one (3×7), her wisdom teeth have grown up by this stage, and her teeth are completely developed.

"By the age of twenty eight (4×7), her vital energy and blood become substantial, her extremities become strong, the developement of the tissues and hair of her whole body are flourishing. In this stage, her body is in the most strong condition.

"The physique of a woman turns from prosperity to decline gradually after the age of thirty five (5×7). So, by this time, her Yangming channel turns to debility, her face becomes withered, and her hair begins to fall.

"By the age of forty two (6×7), her three Yang channels (Taiyang, Yangming and Shaoyang)all begin to decline. By this time, her face complexion becomes wane, and her hair begins to turn white.

"After the age of forty nine(7×7), her Ren and Chong channels are both declining, her menstruation severs as her Taingui being exhausted. Her physique turns old and feeble, and by then, she can no more conceive."

丈夫八岁，肾气实〔《圣济总录》引“实”作“盛”〕，发长齿更。二八，肾气盛，天癸至〔三字衍〕，精气溢泻，阴阳和，故能有子。三八，肾气平均，筋骨劲强，故真牙生而长极。四八，筋骨隆盛，肌肉满壮。五八，肾气衰，发堕齿槁。六八，阳气衰竭于上、面焦，发鬓颁白〔《太平圣惠方》引无“颁”字〕。七八，肝气衰，筋不能动，天癸竭，精少，肾藏衰，形体皆极。八八，则齿发去。肾者主水，受五藏六府之精而藏之，故五藏盛，乃能泻。今五藏皆衰，筋骨解堕，天癸尽矣。故发鬓白，身体重，行步不正，而无子耳。

"For a man, his kidney energy becomes prosperous by the age of eight. By then, his hair developes and his permanent teeth emerge.

"His kidney energy becomes prosperous by the age of sixteen (2×8). he it is filled with vital energy and is able to let out sperm. If he conducts sexual intercourse with a woman, he

might have a chid.

"By the age of twenty four (3×8), his kidney energy is well developed to reach the state of an adult. By this time, his extremities are strong, his wisdom teeth have grown up, and all his teeth are completely developed.

"By the age of thirty two (4×8), his whole body has developed to its best condition, and his extremities and muscles are very strong.

"By the age of forty (5×8), his kidney energy turns gradually from prosperous to decline. As a result, his hairs begin to fall and teeth begin to wither.

"By the age of forty eight (6×8), his kidney energy declines even more. As the kidney energy is the source of Yang energy, the Yang energy of the whole body begins to decline due to the decline of kidney energy. As a result, his complexion becomes withered and his hair becomes white.

"After the age of fifty six (7×8), his liver energy declines in the wake of the deficiency of the kidney energy 〔the liver energy (wood) stems from kidney energy (water)〕. As liver determins the condition of the tendon, the deficiency of kidney energy will cause malnourishment to tendons which will become rigid and fail to act so nimbly.

"After the age of sixty four (8×8), his Tiangui being exhausted, his essence and vital energy being reduced, and his kidney energy becomes weak. As kidney determines the condition of the bone, the debility of kidney causes the weakness of the tendons and bones. Thus, at this stage, his essence and vital energy turn to the utmost decline, his teeth fall off, and every part of his body becomes decrepit.

"The kidney energy is the congenital energy of human body, but it can only bring its functions into play when it is nourished by the postnatal energy. The essence of the five solid organs and six hollow organs are originated from the essence and energy of water and cereals. It is only after the receiving and storing the essence of water and cereals of the five solid and the six hollow organs in advance, can the organs provide the energy for kidney. Kidney associates with water, it receives and stores the essence and energy come from the five solid and six hollow organs. Therefore, the kidney can only spread its essence and energy to the whole body when the five solid and six hollow organs are substantially filled.

"As one's five viscera are then all declining, the tendons and bones are all becoming weak, and the Taingui is also exhausted, his hair turns white, his body becomes clumsy, unable to walk straight, and all his other physiologlcal functions are declining. So, it is imposible for him to have child anymore."

帝曰：有其年已老而有子者何也？岐伯曰：此其天寿过度，气脉常通，而肾气有余也。此虽有子，男不过尽八八，女不过尽七七，而天地之精气皆竭矣。

The Emperor asked: "Someone is able to have a child even he is old, and what is the reason?" Qibo answered: "This kind of people has a richer natural endowment of primordial kidney energy, and has a better postnatal recuperation to health, although they are aged, yet their channel-energies are still not declining, so, there is still possibility for them to have

children. Nevertheless, for a man, the age for having a child can not exceed sixty four (8×8), and for a woman, can not exceed the age of forty nine (7×7). When the essence and vital energy of a man or woman being exhausted, it is also impossible for them to have any child."

帝曰：夫道者年皆百数，能有子乎？岐伯曰：夫道者能却老而全形，身年虽寿，能生子也。

The Emperor said: "Since people who are good at preserving health can live to the age of one hundred years old, can a person of one hundred years old to have any child?" Qibo answered: "For those who are good at preserving health, although they reach the age of one hundred years old, as they can keep their body in a good condition to postpone senility, preserve their physique from declining, they still can have children."

黄帝曰：余闻上古有真人者，提挈天地，把握阴阳，呼吸精气，独立守神，肌肉若一，故能寿敝〔沈祖绵曰："敝字误疑敌字也"〕天地，无有终时，此其道生。

The Emperor said: "As I am told that in ancient times, some people who were very good at preserving their health, reaching the level of being a 'perfect man'. All their behaviours adapted to the change of nature quite at ease, they could master the law of the wax and wane of Ying and Yang. They respired the refined energy, guarding the spirit independently and thus their muscles would be an integrated whole. Since they could modulate their essence and vital energy to adapt their physique and spirit, therefore, their life would be everlasting, and could survive for ever like the heaven and earth. This is mainly because they could practise the way of preserving health properly.

中古之时，有至人者，淳德全道，和于阴阳，调于四时，去世离俗，积精全神，游行天地之间，视听八达之外，此盖益其寿命而强者也，亦归于真人。

"In the middle ancient times, some people who were good at preserving health reaching the level of being a 'supreme man'. They studied and practised the way of preserving health whole heartedly with a pure and honest moral character. They could keep their behaviours and minds to fit the law of the wax and wane of Yin and Yang and the sequent weather changes of the seasons. They were able to maintain their primordial energy concentratively by freeing themselves from wordly turmoil so as they could keep their physique strong, their spirit abundant, and their ears and eyes acute. They travelled extensively and to hear and see things in distant places. This kind of people could certainly prolong their life span. Their level of cultivating health had almost attained the status of a 'perfect man'.

其次有圣人者，处天地之和，从八风之理，适嗜欲，于世俗之间，无恚嗔之心，行不欲离于世，被服章〔林校云"被服章"三字疑衍〕，举不欲观于俗，外不劳形于事，内无思想之患，以恬愉为务，以自得为功，形体不敝，精神不散，亦可以百数〔"亦"字疑脱"年"字，王注："年登百数"〕。

"Next, some people who were good at preserving health to the level of being a 'Sage'. They lived quietly and comfortably in the natural environment of the universe, they follow the rule of the eight winds (different winds from all directions) and could avoid being hurt by them. They regulated their eating, drinking and daily life in a moderate style when lived to-

gether with common people. Their temperaments were stable and calm without indignation and fluctuation of mood. In outward appearance, they did not divorce from the reality of their daily life, they worked in the office with office dresses like others, but they dealt with things differently from that of common people. They never did excessive physical labour or engaged in any excessive deliberation to cause worry, but always kept their mind in a cheerful mood and contented with their own circumstances. It was precisely because of these facts, they could cultivated themselves to have strong bodies, and kept their spirit from dissipating, and thus, their lives could be lasted to one hundred years old.

其次有贤人者，法则天地，象似日月，辨〔"辩"应作"辨"〕列星辰，逆从阴阳，分别四时，将从上古合同于道，亦可使益寿而有极时。

"Next, those who could preserve their health to the state of being a 'Wise and good man'. They could master and apply the way of preserving health in accordance with the variation of heaven and earth, such as with the different location of the sun, the waxing and waning of the moon, the distribution of stars, the mutual contradiction of Yin and Yang and the alternation of the four seasons. They mastered and practised the ways of preserving health, sought to tally with the ways of preserving health in ancient times, so they could also prolong their lives to the maximum limit."

四气调神大论篇第二

Chapter 2
Si Qi Tiao Shen Da Lun
(On Preserving Health in Accordance with the Four Seasons)

春三月，此谓发陈，天地俱生，万物以荣，夜卧早起，广步于庭，被发缓形，以使〔《病沅》卷十五《肝病候》'使'下有"春"字〕志生，生而勿杀，予而勿夺，赏而勿罚，此春气之应，养生〔《类说》卷三十七"养生"作"生养"〕之道也。逆之则伤肝，夏为寒变，奉长者少。

In The period of the three months in spring is the time of birth and spread. Grasses and trees are becoming vivid and all living things in the world become flourishing with a new dynamic atmosphere. Since a man is one of the living things in the universe, he can by no means be excluded. In order to keep in accordance with the law of the variation of the seasonal sequence, one should go to bed when night comes and gets up early in the morning. In the morning, he should breathe the fresh air while walking in the yard to exercise his tendons and bones and loosen his hair to make the whole body comfortable along with the generating of spring energy. Since spring is the season of generation, one must not wrest the faculty of growth. What one should do is to help surviving and not killing, to donate but not to wrest, to award and not to punish so as to correspond the property of spring energy and fit in the way of preserving one's health. If this principle is violated by a man, his liver will be hurt, as liver associates with the wood, and woods are prosperous in spring. If one fails to adapt to the property of spring energy which is "generation" and thus hurts his liver, he will contract cold syndrome in summer. This is because his adaptability to summer has been weaken due to his inability of following the property of spring energy which is "generation" to preserve health. In this case, it is called "inadequate of offering to growth".

夏三月，此谓蕃秀，天地气交，万物华实，夜卧早起，无厌于日，使志无怒，使华英成秀，使气得泄，若所爱在外，此夏气之应，养长之道也。逆之则伤心，秋为痎疟，奉收者少，冬至重病〔柯逢时曰："依例'冬至'四字衍"〕。

The period of three months of summer is called the season of flourishing as all the living things in the world are prosperous and beautiful. On Summer Solstice, Yang energy reaches its submit and Yin energy begins to emerge, thus, the intercourse Yin and Yang energies occurs the at this time. As Yang energy forms the vital energy of things and Yin energy shapes up things, the combination of vital energy and the shaping energy cause all living things on earth come into blossoming and yielding fruits. In the course of intercrossing heaven-energy and earth-energy, one should, like in spring time, sleep when night comes and gets up early

in the morning. He should not detest the sun shine nor to get angry often, so as to correspond to the property of summer energy of 'growth' that promotes the growing of the flowers and fruits. Ones sweat should be perspired for letting off the Yang energy to avoid the heat being stagnated, in other words 'be keen on the exterior'. These are the ways of preserving health in summer. If these principles are violated by a man, his heart will be hurt, as heart associates with fire and fire is vigorous in summer. If one fails to adapt to the property of summer energy which is 'growth', his heart will be hurt, and he will contract malaria in autumn. This is because his adaptability to autumn energy has been weaken due to his inability of following the property of summer energy which is 'growth' to preserve health. In this case, it is called "inadequate of offering to harvesting".

秋三月，此谓容平，天气以急，地气以明，早卧早起，与鸡俱兴，使志安宁，以缓秋刑〔熊本“刑”作“形”〕，收敛神气，使秋气平，无外其志，使肺气清，此秋气之应，养收之道也，逆之则伤肺，冬为飧泄，奉藏者少。

In the three months of autumn, the shapes of all living things on earth become mature naturally and are ready to be harvested. In autumn, the wind is vigourous and rapid, the environment on earth is clear and bright, so during this period, one should go to bed early to stay away from the chillness, get up early to appreciate the crisp air of autumn, keep the spirit tranquil and stable to separate oneself from the sough of autumn by means of restraining the spirit and energy internally and guard the mind against anxiety and impetuosity. In this way, ones tranquillity can still be manitained even in the sough of autumn atmosphere, and the breath of lung can be kept even as well. If these principles are violated by a man, his lung will be hurt, as lung associates with metal and the metal prospers in autumn. If one fails to adapt to the property of autumn energy which is 'harvesting', one will apt to contract lienteric diarrhea with watery stool containing undigested food in winter. This is because his adaptability to winter energy has been weakened due to his inability of following the property of autumn energy which is 'harvesting' to preserve health. In this case, it is called "inadequate of offering to storing".

冬三月，此谓闭藏，水冰地坼，无扰乎阳，早卧晚起，必待日光，使志若伏若匿〔《病沅》“伏”下无“若”字〕，若有私意，若已有得，去寒就温，无泄皮肤、使气亟夺，此冬气之应，养藏之道也。逆之则伤肾，春为痿厥，奉生者少。

In the three months of winter, all grasses and most of the trees are withered, the insects are in hibernation, the water ices up and the ground is frozen with gaps. Things mostly are shut up or go into hiding to guard against the cold. It is called the season of 'shutting and storing'. In this period, one should be kept warm in the room, dress warmly and take strict prevention against the cold, so that the Yang energy may not be disturbed; he should go to bed early in night and get up late to wait for contacting the sunlight; keep the spirit hiding and subsiding, like having a private consideration in heart but not revealing or seem to have a definite idea in mind already for meeting the situation. Since the weather is cold in winter, one should avoid the cold and move toward warmness, prevent the skin from much perspir-

ing to guard against the consumption or exhaustion of Yang energy. These are the ways of preserving health in winter. If these principles are violated by a man, his kidney will be hurt, as the kidney associates with water and water is prosperous in winter. If one fails to adapt to the property of winter energy which is 'storing', he will be apt to contract muscular flaccidity and coldness of the extremities in spring. This is because his adaptability to spring energy has been weaken due to his inability of following the property of winter energy which is "shutting and storing" to preserve health. In this case, it is called 'inadequate of offering to birth'.

天气，清净光明者也，藏德不止，故不下也。天明〔《易·蒙》郑注："天明即天蒙〕则日月不明，邪害空窍，阳气者闭塞，地气者冒明，云雾不精，则上应白〔《太素》"白"作'甘'〕露不下。交通不表，万物命故不施，不施则名木多死。恶气不发，风雨不节，白露不下，则苑藁不荣。贼风数至，暴雨数起，天地四时不相保，与道相失，则未央绝灭。唯圣人从之，故身无奇病，万物不失，生气不竭。

The energy of heaven is clear and bright. It continuously promotes the birth, growth, getting sick and getting old of all things and human beings. The vitality of its clearness and brightness will never cease, therefore, it will not decline either.

If the sky is not brignt, the sun, moon and the whole earth must be dark and the functional activities of vital energy will be obstructed like the hollow orifices of human body being obstructed when being encroached by the evil factors. The intercrossing between the energies of heaven and earth depends on the motions and illuminations of the sun and moon, if the sun and moon cease to illuminate, the heaven energy will be obstructed and fails to descend. As a result, the sky will be overcast with clouds and mists, the energy of earth will fail to ascend to respond the energy of heaven and the due will not be able to fall.

The growth and developement of all things on earth depend on the intercrossing of the energies of Yin and Yang. If the two energies fail to communicate, all things on earth will lose their source of nourishment. Under such circumstance, most of the big trees will die. Besides, some abnormal change will happen in the world and the weather sequence of the four seasons will be confusing: the weather will not be severe in autumn and not be bitterly cold in winter, the wind and rain won't be regular in spring, and no dew will occur in summer. Since the Yin and Yang energies being maladjusted, the four seasons will lose their regular patterns, they can no more help the birth and growing of all things, and all things on earth will die young.

The sages know the hows and whys of the viarition of Yin and Yang, so they can avoid queer diseases even under the condition of sudden change of the environment. As they can adapt to the mechanism of existence like other things on earth, so their vital energy will never be exhausted.

逆春气，则少阳不生，肝气内变。逆夏气，则太阳不长，心气内洞〔《太平圣惠方》引"洞"作"动"〕。逆秋气，则太阴〔按"太阴与下逆冬气"少阴"颠倒，应改正过来〕不收，肺气焦满。逆冬气，则少阴不藏，肾气独沉〔《外台》卷十六引《删繁》，林校引《太素》并

作“沉浊”〕。夫四时阴阳者，万物之根本也，所以圣人春夏养阳，秋冬养阴，以从其根，故与万物沉浮于生长之门。逆其根，则伐其本，坏其真矣。故阴阳四时〔《甲乙》“阴阳”下无“四时”二字〕者，万物之终始也，死生之本也，逆之则灾害生，从之则苛疾不起，是谓得道。道者，圣人行之，愚者佩〔《类说》引“佩”作“背”〕之。从阴阳则生，逆之则死，从之则治，逆之则乱。反顺为逆，是谓内〔《外台》引“内”作“关”〕格。

If the principle of preserving health in spring being violated, one's Shaoyang energy will not be able to bring the function of generation into full play. Thus, the kidney energy will become worse interally.

If the principle of preserving health being violated in summer, one's Taiyang energy will not be able to bring the function of growth into full play. Thus, the heart energy will be stirring inside.

If the principle of preserving health being violated in autumn, one's Shaoyin energy will not be able to bring the function of harvesting into full play. Thus, the distention of lung energy will occur.

If the principle of preserving health being violated in winter, one's Taiyin energy will not be able to bring the function of storing into full play. As the Taiyin energy connects with the kidney internally, so when Taiyin fails to store, the kidney energy will degenerate and its functions will become weak.

The energies of all things on earth are born in spring, grow in summer, yield in autumn and hide in winter, they are all promoted by the law of variation of Yin and Yang energies of the four seasons. So Yin and Yang energies of the four seasons are the root-energies of birth and growth of all things. So the sages maintain the heart and liver which is the Yang energy in spring and summer and maintain the lung and kidney which is the Yin energy in autumn and winter to keep consistent with the roots, so as they can preserve them perfectly. Human beings, like all things on earth, also submit to the law of Yin and Yang energies variation, when one runs counter to the law which is the root, his origin of life will be cut and his primordial energy will be spoiled. Therefore, the law of Yin and Yang energies variation dominates the beginning and end and decide the birth and death of everything. If the law of Yin and Yang energies variation is violated by a man, diseases will occur frequently, but if it is well adapted, no strange diseases will happen. The one who can keep this law well adapted, he is actually the one who has mastered the proper way of preserving health. Commonly, only the sages can follow the law and the foolish people run counter to it. In a word, man will survive when following the law, and dies when acts against it. If the Yang energy fails to enter into the body and Yin energy can not come out from the body, the favorable condition of health will turn to the adversity, the contradiction between exterior and interior will cause the disease of mutual excluding of Yin and Yang.

是故圣人不治已病治未病，不治已乱治未乱，此之谓也。夫病已成而后药之，乱已成而后治之，譬犹渴而穿井，斗而铸锥〔《太素》“锥”作“兵”〕，不亦晚乎！

When a sage treats a patient, precaution is always emphasized, and often uses preven-

tive measures in calming down the disturbances. If the disease is treated after it has already been formed, or try to calm down the disturbance after it has already taken shape, it will be too late, just like to dig a well until one is thirsty, or to cast the weapon after the war has already broken out.

生气通天论篇第三

Chapter 3
Sheng Qi Tong Tian Lun
(On the Human Vital Energy Connecting with Nature)

黄帝曰：夫自古通天者生之本，本于阴阳。天地之间，六合之内，其气九州九窍〔俞樾说："九窍是衍文，九州即九窍，古窍为州"〕、五藏、十二节，皆通乎天气，其生五、其气三，数犯此者，则邪气伤人，此寿命之本也。

The Emperor said: "Since ancient time, it is considered that the existence of men has depended upon the communications of the variation of Yin and Yang energies, thus, human life is based on Yin and Yang.

"All things on the earth and in the space communicate with the Yin and Yang energies. Human being is a small universe as human body has everything that the universe has. In the universe, there are nine states (namely Ji, Yan, Qing, Xu, Yang, Jing, Yu, Liang and Yong), and man has nine orifices (seven orifices: two ears, two eyes, two nosetrils, and one mouth; two Yin orifices: external urethral orifice and the anus); there are five musical tones in the universe, man has five solid organs responsible for storing the mental activities (liver stores soul, heart stores spirit, spleen stores consciousness, lung stores inferior spirit, kidney stores will); there are twelve solar terms in the universe, and man has twelve channels. The Yin and Yang energies of human being correspond with the Yin and Yang energies of the universe, and the Yin and Yang energies of all things (including men) are communicating with that of the universe.

"The survival of a man depends on the Yin and Yang energies and depends on the five elements (metal, wood, water, fire and earth), it is the so called 'life depends on five'. The five elements on earth correspond to the three Yins (cold, dryness and wetness) and the three Yangs (wind, fire and summer heat), it is the so called 'energies depend on the three'. If one violates the principles of preserving health frequently, his health will be hurt by the evil factors and contracts diseases. Therefore, Yin and Yang energies are the foundation of life.

"苍天之气，清净则志意治，顺之则阳气固，虽有贼邪，弗能害也，此因时之序。故圣人传精神，服天气，而通神明。失之则内闭九窍，外壅肌肉，卫气散解，此谓自伤，气之削也。

When the human energy is connected with that of the universe, the human temperament will be fresh and cool in a calm circumstance where there is no strong wind and rain-storm. With the calm circumstance, one can keep his spirit quiet and clear as the blue sky, refrain from the disturbances of overjoy and violent rage. By this time, his bodily Yang energy is substantial, and will not be hurt even though being attacked by evil factors. This is due to

his ability of adapting the sequence and variations of the four seasons to preserve his health in a good way.

"Therefore, as a sage can keep his essence of life and energy in concert with the Yang energy of heaven, thus can communicate his energy with the divinity of heaven. But, unfortunately, most people run in the opposite direction to it, so, whenever he is assaulted by evil factors, his nine orifices become obstructed internally, and his muscle contracts disease of stagnation externally, even his Wei-energy becomes dispersed. This is due to his inability of adapting to the sequence and variations of the four seasons.

阳气者若天与日，失其所，则折寿而不彰，故天运当以日光明，是故阳因而上卫外者也。

"There is Yang energy in human body like there is sun in the sky. When the sun is not at its proper position, the heaven and earth will become dark, and when the Yang energy of a man is not at his proper position, he will die early. So the unceasing operation of heaven depends on the brightness of the sun, and the bodily health of a man depends on the clear and floating of Yang energy which guards against outside.

因于寒，欲如运枢，起居如惊〔吴本"惊"作"警"〕，神气乃浮。因于暑，汗，烦则喘喝，静则多言，体若燔炭，汗出而散。因于湿，首如裹，湿热不攘，大筋緛短，小筋弛长，緛短为拘，弛长为痿。因于气，为肿，四维相代，阳气乃竭。

"When a man is invaded by cold, he will be disquieted and restless like being on alert, his spirit and energy excrete outside and his Yang energy becomes unstable.

"When a man is invaded by heat, he will be sweating a lot, irritable and breathe rapidly with noise. If the heat invades to affect the spirit, he will have the syndromes of short of breath, gasp, thirst, polylogia and his body will be hot like the burning charcoal. The stagnated heat-evil can only be dispersed by perspiration.

"If the disease stems from the wetness-evil, one's head will feel heavy like being wraped. The prolonged wetness will turn to heat. It should be eliminated in time, otherwise, the heat will hurt the Yin blood to cause malnourishment to the tendons, making the large tendons become rigid and cramps occur, or making the small ones relaxation and flaccidities occur.

"When a man is invaded by the wind-evil, swelling will occur, and the four extremities will be swelling alternately which shows the exhaustion of the Yang energy.

阳气者，烦劳则张，精绝，辟积于夏，使人煎厥。目盲不可以视，耳闭不可以听，溃溃乎若坏都，汩汩乎不可止。阳气者，大怒则形气绝；而血菀于上，使人薄厥。有伤于筋，纵，其若不容，汗出偏沮，使人偏枯。汗出见湿，乃生痤疿。高〔《太素》"高"作"膏"〕梁之变，足生大丁，受如持虚〔《素问病机气宜保命集》卷二十六引作"受持如虚"〕。劳汗当风，寒薄为皶，郁乃痤。

"When one is over-worked, the Yang energy in his body will become hyperactive and excretes outside causing the exhaustion of Yin. If the disease is protracted, and the weather is hot in summer, the disease of anterior jue will occur. The disease is characterized by the syndromes of hearing nothing as if the ears are being stopped, and seeing nothing as if the

eyes are dim-sighted, like the dash of water in swift and irresistible momentum which can hardly be controlled.

"The Yang energy will rush upward when one is in a great rage, and the blood will go upward in the wake of it. If the blood stagnates in the chest, the physique and the activating vital energy will become obstructed. In this case, the confusion of vital energy and blood is called syncope due to emotional upset.

"If the tendon is hurt, it will be slow in contracting and can not be used wilfully.

"If one side of the body of a man is usually obstructed and no sweat appears when one should perspire, he might contract hemiparalysis in the near future.

"When one is perspiring and sweat pores are opened, if by this time, he takes a cold bath, the evils of wetness and heat will be stagnated within the muscular striae. If will cause furuncle when the case is serious and cause prickly heat when the case is slight.

"The one who is addicted to delicious food often has stagnated heat inside and is apt to contract cellulitis and the stagnated heat stemmed from asthenia.

"When one sits or lies against the wind and perspires after doing hard labour, the cold-evil may invade his skin and muscular striae. It will cause comedo when the case is slight, and cause sore when the case is serious.

精气者，精则养神，柔则养筋。开阖不得，寒气从之，乃生大偻。陷脉为瘘，留连肉腠。俞气化薄，传为善畏，及为惊骇。营气不从，逆于肉（莫校本"肉"一作"内"）理，乃生痈肿。魄汗未尽，形弱而气烁、穴俞以闭，发为风疟。

"When the Yang energy is within one's body and brings its delicate function into play, it will nourish the vitality internally and soften the tendon externally.

"It is normal when the skin straie of a man opens in spring and close in winter. If it does not open when it should open and does not close when it should close, it will leave the opportunity for the cold-evil to invade. When the cold-evil penetrates deep and damages the Yang energy, he may contract hunchback. This is because of the damaged Yang energy can no more soften the tendons.

"When the cold-evil enters into one's channels, it will cause stagnation of the blood. When the cold-evil and blood accumulate and remain in the muscle straie for a long time, scrofula may be contracted.

"When the energy of the channel system is in debility, the cold-evil will invade the solid and hollow organs through the channels. As the solid organs take charge of the mental activities, so when invaded by the cold-evil, one's spirit will lost its quietness and occur the syndromes of timorousness (due to heart) and timidness (due to liver). This is because of the damaged Yang energy can no more support the spirit.

"If the Yang energy flows reversely due to the invasion of the evil energy, the blood will stagnate in the striae of skin. The stagnation of blood will cause the accumulation of heat, as time passes it will suppurate and form a carbuncle.

"If one is attacked by the wind-cold evil when his sweat is not thoroughly perspired, his

shu-points on the channels will be closed and cause the heat stagnated in it. When both the heat and cold attack simultaneously, wind-type malaria will happen.

故风者，百病之始也，清净则肉腠闭拒，虽有大风苛毒，弗之能害，此因时之序也。

"Therefore, wind is the main source of various diseases, But how can the wind-evil be resisted? The clue is to keep one's physique and spirit quiet and not being bothered by material concerns, that his Yang energy may be substantial and his striae of skin dense. When his striae of skin is dense, he will be able to resist the strong wind-evil and severe toxin. It is important to adapt to the weather sequence to nurse one's physique and spirit, that is, to preserve health in accordance with the law of Yin and Yang.

"故病久则传化，上下不并，良医弗为。故阳〔熊本"阳"下有"气"字〕畜〔（滑抄本"畜"作"蓄"）〕积病死，而阳气当隔，隔者当泻，不亟正治，粗乃败之。故阳气者，一日而主外，平旦人〔"人"下脱"阳"字，王注与《学医随笔》俱引有"阳"字〕气生，日中而阳气隆，日西而阳气已虚。气门乃闭。是故暮而收拒，无扰筋骨，无见雾露，反此三时，形乃困薄。

"When a disease is protracted, the evil factors will be transmitted to interior and change will take place. When the condition is serious, the Yin and Yang energies will be unable to communicate with eachother, which will make even a good doctor can do nothing with it.

"Due to the inability of communcating between the Yin and Yang energies, the Yang energy will be accumulated, and the patient will be seized by fatal disease and die suddenly. Under such circumstance, the patient should be treated with rapid purgation. If the treatment is delayed, the patient will die within a few days.

"The Yang energy determines the exterior in day time. The Yang energy of man begins to emerge in early morning, being prosperous at noon and become weak in the dusk, henceforth, the entrance of energy (the oppening of sweat gland) closes in the wake of it. This shows when one takes good care of his spirit and energy, he should not only keep in conformity with the growth and decline of Yin and Yang energies in a day. So in the dusk, one should restrain his Yang energy, should not fatigue his extremities by excessive working so as not to disturb the Yang energy, and not to contact mists and dews by staying outdoor so as to avoid the invasion of cold-wetness evil. If one fails to adapt the three different times of the day, fails to use his Yang energy in day time, but fatigues his Yang energy by night instead, his bodily health will be disturbed by the invasion of the evil factors."

岐伯曰：阴者，藏精而起亟〔"起亟"，吴注本作"为守"〕也；阳者，卫外而为固也，阴不胜其阳，则脉流薄疾，并〔《素问病机宜保命集》引作"病"〕乃狂。阳不胜其阴，则五藏气争〔"争"疑系"静"之坏字，阳不胜阴，阴胜则静，阳及运行，郁滞为病，故九窍不通〕，九窍不通。是以圣人陈阴阳，筋脉和同，骨髓坚固，气血皆从。如是则内外调和，邪不能害，耳目聪明，气立如故。

Qibo said: "Yin is to store the essence of life and the vital energy is watching inside, and Yang is to defend the periphery of the body and is guarding outside. If the Yang energy has some activities outside, Yin energy will correspond from inside. If the Yin energy is insuffi-

cient while the Yang energy is excessive to cause Yin inferior to Yang, the flow of channel energy will be forced to become faster and stronger, it may cause mania; if the Yin energy is excessive and the Yang energy is insufficient, causing the Yang inferior to Yin, the energy of the five viscera will be stagnated to form the obstruction of the nine orifices.

"However, the sages can arrange his Yin energy and Yang energy properly to each of its suitable state, keep the tendons and channles in a hormonious condition, make the bone and marrow substantial, and can keep the vital energy and blood each persues its own way. In this way, one may keep his internal and external condition of Yin and Yang energies in harmony, and his health will remain unharmed even when the evil factors invade, his eyes and ears will remain sharp, and moreover, he can frequently maintain his primordial energy firmly inside.

风客淫气，精乃亡，邪伤肝也。因而饱食，筋脉横解，肠澼为痔。因而大饮，则气逆。因而强力，肾气乃伤，高骨乃坏。

"Owning to the wind associates with the liver (liver correspond to the wind and wood), when one is hurt by excessive wind-evil, the essence of life and blood will suffer severe damage. As blood is stored in the liver, the wind-evil will hurt the liver too.

"When eat one's fill, the stomach and intestine are full, the tendons will become loose. If the instestine store up with the undigested food usually, the tendons will be kept loose constantly, and it will cause bloody stool or hemorrhoid.

"When liquor is taken excessively, the lung-energy will run up reversely.

"When one gives way to his carnal desires, and practices sexual intercourse with difficulty, his kidney will be hurt to wither up the marrow and his lumbar vertebra will be damaged.

凡阴阳之要，阳密乃固〔《太素》作"阴密阳固"〕，两者不和，若春无秋，若冬无夏，因而和之，是谓圣度。故阳强不能密，阴气乃绝，阴平阳秘，精神乃治，阴阳离决，精气乃绝。

"The essentials of the communication of Yin and Yang rest in the denseness of the Yin energy and the firmness of the Yang energy. If the Yin and Yang being inharmonious, it will like to have no autumn but has only spring, no summer but has only winter in a year. Under such circumstance, all living things on earth will not be able to exist and reproduce according to the law of birth, growth, developement, harvesting and storing in due seasons. Since only a sage can harmonize the Yin and Yang energies in a proper way, so it is considered to be the standing order of the sage.

"Therefore, if the Yang energy is too strong and loses its function of defending outside, the Yin essence will be let out due to the Yang's failure of guarding outside. When the Yin essence is consumed, it will soon die out.

"If the Yin and Yang energies of a man being kept in a state of equilibrium, his body will be strong and his spirit sound, if his Yin and Yang energies fail to communicate, his vital energy will be declined and finally exhausted.

因于露风，乃生寒热。是以春伤于风，邪气留连〔"连"作"夏"，属下读，为"夏乃为

洞泄"〕，乃为洞泄。夏伤于暑，秋为痎疟，秋伤于湿，上〔《类说》引"上"作"冬"〕逆而咳，发为痿厥。冬伤于寒，春必温〔明抄本"温病"作"病温"〕病。四时之气，更伤五藏。

"If one contracts a disease stemmed from the exposure to dew and wind, cold and heat will occur. As the dew is Yin-evil and the wind is Yang-evil, and as Yin-evil produces cold, and Yang-evil produces heat, thus, the syndrome of cold and heat will occur.

"When the body is hurt by wind-evil in spring, and the disease comes on immediately, it is the exogenous disease, but if the disease does not comes on immediately but retains inside, it will become diarrhea with indigested food in summer.

"When one is hurt by summer-heat evil in summer, and the disease come on immediately, it is the summer-heat disease; If the disease does not come on immediately, but incubates inside, malaria will occur in autumn.

"When one is hurt by the wetness-evil which runs up adversely to evade the lung in autumn, if the wetness-evil breaks out internally, cough will occur in winter; if it breaks out externally, the tendons will be flaccid and weak to form muscular flaccidity and coldness of the extremities in winter.

"When the body is hurt by cold-evil in winter and the disease comes on immediately, it is the exogenous cold-evil disease. If the disease does not come on immediately and the cold-evil incubates inside, the cold-evil will turn into seasonal febrile disease when the Yang energy ascends in spring.

"When the weathers of the four seasons are warm in spring, hot in summer, cool in autumn and cold in winter in their normal conditions, man will not get sick, If one or more of the weather conditions is particularly stressed to be abnormal, it will not only damage the activation of production, circulation and function of the vital energy, but also will damage the five viscera of a man.

阴之所生，本在五味，阴之五宫，伤在五味。是故味过于酸，肝气以津，脾气乃绝。味过于咸，大骨气劳，短肌，心气抑。味过于甘，心气喘满，色黑，肾气不衡〔《云笈七签》引"衡"作"卫"〕。味过于苦，脾气不濡，胃气乃厚。味过于辛，筋脉沮弛，精神乃央。是故谨和五味，骨正筋柔，气血以流，腠理以密，如是则骨气以精。谨道如法，长有天命。

"The nourishments of the five viscera are stemmed from the five tastes (acrid, sweet, sour, bitter and salty which may be apprehended as tastes of food), but when the five tastes are taken excessively, they will damage the five viscera.

"The sour taste acts on the liver, if sour taste is taken excessively, it will make the liver to have too much body fluid which will cause sthenia of liver-energy. The sthenia of liver will restrict the spleen-earth and make the spleen energy vanishing.

"The salty taste acts on the kidney. As kidney determines the condition of the bone, and salty taste can soften the hardness and is superior to the blood, so when the salty taste is taken too much, it will damage the bone and the muscle. If the kidney-water is abundant to override the heart-fire, the heart energy will be restrained.

"The sweet taste acts on the spleen, and the property of sweet taste is sluggish and

greasy. If the sweet taste is excessively taken, dypsnea will happen. When the spleen is abnormal, it will restrict the kidney-water and cause it to become black (the colour of the kidney). When the kidney water is restricted, the kidney energy will be abnormal to become ill.

"The bitter taste acts on the heart, if the bitter taste is taken excessively, the heart will be hurt. When the heart fire is hurt, the spleen-earth will fail to be moistened (the fire fails to warm the earth). When the spleen is not moistened, it can no more do the transportation work for the stomach, thus, the dry-evil of the stomach will become abundant and the disease of the distension of the stomach energy will happen.

"The acrid taste acts on the lung, if the acrid taste is taken exessively, the lung energy will become abundant, and the abundant lung-metal will restrict the liver wood. As liver determines the condition of the tendons, when the liver is restricted, the tendons will become loose. Due to the acrid taste also has the function of dispersing, the excessive taking of acrid taste will consume the spirit as well.

"Therefore, if the five tastes are adjusted in a harmonious condition without taking them excessively, the whole body will obtain ample source of nourishment, and the tendons, bones, energies, blood and striae of skin will be kept in a strong and normal condition. Thus, the one who is good at adjusting the five tastes can live a long life."

金匮真言论篇第四

Chapten 4
Jin Gui Zhen Yan Lun
(The Truth in the Collections of Books of Golden Chamber)

黄帝问曰：天有八风，经有五风，何谓？岐伯对曰：八风发邪〔《太素》"邪"下有"气"字〕，以为〔《太素》无"以为"二字，"经风"二字属下读，即"经风触五藏"〕经风，触五藏，邪气发病。所谓得四时之胜者，春胜长夏，长夏胜冬，冬胜夏，夏胜秋，秋胜春，所谓四时之胜也〔所谓得四时 32 字，柯逢时说"是衍文"〕。

Yellow Emperor said: "In heaven, there are winds from eight directions, but for man, there are only winds of the five viscera, and what is the reason?"

Qibo answered: "All the eight winds are evil winds that may hurt the human body. If one's channels being affected by the evil wind, it will further invade the viscera. When the viscera are touched by the evil wind through channels, one will contract disease and the winds of the five viscera will occur.

东风生于春，在病肝，俞在颈项；南风生于夏，病在心，俞在胸胁；西方生于秋，病在肺，俞在肩背；北风生于冬，病在肾，俞在腰股；中央为土，病在脾，俞在脊。

"The east wind occurs in spring, and the wind is normal. If the liver energy (liver energy associates with spring) of a man declines, he will be hurt by the wind-evil and contracts disease, what is more, his shu-points will be damaged first. As liver-shu is on the neck, so the disease will come about on the neck. The south wind occurs in summer, and the wind is normal. If the heart energy (heart associates with summer) of a man declines, his shu-points will be hurt first. As the heart-shu is on the chest and hypochondria, so the disease will occur on his chest and hypochondria. The west wind occurs in autumn and the wind is normal. If the lung energy (lung associates with autumn) of a man declines, his shu-points will be hurt first. As the lung-shu is on the shoulder and back, the disease will occur on his shoulder and back. The north wind occurs in winter and the wind is normal. If the kidney energy (kidney associates with winter) of a man declines, his shu-points will be hurt first. As the kidney shu is on the loins, the disease will occur on his loins. The centrality associates to earth and its condition is determined by spleen. If one's spleen energy declines, his shu-points will be hurt first. As the spleen-shu is on the spine, so the disease will occur on the spine. Although they are the shu-points of the five viscera which is being affected, but when take a step further, they will become the disease of the five viscera.

故春气者病在头，夏气者病在藏，秋气者病在肩背，冬气者病在四支。

"Thus, the disease caused by spring-evil is on the head, as liver associates with spring

and the shu-point of liver is on the neck which belongs to the head; the disease caused by summer evil is on the chest and hypochondria as heart associates with summer and the shu point of heart is on the chest and hypochondria which accomodates the viscera; the disease caused by autumn-evil is on the shoulder and back, as lung associates with autumn and the shu point of lung is on the shoulder and back; the disease caused by winter-evil is on the extremities as kidney associates to winter and the shu point of kidney is on the loins, and the extremities are the terminals of the loins.

故春善病鼽衄，仲夏善病胸胁，长夏善病洞泄寒中，秋善病风疟，冬善病痹厥。

"Thus, in spring, one is apt to contract the syndrome of running nose and nasal hemorrhage, as the disease of spring energy is on the head. In midsummer, one is apt to contract the disease on chest and hypochondria as midsummer associates with heart, and the shu point of heart is on the chest and hypochondria. In long summer, one is apt to contract the disease of cold in the spleen and stomach as the spleen associates with long summer and also activate the wetness. When the wetness-evil does not transformed into heat syndrome and the spleen fails to operate, disease of cold in the spleen and stomach will occur. In autumn, one is apt to contract the wind-typed malaria as the disease of autumn energy in on the shoulder and back, when the shoulder and back is invaded by the wind-evil, it will retain in the acupoint Fengfu (Windy Massion), and when the healthy energy and the evil energy are conflicting with each other, wind-typed malaria will occur. In winter, one is apt to contract arthralgia-syndrome of ineffectness and coldness of the limbs as the Yang energy is being shut inside, and the channels of the extremities are easy to be invaded by the cold in winter.

故冬不按跻，春不〔明抄本"不"上无"春"字〕鼽衄，春不病颈项，仲夏不病胸胁，长夏不病洞泄寒中，秋不病风疟，冬不病痹厥。飧泄，而汗出也〔《类说》引无"飧泄"以下六字，林校谓此六字疑剩〕。

"As Yang energy is shut and being kept inside in winter, so, it is advisable not to massage or do any calisthenics in winter as they would arouse the Yang energy. If one's Yang energy is well preserved in winter, the syndrome of having a running nose, nasal hemorrhage and neck diseases may be avoided in spring, the disease in chest and hypochondria may be avoided in midsummer, the syndrome of cold-evil retaining in spleen and stomach may be avoided in long summer, the wind-typed malaria may be avoided in autumn, and arthralgia syndrome, coldness of extremities may be avoided in winter.

夫精者，身之本也。故藏〔于鬯说："藏上当脱'冬'字"〕于精者，春不病温。夏暑汗不出者，秋成风疟。此平人脉法〔此平人之脉也，疑为衍文〕也。

"The essence of life is the vital energy of a human body, and the vital energy is the foundation of man. When one's vital energy is abundant in winter, be can hardly be affected by evil, and the seasonal febrile disease will not be contracted in spring. In summer, if one fails to perspire when there should be a sweating, the evil energy will be shut inside, and one will contract wind-type malaria in autumn.

故曰：阴中有阴，阳中有阳。平旦至日中，天之阳，阳中之阳也；日中至黄昏，天之阳，

阳中之阴也。合夜至鸡鸣，天之阴，阴中之阴也；鸡鸣至平旦，天之阴，阴中之阳也。故人亦应之。

"Yin associates with the interior, and when the Yin energy stays inside, it is Yin in the Yin; Yang associates with the exterior, and when the Yang energy stays outside, it is Yang in the Yang. Take the elapse of day and night for example, the Yang energy emerges in the morning (6 AM) and becomes most prosperous at noon (12 PM), so it is the period of Yang in the Yang of the nature; the period of from noon to dusk (12 PM-6PM) still belongs to the day-time, but the dusk is the time when the Yin energy begins to emerge, so it is the period of Yin in the Yang; in the period of from dusk to cock- crow (6PM-12AM), it belongs to the night-time, and it is also the period of Yin from emergence to most prosperous stage, so, it is called the Yin of heaven, or Yin in the Yin of the nature; the period from cock crow to early morning (12AM-6AM), although it belongs to the night-time, but the morning is the time when the Yang energy begin to emerge, it is called the Yin of the nature and also called the Yang in Yin, and human being corresponds to the universe.

夫言人之阴阳，则外为阳，内为阴。言人身之阴阳，则背为阳，腹为阴。言人身之藏府中阴阳，则藏者为阴，府者为阳。肝心脾肺肾五藏皆为阴，胆胃大肠小肠膀胱三焦六府皆为阳。所以欲知阴中之阴阳中之阳者何也？为冬病在阴，夏病在阳，春病在阴，秋病在阳，皆视其所在，为施针石也。故背为阳，阳中之阳，心也；背为阳，阳中之阴，肺也。腹为阴，阴中之阴，肾也；腹为阴，阴中之阳，肝也；腹为阴，阴中之至阴，脾也。此皆阴阳表里内外雌雄相输应也，故以应天之阴阳也。

"In human body there are also Yin and Yang. For instance, from the view of interior and exterior, the exterior part of the body is Yang, and the interior part is Yin; from the view of front and rear, the back of the body is Yang, and the abdomen is Yin; from the view of solid and hollow organs, the five solid organs (heart, liver, spleen, lung and kidney) are all Yin and the six hollow organs (stomach, gallbladder, large intestine, small intestine, bladder and triple warmer) are all Yang.

"The reason for one to know the principles of Yin in the Yin and Yang in the Yang is for analysing the condition of diseases according to the five viscera and the four seasons. For instance, when one contracts the disease of kidney in winter, as the kidney is Yin and it is situated below, the disease is of Yin in the Yin; when one contracts the disease of heart in summer, as the heart is Yang and is situated above, it is the disease of Yang in the Yang; when one contracts the disease of liver in spring, as the liver is Yang and is situated in the middle warmer, it is the disease of Yang in the Yin; when one contracts the disease of lung in autumn, as lung is Yin and is situated above, it is the disease of Yin in the Yang. When treating the diseases of different solid organs in various seasons with needles and stones, one should comply with the condition of Yin and Yang situation.

"As the back of the body is Yang, the heart corresponds to fire, and the heart is situated on the upper part of the body, i. e., Yang situates on the position of Yang, so heart is the Yang in the Yang. As the abdomin is Yin, the kidney corresponds to water and situates bel-

low, i. e. , Yin situates on the position of Yin, so kidney is Yin in the Yin. As the abdomin is Yin, the liver corresponds to the wood, and the liver situates on the position of the middle warmer, i. e. , Yang situates on the position of Yin, so liver is Yang in the Yin. As the abdomin is Yin, the spleen corresponds to the earth, and spleen situates on the position of Taiyin, so the spleen is the extreme-Yin in the Yin.

"These statments above show the mutual connections of the solid and hollow (male and female) organs and the channel-liaisions of the human body and the endless circulations of the superficies and interior which corresponds the coming and going of the four seasons and the day and night, and the Yin and Yang of a human body corresponds with the Yin and Yang of the universe.

帝曰：五藏应四时，各有收受〔朝本作"攸"，"攸"有"所"义，"受"作"用"解〕乎？岐伯曰：有。东方青色，入通于肝。开窍于目，藏精于肝，其病发惊骇。其味酸，其类草〔沈祖绵说，"草"字衍〕木，其畜鸡，其谷麦，其应四时，上为岁星，是以春气在头也，其音角，其数八，是以知病之在筋也〔"是以"八字系错出应据《素问识》删〕，其臭臊。

Yellow Emperor asked: "Since the five viscera correspond with the four seasons, can all the five viscera be applied in the energies of the four seasons and the energies of Yin and Yang?"

Qibo answered: "Yes, Yang emerges in the east and the colour of east is green, the human liver is also green and corresponds to wood, as the energy of universe is connected with the human energy, so the east energy communicates with the liver. The liver channel gets access to the brain and connecting the eyes, so eyes are the orificcs of the liver. The Yin essence is stored in the liver where the soul lies, one's soul will be uneasy when the liver is ill and panic will occur. The taste of wood is sour, wood is also of the grass kind, so it belongs to the category of wood; Cock associates with wood, for the cock crows at the early morning just like the sun emerges in the east in the morning, so, in livestock, the liver corresponds to cock. Wheat is the crop that emerges in spring, so in crop, the liver corresponds with wheat. In the position of the four seasonal operations, the liver-wood corresponds with the position of the Sui star (the ancient name of Jupiter). In nature, the Yang energy is ascending, and in human body, the Yang energy ascends in spring, so the energy of spring of a man is in the head. In the five tones, the corresponding tone of liver is Jue (the third tone of the five tones,). The corresponding fulfil-number of liver is eight. In the five odours, the odour of liver is stink.

南方赤色，入通于心，开窍于耳〔"耳"误，应作"舌"〕，藏精于心，故病在五藏，其味苦，其类火，其畜羊，其谷黍，其应四时，上为荧惑星，是以知病之在脉也，其音征，其数七，其臭焦。

"The colour of the south is red, it corresponds with the fire, and the heart is also corresponds with the fire, so, the south energy communicates with the heart and stores its essence in the heart, the heart's orifices are in the tongue. The energies of the five viscera are dominated by the heart, so when the heart is ill, it will cause the diseases of the energies

of the five viscera. The taste of fire is bitter and it is also the extended energy of the fire, the heart corresponds with the fire, so, in taste, the heart is bitter, and in category, it belongs to the fire. Sheep is a livestock of fire. The broomcorn millet is red, so in crops, liver corresponds to broomcorn millet. In the positon of seasonal operation, the heart corresponds to Yinghuo star (the ancient name of Mars). As the heart controls the blood and the blood circulates in the vessels, so the disease of heart is in the vessels. The tone of heart is Zhi (the fourth tone in the five tones). The corresponding fulfil-number of heart is seven. In the five odours, the odour of the heart is of scorching.

中央黄色，入通于脾，开窍于口，藏精于脾，故病在舌本，其味甘，其类土，其畜牛，其谷稷，其应四时，上为镇星，是以知病之在肉也，其音宫，其数五，其臭香。

"Yellow is the colour of the centrality, and spleen which corresponds with the earth is also yellow, so the energy of centrality communicates with the spleen and stores its essence in the spleen. The mouth takes in the cereals, which enters into the stomach first, as stomach is the hollow organ of spleen, so the orifice of spleen is the mouth. Spleen energy connects the tongue, so the disease of spleen is in the tongue proper. The taste of the earth is sweet, as all sweets will nourish the spleen, so the taste of the earth is sweet. Millet is the elder one among crops and the millet is yellow, so in crops, the spleen corresponds with the millet. Cow is a livestock on earth, so, in livestock, spleen corresponds with the cow. Spleen corresponds with the earth, so in category, it belongs to earth. In the position of seasonal operation, it corresponds with Zhen star (the ancient name of Saturn). The spleen activates on the muscle, so the disease of spleen is in the muscle. In the five tones, the tone of spleen is Gong (the first tone in the five tones). The corresponding fulfil-number of the spleen is five. In the five odours, the odour of spleen is fragrance.

西方白色，入通于肺，开窍于鼻，藏精于肺，故病在背，其味辛，其类金，其畜马，其谷稻，其应四时，上为太白星，是以知病之在皮毛也，其音商，其数九，其臭腥。

"White is the colour of the west. The lung corresponds with the metal and is white, so the west energy communicates with the lung and stores its essence in the lung. The nose leads to the lung, so the orifice of lung is the nose. As the disease of autumn is on the shoulder and back, so the disease of lung is at the back. Acridness is the taste of the metal, so the taste of lung is acridness. The lung corresponds with the metal, so in category, it belongs to the metal. The horse is the livestock corresponds with the metal, so in livestock, lung corresponds with the horse. The paddy rice yields in autumn, so, in crops, the lung corresponds with the paddy. In the position of seasonal operation, the lung corresponds with the position of Taibai star (the ancient name of Venus). The lung determines the condition of the skin and hair, so the disease of lung is on the skin and hair. The tone of lung is Shang (the second tone in the five tones). The corresponding fulfil-number of lung is nine. In the five odours, the odour of lung is stinking.

北方黑色，入通于肾，开窍于二阴，藏精于肾，故病在谿，其味咸，其类水，其畜彘，其谷豆，其应四时，上为辰星，是以知病之在骨也。其音羽，其数六，其臭腐。

"Black is the colour of the north, the kidney corresponds with the water and stores its essence in the kidney. The openings of the kidney are the two lower orifices (front and rear orifices). The interpaces at the junctions of muscles of the body correspond to the bone, so the kidney disease is in the interpaces at the junctions of bones. Salty is the taste of water, so, in taste, the kidney is salty. Kidney corresponds with water, so it belongs to the category of water. Pig is the livestock corresponds with water, so, in livestock, kidney corresponds with the pig. The colour of the bean (black soya-bean) is black, so, in crops, the kidney corresponds with the bean. In the position of seasonal operation, the kidney corresponds to the position of Chen star (the ancient name of Mercury). Kidney corresponds to the bone, so the disease of kidney is in the bone. The tone of kidney is Yu (the fifth tone in the five tones). The fulfil-number of kidney is six. In the five ordours, the ordour of kidney is rancid.

故善为脉者，谨察五藏六府，一逆一从〔《太素》无两“一”字，“逆从”二字属上读〕，阴阳、表里、雌雄之纪，藏之心意，合心〔《太素》“心”作“之”〕于精。非其人勿教，非其真〔《太素》“真”作“人”〕勿授，是谓得道。

"Those who are keen in palpation of the pulse in diagnosis must investigate carefully to know whether the five viscera are agreeable with the energy and blood, the comprehensive condition of Yin and Yang, superfice and interior, male and female to the exquisite extent by deep consideralion, and at the same time, be familiar with the principles and be skillful in treating. When one is proficient in such a degree, he may select and teach someone and hand down the knowledge. It is only the person with such an achievement is deserved to be the one who has realy known the essentials of diagnosis."

阴阳应象大论篇第五

Chapter 5

Yin Yang Ying Xiang Da Lun

(The Corresponding Relation Between the Yin and Yang of Man and All Things and That of the Four Seasons)

黄帝曰：阴阳者，天地之道也，万物之纲纪，变化之父母，生杀之本始，神明之府也，治病必求于本。故积阳为天，积阴为地。阴静阳躁，阳生阴长，阳杀〔《类说》卷三十七引"杀"作"发"〕阴藏。阳化气，阴成形。寒极生热，热极生寒。寒气生浊，热气生清。清气在下，则生飧泄；浊气在上，则生䐜胀。此阴阳反作，病之逆从也。

Yellow Emperor said: "Yin corresponds to motionless and its energy symbolizes the earth, Yang corresponds to motion and its energy symbolizes the heaven, so, Yin and Yang are the ways of heaven and earth. As the birth, growth, developement, harvesting and storing of all things are all carried out according to the rule of growth and decline of Yin and Yang, so, Yin and Yang are the guiding principles of all things. In the mutual victory or defeat of Yin and Yang, the situation will be of numerous varieties, so, Yin and Yang are the parrents of variations. Yin grows while Yang is in vigour and Yin becomes deficient while Yang is weakened. From birth to death of all things are following the principle of Yin and Yang, so Yin and Yang are the foundation of to born and to kill. When the Yin and Yang are harmonized, the spirit will emerge, so Yin and Yang are the mansions of spirit.

"Thus, when treating a disease, one must base on Yin and Yang, that is to seek the orientation and developement of the disease from the variation of Yin and Yang to determine the guiding principle of treating.

"Heaven situates on up above, it is the accumulation of lucid Yang above; earth situates in down below, it is the accumulation of turbid Yin below. Yin associates with calmness, and Yang associates with impetuous movement. Yang associates with birth (like in spring) and Yin associates with growth (like in summer), Yang associates with developement (like in autumn), and Yin assooiates with hiding (like in winter). Yang has the function of activating the vital energy, and Yin has the function of shaping up the bodies of all things.

"As things which have reached their extremes turn into their opposites, extreme cold will bring on heat and extreme heat will bring on cold. Cold has the function of condensing which causes descending, and thereby turbidity is produced; heat has the function of dispersing which causes ascending, and thereby lucidity is produced. In pathology, when the lucid energy in the body is staying below, the heat-evil will be forced to descend to disturb the functional activities of spleen and stomach and the watery diarrhea with indigested food will

occur, if the tubid energy is staying above, the Yin-evil will rush up reversely to cause the obstruction of functional activities of vital energy and the flatulence will occur. These are the agreeable or adverse pathological changes caused by the abnormal conditions of Yin and Yang.

故清阳为天，浊阴为地；地气上为云，天气下为雨；雨出地气，云出天气。故清阳出上窍，浊阴出下窍；清阳发腠理，浊阴走五藏；清阳实四支，浊阴归六府。

"The energy of lucid Yang accumulates above to form heaven, and the energy of turbid Yin deposits below to form the earth. The earth energy ascends to become cloud by the evapouration of heaven energy. The heaven energy becomes rain when it descends. Thus, although the rain falls from heaven, yet it is transformed by the earth energy; although the cloud is formed from the earth energy, yet it depends on the evaporation by the heaven energy, and these are the relations of mutual functions of Yin and Yang.

Yang determines the energy which is ascending, so the lucid Yang gets out from the upper orifices of a man; Yin determines the shape and is descending, so the turbid Yin gets out from the lower orifices of a man. Yang has the function of guarding the exterior, so the lucid Yang is being sent off from the striae of skin; Yin has the function of watching the interior, so the turbid Yin moves about in the five viscera inside. As all Yangs stem from the four limbs, so the lucid Yang reinforces the four limbs; the six hollow organs transport and digest food to nourish the body, so the turbid Yin stabilizes in the six hollow organs. This is the physiological function of Yin and Yang.

水为阴，火为阳。阳为气，阴为味。味归形，形归气，气归精，精归化；精食气，形食味，化生精，气生形。味伤形，气伤精；精化为气，气伤于味。

"The property of water is cold and motionless, so it corresponds to Yin; the property of fire is hot and up-flaming, so it corresponds to Yang. The lucid Yang is ascending, so it is energy, the turbid Yin is substantial, so it is taste (food).

Man takes in food of five tastes and absorb its essence to nourish the body, so the food finally goes to the physique (including the bodily viscera, muscle, vessel, tendon and bone), when the physique is well nourished, the healthy energy will become substantial. The healthy energy can further produce the essence of life which can promote the living and transformation of all living things. The emergence of the essence of life depends on the healthy erengy, and the shaping up of the physique depends on the food (taste). The food, when being digested and transformed, it turns into the essence of life which can finally substantialize the physique.

"Although tastes can nourish the physique, but if the five tastes are taken excessively, it will hurt the physique; although the energy can promote the emergence of the essence, but if the energy becomes over-abundant, it will hurt the essence. When the essence of blood is abundant, it can be activated to become energy, but when the five tastes are excessively taken so as to hurt the physique, the energy will also be hurt indirectly, so, the energy can also be hurt by the tastes.

阴味出下窍，阳气出上窍。味厚者为阴，薄为阴之阳。气厚者为阳，薄为阳之阴。味厚则泄，薄则通。气薄则发〔李杲说：“‘发’作‘渗’”〕泄，厚则发热。壮火之气衰，少火之气壮，壮火食气，气食少火，壮火散气，少火生气。气味，辛甘发散为阳，酸苦涌泄为阴。

"Yin determines the taste which is substantial, so it is excreted from the lower orifices; Yang being the energy which is invisible, so it is breathed out through the upper orifices.

"Taste associates with Yin, when the taste is heavy, it belongs to Yin, when the taste is light, it belongs to Yang in Yin. The energy associates with Yang, when the energy is thick, it belongs to the pure Yang, when the energy is thin, it belongs to Yin in Yang.

"The property of Yin is cold and Yin moistens things below. The heavy taste is pure Yin, so it causes diarrhea; the light taste is Yang in Yin, so it causes the unimpediment of the stomach and intestine. The property of Yang is hot and Yang is flaming upwards, the thick energy is of pure Yang, so it produces heat, the thin energy is Yin in Yang which can ooze out the evil energy.

"As sthenic-fire which is the fire in hyperactivity consumes the vital energy and causes the wane of it, the medium-fire which is the normal fire nourishes the vital energy, so it makes the energy healthy and strong. Since sthenic-fire consumes the vital energy, so it can check one's vital energy and disperse it. The medium-fire nourishes the vital energy, so one will be nourished by it and the medium fire can cause the emergence of vital energy.

"In the tastes of Yin and Yang : the tastes of acrid and sweet have the functions of dispersing (sweet for moderating and acrid with sweet for dispersing), they associates with Yang. The tastes of bitter and sour have the function of causing vomit and diarrhea (bitter for diarrhea, sour for astringency, and sour with bitter for vomitting and discharging), they associate with Yin.

阴胜则阳病，阳胜则阴病。阳胜则热，阴胜则寒。重寒则热，重热则寒。寒伤形，热伤气。气伤痛，形伤肿。故先痛而后肿者，气伤形也；先肿而后痛者，形伤气也。风胜则动〔《类说》引“动”作“痛”〕，热胜则肿，燥胜则干，寒胜则浮〔《太素》“浮”作胕〕，湿胜则濡泻。

"The Yin and Yang within a human body must always be kept in balance. The over-abundance of Yin will cause Yang diseases, and the over-abundance of Yang will cause Yin diseases. The over-abundance of Yang will bring about heat evil, and the abundance of Yin will bring about cold-evil. But things will develope into the opposite direction when they become extreme, so the extreme heat may cause cold, and the extreme cold may cause heat.

"Cold is Yin-evil and heat is Yang-evil, Yang produces the vital energy and Yin shapes up the physique. So it is cold-evil that hurts the physique and heat-evil that hurts the vital energy. When one's energy is hurt, his channel energy will be stagnated and cause pain, when one's physique is hurt, his muscle will be cloggy and cause swelling. So, when the patient suffers from pain first and then suffers from swelling is due to the disease of vital energy which hurts the physique; when the patient suffers from the swelling first and then becomes painful, it is due to the damage of the physique which affects the vital energy.

"The property of wind is stirring, when the wind-evil is partial predominating, shaking and trembling of the patient will happen. When the heat-evil is partial predominating, it will stagnat inside and hurt the muscle to cause swelling. When the dry evil is partial predominating, the body fluid will be consumed and cause dryness. When the cold-evil is partial predominating, it will cause the debility of the Yang energy which fails to circulate and brings about edema. When the wetness-evil is partial predominating, the water and fluid will run downwards and cause diarrhea.

天有四时五行〔"五行"二字误窜，应在"以生寒暑"句上。王注："故云五行以生寒暑燥湿风五气也"〕，以生长收藏，以生寒暑燥湿风。人有五藏，化五气，以生喜怒悲忧恐。故喜怒伤气，寒暑伤形。暴怒伤阴，暴喜伤阳。厥气上行，满脉去形。喜怒不节，寒暑过度，生乃不固。故重阴必阳，重阳必阴。故曰：冬伤于寒，春必温〔胡本，讹本、赵本、吴本"温病"并作"病温"〕病；春伤于风，夏生飧泄；夏伤于暑，秋必痎疟；秋伤于湿，冬生〔《济生拔萃》引"生"作"必"〕咳嗽。

"In nature, there are the elapse of four seasons, and the changes of five elements produce the five energies, i. e., cold, heat, dryness, wetness and wind, and thereby to promote the birth, growth, harvesting and storing of all things. As the nature and man combine into one, there are five viscera for man correspondently. The five viscera of man produce the five energies which appear to be overjoy, anger, melancholy, anxiety and terror respectively.

"The excitation of moods like overjoy, anger etc. may damage the viscera, so it hurts the vital energy of a man. The sudden change of different weather, such as cold, heat, etc. may invade the muscle and skin, thus, it hurts the physique of a man.

"Violent rage makes the vital energy flows reversely and force the blood to run upwards and causes blood stagnation above, as a result, the Yin is hurt. Violent overjoy causes the vital energy to slow down and descend, as a result, the Yang is hurt.

"When the cold-evil attack the brain, the blood goes upwards together with the energy to cause the channels and vessels to fill up with blood. When the blood is overflowed, hemiparalysis of the body will occur.

"All the stimulation of overjoy or anger without temperance, and all the abnormal change of the cold and hot weather can damage the true energy of a man and shorten his life span.

"Therefore, excessive Yin will be changed into Yang, and excessive Yang will be changed into Yin.

"When the body is affected by cold-evil in winter, and the disease does not come on immediately, the cold-evil will hide inside, and tranforms into heat to become seasonal febrile disease in spring when Yang grows. When the body is affected by wind-evil in spring, as the wind-evil communicates with the liver, its energy will become abundant through the wind. When the liver is over-abundant, the spleen will be restricted. When the spleen fails to transport and digest the food, watery diarrhea with indigested food will occur in summer.

When the body is affected by summer-heat evil in summer and the disease does not come on immediately, the summer heat will hide inside, and when the body is invaded by the cold-evil in autumn, the contention of cold and heat against each other will cause malaria in autumn. When the body is affected by wet-evil in autumn, the wetness-evil will go up adversely to attack the lung, cough will occur in winter when the cold begins to evade."

帝曰：余闻上古圣人，论理人形，列别藏府，端络经脉，会通六合，各从其经；气穴所发，各有处名；谿谷属骨，皆有所起；分部逆从，各有条理；四时阴阳，尽有经纪，外内之应，皆有表里，其信然乎？

Yellow Emperor said: "I am told when the sages discribed the human body in ancient times, they always enumerated the positions of the five solid and six hollow organs respectively, pointed out the starting points and terminals of the twelve channels and the locations they pass through, divided the superficies and interiors of the three Yang channels and the three Yin channels into six coincidences (the Hand and Foot Shaoyin coincid with Taiyang channels, the Hand and Foot Taiyin coincide with Yangming channels and the Hand and Foot Jueyin coincide with Shaoyang channels), and each of them has accessible passage. The energy-points for affecting the channels are all located on specific positions and are all having their definite names. As the Xigu (Stream Valley) points locate between the joint of bones, so they belong to the bone, they are all having their starting points and terminals. The superficial collaterals on skin which belong to the twelve channels are in agreeable or adversed direction. The Yin and Yang change of the four seasons are all in a regular pattern and the superficies (Yang channels) and interiors (Yin channels) of a human body are corresponding. Are these versions correct?"

岐伯对曰：东方生风，风生木，木生酸，酸生肝，肝生筋，筋生心，肝主目。其在天为玄，在人为道、在地为化。化生五味，道生智，玄生神。神在天为风，在地为木、在体为筋，在藏为肝，在色为苍，在音为角，在声为呼，在变动为握，在窍为目，在味为酸，在志为怒。怒伤肝、悲胜怒；风伤筋，燥胜风；酸伤筋，辛胜酸。

Qibo answered: "The east corresponds to spring when the Yang energy begins to generate, as the Yang energy ascends and disperses to become wind, so the east produces the wind. The wind causes the wood to become flourishing, so, the wind produces the wood. Wood is one of the five elements, it produces sour in accordance with the earth energy, and produces the liver in accordance with the wood energy, so, the sour produces the liver. Liver maintain the tendons, so, liver produces the tendons. As tendon is produced from the liver, liver associates with the wood, and wood can produce fire, so the tendon produces the heart (heart corresponds to the fire). The liver energy communicates with the eyes, so, the liver determines the condition of the eyes.

"The heaven has its subtle effect of developement, and man has his ways of adapting to the variations of Yin and Yang, and the earth has its function of activating the growth of all things on earth. As the growth of all things are activated, the five tastes are produced, in the course of adapting the change of all things, the wisdom produced, and under the subtle

effect of developement, the deity produced. The deity takes charge of winds in heaven, takes charge on wood on earth, takes charge of tendons in human body, and takes charge of the liver in the five viscera.

"The colour of woods is green, in the five tones, it is Jue (the third tone), in sounds, it is shouting, in variations, it is grip. The eyes are the orificies of the liver, the taste of liver-wood is sour, the emotion of liver is anger, excessive anger will hurt the liver, but sorrow can overcome the anger (sorrow is the emotion of lung, and metal can restrict the wood). Excessive wind will hurt the tendon, but dryness can overcome the wind (dryness corresponds to the metal, and metal can restrict the wood); excessive sour food taken will hurt the tendon, but acridness can overcome the sourness (acrid corresponds to the metal and metal can restrict the wood).

南方生热，热生火，火生苦，苦生心，心生血，血生脾，心主舌。其在天为热，在地为火，在体为脉，在藏为心，在色为赤，在音为征，在声为笑，在变动为忧，在窍为舌，在味为苦，在志为喜。喜伤心，恐胜喜；热伤气，寒胜热；苦伤气，咸胜苦。

"The south corresponds to summer, and heat is produced in the land of fire in summer, the fire can be transformed into bitterness which is the taste of heart. The heart determines the condition of blood, which generates the spleen (fire generates the earth). As the tongue is the symptoms of trend for heart, therefore, the heart associates with the tongue.

"In the six weathers of heaven, the south is heat, in the five elements on earth (wood, fire, earth, metal and water), it is fire, in the human body, it is channel, in the five viscera (heart, liver, spleen, lung and kidney), it is heart, in the five colours (green, red, yellow, white and black), it is red, in the five tones, it is Zhi (the fourth tone), in sounds, it is laughing, in the variations of emotion, it is melancholy, in the orificies, it is the tongue, in tastes, it is bitterness, in the emotional actions, it is overjoy; excessive overjoy may hurt the heart, but terror can overcome the overjoy (terror is the emotion of kidney, and water can restrict the fire); excessive heat, on the contrary, can damage the vital energy (sthenic-fire consumes vital energy), cold can overcome the heat (cold water can overcome the fire energy); bitterness is the taste of fire, excessive bitterness can also consume the energy, and saltiness can overcome the bitterness (the taste of kidney is salty, and water can restrict fire).

中央生湿，湿生土，土生甘，甘生脾，脾生肉，肉生肺，脾主口。其在天为湿，在地为土，在体为肉，在藏为脾，在色为黄，在音为宫，在声为歌，在变动为哕，在窍为口，在味为甘，在志为思。思伤脾，怒胜思；湿伤肉，风胜湿；甘伤肉，酸胜甘。

"The centrality corresponds to the earth which produces the wetness, wetness is invisible and the earth is visible, as the visible things are produced from the invisibles, so wetness produces the earth. Earth associates with the farm, and crops in farm produces sweet, so the earth produces the sweet. The spleen controls the muscle, spleen-earth produces the lung-metal. Mouth is the orifice of spleen, so spleen associates with the mouth.

"In the six kinds of weather in heaven, centrality is wetness, in the five elements on

earth, it is earth, in human body, it is muscle, in the five viscera, it is spleen, in the five colours, it is yellow, in the five tones, it is Gong (the first tone), in sounds, it is singing, when the energy becomes adverse, it is hiccup, in the nine orificies, it is mouth, in the five tastes, it is sweetness, in emotions, it is anxiety. Excessive anxiety may hurt the spleen, but anger can overcome anxiety (anger is the emotion of liver, and the wood can restrict the earth), excessive wetness may hurt the muscle, but wind can overcome the wetness (wind associates with the wood, and wood can restrict the earth), excessive sweetness may hurt the muscle, but sour can overcome the sweetness (sour associates with the wood, and wood can restrict the earth).

西方生燥，燥生金，金生辛，辛生肺，肺生皮毛，皮毛生肾，肺主鼻。其在天为燥，在地为金，在体为皮毛，在藏为肺，在色为白，在音为商，在声为哭，在变动为咳，在窍为鼻，在味为辛，在志为忧，忧伤肺，喜胜忧；热〔据林校引《太素》“热”为“燥”〕伤皮毛，寒胜热；辛伤皮毛，苦胜辛。

"The west corresponds with dryness-metal, so the west produces the dryness, dryness is invisible and metal is visible, as the invisible things are produced from the invisibles, so dryness produces metal. The taste of metal is acrid, so metal produces acridness, lung associates with metal, so the acridness produces the lung. Lung determines the condition of hair and skin, so lung-metal produces the hair and skin. Lung-metal produces the kidney-water, so the hair and skin produces the kidney. The orifice of lung is nose, so the lung associates with the nose.

"In the six kinds of weather on heaven, the west is dryness, in the five elements on earth, it is metal, in human body, it associates with the hair and skin, in the five colours, it is white, in the five viscera, it is lung, in the five tones, it is Shang (the second tone), in sounds, it is crying, when the breath is adversing, it is cough, in the nine orifices, it is nose, in the five tastes, it is acridness, in emotions, it is melancholy, excessive melancholy may hurt the lung, but overjoy can overcome the melancholy (fire can restrict the metal), excessive dryness may hurt the hair and skin, and cold can overcome the heat.

北方生寒，寒生水，水生咸，咸生肾，肾生骨髓，髓生肝，肾主耳。其在天为寒，在地为水，在体为骨，在藏为肾，在色为黑，在音为羽，在声为呻，在变动为栗，在窍为耳，在味为咸，在志为恐。恐伤肾，思胜恐；寒伤血〔林校引《太素》“血”作“骨”〕，燥〔林校引《太素》“燥”作“湿”〕胜寒；咸伤血〔林校引《太素》“血”作“骨”〕，甘胜咸。

"The north corresponds to cold-water, cold is invisible and water is visible, as visible things are produces from the invisibles, so, water is produced from the cold. The taste of kidney is salty, so water produces the saltiness, and saltiness produces kidney, when the kidney obtains the water essence, it produces fat, fat produces marrow, so the kidney produces the marrow. The kidney water produces the liver-wood, the orifices of kidney are ears, so, kidney associates with the ears.

"In the six kinds of weathers in heaven, the north is cold, in the five elements on earth, it is water, in human body, it is bone, in the five viscera, it is kidney, in the five colours, it

is black, in the five tones, it is Yu (the fifth tone), in sounds, it is groaning (groaning is the sound of kidney), when it is reversed, shiver occur, the orifices of kidney are the ears, in the five tastes it is saltiness, in emotions, it is terror. Excessive terror may hurt the kidney, but anxiety can overcome the terror (earth can restrict the water). Excessive cold may hurt the bone and wetness may overcome the cold. Excessive saltiness may hurt the bone, but sweetness can overcome the saltiness (sweet is the taste of spleen).

故曰：天地者，万物之上下也；阴阳者，血气之男女也；左右者，阴阳之道路也；水火者，阴阳之征兆也；阴阳者，万物之能始也。故曰：阴在内。阳之守也；阳在外，阴之使也。

"All things situate between the heaven and earth, and they are relying on the energies of heaven and earth for existence. The heaven up above is Yang and the earth down below is Yin, so the heaven and earth are the ups and downs of all things. All things are born in accordance with the change of Yin and Yang of heaven and earth. For human being, those who draw support from Yang energy abundantly are men and are of vital energy, those who draw support from Yin energy abundantly are women and are of blood, so the Yin and Yang are the man and woman of energy and blood. Within the three dimensions of heaven and earth, east and south being the left, which is Yang; west and north being the right which is Yin. Yang associates with ascent and Yin associates with descent, thus, left and right are the routs for ascent and descent of Yin and Yang. The variations of Yin and Yang are invisible, but they can be observed through the change of water (corresponds to Yin) and fire (corresponds to Yang), so water and fire are the symptoms of Yin and Yang. Yin grows while Yang is in vigour, and Yin becomes deficient while Yang is weakened. All things are adhering to this law in the course of life from birth to death, so Yin and Yang are the initiators of all things. In a human body, Yin resides inside and Yang guarding outside. It is only when Yang guarding outside can Yin defend inside without dispersing; and it is only due to the Yin defending inside, can Yang operates outside. This is the case of mutual action of Yin and Yang."

帝曰：法阴阳奈何？岐伯曰：阳胜则身热，腠理闭，喘粗为之俯仰，汗不出而热，齿乾以烦冤，腹满死，能冬不能夏。阴胜则身寒，汗出，身常清，数栗〔《阴证略例：阴毒三阴混说》"栗"引作"躁"〕而寒，寒则厥，厥则腹满死，能夏不能冬。此阴阳更胜之变，病之形能也。

Yellow Emperor asked: "How can a man regulate the Yin and Yang of his own according to the operations of Yin and Yang of heaven and earth?" Qibo answered: "Overabundance of Yang should bring about the heat of the body and the openning of the striae of skin to cause sweating, but why it is when the body is hot, that the striae of skin is closed and no sweat appears? It is because the body fluid has become dry due to the scorching by the overabundance of Yang, and the sweat lost its source so as to have no perspiration occur. The dry up of body fluid is also evidenced by the dryness of the front teeth. When the Yang energy is partial over-abundant, it will make the patient gasp rapidly with continuous bending and lifting of head; when the heat-evil stagnated inside of the body, it will make the patient irritable

and depressed; the excessive heat may also cause the fullness of the abdomen of the patient. These are the fatal disease due to partial overabundance of Yang or even of pure Yang without Yin. If this kind of disease being encountered in the cold winter, the patient can still barely survive, but if it occurs in summer, the patient will surely die.

"When the Yin energy of the patient is partial overabundant, his Yang energy must be deficient, and his Wei-energy will be weakened, so his striae of skin becomes loose, his body perspires and often feels restless or even falls into coma. The patient may also feel the fullness of abdomen due to the stagnation of cold-evil. These are the fatal diseases of partial overabundance of Yin energy while the Yang energy being cut off. In this case, the patient can still barely survive when the disease occurs in winter, but will certainly die when the disease occurs in summer. The above statements show the symptom of the pathological change of Yin and Yang imbalance."

帝曰：调此二者奈何？岐伯曰：能知七损八益，则二者可调；不知用此，则早衰之节〔《甲乙》无"之节"二字〕也。年四十，而阴气自半也，起居衰矣；年五十，体重，耳目不聪明矣；年六十，阴痿，气大衰，九窍不利，下虚上实，涕泣俱出矣。故曰：知之则强，不知则老，故同出而名异耳。智者察同，愚者察异。愚者不足，智者有余，有余则耳目聪明，身体轻强，老者复壮，壮者益治。是以圣人为无为之事，乐恬憺之能，从欲快志于虚无之守，故寿命无穷，与天地终，此圣人之治身也。

Yellow asked: "But how to regulate properly the energies of Yin and Yang?" Qibo answered: "If one can regulate the Yin and Yang according to the physiological rule of seven disadvantages and eight advantages of men and women, one will promise longevity, if one can not do it properly, one would become early ageing.

"The Tiangui (substance origins from the kidney essence necessary for regulation of growth and reproduction) of man exhausts at the age of 64 (8×8). When he is 40 (5×8), only half of his Yin energy is left over, and his actions in daily life become weak. When he is 50, his blood and energy decline and his body becomes clumsy. As the essence and blood are insufficient to nourish oneself, his eyes and ears are no more accute. At the age of 60 which is approaching 64 (8×8), his Tiangui becomes exhausted, his kidney being declined and he becomes impotent. The kidney energy is the primordial true energy, when it is declined, the solid and hollow organs energies will all be weakened and can no more nourish the nine orifices and they will be no more facile. Since the Yang energy below is feeble and the Yin energy above is overabundant, it causes the tears to come out. This is the case when one fails to regulate the Yin and Yang properly and causes early ageing.

"Therefore, when one knows how to regulate the Yin and Yang properly will make his body strong, and his body will become decrepit and senile when not knowing how to regulate it. All the people live by drawing support from the energies of heaven and earth, but some of them live a long life and some die early due to their different achievments of health protecting. This is because a wise man can preserve his health before senility while a stupid man can only discover the fact after his senility has occurred. Thus, a wise man can remain strong

constantly and have enough essence and blood to spare, while a stupid man is always short of essence and blood. When one's essence and blood are ample, his body will be healthy and strong, his eyes and ears will be able to see and hear clearly, for an aged man, he can still have a strong body, for a young man, he will be even stronger.

"So the sages do nothing that is unprofitable to health preserving, find pleasure in the mode of indifferent to fame and gain and free from distracting thoughts, follow what the heart desire leisurely and take delight in the state of having no desire, so that their life may be endless and ever-lasting as the heaven and earth. This is the way of the sages to preserve health.

天不足西北，故西〔《太素》“西”下无“北”字〕北方阴也，而人右耳目不如左明也。地不满东南，故东〔《太素》“东”下无“南”字〕南方阳也，而人左手足不如右强也。帝曰：何以然？岐伯曰：东方阳也，阳者其精并于上，并于上则上明〔《类说》“明”引作“盛”〕而下虚，故使耳目聪明而手足不便也。西方阴也，阴者其精并于下，并于下则下盛而上虚，故其耳目不聪明而手足便也。故俱感于邪，其在上则右甚，在下则左甚，此天地阴阳所不能全也，故邪居之。

"The sky is lacking in north-west, and west corresponds to Yin, so the right eyes and ears of a man are not so acute as the left ones. The earth is not full in south-east, and east is Yang, so the left hand and foot of a man are not so strong as the right ones. This is to show the human body is matching the heaven and earth, and they are not perfect."

The Yellow Emperor asked: "Why is it so?" Qibo answered: "The east corresponds to Yang, when both Yang and the its essence staying above, the lower part of the body must be in debility, thus making the ears and eyes acute but the hands and feet not so facile. The west corresponds to Yin, when both Yin and its essence staying below, the upper part must be in debility making the ears and eyes not so acute but the hands and feet nimble. It is precisely because of the phenomena of Yin, Yang and essence being partial overabundant in the upper part or the lower part of the body, so as to cause the body to become overabundant above and in debility below or the vice versa. When evil is contracted, different cases may occur, such as in the upper part diseases of 'Yin and its essence both staying below and cause debility of the upper part', the disease in the right side is more serious than that of the left side (right corresponds to Yin), in the lower part diseases of 'Yang and its essence both staying above to cause debility of the lower part', the disease in the left side is more serious that that of the right side (left corresponds to Yang). This is because of the human, heaven and earth are not perfect in every way, and the evil energy takes advantage of the debility to reside.

故天有精，地有形，天有八纪，地有五里〔《太素》作“理”〕，故能为万物之父母。清阳上天，浊阴归地，是故天地之动静，神明之纲纪，故能以生长收藏，终而复始。惟贤人上配天以养头，下象地以养足，中傍人事以养五藏。天气通于肺，地气通于嗌〔《太素》“嗌”作“咽”〕，风气通〔《外台》引《删繁》“通”作“应”〕于肝，雷气通〔《外台》引《删繁》“通”作“动”〕于心，谷气通〔《外台》引《删繁》“通”作“感”〕于脾，雨气通

〔《外台》引《删繁》"通"作"润"〕于肾。六经为川，肠胃为海，九窍为水注之气〔《医说》引无"注之气"三字〕。以天地为之阴阳，阳〔"阳"应作"人"，王注："夫人汗泄於皮肤者"，似王所据本原作"人"〕之汗，以天地之雨名之；阳之气，以天地之疾风名之。暴气象雷，逆气象阳。故治不法天之纪，不用地之理，则灾害至矣。

"The reason of the heaven and earth can be the parents of all things is that the heaven has its invisible refined energy and the earth has its visible substance. The heaven has eight weather terms (i. e. the Beginning of Spring, the Spring Equinox, the Beginning of Summer, the Summer Solstice, the Beginning of Autumn, the Autumn Equinox, the Beginning of Winter and the Winter Solstice), and the earth has the distribution of five elements to be the guiding principle to breed all things. all the changes of heaven, earth, Yin and Yang are having their regular pattern, all things adhere to the regular law of birth, growth, harvesting and hiding.

"It is only the wise men can follow the law of light lucid energy of heaven to nourish his head which is above, and learn from the phenomenen of earth turbid energy to nourish his feet which is below, in the middle, he can regulate his eating and drinking, suits his motions and mind to nourish his five viscera.

"The lung situates on the upper part of the body and takes charge of respiration, so the heaven energy comunicates with the lung, the larygopharynx is the exit of the stomach which receives the cereals, so the earth energy communicates with the larygopharynx, As the wind energy produces the liver wood, so the wind energy corresponds with the liver; as the heart associates with the fire, and the thunder also associates with the fire, since like draws to like, so the thunder energy plays a part in the heart; the spleen takes charge of transporting and digesting the cereals, so, the energy of essential substance from cereal communicates with the spleen; the kidney is a solid organ of water, so the rain energy can moisten the kidney.

"The six channels of a man are like rivers in circulating, and the stomach and intestine which hold the cereals are like sea that contains everything. The refined energy of water connects the upper orifices, and the turbid energy of water connects the lower orifices. Since the tear, nasal mucus, saliva, urine and excrement all belong to the water, so the orifices are like the water flow.

"Take Yin and Yang of heaven and earth to analogize the Yin and Yang of a human body: when the Yin and Yang of heaven and earth combine, it becomes rain; when the vital energy and blood of a man merge, it causes sweating, so the sweat of man' is named as rain. The Yang energy circulates all through the body, and the wind energy spreads all over the land, so the 'energy of man' is named as the wind of heaven and earth. The violent-tempered energy of a man is like the burst of thunder, and the reversed energy of a man resembles the ascending of Yang.

"The life activity of a man has a close bearing with the heaven energy. When in treating a disease, one must follow the law and discipline of heaven and earth, otherwise, the

patient's life activity would be damaged, and calamity will occur immediately.

故邪风之至，疾如风雨，故善〔《千金》“治”下有“病”字〕治者治皮毛，其次治肌肤，其次治筋脉，其次治六府，其次治五藏。治〔《千金》“治”作“至”〕五藏者，半死半生〔《千金》无“半生”二字〕也。故天之邪气，感则害人五藏；水谷之寒热，感则害于六府；地之湿气，感则害皮肉筋脉。

"The arrival of evil-wind is like a sudden storm or tempest. When the evil-wind invades, it invades the skin and hair first, so it is important for a keen physician to treat at the begining of the invasion of skin and hair. If the evil-wind is not treated in time, it will further invade the muscle, so, it is the muscle that should be treated next. If the muscle is not treated in time, the wind-evil will further invade the tendons and the channels, so next, the tendons and channels should be treated. If the tendons and channels are not treated in time again, the wind-evil will further invade the five viscera, so next, the viscera should be treated. But, by the time when treating the wind-evil in the five viscera, it is hard to anticipate the curative effect, as the surviving rate of the patient is only 50%.

"Therefore, the evil energy from heaven often invades the human body from the exterior first, and then to the interior, shallowly first, then to the depth, and finally to the five solid organs. When the food or drink of improper temperature is taken into the stomach, it may cause disease of stomach and intestine, so the food can hurt the six hollow organs. The wet-evil retained in the body after invasion will make the Wei-energy and Ying-energy fail to operate properly and will damage the skin, muscle, tendon and channel.

故善用针者，从阴引阳，从阳引阴，以右治左，以左治右，以我知彼，以表知里，以观过与不及之理，见微得〔周本“得”作“则”〕过，用之不殆。

"So, he who is good at the acupuncture treatment must know the principle of Yin and Yang. As the Yin and Yang, vital energy and blood, channels and collaterals are linking each other, the evil that invades Yang can occur in Yin as well, so in acupuncture treatment, the evil in Yang can be drawn through Yin; the evil that invades Yin can occur in Yang as well, so the evil in Yin can be drawn through Yang also. By the same reason, disease on the left side can be treated from the right, and vice versa. Besides, in investigating a syndrome, the interior-syndrome can also be inferred through the superficies-syndrome. What is more important is to have the ability to analyse the asthenia and sthenia, heathy and evil energies of Yin and Yang and determine the location of the disease from the symptoms occurred. When a physician can diagnosis properly according to the principles of Yin and Yang, to know whether the disease is severe or slight, the patient will be unlikely to be left into danger due to misdiagnosis.

善诊者，察色按脉，先别阴阳。审清浊，而知部分；视喘息，听音声，而知〔《甲乙》“知”下有“病”字〕所苦；观权衡规矩，而知病所主〔《甲乙》“主”作“生”〕；按尺寸，观浮沉滑涩，而知病所生〔《类说》引“生”作“在”〕。以治无过，以诊则不失矣。

"He who is good at diagnosis always observes the complexion of the patient and palpates the pulse first, to distinguish whether the disease belongs to Yang or Yin (such as the red

complexion represents Yang, white complexion represents Yin, floating pulse shows Yang and deep pulse shows Yin, etc); infer in which channel the disease exists by observing the colour and the lucid or turbid complexion of the patient (such as the lucid is Yang, the turbid is Yin, the disease can be inferred from the five colours of the five parts of the face); distinguish to which solid organ the disease associates with from the pulse condition of the various seasons (such as spring determines the condition of liver, summer determines the condition of the heart, etc.); observe the condition of dyspnea and listen to the sound to infer the pain of the patient; feel the Chi and Cun pulse condition of the patient to know whether the disease is in the superficies or in the interior, in Yin or in Yang according to the floating, deep, slippery, choppy pulse conditions and treat the disease accordingly. In this way, the diagnosis may not be mistaken.

故曰：病之始起也，可刺而已；其盛，可待衰而已。故因其轻而扬之，因其重而减之，因其衰而彰之。形不足者，温之以气〔以气以味；柯校本“以气”作“以味，“以味”作“以气”按柯校“气味两字互易”〕；精不足者，补之以味〔应作“气”〕。其高者，因而越之；其下者，引而竭之；中满者，泻之于内；其有邪者，渍形〔《太素》作“清”〕以为汗；其在皮者，汗而发之，其慓悍者，按而收之；其实者，散而写之。审其阴阳，以别柔刚，阳病治阴，阴病治阳。定其血气，各守其乡，血实宜决之，气虚宜掣引之

“So, at the beginning, when the evil is still at the superficies, the disease can be cured by the pricking of needle for purging the evil; if the evil is overabundant, the needle should be retained after pricking to allow the evil-energy to decline automatically.

“When the disease is not at all serious and is on the superficies, it can be expelled by diaphoretic agent; when the disease is serious with internal sthenia, it can be discharged by excrement with purgative agent; when the disease is caused by deficiency of vital energy and blood, the vital energy and blood can be resumed by tonic therapy.

“As the physique is Yang, and the essence is Yin, the energy is Yang and the taste is Yin, the deficiency of the physique is a sign of the decline of Yang, it should be warmed with heavy taste, deficiency of essence shows the decline of Yin, it should be replenished by qifen drugs.

“When the evil is above the diaphram, emetic therapy can be used; when the evil is in the abdomen, purgation therapy can be used; when there is an abdominal flatulence, therapy of promoting digestion can be used.

“If the invasion of evil is deeper, the evil can be dispersed through sweat by hot-bathing; when the evil is on the skin and hair, it can be dispersed by diaphoresis; if the disease comes on suddenly with pain, massage can be used to calm its energy; when the disease associates with sthenia syndrome, it should be treated with dispersing therapy, and when the disease associates with the Yin sthenia sysndrome, it should be treated with purgative therapy.

“Investigate whether the disease belongs to Yin or Yang, and determine the case of disease and the way of treatment from the rigid or soft phenomenon.

"To the case of overabundance of Yang and Yin deficiency, Yin should be nourished, to the case of overabundance of Yin and Yang-deficiency, Yang should be strengthened, so that the energies of Yin and Yang may be balanced.

"Calm the blood and vital energy, so that they may remain in their own position without moving rashly.

"Sthenia means the sthenia of evil, and deficiency means the deficiency of healthy energy. When the blood is sthenic, the evil should be discharged by pricking when out letting the blood; deficiency of vital energy is the asthenia of channels and collaterals, so the energy should be drawn from the channel which is not deficient, to replenish the deficiency."

阴阳离合论篇第六

Chapter 6
Yin Yang Li He Lun
(The Individual Activities and the Mutual Functionings of Yin and Yang)

黄帝问曰：余闻天为阳，地为阴，日为阳，月为阴，大小月三百六十〔《太素》“六十”有“五”字〕日成一岁，人亦应之。今三阴三阳，不应阴阳，其故何也？岐伯对曰：阴阳者，数之可十，推之可百，数之可千，推之可万，万之大不〔按《素问玄机原病式》引无“大”字〕可胜数，然其要一也。

Yellow Emperor asked："I was told that the heaven is Yang and the earth is Yin，the sun is Yang and the moon is Yin. The year of 365 days is formed by the lunar months of 29 and 30 days，and man is corresponding with the change of the Yin and Yang of the four seasons. But now the three Yins and Yangs of human body do not tally with the Yin and Yang of heaven and earth，and why is it so?"

Qibo answerd："Yin or Yang is only a name which has no shape. It can be applied to everything，can be counted from one to ten，can be inferred from ten to one hundred，can be counted from one hundred to one thousand，and inferred from one thousand to ten thousand and even to innumerrable number. Although its change is infinite，but the process of Yin and Yang developement which is the unity opposites of things in the course of developement being one.

天覆地载，万物方生，未出地者，命曰阴处，名曰阴中之阴；则出地者，命曰阴中之阳。阳予之正，阴为之主。故生因春，长因夏，收因秋，藏因冬，失常则天地四塞。阴阳之变，其在人者，亦数之可数〔《太素》“数”作“散”，杨注：“散，分也”〕。

"With the ceiling of heaven above and the load of earth below，all living things survive by the descending of heaven energy and the ascending of earth energy. The heaven is Yang which associates with movement，the earth is Yin which associates with motionless. All things that concealed under earth are in the position of static Yin，they are called the component parts of Yin in Yin；all things that appear above the ground level are of Yin that reveal outside，they are called the component parts of Yang in Yin.

"Yang is to spread the healthy energy of coldness and warmness，Yin is to take charge of the vitality of all things. So the birth of all things is owning to the warmness of the spring energy，the growth of all things is a result of the hotness of summer energy，the harvesting of all things is due to the elimination and kill of the autumn energy，and the shut and hiding of all things are by the virtue of the coldness of winter energy. These are the regular pattern

of the four seasonal weather change and the birth, growth, harvesting and hiding of all things. If this normal condition is diverged, the heaven and earth will not be harmonious and the Yin and Yang will be obstructed from each other. The change of a human body can also be inferred from the phenomena of nature."

帝曰：愿闻三阴三阳之离合也。岐伯曰：圣人南面而立，前曰广明，后曰太冲，太冲之地，名曰少阴，少阴之上，名曰太阳，太阳根起于至阴，结于命门，名曰阴中之阳。中身而上，名曰广明，广明之下，名曰太阴，太阴之前，名曰阳明，阳明根起于厉兑，名曰阴中之阳。厥阴之表，名曰少阳，少阳根起于窍阴，名曰阴中之少阳。是故三阳之离合也，太阳为开，阳明为阖，少阳为枢。三经者，不得相失也，搏而勿浮，命曰一阳。

Yellow Emperor said: "I like to know the individual activities and mutual functionings of the three Yins and the three Yangs." Qibo said: "When a sage stands facing the south, in the front is Yang and it is called Guangmin (Yang being abundant), while the rear is Yin and it is called Tai chong, The Taichong channel starts from the kidney channel of Foot-Shaoyin, above the kidney channel of Foot-Shaoyin is the Urinary Bladder Channel of Foot-Taiyang. The lower terminal of Foot-Taiyang starts from the Zhiyin point of the foot , and its upper terminal connects the Jingming point on the face (the eye). The Taiyang channel coincides with the Shaoyin channel, and the Taiyang channel and the Shaoyin channel are being the superficies and the interior, so the Taiyang channel is called a component part of Yang in Yin.

"In the upper part of the body, Yang is overabundant, so it is called Guangming. Below the Guangming is the location of Taiyin-spleen, as the lower part of the body associates with Yin, so it is called Taiyin. In front of the Taiyin is the location of the Yangming-stomach, as the front associates with Yang, so it is called Yangming. The lower terminal of Yangming channel starts from the Lidui point of the foot, as Yangming channel and Taiyin channel are being the superficies and interior, so it is called a component part of Yang in Yin.

"The Jueyin and Shaoyang channels are being the superficies and interior, Jueyin in the exhaustion of Yin, which causes the Yang to emerge, as the Yang is newly born, it is called Shaoyang. The lower end of Shaoyang channel starts from the Qiaoyin point of the foot, as Shaoyang channel and Jueyin channel are being the superficies and the interior, and also is in the stage of initial birth of Yang energy, so it is called a component part of Shaoyang in Yin.

"So the activities and mutual functionings of the three Yangs are: The Taiyang controls the superficies, it spreads the Yang energy to guard the exterior, so it is open; Yangming controls the interior, it recieves the Yang energy to support the viscera, so it is close; the Shaoyang situates at the location of half superficies and half interior to transport between the exterior and the interior, so it is the pivot. The mutual functions of open, close and pivot of the three Yangs must not be lacking, its pulse condition should be a little bit slippery and not floating. When the energies of the three Yangs being harmonious and unified, the condition is called one Yang. In a word, the open, close and pivot are the activities of the three Yang channels, and the mutual actions of regulating and unifying are the mutual functions of the three Yang channels."

帝曰：愿闻三阴。岐伯曰：外者为阳，内者为阴，然则中为阴，其冲在下，名曰太阴，太阴根起于隐白，名曰阴中之阴。太阴之后，名曰少阴，少阴根起于涌泉，名曰阴中之少阴。少阴之前，名曰厥阴，厥阴根起于大敦，阴之绝阳，名曰阴之绝阴。是故三阴之离合也，太阴为开，厥阴为阖，少阴为枢。三经者，不得相失也，博而勿沉，名曰一阴。

Yellow Emperor said: "What about the individual activities and mutual functionings conditions of the three Yins' channels?" Qibo said: "Yang guards the muscle and superficies outside, and Yin nourishes the viscera inside. As the 'inside' is also Yin, and the Chong channel is below the Yin, so it is called Taiyin Channel, The Taiyin channel starts from the Yinbai (Hidden White) point on the foot, so it is called a component part of Yin in Yin.

"Behind the Taiyang-spleen is the location of Shaoyin-Kidney. The terminal of Shaoyin channel starts from the Yongquan (Pouring Spring) point of the foot, it is called a component part of Shaoyin in Yin.

"In front of the Shaoyin-kidney channel is the location of the Jueyin-liver channel, the root of the Jueyin channel starts from the Dadun (Great Mound) point of the foot. Since this channel is of pure Yin without Yang, so it is the exhausted Yang in Yin, as Yin is exhausted here, it is also called exhausted Yin in Yin.

"Therefore the condition of individual activities and mutual functions of the three Yins are: Taiyin is the superficies of the three Yins, if locates in the middle to spread Yin-energy and irrigates the surroundings, so it is open; Jueyin collects the Yin energy and transmits it to the interior, so it is close. Shaoyin is the kidney, when the kidney-energy is ample, the liver and spleen will bring their functions of open and close into a full play, so it is the pivot. The functions of these channels are complementing each other and none of them should be lacking. Its pulse condition should be of slight slippery and must not be over-floating. In this way, the energies of the three Yins will be harmonious and integrated, so it is called one Yin. The open, close and pivot are the activities of the three Yin channels, and they are supplementing each other, keeping harmony and integrity are the mutual functions of the three Yin channels. These are the general condition of the three Yin channels.

阴阳153153，积传为一周，气里形表而为相成也。

"The energies of Yin and Yang operate and move to and fro unceasingly in the body. It circulates one cycle by a day and night and goes round and starts again. This is the over-all condition of the energy which moves inside and manifest outside of the body, which is completed by the mutual actions of the interior and the exterior."

阴阳别论篇第七

Chapter 7
Yin Yang Bie Lun
(The Yin and Yang of Pulse Condition)

黄帝问曰：人有四经十二从，何谓？岐伯对曰：四经应四时，十二从应十二月，十二月应二十脉。

Yellow Emperor asked："A man has four channels and twelve equivalences, and what are the implications of them?" Qibo answered："The four channels are the four solid organs which correspond to the four seasons; the twelve equivalences are the twelve two-hour periods, the twelve two-hour periods correspond to the twelve meridians (The four channels are of liver, heart, lung and kidney, as the spleen does not correspond to one season only, so it is not mentioned. The liver channel corresponds to spring, the heart channel corresponds to summer, the lung channel corresponds to autumm, and the kindney channel corresponds to winter.) The twelve-hour periods correspond to the twelve months, such as correspond to Yin, Mao and Chen months in spring, to Si, Wu and Wei months in summer, to Shen, You, and Xu months in autumn and to Hai, Zi and Chou months in winter. The twelve months correspond to the twelve channels, such as the Hand Taiyin channel corresponds to the lunar first month, the Hand Yangming corresponds to the second month, the Foot Yangming Corresponds to the third month, the Foot Taiyin corresponds to the forth month, the Hand Shaoyin corresponds to the fifth month, the Hand Taiyang corresponds to the sixth month, the Foot Taiyang corresponds to the seventh month, the Foot Shaoyin corresponds to the eigth month, the Hand Jueyin corresponds to the ninth month, the Hand Shaoyang corresponds to the tenth month, the Foot Shaoyang corresponds to the eleventh month and the Foot Jueyin corresponds to the twelfth month.

脉有阴阳，知阳者知阴，知阴者知阳。凡阳有五，五五二十五阳。所谓阴者，真藏也，见则为败，败必死也。所谓阳者，胃脘之阳也。别于阳者，知病处也；别于阴者，知死生之期。三阳在头，三阴在手，所谓一也。别于阳者，知病忌时；别于阴者，知死生之期。谨熟阴阳，无与众谋。

"The pulse of Yin and Yang may be divided into position of Yin for Yang (such as floating, deep, slow or rapid pulse) and belonging to the Yin or Yang viscera (such as belonging to the solid organs or the hollow organs). Although the Yin and Yang pulse are different, yet they should be integrated and be kept consistent anywhere, and they must be in equilibrium. If one of the Yin and Yang being abnormal, the other one will be out of order, if Yang being over-abundant, then Yin must be in debility, and if Yin being over-abundant, then

Yang must be in debility. Thus, when one knows the condition of Yin, one can also know the condition of Yang, and when one knows the condition of Yang, he can also know the condition of Yin.

"In each of the five solid organs (heart, liver, spleen, lung and kidney), there is the Yang pulse for moderating. The pulses of the five solid organs correspond to the four seasons, and in each corresponding season occurs the pulse of its own with moderating stomach-energy. At the same time, in the other solid organs occur concurrently the pulse condition of the solid organs corresponds to the relevant season, such as in spring, the liver pulse is slightly wiry, and in the four solid organs of heart, spleen, lung and kidney also occur the moderating stomach pulse which are slightly wiry. Thus, there are five solid organs, and each of them has five different pulses in the different five seasons, and five times five are the twenty five Yang pulses.

"Yin indicates the pulse condition of indicating the exhaustion of visceral energy which is of entirely no stomach-energy. It may occur in all the pulses of the five solid organs. In clinic, most of them represent the syndrome of corruption. As the viscera-energy is corrupted and the stomach-energy is severed, the patient will surely die.

"Yang indicates the Yang of the gastric cavity which is also the stomach-energy. The stomach is the sea of water and cereal which receives the food, it takes charge of digesting the food to nourish the viscera, bones and the extremities, so all the channels of the five viscera depend on the nourishment of the stomach-energy.

"In pulse palpating, when one discovers the stomach-energy (the Yang energy) in a certain viscera is abnormal, he can ascertain that the disease is in the said viscera, so when Yang is abnormal, the location of disease can be indicated; when the pulse shows the visceral-energy and stomach-energy in certain viscera is exhausted, the time of the patient's death can be anticipated, so when the pwlse condition indicating the exhaustion of visceral energy is seen, the date of death can be scheduled.

"When the three Yangs (of which the stomach-energy dominates) on the head and the three Yins (of which the lung-energy dominates) on the hands being kept harmony, a normal physiological function of a man can be maintained (the three Yangs on head indicate the Renying pulse of the cervical arteries latereal to the thyroid cartilage reflecting the stomach-energy; the three Yins on hand indicate the Cunkou pulse along the radial artery proximal to the wrest reflecting the lung energy).

"In observing the pulse condition, one can know the taboo date of the disease, when the moderating stomach-energy of a certain solid organ is missing (such as the taboos of the liver disease are Geng and Xin, the taboos of the lung disease are Bing and Ding, etc.). So one can know the taboo date for the disease when Yang is abnormal, and one can know the date of death or survival when Yin is abnormal.

"When one knows well the principles of Yin and Yang and the Yin, Yang in the pulse, he can determine the proper treatment in the clinic without consulting others.

所谓阴阳者，去者为阴，至者为阳；静者为阴，动者为阳；迟者为阴，数者为阳。凡持真脉之藏脉者，肝至悬急，十八日死，心至悬绝，九日死，肺至悬绝，十二日死；肾至悬绝，七日死；脾死悬绝，四日死。

"In distinguishing the Yin, Yang from the pulse condition, all the going, calm and slow pulses belong to Yin, and all the coming, mobile and rapid pulses belong to Yang.

When the stomach-energy is exhausted in the liver pulse which is different from other viscera pulse, the patient will die in eighteen days; when the stomach-energy is exhausted in the heart pulse, which is different from other viscera pulse, the patient will die in nine days; when the stomach-energy is exhausted in the lung pulse which is different from other viscera pulse, the patient will die in twelve days; when the stomach-energy is exhausted in the kidney pulse which is different from other viscera pulse, the patient will die in seven days; when the stomach-energy is exhausted in the spleen pulse which is different from other viscera pulse, the patient will die in four days.

曰：二阳之病发心脾，有不得隐曲，女子不月；其传为风消，其传为息贲者，死不治。

"The disease of second Yang indicates the disease of Yangming stomach and large intestine, when one feels depressed, it will affect the functions of transportation and digestion of the spleen (anxiety hurts the spleen), and can also suppress the heart-energy; when the spleen is out of order, the stomach will be unable to digest the food, causing one to lose the source of nutrition, and when the heart-enerty is suppressed, it will be unable to transform the nutritive substances absorbed by the stomach and intestine into blood, and for a woman, her menstruation will stop. So the diseases of second Yang break out from the heart and spleen. If the disease protracts, the muscle will become emaciated due to the stomach fails to support the essence of the food, besides, the lung will be scorched by the heart-fire due to the faliure of the stomach fluid moistening the lung, in this case, dyspnea and the up-reversing of breath will occur. Since both the solid and hollow organs are damaged, the patient will certainly die.

曰：三阳为病发寒热，下为痈肿，及为痿厥腨痟；其传为索泽，其传为颓疝。

"The disease of the third Yang indicates the Taiyang disease. The Taiyang channel takes charge of the superficies, when the evil first invades a man, it is on the superficies, and when the healthy and evil energies contend, cold-heat will occur; if the evil stagnates between the muscle and the striae of skin, carbuncle will occur; when the evil hurts the Foot Taiyang bladder channel, the calf muscle where the channel passes will become painful, the foot will also become flaccid and cold. If the disease being protracted, the body fluid will become dry up due to the scorching of heat, the skin will become dry up due to the scorching of heat, the skin will become coarse and split open as it fails to be moistened, and when the wetness-heat pour down to invade the scrotum, hernia will occur.

曰：一阳发病，少气善咳善泄；其传为心掣，其传为隔。

"The disease of the first Yang indicates the disease of Shaoyang. Shaoyang is the stage of Yang newly born when the Yang is tiny, and Yang will be even tiny when the disease is

contracted. The Shaoyang being the prime minister-fire, when the fire scorch the lung-metal, cough will occur. The large intestine and the lung being the superficies and the interior, when the adverse rising lung energy being hurt, the energy of the large intestine will be unstable, and diarrhea will occur. As the prime minister-fire is vigorous inside, the heart will be affected and become uneasy. As the wood fire restricts the spleen and stomach, the food intake will be obstructed and cause dysphagia.

二阳一阴发病，主惊骇背痛，善噫善欠，名曰风厥。

"The disease of the second Yang and first Yin indicates the disease of Yangming and Jueyin. As the Jueyin liver disease appears to be terror, and the Yangming disease occurs on the tendon of the spine, so, backache will occur. When the Yangming stomach is hurt by the wind-evil, often belching and yawn will occur. The above syndromes of adverse rising of lung-energy caused by the disease of liver and stomach affected by wind are called Jue-syndromes of wind.

二阴一阳发病，善胀心满善气。

"The disease of the second Yin and first Yang indicates the diseases of Shaoyin (kidney) and Shaoyang (gallbladder). When the gallbladder energy is over-abundant, it will restrict the spleen earth to cause the spleen become ill and distending. In the disease of Shaoyin, the channels of heart and kidney fail to communicate, so the fullness of heart is felt with often deep sighing.

三阳三阴发病，为偏枯、痿易、四支不举。

"The disease of the third Yang and third Yin indicates the disease of Taiyang and Taiyin. As the Taiyang takes charge of the energy, when the Yang energy is in debility, hemiplegia will occur; as Taiyin takes charge of the blood, when the Yin blood fails to nourish the tendon, the tendon will be in flaccidity and out of order, as the spleen takes charge of the four limbs, when the spleen is ill, the four limbs will be unable to lift up.

鼓一阳曰钩〔能志聪说："钩"当作"弦"，下文"弦"当作"钩"〕鼓一阴曰毛，鼓阳胜急曰弦〔当作钩〕，鼓阳〔"阳"象上误，疑当作"阴"〕至而绝曰石，阴阳相过曰溜。

"When there is a mild energy stirring in the pulse which appears to be straight and long, it is called the 'wiry pulse'; When there is a Yin energy stirring in the pulse which is light, empty and floating, it is called the 'feather pulse'; when the rapid pulse of Yang is abundant which begins strongly and ends weakly, it is called the 'hook pulse'; when in the pulse, the Yang energy is deep lying low and is about to sever, and the pulse is sunken, it is called the 'stone pulse'; when in the pulse, the Yin and Yang energies are soft and harmonious, and the pulse is moderate, it is called the 'flowing pulse'.

阴争于内，阳扰于外，魄汗未藏，四逆而起，起则熏〔"熏"应作"动"，"动"作"伤解，杨上善说"内伤于肺"〕肺，使人喘鸣。阴之所生，和本曰和〔《太素》"和"作"味"，杨上善说："和气之本曰五味也"〕是故刚与刚，阳气破散，阴气乃消亡。淖则刚柔不和，经气乃绝。

"When Yin is contending inside and Yang is disturbing outside, Yin and Yang will be

out of balance. When Yang is not dense outside, the sweat gland will be wide open, and continuous sweating will occur, When Yin is out of order inside, the Yin essence will be out let and cause coldness of the extremities. When the heat of Yang hurts the lung, it will cause dyspnea and bronchial asthma.

"As Yin depends on the harmony of Yin and Yang to generate all things, so the generation of Yin of the five solid organs all depends on the nourishments of the five tastes.

When Yang is over-abundant all by itself and fails to keep harmony with Yin, it is the situation of 'vigorous with vigorous', which is called the single Yang. When the single Yang is broken and dispersed outside, Yin will be withered away in the wake of it.

"Excessive Yin causes the over-abundance of cold-wetness, when Yin being over-abundant all by itself without keeping harmony with Yang, it is called the single Yin, as the single Yin can not promote the birth and growth of all things, the channel-energy will be severed.

死阴之属，不过三日而死；生阳之属，不过四日而死〔周本"死"作"生"，《太素》"死"作"已"，"已"谓病愈〕。所谓生阳死阴者，肝之心谓之生阳，心之肺谓之死阴，肺之肾谓之重阴，肾之脾谓之辟阴，死不治。

"When the five-solid organs passes on from one to another to subjugate, it is called the 'dead Yin'; when the five solid organs pass on from one to another to generate, it is called the 'living Yang'. The patient with dead Yin will die in three days, and that with living Yang will be recovered and survive in four days.

"The meaning of living Yang and dead Yin are: when the liver passes on to the heart (wood generates fire), it is called the living Yang, when the heart passess on to the lung (fire restricts metal), it is called the 'dead Yin'; when the lung passes to the kidney, both the organs are of Yin, and the two Yins' combining causes the disease to become serious, so it is called the 'double Yin'; when the kidney passes to the spleen, that is, the kidney water bully the spleen earth reversely, it causes the spleen earth to become declined and severed, the disease will become even serious, in this case, it is called the excluding Yin, the patient will die without being cured.

结阳者，肿四支。结阴者。便血一升，再结二升，三结三升。阴阳结斜，多阴少阳曰石水，少腹肿。二阳结谓之消，三阳结谓之隔，三阴结谓之水，一阴一阳结谓之喉痹。阴搏阳别〔《济生方》卷七引作"阳搏阴别"〕谓之有子。阴阳虚肠辟死。阳加于阴谓之汗。阴虚阳搏谓之崩。

"Yang indicates the three Hand and Foot channels, as the Yang channels act on the superficies of the four extremities, whenever there is a stagnation of evil, the energy and blood will become sluggish in the extremities and causes swelling of the limbs.

"The blood belongs to Yin, since the Yin channel stagnates, it will affect the circulation of the blood, when the blood fails to circulate outside, it will be accumulated and seeped into the intestine to cause hematochezia; when the Yin channel stagnates further, the bloody stool will come to two litres, if the disease is getting even worse, the bloody stool will come

to three litres.

"In the stagnation of evil in Yin and Yang, when Yin is more and Yang is less, then Yang will be in debility. Since the bladder loses its function to evaporate the body fluid, it will cause accumulation of the fluid which is called the water of stone. The lower abdomen will be swelling on account of it.

"The second Yang indicates the Yangming channel and the stomach, if there is a heat stagnated in the large intestine and stomach, the water and cereal will be consumed rapidly to contract diabetes and the patient gets hungry no sooner than the food has been taken.

"The third Yang indicates the Taiyang small intestine and the bladder channels. When there is a stagnated heat in the small intestine and bladder, the stool and urine will be blocked.

"The third Yin indicates the Taiyin lung and spleen channels. When there is a stagnated heat in the lung and spleen, they can no more transport the body fluid, as the fluid stagnates, edema will occur.

"The first Yin indicates the Jueyin liver and pericardium, the first Yang indicates the Shaoyang of gallbladder and the triple warmer, both the two channels associate with fire, when it moves, wind will produce. When the wind joins the fire, it will scorch the body fluid and sore throat will occur.

"When the pulsation of Cun pulse of Yang is different from that of Chi pulse of Yin, it is the pulse condition of the pregnacy of a woman.

"When both the Yin and Yang pulses are in debility with bloody stool in bubble, it is the severing of the true energy, the patient will die certainly.

"When Yang is more abundant than Yin, the Yang energy will force the Yin fluid to discharge and cause sweating.

"When Yang is contending, it is the over-abundant of Yang, when Yin is in debility and Yang is over-abundant, the blood will be forced to run rashly and cause metrorrhagia.

三阴俱搏，二十日夜半死。二阴俱搏，十三日夕时死。一阴俱搏，十日〔吴本，周本，朝本“十日”下并有“平旦”二字〕死。三阳俱搏且鼓，三日死。三阴三阳俱搏，心腹满，发尽，不得隐曲，五日死。二阳俱搏，其病温〔胡本，朝本“温”并作“滥”〕，死不治，不过十日死。

"When the pulses of the third Yin (lung and spleen) all pulsate under the fingers, the patient will die at midnight of the twentieth day. When the pulses of the second Yin (heart and kidney) all pulsate under the fingers, the patient will die in the evening of the thirteenth day. When the pulses of the first Yin (pericardium and liver) all pulsate under the fingers, the patient will die in the early morning of the tenth day. When the pulses of the third Yang (bladder and small intestine) all pulsate under the fingers, and the beats are stirring vigorously, the patient will die on the third day. When the pulses of the third Yin and the third Yang all pulsate under the fingers, the patient will feel fullness and flatulence of the abdomen and heart, suffering from pain and the retention of faeces and urine, he will die on the fifth day.

When the pulses of the second Yin (stomach and large intestine) all pulsate under the fingers, it means that the channel-energy has already dispersed which can by no means be cured, the patient will die within ten days."

灵兰秘典论篇第八

Chapter 8
Ling Lan Mi Dian Lun
(The Confidential Collections in the Royal Library about the Functions of the Twelve Viscera)

黄帝问曰：愿闻十二藏之相使，贵贱何如？岐伯对曰：悉乎哉问也，请遂言之。心者，君主之官也，神明出焉。肺者，相傅之官，治节出焉。肝者，将军之官，谋虑出焉。胆者，中正之官，决断出焉。膻中者，臣使之官，喜乐出焉。脾胃〔《五行大义》引无“胃”字〕者，仓廪之官，五味出焉。大肠者，传道之官，变化出焉。小肠者，受盛之官，化物出焉。肾者，作强之官，伎巧出焉。三焦者，决渎之官，水道出焉。膀胱者，州都之官，津液藏焉，气化则能出矣。凡此十二官者，不得相失也。故主明则下安，以此养生则寿，殁世不殆，以为天下则大昌。主不明则十二官危，使道闭塞而不通，形乃大伤，以此养生则殃，以为天下者，其宗大危，戒之戒之！

The Yellow Emperor asked: "I would like you to tell me the mutual relations between the twelve viscera in human body and their principal and subordinate status in functions."

Qibo answered: "What an exhaustive question you have asked: Now, let me tell you: The heart is the supreme commander or the monarch of the human body, it dominates the spirit, ideology and thought of man.

"The lung governs the various vessels and regulates the energy of the whole body, like a prime minister assisting the king to reign the country.

"The liver is a vigorous viscera, its emotion is anger, it is like a general who is valiant and resourceful.

"The gallbladder is like an impartial judge who makes one to judge what is right and what is wrong.

"The Tan Zhong (indicating the pericadium here) is like a butler of the king who can transmit the joyfulness of the heart through it.

"The spleen is like an officer who is in charge of the granary, it takes charge of the digesting, absorbing, spreading and storing of the essence of food.

"The large intestine is the route for transmitting the drosses, it transforms the drosses into faeces and then excretes them to the outside of the body.

"The small intestine receives the food from the stomach, it digests the food further, divides them into the essence and the dregs, then asborbs the essence and transmits the dregs to the large intestine.

"The kidney is an organ with strong functions, when the essence and energy in the kid-

ney are abundant, the body will be strong and the person is skillful and wise in doing things.

"The triple warmer takes the office of dredging water in the watercourse of the whole body, it takes charge of the activity of the vital energy of the body fluid and the regulation and the dredging of the fluid.

"The bladder takes the office of gathering, it stores the water and fluid, after the body fluid is transformed into water by the activating of vital energy, it can be excreted.

"The above twelve viscera must be coordinating and supplementing to each other. As the heart is the monarch in the organs, it dominates the functions of the various viscera, so when the function of heart is strong and healthy, under its unified leadership, all the functions of the various viscera will be normal, the body will be healthy and the man will live a long life, and in his life long days, no serious disease would occur. It is just like the condition in a country, when the monarch is wise and able and all the work in various departments are in concert, the country will be prosperous and powerful, but when the monarch is thick-headed, that is, when the function of the heart is incapable, the mutual relations between the viscera in the body will be damaged, the body will suffer great injury to affect one's health and the length of life. In a country, the political power will be unstable and every thing in the country will be out of order. It is advisable for one to pay attention to it greatly.

至道在微，变化无穷，孰知其原！窘乎哉，消者瞿瞿，孰知其要！闵闵之当，孰者为良！恍惚之数，生于毫厘，毫厘之数，起于度量，千之万之，可以益大，推之大之，其形乃制。

"The principle of health-preserving is rather delicate, one can by no means to understand its origin unless by looking into it carefully.

"Since the principle of health-preserving is subtle and hard to comprehend, one can hardly decide what is right among the essentials although by painstaking pondering during study. It is only by explicit analysis through weighing the conditions can one understand the essence of heart which is the dominator of the whole body and the importance of heart to the twelve organs.

"Any tiny substance in the nature, though it is invisible to the naked eye, yet it is an existing matter anyway. When they are assembled together to have a size of about a milimeter, they become visible, and their size and weight can be measured by calculation. When the tiny substances being accumulated and expanded to a certain extent, it forms the human body."

黄帝曰：善哉，余闻精光之道，大圣之业，而宣明大道，非斋戒择吉日，不敢受也。黄帝乃择吉日良兆，而藏灵兰之室，以传保焉。

Yellow Emperor said: "Very good. I am told that all principles pure and bright (indicating the way of preserving health here) are from the sages. I should fast and select an auspicious day to accept it". So Yellow Emperor selected an auspicious day with good omen and kept the conversation in written material in the royal library for storing and handing down.

六节藏象论篇第九

Chapter 9
Liu Jie Zang Xiang Lun
(The Close Relation Between the Viscera in Human Body with the Environment of the Outside World)

黄帝问曰：余闻天以六六之节，以成一岁，人以九九制会，计人亦有三百六十五节，以为天地久矣。不知其所谓也？岐伯对曰：昭乎哉问也，请遂言之。夫六六之节，九九制会者，所以正天之度，气之数也。天度者，所以制日月之行也；气数者，所以纪化生之用也。天为阳，地为阴；日为阳，月为阴；行有分纪，周有道理，日行一度，月行十三度而有奇焉，故大小月三百六十五日而成岁，积气余而盈闰矣。立端于始，表正于中，推余于终，而天度毕矣。

Yellow Emperor asked: " I am told that with the combination of of heaven's decimal cycle (Jia, Yi, Bing, Ding, Wu, Ji, Geng, Xin, Ren and Gui) and the earth's twelve duodecimal cycle (Zi, Chou, Yin, Mao, Chen, Si, Wu, Wei, Shen, You, Xiu and Hai) it makes a cycle of sixty days and six cycles make a year; the earth with its ninety days in a season to commiunicate with the heaven; and man has the 365 acupoints to correspond with the number of heaven and earth. This version has long been disseminated, but why is it so?"

Qibo answered: " What a brilliant question you have asked: Now let me explain it to you: The six and six number is to set the degree of heaven, and the nine and nine number is to illustrate the earth energy in generating all things. The degree of heaven is the criterion of the motion of sun and moon, and the number of earth-energy is the outline of its periodic cycle in generating and promoting growth of all things.

" The heaven is Yang and the earth is Yin; the Sun is Yang and the moon is Yin. The revolution of sun and moon are all according to regular degrees, and the speed of their revolution are subjected to a certain rule. The complete cycle of heaven is three hundred sixty five degrees. The sun moves one degree in a day and night, the moon moves thirteen and seven and nineteenth degrees in a day and night. It takes three hundred and sixth five days odd for the moon to travel the complete cycle, and twenty nine days odd for the moon to travel the complete cycle. It is stipulated that the days for the moon to travel the complete cycle is a month, and the days for the sun to travel the complete cycle is a year. When adding all the big and small months of the year, there are three hundred and sixty five days with some remainder (the complete cycle is three hundred and sixty five and one fourth degrees). With the six days of the six small months which are lacking in the year and the remainder days stated above, we add two leap months in five years so that the degree of heaven

may be fitted.

" Set up an erect wooden pole on the ground, measure the various length of the sun's shadow from the day of Winter Solstice or Summer Soltice daily to calculate the revolving degree of the sun and moon, and in addition with the remainder, then, the calculation of the degree of heaven can be accomplished."

帝曰：余已闻天度矣，愿闻气数何以合之？岐伯曰：天以六六为节，地以九九制会，天有十日，日六竟而周甲，甲六复而终岁，三百六十日法也。夫自古通天者，生之本，本于阴阳，其气九州九窍〔"九窍"二字是衍文〕，皆通乎天气，故其生五，其气三，三而成天，三而成地，三而成人，三而三之，合则为九，九分为九野，九野为九藏，故形藏四，神藏五，合为九藏以应之也。

Yellow Emperor said: " Now I have heard the essentials of the degree of heaven, but I want to hear further how the number of earth being in concert with the heaven's degree." Qibo answered: " The heaven takes the number of six to be the criterion and the earth communicates the heaven with the number of nine. When the ten decimal cycle of heaven in combination with the twelve duodecimal cycle of earth (becoming Jia Zi, Yi Chou....) it makes a cycle of sixty days, and six cycles make a year, and this is the way of calculating the three hundred and sixty days in a year.

" Since ancient time, all who know the principle of heaven, take the heaven as the source of life, in other words, all lives on earth stem from Yin and Yang. the earth-energy of all the prefectures (the various districts on earth) are communicating with the heaven energy.

" Thus, there is a version of the five elements (wood, fire, earth, metal, water) and the three energies (three Yin energies and three Yang energies).

" There are three energies in heaven, three energies on earth, and three energies for man, and the sum will aggregate to nine. On earth, there are nine prefectures, and for man, there are nine viscera, that is, the four organs which store substances (stomach, large intestine, small intestine, bladder) and the five organs which store the spirits (lung stores inferior spirit, liver stores soul, heart stores spirit, spleen stores consciousness, kidney stores will), and the number of nine viscera correspond with the number of six and six of heaven."

帝曰：余已闻六六〔"六六"之下，似脱"之节"二字〕九九之会也。夫子言积气盈闰，愿闻何谓气？请夫子发蒙解惑焉。岐伯曰：此上帝所秘，先师传之也。帝曰：请遂闻之。岐伯曰：五日谓之候，三候谓之气，六气谓之时，四时谓之岁，而各从其主治焉。五运相袭，而皆治之，终朞之日，周而复始；时立气布，如环无端，候亦同法。故曰：不知年之所加，气之盛衰，虚实之所起，不可以为工矣。

Yellow said: " Now I understand the meaning of the correspondance of six and six with nine and nine. You have mentioned the remainder days of the solar terms are accumulated into the leap months, but what is the solar term? Please enlighten my ignorance and untie my perplexity." Qibo said: " This is what the preceding emperors would not tell, and was imparted to me by my teacher." Yellow Emperor said: " I hope you can tell me all about it."

Qibo said: " There are five days for a pentad and three pentads make a solar term; six solar terms (ninety days) make a season, and four seasons make a year. In each year, there is an element-energy dominanting the year (such as the earth-element dominates the year of Jia Zi), and the five element-energy dominating alternately in a regular order. When treating, one must suit the dominating element energy in various periods. After an element dominates the period of one year , the next element will be dominating in next year, after five years which is of sixty months, it is a cycle of Jia Zi. The energies of the five elements are dominating one after another and go round and begin again. It is divided into five parts in a year, and each of the five elements dominates one season (wood dominates spring, fire dominates summer, earth dominates long summer, metal dominates autumn, water dominates winter). Thus, each of the four seasons are disseminating on due time the energy of its corresponding element. When reducing the scope into a pentad, it is also divided into five, and the way of division is the same with that in a year. Thus, when treating a disease, if one is ignorant about the period of the arrival of the energy of wind, cold, heat, wetness and fire in the year, and know not the principle of asthenia and sthenia induced by the going beyond or falling short of energies of the five elements, he will be unable to master the rule of the pathological change in the usual enviroment, and is uncapable to be a physician. "

帝曰：五运之〔"之"应作"终"〕始，如环无端，其太过不及何如？岐伯曰：五气更立，各有所胜，盛虚之变，此其常也。帝曰：平气何如？岐伯曰：无过者也。帝曰：太过不及奈何？岐伯曰：在经有也。帝曰：何谓所胜？岐伯曰：春胜长夏，长夏胜冬，冬胜夏，夏胜秋，秋胜春，所谓得五行时之胜，各以气命其藏。帝曰：何以知其胜？岐伯曰：求其至也，皆归始春，未至而至，此谓太过，则薄所不胜，而乘所胜也，命曰气淫；不分邪僻内生工不能禁。（王注：此十字文义不伦，应古人错简。）至而不至，此谓不及，则所胜妄行，而所生受病，所不胜簿之也，命曰气迫。所谓求其至者，气至之时也，谨候其时，气可与期。失时反候。五治不分，邪僻内生，工不能禁也。

Yellow Emperor said: " Now I understand the condition of the energies of the five elements dominating the year, and they are going round and begin again like a ring without terminal. But when the element-energy is dominating the year, what will be the condition when they are going beyond or falling short?" Qibo said: " The dominating year of the five elements is in succession and alters once a year. In the period of dominating, there often occurs the case of going beyond or falling short, so in the operation of energy in a year, it often has victory or defeat. When being victorious, it is over-abundant or going beyond, when being defeated, it is in debility of falling short. In this case, their energies will be out of balance which will affect the health of human being, and the pathological change of man will be an in evitable phenomenon when the operation of heaven is abnormal. "

Yellow Emperor said: " What is the case of energy in common condition?" Qibo said: " When the energy appears on due time without going beyond and falling short, it is the common condition. "

Yellow Emperor said: " What is the case when the energy is going beyond or falling

short?" Qibo said: " It was recorded in the classics. "

Yellow asked: " What do you mean by overcoming?" Qibo said: " The fact of victory or defeat of the four seasons is based on the principle of the overcome and restrict of the five elements, and the victorious energy will restrict the defeated declining energy, such as spring overcomes the long summer, that is, the wood restricts earth; the long summer overcomes winter, that is, the earth restricts water; the winter overcomes summer, that is water restricts fire; the summer overcomes autumn, that is, fire restricts metal; the autumn overcomes spring, that is, metal restricts wood. The viscera are nominated respectively according to the energy of the four seasons and the five-element energy of which the viscera stored. This is the condition of the overcoming of the five-element energy of spring, summer, long summer, autumn and winter. Besides, when the energies are dominating the seasons, the dominating element-energy stores in the correspondant viscera of man, such as, the spring wood energy stores in liver, the summer fire energy stores in heart, the long summer earth energy stores in spleen, the autumn metal energy stores in lung, and winter water energy stores in kidney. "

Yellow Emperor asked: " How can we know when the energy is overcoming?" Qibo said: " One can discover it by comparing the solar term with the arriving time of the stored energy of the viscera. The Beginning of spring is the first solar term of the year, and it is also the time for the stored energy of viscera begin to arrive. If the stored element energy arrives prior to the solar term of Beginning of spring, it is the case of the stored element-energy being over-abundant which is going beyond. When the stored energy is over-abundant, it will invade the element energy which overcomes itself and restricts the element-energy further which it overcomes (such as, if the wood energy is abundant and the metal energy is in debility, then the wood, on the contrary, will bully the metal, and at the same time, restrics earth even more). In this case, it is called the 'mixing of the solar term's energy with the going beyond stored energy'. When the normal physiology of man is interrupted by the confussion of the weather, internal disease will occur, and the affection seduced by the abnormal weather can by no means be prevented by a physician.

" If the stored element-energy of the viscera does not come in the due solar term, it is called the falling short, the element-energy which is then in debility will be unable to control the element-energy which it used to overcome and cause it to run rashly. Besides, the energy which is then in debility can no more support its generation energy and cause the decline of it, and the energy which is in debility itself will be persecuted by the energy that restricts it, such as, when wood energy is in debility, earth energy will run rashly, as water is restricted by earth, even more water will be unable to support the wood. (wood is the son of water) the wood energy will be restricted by metal with intensification. In this case, it is called the 'pressing between energies'.

" The condition above shows the going beyond and falling short of energy are determinded by the time of arrival of element-energy of the viscera, one should examine carefully

whether it is in conform with the time of the solar term then. If the stored element-energy is not conform with the arriving time, and its correspondant relation with the five elements can hardly be sorted out for treating, it shows the evil energy inside has been formed and a physician can do nothing with it."

帝曰：有不袭乎？岐伯曰：苍天之气，不得无常也。气之不袭，是谓非常，非常则变矣。帝曰：非常而变奈何？岐伯曰：变至则病，所胜则微，所不胜则甚，因而重感于邪则死矣，故非其时则微，当其时则甚也。

Yellow Emperor asked: "Is there any case of the five elements energies not dominating according to the regular pattern of succession?" Qibo answewed: "The energies of heaven become prosperous alternately in various seasons and they are dominating in sequence in a regular pattern. When it is out of order, it should be considered to be abnormal. When the seasonal energy becomes abnormal, the weather will change and calamities will happen."

Yellow Emperor asked: "What will be the condition if the abnormal change happens?" Qibo answered: "Man will contract disease on account of it. If there is change in the energy which can be overcome by the dominating energy, the disease will be slight, but if there is change in the energy which can not be overcome by the dominating energy, the disease will be serious (such as when the spring wood dominating the season, and the earth energy is changing, as the wood can restrict the earth, so the disease is slight; but if the metal energy is changing, as wood is restricted by metal, so the disease will be serious). If the patient is invaded by evil energy during this period, he will die. Therefore, when the energy undergoes change, when the dominating energy is able to restrict the changing energy, the disease will be slight, but if the dominating energy is unable to restrict the changing energy, the disease will be serious."

帝曰：善！余闻气合而有形，因变以正名，天地之运，阴阳之化，其于万物，孰少孰多，可得闻乎？岐伯曰：悉哉问也！天至广不可度，地至大不可量，大神灵问，请陈其方。草生五色，五色之变，不可胜视，草生五味，五味之美，不可胜极，嗜欲不同，各有所通。天食人以五气，地食人以五味，五气入鼻，藏于心肺，上使五色修明，音声能彰；五味入口，藏于肠〔"肠"字衍〕胃，味有所藏，以养五气，气和而生，津液相成，神乃自生。

Yellow Emperor said: "Good! I am told that when the energies of heaven and earth combine, it generates all things, All things are being shaped up through change and birth, and their names were ascertained according to its form. In the course of transforming and generating all things by Yin and Yang of heaven and earth, which one of them is more functional and which one is less?"

Qibo answered: "What an exhaustive question you have asked! The heaven and earth are so spacious that they are hard to measure, so I can not answer your profound question in detail, but I can tell you in a concise way. There are five colours in herbs, but the variations of the five colours are too numerous to see; there are five tastes in herbs, but the various combinations, from the five tastes are too many for one to taste all over. The desire and addiction for every one are different, and the preferences for different people are not the same.

The heaven provides the human being with five energies (such as the wind-energy which enters into the liver, the heat-energy which enters into the heart, the wet-energy which enters into the spleen, the dry-energy which enters into the lung, and the cold-energy which enters into the kidney), and the earth provides the human being with five tastes (such as the sour taste which enters into the liver, the bitter taste which enters into the heart, the sweet taste which enters into the spleen, the acrid taste which enters into the lung, and the salty taste which enters into the kidney). The five energies from heaven enter into the body through the nose and being stored in the heart and lung, as the heart associates with the blood and vessels, the energies will nourish one's complexion and cause it bright and moist in a fine colour, and as the lung associates with the voice, the energies will cause the voice loud and clear. The five tastes of foods from the earth enter into the body through the mouth and being stored in the stomach, when being digested, their essence will be transported and spread to nourish the energies of the five viscera, when the energies are being transformed and converted, it will give vitality, with the function of the saliva in addition, the spirit and energy of man will become prosperous naturely."

帝曰：藏象何如？岐伯曰：心者，生之本，神之变〔林校引全本“变”作“处”，按《五行大义》，引“变”作“处”〕也；其华在面，其充在血脉，为阳中之太阳，通于夏气。肺者，气之本，魄之处也；其华在毛，其充在皮，为阳中之太阴〔林校引《甲乙》、《太素》“太阴”作“少阴”〕，通于秋气。肾者，主蛰，封藏之本，精之处也；其华在发，其充在骨，为阴中之少阴〔林校引《甲乙》、《太素》“少阴”作“太阴”〕，通于冬气。肝者，罢极之本，魂之居也；其华在爪，其充在筋，以生血气，其味酸，其色苍〔滑本无“以生”十字〕，此为阳中〔林校本及《甲乙》、《太素》“阳中”并作“阴中”〕之少阳，通于春气。脾胃大肠小肠三焦膀胱者〔《五行大义》、《云笈七签》引并无“胃大肠小肠膀胱”九字〕，仓廪之本，营之居也，名曰器，能化糟粕，转味而入出者也；其华在唇四白，其充在肌，其味甘，其色黄〔林校云：“其味甘，其色黄”六字当去〕，此至阴之类，通于土气。凡十一藏取决于胆也〔(此句九字，疑为后人所增〕。

Yellow Emperor asked: "What are the outer appearances like when the viscera corresponding to heaven, earth, Yin and Yang?"

Qibo answered: "The heart is the base of life and the place where the wisdom and mind locate, its quintessence appears on the face, and its function is to fill the blood in the vessel. As the heart associates with the fire and is the Taiyang of Yang, so its energy communicates with summer.

"The lung is the base of a man's breath and the place where the inferior spirit of a man locates, its quintessence appears in the soft hair of the body, its function is to enrich the surface of the skin. As the lung associates with metal, it is the surface of the skin. As the lung associates with metal, it is the Shaoyin in Yang, and its energy communicates with the autumn energy.

"The kidney is the place where the true Yin and true Yang of a man hibernate, it is the base of hiding and the place for storing the refined energy, its quintessence appears on the

hair, and its function is to enrich the marrow of bone. As the kidney associates with water, it is the Taiyin in Yin, and its energy communicates with winter.

"The livei is the base of the four limbs, it is the place where the soul lies, its quintessence appears on the nails, its function is to enrich the tendons. The liver is also the place for storing the blood, so it can generate the blood. The taste of liver is sour, and its colour is green. As liver associates with wood, it is the Shaoyang in Yin and it communicates with spring.

"The spleen is the base of storing water and cereal, it is the place where the Ying energy generates. It is called the 'transfer and transform' which means it can discharge the dross of the food, that is, to transform the five tastes and take change of the absorption and the excretion. As the lips are the extention of the muscle, the spleen's quintessence appear on all sides of the lips, its function is to enrich the muscle. As the spleen associates with earth, it belongs to the extreme Yin, and its energy communicates with earth.

故人迎一盛，病在少阳，二盛病在太阳，三盛病在阳明，四盛已上为格阳。寸口一盛，病在厥阴，二盛病在少阴，三盛病在太阴，四盛已上为关阴。人迎与寸口俱盛四倍已上为关格，关格之脉赢〔胡本、赵本、吴本、明抄本，周本“赢”并作“羸”〕，不能极于天地之精气，则死矣。

"When the Renying pulse (the pulse of the cervical arteries lateral to the thyroid cartilage, reflecting the condition of the stomach) becomes acute, one fold greater than the Cunkou pulse (along the radial artery proximal to the wrist), the disease is in the Shaoyang, when Renying pulse becomes acute two fold greater than Cunkou pulse, the disease is in the Taiyang, when the Renying pulse becomes acute three fold greater than the Cunkou pulse, the disease is in the Yangming, when the Renying pulse becomes acute more than four fold greater than the Cunkou pulse, it indicates that Yang is abundant to the utmost which can no more communicate with Yin, and in this case, it is called 'Yang being rejected'.

" When the Cunkou pulse is one fold greater then the Renying pulse, the disease is in the Jueyin, when the Cunkou pulse is two fold greater than the Renying pulse, the disease is in the Shaoyin, when the Cunkou pulse is three fold greater than the Renying pulse, the disease is in the Taiyin, when the Cunkou pulse is more than four fold greater than the Renying pulse, Yin is abundant to the utmost, and Yang energy can no more communicate with it, and in this case, it is called 'Yin being closed'.

" If the Renying pulse and the Cunkou pulse are four fold greater than their normal condition, it indicates both Yin and Yang are in utmost over-abundance to cause the severing of them which is called 'Guange' (fails in mutual supporting) The Guange pulse is so decline failing to communcate with the essence of heaven and earth. The patient with this pulse will die. "

五藏生成篇第十

Chapter 10
Wu Zang Sheng Cheng Pian
(The Functions of the Five Viscera to Human Body and Their Mutual Relations)

心之合脉也。其荣色也，其主肾也。肺之合皮也，其荣毛也，其主心也。肝之合筋也，其荣爪也，其主肺也。脾之合肉也，其荣唇也，其主肝也。肾之合骨也，其荣发也，其主脾也。

The specific functions of the heart and the vessel are related, the quintessence of the heart is reflected on the complexion, and the heart is controlled by the kidney.

The specific functions of the lung and the skin are related, the quintessence of the lung is reflected on the soft hair, and the lung is controlled by the heart.

The specific functions of the liver and the tendon are related, the quintessence of liver is reflected on the nail, and liver is controlled by the lung.

The specific functions of spleen and muscle are related, the quintessence of the spleen is reflected on the lips, and the spleen is controlled by the liver.

The specific functions of kidney and bone are related, the quintessence of the kidney is reflected on the hair, and the kidney is controlled by the spleen.

是故多食咸，则脉凝泣而变色；多食苦，则皮槁而毛拔；多食辛，则筋急而爪枯；多食酸，则肉胝䐢而唇揭；多食甘，则骨痛而发落，此五味之所伤也。故心欲苦，肺欲辛，肝欲酸，脾欲甘，肾欲咸，此五味之所合也。

So, when the salty food is excessively taken, it will cause the stagnation of blood and the eclipse of one's complexion; when the bitter food is excessively taken, it will cause the dryness of the skin and the falling of hair; when the acrid food is excessively taken, it will cause cramp of the tendons and the withering of the nails; when the sour food is excessively taken, it will cause the skin to become tough and thick and the lips wrinkle and shrink; when the sweet food is excessively taken, it will cause the bone pain and the falling of hair. These are the conditions of the partiality for a particular taste. So, the heart prefers the bitter taste, the lung prefers the acrid taste, the liver prefers the sour taste, the spleen prefers the sweet taste, and the kidney prefers the salty taste. These are the corresponding relations between the five tastes and the five viscera.

五藏之气，故色见青如草兹〔《脉经》《千金方》并作“滋”《说文通训。定声》“兹”，黑也〕者死，黄如枳实者死，黑如炲〔《千金翼方》“炲”下有“煤”字〕者死，赤如衃血者死，白如枯骨者死，此五色之见死也。

When the quintessence of the five viscera reflected on the complexion appears to be

green and black like the dead grass in dark, the patient will die; when it appears to be yellow like the fruit of unriped citron, the patient will die; when it appears to be black like coal, the patient will die; when it appears to be red like blood in stagnation, the patient will die; when it appears to be white as a piece of dry bone, the patient will die. These are the five colours for distinguishing the fatal diseases.

青如翠羽者生，赤如鸡冠者生，黄如蟹腹者生，白如豕膏者生，黑如乌羽者生，此五色之见生也。生于心，如以缟裹朱；生于肺，如以缟裹红；生于肝，如以缟裹绀；生于脾，如以缟裹栝楼实，生于肾，如以缟裹紫，此五脏所生之外〔《太素》"之"下无"外"字〕荣也。

When the quintessence of the five viscera reflected on the complexion appears to be green like a bird's green feather, the patient will live; when it appears to be red like a cockcomb, the patient will live; when it appears to be yellow like the belly of a crab, the patient will live; when it appears to be white like lard, the patient will live; when it appears to be black like the feather of a crow, the patient will live. These are the five colours for distinguishing the vitality of man. The colour of vitality in heart is like the cinnabar wrapped in white thin silk; the colour of vitality in lung is like something red wrapped in white thin silk; the colour of vitality in liver is like something reddish-black wrapped in white thin silk; the colour of vitality of spleen is like trichosanthes seed (reddish-yellow) wrapped in white thin silk; the colour of vitality of kidney is like something purple wrapped in white thin silk. These are the appearance of vitalities of the five viscera.

色味当五藏：白当肺、辛，赤当心、苦，青当肝、酸，黄当脾、甘，黑当肾、咸。故白当皮，赤当脉，青当筋，黄当肉，黑当骨。

The five colours and the five tastes are conform with the five viscera. White conforms with the lung and acridness, red conforms with the heart and bitterness. green conforms with the liver and sour taste, yellow conforms with the spleen and sweet taste, black conforms with the kidney and the salty taste. So white also conforms with the skin, red also conforms with the vessel, green also conforms with the tendon, yellow also conforms with the muscle, and black also conforms with the bone.

诸脉者皆属于目，诸髓者皆属于脑，诸筋者皆属于节〔《太素》作肝〕，诸血者皆属于心，诸气者皆属于肺，此四支八谿之朝夕也。

All channels of man lead to the eyes, all the marrows lead to the brain, all tendons lead to the liver, all the blood lead to the heart, all the air in respiration lead to the lung. The air, blood, tendons and vessels are like the ebb and flow of the tide pouring to the elbows, armpits, hips, popliteal fossa and the four extremities.

故人卧血归于肝，肝〔《伤寒论》、《宣明论方》并引作"目"〕受血而能视，足受血而能步，掌受血而能握，指受血而能摄。卧出而风吹之，血凝于肤者为痹，凝于脉者为泣，凝于足者为厥，此三者，血行而不得反其空，故为痹厥也。人有大谷十二分，小谿三百五十四名，少十二俞〔《太素》作"关"〕，此皆卫气之所留止，邪气之所客也，针石缘而去之。

When a man lies down, his blood turns towards the liver. The blood can nourish the extremities and all parts of the body, so, when the eyes obtain the blood, they can see, when

the feet obtain the blood, they can walk, when the palms obtain the blood, they can hold things, when the fingers obtain the blood, they can fetch things. When one walks away to outside immediately after sleeping and is invaded by the blow of wind, if the blood stagnation is on the surface of skin, bi-syndrome (a syndrome marked by arthralgia, numbness and dyskinesia of the limbs) will occur; when the blood stagnation is in the channels, it will cause the retardation of the blood flow; when the blood stagnation is in the feet, it will cause coldness of the lower extremities. All the three kinds of diseases are due to the inability of the blood to flow back to the channel's circulation. There are twelve main joints in the four extremities and three hundred and fifty four small bone joints in human body, excluding the shu points in the twelve channels. All of them are the places for the Wei-energy to stay, and they are also the places for the evil-energy to reside, when one is atacked by the evil-energy, it should be removed by acupuncture or by the therapy of stone needle.

诊病之始，五决为纪，欲知其始，先建其母。所谓五决者，五脉也。

At the beginning of the diagnosis, one should take the five determinations as the outline, When treating the disease, one must know which viscera the disease comes from, and investigates the condition of the stomach-energy of the said viscera. If the stomach-energy of a certain viscera is deficient, one should set up its stomach-energy which is the mother of all other viscera energies first (earth is the mother of all things, and stomach associates with earth). The so called five determinations are actually the pulse conditions of the five viscera.

是以头痛巅疾，下虚上实，过在足少阴、巨阳，甚则入肾。徇蒙招尤〔《妇人良方》“尤”并作“摇”〕，目冥耳聋，下实上虚，过在足少阳、厥阴，甚则入肝。腹满旗胀，支鬲胠〔《太素》“胠”下无“胁”字〕胁，下厥〔《甲乙》“厥”作“病”〕上冒，过在足太阴、阳明。咳嗽上气，厥在胸中〔《甲乙》作“胸中痛”〕，过在手阳明、太阴。心烦头痛，病在鬲中〔病在鬲中：《甲乙》作“支满，腰脊相引而痛”〕。过在手巨阳、少阴。

Headache and other disease on head belong to the category of asthenia of healthy-energy in the lower part and sthenia of evil-energy in the upper, the disease is in the Foot Shaoyin and Taiyang channels, if the disease turns to the worse, it will be transmitted into the kidney. Presbyopia with shaking head when the attack is acute, or dim-sighted in eyes and deafness in ears when protracted, it belongs to the category of sthenia of the lower part and asthenia in the upper, the disease is in the Foot Shaoyang and Jueyin channels, if the disease turns to the worse, it will be transmitted into the liver. When one has fullness and intension of the abdomen and his armpits like being propped, feels cold in the lower part of the body and feels dizzy in the upper, the disease is in the Foot Taiyin and Yangming channels. When ones has cough with rapid respiration and feeling sick in the chest, the disease is in the Hand Yangming and Taiyin channels. When one has pain in the chest, and pain along the spinal column like tearing, the disease is in the Hand Taiyang and Shaoyin channels.

夫脉之小大滑涩浮沉，可以指别；五藏之象，可以类推；五藏相音，可以意识；五色微诊可以目察。能合脉色，可以万全。赤，脉之至也，喘而坚，诊曰〔《太素》“曰”作“之”〕有〔《甲乙》“有”作“为”〕积气在中，时害于食，名曰心痹，得之外疾〔能琦说：“外疾二

字是衍文”〕思虑而心虚，故邪从之。白，脉之至也，喘而浮，上虚下实，惊〔按：“惊”字误窜，似应在“喘而虚”句下〕，有积气在胸中，喘而虚，名曰肺痹，寒热，得之醉而使内也。青，脉之至也，长而〔《甲乙》“而”下有“弦”字〕左右弹，有积气在心下支胠，名曰肝痹，得之寒湿，与疝同法，腰痛足清头痛。黄，脉之至也，大而虚，有积气在腹中，有厥气，名曰厥疝，女子同法，得之疾使〔《中藏经》无“疾使”二字〕四支汗出当风。黑，脉之至也，上〔按：“上”字误，应为“下”〕坚而大，有积气在小腹与阴，名曰肾痹，得之沐浴清水而卧。

The pulse in the condition of weak, strong, slippery, choppy, floating or sunken, can be distinguished by the palpation of the fingers, The energies and phenomena of the five viscera, can be inferred by analogy. The sound responded by the five viscera, can be conceived mentally and analysable. Although the five colours are exquisite to differentiate, yet they can be observed by eyes. If one combines the methods of applying the colour and pulse condition, he can absolutely be certain about his diagnosis.

If the patient's complexion appears to be red, the pulse is rapid and full, it is, according to diagnosis, the evil-energy stagnates in the abdomen, and will often hinder the food and drink, this kind of disease is called the cardiac bi-syndrome; it is due to the heart-energy being hurt by the worriness, and the evil-energy takes advantage of its debility to invade.

If the patient's complexion appears to be white, and the pulse is rapid and floating, it is because the lung is asthenic, and the heart-fire is sthenic, as the heart is under the lung, so, it is asthenia in the upper part and sthenia in the lower. When the heart-fire is over-abundant, the mind will be distracted to cause fright. The disease is called lung bi-syndrome, which is caused by cold and heat and the conducting sex intercourse after being drunken.

If the patient's complexion appears to be green, and the pulse is long and over-flowing, and flicks the fingers in the left and right sides, it shows there is coldness of the liver which causes the evil-energy stagnates under the heart propping the armpits, the disease is called the hepatic bi-syndrome, and is caused by cold-wetness which is the same case of causing hernia. Besides, the syndromes of lumbago, cold feet and headache will also occur.

If the patient's complexion appears to be yellow, the pulse is heavy but empty, it is the evil-energy stagnated in the abdomen and the patient feels the adverseness of the vital energy. As hernia belongs to the disease of liver, and wood restricts earth, the disease relates to liver, so, it is called hernia syncope instead of spleen bi-syndrome. For a woman, when she is contracted with the hernia syncope of adverseness of vital energy with pain, it is caused by the invasion of wind-evil after perspiration when the four limbs are fatigue.

If the patient's complexion appears to be black, the pulse is firm and heavy, it is the evil-energy being stagnated in the lower abdomen and the external genital organ or the external urethral orifice, and it is called the kidney bi-syndrome; the disease is caused by sleeping immediately after a cold bath.

凡相五色之奇脉〔《千金翼方》无“之奇脉”〕，面黄目青，面黄目赤，面黄目白，面黄目黑者，皆不死也。面青目赤，面赤目白，面青目黑，面黑目白，面赤目青，皆死也。

In observing the five colours of the complexion, when it appears to be yellow, which is the outer appearance of the stomach-energy, the patient will survive, such as yellow face with green eyes, yellow face with red eyes, yellow face with white eyes, or yellow face with black eyes, they are all not the symtoms of death. When the patient's complexion is green with red eyes, red with white eyes , green with black eyes, black with white eyes , and red with green eyes, it shows the stomach energy has been exhausted, so, they all are the symtoms of death.

五藏别论篇第十一

Chapter 11
Wu Zang Bie Lun
(The Different Functions Between the Hollow Organs and the Extraordinary Hollow Organs for Digestion and Elimination)

黄帝问曰：余闻方士，或以脑髓为藏〔《太素》“为藏”下有“或以为府”四字〕，或以肠胃为藏，或以为府，敢问更相反，皆自谓是，不知其道，愿闻其说。

Yellow Emperor asked: “I have heard different comments from diffent physicians, some take the brain and the spine cord as solid organs, some take them as hollow organs; some take the intestine and stomach as solid organs, some take them as hollow organs. They hold different opinions, but all insist on what they said is right. I don't know the reasons of their different comments, and I hope you can tell me.”

岐伯对曰：脑髓骨脉胆女子胞，此六者，地气之所生也，皆藏于阴而象于地，故藏而不写，名曰奇恒之府。夫胃、大肠、小肠、三焦、膀胱，此五者，天气之所生也，其气象天，故写而不藏，此受五藏浊气，名曰传化之府，此不能久留输写者也。魄门亦为五藏，使水谷不得久藏。所谓五藏者，藏精气而不写也，故满而不能实。六府者，传化物而不藏，故实而不能满也。所以然者，水谷入口，则胃实而肠虚；食下，则肠实而胃虚，故曰实而不满，满而不实也〔明抄：无“满而不实”四字〕。

Qibo answered: “The six organs of brain and spine cord, bone, vessel, gallbladder and womb of a woman are generated in accordance with the earth-energy, they store the essence and blood, like the thickness of the earth which loads all things. Their function is to store the essence and energy to nourish the body without letting it out to the outside of the body, and they are called the ‘Extraordinary Hollow Organs’.

“The five organs of stomach, large intestine, small intestine, triple warmer and bladder are generated in accordance with the heaven-energy, they work unceasingly, like the heaven opperating without stopping. They discharge without storing, and they are called the ‘Hollow Organs for Digestion and Elimination’.

“This is to say the water, cereal and turbid-energy they received can not be retained in the body long, but, after being decomposed, the essence being transported and the dross being discharged respectively.

“The anus, which is supposed to be the sixth hollow organs also has the function of preventing the dross to remain in the body long.

“The function of the five solid organs is to store the essence without discharging, although they are filled often yet they are not substantialized. They are not like the stomach

and intesline which are often substantialized with water and cereal.

" The function of the six hollow organs is to digest, absorb and transport the food, so, although they are often substantial, yet they can not be filled like the five solid organs. When the food is taken through the mouth, the stomach may be substantialized, but the intestine is then empty, and when the food enters into the intestine, the intestine is substantial, but the stomach is then empty. "

帝曰：气口何以独为五藏主〔《太素》"主"下有"气"字〕？岐伯曰：胃者，水谷之海，六府之大源也。五味入口，藏于胃以养五藏气。气口亦〔《何校云："'亦'当作'手'"》〕太阴也，是以五藏六府之气味〔明抄、《类说》"气"下皆无"味"字〕，皆出于胃，变见于气口。故五气入鼻，藏于心肺〔《类说》引"于"下无"心"字〕，心肺有病，而鼻为之不利也。凡治病必察其下，适其脉，观其志意，与其病也。

Yellow Emperor asked: " When one inspects only the pulse condition of Cun Kou by palpation, how can he know the conditions of the energies of the five solid organs, six hollow organs and the twelve channels?"

Qibo said: " The stomach is the sea of water and the source of the six hollow organs. All the five tastes are taken through the mouth, are stored in the stomach, and then being digested and transported by the spleen to nourish the blood and energy of the viscera. Qikou (Cunkou) pulse belongs to the Hand Taiyin lung channel, and the lung channel is dominating all the pulses. So, all energies of the five solid organs and the hollow organs are stemmed from the stomach, and their variations are all reflected on the Qikou pulse. When the five odours (foul, scorched, sweet, stink and rancid) enter the lung through the nose and cause the disease of lung, the function of the nose will be reduced.

" When one treats a disease, he must know first the urine and stool conditions, distinguishes and analyses the pulse condition, observes the spirit and the pathosis of the patient.

拘于鬼神者，不可与言至德〔《太素》"德"作"治"〕，恶于针石者，不可与言至巧，病〔《太素》"病"上有"治"字〕不许治者，病必不〔《太素》作"不必"〕治，治之无功矣。

" If the patient is very superstitious in believing in goasts and gods, it is not necessary to tell him the theory of treating; if the patient detests extremely the acupuncture and stone therapy, it is not necessary to tell him the skill related to the treating; if the patient is reluctant to be treated, it is not necessary to treat him with difficulty. In such case, no expected curative effect can be harvested by any treatment. "

异法方宜论篇第十二

Chapter 12
Yi Fa Fang Yi Lun
(Discriminative Treating for Patients of Different Regions)

黄帝问曰：医之治病也，一病而治各不同，皆愈何也？岐伯对曰：地势使然也。故东方之域，天地之所始生也，鱼盐之地，海滨〔《医心方》并作“浜海”〕傍水，其民食鱼而嗜咸，皆安其处，美其食，鱼者使人〔《本草衍义》引无“使人”〕热中，盐〔按“盐”误应作“咸”〕者胜血，故其民皆黑色疏理，其病皆为痈疡〔《甲乙》“疡”作“肿”〕，其治宜砭石，故砭石者，亦从东方来。

Yellow Emperor asked: " When the same kind of diseases are treated by different physicians with different ways, the diseases can all be cured, and what is the reason?" Qibo answered: " It is due to the different conditions of the localities.

" In the eastern district, where the weather is warm like spring time, and the district is near the sea and water. As the district is rich in producing fish and salt, the local people like to eat fish and salt, and they are accustomed to live in the district and enjoy their food. But when fish is excessively taken, it will cause the heat-evil to retain in the stomach and intestine; when salt is excessively taken, it will hurt the blood of a man. Most of the local people there are black in skin and loose in striae, and their diseases are mostly of carbuncle kind. It is suitable to treat the disease with stone therapy (to prick with stone), so, the stone therapy is transmitted from the east.

西方者，金玉之域，沙石之处，天地之所收引也。其民陵〔《后汉书·西羌传》引“陵”作“山”〕居而多风，水土刚强，其民不衣而褐荐，其民华食而脂肥，故邪不能伤其形体，其病〔《太素》“病”下并有“皆”字〕生于内，其治宜毒药，故毒药者，亦从西方来。

" In the western district of mostly desert and stone, where the gold and jade are richly produced, the weather is restraint like autumn. The inhabitants are living by the mountain and the climate is rather stubborn with wind and dust usually. The local people do not wear silk and thin cotton, but mostly in coarse cotton and straw mat. They are particular about delicious food which may cause them to become fleshy. In this case, although their bodies can hardly be hurt by the exogenous evil, but are apt to suffer from visceral illness due to food and emotions. In treating the disease, drug is necessary, thus the drug therapy is transmitted from the west.

北方者，天地所闭藏之域也，其地高陵居，风寒冰冽〔《医心方》“冽”并作“冻”〕，其民乐野处而乳食，藏寒生满病〔《本草纲目》引作“其病藏寒生满”〕其治宜灸焫，故灸焫者，亦从北方来。

" In the northern district of mostly highland, where the weather is cold, shutting and hiding like winter, the people there live in the mountains and hills, and the cold wind often sweeps the frozen land. The local people like to stay in the wilderness to drink the milk of cow and sheep. In this case, their viscera can easily contract cold and occur the disease of abdominal distention. In treating the disease, moxibustion therapy should be used, thus the moxibustion therapy is transmitted from the north.

南方者，天地所长养，阳之所盛处〔俞樾说："应作'盛阳之所处'"〕也，其地下，水土弱，雾露之所聚也，其民嗜酸而食胕〔《甲乙》作"臊"，俞樾说："胕"即"腐"字〕。故其民皆致理而赤色，其病挛痹，其治宜微针。故九针者，亦从南方来。

" In the southern district of mostly lowland where the weather is hot like summer with abundant Yang energy to breed all things, due and rain are plenty and the climate is delicate. The people there prefer to eat sour and stinking food; their skin are dense and red, and they often contract the disease of spasm and wet-type arthralgia. In treating the disease, acupuncture therapy of nine kinds of needle is suitable. So, the acupuncture therapy of nine kinds of nedele is transmittd from the south.

中央者，其地平以湿，天地所以生万物也众〔《太素》、《医心方》并作"天地所生物色者众"〕，其民食杂而不劳，故其病多痿厥寒热，其治宜导引按跷，故导引按跷者，亦从中央出也。故圣人杂合以治，各得其所〔"所"字衍〕宜，故治所以异而病皆愈者，得病之情，知治之大体也。

"In the central district of mostly level land with wetness where the natural products are abundant, the people there have plenty of food to eat without trouble and suffering hardships. So, most of the diseases the people contract are muscular flaccidity and coldness of extremities, and also cold and heat. In treating the diseases, limb-exercise and massage should be applied. So, the therapies of limb-exercise and massage are transmitted from the centrality.

"Since a keen physician can gather all kinds of threapies and treat properly according to the specific condition of the disease, so, although the treatments to the same disease are different, they can all cure the diseases. "

移精变气论篇第十三

Chapter 13
Yi Jing Bian Qi Lun
(On the Therapy of Transfering Thought and Spirit)

黄帝问曰：余闻古之治病，惟其移精变气，可祝由而已。今世治病，毒药治其内，针石治其外，或愈或不愈，何也？

Yellow asked："I am told that in ancient times，when a physician treated a disease，he only transfered the patient's thought and spirit to sever the source of the disease. In nowadays，the patient is treated with drugs internally and acupuncture externally. Nevertheless，some of the diseases are cured，but some of them can not be cure and why is it so？"

岐伯对曰：往古人〔《太素》"人"下有"民"字〕居禽兽之间，动作以避寒，阴居以避暑，内无眷慕之累，外无伸官〔《太素》"伸官"作"由宦"〕之形，此恬憺之世，邪不能〔《太素》"不"下无"能"字〕深入也。故毒药不能〔无"能"字〕治其内，针石不能治其外，故可移精〔杨、王两注："移精"下有"变气"二字〕祝由而已。当今之世不然，忧患缘其内，苦形伤其外，又失四时之从，逆寒暑之宜，贼风数至，虚邪朝夕，内至五藏骨髓，外伤空窍肌肤〔《医垒元戎》"肤"作"肉"〕，所以小病必甚，大病必死，故祝由不能已也。

Qibo answered："In ancient times，people lived in the cave of the wilderness surrounded with birds and beasts，they drove away the coldness by the motion of themselves，and evaded the hot summer by living in the shade. They had no burden in heart in admiring the fame and gain，and had no fatigue in the body for seeking a high position，thus，one can hardly be invaded by exogenous evil in this calm and plain environment. So，when one contracted disease，both drugs for curing inside and acupuncture for curing outside were not neccessary，but only transferred the patient's emotion and spirit to sever the source of the disease would be enough.

"But the case in nowadays is different，people are often bothered by anxiety in the heart inside，and hurt by the toil of the body outside，together with the careless of the patient to violet the changing rule of the weather sequence of the four seasons，and the coldness and heat of morning and evening，When the thief-evil invades unceasingly，the patient's viscera and bone marrow will be hurt inside，and the orifices and muscle will be hurt outside. If the disease contracted is a slight one，it will surely turn into a serious disease，if the disease contracted is a serious one，the patient will surely die. Therefore，the disease nowadays can not be cured by severing the source of the disease only."

帝曰：善。余欲临病人，观死生，决嫌疑，欲知其要，如日月光，可得闻乎？岐伯曰：色脉者，上帝之所贵也，先师之所传也。上古〔《太素》"上古"之下有"之时"二字，"使"下

无“僦”字〕使僦贷季，理色脉而通神明，合之金木水火土四时〔《太素》“四时”下有“阴阳”二字〕，八风六合，不离其常，变化相移，以观其妙，以知其要〔按此四字似衍〕，欲知其要，则色脉是矣。色以应日，脉以应月，常求其要，则其要也。夫色〔《太素》“色”下有“脉”字〕之变化，以应四时之脉，此上帝之所贵，以合于神明也。所以远死而近生，生道以长，命曰圣王。中古之治病，至〔《太素》“至”上有“病”字〕而治之，汤液十日，以去八风五痹之病，十日不已，治以草苏草荄之枝，本末为助〔《太素》“助”作“眇”〕，标本已得，邪气乃服。暮世之治病也则不然，治不本四时，不知日月，不审逆从，病形已成，乃欲微针治其外，汤液治其内，粗工兇兇〔《太素》作“凶凶”按“凶”，“兇”之借字，与“匈”通，“匈匈”有“灌哗”之意〕，以为可攻，故〔《太素》“故”作“旧”〕病未已，新病复起。

Yellow Emperor said: “Good, I hope when I diagnose a patient, I can distinguish whether the disease is slight or serious, decide the doubtful point of the disease and master the essentials of the disease clearly as being illuminated by the sun and moon. Can you tell me what shall I do?” Qibo said: “The former kings attached importance to the inspection of the conditon of complexion and the pulse, and it was handed down by teachers in the past.

“In ancient times, there was a physician whose name was Daiji. He studied the principle of complexion and pulse to the degree of communicating with the deity, he could connect them to the five elements of metal, wood, water, fire and earth, the four seasons, Yin and Yang, evil-winds of all directions and the three dimensions, not divorcing from the principle of the regular rule of complexion and pulse, and he can also observe the profound essence from their mutual changing. So, it is important for one to observe the complexion and pulse conditions to know the essentials of the disease.

“The complexion is like the sun, which has different conditions in the fine days and the cloudy days, and the pulse is like the moon, which has different conditions of wax and wane. It is very important in diagnosis to observe carefully the brightness and darkness of the complexion, and the difference of sthenia and asthenia of the pulse. In a word, the variation of complexion and pulse correspond with the variations of the energies of the four seasons. The former kings attached great importance to the principle, as it is in conformity with the deity. If one can master the diagnosis like this, he can help the patient to avoid death and become surviving. When the life of the patient is prolonged, he will praise you as a king of sages.

“In middle ancient times, the physician often treated the patient when the disease had occured, he treated with decoction for ten days to remove arthralgia and wind-evil; if the patient was not cured in ten days, herbal medicine was applied. It is very important to treat with herbal medicine, and the cooperation of the patient is very important as well. In this case, the evil-energy can be subdued, and the disease can be healed.

“But the physicians in later generations treat the patients in different ways, they do not treat according to the weather variations of the four seasons, they neglect the importance of the complexion and pulse, and do not distinguish the agreeable or adverse condition of the complexion and pulse, but make use of the decoction and acupuncture to treat inside and outside respectively after the disease has already shaped up. He boasts of his curative effect

about his treating, supposing that the disease can surely be cured, but finally, the former disease is still remaining , and some new diseases are added."

帝曰：愿闻要道。岐伯曰：治之要极，无失色、脉；用之不惑，治之大则。逆从到〔吴本“到”作“倒”〕行，标本不得，亡神失国〔疑“亡神”句上脱“如使辅君”四字〕。去故就新，乃得真人。帝曰：余闻其要于夫子矣，夫子言不离色、脉，此余之所〔滑抄本“所”下有“未”字〕知也。岐伯曰：治之极于一。帝曰：何谓一？岐伯曰：一者因〔滑抄本“因”下有“而”字，主注：“因问而得之”〕得之。帝曰：奈何？岐伯曰：闭户塞牖，系之病者，数问其情，以从其意，得神者昌，失神者亡。帝曰：善。

Yellow Emperor said: "I want to hear some fundamental theory about the treatment." Qibo said: "The most important crux of treating is to abide with the inspection of patient's complexion and his pulse condition, and insist on this highest principle. If the source of the disease in comprehended in a wrong sequence, or fail to obtain the cooperation of the patient, the treatment will not succeed. When one assists a king to rule the country like this, the country will be subjugated. In treating, one must remove the old disease first, and then treat the disease contracted recently, the one who can treat in this way is supposed to obtain the impartation of a keen physician."

Yellow Emperor said: "Now I have heard the fundamental principle of treating, and the centre of your words is not to divorce from the inspection of the complexion and pulse condition in treating, which I have not heard before." Qibo said: "There is another important crux." Yellow Emperor asked: "What is it?" Qibo said: "It is the diagnosis by inquiring." Yellow Emperor asked: "How to do it?" Qibo said: "The patient should be left alone in the room, the windows and doors should be shut to eliminate all the misgiving of the patient, and ask him about the condition of disease confidentially in detail. After inquiring, refer to the conditions of his complexion and pulse, if the complexion of the patient is lustrous, and the pulse beat is calm, it is called the 'spiritedness', the disease can be healed. When the complexion of the patient has no lustre, and his pulse fails to correspond with seasonal variations, it is called the 'depletion of spirit', the disease can by no means be cured." Yellow Emperor said: "Good. I suppose what you have said is correct."

汤液醪醴论篇第十四

Chapter 14
Tang Ye Lao Li Lun
(On the Rice Soup，Turbid Wine and Sweet Wine)

黄帝问曰：为五谷汤液及醪醴奈何？岐伯对曰：必〔《圣济经》“必”作“醞”〕以稻米，炊之稻薪，稻米者完，稻薪者坚。帝曰：何以然？岐伯曰：此得天地〔《知古今篇》“天”下无“地”字〕之和，高下之宜，故能至完，伐取得时，故能至坚也。

Yellow Emperor asked：“ What is the method of making the rice soup，turbid wine and the sweet wine with five cereals?” Qibo answewed：“ Keep the paddy rice in fermentation and the rice stalk as the fuel，as the energy of the paddy rice is complete with that of all seasons and orientations，and the rice stalk is tough. ” Yellow Emperor asked：“ Why is it so?” Qibo answered：“ The paddy rice receives the harmonious energy of the heaven and grows in the land of proper altitude in centrality，so，it receives the energy which is most complete as it is harvested in the appropriate season，and the rice stalk is most tough. ”

帝曰：上古圣人作汤液醪醴，为而不用何也？岐伯曰：自〔《太素》“自”作“上”〕古圣人之作汤液醪醴者，以为备耳，夫上古作汤液，故为而弗服也。中古之世，道德稍衰，邪气时至，服之万全。帝曰：今之世不必已何也？岐伯曰：当今之世，必齐毒药攻其中，鑱石针艾治其外也。帝曰：形弊血尽而功不立者何？岐伯曰：神不使也。帝曰：何谓神不使？岐伯曰：针石，道也。精神不进〔《太素》“进”作“越”〕，志意不治〔《太素》“治”作“散”〕，故病不可愈。今精坏神去，荣卫不可复收。何者？嗜欲无穷，而忧患不止，精气弛坏，荣泣卫除，故神去之而病不愈也。

Yellow said：“ In ancient times，the rice soup，turbid wine and sweet wine prepared by the physicians were used in sacrifices or entertaining guests but seldom used in treating disease，and why was it so?” Qibo answered：“ In ancient times，the rice soup，turbid wine and sweet wine prepared were only used in contingency，so，they were rarely used in treating disease.

“In the middle ancient times，the people paid less attention to health-preserving and their bodies became weaker，but when the exogenous evil took advantage to invade，after some rice soup，turbid wine or sweet wine were taken by the patient，the disease was cured. ”

Yellow Emperor asked：“ In nowadays，when people contract disease，although some rice soup，turbid wine or sweet wine were taken，the disease is not surely to be cured，and why is it?” Qibo said：“ In nowadays，when people contract disease，it is neccessary to treat them with medicine internally or with acupuncture stone pricking or moxibustion externally to cure the disease. ”

Yellow Emperor said: " When the body of the patient is declined, his blood and energy are exhausted, why is it that the treating is ineffective?" Qibo said: " This is because the spirit of the patient can no more play the role it should play. " Yellow Emperor asked: " What do you mean by that?" Qibo said: " The acupuncture and stone therapy can only conduct the blood and energy, but can do nothing to the spirit and consciousness of the patient . If the spirit and the energy of the patient are disappearing, his will and consciousness are dispersing, the disease can by no means be cured. Since now the patient's spirit is declining, and his energy is dispersing, the functions of his Rong-energy inside of the vessels for nourishing the whole body and the Wei-energy outside of the vessels for moisturing the skin and striae can no more be recovered. The reason of the disease being developed into such a serious condition is the patient's excessive indulging of sexual desire, together with endless anxieties to worry his heart, so as causing his spirit and energy be on the wane, his Rong-energy in blood exhausted, and the Wei-energy diminishing. Since his spirit and energy are divorcing from the body, his disease will not be cured. "

帝曰：夫病之始生也，极微极精，必先入结〔《太素》“入结”作“舍”〕于皮肤。今良工皆称曰病成，名曰逆，则针石不能治，良药不能及也。今良工皆得其〔《太素》作“持”〕法，守其数，亲戚兄弟远近音声日闻于耳，五色日见于目，而病不愈者，亦何暇〔《太素》“何暇”作“可谓”〕不早乎？岐伯曰：病为本、工为标、标本不得，邪气不服，此之谓也。

Yellow Emperor said: " When the disease was in the initial stage, it was quite superficial and simple, the evil was only hiding in the skin and the disease should have been cured easily. But the physician then ascertained that the disease had already shaped up, which should be treated earlier, so, both acupuncture and decoction would be effective. But in fact, many physicians at the present know well the way of the treatment, many relatives and friends are keeping the patient accompany to look after him, hearing his voice and watching his complexion every day, how can one say that the treatment is not early enough?"

Qibo said: " The patient is the root and the physician is the branch, they must be compatible. Of course, the cooperation of the patient is neccessary, but only the cooperation of the patient without a good physician is not enough, it also called incompatible of the root and branch, and the evil can not be removed either. "

帝曰：其有不从毫毛而生〔金刻本、胡本、之头本、赵本、周本“而生”二字至乙，“而字属下读，《太素》“其”下有“病”字〕五藏阳〔《太素》“阳”作“伤”〕以竭也，津液充郭〔《太素》作“虚廓”〕，其魄独居，孤精于内，气耗于外，形不可〔《太素》“形不可”作“形别不”〕与衣相保，此四极急而动中，是气拒于内，而形施于外，治之奈何？岐伯曰：平治于权衡，去宛陈莝，微动四极，温衣〔滑抄本“衣”作“之”〕，缪刺其处，以复其形。开鬼〔按“鬼”疑为“魄”之坏字〕门，洁净府，精以时服，五阳已布，疏涤五藏，故精自生，形自盛，骨肉相保，巨气乃平。帝曰：善。

Yellow Emperor said: " Some of the diseases are not initiated from the surface of the body but from the injury of the five viscera directly. Their symptoms appear to be the emptiness of the body fluid, the withering of the spiritual activities, consumption of the essence

and blood inside, and the dispersion of the Wei-energy outside. The patient is emaciated and tender to have no more suitable dress to fit the body, and later, occurs the cramping of the four limbs and the weavering of the middle-energy. In short, the vital energy of the viscera are weary inside and the physique is in insubstantiality outside. How should this kind of patient be treated?"

Qibo said: "In treating, one should harmonize the two Yin and Yang channels of the solid and hollow organs, remove the stagnated blood and eliminate the accumulated water, make the patient to excercise his extremities slightly, to cause the Yang energy to spread gradually; then, try to make the patient to perspire thoroughly, and keep his urination unobstructed, besides, give the patient, according to the condition, some medicine on due time. When the Yang-energy in the five viscera of the patient being spread, the stagnations in the five viscera being cleared, his essence and energy will be sure to regenerate, his body will certain become strong, his bone and muscle will supplement each other again, and his stagnated energy inside will be removed naturally." Yellow Emperor said: "Good!"

玉版论要篇第十五

Chapter 15
Yu Ban Lun Yao
(Methods of Palpation for Measuring and Distinguishing the Disease Recorded on the Jade Tablet)

黄帝问曰：余闻揆度奇恒，所指不同，用之奈何？岐伯对曰：揆度者，度病之浅深也。奇恒者，奇恒者，言奇病也。请〔林校引全本“请”作“谓”〕言道之至数，五色脉变、揆度奇恒，道在于一。神转不回，回〔《太素》“回”作“迴”〕则不转，乃失其机，至数之要，迫近以微，著之玉版，命曰合玉〔俞樾说：“合”字衍〕机。

Yellow Emperor asked: “ I am told the two methods for measuring and distinguishing disease by palpation are different, how can they be applied in relation with each other?” Qibo answerd; ”Measuring is to estimate the degree of seriousness of the disease, and distinguishing is to identify the irregular disease. I suppose the variations of the complexion and the pulse condition are the axioms of diagnosis. The main point of measuring and distinguishing is to take hold of the corresponding relation between the complexion and the pulse condition.

The energy and blood of a human body is always operatng. If it stops, the vitality will be lost. This principle is very important and is recorded on the jade tablet, which is called the principle of preserving health recorded on the jade tablet.

容〔《太素》“容”作“客”〕色见上下左右，各在其要，其色见浅者，汤液主治，十日已。其见深者，必齐主治，二十一日已。其见大深者，醪酒〔“酒”应作“醴”〕主治，百日已。色夭〔《太素》“夭”作“赤”〕面脱，不治。百日尽已〔按“百日”上疑脱“色不夭面不脱”二字〕。脉短气绝死。病温虚甚死。

“The colour other than the energy of the corresponding viscera in the complexion is called the guest colour. It appears on the different position of the upper, lower, right or left side of the nose, and one should inspect its variation in different shades carefully. when the guest colour appears to be light, it indicates the disease is slight, which can be cured in about ten days by treating with decoction of the five grains; when the guest colour is heavy, it is neccessary to treat with medical decoction, and the disease can be cured in about twenty one days. If the guest colour appears to be very dark, it shows the disease is very serious, which is neccessary to treat with tincture, and it may be cured in about one hundred days. If the complexion of the patient is red, which shows the absense of stomach-energy which is yellow, and his face is thin, the disease can by no means to be cured, If the complexion of the patient is not red, and the face is not thin, the disease can be healed after one hundred days.

“Besides, if the patient's pulse is short, failing to reach both the position of Guan and

Chi pulses, it indicates the severing of Yin and Yang energies, and the patient will die. If the disease contracted is seasonal febrile disease and the vital energy is in utmost deficiency, the patient will die.

色见上下左右，各在其要，上为逆，下为从。女子右为逆，左为从；男子左为逆，右为从。易，重阳死，重阴死。阴阳反他，治在权衡相夺，奇恒事也，揆度事也。

"One should observe carefully the guest colour appears on the upper, lower, left or right side of the nose to discover its movement. When it moves upwards, it is in the reverse direction, when it moves downwards, it is in the agreeable direction; for a women, when the guest colour is moving from right to left, it is reversing, when it is moving from left to right, it is agreeable; for a man, if the guest colour is moving from left to right, it is reversing, when it is moving from right to left, it is agreeable. If the moving direction of the man and woman is alternating to change from agreeable to reversing, for a man, it is double Yang, and for a woman, it is double Yin. Both patients with double Yang or double Yin are apt to die.

"As to the patient whose Yin and Yang is different with others, should be treated by weighing the comparative importance to reverse the abnormal condition to become normal. Since this is an irregular disease, one must diagnose it with great care.

搏脉，痹躄。寒热之交。脉孤为消气〔《太素》"消"下无"气"字〕，虚泄〔《太素》作"虚与泄"〕为夺血。孤为逆，虚为从。行奇恒之法，以〔"以"误，应作"从"〕太阴始。行所不胜曰逆，逆则死；行所胜曰从，从则活。八风四时之胜，终而复始，逆行一过，不复可数，论〔《太素》"论"作"诊"〕要毕矣。

"When the pulses beat under the fingers, and the disease reflected as the bi-syndrome (a syndrome marked by arthralgia and numbness and dyskinesia of the limbs) or flaccidity of feet, they are all caused by the simultaneous occurrng of cold and heat energies. If the pulse appears to be solitary, it shows the Yang-energy is damaged inside; if the pulse appears to be feeble, it is the syndrome of diarrhea and consumption of blood. All the solitary pulses which show the stomach energy in absence are adversing and are of unfavourable prognosis; all the deficient pulses are agreeable and are of favourable prognosis.

"When applying the method of distinguishing, one should begin to palpate from the Cun Kou pulse of Hand Taiyin channel. When the visceral pulse has the trait of another visceral pulse which is overcoming, such as, when the liver (wood) pulse has the trait of lung (meal) pulse, when the lung pulse has the trait of heart (fire) pulse, when the heart pulse has the trait of kidney (water) pulse, when the kidney pulse has the trait of the spleen (earth) pulse, or when the spleen pulse has the trait of the liver (wood) pulse, it is the adverse pulse, and the patient will die. When the visceral pulse has the trait of another visceral pulse except that which is overcoming, such as, when the liver (wood) pulse has the trait of the kidney (water), heart (fire) or spleen (earth) pulse; when the heart (fire) pulse has the trait of the lung (metal), spleen (earth) or liver (wood) pulse, etc, it is the agreeable pulse, and the patient will survive.

"Each wind from various directions is dominating a season, such as, the east wind dominates spring, and the east associated wood overcomes earth; the south wind dominates summer, and the south-associated fire overcomes metal; the west wind wind dominates autumn, and the west-associated metal overcomes wood; the north wind dominates winter, and the north-associated water overcomes fire. They repeat in cycles, go round and begin again.

"If the weather of the four-season becomes abnormal, it must not be inferred by the common practice. These are the entire essentials of the measuring and distinguishing."

诊要经终论篇第十六

Chapter 16
Zhen Yao Jing Zhong Lun
(The Essentials of Diagnosis and the Symptoms of the Severing of the Twelve Channels)

黄帝问曰：诊要何如？岐伯对曰：正月二月，天气始方，地气始发，人气在肝。三月四月，天气正方，地气定发，人气在脾。五月六月，天气盛、地气高、人气在头。七月八月，阴气始杀，人气在肺。九月十月，阴气始冰〔王注“冰”作“凝”〕，地气始闭，人气在心。十一月十二月，冰复，地气合，人气在肾。

Yellow Emperor asked:" What are the essentials of diagnosis?" Qibo answered:" In the first and second lunar months ,the heaven energy begins to ascend, and the earth-energy begins to start up, by this time, the energy of man is in the liver.

"In the third and fourth lunar month, the heaven-energy is developing and the earth-energy is growing, at this time, the energy of man is in the spleen.

"In the fifth and sixth lunar month, the heaven energy is abundant and the earth-energy is ascending, at this time, the energy of man is on the head.

"In the seventh and eighth luner month, the solemn and killing weather begin to occur, at this time, the energy of man is in the lung.

"In the ninth and tenth lunar months, the Yin-energy becomes stagnated and the earth-energy begins to shut and hide, at this time, the energy of man is in the heart.

"In the eleventh and twelve lunar month, the land is ice bounded and the earth-energy is sealed, at this time, the energy of man is in the kidney.

故春刺散俞，及与分理，血出而止，甚者传气，间者环〔林校引《太素》“也”作“已”〕也。夏刺络俞，见血而止，尽气闭环，痛病必下，秋刺皮肤，循理，上下同法，神变而止。冬刺俞窍于〔《甲乙》“于”上有“及”字〕分理，甚者直下，间者散下，春夏秋冬，各有所刺，法其所在。

"When treating in spring, one should prick the scattered shu-points to reach the position of the muscle adhering to the bone, and stop the pricking immediately when the blood is seen. If the disease is serious, when the energy being dredged after pricking, the disease will be recovered gradually; if the disease is slight, it will be removed immediately.

"In summer, one should prick the shu-points of the minute collaterals, stop the pricking immediately when blood is seen. When the evil-energy is removed, the hole of the acupoint is closed, the pain will be eliminated.

"In autumn, one should prick the skin, but rub and press the vein of muscle to dispel

the energy and blood first. The depth of pricking should be controlled like that stated above, to the extent that blood is seen. Observe the expression of the patient and stop the pricking whenever the complexion of the patient is changing.

"In winter, one should prick the shu-points deeply to reach the position of the muscle adhering to the bone. When the disease is serious, the pricking should be deep and direct without rubbing and pressing the vein of the muscle; when the disease is slight, direct pricking is not neccessary, but can prick up and down or left and right in a flexible way.

"In short, the ways of pricking in the four seasons are different, and the pricking in the four seasons are each having their different positions.

春刺夏分，脉乱气微，入淫骨髓，病不能愈，令人不嗜食，又且少气。春刺秋分，筋挛逆气，环为咳嗽，病不愈，令人时惊，又且哭。春刺冬分，邪气著藏，令人胀〔《四时刺逆从论》"胀"上脱"腹"字〕，病不愈。又且欲言语。

夏刺春分，病不愈，令人解堕。夏刺秋分，病不愈，令人心中欲无言，惕惕如人将捕之。夏刺冬分，病不愈，令人少气〔"少"疑作"上"〕，时欲怒。

秋刺春分，病不已，令人惕然，欲有所为，起而忘之。秋刺夏分，病不已，令人益嗜卧，又且善梦。秋刺冬分，病不已，令人洒洒时寒。

冬刺春分，病不已，令人欲卧不能眠，眠而有见。冬刺夏分，病不愈，气上，发为诸痹。冬刺秋分，病不已，令人善渴。

"When one pricks the position of summer by mistake in spring, disorder of the pulse and the decline of energy will happen, and the evil-energy will invade into the bone marrow. The disease will not be healed and causes the patient to have no appetite and the deficiency of energy.

"When one pricks the position of autumn by mistake in spring, convulsion and adverseness of vital energy will occur, and cough will come in the wake of it. The disease will not be healed, and the patient will sometime becomes startled, and sometimes he wants to cry.

"When one pricks the winter position by mistake in spring, the evil-energy will harbour deep in the viscera to cause the distension of abdomen of the patient. The disease will not be healed, and cause the patient to become talkative.

When one pricks the position of spring in summer, the disease will not be healed, and the patient will become tired, weary and weak.

"When one pricks the position of autumn by mistake in summer, the disease will not be healed, the patient will be unwilling to talk by heart, and often feels uneasy as if some-one is trying to arrest him.

"When one pricks the position of winter by mistake in summer, the disease will not be healed, the adverseness of vital energy of the patient will occur, and he is apt to get angry.

"When one pricks the position of spring by mistake in autumn, the disease will not be healed and the patient will be restless, when he wants to do something, he forgets what he wants to do right away.

"When one pricks the position of summer by mistake in autumn, the disease will not be

healed, and the patient will become more and more addicted to sleep with dream.

"When one pricks the position of winter by mistake in autumn, the disease will not be healed, and the patient often feels chilly.

"When one pricks the position of spring by mistake in winter, the disease will not be healed, the patient can not fall into sleep even when he is very tired, even if he has fallen into sleep, it is like something being seen in dream.

"When one pricks the position of summer by mistake in winter, the disease will not be healed, adverseness of vital energy of the patient and also the bi-syndrome or numbness will occur.

"When one pricks the position of autumn by mistake in winter, the disease will not be healed, and the patient will often be thirsty.

凡刺胸腹者，必避五藏。中心者环死，中脾者五日死，中肾者七日死，中肺者五日死，中鬲者，皆为伤中，其病虽愈，不过一岁必死。刺避五藏者，知逆从也。所谓从者，鬲与〔"鬲"上疑脱"知"字〕脾肾之处，不知者反之。刺胸腹者，必以布憿著之，乃从单布上刺，刺之不愈复刺。刺针必肃，刺肿摇针，经刺勿摇，此刺之道也。

"When one pricks on the chest of abdomen of the patient, he should pay attention to avoid hurting the viscera. If the heart is pricked, the patient will die in one day; if the spleen is pricked, the patient will die in five days; if the kidney is pricked, the patient will die in seven days, if the diaphram is pricked, which is called hurting the middle, although the disease can turn to the better temporarily, but due to the disorder of the visceral energy, the patient will die in a year.

"The crux for one to keep away from the viscera in pricking is to know the adverse and agreeable ways in pricking. The so called agreeable way is to know the positions of the organs of diaphram, spleen, kidney etc., and one should take good care to avoid them; if one does not know their positions and does not avoid them, the five viscera can easily be hurt, which is called the adverse way. So it is neccessary before pricking the chest or abdomen to wind the chest or abdomen with cloth to avoid hurting the viscera by deep pricking. If the pricking has no curative effect, it should be pricked again.

"In pricking, the inserting of needle should be quick in action; when treating a disease of swelling, the method of rotating the needle to remove the evil may be applied; if the pricking is on the channel, rotating method is not neccessary. These are the essentials of acupuncture."

帝曰：愿闻十二经脉之终奈何？岐伯曰：太阳之脉，其终也，戴眼，反折瘈瘲，其色白〔明抄本"白"作"黑"〕，绝汗乃出，出则死矣。少阳终者，耳聋，百节皆纵，目睘〔《甲乙》校注云："一本无"睘"字，按《灵枢经·经始篇》作"目系绝"〕绝系，绝〔"系"字衍，上"系"字连"绝"字之头，应作"系绝一日半死"〕系一日半死，其死也〔《难经·二十四难杨注引无"死也"二字》〕，色先〔"先"字衍〕青白，乃死矣。阳明终者，口目动作，善惊，妄言，色黄，其上下经盛，不仁〔《灵枢·终始》"仁"作"行"字〕，则终矣。少阴终者，面黑，齿长而垢，腹胀闭，上下不通而终矣。太阴终者，腹胀闭不得息，善噫〔《难

经·二十四难》虞注引无“善噫”二字，似衍〕善呕，呕则逆，逆则面赤，不逆〔“逆”字误，应作“呕”〕则上下不通，不通则面黑，皮毛焦而终矣。厥阴终者，中热嗌乾，善溺心烦，甚则舌卷卵上缩而终矣。此十二经之所败也。

Yellow Emperor asked:“ What are the conditions about the severing of the twelve channels?”

Qibo answered:“ In the severing of the Taiyang channel, the patient will look up staring continuously with the two eyes, the back of the body is like a bow bending in the opposite direction, the extremities are cramping with the severing of sweat, and when the severing of sweat occurs, the patient will die.

“In the severing of the Shaoyang channel, the patient will become deaf, the joints of the whole body become loose, the connection of visual scene severs, and when it severs, the patient will die in one and half days. Just before dying, there occurs the green and white colours in the patient's complexion, and then dies immediately.

“In the severing of the Yangming channel, the mouth and the ears of the patient will be wide open; he is frightened extremely, ramble in his statement with yellow complexion, if the Hand and Foot channels are in hyperirritability which fail to keep operating, the patient will die.

“In the severing of the Shaoyin channel, the patient appears to have black complexion, his teeth feel like longer with plenty tartars, and his abdomen is feeling fullness and has retention of feces and urine. When his upper part and the lower part fail to communicate with each other, the patient will die.

“In the severing of the Taiyin channel, the patient will be feeling distending and blocking in the abdomen, difficult in respiration and vomit often, the vomiting causes the adverseness of the energy, and the adverseness of energy causes the complexion to become red. If the vomiting stops, the communication between the upper part and the lower part of the body will be blocked, then, the complexion of the patient will become black, and his skin and its fine soft hair will be withered extremely, in this condition, the patient will die.

“In the severing of the Jueyin channel, the chest of the patient will become hot with dryness of his throat, frequency of urination and restless. When the disease is serious, the symptoms of curled tongue and retracted testes will occur , and in this case, the patient will die. These are the symptoms of the severing of the twelve channels.”

脉要精微论篇第十七

Chapter 17
Mai Yao Jing Wei Lun
(The Essentials and Fundamentals of Diagnostic Palpation)

黄帝问曰：诊法何如？岐伯对曰：诊法常以平旦，阴气未动，阳气未散，饮食未进，经脉未盛，络脉调匀，气血未乱，故乃可诊有过之脉。

Yellow Emperor asked: "What is the diagnostic method in pulse palpation?" Qibo answered: "The palpation of pulse should be carried on in early morning, when the Yang-energy has not yet been stirred, the Yin-energy has not yet been dispersed thoroughly, the food and drink of man have not yet been taken, the channel-energy then is not in hyperactivity, the energies of the collateral branches of the large channels are in harmony and the energy and blood have not been disturbed. In this situation can the pulse condition be diagnosed effectively.

切脉动静而视精明，察五色，观五藏有余不足，六府强弱，形之〔《类说》引"之"作"气"〕盛衰，以此参伍决死生之分。

"At the same time of diagnosing the dynamic and static variations of the patient's pulse, his pupils and complexion should be inspected, so as to distinguish whether his energies of the five viscera are abundant or not, his six hollow organs are strong or not, his physique and energy are prosperous or not. When these aspects are considered comprehensively, one can judge the date of the death or survival of the patient.

夫脉者，血之府也，长则气治，短则气病，数则烦心，大则病进，上盛则气高〔林校本引全本引"高"作"鬲"〕，下盛则气胀，代则气衰，细则气少，濇则心〔金刻本"心"作"气"〕痛，浑浑革〔《脉经》、《千金》"革"下并重"革"字，"至"字属下之头〕至如涌泉。病进而色弊〔《脉经》、《千金》"色"并作"危"，《千金》"弊"下重"弊"字〕，绵绵〔《千金》"绵绵"作"绰绰，孙鼎说："弊弊者，弓弦已坏之意，绰绰者弦绝之声"〕其去如弦绝，死。

"The vessel is the place where the blood assembles, and the circulation of blood depends on the guidance of the energy. The long pulse shows the functional activities of vital energy is normal; the short pulse shows the patient to have qifen syndrome; the rapid pulse shows the feverish sensation accompanied with restlessness of the patient; the large pulse shows the disease is turning to the worse.

"If the pulse for the upper of the body is over-abundant, it shows the evil-energy is stagnated in the chest, if the pulse for the lower part of the body is overabundant, it shows the evil-energy is expanding in the abdomen; the intermittent pulse shows the debility of the

energy, the thready pulse shows the patient to have less evil-energy, the uneven pulse shows the patient is painful due to evil-energy.

"When the coming of the pulse is strong like water gushing from the spring, it shows the disease is turning to the worse to become dangerous; if the coming of the pulse seems to exist and again not to exist, and its going is like a piece of broken string, the patient will sure to die.

夫精明〔《千金翼方》无"精明"二字〕五色者，气之华也，赤欲如白〔《脉经》、《千金》引"白"并作"帛"〕裹朱，不欲如赭；白欲如鹅羽，不欲如盐；青欲如苍璧之泽，不欲如蓝；黄欲如罗裹雄黄，不欲如黄土；黑欲如重漆色，不欲如地苍〔《脉经》、《千金》"地苍"并作"炭"〕。五色精微象见矣，其寿不久也。夫精明者，所以视万物，别白黑，审短长。以长为短，以白为黑，如是则精衰矣。

"The five-colour of the complexion is the outer appearance of the vital energy, when it is red, it should like the cinnabar wrapped in a piece of white thin silk which can be seen indistinctly with ruddy colour, and does not like ochre in purplish red; when it is white, it should like the goose feather with brightness, and does not like salt which is white with mixed dark dregs; when it is green, it should be green like jade with lustre, and does not like indigo-blue in dark-green; when it is yellow, it should like realgar wrapped in a piece of white thin silk in reddish-yellow, and does not like earth in yellow with residue; when it is black, it should like black paint with moistening bright, and does not like charcoal in withering dark. If the decayed phenomena of the five colours appear, the life of the patient will not last long.

"The eyes of a man are for observing things, distinguishing the black, white and the length. If one can no more distinguish the length and the black and white, his vital energy has already been exhausted.

五藏者，中之守也，中盛藏满，气胜伤恐者〔《三因方》引无此五字〕，声如从室中言，是中气之湿也。言而微，终日乃复言〔于弁说："曰"字衍〕者，此夺气也。衣被不敛，言语善恶，不避亲疏者，此神明之乱也。仓廪不藏者，是门户不要也。水泉不止者，是膀胱不藏也。得守者生，失守者死。

"The functions of the five viscera are storing the essence of men and guard it inside. If the energy of the abdomen is over-abundant, the energy stored inside will be filling, the voice of the patient will be harsh and turbid, like being sent out from a room, as the middle warmer energy is covered by the wetness-evil; if the voice of the patient is low, repeating again and again when talking, it shows the healthy-energy is declined evidently; if the patient can not tidy up his belongings, rambles in his statement, can not distinguish people in close or distant relation, it is obvious that his consciousness has become disordered; if the stomach and intestine of the patient can hardly hold the water and cereal with fecal incontinence, it is asthenia of kidney which fails to confine; if there is incontinence of urine, it is due to the inability of the shut and store of the bladder. In short, if the five viscera are able to play their roles of guarding inside, the health of the patient can be restored, otherwise, the patient will soon die.

夫五藏者，身之强也。头者，精明〔《类说》“精明”引作“精神”〕之府，头倾视深，精神将夺矣。背者胸中〔《类说》、《天中记》引“胸”下并无“中”字〕之府，背曲肩随，府〔《类说》“府”并作“胸”〕将坏矣。腰者肾之府，转摇〔《类说》引“摇”作“腰”〕不能，肾将惫〔《天中记》引“惫”作“败”〕矣。膝者筋之府，屈伸不能，行则偻附，筋将惫矣。骨者髓〔按骨髓二字误倒应作“髓者骨之府”〕之府，不能久立，行则振掉，骨将惫矣，得强则生，失强则死。

"The five viscera are the foundation of the bodily health, and the head is where the spirit locates, if the head hangs down or tilts with eyes caving in, it shows the spirit will decline soon; as the five viscera locate in the chest and abdomen, and all the shu-points of viscera are on the back, so the energies of the viscera appear on the back, if the back is bent and the shoulder drooped, it shows the viscera will decline soon; the kidney energy appears on the loin, if the loin can not be turning, the kidney-energy will soon be exhausted; the tendon-energy appears on the knees, if the knees bend and stretch with difficulty, the back of the patient will be hunched and his head will hang down while walking, it shows the tendons will soon be worn out; the energy of bone appears in the marrow, if one can not stand long, wavering while walking, it shows the bone will be degenerated. In short, if the viscera can turn strong from weakness, the patient's life can be preserved, otherwise, he will die."

岐伯曰：反四时者，有余为精，不足为消。应太过，不足为精；应不足，有余为消。阴阳不相应，病名曰关格。

Qibo said: " The human viscera are corresponding with the four seasons, if they behave against the four seasons, the visceral essence and energy of the patient will be over-abundant, the substances in the six hollow organs for to convert and transport will be not be enough; if the correspondence of them is excessive, the essence and energy of the viscera, on the contrary, will become deficient; then the substances for to convert and transport will become more than enough. Both the cases are the inadaptability of Yin and Yang, and the disease is called 'Guange'."

帝曰：脉其〔《甲乙》“其”作“有”〕四时动奈何？知病之所在奈何？知病之所变奈何？知病乍在内奈何？知病乍在外奈何？请问此五者，可得闻乎？岐伯曰：：请言其与天运转大〔《太素》无“大”字〕也。万物之外〔《甲乙》无此四字〕，六合之内，天地之变，阴阳之应，彼春之暖〔林校引全本作“缓”〕，为之夏暑，彼秋之忿〔《太素》作“急”〕，为冬之怒，四变之动，脉与之上下，以春应中规〔《阴阳应象大论》王注引“中规”下有“言阳气柔软”五字〕，夏应中矩〔《阴阳应象大论》王注引“中矩”下有“言阳气盛强”五字〕，秋应中衡〔《阴阳应象大论》王注引“中衡”下有“言阴升阳降，气有高下“九字”〕，冬应中权〔《阴阳应象大论》王注引“中权”下有“言阳气居下也”六字〕是故冬至四十五日，阳气微上，阴气微下；夏至四十五日，阴气微上，阳气微下。阴阳有时，与脉为期，期而相失，知〔金刻本、之头本、赵本、吴本“知”并作“如”〕脉所分，分之有期，故知死时。微妙在脉，不可不察，察之有纪，从阴阳始，始之有经，从五行生，生之有度，四时为宜〔《太素》“宜”作“数”〕，补写勿失，与天地如一，得一之情，以知死生。是故声合五音，色合五行，脉合阴阳。

Yellow Emperor asked: " What is the condition of pulse variation in the four seasons? How to locate the disease from palpation? How to know the variations of the disease from palpation? How to know the disease is suddenly inside by palpation? How to know the disease is suddenly outside by palpation? Can you tell me the answers of these five questions?"

Qibo answered: " Let me tell you the relation between variations about the five aspects and the operations of heaven. The natural variations and the reflections of Yin and Yang in heaven and earth are like the relaxed spring weather developes into the scorching heat of summer and the vigorous and urgent autumn weather developes into the severe coldness in winter. The coming and going and the ups and downs of the pulse are corresponding with the variations of the four seasons: the spring pulse in correspondence should like a pair of compasses with a soft Yang energy ; the summer pulse in correspondence should like a ruler with a strong and abundant Yang-energy; the autumn pulse in correspondence should like a balance with ascending Yin and decending Yang in different levels; and the winter pulse in correspondance should like a scale with Yang energy abiding low.

"The conditions of Yin and Yang in the four seasons are: the first Yang generates on the winter solstice, and on the forty-fifth day after it, the Yang-energy ascends slightly and the Yin-energy descends slightly; the first Yin generates on summer solstice and on the forty-fifth day after it, the Yin-energy ascends slightly, and the Yang-energy descends slightly, the ascending and descending of Yin and Yang are having their definite time which are in conformity with the variation of the pulse condition. If the pulse condition does not agree with the four seasons, one will know to which viscera the disease belongs, and the date of the patient's death can be deduced according to the abundance and debility of the viscera. The condition of pulse is most subtle which must be observed carefully. In observation, one should follow certain essentials and start from Yin and Yang. In observing Yin and Yang, some main points must be followed as well. Yin and Yang are generated with the help of the five elements under the specific rule of the variations of the four seasons. When treating a disease, one must follow the rule and must not divorce from it, and at the same time, connect the pulse conditions and the variations of Yin and Yang of heaven and earth. If one can master indeed the crux of the comprehensive consideration, one will be able to predict the death or survival of the patient.

"In short, the human voice is corresponding with the five tones (Gong, Shang, Jue, Zhi and Yu), the complexion of a man is corresponding with the five elements, and the pulse variations of a man are corresponding with Yin and Yang, heaven and earth, and the four seasons.

是知〔《明抄本“知”作“故”》〕阴盛则梦涉大水恐惧，阳盛则梦大火燔灼，阴阳俱盛则梦相杀毁伤；上盛则梦飞〔《太素》“飞”下有“扬”字〕，下盛则梦堕〔《太素》“堕”下有“坠”字〕；甚饱则梦予，甚饥则梦取；肝气盛则梦怒，肺气盛则梦哭〔《太素》“哭”作“哀”〕；短虫多则梦聚众，长虫多则梦相击毁伤。

"When one's Yin-energy is over-abundant, he will dream that he is wading across a riv-

er and is frightened. When his Yang-energy is over-abundant, he will dream that a big fire is burning.

"When both his Yin and Yang are over-abundant, he will dream that people are slaughtering each other.

"When the energy is over-abundant in the upper of the body, he will dream that he is flying upward, when the over-abundance is in the lower part, he will dream that he is dropping down. When eats his fill excessively, he will dream that he is giving things to others. When he is excessively hungry, he will dream that he is taking foods from others. When his liver-energy is over-abundant, he will dream that he is getting angry. When his lung-energy is over-abundant, he will dream that he is in grieve.

"When there are plenty pinworms in the abdomen, he will dream that many people are assembling. When there are many roundworms in the abdomen, he will dream that he is hurt in fighting with others.

是故持脉有道，虚静为保〔《甲乙》“保”作“宝”〕。春日浮，如鱼之游在波〔《太素》“波”作“皮”，谓浮而未显〕；夏日在肤，泛泛〔《太素》作“沉沉”〕乎万物有余；秋日下肤，蛰虫将去；冬日在骨，蛰虫周〔《太素》“周”作“固”〕密，君子居室。故曰：知内者按而纪之，知外者终而始之，此六者，持脉之大法。

"So, one should have a knack in palpation, and it is valuable only when one is modest and calm in palpating. The pulses are different in various seasons: in spring, the pulse is up floating like fish swimming under the water surface; in summer, the pulse is on the skin and is abundant like filling with things; in autumn, the pulse sink slightly to be under the skin like a hibernating worm entering into the hole; in winter, the pulse sinks to the bone, like a hibernating worm hiding in the hole or man lives in the inner chamber. So, if one wants to know the interior of the pulse, one must palpate deeply to know its essentials. When one wants to know the superficies of the pulse, he must emphasize on seeking the source of the disease according to its condition. The six points concerning spring, summer, autumn, winter, interior, and superficies stated above are the main points of diagnostic palpation.

心脉搏坚而长，当病舌卷〔《中藏经》“卷”作“强”〕不能言；其耎〔《千金》“耎”作“濡”，谓力量不及〕而散者，当消环自已。肺脉搏坚而长，当病唾血；其耎而散者，当病灌〔《千金》“灌”作“漏”〕汗，至今不复散发〔据杨注“散发”二字乃衍文，应删〕也。肝脉搏坚而长，色不青，当病坠若搏，因血在胁下，令人喘〔《太素》作“善喘”〕逆；其耎而散色泽者，当病溢饮，溢饮者，渴〔《脉经》“喝”作“湿”〕暴多饮，而易〔《千金》“易”作“溢”〕入肌皮肠胃之外也。胃脉搏坚而长，其色赤，当病折髀；其耎而散者，当病食痹〔按“痹”误，应为“痞”，“痞”，痛也〕。脾脉搏坚而长，其色黄，当病少气；其耎而散色不泽者，当病足骱肿，若水状也。肾脉搏坚而长，其色黄而赤者，当病折腰；其耎而散者，当病少血，至今不复〔《脉经》无此四字〕也。

"When the heart pulse is vigorous and long, it shows the fire is over-abundant in the heart-channel which causes the syndrome of stiff tongue and speechlessness; if the pulse is weak and scattered, the patient will feel deficiency of heart-energy, but after the channels

transmit in sequence, and when it returns to the original position after one cycle, the patient will be recovered.

"When the lung pulse is vigorous and long, it shows the fire is over-abundant in the lung channel to cause blood-spitting; if the pulse is weak and scattered, it is the deficiency of lung-energy , and the skin and hair will be unstable with plenty sweat, and in this case, the bodily strength can hardly be restored.

"When the liver pulse is vigorous and long and the complexion of the patient is not green, it is the syndrome of trauma caused by falling or striking; as the stagnated blood is under the flanks, it causes the patient to respire rapidly, but if the pulse is floating, hot and dispersed, and the complexion is smooth and moist, it is the disease of anasarca (the fluid stagnated in the skin and extremities) which is caused by wetness accumulated inside and too much drinking; as the stagnated liver-energy can not be dispersed, it makes the fluid floating between the muscle and the skin, and also to the outside of the stomach and intestine.

"When the stomach pulse is vigorous and long, and the patient has red complexion, his spleen will be painful greatly; if the pulse is weak and scattered, it is the deficiency of stomach-energy and the disease of stomach after food-intake.

"When the spleen pulse is vigorous and long with yellow complexion of the patient, it is the spleen pulse fails to keep slow and moderate, and the spleen-energy fails to transport, and the syndrome of short of energy will occur in the wake of it; if the pulse is floating. weak and scattered and the complexion is not smooth and lustrous, edema of the shank will occur, and it will be swelling like being filled with water.

"When the kidney pulse is vigorous and long and the patient has yellowish-red complexion, the loin of the patient will suffer great pain; if the pulse is floating. weak and scattered, it is the deficiency of the essence and blood."

帝曰：诊得心脉而急，此为何病？病形何如？岐伯曰：病名心疝，少腹当有形也。帝曰：何以言之？岐伯曰：心为牡藏，小肠为之使，故曰少腹当有形也。帝曰：诊得胃脉，病形何如？岐伯曰：胃脉实则胀，虚则泄。

Yellow Emperor asked: "When knowing the heart pulse is tight by palpation, what is the disease, and what is the disease like?" Qibo answered: "It is called the heart-channel colic, and there will be blocks occur in the lower abdomen." Yellow Emperor asked: "Why is it so?" Qibo answered: "The heart is a solid organ of Yang, and heart is the superficies and interior with the small intestine, as the small intestine is in the lower abdomen, thus, blocks will occur in the lower abdomen."

Yellow Emperor asked: "When knowing the disease is in the stomach-energy through palapation, what are the syndromes like?" Qibo answered: "If the pulse of stomach is of sthenia, the disease is flatuence and fullness of the abdomen; if the pulse of stomach is of asthenia, it is diarrhea."

帝曰：病成而变何谓？岐伯曰：风成为寒热，瘅成为消中，厥成为巅疾，久风为飧泄，脉风成为疠，病之变化，不可胜数。

Yellow Emperor asked: "What is the reason of forming the disease and what is the condition of its variation?" Qibo answered: "The disease will become cold and heat syndrome due to wind-evil; will become diabetes involving the middle warmer due to heat-evil; will become mania due to the continuous adverseness of the vital energy; when the wind-evil of wood staying inside for a long time, it will restrict the spleen earth and lienteric diarrhea will occur; as the wind-cold evil has invaded into the pulse, and can not be removed for a long time, it will turn into the syndrome of leprocy. The variations of the diseases are tremendous which can hardly be counted."

帝曰：诸痈肿筋骨痛，此皆安生？岐伯曰：此寒气之肿〔按：肿应作钟，犹言聚也〕，八风之变也。帝曰：治之奈何？岐伯曰：此四时之病，以其胜治之愈也。

Yellow Emperor asked: "How do the disease of carbuncle, spasm of tendon and the pain of bone occur?" Qibo said: "Thay are caused by the accumulation of cold-evil and the invasion of the wind-evil." Yellow Emperor asked: "How to treat them?" Qibo answered: "The diseases are caused by the evils of the four seasons, they can be cured by using the method of sequential overcoming of the five elements."

帝曰：有故病五藏发动，因伤脉色，各何以知其久暴至〔按："至"字衍〕之病乎？岐伯曰：悉乎哉问也！征其脉小色不夺者，新病也；征其脉不夺其色夺者，此久病也；征其脉与五色俱夺者，此久病也；征其脉与五色俱不夺者，新病也。肝〔《太素》"肝"上有"故"字〕与肾脉并至，其色苍赤，当病毁〔《太素》"毁"作"击"〕伤，不见血，已见血，湿若中水也。

Yellow Emperor asked: "When the viscera of some patients with old disease being stirred, it often effects his pulse and complexion, how can we know the disease is an old one or a new one?" Qibo answered: "What a meticulous question you have asked. You can distinguish it by watching the patient's complexion. Generally speaking, if the pulse is weak but the complexion remians unchanged, it is a new disease; if the pulse remanis unchanged, but the complexion is haggard without lustre, it is an old disease; if both the pulse and complexion are far from satisfaction, it is a protracted disease; if both the complexion and pulse are good, it is a new disease. When the liver pulse and the kidney pulse appear to be sunken and wiry, and the skin appears to be purplish red, it is caused by strikes, no matter whether or not the blood is seen, the body will sure to become swelling like edema with stagnated blood.

尺内两傍，则季胁也。尺外以候肾，〔柯校本"肾"作"背"〕，尺里以候腹中附上，左外以候肝，内以候鬲；右外以候胃，内以候脾。上附上，右外以候肺，内以候胸中，左外以候心，内以候膻中。前以〔《太素》无"以"字〕候前，后以〔《太素》无"以"字〕候后。上竟上者，胸喉〔《三因方》"胸喉"有"头项"二字〕中事也；下竟下者，少腹腰股膝胫足中事也。

"When palpating the two sides of the Chi pulse, it is to detect the disease of chest and ribs. When palpating the Chi pulse slightly, it is to detect the back, when palpate heavily, it is to detect the abdomen. As to the middle part of the Chi pulse, when palpating the left side

slightly, it is to detect the liver, and when palpating heavily, it is to detect the diaphram; when palpating the right side slightly, it is to detect the stomach, and when palpating heavily, it is to detect the spleen. As to the upper part of the Chi pulse, when palpating the right side slightly, it is to detect the lung, when palpating heavily, it is to detect the chest; when palpating the left side slightly, it is to detect the heart, and when palpating heavily it is to detect the Tanzhong. When palpating the demarcation of the Yin channel of the inner side of the arm, it is to detect the abdomen, when palpating the demarcation of Yang channel of the outer side of the arm, it is to detect the back. When palpating the terminal of the upper section, it is to detect the disease of the head, neck chest and throat, when palpating the terminal of the lower section, it is to detect the disease of lower abdomen, loin, thigh, knee, shank and foot.

粗大者，阴不足阳不余，为热中也。来疾去徐，上实下虚，为厥巅疾〔“疾”下有“者”字〕；来徐去疾，上虚下实，为恶风也。故中恶风者，阳气受也〔《太素》无此九字〕。有脉俱沉细数者，少阴厥也。沉细数散〔“数”字衍，《太素》杨注：“沉细阴也，散为散，故病寒热”〕者，寒热也。浮而散者为眴仆。诸浮不躁〔柯校“不”作“而”〕者皆在阳，则为热；其有躁者在〔《太素》“有”作“右”，“在”下有“左”字〕手。诸细而沈者皆在阴，则为骨痛；其有静者在足。数动一代者，病在阳〔按“阳”应用“阴”〕之脉也，泄〔《太素》“泄”上有“溏”字〕及便脓血。诸过者切之〔《甲乙》无此五字〕，濇者阳气有余也，滑者阴气有余也。阳气有余为身热无汗，阴气有余为多汗身寒，阴阳有余则无汗而寒。推而外之，内而不外，有心腹积也。推而内之，外而不内，身〔《太素》“有”上无“身”字〕有热也。推而上之，上而不下，腰足清也。推而下之，下而不上，头项痛也。按之至骨，脉气少者，腰脊痛而身〔《太素》“身”下有“寒”字〕有痹也。

“When the pulse condition is overflowing, it is deficient of Yin and abundant of Yang, and it occurs in the internal heat-syndrome. When the pulse is rapid in coming and slow in going; it is the sthenia in the upper part and asthenia in the lower, and it occurs in the evil-wind syndrome.

“When the pulse condition is sunken, fine and rapid, it is the cold and heat syndromes, when the pulse is floating and scattered, it is the disease of dizziness which will cause falling, when the pulse is floating and impetuous, the disease is on the superficies, and the patient will have a fever; when the hyperirritability is in the right collateral, the disease is in the left hand. When the pulse is fine and sunken, the disease is in the interior, and the joints of bone will become painfull . If the pulse is fine, sunken and calm, then, the disease is in the three Foot channels. When the pulse is intermittent, the disease is in the Yin channel, and the syndrome of diarrhea with loose stool and bloody stool will occur.

“When the pulse is rough, it shows the Yang-energy is more than enough; when the pulse is slippery, it shows the Yin-energy is more than enough. When the Yang-energy is more than enough, the body will be hot without sweat; when the Yin-energy is more than enough, the body will be cold with plenty of sweat; when both the Yin-energy and Yang-energy are more than enough, the patient will be cold without sweat.

"There is another method of inspecting the diseases: when the disease appears to be a syndrome of superficies of which its pulse should be floating, but a sunken and slow pulse is seen, it shows the disease is accumulated in the heart and abdomen; when it appears to be a disease of the interior, of which its pulse should be sunken, but a floating and rapid pulse is seen, it shows it is the internal heat-syndrome; when detecting the upper part of the body, if only the pulse for the upper part is prominent, and that for the lower part is quite little, it is the syndrome of chillness of loin and feet; when detecing the lower part of the body, if only the pulse for the lower part is prominent, and that for the upper part is in debility, it is the syndrome of pain of the head and neck. If the palpation is heavy reaching the bone, yet the channel-energy is still little, it is the syndrome of pain in the loin and spine with cold-type arthalgia."

平人气象论篇第十八

Chapter 18
Ping Ren Qi Xiang Lun
(On the Normal Pulse of a Person)

黄帝问曰：平人何如？岐伯对曰：人一呼脉再动，一吸脉亦再动，呼吸定息脉五动，闰〔《外科精义》引“闰”作“为”〕以太息，命曰平人。平人者不病也。常以不病〔《甲乙》“不病”下有“之人以”三字〕调病人，医不病，故为病人平息以调之为法。

Yellow Emperor asked："What is the pulse beat condition of a normal person like?" Qibo answered："The pulse of a normal person beats twice in an exhalation, and twice in an inhalation, and an inhalation and an exhalation is called one respiration. Sometimes, a pulse beat occurs in the interval of the end of inhalation and the beginning of exhalation. The condition of the pulse beat five times in a respiration is the longer respiration of the person. People of four or five times of pulse beats in a respiration is called a normal person who has no disease.

"In diagnostic palpation, one should measure the patient's pulse with the standard of a normal healthy person who has no disease to check the variation of the pulse beats of the patient's pulse beats with the breathing of a normal person. This is the rule of diagnostic palpation.

人一呼脉一动，一吸脉一动〔《太素》“动”下有“者”字〕，曰少气。人一呼脉三动，一吸脉三动而躁，尺热曰病温，尺不热脉滑曰病风，脉濇曰痹〔《甲乙》无“脉濇曰痹”四字〕。人一呼脉四动以上〔《太素》“动”作“至”，无“以上”二字〕曰死，脉绝不至曰死，乍疏乍数曰死。

"If the pulse of the patient beats once in an exhaltion and once in an inhalation, it shows the healthy-energy of the patient is declined.

"If the pulse beats three times in an exhalation and three times in an inhalation, and the pulse is rapid with hyperirritability, and at the same time the skin by the Chi-fu is hot like burning, it is the seasonal febrile disease; if the skin by the Chi-fu is not hot, and the pulse is slippery, it is the disease of wind-evil.

"If the pulse beats four times in an exhalation, ie. eight times or more in a respiration, or the pulse beats stop without reappearing, or the pulses beat rapidly and slowly by turns without a regular pattern, the patient will die.

平人之常气禀于胃〔《甲乙》作“人常禀气于胃”〕，胃〔《太机真藏论》王注引“胃”下有“气”字〕者，平人之常气也。人无胃气曰逆，逆者〔《太素》“者”作“曰”〕死。

"The normal pulse energy stems from the stomach, and the stomach-energy is the nor-

mal pulse energy of a normal person. If the stomach-energy is absent in one's pulse, it is called the adverse condition, which may cause the death of the patient,

春胃微弦曰平，弦多胃少曰肝病，但弦无胃曰死，胃而有毛〔《脉经》作“有胃而毛”，“毛”为轻而浮滑之脉乃秋平之象〕曰秋病，毛甚曰今病，藏真散于肝，肝藏筋膜之气也。夏胃微钩曰平，钩多胃少曰心病，但钩无胃曰死，胃而有石曰冬病，石甚曰今病，藏真通于心，心藏血脉之气也。长夏胃微软弱曰平，弱多胃少曰脾病，但代〔按“代”字误，应作“弱”〕无胃曰死，软弱有石曰冬病，弱〔《千金》“弱”作“名”〕甚曰今病，藏真濡于脾，脾藏肌肉之气也。秋胃微毛曰平，毛多胃少曰肺病，但毛无胃曰死，毛〔明抄本，吴注本“毛”并作“胃”〕而有弦曰春病，弦甚曰今病，藏真高于肺，以行荣卫阴阳也。冬胃微石曰平，石多胃少曰肾病，但石无胃曰死，石而有钩曰夏病，钩甚曰今病，藏真下于肾，肾藏骨髓之气也。

"The pulse condition in spring is wiry with moderate stomach-energy is called the normal pulse of spring, if the wiry condition is outstanding with little stomach-energy, it is the diseases pulse of liver; if only the wiry pulse condition is seen without any stomach-energy, the patient will die; if in the stomach-energy has, in addition, the light, floating or slippery pulse which is a typical autumn pulse, the patient will contract disease in autumn, but if the floating and slippery condition is outstanding, the disease will occur immediately. In clinic observation, one should notice that spring is the season for the heathy energies of viscera spreading on the liver, and liver is to store the energy of aponeurosis mainly.

"The pulse condition in summer is hooked with moderate stomach-energy which is called the normal pulse of summer, if the hooked pulse condition is outstanding with little stomach energy, it is the diseased pulse of heart; if only the hooked condition is seen without any stomach-energy, the patient will die; if in the stomach-energy has, in addition, the stony pulse which is the typical winter pulse, the patient will contract disaese in winter, but if the stony condition is outstanding, the disease will occur immediately. In clinic observation, one should notice that summer is the season for the true energies of five viscera to communicate with the heart, and the heart is to store the energy of the blood mainly.

"The pulse condition in long summer is soft and weak with moderate stomach-energy which is called the normal pulse of long summer; if the weak and soft condition is outstanding with little stomach-energy, it is the diseased pulse of spleen, if only the soft and weak condition is seen without any stomach energy, the patient will die; if in the soft and weak pluse has in addition the stony pulse, which is a typical winter pulse, the patient will contract disease in winter, but if the soft and weak condition of the pulse is outstanding, the disease will occur immediately. In clinic observation, one should notice that long summer is the season for the healthy energies of five viscera to nourish the spleen, and the spleen is to store the muscular-energy mainly.

"The pulse condition in autumn is floating and scattering with moderating stomach-energy, it is called the normal pulse of autumn; if the floating and scattering condition is prominent with little stomach-energy, it is the diseased pulse of lung; if only the floating and scattering condition is seen without any stomach-energy, the patient will die. If the wiry pulse

condition occurs with the stomach-energy, the patient will contract disease in spring, but if the wiry condition is outstanding, the disease will occur immediately. In clinic observation, one should notice that autumn is the season when the healthy energies of five viscera reaching up to communicate with the lung, and the lung is to store the energies of skin and hair mainly.

"The pulse condition in winter is sunken and stony with moderating stomach-energy, which is called the normal pulse of winter; if the sunken and stony condition is prominent with little stomach-energy, it is diseased pulse of kidney; if only the sunken and stony pulse is seen without any stomach energy, the patient will die; if the hooked condition is seen in addition to the sunken and stony pulse, the patient will contract disease in summer, if the hooked condition is outstanding, the disease will occur immediately. In clinic observation one should notice that winter is the season for the healthy energies of five viscera to store in the kidney, and kidney is to store the energy of bone marrow mainly.

胃之大络，名曰虚里，贯鬲络肺，出于左乳下，其动应衣〔《甲乙》"衣"作"手"〕，脉〔《甲乙》"脉"下有"之"字〕宗气也。盛喘数绝〔按"喘"似应作"搏"，"绝"涉下误，疑应作"疾"〕者，则病在中；结而横，有积矣；绝不至日死。乳之下其动应衣，宗气泄也〔林校引全本及《甲乙》无"乳之下"十一字〕。

"The large collateral of the stomach channel is called 'Xuli' which turns up under the left breast, passing through the diaphram and reaching up to connect the lung, and one can feel its pulsation with hand. It is the place where the Zong energy of channels locates.

"If the beat of Xuli is violent and rapid, it shows the disease is in the Tanzhong; if the beats are behind time occasionally and its position shifting to the side, it shows there are blocks in the body; if the pulse severs and fails to return, the patient will die.

欲知〔《脉经》、《千金》并无"欲知"二字〕寸口太过与不及，寸口之〔"之"系衍〕脉中手短者，曰头痛。寸口脉中手长者，曰足胫痛。寸口脉中手促上击〔《甲乙》"击"作"数"〕者，曰肩背痛。寸口脉沈而坚者，曰病在中。寸口脉浮而盛者，曰病在外。寸口脉沈而弱，曰寒热及疝瘕少腹痛。寸口脉沉而横，曰胁下有积〔《甲乙》《千金》"有积"并作"及"字〕，腹中有横积痛。寸口脉沉〔《甲乙》"沉"作"浮"，"喘"乃"搏"之误字〕而喘，曰寒热。脉盛滑坚者，曰病在外，脉小实而坚者，病在内。脉小弱以濇，谓之久病。脉滑浮而疾者，谓之新病。脉急者，曰疝瘕少腹痛。脉滑曰风，脉濇曰痹。缓而滑曰热中。盛而紧曰胀。脉从阴阳，病易已；脉逆阴阳，病难已。脉得四时之顺，曰病无他；脉反四时及不间藏〔《太素》"四时"下无"及不间藏"四字〕，曰难已。

"As to the knowing of the going beyond and falling short of the Cunkou pulse through palpation, when the Cunkou pulse under the fingers is short, the evil is in the upper part, and the disease may appear to be headach; when the Cunkou pulse under the fingers is long, the evil is in the lower part, and the disease may appear to be pain in the tibia and foot; when the Cunkou pulse beats are short and urgent, bouncing up to hit the fingers, it is over abundant of Yang in the upper part, and the disease may appear to be pain of the shoulder and back; when the pulse is sunken and tight, the disease is in the interior; when the pulse

is floating and strong, the disease is in the superficies; when the pulse under the fingers is sunken and weak, it shows the cold-evil attacks the Shaoyin and Jueyin channel to cause chillness and fever and pain of the lower abdomen; when the Cunkou pulse is sunken and slanting, it shows there are blocks in the hypochondrium the thorax and abdomen which cause pain; when the pulse under the finger is floating, it is the cold and heat syndrome.

"When the pulse is strong, slippery and tight, it shows a serious disease is in the six hollow organs; when the pulse is tiny, substantial and firm, it shows a more serious disease is in the five viscera.

"When the pulse is tiny, weak and rough in coming, it shows the disease is protracted; when the pulse is floating, slippery in coming, it is a disease contracted rescently.

When the pulse is tight and hasty in coming it shows syndromes of chillness and fever and the pain in the lower abdomen. When the pulse is slippery and fluent in coming, it is the disease of wind-evil. When the pulse is rough and stagnated in coming, it is the bi-syndrome; when the pulse is slow and slippery in coming, it is the disease of retention of heat-evil in the middle warmer. When the pulse is strong and tight in coming, it shows the distension of the abdomen.

"When the pulse is agreeable with Yin and Yang, the disease is apt to be cured, otherwise, the disease can hardly be cured. When the pulse is corresponded with the four seasons, it is the case of agreeableness, the disease contracted will be of no danger, but when the pulse reverses against the four seasons, the disease can hardly be cured.

臂多青脉，曰脱血。尺脉缓〔"脉缓"二字误倒，本句应作"尺缓脉濇"〕濇，谓之解㑊。安卧脉盛，谓之脱血。尺濇脉滑，谓之多汗。尺寒脉细，谓之后世。脉尺粗常热者，谓之热中。

"When plenty of blue veins are seen in the arm where Renying and Cunkou locate, it is due to the blood loss. When the Chi pulse is slow and stagnated, it is the obstruction of wetness-evil inside to cause fatigue and sleepiness. When the skin by the Chi pulse is hot and the pulse is strong in coming, it shows serious blood loss; when the skin by the Chi pulse is choppy and the pulse is slippery in coming, it is the deficiency of Yin, and the patient will have plenty of sweat; when the skin by the Chi pulse is cold and the pulse is thin, it is the asthenia-cold of the spleen and stomach which causes diarrhea; when the skin by the Chi pulse is rough and the pulse-energy appears to be hot often, it is the heat syndrome in the interior caused by Yin-deficiency.

肝见庚辛死，心见壬癸死，脾见甲乙死，肺见丙丁死，肾见戊已死，是谓真藏见皆死。

"When the liver pulse condition is indicating the exhaustion of the visceral-energy, the patient will die on the days of Geng and Xin (the five-element related day of overcoming). When the heart pulse condition is indicating the exhaustion of the visceral energy, the patient will die on the days of Ren and Gui. When the spleen pulse condition is indicating the exhaustion of the visceral-energy, the patient will die on the days of Jia and Yi. When the lung pulse condition is indicating the exhaustion of the visceral energy, the patient will die on

the days of Bing and Ding. When the kidney pulse condition is indicating the exhaustion of the visceral-energy, the patient will die on the days of Wu and Ji. These are the dates of the patient's death after the pulse condition is indicating the exhaustion of the visceral-energy.

颈脉动喘疾〔《太素》乙作“疾喘”〕欬，曰水。目里〔金刻本、赵本、吴本“里”并作“裹”〕微肿如卧蚕起之状，曰水。溺黄赤〔《太素》“黄”下无“赤”字〕安卧者，黄疸。已食〔王注所据本“已食”作“食已”〕如饥者，胃疸。面肿曰风，足胫肿曰水，目黄者曰黄疸妇人手〔林校引全本“手”作“足”〕少阴脉动甚者，姙子也。

“When the patient's pulse of the neck is pulsating severely, and together with the syndrome of rapid breathing and cough, it is the disease associated with water. When the eyelid is swelling like the silkworm lying torpid, it is also the disease associated with water.

“When the urine is yellow and the patient is often sleepy, it is the jaundice; when still feeling hungry after food intake, it is the syndrome of diabetes involving the middle warmer.

“When the edema is on the face, it is the disease associated with wind, when the edema is in the tibia of foot, it is associated with water. When the eyeball is yellow, it is jaundice.

“When the Foot Shaoyin channel of a woman pulsates violently, it is the phenomenon of pregnacy.

脉有逆从，四时未有藏形，春夏而脉瘦，秋冬而脉浮大，命曰逆四时也。风热而脉静，泄而脱血脉实，病在中，脉虚，病在外，脉濇坚者，皆难治，命曰反四时也〔明抄本“反”下无“四时”二字。〕。

“Sometimes, the appearance of pulse condition may reverse against the four seasons, that is, when other pulse condition appears instead of the normal pulse condition which should appear in due season, such as the lean and small pulse appear in spring and summer, or the floating and full pulse appears in autumn and winter , they are all against the normal condition. In these cases, they are called the adverse pulse condition against the four seasons.

“In the disease of wind-heat, of which the pulse condition should be irritable, but, on the contrary, it appears to be calm; in the disease of diarrhea and blood lose, of which the pulse condition should be asthenic, but on the contrary, it appears to be sthenic; when the disease is in the interior of which the pulse condition should be sthenic, but on the contrary, it appears to be asthenic, when the disease is in the exterior, of which the pulse condition should be floating and slippery, but on the contrary, it appears to be rough and firm, in all the above cases, the diseases can hardly be cured, as they are against the normal rule.

人以水谷为本，故人绝水谷则死，脉无胃气亦死。所谓无胃气者，但得真藏脉不得胃气也。所谓脉不得胃气者，肝不弦肾不石也。

“The foundation of human life is water and cereals. When they are being severed, the patient will die. When the stomach-energy is absent in the pulse, the patient will also die. The so called the absence of stomach-energy is that when the pulse condition indicating the exhaustion of visceral energy appears without any moderating stomach-energy. In this case, the wiry pulse of liver in spring can no more be called the wiry pulse, and the sunken pulse

of kidney in winter can no more be called the suncken pulse.

太阳脉至〔据《难经·七难》"太阳"等八字应在"阳明脉至，浮大而短"之后〕，洪大以长；少阳脉至，乍数乍疏，乍短乍长；阳明脉至，浮大而短。

"The Shaoyang channel dominates in the first and second months of the lunar month, the coming of pulse then is suddenly close and suddenly loose, suddenly short and suddenly long; the Yangming channel dominates in the third and fourth months of the lunar month, the coming of the pulse then is floating, large and short; the Taiyang channel dominates in the fifth and sixth months of the lunar month, the coming of the pulse then is full and long.

夫平〔《甲乙》"心脉"上无"夫平"二字〕心脉来，累累〔《甲乙》"累累"下有"然"字〕如连珠，如循琅玕，曰心平。夏以胃气为本。病心脉来，喘喘连属，其中微曲，曰心病。死心脉来，前曲后居，如操带钩，曰心〔《甲乙》"曰"下无"心"字〕死。

"When the heart pulse with stomach energy comes, it is like pearls in consecution, rolling continuously and is smooth like stroking a piece of marble, it is the normal pulse condition of heart, and the stomach-energy is the fundamental energy of summer. When the pulse is very rapid with slightly crooked, it is the diseased pulse of heart. If the pulse is crooked in coming and then stay still like holding a hook without easing up, it is the heart pulse indicating death.

平肺脉来，厌厌聂聂，如落榆荚，曰肺平，秋以胃气为本。病肺脉来，不上不下〔《病沅》"不上不下"作"上下"连下读〕，如循鸡羽，曰肺病。死肺脉来，如物〔据《太素》杨注"物"当作"芥"〕之浮，如风吹毛，曰肺死。

"When the coming of the lung pulse with stomach-energy which is light, floating and soft like an elm leaf blowing in wind, it is the normal pulse condition of lung, the stomach-energy is the fundamental energy of autumn. When the pulse is rough like stroking the firm and sturdy feathers of a cock, it is the diseased pulse of lung; if the coming of the pulse is like weeds floating on the water or a piece of feather floating like being blown in the wind, it is the lung pulse indicating death.

平肝脉来，软弱招招，如揭〔《千金》"揭"下无"长"字〕长竿末梢，曰肝平，春以胃气为本。病肝脉来，盈实而滑，如循长竿〔于鬯说："'竿'字当是笄之坏文，长笄者指因冠之笄〕，曰肝病。死肝脉来，急益劲，如新张弓弦，曰肝死。

"When the coming of the liver pulse with stomach-energy is like holding a pole with a soft and long terminal, it is the normal pulse condition of liver, and the stomach-energy is its fundamental energy in spring. When the pulse is substantial and slippery like stroking a headgear clipper, it is the diseased pulse of the liver; if the coming of the pulse is wiry and stiff like pulling a new bow with a tight and hard string, it is the liver pulse indicating death.

平脾脉来，和柔相离，如鸡〔《甲乙》"鸡"下并有"足"字〕践地，曰脾平。长夏以胃气为本。病脾脉来，实而盈数，如鸡举足，曰脾病。死脾脉来，锐坚如乌之喙，如鸟之距，如屋之漏，如水之流〔《脉经》"流"作"溜"〕，曰脾死。

"When the coming of the spleen pulse with stomach-energy is mild but adhering with energy, likes a cock's claws falling leisurely on the ground when walking, it is the normal

pulse condition of spleen, and the stomach-energy is its fundamental energy in long summer. When the coming of the pulse is substantial and rapid, like a cock running swiftly, it is the diseased pulse of the spleen; if the coming of the pulse is wiry and hard, firm and sharp like the beak or claw of a crow, or like the rain drops in a leaking room with uncertain intervals, or like flowing water that never comes back again, they are all the spleen pulse indicating death.

平肾脉来，喘喘累累如钩，〔《太素》〕"钩"作"旬"，按"旬"古与"营"通，"营"为莹之假字，"莹"石似玉也〕按之而坚，曰肾平，冬以胃气为本。病肾脉来，如〔"如"上脱"形"字，王注："形同引葛"〕引葛，按之益坚，曰肾病。死肾脉来，发如夺〔《难经》《千金》"夺"并作"解"，《千金》校语说解索者，动数而随散乱，无复次绪也〕索，辟辟如弹石，曰肾死。

"When the coming of the kidney pulse with stomanch-energy is continuous, tiny, firm, smooth, and is hard as stone when being pressed, it is the normal pulse condition of kidney, and the stomach-energy is its fundamental energy in winter. When the coming of the pulse is sunken and tight, like hauling a rattan vein, it is the diseased pulse of the kidney. If the pulse is rapid and disorderly heavy and hard like marble, it is the kidney pulse indicating death."

玉机真藏论篇第十九

Chapter 19
Yu Ji Zhen Zang Lun
(The Valuable Collection of the Jade Plate on the Pulse Condition Indicating the Exhaustion of the Visceral-energy)

黄帝问曰：春脉如弦，何如而弦？岐伯对曰：春脉者肝〔《脉经》《甲乙》《千金》“脉”下并无“者”字，下“夏、秋、冬”同《太素》《四时脉形论》“肝”下有“脉”字〕也，东方木也，万物之所以始生也，故其气来，软弱轻〔《太素》“软”作“濡”，“轻”作“软”〕虚而滑，端直以长，故曰弦，反此者病。帝曰：何如而反？”岐伯曰：“其气来实而强〔《千金》“强”作“弦”〕，此谓太过，病在外；其气来不实而微，此谓不及，病在中。”帝曰：“春脉太过与不及，其病皆何如？”岐伯曰：“太过则令人善忘〔《气交变大论》林校引“善忘”作“善怒”〕，忽忽眩冒而巅疾；其不及，则令人胸痛引背，下则〔明抄“两胁”上无“下则”二字〕两胁胠满。”

Yellow Emperor asked: “The pulse condition of spring is wiry, but what is wiry like?”

Qibo answered: “The pulse of spring is liver pulse, it associates with wood of east, which has the scene of vitality of all things; as the pulse condition is moist, soft, weak, empty and slippery, straight and long, so it is called wiry. If the condition is on the contrary, it is the diseased pulse.”

Yellow Emperor asked: “What is the condition when it is on the contrary?” Qibo answered: “When the condition of the pulse-energy is substantial and wiry in coming, it is the condition of going beyond, which is the disease in the exterior; if the pulse energy is not substantial and weak, it is the condition of falling short, which shows the disease is in the interior.” Yellow Emperor asked: “What syndromes will occur when the pulse condition of spring is going beyond or falling short?” Qibo answered: “One will often get angry and feel dizziness and headache when it is going beyond; one will feel pain in the chest like the back being dragged, and distension of the lateral sides of the thorax when it is falling short.”

帝曰：“善，夏脉如钩，何如而钩？”岐伯曰：“夏脉者心也，南方火也，万物之所以盛长也，故其气来盛去衰，故曰钩，反此者病。”帝曰：“何如而反？”岐伯曰：“其气来盛去亦盛，此谓太过，病在外；其气来不盛去反盛，此谓不及，病在中”。帝曰：“夏脉太过与不及，其病皆何如？”岐伯曰：“太过则令人身热而肤〔《太素》《甲乙》“肤”并作“骨”〕痛，为浸淫；其不及则令人烦心〔《中藏经》“心”作“躁”〕，上见欬唾〔《中藏经》“见”作“为”，《太素》“欬”作“噬”〕，下为气泄。”

Yellow Emperor said: “Good”, The pulse condition of summer is like a hook, but what is a hooked pulse?” Qibo answered: “The pulse of summer is the heart pulse, it associates

with fire of south, which has the scene of flourishing of all things; as the coming of the pulse-energy is abundant, but becomes deficient when going like the image of a hook, it is called the hooked pulse, if the condition is on the contrary, it is the diseased pulse."

Yellow Emperor asked: "What is the condition when it is on the contrary?" Qibo answered: "When the pulse energy is abundant in coming, and also abundant in going, it is going beyond which shows the disease is in the exterior; if the pulse energy is not abundant in coming but becomes abundant when going, it is falling short which shows the disease is in the interior." Yellow Emperor asked: "What are the diseases of going beyond and falling short in summer?" Qibo answered: "One will have fever, pain in bone and erosion of sore when it is going beyond; feeling oppressed over the chest, chewing saliva in the upper part and breaking wind in the lower when it is falling short."

帝曰：善。秋脉如浮，何如而浮？岐伯曰：秋脉者肺也，西方金也，万物之所以收成也，故其气来，轻虚以浮，来急去散，故曰浮，反此者病。帝曰：何如而反？岐伯曰：其气来，毛布中央坚，两傍虚，此谓太过，病在外；其气来，毛而微，此谓不及，病在中。帝曰：秋脉太过与不及，其病皆何如？岐伯曰：太过则令人逆气而背痛，愠愠然；其不及，则令人喘，呼吸少气而欬，上气见血，下闻病音。

Yellow Emperor said: "Good , The pulse condition of autumn is floating, but what is floating like?" Qibo answered: "The pulse of autumn is the pulse of lung, it associates with the metal of west, which has the scene of harvesting of all things; as the pulse energy is light, feeble, floating and hasty in coming, but becomes scattered when going, it is called the floating pulse. If the condition is on the contrary, it is the diseased pulse."

Yellow Emperor asked: "What is the condition when it is on the contrary?" Qibo answered: "When the pulse is floating and soft with firmness in the central part but being empty on both sides in coming, it is going beyond, which shows the disease is in the exterior; when the pulse energy is floating, soft and tiny in coming, it is falling short which shows the disease is in the interior." Yellow Emperor asked: "What diseases will occur when it is going beyond or falling short?" Qibo answered: "One will feel adverseness of vital energy, pain on the back, feeling dull and depressed when going beyond: to have rapid breathing and cough, hemorrhage due to adverseness of vital energy in the upper part of the body and the sound of rapid respiration can be heard on the lower part of the chest when falling short."

帝曰：善。冬脉如营，〔《难经·十五难》"营"作"石"，按"营"为"莹"之借字〕何如而营？岐伯曰：冬脉者肾也，北方水也，万物之所以合藏〔滑抄本，"合"作"含"，《太素》"所以"下无"合"字〕也，故其气来沉以〔《甲乙》"搏"作"濡"〕搏，故曰营，反此者病。帝曰：何如而反？岐伯曰：其气来〔《脉经》"气"下无"来"字〕如弹石者，此谓太过，病在外；其去如数〔《太素》"数"作"毛"〕者，此谓不及，病在中。帝曰：冬脉太过与不及，其病皆何如？岐伯曰：太过则令人解㑊，脊脉〔《太素》"脊脉"作"腹"〕痛，而少气不欲言；其不及则令人心悬如病饥，眇中清，脊中痛，少腹满，小便变〔《脉经》"变"作"黄赤"〕。帝曰：善。

Yellow Emperor said: "Good. The pulse condition of winter is stony, but what is stony

like?" Qibo answered: "The pulse of winter is the pulse of kidney, it associates with water of north with the scene of shutting and hiding of all things; as the coming of the pulse energy is sunken and moist, so it is called the stony pulse. If the condition is on the contrary, it is the diseased pulse."

Yellow Emperor asked: "What is the condition of the pulse when it is on the contrary?" Qibo answered: "When the pulse is hitting the fingers like marble, it is going beyond, it shows the disease is in the exterior; if the pulse condition is floating and soft, it is falling short which shows the disease is in the interior." Yellow Emperor said: "What disease will occur when the winter pulse is going beyond or falling short?" Qibo answered: "One will be feeling fatigue, pain of the abdomen and speechless when going beyond; and one's heart will be suspending like getting hungry, feeling cool in the empty and soft part beneath the hypochondrium, pain in the spine, distension of the lower abdomen and with deep-coloured urine when falling short." Yellow Emperor said: "Good!"

帝曰：四时之序，逆从之变异也，然脾脉独何主？岐伯曰：脾脉〔《脉经》"脾"下无"脉"字〕者土也，孤藏以灌四傍者也。帝曰：然则脾〔《太素》"脾"下有"之"字〕善恶，可得见之乎？岐伯曰：善者不可得〔《太素》《脉经》《甲乙》"不可"下并无"得"字〕见，恶者可见。帝曰：恶者何如可见？岐伯曰：其来如水之流者，此谓太过，病在外；如鸟之喙〔《太素》"如"上有"其来"二字《难经》作"啄"〕者，此谓不及，病在中。帝曰：夫子言脾为孤藏，中央土以灌四傍，其太过与不及，其病皆何如？岐伯曰：太过则令人四支〔《脉经》《千金》"四支"下并有"沉重"二字〕不举；其不及则令人九窍〔《脉经》《千金》"九窍"下并有"壅塞"二字〕不通，名曰重强。

Yellow Emperor said: "The sequence of the four seasons is the source for indicating the agreeable and adversed change of the pulse condition, but which season the spleen dominates?" Qibo answered: "The spleen associates with earth and it is a solitary viscus which has the function of moistening all around and other viscera."

Yellow Emperor asked: "Can we distinguish whether or not the function of the spleen is normal?" Qibo answered: "It can hardly be distinguished through the normal spleen pulse, but it can be distinguished through the diseased pulse: "Yellow Emperor said: "What is the diseased pulse like?" Qibo answered: "When the coming of the pulse is like flowing water, it is going beyond, which shows the disease is in the exterior; when the coming of the pulse is like a bird pecking at the grain, it is falling short which shows the disease is in the interior." Yellow Emperor said: "Since, as you have said, the spleen is a solitary viscus which situates in the centrality for moistening all around and other viscera, what disease will occur when it is going beyond or falling short?" Qibo answered: "One will feel heavinese of the extremities and difficulty in lifting when going beyond; and one's nine orifices will be obstructed and the body will become clumbsy when falling short."

帝瞿〔明抄本"瞿"作"矍"〕然而起，再拜而稽首曰：善。吾得脉之大要，天下至数，五色〔《太素》"脉"上无"五色"二字〕脉变，揆度奇恒，道在于一，神转不廻，廻则不转，乃失其机，至数之要，迫近以微，著之玉版，藏之藏府〔《太素》"藏府"作"于府"〕，每旦

读之，名曰玉机。

Yellow Emperor stood up in amazement, made a bow and said: "Very good! Now I understand the fundamental essentials of palpation and the maxim in the world. The essentials of diagnosing through palpation for to observe the normal and abnormal pulse condition is to keep in line with the principle of the unceasing and forth-going operation of vitality, if it stops, the least of life will be lost. This is a very important and profound truth which should be recorded on a plate of jade and be kept in the inner mansion for to recite every morning. Its name should be called the 'Plate of Jade'".

五脏受气于其所生，传之于其所胜，气舍于其〔"其"疑衍〕所生，死于其所不胜。病之且死，必先传行至其所不胜，病乃死，此言气之逆行也，故死〔此二字疑衍〕。肝受气于心，传之于脾，气舍于肾，至肺而死。心受气于脾，传之于肺，气舍于肝，至肾而死。脾受气于肺，传之于肾，气舍于心，至肝而死。肺受气于肾，传之于肝，气舍于脾，至心而死。肾受气于肝，传之于心，气舍于肺，至脾而死，此皆逆死〔按"逆死"似应作"逆行"〕也。一日一夜五分之，此所以占死〔《甲乙》"生"作"者"〕生之早暮也。

"The evil-energy of a certain viscera originates from the viscera that it produces (such as liver's evil-energy originates from heart), transmits to the viscera which it restricts (such as the evil-energy is transmitted from liver to spleen), retains in the viscera that produces it (such as the liver's evil-energy retains in the kidney), and the patient will die when the transmission reaches the viscera that restricts it (such as, when the evil-energy being transmitted to the lung, the patient will die). The patient will die only after the visceral-energy being transmitted to the vsicera that restricts it, and this is the adverse direction of the transmission of the evil-energy.

"For instance, the liver's evil-energy originates from the heart, then being transmitted to the spleen, and then, being retained in the kidney, when the transmission reaches the lung, the patient will die. The heart's evil-energy originates from the spleen, then being transmitted to the lung and retained in the liver, when the transmission reaches the kidney, the patient will die. The spleen's evil-energy originates from the lung, then being transmitted to the kidney, and then retained in the heart, when the transmission reaches the liver, the patient will die. The lung's evil-energy originates from the kidney, then being transmitted to the liver and retained in the spleen, when the transmission reaches the heart, the patient will die. The kidney's evil-energy originates from the liver, then being transmitted to the heart and retained in the lung, when the transmission reaches the spleen, the patient will die. These are the conditions of the adversed drive of the evil-energies. When divide the day and night hours into five parts to associate the five viscera respectively, the hour of the patient's death can be probably estimated (when the transmission of the the spleen's evil-energy reaches the liver, the patient will die in the morning, will die in the forenoon when the lung's evil-energy reaches the heart, will die at noon when the kidney's evil-energy reaches the lung, will die in the night when the heart's evil-energy reaches the kidney)."

黄帝曰：五藏相通，移皆有次，五藏有病，则各传其所胜。不治，法〔《标本病传论》王

注引作“或”〕三月若六月，若三日若六日，传五藏〔《标本病传论》王注引“传”下无“五藏”二字，《类说》引“而”作“皆”〕而当死，是顺传所胜之次〔林校引《素问》及《甲乙》并无此七字〕。故曰：别于阳者，知病从来；别于阴者，知死生之期，言知〔《甲乙》“言”下无“知”字〕至其所困而死。

Yellow Emperor said："The five viscera are communicating with each other，and the transmission of the evil-energies are of regular sequence. If one of the five viscera is ill，its evil-energy will be transmitted to the viscera it restricts；if the treating is not in time，such a transmission will cause death of the patient in three to six months when the time is long，and three to six days when the time is short. Thus，when one can distinguish the superficial lesion，he can know in which channel the disease locates. When one can distinguish the interior-syndrome，he can know the critical day of the disease，that is，when the viscera being distressed by the evils，it is the date of the patient's death.

是故风者百病之长也，今风寒客于人，使人毫毛毕直，皮肤闭而为热，当是之时，可汗而发也；或痹不仁肿痛，当是之时，可汤熨及火灸刺而去〔《圣济总录》引“刺”下无“而去”二字〕之。弗治，病〔“病”字误移，似应在“名曰”上，病名曰肺痹〕入舍于肺，名曰肺痹，发欬上气，弗治，肺即传而行之肝〔《脉乐大典》引作“肺传之肝”〕，病名曰肝痹，一名曰厥，胁痛出食，当是之时，可按若刺耳。弗治，肝传之脾，病名曰脾风，发瘅，腹中热，烦心出黄，当此之时，可按可药可浴。弗治，脾传之肾，疝名曰疝瘕，少腹冤热而痛，出白〔《甲乙》作“汗出”〕，一名曰蛊，当此之时，可按可药。弗治，肾传之心，病〔熊本“引”下无“而”字。再“筋脉相引而急”与下“病名曰瘛”误倒，《圣济经》吴注引“肾传之心，是为心瘛”〕筋脉相引而急，病名曰瘛，当此之药，可灸可药。弗治，满十日，法当死。肾因传之心，心即复反传而行之肺，发寒热，法当三岁〔滑寿说：“三岁当作三日”〕死，此病之次也。

"diseases elicid by wind evil is in the first place of all diseases.

"When the wind-cold evil invades the human body，it causes the standing up of the soft hairs ，obstruction of the skin and interior fever of a man inside. By this time，it can be cured by the sweating method. If the treating is not in time，syndromes of numbness and swelling will occur，by this time，they can be cured by therapies of hot press，fire，moxibustion and acupuncture. If the treating is delayed，the evil-energy will be transmitted and retained in lung to cause lung-bi-syndrome，and cough and adverseness of lung energy will occur. If the disease is not treated again，the evil-energy will be transmitted from lung to liver to cause hepatic bi-syndrome，hypochondriac pain and loss of appetite . By this time it can be treated with massage and acupuncture，if the treating is delayed，the evil-energy will be transmitted from liver to spleen to cause splenic wind-syndrome，jaundice，hotness of the abdomen，irritability and yellow urine，By this time，it can be treated with massage，medicine and hot bath，if it is not treated again，the evil-energy will be transmitted from spleen to kidney to cause the syndrome of retention of evils in the lower warmer，and the heat will be accumulated in the lower abdomen to cause pain and sweating. This disease is called the syndrome of tympanites due to the parasitic infestation. By this time，it can be treated with

massage and medicine. If the treating is delayed again, the evil-energy will be transmitted from kidney to heart to cause the syndrome of spasm of muscle and tendons which is called convulsion. By this time, it can be treated with moxa cone moxibustion and medicine. If the disease in not healed, the patient will die after ten days. If the evil-energy is transmitted from kidney to heart, and then being transmitted reversely to lung with fever and cold, the patient will die in three days. This is the sequence of the transmission of the disease.

然其卒发者，不必治于传，或其传化有不以次，不以次入〔《甲乙》无“不以次入”四字，“者”字连上读〕者，忧恐悲喜怒，令不得其次，故令人〔《甲乙》“人”下无“有”字，“大”疑作“卒”〕有大病矣。因而喜大虚〔“大虚”二字似衍〕则肾气乘矣，怒则肝气乘矣〔张志聪说：“肝”应作“肺”〕，悲则肺气乘〔张志聪说：“悲应作“思”，“肺”应作“肝”〕矣，恐则脾气乘矣，忧则心气乘矣，此其道也。故病有五〔据林校引文，“五”下有“变”字〕，五五二十五变，及〔胡本、赵本、吴本明抄本“及”并作“反”〕其传化。传，乘之名也。

“If the disease comes abruptly, it is not necessary to follow the regular sequence in treating, as the transmission is not necessarily of regular sequence. The five emotional activities of melancholy, terror, sorrow, overjoy and anger can cause the evil-energy to transmit not according to the regular sequence and cause the disease to be occurred all of a sudden.

“Such as, overjoy may hurt the heart, and the kidney energy which restricts the heart may take advantage to invade. Anger hurts the liver, and the lung energy which restricts the liver may take advantage to invade. Anxiety hurts the spleen, and the liver-energy which restricts the spleen may take advantage to invade. Terror hurts the kidney, and the spleen-energy which restricts the kidney may take advantage to invade. Melancholy hurts the lung, and the heart-energy which restricts the kidney may take advantage to invade. These are the rules that the disease does not follow the regular sequence. Thus, although there are five variations of the disease, but they can turn out to be twenty-five variations which are on the contrary of the normal transmission. Transmission is the byname of ‘invasion’.

大骨枯稿，大肉陷下，胸中气满，喘息不便，其气动形，期六月死，真藏脉〔《太素》“藏”下无“脉”字〕见，乃予之期日。大骨枯稿，大肉陷下，胸中气满，喘息不便，内痛引肩项，期一月死，真藏见，乃予之期日。大骨枯稿，大肉陷下，胸中气满，喘息不便，内痛引肩项，身热脱肉破䐃，真藏见，十月〔明抄本，“月”作“日”〕之内死。大骨枯稿，大肉陷下，肩髓内〔吴本“内”作“肉”，《太素》“髓”作“隋”〕消，动作益衰，真藏〔《太素》“来”作“未”〕来见，期一岁死，见其真藏，乃予之期日。大骨枯稿，大肉陷下胸中气满，腹内痛，心中不便，肩项〔“肩项”二字似蒙上节“内痛引肩项”衍。“身热”二字属下之头〕身热，破䐃脱肉，目匡〔明抄本“匡”作“眶”〕陷，真藏见，目不见人，立死，其见人者，至其所不胜之时〔于鬯说“时”应作“日”〕则死。

When the large bones of the patient are withered, his large muscles become thin and subsided with fullness of breath in the chest, restless with rapid breathing to cause the shaking of the shoulder and chest, the patient will die in about six months. Whenever the pulse condition indicating the exhaustion of the lung energy is seen, the date of the patient's death can be predicted.

"When the large bones of the patient are withered, his large muscles are thin and subsided with fullness of breath in the chest and rapid breathing to cause pain of heart and the uneasiness of the shoulder and neck, the patient will die in about one month. Whenever the pulse condition indicating the exhaustion of the spleen-energy is seen, the date of the patient's death can be predicted.

"When the large bones of the patient are withered, his large muscles are thin and subsided with fullness of breath in the chest and rapid breathing, the patient will have pain of the abdomen causing the ups and downs of the shoulder and neck, to have fever all over the body, being emaciated in muscles with the protruding muscles of the joints of elbows and knees being worn out, if, by this time, the pulse condition indicating the exhaustion of the visceral-energy is seen, the patient will die within ten days.

"When the large bones of the patient are withered, his large muscles are thin and subsided, his two shoulder are sinking, his muscles are declining, and he is feeble in action, if, by this time, the exhaustion of the kidney-energy is not seen, the patient will die in about one year; when the exhaustion of the kidney-energy is seen, the date of the patient's death can be predicted.

"When the large bones of the patient are withered, his large muscles are thin and subsided, moreover, with the distension of the chest, pain in the abdomen, restless and fever all over the body, worn out of poplitea, wearing down of the muscles, sinking of the eyesocket, if by this time, the pulse indicating the exhaustion of the liver-energy is seen, and the patient can not see anything, he will die very soon. If the patient still can see something, he will die later until his bodily resistance being lost.

急虚身中卒至，五藏绝闭，脉道不通，气不往来，譬于堕溺，不可为期。其脉绝不来，若人一息〔《甲乙》"若"下无"人"字，按"若"有"或"义，"息"字误，似应作"吸"〕五六至，其形肉不脱，真藏虽不〔于鬯说："'不'字疑因下'不'字而误，《三部九候论》'形肉已脱，九候虽调，犹死'"〕见，犹死也。

"When the healthy-energy becomes asthenic all of a sudden, and the exogenous evil invades the body abruptly to make the five viscera blocked, the channels obstructed, and the communication of air severed, like a man falling down or drowned in the water, one can, in such a sudden affection, hardly predict the date of the patient's death. If the pulse severs and not coming back, or five or six pulsations in an inhalation, the muscles being disjointed from the body, in this case, even no exhaustion of the visceral-energy is seen, the patient will die soon also.

真肝脉至，中〔《千金》"中"作"内外急"犹言浮中沉，三候皆坚动〕外急如循刀刃，责责然，如按琴瑟弦〔《病沅》作"如新张弓弦"〕，色青白不泽，毛折，乃死。真心脉至，坚〔《病沅》"坚"作"牢"〕而搏，如循薏苡子〔《太素》"苡"下无"子"字〕累累然，色赤黑不泽，毛折，乃死。真肺脉至，大而虚，如以毛羽中人肤〔《三部九候论》王注引"如"下无"以"字，《太素》"肤"下有'然"字〕，色白赤不泽，毛折，乃死。真肾脉至，搏而绝〔《太平圣惠方》"搏而绝"作"坚而沉"〕，如指〔滑本"如"下无"指"字〕弹石辟辟然，色

黑黄不泽，毛折，乃死。真脾脉至，弱而乍数乍疏〔《千金》“乍数乍疏”并作“乍疏乍散”〕，色黄青不泽，毛折，乃死。诸真藏脉见者，皆死不治也。

"When the coming of the pulse indicating the exhaustion of the liver-energy of the patient is vigorous regardless in light, moderate or heavy pressure, like the sound of rubbing the blade of a broad sword, or being tight like the string of a bow which has just been pulled, the patient's complexion is evidently green and white without lustre, and his soft hair is also withering, the patient will die. When the pulse indicating the exhaustion of the heart-energy is firm and hitting the fingers like touching the Job's-tears which are tiny and firm, and the patient's complexion is evidently reddish-black without any lustre with withering soft hairs, the patient will die. When the coming of the pulse indicating the exhaustion of the lung-energy is full but very feeble like a feather touching the skin of man, and the patient's complexion is evidently red and pale without any lustre with withering soft hair, the patient will die. When the coming of the pulse indicating the exhaustion of the kidney energy is firm and sunken, very hard like marble, the complexion of the patient is evidently dark yellow without any lustre and his soft hairs are withering, the patient will die. When the coming of the pulse indicating the exhaustion of the spleen-energy is weak and scattering, and the patient's complexion is evidently yellowish-green without any lustre with withering soft hairs, the patient will die. In a word, whenever the pulse indicating the exhaustion of the visceral-energy is seen, it shows a fatal disease."

黄帝曰：见真藏曰死，何也？岐伯曰：五藏者，皆禀气于胃，胃者五藏之本也，藏气〔《太素》“藏气者”作“五藏”〕者，不能自致于手太阴，必因于胃气，乃至于手太阴也〔《甲乙》无“乃至”七字〕，故五藏各以其时，自为而至于手太阴也。故邪气胜者，精气衰也，故病甚者，胃气不能与之俱至于手太阴，故真藏之气独见，独见者病胜藏也，故曰死。帝曰：善。

Yellow Emperor said: "The patient will die when the exhaustion of the visceral-energy appears, but why is it so?" Qibo answered: "The nourishment of the energies of the five viscera depends on the refined substance of water and cereals of the stomach, so, stomach is the root of the five viscera. The energies of the five viscera can not reach the Cunkou of the Hand Taiyin Channel directly, but it can reach with the help of the stomach-energy. The pulse conditions of the five viscera can only appear on the Cunkou when being abundant with the help of the stomach-energy. If the evil-energy is overabundant, the healthy-energy will decline naturally; so when the evil-energy is critical, the stomch-energy will be unable to reach to Hand Taiyin simultaneously with the visceral-energy. In this case, the pulse indicating the exhaustion of the visceral energy (without any stomach energy) will be appearing on Cunkou alone. The 'appearing alone' shows the evil-energy has overcome the visceral-energy, and the patient will die." Yellow said: "Good."

黄帝曰：凡治病，察其形气色泽，脉之盛衰，病之新故，乃治之无后其时。形气相得，谓之可治；色泽以浮，谓之易已；脉从四时，谓之可治；脉弱以滑，是有胃气，命曰易治，取〔《太素》“取”作“趣”，《甲乙》作“治之趣之，无后其时”〕之以时。形气相失，谓之难治；

色夭不泽，谓之难已；脉实以坚，谓之益甚；脉逆四时，为不可治〔《甲乙》并作“谓之不治”〕。必察四难而明告之。

Yellow Emperor said: “The routine of treating a patient is: inspect first the body, breath and complexion of the patient, the asthenia and sthenia of the pulse condition, to know whether the disease is newly contracted or a protracted one, then, begin the treating, and one must not miss the opportunity of treating.

“When the body and breath of the patient are matching, the disease can be cured, when the complexion of the patient is moist, the disease can be cured easily. When the pulse condition is fitting the four seasons, the disease is curable, when the coming of the pulse is weak and fluent, it shows the stomach-energy is existing, the disease can be cured easily, all the cases above are the diseases which can be cured or can be cured easily provided that the treatment is in time. When the body and breath of the patient is not matching, the disease is difficult to be cured, when the complexion of the patient is withered without any lustre, the disease can hardly be cured. When the pulse is substantial and firm, it is an aggravated disease, if the pulse does not fit the four seasons, it is an incurable disease. One must find out the four difficult cases and tell the patient clearly.

所谓逆四时者，春得肺脉，夏得肾脉，秋得心脉，冬得脾脉，其至皆悬绝沉濇者，命曰逆。四时未有藏形，于〔《太素》无“于”字〕春夏而脉沉濇，秋冬而脉浮大，名曰逆四时也。

“The so called the adversed pulse condition to the four seasons are: when the lung pulse is seen in spring, when the kidney pulse is seen in summer, when the heart pulse is seen in autumn, and when the spleen pulse is seen in winter. All the coming of the pulses above are of ‘appearing alone’ indicating the exhaution of the visceral-energy, (it appears alone, sunken and rough with no stomach-energy). They are all the adversed pulse condition.

“When there is no pulse indicating the exhaustion of the viseral-energy occurs in the four seasons, but sunken and rough pulse conditions occur in spring and summer instead, or the floating and full pulse condition occur in autumn and winter instead, they are all called the adverse pluse condition which are against the four seasons.

病热脉静〔“脉”下有“青”字〕，泄而〔《千金》“而”作“利”〕脉大，脱血而脉实，病在中脉实坚，病在外脉不实坚者，皆〔《甲乙》“皆”下有“为”字〕难治。

“When in the disease of heat-syndrome, but the pulse condition, on the contrary, is cool and calm; when in the diarrhea, but the pulse condition, on the contrary, is full; when the patient collapses due to massive hemorrhage, but the pulse condition, on the contrary, is substantial; when the disease is in the interior, but the pulse condition, on the contrary, is firm, when the disease is in the exterior, but the pulse condition, on the contrary is neither substantial nor firm; they are all the cases of the adverseness of pulse condition, and these diseases can hardly be cured.”

黄帝曰：余闻虚实以决死生，愿闻其情。岐伯曰：五实死，五虚〔《儒门事亲》“实”、“虚”下并有“者”字〕死。帝曰：愿闻五实五虚。岐伯曰：脉盛、皮热、腹胀、前后不通、

闷瞀，此谓五实。脉细、皮寒、气少、泄利前后，〔《卫生宝鉴》引无“前后”二字〕饮食不入，此谓五虚。帝曰：其时有生者，何也？岐伯曰：浆粥入胃，泄注止〔“注”字误，应作“利”〕，则虚者活，身汗得后利，则实者活，此其候也。

Yellow Emperor said: “I am told that one can predict the patient’s death or survival according to astheria and sthenia of the patient. I hope you can tell me the reason.”

Qibo answered: “When the sthenia-syndrome of the five viscera or the asthenia-syndrome of the five viscera being contracted, the patient will die.” Yellow Emperor said: “Please tell me what is the sthenia-syndrome and asthenia-syndrome of the five viscera.” Qibo said: “When the coming of the pulse is flourishing, the skin of the patient is hot, with distension and fullness of the abdomen, retention of feces and urine, and also with mental confusion, it is called the sthenia-syndrome of five viscera. When the pulse condition is very fine, cold of skin, short of breath, diarrhea and poor appetite, it is called the asthenia-syndrome of five viscera.” Yellow Emperor said: “Some of the patients who contracted with sthenia and asthenia syndrome of five viscera were finally healed, and what is the reason?” Qibo answered: “If the patient of asthenia of five viscera takes some gruel or thick fluid to restore his stomach-energy gradually, and his diarrhea being stopped, he may be recovered; if the patient of sthenia-syndrome of five viscera is sweating, and his stool being unobstructed, his superfices and interior become harmony, the disease can also be healed. This is the principle of predicting the death and survival of the patient according to asthenia and sthenia.”

三部九候论篇第二十

Chapter 20
San Bu Jiu Hou Lun
(On the Three Parts and the Nine Sub-parts of Pulse)

黄帝问曰：余闻九针〔《太平圣惠方》引作“候”〕于夫子，众多博大，不可胜数。余愿闻要道〔林校引全元起本“道”作“地”〕，以属子孙，传之后世，著之骨髓，藏之肝肺，歃血而受，不敢妄泄，令合天道〔“道”林校引作“地”〕，必有始终，上应天光星历纪，下副四时五行。贵贱更互（胡本、赵本“互”并作“立”）冬阴夏阳，以人应之奈何？愿闻其方。

Yellow Emperor asked: “The principle of nine sub-parts of pulse I have heard was abundant and vast to me, which can hardly be related in full. I hope to hear some more about the principle which are important, so that I can enjoin my descendants to hand down to the future generations. I will firmly bear them mind, and swear not to disclose them out carelessly. I will keep them in compatible with the heaven and earth from beginning to end and let it correspond with the numbers of the sun, moon, star and the solar terms above, and in accordance with the variation of the four seasons and the five elements below. Since there are different conditions of abundance and decline in the five elements, and in the four seasons, winter is Yin and summer is Yang, how can a man adapt these natural laws? I hope you can tell me if there is any method.

岐伯对曰：妙乎哉问也！此天地之至数。帝曰：愿闻天地之至数，合于人形，血气通〔按“通”字误倒，应作“通血气”〕，决死生，为之奈何？岐伯曰：天地之至数，始于一，终于九焉。一者〔明抄本“者”作“曰”〕天，二者〔应作“曰”〕地，三者〔应作“曰”〕人，因而三之，三三者九，以应九野，故人〔《类说》引“人”作“脉”〕有三部，部有三候，以决死生，以处百病，以调虚实，而除邪疾。

Qibo said: “What a good question you have asked, it is the axiom of heaven and earth.”

Yellow Emperor said: “I hope you can tell me the axiom of heaven and earth so that it may be in confromity with the human body, dredging the blood and energy, and enable one to distinguish the death and survival of the patient. But how can this be achieved?” Qibo said: “The numbers of heaven and earth begin from one and end in nine.

“One is Yang and it stands for heaven, two is Yin and it stands for earth, as men lives between heaven and earth, so three stands for man, since the heaven, earth and man are three, three times three is nine which is corresponding with the number of the nine prefectures.

“Thus, there are three parts in the pulse, and each of them has three sub-parts which are the foundations for to distinguish the death and survival of the patient, diagnose all kinds

of disease, adjust the asthenia and sthenia, and remove diseases."

帝曰：何谓三部？岐伯曰：有下部，有中部，有上部，部各有三候，三候者，有天有地有人也，必指而导之，乃以为真。上部天〔"上部天至下部人，足太阴也"〕，两额之动脉；上部地，两颊之动脉；上部人，耳前之动脉。中部天，手太阴也；中部地，手阳明也；中部人，手少阴也。下部天，足厥阴也；下部地，足少阴也；下部人，足太阴也。故下部之天以候肝，地以候肾，人以候脾胃之气。

Yellow Emperor asked: "What are the three parts?" Qibo said: "The three parts are the lower part, the middle part and the upper part, and each of them has three sub-parts which are represented by heaven, earth and man respectively, and one can only understand them with the instruction of others.

The upper part of heaven represents the arteries of the two sides of the forehead, the upper part of earth represents the arteries of the two cheeks, the upper part of man represents the arteries of the two ears; the middle part of heaven is Hand Taiyin, the middle part of earth is Hand Yangming, the middle part of man is Hand Shaoyin; the lower part of heaven is Foot Jueyin, the lower part of earth is Foot Shaoyin, the lower part of man is Foot Taiyin.

"The heaven sub-part of the lower part can be used to diagnose the energy of liver, the earth sub-part of the lower part can be used to diagnose the energy of kidney, and the man sub-part of the lower part can be used to diagnose the stomach and spleen."

帝曰：中部之候奈何？岐伯曰：亦有天，亦有地，亦有人。天以候肺，地以候胸中之气，人以候心。帝曰：上部以何候之？岐伯曰：亦有天，亦有地，亦有人。天以候头角之气，地以候口齿之气，人以候耳目之气。三部者，各有天，各有地，各有人，三而成天，三而成地，三而成人，三而三之，合则为九，九分为九野，九野为九藏。故神藏五，形藏四，合为九藏。五藏已败，其色必夭，夭必死矣。

Yellow Emperor asked: "What is the condition of the middle part?" Qibo said: "There are also three sub-parts of heaven, earth, and man in the middle part. The heaven sub-part of the middle part can be used to diagnose the energy of the lung, the earth sub-part of the middle part can be used to diagnose the energy of the chest, the man sub-part of the middle part can be used to diagnose the energy of the heart."

Yellow Emperor asked: "What is the condition of the upper part?" Qibo said: "There are also three sub-parts in the upper part. The heaven sub-part of the upper part can be used to diagnose the energy of the corner of the forehead, the earth sub-part of the upper part can be used to diagnose the energies of the mouth and teeth, the man sub-part of the upper part can be used to diagnose the energies of the ears and eyes.

"In a word, in each of the three parts, there are heaven, earth and man respectively; there are three sub-parts of heaven, three sub-parts of earth and three sub-parts of man. Three times three, there are all together nine sub-parts. The nine sub-parts of pulse correspond to the nine prefectures of earth, and the nine prefectures correspond to the nine organs of man, ie., the five spirit-storing organs of liver, lung, heart, spleen and kidney and the

four substantial-storing organs of stomach, large intestine, small intestine and bladder. If the five viscera decline, the complexion will be withered and dark, and the patient will die."

帝曰：以候奈何？岐伯曰：必先度其形之肥瘦，以调其气之虚实，实则写之，虚则补之。必先去其血脉，而后调之，无问其病，以平〔《原病式》引'以平"上有"五藏"二字〕为期。

Yellow Emperor asked: "What is the method of examining a patient?" Qibo said: "One must estimate first whether the body of the patient is fat or thin so as may adjust the asthenia or sthenia of his energy. When the patient's energy is of sthenia, the surplus should be discharged; when the patient's energy is of asthenia, the insufficiency should be made up. Before adjusting, the patient's blood stasis must be removed. In treating, no matter what the disease is, the five viscera should be kept in equilibrium."

帝曰：决死生奈何？岐伯曰：形盛脉细，少气不足以息者危〔林校引全本及《甲乙》、《脉经》"危"作"死"〕。形瘦脉大，胸中多气者死，形气相得者生，参伍不调者病。三部九候皆相失者死。上下左右之脉相应如参舂者病甚。上下左右相失不可数者死。中部之候虽独调，与众相失者死，中部之候相减者死。目内陷者死。

Yellow Emperor asked: "How to distinguish the death and survival of the patient?" Qibo said: "When the body of the patient is strong, but his pulse is fine instead, short of breath as if his breathing is discontinuous, it shows the patient will die. When the body of the patient is thin, but his pulse is full instead, with plenty breath in his chest, it also shows the patient will die. When the pulse beats are disorderly and disharmonious, it shows the disease is existing. If the three parts and the nine sub-parts of the pulse are all irregular, it shows the patient will die; when the upper and lower, left and right pulses are corresponding but with uneven movement, up and down like a pestle in the mortar and in large and rapid beats, it shows the disease is serious. When the upper and lower, left and right pulses are disharmonious to cause one unable to count the number of pulsation in an inhalation, it is the symptom of patient's death. When the pulse of the middle part is harmonious by itself, but the pulses indicating the various viscera of the upper part and the lower are irregular, it is also the symptom of the patient's death; when the pulse of the middle part is lesser than that of the upper and lower parts, it is also the symptom of death. When the eyesocket of the patient is sunken, it is the symptom of decline of vital energy, the patient will die."

帝曰：何以知病之所在？岐伯曰：察九候，独小者病，独大者病，独疾者病，独迟者病，独热者病，独寒者病，独陷下者病。以左手足上，上〔《甲乙》"去"上无"上"字，按"以左手"两句，亡名氏《脉经》作"以左手去足内踝上五寸微指按之"文义较明显〕去踝五寸按之，庶右手足当踝而弹之，其应过五寸以上蠕蠕然者不病；其应疾中手浑浑然者病；中手徐徐然者病；其应上不能至五寸，弹之不应〔亡名氏《脉经》"不应"下有"手"字〕者死。是以脱肉身不去者死。中部乍疏乍数者死。其脉代〔孙鼎宜说："'代'当作'大'"〕而钩者，病在络脉。九候之相应也，上下若一，不得相失。一候后则病，二候后则病甚，三候后则病危，所谓后者，应〔亡名氏《脉经》"应"上有"上中下"三字〕不俱也。察其府藏〔《太素》作"病"〕，以知死生之期。必先知经脉，然后知病脉，真藏脉见者胜〔《甲乙》"者胜"

作“邪胜者”〕死。足太阳气绝者，其足不可屈伸，死必戴眼。

Yellow Emperor asked: “How can one know where the disease locates?” Qibo said: “When one of the nine sub-parts is solely tiny, solely large, solely rapid, solely slow, solely hot (slippery), solely cold (rough), or solely subsided (sunken or hidden), there are all the symptoms of disease.

“When one presses lightly the location of five cun (inches) above the foot inner ankle with the left hand, and flick the ankle slightly with the right hand, when the vigorous beats of the pulse beyond the range of five cun is felt, it shows the patient has no disease; if the coming of the energy is hasty, but weak when responding the fingers, it shows the disease is existing. When there is no respond after flicking within the range of five cun above, it is the symptom of death.

“If the muscle is substantial, but the pulse fails to come and go. it is the symptom of death. When the pulse of the middle part is close and loose at intervals, and the channel-energy is scattered and disorderly, it is also the symptom of death. When the pulse of the upper part is large and hooked, it shows the disease is in the channel and collateral.

“The nine sub-parts should be harmonious and be in accordance with each other and must not be uneven, if one of them in the nine parts is not corresponding, it is the symptom of disease; when two of them are not corresponding, the disease is serious; when three of them are not corresponding, the patient is in danger. The so called not corresponding means the three parts of the upper, middle and the lower fail to keep identical. When the diseased viscera is examined, the time of the patient's death or survival can be anticipated. One must know the condition of the normal pulse first, then can he know what is a diseased pulse. When the pulse indicating the exhaustion of the visceral-energy is seen and the evil-energy is abundant, the patient will die. When the channel-energy of Foot Taiyang is severing, the patient will find difficulty to bend and stretch his feet, and his eyes will certainly be looking up when dying.”

帝曰：冬阴夏阳奈何？岐伯说：九候之脉，皆沈细悬绝者为阴，主冬，故以夜半死。盛躁喘数者为阳，主夏，故以日中死。是故寒热病〔《太素》、《脉经》“热”下并无“病”字〕者，以平旦死。热中及热病者，以日中死。病风者，以日夕死。病水者，以夜半死。其脉乍疏乍数乍迟乍疾者，日〔《太素》、《甲乙》、《脉经》“日”上并有“以”字〕乘四季死。形肉已脱，九候虽调，犹死。七诊虽见，九候皆从者不死，所言不死者，风气之病，及经月〔《太素》“月”作“间”杨注：经脉间轻病〕之病，似七诊之病而非也，故言不死。若有七诊之病，其脉候亦败者死矣。必发哕噫〔按“噫”字疑衍〕。必审问其所始病〔《太素》作“其故所始作病”〕，与今之所方病，而后各〔《太素》、《甲乙》“后”下并无“各”字〕切循其脉，视其经络浮沉，以上下逆从循之。其脉疾者不〔不字疑衍〕病，其脉迟者病，脉不往〔《甲乙》“往”下有“不”字〕来者死。皮肤著者死。

Yellow Emperor asked: “What do you mean by winter is Yin and summer is Yang?” Qibo said: “When the pulse conditions of the nine sub-parts are all of sunken, fine, wiry and severing, it is Yin like in the winter, the patient of such disease will die at midnight. If the

pulse conditions of the nine sub-parts are all of vigorous and, fast in beating, it is Yang like in the summer, the patient of such disease will die at noon. When the cold-syndrome and heat-syndrome occur alternately, the patient will die at dawn when the Yin and Yang intercourse. When the heat is both in the interior and the superficies, the patient will die at noon when Yang is extreme.

"When being attacked by wind-evil, the patient will die in the two-hour period of Shen (3: 00-5: 00 PM) and You (5: 00-7: 00 PM). When being attacked by the retention of fluid, the patient will die at midnight when Yin is extreme. If the pulse is loose and close, slow and fast at intervals, it shows the spleen-energy is severed inside, the patient will die in the two-hour period of Chen (7: 00-9: 00 AM), Xiu (7: 00-9: 00 PM), Chou (1: 00-300 AM) and Wei (1: 00-3: 00 PM).

"If the muscle is divorced from the body, even though the nine sub-parts are in harmony, it is also the symptom of death. If the seven kinds of pulse of palpation (one of the nine sub-parts is solely tiny, solely full, solely fast, solely slow, solely hot, solely cold or solely subsided) appears, but the nine-sub-parts are fitting the four seasons, the patient may not die, and the disease is not fatal. Such as in the wind syndrome or the disease between the channels, although pulse condition is much alike the seven kinds of diseased pulse, yet they are not exactly the same, so, it is not the symptom of death. If the seven kinds of the diseased pulse are seen and the sub-parts are also of corrupt appearance, it is the symptom of death, and the patient will sure to hiccup when dying.

"Therefore, when treating, one must ask the patient in detail about the condition of the disease in the beginning and the present first, and then, palpate the pulse, inspect the floating and the sinking of the channel, and the adversed and agreeable condition of the upper and the lower part of the patient. When the pulse is fluent in coming, no disease is existing; when the pulse fails to go and come, it is the symptom of death; when the muscle is divorced from the body, when the disease is protracted, and the skin is attaching the bone, it is also the symptom of death."

帝曰：其可治者奈何？岐伯曰：经病者治其经，孙络病者治其孙络血，血病身有痛者治其经络。其病者在奇邪，奇邪之脉则缪刺之。留瘦不移，节而刺之。上实下虚，切而从之，索其结络脉，刺出其血，以见通〔《太素》"以"以下无"见"字〕《甲乙》"以见通之"作"以通其气"〕之。瞳子高者，太阳不足，戴眼者，太阳已绝，此决死生之要，不可不察也。手指及手外踝上五指留针（此"手指"十一字据王注是错简文）。

Yellow Emperor asked: "How to treat the disease when it is a curable one?" Qibo said: "When the disease is in the channel, prick the channel; when the disease is in the minute collateral, prick the minute collateral until it bleeds; when the disease is associated with the blood with syndrome of pain, prick the channel and the minute collateral. If the evils retain in the large collateral, apply collaterals insertion of pricking the left when the disease is in the right, and pricking the right when the disease is in the left. When the patient is skinny due to the protracted disease with unchanged syndrome, one should prick the joint where the

evil energy harbours. When the patient is sthenic in the upper part and is asthenic in the lower, one must palpate first and then treat with acupuncture, seek the stagnated location of the channels and collaterals, and prick until bleeding to dredge the energy. When the eyes of the patient is looking upward and staring continuously, it shows the energy of Taiyin channel has been severed. These are the important knacks for distinguishing the death or survival of the patient which should be observed carefully."

经脉别论篇第二十一

Chapter 21
Jing Mai Bie Lun
(Further Comments On Channel)

黄帝问曰：人之居处动静勇怯，脉亦为之变乎？岐伯对曰：凡人之惊恐恚劳动静，皆为变也。是以夜行则喘〔防鼎宜说："'喘'当作'惴'形误（下同）"〕出于肾，淫气病肺。有所堕恐〔"恐"字误，似应作"坠"，〕，喘〔当作"惴"〕出于肝，淫气害脾。有所惊恐，喘〔当作"惴"〕出于肺，淫气伤心。度水跌仆，喘〔当作"惴"〕出于肾与骨〔《难经》虞注引"骨"作"胃"〕，当是之时，勇者气行则已，怯者则着〔胡本、之头本"着"并作"著"，按《国语·晋语》韦注"著，附也"附有"随义"）〕而为病也。故曰：诊病之道，观人勇怯骨〔《素问校讹》引古抄本"骨"作"肌"〕肉皮肤，能知其情，以为诊法也。

Yellow Emperor asked: "Since men live in different environments and labour in different extents with different moods, will their channels, blood and energies change along with different situations?" Qibo answered: "The channel, blood and energy of a man will be affected and changed by terror, fright, anger, fatigue, motion and stillness. So, when one travels at night, fright will stem from the kidney, when the energy is over-abundant and moves rashly, it will hurt the lung. When one falls down, fright will stem from the liver, when the energy is over-abundant and moves rashly, it will hurt the spleen. When one is terrified greatly, terror will stem from the lung. When the energy is abundant and runs rashly, it will hurt the heart. If one wades across a river or falls, fright will stem from the kidney and stomach. Under these situations, if one has a strong body, his energy can be dredged, and his sickness can be recovered; if his body is weak, the evil energy will hurt the body in the wake of it. So, when treating, one should examine whether the body of the patient is strong or weak, and the appearance of his skin and muscle to know where the disease stems from, and this is the method of diagnosing a disease.

故饮食饱甚，汗出〔按《难经》虞引注"汗出"作"必伤"〕于胃；惊而夺精，汗出〔应作必伤〕于心；持重远行，汗出〔应作"必伤"〕于肾；疾走恐惧，汗出〔应作"必伤"〕于肝；摇体〔《医说》引"体"作"动"〕劳苦，汗出〔应作"必伤"〕于脾。故春秋冬夏四时阴阳，生病起于过用，此为常也。

"Therefore, when one eats too much, his stomach will certainly be hurt. When one is frightened, his heart will certainly be hurt. When one carries a heavy thing and travels far, his kidney will certainly be hurt. When one is walking rapidly with terror, his liver will certainly be hurt. When one waves with fatigue, his spleen will certainly be hurt.

"So, during the variations of Yin and Yang in the four seasons of spring, autumn, win-

ter and summer, most diseases are certainly due to the excessiveness of physical labour, food and drink, fatigue and the consumption of spirit.

食气入胃，散精于肝，淫气于筋。食气入胃，浊气归心〔沈思敏说：“‘心’字误，应作‘脾’”〕，淫精于脉。脉气流经，经气归于肺，肺朝百脉，输精于皮毛。毛〔《素问入气运气论奥》引“脉”上无“毛”字〕脉合精，行气于府。府精神明，留于四藏，气归于权衡，权衡以平，气口成寸，以决死生。

When the food enters into the stomach, after being digested, part of it which is the refined substance is transported to the liver to moisture the tendons of the whole body.

"Another part of it which is the essential substance from cereals is poured into the spleen and being soaked into the channel and blood.

"The channel-energy circulates in the channels and goes up to the lung. After the various channel-energies being converged in the lung, they are transported to the skin and hair.

"When the channel-energy and the refined energy combines, it flows into the six hollow organs, and the body fluids of the six hollow organs flow to the heart, liver, spleen and kidney.

"The spreading of the refined energy depends on the lung, and the condition of the lung is expressed on the pulse of Cunkou. One can distinguish whether the patient's disease is curable or not according to the pulse condition of Cunkou.

饮入于胃，游溢精气，上输于脾。脾气散精，上归于肺，通调水道，下输膀胱。水精四布，五经并行，合于四时五藏阴阳揆度〔林校引别本作“动静”〕，以为常也。

"When the water enters the stomach, it evaporates the refined energy and spread it to the spleen above; and the spleen spreads the essence into the lung above; the lung energy communicates with the water way, and transports the essence to the bladder. In this way, with the production, circulation activity of the vital energy and the promotion of the water, the refined energy spreads to the skin and hair of the whole body, they circulate in the channels of the five viscera and being kept in accordance with the variations of the motion and motionless of Yin and Yang of five viscera in the different seasons, and this is the normal condition of the channels.

太阳藏独至，厥喘虚气逆，是阴不足阳有余也，表里当俱写，取之下俞。阳明藏独至，是阳气重并也，当写阳补阴，取之下俞。少阳藏独至，是厥气也，跃前卒大，取之下俞。少阳独至者，一阳之过也。太阴藏搏〔四库本“博者”作“独至”〕者，用心省真，五脉气少，胃气不平，三阴〔按“三阴”下似脱“之过”〕也，宜治其下俞，补阳写阴。一阳〔林校云：“‘一阳’乃‘二阳’之误”〕独啸，少阳〔林校引全本“少阳”作“少阴”〕厥也，阳并于上，四脉争张，气归于肾，宜治其经络，写阳补阴，一阴〔按“一阴”下脱“独”字〕至，厥阴之治也，真虚痟心，厥气留薄，发为白〔“白”应作“自”〕汗，调食和药，治在下俞。

"When the channel of Taiyang is solely over-abundant, adverseness of asthenic-energy and dyspnea will occur. This shows Yin is insufficient and Yang is having a surplus, the purgation of superficies and interior should be applied: prick the Shugu (Shu Bone) point of the lower Shu-point of the Bladder Channel and the Taixi (Big Stream) point of the lower

Shupoint of the kidney channel.

"If the Yangming channel is solely over-abundant, and the Yang energy is very abundant and sthenic which should be purged by pricking the Xiangu (Sinking Vallgy) point of the Foot Yangming Channel, and Foot Taiyin Channel should be invigorated by pricking the Taibai (Grand White) point.

"If the Shaoyang Channel is solely over-abuudant, chaotic energy will occur, so the Shaoyang Channel which is in front of the Yangjiao Channel becomes large suddenly, and one should prick the Linqi (Fall Tears) point of the Shaoyang Channel.

"When the Shaoyang Channel is solely over-abundant, it shows the Shaoyang is excessive. When the Taiyin Channel is solely over-abundant, it should be examined carefully: if the channel-energies of the five visera are reducing, and the stomach-energy can not be kept in order, it is because the Taiyin is excessive, In treating, the Foot Yangming Channel should be invigorated by pricking the Xiangu (Sinking Velley) and the Foot Taiyin channel should be purged by pricking the Taibai (Grand White) point.

"If the second Yin channel is solely over-abundant, it is caused by the cold extremities due to heat-evil of Shaoyin and asthenic Yang above, and the energies of heart, spleen, liver and lung are contending. When the evil-energy is in the kidney, both the superficies and interior on the channel should be treated, the Foot Taiyang Channel should be purged by pricking the Kunlun (Big and High) point on the channel and the Feiyang (Flying up) point on the collateral, and invigorate the Foot Shaoyin Channel by pricking the Fuliu (Repeating Slip) point of the channel and the Dazhong (Big Bell) point on the collateral points.

"If the first Yin Channel is solely over-abundant, it is dominated by the Jueyin Channel, and the healthy energy is insufficient. The patient will feel ache in the heart, and his retained adverse energy will combat with the healthy energy, and he often has spontaneous perspiration. In this case, one should take care of adjusting the food and drink, and treat with medicine in concert. When applying acupuncture, The Taichong (Great Rush) point of Jueyin Channel should be pricked."

帝曰：太阳藏何象？岐伯曰：象三阳而浮也。帝曰：少阳藏何象？岐伯曰：象一阳也，一阳藏者，滑而不实也。帝曰：阳明藏何象？岐伯曰：象大浮〔林校引《太素》及全元起本"大浮"上有"心之"二字〕也。太阴藏搏，言伏鼓也。二阴搏至，肾沉不浮也。

Yellow Emperor asked: "What is the pulse condition of the Taiyang Channel like?" Qibo said: "The Taiyang Channel is abundant like that of the three-Yang channels, but at the same time, it is light and floating." Yellow Emperor asked: "What is the condition of the Shaoyang Channel like?" Qibo said: "It is like the first Yang channel which is slippery and not substantial." Yellow Emperor asked: "What is the pulse condition of the Yangming Channel?" Qibo said: "It is large and floating like the heart pulse. When the pulse of the Taiyin Channel pulsates, its pulse condition is sunken and hidden, but it hits the fingers substantially; when the pulse of the second Yin Channel pulsates, it is the appearance of the sunken and not floating like that of the Kidney pulse."

藏气法时论篇第二十二

Chapter 22

Zang Qi Fa Shi Lun

(On the Relation Between Energies of Five Viscera and the Four Seasons)

黄帝问曰：合人形以法四时五行而治，何如而从？何如而逆？得失之意，愿闻其事。岐伯对曰：五行者，金木水火土也，更贵更贱以知死生，以决成败，而定五藏之气，间甚之时，死生之期也。

Yellow Emperor asked: "When one treats the disease integrating the human body and following the law of the four seasons and the five elements, what is the agreeable way and what is the adverse way, which way will be hitting and which way will be missing?" Qibo answered: "The five elements you have said are metal, wood, water, fire and earth, from which one can infer whether the disease is serious or not, whether the treating will be successful or not by the variations of decline and prosperity, producing and restricting of them, so as one can distinguish the prosperity or decline of the five viscera, the serious extent of the disease, and the date of death or survival of the patient."

帝曰：原卒闻之。岐伯曰：肝主春，足厥阴少阳主治，其日甲乙，肝苦急，急食甘以缓之。

Yellow Emperor said: "I hope you can tell me in details." Qibo said: "The liver takes charge of the energy of spring which is the season of wood, there are Yin wood and Yang wood, when liver is in the Foot Jueyin Channel, it is Yin wood, when the gallbladder is in the Foot Shaoyang Channel, it is Yang wood, in spring, these are the two main channels for treating. Jia and Yi associate with wood, so Jia and Yi are the days when liver being prosperous, The characteristic of liver is impetuos which should be moderated with medicine of sweet taste.

心主夏，手少阴太阳主治，其日丙丁，心苦缓，急食酸以收之。

"The heart takes charge of the energy of summer which is the season of fire, there are Yin fire and Yang fire, when the heart is in the Hand Shaoyin Channel, it is Yin fire, when the small intestine is in the Hand Taiyang Channel, it is Yang fire; in summer, these are the two main channels for treating. Bing and Ding associate to the fire, so Bing and Ding are the days when the heart energy being prosperous. The characteristic of heart is dispersing, it should be gathered with medicine of sour taste.

脾主长夏，足太阴阳明主治，其日戊已，脾苦湿，急食苦〔《素问绍识》："'苦'是

‘咸’之误”〕以燥之。

“The spleen takes charge of the energy of long summer which is the season of earth, there are Yin earth and Yang earth, when the spleen is in the Foot Taiyin Channel, it is Yin earth, when the stomach is in the Foot Yangming Channel, it is Yang earth; in long summer, these are the two main channels for treating. Wu and Ji associate with earth, so Wu and Ji are the days when the spleen being prosperous. The characteristic of spleen is wet, it should be dried with medicine of salty taste.

肺主秋，手太阴阳明主治，其日庚辛，肺苦气上逆，急食苦以泄之。

“The lung takes charge of the energy of autumn which is the season of metal, there are Yin metal and Yang metal, when lung is in the Hand Taiyin Channel, it is Yin metal, when the large intestine is in the Hand Yangming Channel, it is the Yang metal; in autumn, these are the two main channels for treating. Geng and Xin associate with metal, so Geng and Xin are the days when lung being prosperous. When the lung energy goes up adversely, it should be purged with medicine of bitter taste.

肾主冬，足少阴太阳主治，其日壬癸，肾苦燥，急食辛以润之，开腠理，致津液，通气也。

“The kidney takes charge of the energy of winter which is the season of water, there are Yin water and Yang water, when the kidney is in the Foot Shaoyin Channel, it is Yin water, when the bladder is in the Foot Taiyang Channel, it is Yang water; in winter, these are the two main channels for treating. Ren and Gui associate with water, so Ren and Gui are the days when kidney being prosperous. The characterstic of kidney disease is dry, it should be moistened with medicine of acrid taste. In a word, when treating the five viscera with the five tastes, it is for to open the striae of skin, circulate the body fluid and dredge the energy.

病在肝，愈于夏，夏不愈，甚于秋，秋不死，持于冬，起于春，禁当风。肝病者，愈在丙丁，丙丁不愈，加于庚辛，庚辛不死，持于壬癸，起于甲乙。肝病者，平旦慧，下晡甚，夜半静。肝欲散，急食辛以散之，用辛补之，酸写之。

“When the disease is in the liver, it could be recovered in summer, if it is not recovered it will become aggravated in autumn, if the patient does not die in autumn, the disease will become protracted in winter, and the patient can only be picked up in spring of next year when the wood energy is prosperous, but the patient must take good care of avoiding wind-evil.

“The patient of liver disease may turn to the better in Bing and Ding days, if the disease is not recovered then, it will become aggravated on Geng and Xin days, if it does not aggravate then, it will be protracting on Ren and Gui days, but will turn to the better until Jia and Yi days.

“The patient with liver disease will turn to the better at dawn, turn to the worse at dusk, become calm down at midnight.

“The evil-energy of liver should be dispersed with acrid medicine, when invigoration is needed, sour medicine should be used to replenish the liver; when purgation is needed,

medicine of acrid taste should be used to clear away the fire of the liver-energy.

病在心，愈在长夏，长夏不愈，甚于冬，冬不死，持于春，起于夏，禁温食热衣。心病者，愈在戊已，戊已不愈，加于壬癸，壬癸不死，持于甲乙，起于丙丁。心病者，日中慧，夜半甚，平旦静。心欲软，急食咸以软之，用咸补之，甘写之。

"When the disease is in the heart, it could be recovered in long summer, if it is not recovered then, it will become aggravated in winter, if the patient does not die in winter, the disease will become protracting in spring of next year, but will turn to the better gradually in summer when the fire is prosperous, but the patient should take good care of not wearing warm clothes, nor taking hot food so that the fire-energy may not grow.

"The patient of heart disease may turn to the better on Wu and Ji days, if it is not recovered then, it will become aggravated on Ren and Gui days, if it is not aggravated then, it will become protracting on Jia and Yi days, but will turn to the better on Bing and Ding days.

"The patient with heart disease will feel better at noon, will become more serious at midnight, but will calm down at dawn.

"The evil-energy of heart should be softened by medicine of salty taste, when invigoration is needed, medicine of salty taste should be used to replenish the heart, when purgation is needed, medicine of sweet taste should be used to purge the heart-energy.

病在脾，愈在秋，秋不愈，甚于春，春不死，持于夏，起于长夏，禁温食〔张琦说："疑当作'冷食'"〕饱食湿地濡衣。脾病者，愈在庚辛，庚辛不愈，加于甲乙，甲乙不死，持于丙丁，起于戊已。脾病者，日昳慧，日出〔《病源》、《脾病候》"日出"作"平旦"林校引《甲乙》亦作"平旦"〕甚，下晡静。脾欲缓，急食甘以缓之，用苦写之，甘补之。

"When the disease is in the spleen, it could be recovered in autumn, it will be aggravated in spring, if the patient does not die in spring, the disease will become protracting in summer, but will turn to the better when earth-energy is prosperous in long summer, but the patient must take good care of not taking cold food, nor to eat his fill and avoid living in wet places or wearing wet clothes.

"The patient with spleen disease will turn to the better on Geng and Xin days, if the disease is not recovered then, it will become aggravated on Jia and Yi danys, if the patient does not die in Jai or Yi days, it will become protracting on Bing and Ding days, but will turn to the better until Wu and Ji days.

"The patient with spleen disease will feel better in the two-hour of Wei (1:00-3:00 PM), the disease will become more serious at dawn, and become calm at dusk.

The evil-energy of spleen should be moderated with sweet medicine, when purgation is needed, medicine of bitter taste should be used to purge the spleen, when invigoration is needed, medicine of sweet taste should be used to replenish the spleen.

病在肺，愈在冬，冬不愈，甚于夏，夏不死，持于长夏，起于秋，禁寒饮食寒衣。肺病者，愈在壬癸，壬癸不愈，加于丙丁，丙丁不死，持于戊已，起于庚辛。肺病者。下晡慧，日中甚，夜半〔《素问识》云："按据前后文例当是'曰昳静'"〕静。肺欲收，急食酸以收之，

用酸补之，辛写之。

“When the disease is in the lung, it could be recovered in winter, if it is not recovered in winter, it will become aggravated in summer next year, if the patient does not die in summer, the disease will become protracting in long summer, but will turn to the better in autumn when metal energy is prosperous in autumn, but the patient must take good care of not taking cold food or drink, nor to wear too little for the weather.

“The patient with lung disease could be recovered on Ren and Gui days, if it is not recovered then, it will become aggravated on Bing and Ding days, if it is not aggravated then, it will become protracting on Wu and Ji days, but will turn to the better on Geng and Xin days.

“The patient with lung disease will feel better at dusk, become more serious at noon, and become calm in the two-hour of Wei (1：00-3：00 PM).

“The evil-energy of lung should be restrained with the medicine of sour taste. When invigoration is needed, medicine of sour taste should be used to replenish the lung; when purgation is needed, medicine of acrid taste should be used to purge the sthenic lung-energy.

病在肾，愈在春，春不愈，甚于长夏，长夏不死，持于秋，起于冬，禁犯焠㶼热食温〔“犯”字衍，伟以“禁当风”，又“温”亦衍文，应据《病沅》《肾候病》删〕炙衣。肾病者，愈在甲乙，甲乙不愈，甚于戊已，戊已不死，持于庚辛，起于壬癸。肾病者，夜半慧，四季〔《病沅》“四季”上有“日乘”二字〕甚，下晡静。肾欲坚，急食苦以坚之，用苦补之，咸写之。

“When the disease is in the kidney, it could be recovered in spring, if it is not recovered in spring, it will become aggravated in long summer, if the patient does not die in long summer, the disease will become protracting in autumn but will turn to the better when the water energy is prosperous in winter, but the patient must take good care of not taking fried and scorched food or food and drink which is too hot, nor to wear the clothes being warmed nearby fire so as not to arouse the dryness-heat syndrome.

“The patient with kidney disease could be recovered on Jia and Yi days, if it is not recovered then, it will turn to the worse on Wu and Ji days, if the patient does not die then, it will become protracting on Geng and Xin days, but will turn to the better until Ren and Gui days.

“The patient with kidney disease will feel better at midnight, will become aggravated in the two-hour of Chen (7：00-9：00 AM), Xu (7：00-9：00 PM), Chou (1：00-3：00 AM) and Wei (1：00-3：00 PM), and become calm at dusk.

“In the kidney disease, the kidney energy should be reinforced with the medicine of bitter taste, when invigoration is needed, medicine of bitter taste should be used to replenish the kidney, when purgation is needed, medicine of salty taste should be used to purge the kidney energy.

夫邪气之客于身也，以胜相加，至其所生而愈，至其所不胜而甚，至于所生而持，自得其位而起，必先定五藏之脉，乃可言间甚之时，死生之期也。

When the evil-energy invades the body, the visceral disease is caused by the day-associated element energy which is overcoming (such as liver wood disease is caused by metal lung energy), it will be recovered on the day of the associated element it produces (liver disease recovers in summer or at the days of Bing and Ding), will be aggravated in the day of the associated element restricts oneself (liver disease becomes aggravated on the days of Geng and Xin, as metal retricts wood), will become stalemated on the day of the associated element that produces itself (liver disease will be stalemated in winter or at the days of Ren and Gui, as water produces wood), will turn to the better when reaching the time of the element that associates to itself (liver disease will turn to the better in spring and liver wood energy is prosporous in spring). One must ascertain the normal pulse condition of the five viscera (ie., liver pulse is wiry, heart pulse is hooked, spleen pulse is slow, lung pulse is floating and kidney pulse is stony) first, then can he infer whether the disease is slight or serious, and the date of the death or survival of the patient.

肝病者，两胁下痛引少腹，令人善怒，虚则目䀮䀮无所见，耳无所闻，善恐，如人将捕之，取其经，厥阴与少阳，气逆，则头痛耳聋不聪〔《云笈七签》引无“不聪”二字〕颊肿。取血者。

“In the liver disease, when the liver is of sthenic, there will be pain over the hypochondrium which affects the lower abdomen, and the patient will get angry often; if the liver is of asthenia, the two eyes of the patient will be dim with obscured views, his two ears can not hear things distinctly, being frightened often like some one is going to arrest him.

“The disease should be treated with pricking the shupoints of the Jueyin and Shaoyang Channels. If the liver-energy is going up adversely, the patient will have the syndromes of pain in eyes, deaf of ears and swelling of cheeks, it should also prick the acupoints of Jueyin and Shaoyang Channels until bleeding.

心病者，胸中痛，胁支〔《甲乙》“支”作“榰”，《尔雅・释言》：“榰”柱也，此言胁胀，如柱撑着也〕满，胁下痛，膺背肩甲〔朝本“甲”作“胛”〕间痛，两臂内痛；虚则胸腹大，胁下与腰〔《脉经》“腰”下有“背”字〕相引而痛，取其经，少阴太阳，舌下血者。其变病刺郄中血者〔《圣济总录》卷一百九十一引“血者”作“出血”〕。

In the heart disease, when the heart is of sthenia, pain in the chest, distention of the hypochondrium, pain under the armpit, pain between the breast, back and upper arms will occur; if the heart is of asthenia, the swelling of chest and abdomen which causes the pain of the hypochondrium, loin and back.

“The disease should be treated with pricking the acupoints of the Shaoyin and Taiyang Channels and also beneath the tongue until bleeding. If the condition of the disease is different from that of the beginning, it should prick Weizhong (Popliteal Centre) until bleeding.

脾病者，身重善肌〔明抄本，朝本“肌”作“饥”，《脾胃论》亦引作“善饥”〕肉痿，足不收行〔林校引《千金》作“足痿不行”〕善瘛，脚下痛；虚则腹满〔《甲乙》“满”作“胀”〕肠鸣，飧泄食不化，取其经，太阴阳明少阴血者〔（沈祖绵说：宜作“取其经太阴阳明之外，少阴血者”）〕。

"In the spleen disease, when the spleen is of sthenia, the patient will feel heavy of the body, apt to get hungry, flaccidity of the legs and unable to lift up when walking and pain of the feet; if the spleen is of asthenia, abdominal flatulence and borborygmus with undigested cereals in the stool will occur.

"The disease should be treated by pricking the lateral sides of the Taiyang and Yangming Channels first, and then, prick the acupoints of the Shaoying Channel until bleeding.

肺病者，喘咳逆气，肩背痛，汗出，尻阴股膝髀〔《云笈七签》引无"髀"字，日本田中清左卫门刻本《素问》旁注谓无"阴"字〕腨胻足皆痛；虚则少气不能报〔《太平圣惠方》"报"作"太"〕息，耳聋〔《太平圣惠方》引作"胸满"〕嗌乾，取其经，太阴足太阳之外厥阴内〔《脉经》、《甲乙》"厥阴内"并有"少阴"二字〕血者。

"In the lung disease, when the lung is of sthenia, cough, respiration, adverseness of vital energy, pain in the back and shoulders, sweating and pain in the buttocks, thigh, calf, tibia and foot will occur; if the lung is of asthenia, the patient will be short of breath, unable to sigh, with fullness of the chest and dryness of the throat.

"When treating the disease, it should prick the lateral sides of the Taiyin and Foot Taiyang Channels, and Shaoyin Channel of the inner lateral side of the Jueyin Channel until bleeding.

肾病者，腹大胫肿〔《脉经》"肿"下有"痛"字〕，喘咳身重，寝汗出，憎风；虚则胸中痛〔《史载之方》引"痛"作"满"〕，大腹〔《太平圣惠方》卷七《肾藏论》引无"大腹"二字〕小腹痛，清厥意不乐，取其经，少阴太阳血者。

"In the kidney disease, when the kidney is of sthenia, the syndrome of swelling and pain of the abdomen and the tibia, cough, rapid respiration, heaviness of the body, night sweat and has an aversion to wind will occur; if the kidney is of asthenia, the patient will feel fullness of the chest, pain of the lower abdomen, and feeling unhappy.

"When treating the disease, one should prick the acupoints of the Shaoyin and Taiyang Channels until bleeding.

肝色青，宜食甘，粳米〔《太素》"米"后有"饭"字〕牛肉枣葵皆甘。心色赤，宜食酸，小豆〔《太素》无此二字〕犬肉李韭皆酸。肺色白，宜食苦，麦羊肉杏薤皆苦。脾色黄，宜食咸，大豆豕肉栗藿皆咸。肾色黑，宜食辛，黄黍鸡肉桃葱皆辛。辛散，酸收，甘缓，苦坚，咸软〔《太素》作"耎"〕。

"The liver associates with the colour of green, its characteristic is urgent when ill, so it should be moderatad with food of sweet taste. Paddy rice, beef, jujube and sunflower are all sweet.

"The heart associates with the colour of red, its characteristic is dispersing when ill, so it should be gathered by taking the food of sour taste. Flax, dog's meat, plum, Chinese chives are all sour.

"The lung associates with the colour of white, its characteristic is adversing of energy when ill, so it should be purged by taking the food of bitter taste. Wheat, mutton, apricot and leek are all bitter.

"The spleen associates with the colour of yellow, its characteristic is wet when ill, so it should be dried by taking the foods of salty taste. Soya-bean, pork, millet and betony are all salty.

"The kidney associates with the colour of black, its characteristic is dry when ill, so it should be moistened by taking the foods of acrid taste. Glutinous millet, chicken, peach and scallion are all acrid.

"The food with acrid taste has the function of dispersing, the food with sour taste has the function of collecting, the food with sweet taste has the function of moderating, the food with bitter taste has the function of drying and the food with salty taste has the function of softening the hardness.

毒药攻邪，五谷为养，五果为助，五畜〔《千金》作“肉”〕为益，五菜为充。气味合而服之，以补精益气。此五〔《太素》“五”下有“味”字〕者，有辛酸甘苦咸，各有所利，或散，或收，或缓，或急〔按“或急”衍〕，或坚，或软，四时五藏，病随〔《太素》“病”下无“随”字〕五味所宜也。

"Poisonous drugs are to expel evils. The five kinds of cereals are to nourish the body, the five kinds of fruits are for supplementing, the five kinds of meats are for invigorating, and the five kinds of vegetables are for recuperating.

"When one takes the tastes of the cereal, fruit, meat and vegetable in combination, it can invigorate the essence and nourish the vital energy.

"The five tastes of acrid, sour, sweet, bitter and salty in various foods have their specific functions of dispersing, collecting, moderating, reinforcing and softening respectively. When treating, it should use the five tastes properly according to the specific conditions of the four seasons and the five viscera."

宣明五气篇第二十三

Chapter 23
Xuan Ming Wu Qi
Expounding on the Energies of Five Viscera

五味所入：酸入肝，辛入肺，苦入心，咸入肾，甘入脾，是谓五入。

When the foods of the five tastes enter into the stomach, they go into various viscera respectively according to their own preferances: sourness enters into the liver, acridness enters into the lung, bitterness enters into the heart, salty taste enters into the kidney and sweetness enters into the spleen. These are the so called the five enterings.

五气〔《太素》卷六《藏府气液》作“五藏气”〕所病：心为〔《太素》“为”作“主”〕噫，肺为咳，肝为语，脾为吞，肾为欠〔《太素》“欠”下无“为嚏”二字〕为嚏，胃为气逆，为哕为恐〔《太素》无“为恐”二字〕，大肠小肠为泄，下焦溢为水，膀胱不利为癃〔《太素》无此四字〕，不约为遗溺，胆为怒，是谓五病。

The syndromes of the five solid-organ energies are: when the heart-energy is depressed, one will eruct, when the lung-energy is not clear, one will cough, when the liver-energy is not dredged, one will have polylogia, when the spleen-energy fails to transport and convert, one's throat will be swallowing, when the kidney-energy is insufficient, one will yawn. The syndromes of the energies of the six hollow organs are: when the stomach-energy is not descending, it will go up adversely and one will hiccup; when the large or small intestine is ill, one will have diarrhea; when the body fluid of the lower warmer flooded into the skin, one will have edema, when the energy of the bladder is not being converted, one will have dysuria, when it is out of control, one will have enuresis, when the energy of gallbladder is ill, one will apt to get angery. These are the disease of the five solid organs and the six hollow organs.

五精所并〔《太素》“五精所并”作“五并”〕：精气并于心则喜，并于肺则悲，并于肝则忧〔张琦说：“忧”当作“怒”〕，并于脾则畏〔疑当作思〕，并于肾则恐，是谓五并，虚而相并者也。

When the refined energies of the five solid organs being merged into one organ, the organ's energy will become sthenic and disease will occur: when the refined energy is merged into the heart, the heart-energy will have a surplus and one will desire for laughing; when it is merged into the lung, the lung-energy will have a surplus and one will become sorrowful; when it is merged into the liver, the liver-energy will become partial overabundant to restrict the spleen and one will be angry; when it is merged into the spleen, the spleen-energy will become partial overabundant and restrict the kidney and one will have anxiety; when it is

merged into the kidney, the kidney-energy will have a surplus and one will be terrified. These are the so called five mergings.

五藏所恶〔《太素》作“五恶”〕：心恶热，肺恶寒，肝恶风，脾恶湿，肾恶燥，是谓五恶〔《太素》作“此五藏气所恶”〕。

The five solid organs have their detestations respectively: the heart is apt to become ill when it is hot so as to hurt the Yin blood, so the heart detests the hotness; the lung is apt to become ill when it is cold so as to obstruct the energy, so, the lung detests the cold; the liver is apt to become ill when invaded by wind to cause the contracture of the tendon, so liver detests the wind; the spleen is apt to become ill when it is wet to cause the swelling of the muscle, so the spleen detests wetness; the kidney is apt to become ill when it is dry to cause the exhaustion of the Yin essence, so the kidney detests dryness, These are the so called detestations of the five solid organs.

五藏化液〔《太素》作“五液”〕：心为汗〔《太素》“为”作“主”下同〕，肺为涕，肝为泪，脾为涎，肾为唾，是谓五液〔《太素》作“此五液所生”〕。

The secretions from the five solid organs are: the heart takes charge of the blood, and sweat is transformed from the blood, so sweat is the secretion of heart; the nose is the orifice of the lung, and nasal discharge is from the nose, so nasal discharge is the secretion of lung; the eyes are the orifices of the liver, and tears are from the eyes, so tears are the secretion of liver; the mouth is the orifice of spleen and serous saliva is from the mouth, so serous saliva is the secretion of spleen. The pulse of Foot Shaoyin is under the tongue, the mucous saliva is from beneath the tongue, so mucous saliva is the secretion of kidney. These are the five kinds of secretions converted and produced from the five solid organs.

五味所禁：辛走气，气病无多食辛〔《太素》作“病在气无食辛”，下血、骨、肉、筋句法同〕；咸〔《太素》“咸”作“苦”〕走血，血病无多食咸；苦〔《太素》“苦”作“咸”〕走骨，骨病无多食苦；甘走肉，肉病无多食甘；酸走筋，筋病无多食酸。是谓五禁，无令多食〔《医说》引无“无令多食”四字〕。

The five kinds of tastes are contraindicated to certain diseases of the five solid organs respectively: the acrid taste affects the energy, so in diseases of energy, one must not take plenty of acrid food; the bitter taste affects the blood, so in diseases of blood, one must not take plenty of bitter food; the salty taste affects the bone, so in diseases of bone, one must not take planty of salty food; the sweet taste affects the muscle, so in the diseases of muscle, one must not take plenty of sweet food; the sour taste affects the tendon, so in diseases of tenden, one must not take plenty of sour food. These are the five kinds of tastes which should be contraindicated.

五病所发：阴病发于骨，阳病发于血，阴病发于肉〔《太素》、《邪传》作“以味病发于气”，按“以味”应据杨注作“五味”〕，阳病发于冬，阴病发于夏，是谓五发。

The five diseases occur in different locations or seasons are: the kidney is a solid organ of Yin and it takes charge of the bone, the disease of kidney stems from the bone marrow; the heart is a solid organ of Yang and it takes charge of the blood, the disease of heart stems

from the blood; the spleen is a solid organ of Yin, it takes charge of the muscle, the disease of spleen stems from the muscle; the liver is a solid organ of Yang, it associates with spring, but its disease stems from winter; the lung is a solid organ of Yin, it associates with autumn, but its disease stems from summer. These are the cases of the diseases of the five solid organs stem from. They are called the five occurrences.

五邪所乱〔《太素》"所乱"作"入"〕：邪入于阳则〔《太素》"则"下有"为"字〕狂，邪入于阴则〔《太素》"则"下有"为血"二字〕痹，搏阳则为巅疾〔《太素》作"邪入于阳搏则为巅疾"〕，搏阴则为瘖，阳入之阴则〔《太素》"则"作"病"〕静，阴出之阳则怒〔《太素》作"病善怒"〕，是谓五乱。

When the five solid organs being invaded by the evil-energy, different affections will occur: when the evils enter into Yang, heat will disturb one's consciousness and mania will occur; when the evils enter into Yin, the circulation of blood will be disturbed, arthralgia due to blood disorder will occur; when the evils enter into Yang to cause adverseness of the vital energy, dian disease will occur; when the evils enter into Yin to cause the damage of Yin-fluid, dumbness of the patient will occur; when the evils turn from Yang to Yin and Yin becomes overabundant, the patient will become calm; when the evils turn from Yin to Yang and Yang becomes overabundant, the patient will get angry often. These are the diseases caused by the five evils.

五邪所见，春得秋脉，夏得冬脉，长夏得春脉，秋得夏脉，冬得长夏脉，名曰阴出之阳〔林校云："按'阴出之阳病善怒'已是前条，此再言之文义不伦，必古文错简"〕，病善怒不治，是谓五邪。皆同命，死不治。

The pulse conditions of the five evils are: when floating pulse of autumn is seen in spring, when stony pulse of winter is seen in summer, when wiry pulse of spring is seen in long summer, when hooked pulse of summer is seen in autumn, and when soft and floating pulse of long summer is seen in winter. These are the conditions of evil pulse which should not occur. If any of them is seen in the four seasons, the disease will not be cured.

五藏所藏：心藏神，肺藏魄、肝藏魂，脾藏意〔《五行大义》引"意"作"志"〕，肾藏志〔《五行大义》"志"作"精"〕，是谓五藏所藏。

There are different storings in the five solid organs: the heart stores mind, the lung stores inferior spirit, the liver stores spirit, the spleen stores will and the kidney stores essence. These are the storings of the five solid organs.

五藏所主：心主脉，肺主皮，肝主筋，脾主肉，肾主骨，是谓五主。

The different functions of the five solid organs are: the heart promotes the circulation of the blood, so the heart takes charge of the vessel; the lung spreads the energy to the surface of the skin, so the lung takes charge of the skin; the liver stores the blood and disperses its essence to nourish the tendon, so liver takes charge of the tendon; the spleen transports and converts the water and cereals to nourish the muscle, so the spleen takes charge of the muscle; the kidney stores the essence and generates the marrow to nourish the bone, so kidney takes charge of the bone. These are the functions of the five solid organs.

五劳所伤：久视伤血，久卧伤气，久坐伤肉，久立伤骨，久行伤筋，是谓五劳所伤。

The five kinds of impairment by overstraining are: protracted watching will overstrain the heart and impair the blood; protracted lying will overstrain the lung and impair the energy; protracted sitting will overstrain the spleen and impair the muscle; protracted standing will overstrain the kidney and impair the bone; protracted walking will overstrain the liver and impair the tendon. These are the five kinds of impairments by overstraining.

五脉应象：肝脉弦，心脉钩，脾脉代，肺脉毛，肾脉石，是谓五藏之脉。

The pulse condition of the five solid organs corresponding to the four seasons are: the liver pulse corresponds to spring and it appears to be wiry; the heart pulse corresponds to summer and it appears to be hooked; the spleen pulse corresponds to long summer and it appears to be intermittent; the lung pulse corresponds to autumn and it appears to be floating; the kidney pulse corresponds to winter and it appears to be stony. These are the pulse condition of the five solid organs.

血气形志篇第二十四

Chapter 24
Xue Qi Xin Zhi
On Blood，Energy，Body and Spirit

夫人之常数，太阳常多血少气，少阳常〔《太素》卷十九《知形志所宜》“少阳”下无“常”字〕少血多气，阳明常多气多血，少阴常少血多气，厥阴常多血少气，太阴常多气少血，此天〔“天”字疑误，据上文应作“人”〕之常数。

The distributed portion of energy and blood in human body is constant. Blood is plenty and energy is little in Taiyang Channel; blood is little and energy is plenty in Shaoyang Channel; both blood and energy are plenty in Yangming Channel; blood is little and energy is plenty in Shaoyin Channel; blood is plenty and energy is little in Jueyin Channel; energy is plenty and blood is little in Taiyin Channel. These are the constant conditions of blood and energy in human body.

足太阳与少阴为表里，少阳与厥阴为表里，阳明与太阴为表里，是为足〔滑抄本“足”下有“之”字〕阴阳也。手太阳与少阴为表里，少阳与心主为表里，阳明与太阴为表里，是为手之阴阳也。今知手足阴阳所苦〔《太素》无此八字〕，凡治病必先去其血，乃去其所苦，伺之所欲，然后写有余，补不足。

The Foot Taiyang Bladder Channel and Foot Shaoyin Kidney Channel are superficies and interior, Foot Shaoyang Gallbladder Channel and Foot Jueyin Liver Channel are superficies and interior, Foot Yangming Stomach Channel and Foot Taiyin Spleen Channel are superficies and interior, these are the relations between the three Yin channels of foot and the three Yang channels of foot. The Hand Taiyang Small Intestine Channel and the Hand Shaoyin Heart Channel are superficies and interior, the Hand Shaoyang Triple Warmer Channel and the Hand Jueyin Pericardium Channel are superficies and interior, the Hand Yangming Large Intestine Channel and the Hand Taiyin Lung Channel are superficies and interior; these are the relations between the three Yin channels of hand and the three Yang channels of hand.

When treating, if the blood is prevailing, it must be pricked to remove the blood to alleviate the pain of the patient first, than examine the will of the patient, find out the asthenic and sthenic condition of the disease and purge the surplus or invigorate the deficiency.

欲知背俞，先度其两乳间，中折之，更以他草度去〔《太素》卷十一《气穴》、《医心方》“去”下并有“其”字〕半已，即以两隅相拄〔朝本“拄”作“柱”〕也。乃举〔《医心方》“举”下有“臂”字〕以度其背，令其一隅居上，齐脊大椎，两隅在下，当其下隅者，肺之俞也；复下一度，心之俞也；复下一度，左〔《太素》《医心方》并作“右”〕角肝之俞也，

右〔《太素》《医心方》并作“左”〕角脾之俞也；复下一度，肾之俞也；是谓五藏之俞，灸刺之度也。

When one wants to know the locations of the shu-points of the five viscera, he can measure the distance between the two nipples of the breast of the patient with a piece of straw and break it to make its length to fit the distance; fold the straw twice and make its four strands to be one forth of the distance between the nipples, than take away one of the four strands and make a triangle with the three strands. Ask the patient to stretch up his arms and put the top angle of the triangle on the acupoint of Dazhui (Big Vertebra) of the patient, and the locations of the two lower angles are the Lung-shu points.

Move the top angle of the triangle to the middle point of the connecting line of the two lung-shu points, the location of the two lower angles of the triangle are heart-shu points, if move the triangle downward again as above, the right lower angle will be the liver-shu point, and the left lower angle will be the spleen-shu point, if move the triangle again as above, the lower left and right angles will be the kidney-shu points. These are the locations of the shu-points of the five viscera, and they are the standing orders of acupuncture and moxibustion.

形乐志苦，病生于脉，治之以灸刺；形乐志乐，病生于肉，治之以针石；形苦志乐，病生于筋，治之以熨引；形苦志苦，病生于咽嗌〔林校引《甲乙经》作“困竭”〕，治之以百〔《甲乙》“百”作“甘”〕药；形数惊恐，经络〔《太素》《医心方》“经络”并作“筋脉”〕不通，病生于不仁，治之以按摩醪药，是谓五形志也。

When the patient is not fatigue in body but is worrying all the time, his disease is due to the obstruction of the channel. It should be treated with acupuncture and moxibustion.

When the body and the spirit of the patient are all at ease, his disease is due to the swelling of muscle. It should be treated by pricking the acupoints with stone needles.

When the patient appears to be weary and fatigue in body but has a joyous mood, his disease is due to the damage of tendons. It should be treated with topical application of heated drugs.

When the patient is weary and fatigue both in body and in spirit, his disease is due to worn out and exhaustion of energy. It should be treated with medicine of sweet taste.

When the patient is being frightened again and again to cause obstruction of the tendons, his disease is due to numbness. It should be treated with massage and tincture.

These are the five kinds of disease of the body and spirit.

刺阳明〔《太素》“刺”上有“故曰”二字〕出血气，刺太阳出血恶气，刺少阳出气恶血，刺太阴出气恶血，刺少阴出气恶血〔《太素》“出气恶血”作“出血气”〕，刺厥阴出血恶气也。

Therefore, when pricking the Yangming Channel, it is permissible to let out the blood and energy; when pricking the Taiyang Channel, only letting out of blood is allowed, while the energy must not be hurt; when pricking the Shaoyang Channel, only the letting out of energy is allowed, while the blood must not be hurt; when pricking the Taiyin Channel, both letting out of blood and the energy are permissible; when pricking the Shaoyin Chan-

nel, only letting out of energy is allowed while the blood must not be hurt; when pricking the Jueyin Channel, only letting out of blood is allowed, while the energy must not be hurt.

宝命全形论篇第二十五

Chapter 25

Bao Ming Quan Xing Lun

(Following the principle of Nature in Treating)

黄帝问曰：天覆地载，万物悉备，莫贵于人，人以天地之气生，四时之法成，君王众庶，尽欲全形，形之疾病〔《太素》卷十九《知针石》作“所疾”〕，莫知其情，留淫日深，著于骨髓，心私虑〔《太素》“虑”作“患”〕之，余欲针除其疾病，为之奈何？

Yellow Emperor asked: Among all things between the heaven and earth, nothing is more precious than man. Man depends on the energies of heaven and earth to exist and grow along with the Law of the four seasons. All people, including Kings and common people, wish to have a healthy body, but occasionally, they feel a bit of unwell and neglect it, and the disease gradually accumulates and finally goes into hiding in the bone marrow which can hardly be removed. This is what I am worrying about, and I wish to alleviate their pains with acupuncture, but how can I do it?".

岐伯对曰：夫盐之味〔袁刻《太素》无“味”字〕咸者，其气令器津泄；弦绝者，其音嘶败〔“败”字衍〕；木敷〔《太素》“敷”作“陈”〕者，其叶发〔“发”是“落”之坏字〕；病深者，其声哕。人有此三〔“三”字疑衍〕者，是谓坏府，毒药无治，短针无取，此皆绝皮伤肉，血气争黑〔《太素》“黑”作“异”〕。

Qibo answered: "In diagnosis, one should pay attention to examine the syndromes that appear : such as, when salt is stored in an utensil, the water can ooze out from it; when the string of an instrument is about to break, it produces a hissing sound; when a tree is ruined and wornout, its leaves become falling; when the disease of a man is in a critical stage, his voice will be like that of vomitting ; under such conditin, it shows that his viscera have been damaged seriously, and both applying medicine and acupuncture will be futile; since the skin, muscle, blood and energy of the patient are disconnecting, his disease can hardly be cured."

帝曰：余念其痛，心为之乱惑，反甚其病，不可更代，百姓闻之，以为残贼，为之奈何。

Yellow said: "I am quite concerned about the diseases of the people, but I have some misgivings: I wish to treat the patient, but if I failed, the disease will turn to the worse, and I could not suffer for them, people may think that I am a cruel man. What shall I do?"

岐伯曰：夫人生于地，悬命于天，天地合气，命之曰人。人能应四时者，天地为之父母。知万物者，谓之天子。天有阴阳，人有十二节；天有寒暑，人有虚实。能经天地阴阳之化者，不失四时；知十二节之理者，圣智不能欺也。能存八动〔“动”疑当作“风”〕之变，五胜更立，能达虚实之数者，独出独入，呿吟至微，秋毫在目。

Qibo said: "Although man lives on earth, but his life can by no means divorce from heaven, when the energies of heaven and earth are combining, it produces man. If a man can adapt to the change of the four seasons, then, all things in nature will become the source of his life. If one can understand every thing, he is fit to be an emperor. Man corresponds with nature: in heaven, there are Yin and Yang, in man, there are twelve large joints of the limbs; in heaven, there are coldness and hotness, in man, there are asthenia and sthenia; so when one can follow the Yin and Yang variations of heaven and earth, he will never violate the law of the four seasons. When one understands the principles of the twelve joints, even a sage can not surpass him. When one is able to examin the Eight Winds, the decline and prosperity of the five elements, and can understand further the law of the asthenic and sthenic change, he will be able to know full well the conditions of the disease and the pain of the patient, even as tiny as a piece of fine hair will not escape his notice."

帝曰：人生有形，不离阴阳，天地合气，别为九野，分为四时，月有小大，日有短长，万物并至，不可胜量，虚实呿吟，敢问其方。

Yellow Emperor said: "Man exists in the form of physical body but he can not divorce from Yin and Yang; all things come to the existing in the world after the combination of energies of heaven and earth. In geography, the earth is divided into nine prefectures; in weather, it is divided into four seasons ; in months, there are the odds months of 30 days and the lunar months of 29 days: in the day time of a day, some of the length are longer and some are shorter; all things come into the world simultaneously and they can hardly be measured. What I intend is to alleviate the pain of the patients only, can you tell me what method of acupuncture should be applied?"

岐伯曰：木得金而伐，火得水而灭，土得木而达〔《素问绍识》谓"达"当作"夺"声误〕，金得火而缺，水得土而绝，万物尽然，不可胜竭。故针有悬布〔明抄本"布"下有"于"字〕天下者五，黔首共余食，莫知之也。一曰治神，二曰知养身〔杨所据本无"知"字，又"身"应作"形"〕，三曰知毒为真，四曰制砭石小大，五曰知府藏血气之诊。五法俱立，各有所先。今末世之刺〔《太平圣惠方》卷九十九《金十经序》引"刺"作"制"〕也，虚者实之，满者泄之，此皆众工所共知也。若夫法天则地，随应而〔四库本"而"作"即"〕动，和之者若响，随之者若影，道无鬼神，独来独往。

Qibo said: "The method of acupuncture can be analysized by the principle of the changes of the five elements: when wood encounters metal, wood will be cut; when fire encounters water, fire will be extinquished; when earth encounters wood, earth will be restrained; when metal encounters fire, metal will be melted; when water encounters earth, water will be halted. The changes are the same in every thing and the examples are too numerous to be enumerated. There are five acupuncture methods which have been published to all, but people care for their meal only and try not to understand them thoroughly. The five methods are: first, concentrate the attention; second, take care of the body; third, knowing the actual property of the medicine; fourth, preparing different sizes of stone needles to meet the need of treating various diseases; fifth, knowing the diagnostic method for the viscera, blood

and energy. Each of the methods has its merits, and one can decide which one should be used first according to the specific situation. At present, the acupuncture therapy is to invigorate when the energy is asthenic, and purge when the energy is overabundant, and it is known to all physicians. If one can apply the acupuncture therapy according to the principle of the variations of Yin and Yang of heaven and earth, the curative effects will be obtained as a matter of course. This is nothing mysterious, when one is serious in accumulating acupuncture knowledges with protracted experience, something uniqueness in his achievement will certainly occur."

帝曰：愿闻其道。

岐伯曰：凡刺之真，必先治神，五藏已定，九候已备〔《甲乙》"备"作"明"〕，后乃存针，众脉不见，众凶弗闻，外内相得，无以形先，可玩往来，乃施于人。人有虚实〔《甲乙》作"虚实之要"〕，五虚勿近，五实勿远，至其当发，间不容瞚。手动若务，针耀而匀，静意视义〔"义"字误，应作"息"〕，观适之变，是谓冥冥，莫知其形，见其乌乌，见其稷稷，从〔于鬯说："从"字盖"徒"字之误〕见其飞，不知其谁〔《太素》"知"作"见"，"谁"作"杂"〕，伏如横弩，起如发机。

Yellow Enperor said: "I would like to know the principles about acupuncture." Qibo said: "The correct method of acupuncture is to concentrate the mind first. The pricking can be applied only after the asthenia and sthenia of the five viscera has been ascertained and the nine sub-parts of the pulse has been made clear. When pricking, one must concentrate his attention, seeing no one even there is someone watching, and hearing nothing even there are noisy disturbances. Examine the pulse condition of the patient, be sure the pulse of the exhausted visceral-energy is existing and must not examine the outer appearance of the patient only. Before pricking, one must understand the syndrome thoroughly to the extent of being mature, and master the condition of the coming and going of the channel-energy. As the pricking is easy in purging and difficult in invigorating, to the patients of the five asthenic diseases (fine pulse, cold skin, short of breath, diarrhea, fail to take food), one must not prick rashly; to the patients of the five sthenic diseases (full pulse, hot skin, distention of abdomen, dysuria and restless), one must not be reluctant to prick. In prickng, when the channel energy is arrived, one must seize the opportunity to prick without delay, not even in the time of a twinkling of an eye. When twisting the needle, one must not have other things in mind to assure the pricking is clean and smooth; after the needle is applied, one must pay attention to the breathing of the patient and examine the expected energy change. The coming and going of the energy is invisible and is quite difficult to trace. It is like birds in different sexes flying in crowds, one can only see the harmonious flying, but can not see the diversity of sexes.

Before the channel-energy arrives, the physician should wait patiently like waiting for a prey, lying with a drawing bow; when the channel-energy arrives, he should prick as quick as pulling the trigger."

帝曰：何如而虚！何如而实？岐伯曰：刺虚者须其实，刺实者须其虚，经气已至，慎守

勿失，深浅在志，远近若一，如临深渊，手如握虎，神无营于众物。

Yellow Emperor said: "How to prick an asthenic disease, and how to prick a sthenic disease?" Qibo said: "When pricking the disease of asthenia, invigorating therapy should be applied, when pricking the disease of sthenia, purge therapy should be applied. When the channel-energy has arrived, one must be cautious not to miss the opportunity. No matter the pricking is deep or shallow, the acupoint is far from or near to the focus, the acupuncture feeling obtained should be of the same. When twisting the needle, one must be very careful as if he is standing upon the edge of an abyss, and be very concentrative as if holding a fierce tiger. In a word, one should concentate his mind, and not being disturbed by other things."

八正神明论篇第二十六

Chaoter 26

Ba Zheng Shen Ming Lun

(The Relation Between the Weather Change of Eight Main Solar Terms and the Purging and Invigorating by Acupuncture)

黄帝问曰：用针之服，必有法则焉，今何法何则？岐伯对曰：法天则（“天则”明抄本作“则天”）地，合以天光。

Yellow Emperor asked："The technique of acupuncture must have some specific rules. What are the rules then?" Qibo said："One can only study and realize then by following the pattern of heaven, earth, Yin and Yang and the celestial bodies of the sun, moon and stars."

帝曰：愿卒闻之。岐伯曰：凡刺之法，必候日月星辰四时八正之气，气定乃刺之。是故天温日明，则人血淖液而卫气浮，故血易写，气易行；天寒日阴，则人血凝泣〔《太素》“凝”作“涘”，《云笈七签》引“泣”作“冱”〕而卫气沉。月始生则血气始精，卫气始行；月郭满，则血气实〔《太素》“实”作“盛”〕，肌肉坚；月郭空，则肌肉减，经络虚，卫气去，形独居。是以因天时而调血气也。是以天〔《甲乙》“天”作“大”下“天温”同〕寒无刺，天温无疑〔《针灸大成》卷二《标幽赋》杨注引“疑”作“灸”〕。月生无写，月满无补，月郭空无治，是谓得时而调之。因天之序，盛虚之时，移光定位，正立而待之故曰：月生而写，是谓藏虚；月满而补，血气扬〔《移精变气论》王注引“扬”作“盈”〕溢，络有留血，命曰重实；月郭空而治，是谓乱经。阴阳相错，真邪不别，沈以留止，外虚内乱，淫邪乃起。

"Yellow Emperor said："I hope you can tell me in detail." Qibo said："Generally, one must examine the energies of the eight main solar terms (the spring equinox, the autumnal equinox, the summer solistice, the winter solistice, the beginning of spring, the beginning of summer, the beginning of autumn and the beginning of winter) and prick after the energy is stabilized.

"If the weather is fine, and the sun is shining bright, the blood of the body will be moist and the Wei-energy will be abundant; if the weather is cold and cloudy, the blood circulation will be dull and stagnated, and the energy will be sunken and hiding. When the moon is newly appeared, the blood and energy of man begin to generate in the wake of it, and the Wei-energy starts to operate with it; when the moon is full, the blood and energy of man will be prosperous and his muscle will be firm and substantial; when the moon is dark, the muscle of man will become emaciated, by this time, his channel and collaterals become asthenic, his Wei-energy is gone, and his body is left all alone. Therefore, when pricking, one must adjust the blood and energy along with the condition of heaven.

"Thus, do not prick when the weather is too cold; do not treat with moxibustion when

the weather is too warm; do not apply purging therapy when the moon is newly appeared; do not apply invigoration therapy when the moon is full; do not treat at all when the moon is dark: and this is the so called the capability of adjusting the energy and blood according to the condition of heaven. One should ascertain the location of the energy according to the moving sequence of the season and the abundant or decline status of blood and energy of a man, and wait attentively for the optimum opportunity for treating.

"If purge is applied when the moon is newly appeared, it is called the 'double asthenia'; when pricking is applied when the moon is dark, it will disturb the channel-energy, and it is called the 'channel confusion'. These maltreatments will cause the disorder of Yin and Yang, confusing of the healthy and the evil-energy, retention of the evils, as a result the syndrome of outer asthenia of the collateral and inner confusion of the channel will occur, and the evil-energy will take advantage to invade."

帝曰：星辰八正何候？

Yellow Emperor said: "What do the stars, eight main solar terms and the four seasons verify?

岐伯曰：星辰者，所以制日月之行也；八正者，所以候八风之虚邪以时至者也；四时者，所以分春秋冬夏之气所在，以时调之也，八正之虚邪，而避之勿犯也。以身之虚，而逢天之虚，两虚相感，其气至骨，入则伤五藏，工候救之，弗能伤也，故曰天忌不可不知也。

Qibo said: "When examining the bearings of the star, it can determine the regular pattern of the abiding route of the sun and moon; when examining the alternation of the regular energies of the eight main solar terms, it can determine the arrival time of the disease which is invaded by the eight winds; when examining the four seasons, it can determine the location of the energies of spring, summer, autumn and winter; when one measures the evil-energy of the eight main solar terms according to the time sequence and try to evade it, the invasion of evil-energy can be avoided. When one is asthenic and being invaded by asthenic evil-energy, the double asthenia will cause the evil-energy to invade the bone. If the physician understands the effects of the weather change and rescue in time, the patient may not be seriously hurt. Otherwise, the evil-energy will penatrate deep into the viscera. Thus, it is neccessary for one to understand the time abstentions associated with heaven."

帝曰：善。其法星辰者，余闻之矣，愿闻法往古者。

岐伯曰：法往古者，先知《针经》也。验于来今者，先知日之寒温、月之虚盛，以候气之浮沉，而调之于身，观其立有验也。观其冥冥者，言形气荣卫之不形于外，而工独之，以日之寒温，月之虚盛，四时气之浮沉，参伍相合而调之，工常先见之，然而不形于外，故曰观于冥冥焉。通于无穷者，可以传于后世也。是故工之所以异也。然而不形见于外，故俱不能见也。视之无形，尝之无味，故谓冥冥，若神仿佛。虚邪者，八正之虚邪气〔"气"字衍〕也。正邪者，身〔《太素》"形"下有"饥"字〕形若用力，汗出，腠理开〔《文选·风赋》善注引"汗出"下无"腠理开"三字〕，逢虚风，其中人也微，故莫知其情，莫见其形，上工救其萌芽，必先见〔《太素》"见"作"知"〕三部九候之气，尽调不败而救之，故曰上工〔《太素》无"上工"二字，"故曰"二字连下读〕。下工〔《太素》"下工"下无救其已成，

救其已败“八字”〕救其已成，救其已败，救其已成者，言不知三部九候之〔《太素》“之”下下有“气以”二字〕相失，因病而败之也。知其所在者，知诊三部九候之病脉处而治之，故曰守其门户焉。莫知其情而见邪形也。

Yellow Emperor said: "Good. Now I have heard the contents of one following the example of the stars, I want to know further how to follow the example of the ancient people." Qibo said: "When one wants to follow the example of the ancient people he must know first the 《Classic of Acupuncture》. If one wants to verify the ancient acupuncture technique at present time, he must know first the heat and coldness of the sun, and the wax and wane of the moon, from which to ascertain the floating and the sinking of the energy, and examine the bodily condition of the patient in integration, then he can see its effect. The so called 'observing in the darkness' is to say, although the changes of blood, energy, Wei-energy and Rong-energy of the patient are not appearing outside, yet the physician can still understand it. This is the result of the synthetic examination of the heat and coldness of the sun, the wax and wane of the moon, and the floating and sinking energies of the weathers of the four seasons. Since the physician can often predict the syndromes when the disease has not been manifested, so it is called 'observing in the darkness'. If a physician can know the disease thoroughly, his experiense may be handed down to the later generations, and this is why a physician is different from common people who can not discover the disease when it is not manifested. Seeing no image when watching, and feeling no taste when tasting, they are the conditions in the darkness, and the disease is like a fairy partly hidden and partly visible which can hardly be fathomed.

"The asthenic evil is the evil-energy of the eight solar terms in the four seasons. The sthenic is the result when one is hungry, becomes sweating after physical labour, and is invaded by asthenic-wind. As the initial sthenic-evil can only hurt the patient slightly, so a common physician does not understand its condition nor even become aware of it.

"A good physician can pay attention to the beginning of the disease and treat it when the three parts and the nine sub-parts of the pulse are still in harmony and have not yet corrupted, thus the disease can be cured more easily. A poor physician can not discover the disease at the beginning, he can only treat the disease when it has already taken shape. He can not discover the disharmony from the pulse-energy of the three parts and the nine sub-parts beforehand, he can only treat afterwards. If a physician can discover the location of the disease from the pulse of the three parts and the nine sub-parts and treat in time, it will guard against the invasion of the evil-energy, so it is called the 'guarding of entrance'. The physician will be bogged into a passive position when he only knows the superficial appearance of the disease instead of knowing its pathology."

帝曰：余闻补写，未得其意。

岐伯曰：写必用方，方者，以气方盛也，以月方满也，以日方温也，以身方定也，以息方吸而内针，乃复候其方吸而转针，乃复候其方呼而徐引针，故曰写必用方，其气而行〔明抄本，“而”并作“易”〕焉。补必用员，员者行也，刺必中其荣，复以吸排针也。故员与方，

非〔《太素》"非"作"排"〕针也。故养神者，必知形之肥瘦，荣卫血气之盛衰。血气者，人之神。不可不谨养。

Yellow Emperor said: " I am told there are purging and invigorating therapeis in acupuncture, but I do not understand their meanings." Qibo said: " In purging, one must master the time of 'just', 'just' means the time when the patient's energy is just flourishing, when the moon is just full, when the weather is just warm, and when the body is just stable to keep away from the disturbance of Yang-energy, the inserting of the needle at the time when the patient just inhales and pull out the needle slowly at the time when the patient just exhales. So in purge therapy, it is neccessary to master 'just' in operation, so that the evil-enegy can be drawn forth, the healthy-energy can be put through, and the disease may be cured.

"In invigorating therapy, 'dredging' is neccessary, dredging means to activate the enegy, and activating means to induct the energy to the location of the focus. When inserting the needle, it must reach the proper position; when withdrawing the needle, it must be during the inhalation of the patient, so as to avoid the discharging of the energy along with the needle. When applying the method of 'just' and 'dredging' in acupuncture, to shift the needle up and down is neccessary.

"Thus, the one who is good at acupuncture must examine first whether the patient is fat or thin, and the prosperous or decline condition of his Wei-energy, Rong-energy, blood and energy. Since the blood and energy are the places where the spirit and vital energy abide, they must be cultivated carefully."

帝曰：妙乎哉论也！合〔《太素》"合"上有"辞"字〕人形于阴阳四时，虚实之应，冥冥之期，其非夫子孰能通之。然夫子数言形与神，何谓形，何谓神，愿卒闻之。

Yellow Emperor saisd: "What a brilliant remark you have made. You have integrated the human body with Yin, Yang and the four seasons, and illustrated the responses of asthenia and sthenia and the condition of the disease which is invisible, if it were not you, who can make such a clear explanation? You have mentioned the physique and spirit many times, but what are physique and spirit? I hope you can tell me in details."

岐伯曰：请言形、形乎形、目冥冥，问其所病，索之于经，慧然〔俞樾说："慧然在前"本作"卒然在前"〕在前，按之不得，不知其情，故曰形。

Qibo siad: "I will tell you about physique first, the so called physique is the outer appearance of the patient. The physician can only see faintly the exterior of the patient which has been exposed, but can not see the reason which is concealed, so, he must ask the patient about the cause of the disease, and then combine it with the outer appearance of the disease and the channel condition obtained from the palpation so as to aquire the comprehensive understanding and make a diagnosis. The condition of the disease can by no means be sorted out if nothing is found in palaption. Since the outer appearance of the patient is visible, so, it is called Physique."

帝曰：何谓神？岐伯曰：请言神，神乎神，耳不闻，目〔服子温说："目"下疑脱"不"

字〕明，心开而志先〔《甲乙》“先”作“光”〕，慧然独悟，口弗能言，俱视独见，适若昏，昭然独明请言神，若风吹云，故曰神。三部九候为之原，九针之论，不必存也。

Yellow Emperor asked："What is spirit?"Qibo said："I wIll tell you about it. A physician of higher level can concentate his mind in treating, he can hear no disturbing noise, can see no irrelevant things, being open minded and is able to comprehend clearly the essence of the disease, which can hardly be expressed by words. When a thing is examined by many people, but only one of them can understand it clearly, then, the thing which was in obscurity just then has become as clear as day, like the clouds are driven away by the wind; this is the so called the spirit. The understanding of spirit is stemmed from the knowing of the three parts and the nine sub-parts of the pulse, and also from one's painstaking efforts. When one can attain this level in treating, he may not rigidly adhere to the theory of the nine kinds of needle in acupuncture therapies."

离合真邪论篇第二十七

Chapter 27
Li He Zhen Xie Lun
(Matters Needing Attention in Acupuncture)

黄帝问曰：余闻九针九篇，夫子乃因而九之，九九八十一篇，余尽通其意矣。经言气之盛衰，左右倾移，以上调下，以左调右，有余不足，补泻于荥输，余知之矣。此皆荣卫之〔《太素》“之”下有“气”字〕倾移，虚实之所生，非邪气从外入于经也。余愿闻邪气之在经也，其病人〔《济生拔萃。窦大师流注指要赋》引无“人”字〕何如？取之奈何？

Yellow Emperor asked: "I have heard about the nine chapters about the nine methods of acupuncture, and you have deduced them with nine times nine into eighty one chapters, and now I understand all their meanings. From the classics, I have known there is overabundant or deficient of energy, diverse pricking to the right side or to the left, contralateral insertion of pricking the upper part to cure the lower disease and pricking the left side to cure the right, invigorating the deficiency or purging the surplus through the five shu-points. I have known that they are due to the unusual deviations of the Rong and Wei-energies and the asthenia and sthenia, and they are not the result of the invasion of the evil-energy to the channels. Now I want to know what symptoms will appear when the evil-energy invades the channels from outside, and what is the method in treating them?"

岐伯对曰：夫圣人之起度数，必应于天地，故天有宿度，地有经水，人有经脉，天地温和，则经水安静；天寒地冻，则经水凝泣；天暑地热，则经水沸溢；卒风暴起，则经水波涌而陇起。夫邪之入于脉也，寒则血凝泣，暑则气〔《太素》“气”下有“血”字〕淖泽，虚邪因而入客，亦如经水之得风也，经之动脉〔王注所据本为“经脉之动”〕，其至也亦时陇起，其行于脉中循循然。其至寸口中手也，时大时小，大则邪至，小则平，其行无常处，在阴与阳，不可为度，从而察之，三部九候，卒然逢之，早遏其路，吸则内针，无充气忤；静以久留，无令邪布；吸则转针，以得气为故；候呼引针，呼尽乃去；大气皆出，故命曰写。

Qibo answered: "The regulations formulated by the sages were certain to conform with the nature. There are three hundred and sixty five degrees and twenty eight constellations in heaven, twelve rivers on earth and twelve channels in man.

"When the heaven and earth are warm, the water in the rivers is calm; when the heaven and earth are cold, the water in the river is stagnated and dull; when the weather is scorching hot, the water in the river is boiled and overflowing; when the violent gale arises, white surges will occur in the river like ridges and furrows.

"When the evil -energy invades the channel, if it is a cold-evil, it will cause the blood to become moist. When the wind-evil invades the channel, it is like water being attacked by

wind, and the pulsation of the channel will be also unsmooth like ridges and furrows, when the evil-energy is making trouble in the pulse, it is like a horizontal bar in the front of a car.

"The feeling under the finger in palpation may be some times strong and sometimes weak, when it is strong, it shows the evil-energy is abundant; when it is weak, it shows the evil-energy is calm. When the evil-energy is prevailing, it has no definite position. It can be concealed in Yang, and can be concealed in Yin, which can hardly be estimated. If one wants to examine it, he must follow the proper sequence and trace it by using the method of palpating the three parts and the nine sub-parts of pulse, When inspecting, if the location of the disease is discovered in the three parts and the nine sub-parts of pulse, the evil-energy must be blocked in time by treating.

"In treating, insert the needle when the patient inhales, do not let the energy become adverse when inserting. After insertion, one should wait patiently for the arrival of the energy, and the needle should be retained longer to avoid the despersion of the evil-energy. Twist the needle at the time of the patient's inhalation, so that one may get the desired feeling of acupuncture. Withdraw the needle slowly at the time of the patient's exhalation, and pull it out at the end of the exhalation. In this way. the accumulated energy under the needle will come out thoroughly, and this is the method of purging."

帝曰：不足者补之，奈何？

岐伯曰：必先扪而循之，切而散之，推而按之，弹而怒〔《难经·七十八难》"怒"作"努"〕之，抓而下之，通而取之，外引其门，以闭其神。呼尽内针，静以久留，以气至为故，如待所贵，不知日暮，其气以至，适而自护，候吸引针，气不得出，各在其处，推阖其门，令神〔《甲乙》"神"作"真"〕气存，大气留止，故命曰补。

Yellow Emperor asked:"How to invgorate the syndrome of deficiency?"Qibo said:"Feel and touch with hand along the acupoints and press with finger tips to disperse the evil-energy, then push and press the skin, snap the acupoints to make the energy filling up and begin the pricking when the channel-energy has been dredged. After the pulling out of the needle, massage the skin to close the needle hole, so as the healthy-energy may be stored inside. The inserting of the needle should be carried out by the end of the patient's exhalation and retain the needle longer quietly for to get the acupucture feeling. When waiting the arrival of the energy after inserting, one should be attentive like waiting an honorable guest, unawaring the day is dark. When the desired feeling of acupuncture is felt, it should be looked after causiously. Pull out the needle at the time of the patient's inhalation, so that the healthy energy may not be discharged, and this is the method of invigoration."

帝曰：候气奈何？

Yellow Emperor asked: " How to wait for the energy after insertion?""

岐伯曰：夫邪去络入于经也，舍〔《太素》作"合"〕于血脉之中，其寒温未相得〔《太素》作"合"〕，如涌波之起也，时来时去，故不常在。故曰方其来也，必按而止之，止而取之，无逢其冲而写之。真气者，经气也，经气太虚，故曰其来不可逢，此之谓也。故曰候邪不审，大气已过，写之则真气脱，脱则不复，邪气复至，而病益蓄，故曰其往不可追，此之

谓也。不可挂以发者〔俞樾说“此六字衍文”〕，待邪之至时而发针写矣，若先若后者，血气已尽，其病不可下〔《太素》“不”下无“可”字〕，故曰知其可取如发机，不知其〔《太素》“其”下有“可”字〕取如扣锥，故曰知机道者不可挂以发，不知机者扣之不发，此之谓也。

Qibo said: “When the evil-energy is kept away from the collaterals, it enters into the channel and retains in the channel. By this time, the evil energy which is either hot or cold, has not yet combined with the healthy energy, the pulse condition is floating and gigantic like turbulent waves, come and go without any definite position.

“So, when the evil-energy comes, it should be blocked first, and then overcome it. Do not apply purging when the evil-energy is flourishing.

“When the true energy, ie., the channel energy is deficient, and at the same time, if purging is applied, the channel energy will become more deficient. This is why the saying goes: ‘it must not purge when the energy is deficient’.

When the evil-energy of the patient is not observed and understood in details, and the accumulated energy under the needle has gone already, if purge is applied, it will cause the prostration of the patient which is hard to restore. in this case, the evil energy will come again and the disease will become aggravated. This is why the saying goes: ‘if the evil energy has gone already, it can not be pursued again’.

“In a word, the insertion should be started after the evil-energy has arrived, if the insertion is earlier or later when the blood and energy is in debility, the disease can hardly be alleviated. Thus, the one who is good at acupuncture, his treating effect is like touching a trigger, while a poor hand in acupuncture, it is like knocking the drumsticks without any response. Therefore, to those who know the essentials, the effect is prompt as in the twinkling of an eye, while to those who know not the essentials can not start up even when the trigger is touched.”

帝曰：补写〔明抄本作“取血”〕奈何？岐伯曰：此攻邪也，疾出以去盛血，而复其真气，此邪新客，溶溶〔《太素》无此二字〕未有定处也，推之则前，引之则止，逆而刺之〔《太素》无此四字〕，温〔“温”误，应作“写”〕血也，刺出其血，其病立已。

Yellow Emperor asked: “How to discharge the blood?” Qibo said: “prick and discharge the overabundant blood is to attack the evil-energy and restore the healthy energy. As the evil-energy has just invaded, it is not stable, so it can be moved foward by pushing or can be retained by stopping, so the overabundant blood can be purged by pricking. When the blood is discharged by purging, the patient will be recovered.”

帝曰：善。然真邪以合，波陇不起，候之奈何？

岐伯曰：审扪〔“扪”字衍〕循三部九候之盛虚而调之，察其左右上下相失及相减者，审其病藏以期之。不知三部者，阴阳不别，天地不分，地以候地，天以候天，人以候人，调之中府，以定三部，故曰刺不知三部九候病脉之处，虽有〔明抄本无“虽有”二字〕大过且至，工不能禁也。诛罚〔滑抄本“罚”作“伐”〕无过，命曰大惑，反乱大经，真不可复，用实为虚，以邪为真，用针无义，反为气贼，夺人正气，以从为逆，荣卫散乱，真气已失，邪独内

著，绝人长命〔按此四字涉下误衍〕，予人夭〔胡本，赵本，明抄本，周本“天”并作“夭”〕殃，不知三部九候，故不能久长。因不知合之四时五行，因加相胜，释邪攻正，绝人长命。邪之新客来也，未有定处，推之则前，引之则止，逢而写之，其病立已。

Yellow Emperor said: “Good. But if the evil-energy combines with the healthy energy but causes no fluctuation in the pulse energy, how can one examine and diagnose it?” Qibo said: “It should be traced along with the asthenia and sthenia of the three parts and the nine sub-parts of the pulse, and examine carefully the left, right, upper and lower parts of the patient to see whether there is any place which is weak or not matching, find out the location where the disease conceals, and prick with needle until the arrival of the energy. Inspect the lower warmer from the pulse of the lower part; inspect the upper warmer from the pulse of the upper part; and inspect the middle warmer from the pulse of the middle part . The pulse conditions of the three parts and the nine sub-parts are all determined by the presence or absence of the stomach energy.

“If one does not understand the pulse condition of the three parts and the nine sub-parts, unable to distinguish Yin and Yang, nor can he discern the upper and the lower part and prick rashly, erroneous treatment may be made, the disease will turn to the worse, and hence, even a good physician can do nothing about it.

“If purge is used when it should not be used, it is called the ‘big perplexing’, it may disturb the channels of the viscera, and the healthy-energy will be difficult to be restored, When one mistakes the sthenic syndrome as the asthenic syndrome, mistakes the evil-energy as the healthy energy, and applies the needle without any rule, the evil-energy will cause damage and hurt the healthy-energy of the patient. In this way, the case of a favourable prognosis will become a case of an unfavourable prognosis, the Rong-energy and the Wei-energy of the patient will be confusing, his healthy-energy will be exhausting, and the evil-energy will become prosperous and cause calamities. A physician who knows not the three parts and the nine sub-parts of the pulse, his treating effect would not last long.

“When one does not know the principle of coordinating the four seasons and the overcoming of each other of the five elements, not knowing the arrival of the host energy and the guest energy of the year, unable to control the evil-energy and allow it attacks the healthy-energy, it may ruin the life of the patient.

“Finally, it should be recapitulated that when the evil-energy invades into the body, it has no certain place of residence, and it can be pushed forward and can be drawn back, if the evil-energy is dealt with a head-on purge, the disease can be eased immediately.”

通评虚实论篇第二十八

Chapter 28
Tong Ping Xu Shi Lun
(On the Asthenia and Sthenia)

黄帝问曰：何谓虚实？岐伯曰：邪气盛则实，精〔《难经·七十五难》虞注引"精"作"真"〕气夺则虚。

Yellow Emperor asked："What is Asthenia and Sthenia?" Qibo answered："When the evil-energy is overabundant, it is sthenia, when the healthy-energy is injured, it is asthenia."

帝曰：虚实何如？岐伯曰：气虚者，肺虚也，气逆者，足寒也，非其时则生，当其时则死。余藏皆如此。

Yellow Emperor asked："What are the conditions of asthenia and sthenia respectively?" Qibo said："The lung takes charge of the energy, when the energy is deficient, it is the asthenia of the lung energy which will cause the adverseness of vital energy and cold feet. If the lung disease encounters the season of summer of which its associated element (fire) is subjugating the lung metal, the patient will die. If other season of which its associated element does not subjugate lung metal is encountered, ie., spring, autumn or winter, the patient will survive. The conditions in other viscera are all the same."

帝曰：何谓重实？岐伯曰：所谓重实者，言大热病，气热脉满，是谓重实。

Yellow Emperor asked："What is double Sthenia?" Qibo answered："When the patient has a high fever with hot evil-energy and a full pulse, it is called the double sthenia."

帝曰：经络俱实何如？何以治之？岐伯曰：经络皆实，是寸〔莫文泉说："按王注'脉急谓脉口'是王本原无'寸'字〕脉急而尺缓也，皆当治之，故曰滑则从，濇则逆也。夫虚实者，皆从其物类〔"类"字衍〕始，故五藏骨肉滑利，可以长久也。

Yellow Emperor asked："What is the condition when both the channel-energy and the collateral-energy are sthenic, and how to treat it?" Qibo said："The so called both the channel-energy and the collateral-energy are sthenic indicates the condition when the pulse is rapid but the skin of antero-lateral side of the forearm is relaxed. In this case, both the channel and the collateral should be treated. When the pulse condition is slippery and flourishing, it is called the favourable condition, when the pulse is choppy which shows the energy and blood are deficient and stagnated, it is called the adverse condition. The condition of asthenia and sthenia of a human body is like that of all other living things, it will survive when the condition of the pulse is slippery and flourishing, and will die when it is choppy and stagnated. When one's viscera, bones and muscle are slippery and flourishing, his life will last

long."

帝曰：络气不足，经气有余，何如？岐伯曰：络气不足，经气有余者，脉口〔《太素》卷三十《经络虚实》"脉"下无"口"字〕热而尺寒也，秋冬为逆，春夏为从，治主病者。

Yellow Emperor asked: " What is the condition when the collateral-energy is deficient but the channel-energy is having a surplus?" Qibo said: When the collateral-energy is deficient and the channel-energy is having a surplus, hot in pulse and cold in the skin of anterolateral side of forearm will appear. If it appears in autumn or winter, it is an adverse condition; if it appears in spring or summer, it is a favourable condition. It is the adverse condition of the main disease which should be treated."

帝曰：经虚络满，何如？岐伯曰：经虚络满者，尺热满脉口〔《太素》"脉"下无"口"字〕寒濇也，此春夏死秋冬生也。

Yellow Emperor asked: " What is the condition when the channel is asthenic but the collateral is sthenic ?" Qibo said: "When the channel-energy is asthenic and the collateral-energy is sthenic, the skin of the anterolateral side of the forearm will be hot and the pulse will be cold. If it appears in spring or summer, the patient will die, if it appears in autumn or winter, the patient can survive."

帝曰：治此者奈何？岐伯曰：络满经虚灸阴刺阳；经满络虚，刺阴灸阳。

Yellow Emperor asked: " How to treat the disease?" Qibo said: "When the collateral-energy is sthenic and the channel-energy is asthenic, treat Yin with moxibustion and prick Yang with needle; when the channel is sthenic and the collateral-energy is asthenic, prick Yin with needle and treat Yang with moxibustion."

帝曰：何谓重虚？岐伯曰：脉气上虚尺虚〔明抄本作"脉虚气虚尺虚"〕，是谓重虚。帝曰：何以治之？岐伯曰：所谓气虚者，言无常也。尺虚者，行步恇然。脉虚者，不象阴〔于鬯说"阴"下脱"阳"字〕也。如此者，滑则生，濇则死也。

Yellow Emperor asked: " What is double asthenia?" Qibo said: "When the pulse energy and the chi pulse (the proximal throbbing of the radial pulse) are all asthenic, it is called the double asthenia."

Yellow Emperor asked: "How to distinguish it?" Qibo said: "The asthenia of energy is due to the deficient energy of Tanzhong (Middle Chest) which cause the patient to have discontinuous speech; the asthenia of chi pulse is due to the weakness of the chi pulse which causes the patient to become timid and infirm in walking; the asthenia of pulse is due to both the energy and blood are weak, and the Yin and Yang are not corresponding. The patient with these syndromes will survive if his pulse is slippery, will die if his pulse is choppy."

帝曰：寒气暴〔《脉经》"暴上"作"上攻"〕上，脉满而实何如？岐伯曰：实而滑则生，实而逆则死。

Yellow Emperor asked: " What does it imply when the cold-evil attack upwards and the pulse is full and sthenic?" Qibo said: " When the pulse condition is sthenic and slippery, it shows the patient will survive, when the pulse condition is sthenic, adverse and choppy, it shows the patient will die."

帝曰：脉实满，手足寒，头热，何如？岐伯曰：春秋则生，冬夏则死。脉浮而濇，濇而身有热者死。

Yellow Emperor asked："What does it imply when the pulse condition is sthenic and full, the hands and feet are cold and the head is hot?" Qibo said："If the syndrome occurs in spring and autumn , the patient will survive, if it occurs in winter or summer, he will die. Besides, when the patient's pulse condition is floating and choppy and he has fever in the body, he will also die."

帝曰：其形〔《脉经》校语引《太素》作"举形"〕尽满何如？岐伯曰：其形尽满者，脉急〔明抄：夹注云：脉下有"口"字〕大坚，尺濇而不应也，如是者，故〔《脉经》校语引《太素》无"故"字〕从则生，逆则死。帝曰：何谓从则生，逆则死？岐伯曰：所谓从者，手足温也；所谓逆者，手足寒也。

Yellow Emperor asked："What about the condition when the patient is asthenic with edema?" Qibo said："In the syndrome of asthenic with edema, the Cunkou pulse of the patient is rapid, large and firm, but the Chi pulse is choppy, and they are not adapting with each other, in this case, if the condition is favourable, the patient will survive, if the condition is adverse, the patient will die." Yellow Emperor asked："What is the favourable condition and what is the adverse condition?" Qibo said："When the hands and feet of the patient are warm, it is the favourable condition, when his hands and feet are cold, it is the adverse condition."

帝曰：乳子而病热，脉悬小者何如？岐伯曰：手足〔林校引《太素》无"手"字〕温则生，寒则死。

Yellow Emperor asked："When one has just given birth to a baby and contracts fever with a very tiny pulse, what does it imply?" Qibo said："The patient may survive when her feet are warm, will die when his feet are cold."

帝曰：乳子中风热〔热字疑衍王注引《正理伤寒论》无"热"字〕，喘鸣肩息者，脉何如？岐伯曰：喘鸣肩息者，脉实大也，缓则生，急则死。

Yellow Emperor asked："When one have given birth to a baby and is attacked by wind-evil, with a syndrome of making sound in respiration, openning her mouth and lifting her shoulders, what will happen to him?" Qibo said："When her pulse condition is floating and slow and her stomach energy is existing, she may survive; if her pulse condition is tiny and rapid, and her visceral energy is exhausted, she will die."

帝曰：肠澼便血何如？岐伯曰：身热则死，寒则生。帝曰：肠澼下白沫何如？岐伯曰：脉沈则生，脉浮则死。帝曰：肠澼下脓血何如？岐伯曰：脉悬绝则死，滑大则生。帝曰：肠澼之属，身不热，脉不悬绝何如？岐伯曰：滑大者曰生，悬濇者曰死，以藏期之。

Yellow Emperor asked："What about the patient with bloody stool and dysentery?" Qibo said："When the patient has dysentery with fever, he will die; when the body of the patient is cold but has no fever, he will survive."

Yellow Emperor asked："What about the patient who has bloody stool together with white foam?" Qibo said："If the pulse is sunken, the patient will survive, if it is floating,

the patient will die."

Yellow Emperor asked: "What about the patient who has bloody stool together with purulence?" Qibo said: "When the pulse condition is tiny and choppy, the patient will die;, when the pulse condition is slippery and gigantic, the patient will survive."

Yellow Emperor asked: "What about if the patient has a fever and his pulse is not tiny and choppy?" Qibo said: "When the pulse is slippery and gigantic, the patient will survive, when the pulse condition is floating and severing, the patient will die, as to the date of his death, it is determined by the day when its associated element is being subjugated."

帝曰：癫疾何如？岐伯曰：脉搏大滑，久自已；脉小坚急，死不治。帝曰：癫疾之脉，虚实何如？岐伯曰：虚则可治，实则死。

Yellow Emperor asked: "What about the patient with the disorder of head (such as head-wind, headache, dizziness, vertigo; boils over the scalp etc., due to the ascent of energy and fire)?" Qibo said: "When the pulse condition is gigantic and slippery, the disease can be cured in a period of time; if the pulse is tiny, firm and rapid, it shows the energy is sthenic and being obstructed, the patient will die." Yellow Emperor asked: "What about the asthenic and sthenic condition of the disorder of the head?" Qibo said: "If the pulse condition is asthenic and slow, the disease is curable, if the pulse condition is sthenic and firm, the patient will die."

帝曰：消瘅虚实何如？岐伯曰：脉实大，病久可治，脉悬小坚〔《脉经》"坚"下有"急"字〕，病久不可治。

Yellow Emperor asked: "What about the asthenic and sthenic condition of diabetes?" Qibo siad: "When the pulse condition is sthenic and gigantic, even though the disease is protracted, it can still be cured, if the pulse condition is very tiny, firm and urgent, and the disease is protracted, it will not be cured."

帝曰：春亟治经络，夏亟治经输；秋亟治六府；冬则闭塞，闭塞者，用〔《甲乙》"用"上有"治"字〕药而少〔《太素》"少"下有"用"字〕针石也。所谓少针石者，非痈疽之谓也，痈疽不得顷时回。痈不知所，按之不应手〔《圣济总录》"应"下无"手"字〕，乍来乍已刺手太阴傍三痏与缨脉各二，掖〔朝本"掖"作"腋"〕痈大热，刺足少阳五；刺而热不止，刺手心主三，刺手太阴经络者，大骨之会各三。暴痈筋软，随分而痛，魄汗不尽，胞气不足，治在经俞。

Yellow Emperor said: "When treating a disease in spring, collateral points should be pricked; in summer, the shu point of the various channels should be pricked; in autumn, the converging points of the six bowels should be pricked; in winter, since it is a season of shutting, when treating, it should apply more medicine and less acupuncture and stone. But to carbuncle, one must not hesitate to treat with needle.

"In the initial stage of a carbuncle, it can hardly be found by pressing, and its location of pain is not definite. In this case, prick three times of the acupoints of lateral side of the Hand Taiyin Channel, and twice in the left and right sides of the neck.

"To the patient of carbuncle beneath the armpit with high fever, the Yuanye (Deep Flu-

id, GB. 22) point of Foot Shaoyang Channel should be pricked for five times; if the fever does not come down after pricking, prick the Tianchi (Celestial Pond, LR. 3) in the palm for three times, and prick the collateral points of Hand Taiyin Channel and the Jianzhen (Upright Shoulder, SI. 9) points for three times each.

"To the disease of acute carbuncle, contraction of tendon, aching of muscle along with swelling and continuous sweating, as they are due to the deficiency of the bladder channel, when treating, shu points of the channel should be pricked.

腹暴〔《甲乙》"暴"下有"痛"字〕满，按之不下，取手太阳经络者，胃之募也，少阴俞去脊椎三寸傍五用员利针。霍乱，刺俞傍五，足阳明及上傍三。刺痫惊脉五，针手〔明抄本"手"上无"针"字〕太阴各五，刺经太阳五，刺手少阴经络傍者一，足阳明一，上踝五寸刺三针。

"When the abdomen distends and aches suddenly and can not be alleviated when being pressed, the collateral points of the Hand Taiyang points (ie. the stomach mu-points) and the Kidney shu-points of Shaoyin Channel should be pricked five times each with the round-sharp needle.

"To the patient who suffers with cholera, the Zhishi (Room of Will BL. 52) points by the two sides of the kidney shu points sould be pricked for five times, and the stomach shu points of Foot Yangming Channel and the Weicang (Stomach Granary BL. 50) points by the two sides of the kidney shu-points should be pricked three times each. To convulsive diseases, there are five points for pricking: prick the Jingqu (Channel Gutter LU. 8) point of Hand Taiyin Channel for five times, prick the Yanggu (Yang Valley SI. 5) point of the Small Intestine Channel of Hand-Taiyang for five times, prick the Zhizheng point (Apart from Channel SI. 7.) by the side of the Hand Shaoyin Channel and collateral once, prick the Jiexi (Opened Hollow ST. 41) point of the Foot Yangming Channel once, and prick the Zhubin (Building for Guest KI. 9) point which is five inches above the foot ankle for three times.

凡治消瘅、仆击、偏枯、痿厥、气满发逆〔《甲乙》作"厥气逆满"〕，肥〔守校本"肥"上有"甘"字〕贵人，则高梁之疾也。隔塞闭绝，上下不通，则暴忧之疾也。暴厥而聋，偏塞闭不通，内气暴薄也。不从内，外中风之病，故瘦留著也。蹠跛，寒风湿之病也。

"The diseases of diabetes, cataplexy, hemiplegia, adverseness of vital energy, abdominal flatulence etc. are mostly suffered by the noble people who enjoy excellent food with too much meat and refined rice. Belching of the patient may stagnate the breath and hinder the communication between the upper part and the lower, and the disease is induced by fury and worry. The disease of excruciating pain over the chest and abdomen with coldness of the limbs which occurs all of a sudden, unconsciousness, deaftness, retention of feces and urine are all caused by the up-coercing of the internal energy. Some of the diseases are not stemmed from inside but by the outside invasion of the wind-evil. When the wind-evil retains inside of the body for long, it will be transformed into heat to cause evident emaciation of the muscle. Some people are slanting to one side when walking, it is due to the contracting of cold-evil or wind-wetness evil."

黄帝曰：黄疸暴痛，癫疾厥狂，久逆之所生也。五藏不平，六府闭塞之所生也。头痛耳鸣，九窍不利，肠胃之所生也。

Yellow Emperor said："Jaundice，drastic pain in all of a sudden，mania，adverseness of vital energy etc. are caused by the protracted up-reversing of the channel energy，The disharmony of the five viscera is caused by the stagnation of of the six hollow organs. The headache，tinnitus and the dullish of the nine orifices are caused by the affection of the stomach and intestine."

太阴阳明论篇第二十九

Chapter 29
Taiyin Yangming Lun
(On the Relations Between the Superficies and Interior of Taiyin and Yangming Channels)

黄帝问曰：太阴〔《甲乙》“太阴”上有“足”字〕阳明为表里，脾胃脉也，生病而异者何也？岐伯对曰：阴阳异位，更虚更实，更逆更从，或从内，或从外，所从不同，故病异名也。

Yellow Emperor asked："The Foot Taiyin Channel of spleen and the Yangming Channel of stomach are the superficies and interior, but their diseases are different, what is the reason?" Qibo answered："The spleen belongs to the Yin channel and the stomach belongs to the Yang channel, the two channels are moving about in different routes, they are different in asthenia and sthenia and in agreeable condition or adverse condition; in the sources of diseases from inside or outside, they are also different, so, they are different in names."

帝曰：愿闻其异状也。岐伯曰：阳者，天气也，主外；阴者，地气也，主内。故阳道实，阴道虚。故犯贼风虚邪者，阳受之；食饮不节，起居不时者，阴受之。阳受之则入六府，阴受之则入五藏。入六府，则身热不时卧〔《甲乙》作“不得眠”〕，上为喘呼；入五藏，则䐜满闭塞，下为飧泄，久为肠澼。故喉主天气，咽主地气。故阳受风气，阴受湿气。故阴气从足上行至头，而下行循臂至指端；阳气从手上行至头，而下行至足。故曰阳病者上行极而下〔《太素》、《云笈七签》“下”下并有“行”字〕，阴病者下行极而上〔《太素》《云笈七签》“上”下并有“行”字〕。故伤于风者，上先受之；伤于湿者，下先受之。

Yellow Emperor said: "I hope you can tell me about the different conditions." Qibo said："Yang is like heaven, guarding the exterior of human body, Yin is like earth, protecting the interior of human body. As Yang is firm and Yin is gentle, Yang is often sthenic and Yin is often asthenic. Therefore, when the thief-wind and the debilitating evil invades the body, Yang will be affected first; when one is careless about food and drink or being irregular in daily life, Yin will be injured. If the exterior of the body contracts disease, it will be transmitted to the six hollow organs; if the interior of the body contracts disease, it will be transmitted to the five solid organs. If the evil-energy enters into the six hollow organs, one will have fever, unable to sleep and respires rapidly; if the disease is in the five solid organs, the patient will have distention of abdomen and feel depressive, have lienteric diarrhea, and, after a certain period, it will become dysentery. The throat takes charge of respiration, so it associates with the energy of heaven; the pharynx takes charge of the intake of food, so it associates with the energy of earth. The wind is Yang-evil, when the wind-evil invades the

body, Yang will be infected; the wetness is Yin-evil, when the wetness-evil invades the body, Yin will be infected.

"The channels of three Yin go upwards from the feet to the head, and go downwards from the head to the arms and then to the finger tips of hands. The channels of the three Yang go upwards from hands to the head, and then go downwards to the feet. So, the evil-energy of Yang channel goes upwards to the extreme hight first, and then goes downwards; the evil-energy of Yin channel goes downwards to the extreme bottom first, and then goes upwards. Thus, when one contracts wind-evil from outside, it is mostly on the upper part, when he contracts wetness-evil, it is mostly on the lower part."

黄帝：脾病而四支不用何也？岐伯曰：四支皆禀气于胃，而不得至经〔《太素》作"径至"，"径"有"直"义〕，必因于脾，乃得禀也。今脾病不能为胃行其津〔读本、赵本、吴本"津"并作"精"〕液，四支不得禀水谷气，气〔元残一、赵本、吴本、明抄本"日"上并无"气"字〕日以衰，脉道不利〔《甲乙》"利"作"通"〕，筋骨肌肉，皆无气以生，故不用焉。

Yellow Emperor asked; "The four limbs can not move normally when the spleen is ill, and what is the reason?" Qibo said: "All the four limbs are nourished by the stomach-energy, but the stomach-energy can not reach the four limbs directly. The essence of water and cereals can only reach the four limbs after being converted by the spleen. Now, since the spleen is ill, the essence of water and cereals of stomach can no more be sent to the four limbs, and they will become weaker and weaker day after day. As the channels are obstructed, the patient's tendons, bones and muscles can not be enriched due to malnourishment, the four limbs will not be able to move normally."

帝曰：脾不主时何〔《太素》"脾"下有"之"字〕也？岐伯曰：脾者土也，治中央〔《甲乙》作"土者中央"〕，常以四时长四藏，各十八日寄治，不得独主于时也。脾藏者常著胃〔《太素》作"脾藏有常著"，按"者"作"有"似误，本句应作"脾藏者，常著土之精也"〕土之精也，土者生〔《太素》"生"作"主"〕万物而法天地，故上下至头足，不得主时也。

Yellow Emperor asked: "What is the reason that the spleen can not dominate a single season specifically?" Qibo said: "The spleen associates to earth and locates at the centrality. As it associates to earth, it symbolizes the earth-energy to promote the growth of all living things; as it locates at the centrality, it spreads the body fluid to nourish the other four viscera. In all the four seasons, the four viscera depend on the spleen to get nourishments, so, at the end of each of the four seasons, there are eighteen days out of the ninty days for the spleen to become prosperous and dominating, and thus, the spleen does not dominate an individual season. As the spleen often activates the body fluid for the stomach and nourish the four limbs and bones of the body, it takes effect on the head, foot and everywhere of the body, like the heaven and earth producing and promoting the growth of everything, it does not dominate an individual season specifically."

帝曰：脾与胃以膜相连耳，而能为之行其津液何也？岐伯曰：足太阴者三阴也，其脉贯胃属脾络嗌，故太阴为之行气于三阴。阳明者表也，五藏六府之海也，亦为之行气于三阳。藏

府各因其经而受气于阳明，故为胃行其津液，四支不得禀水谷气〔丹波元坚说“四支”以下二十八字与上文复，正是衍文〕，日以益衰，阴道不利，筋骨肌肉无气以生，故不用焉。

Yellow Emperor asked: " Since there is only a piece of membrane connecting the spleen and the stomach, how can the spleen transport the body fluid for the stomach?" Qibo said: "The Foot Taiyin Channel of Spleen which is the third Yin whose channel is surrounding the stomach, connecting the spleen and clipping the throat, so, the Yangming energy can be transported by the Taiyin Channel, and makes it enter into the three Yin channels of Hand and Foot; the Foot Yangming Channel of stomach is the superficies of the Foot Taiyin Channel of spleen and is also the sea of nutrition of the five solid organs and the six hollow organs, so, the Stomach Channel can also transport the energy of Taiyin into the three Yang channels of Hand and Foot. Since the five solid organs and the six hollow organs can all receive the essence of water and cereals of Yangming with the help of the Spleen Channel, so, the spleen is capable of transporting the body fluid for the stomach."

阳明脉解篇第三十

Chapter 30
Yangming Mai Jie
(The Explanation on the Yangming Channel)

黄帝问曰：足阳明之脉病，恶人与火，闻木音则惕然而惊，钟鼓不为动，闻木音而惊何也？愿闻其故。岐伯对曰：阳明者胃脉也，胃者土也，故闻木音而惊者，土恶木也。帝曰：善。其恶火何也？岐伯曰：阳明主肉，其脉血气盛，邪客之则热，热甚则恶火。

Yellow Emperor asked:"The patient with the disease of Foot Yangming detests man and fire, and become frightened when hearing a sound made by wood, but has no response when hearing the sound of a bell. Why is he afraid of the sound of wood only? I want to know the reason." Qibo answered: " The Foot Yangming is a stomach channel, in the five elements, it belongs to earth, as the earth detests the subjugation from the wood, the patient will be frightened when hearing the sound of wood."

Yellow Emperor said: " Good. But why he detests the fire?" Qibo said: " Yangming takes charge of the muscle, and Yangming Channel is abundant with blood and energy, when it is injured by the exogenous evils, Yang energy will be obstructed and the blood is stagnated to produce heat, when the heat in the body is excessive, the patient will detest fire."

帝曰：其恶人何也？岐伯曰：阳明厥则喘而惋〔《甲乙》作闷〕，惋则恶人。帝曰：或喘而死者，或喘而生者，何也？岐伯曰：厥逆连藏则死，连经则生。

Yellow Emperor asked: " Why he detests man?" Qibo said: "When Jueni (coldness of limbs, pain over the chest and abdomen, and temporary suspension of consciousness) of Yangming occurs, the patient will have dyspnea and feels disquieted, so he detests man."

Yellow Emperor asked: " Some patient died due to jueni and dyspnea, but some can still survive despite of them, and why is it so?" Qibo said: " If Jueni has reached the viscera and the patient has dyspnea, he will die; if Jueni has only reached the channel, he can survive although he has dyspnea."

帝曰：善。病甚〔《太素》"病甚"上有"阳明"二字〕则弃衣而走，登高而歌，或至不食数日，逾垣上屋，所上之处〔《太素》"所上"下无"之处"二字〕，皆非其素所能也，病反能者何也？岐伯曰：四支者，诸阳之本也，阳盛则四支实，实则能登高〔《甲乙》"登高"下有"高歌"二字〕也。

Yellow Emperor said: " Good. Some patient with a serious disease of Yangming, takes off his clothes and run about here and there, sings loudly at a high place; sometimes he eats nothing for several days, jumps up on the walls and roofs. He could not do such things usually, but he is able to do them when he is ill, and why is it so?" Qibo said: " The four ex-

tremities are the foundations of all Yangs, when the Yang energy is overabundant, the extremities will be sthenic, and when the extremities are sthenic, the patient will be able to climb up to a high place."

帝曰：其弃衣而走者何也？岐伯曰：热盛于身，故弃衣欲〔《太素》"欲"作"而"〕走也。

Yellow Emperor asked: " Why the patient takes off his clothes and run about?" Qibo said: " When the heat-evil is partial overabundant in the body, the patient is apt to take off his clothes and run about."

帝曰：其妄言〔《太素》"其"下无"妄言"二字〕骂詈，不避亲疏而歌者何也？岐伯曰：阳盛则使人妄言〔《甲乙》"则使人"作"故"字，"妄言"二字应删〕骂詈不避亲疏，而不欲食，不欲食，故妄走〔明抄本"不欲食"以下九字作"歌"〕也。

Yellow Emperor asked: " Some patients abuse others without distinction of friends and enemies and sometimes sing loudly at will, and why is it?" Qibo said: " When the Yang energy is partial overabundant in the body, it will cause the patient to become confusing in consciousness, that is why he abuses others wantonly and sings at will."

热论篇第三十一

Chapter 31
Re Lun
(On Febrile Disease)

黄帝问曰：今夫热病者。皆伤寒之类也。或愈或死。其死皆以六七日之间。其愈皆以十日以上者何也？不知其解。愿闻其故。

Yellow Emperor asked："Generally，the febrile disease is one of the exognenous diseases，some of the patients has restored to health，but some of them died. Those who died were on the sixth or seventh day，and those who recovered were after ten days，why is it so? I don't understand it，and I hope you can tell me."

岐伯对曰：巨阳者，诸阳之属也，其脉连于风府，故为诸阳主气也。人之伤于寒也，则为病热，热虽甚不死；其两感于寒而病者，必不免于死。

Qibo answered："The Foot Taiyang Channel is the place where all the Yangs converge，its channel connects the Fengfu (Windy Mansion) point of the Du (in the middle of back) Channel；as the Du Channel sees to all the Yang channels of the body，so，Foot Taiyang can dominate the energies of all the Yang channels. When one is invaded by the wind-evil，he will have a fever，but if he only has a fever，he will not die even the fever is severe；but if both the Yang and Yin channels are invaded by the cold-evil at the same time and cause disease，the patient will die."

帝曰：愿闻其状。岐伯曰：伤寒一日，巨阳受之，故头项痛腰脊强〔按《史载之方》引“脊”作“背”〕；二日阳明受之，阳明主肉〔《外台》、《伤寒补亡论》引“主”下并有“肌”字〕，其脉侠鼻络于目，故身热目疼〔《病论》“身”作“肉”字《太素》“热”下无“目疼”二字〕而鼻乾，不得卧也；三日少阳受之，少阳主胆〔《太素》《甲乙》《病论》“胆”并作“骨”字〕，其脉循胁络于耳，故胸胁痛而耳聋，三阳经络皆受其病，而未入于藏〔明抄本“藏”作“府”〕者，故可汗而已；四日太阴受之，太阴脉布胃中络于嗌，故腹满而嗌乾；五日少阴受之，少阴脉贯肾络于肺，系舌本，故口燥〔《太素》《病论》“燥”并作“热”〕舌乾而渴；六日厥阴受之，厥阴脉循阴器而络于肝，故烦满而囊缩，三阴三阳、五藏六府皆受〔《太素》《病论》“皆”下并无“受”字〕病，荣卫不行，五〔《太素》“五”作“府”〕藏不通则死矣。

Yellow Emperor said："I hope to hear about the syndromes of the exogenous febrile disease." Qibo said："On the first day when the patient contracts the exogenous febrile disease，the Taiyang Channel is infected by the cold-evil，he will feel pain on the head，back and loins.

"On the second day，the evil is transmitted into the Yangming Channel. The Yangming

Channel takes charge of the muscle, in its course of running, it clips the nose and surrounds the eyes, so the evil will cause the muscle to become hot, the dryness of nose and sleepiness.

"On the third day, the evil is transmitted to Shaoyang. The Shaoyang Channel takes charge of the bone, it runs along the two lateral sides of the thorax and surrounds the two ears, so the evil will cause pain of the chest and hypochodrium, and deafness of the ear. If all the three Yang channels are infected but the evil has not yet entered into the hollow organs, the disease can be cured by diaphoresis.

"On the fourth day, the evil is transmitted into the Taiyin Channel which is spreading over the stomach and surrounding the pharynx, so the evil will cause the distention of the abdomen and dryness of the pharynx of the patient.

"On the fifth day, the evil is transmitted into the Shaoyin Channel. The Shaoyin Channel is connecting the kidney and the lung, and linking the root of tongue, so, the evil will cause hotness of the mouth, dryness of the tongue and thirsty of the patient.

"On the sixth day, the evil is transmitted to the Jueyin Channel. The Jueyin Channel is running around the external genitals and surrounding the liver, the evil will cause the contracting of the scrotum and boring of the patient.

"If all the three Yin and Yang channels, the five solid organs and the six hollow organs are all infected, both the Rong and Wei energies are obstructed, and the solid and hollow organs are impeded, the patient will die.

其不两感于寒者，七日巨阳病衰，头痛少愈；八日阳明病衰，身热少愈；九日少阳病衰、耳聋微闻；十日太阴病衰、腹减如故，则思饮食；十一日少阴病衰〔《太素》"衰"作"愈"〕、渴止不满〔《甲乙》《伤寒补亡论》引"谒止"下并无"不满"二字〕，舌乾已而嚏；十二日厥阴病衰，囊纵少腹微下，大气皆去，病日已矣。帝曰：治之奈何？岐伯曰：治之各通其藏脉〔何校本"脉"作"腑"〕，病日衰已矣。其〔《病论》"其"下有"病"字〕未满三日者，可汗而已；其满三日者〔《病论》作"其病三日过者"〕，可泄而已。

"If the patient's Yang channel and Yin channel are not being infected by the cold-evil at the same time, then, on the seventh day, the disease of Taiyang will turn to the better and the headache will be somewhat alleviated; on the eighth day, the disease of Yangming will turn to the better and the fever of the body will come down slightly; on the ninth day, the disease of shaoyang will turn to the better, the deafness ameliorated and the patient can hear something; on the tenth day, the disease of Taiyin will turn to the better, the swelling abdomen of the patient will become normal as usual and he wants to eat; on the eleventh day, the disease of Shaoyin will turn to the better, the patient is no more thirsty nor with dryness of tongue, and he often sneezes. On the twelfth day, the disease of Jueyin will be recovered, the scrotum becomes relaxed, the lower abdomen becomes comfortable, the evils are all recessive and the patient is recovered thoroughly."

Yellow Emperor asked: "How to treat it?" Qibo answered: "It should base on the conditions of the solid and hollow organs of various channels and treat respectively to cause the disease decline day after day. To the disease which has been infected in less than three days,

it can be cured by diaphoresis; to the disease which has been infected for more than three days, it can be cured by purgation."

帝曰：热病已愈，时有所遗者何也？岐伯曰：诸遗者，热甚而强食之，故有所遗也〔按此五字涉下疑衍〕，若此者，皆病已衰，而热有所藏，因其谷气相薄〔《伤寒补亡论》引"薄"作"搏"〕，两热相合，故有所遗也。帝曰：善。治遗奈何？岐伯曰：视其虚实，调其逆从，可使必已矣〔《甲乙》"必"作"立"〕。帝曰：病热当何禁之？岐伯曰：病热少愈，食肉则复，多食则遗，此其禁也。

Yellow Emperor asked: "After the febrile disease is cured, there often occurs the remainder heat which has not been cleared away thoroughly, and why is it?" Qibo said: "The remainder heat is due to the patient's taking food with difficulty when the fever was severe. In this case, although the disease has been alleviated, but there is still some remainder heat which entangles with the energy of water and cereals to cause it to retain." Yellow Emperor said: "Good. But how to treat the remainder heat?" Qibo said: "To treat respectively according to the asthenic or sthenic, agreeable or adverse conditions of the disease, and the disease can be cured."

Yellow Emperor asked: "What are the contraindications when one contracts the febrile disease?" Qibo said: "When the febrile disease of the patient turns to the better, if meat is taken, the disease will recur; if plenty of cereals are taken, the remainder heat will retain as well. These are the contraindications of the febrile disease."

帝曰：其病两感于寒者，其脉应与其病形何如？岐伯曰：两感于寒者，病一日则巨阳与少阴俱病，则头痛口乾而烦满〔《外台》、《伤寒补亡论》并作"烦满而渴"〕；二日则阳明与太阴俱病，则腹满〔《太素》"腹"作"肠"〕身热，不欲食，谵言；三日则少阳与厥阴俱病，则耳聋囊缩而厥，水浆不入，不知人，六日死。帝曰：五藏已伤，六府不通，荣卫不行，如是之后，三日乃死何也？岐伯曰：阳明者，十二经脉之长也，其血气盛〔《伤寒总病论》引"血"作"邪"〕，故不知人，三日其气乃尽，故死矣。

Yellow Emperor asked: "What are the pulse conditions and syndromes of the patient who contracts cold-evil in both Yin and Yang channels?" Qibo said: "The conditions of the patient who contracts cold-evil in both Yin and Yang channels are: on the first day when both the Taiyang and the Shaoyin channels are infected, the patient will have the syndromes of headache, dryness of mouth, restless and thirst: on the second day when both the Yangming and the Taiyin are infected, the syndromes of fullness of intestine, fever, detesting food, and incoherent speech will occur; on the third day when both Shaoyang and Jueyin channels are infected, the syndromes of deafness of the ears, contraction of the scrotum and Jueni will occur. If the patient refuses to drink and becomes loss or partial loss of consciousness, he will die on the sixth day."

Yellow Emperor said: "When the disease comes to the stage of all the five viscera being injured, the six hollow organs impeded, the Rong and Wei energies are disharmonious, some of the patients die on the third day, and why is it?" Qibo said: "The Yangming Channel is the most important one in the twelve channels, when the evil-energy is overabundant in

Yangming Channel, the patient is apt to lose his consciousness. After three days of the evil's attack, the energy of the Yangming Channel will be exhausted, and the patient will die.

凡病伤寒而成温〔《外台》卷四《温病论》"温"下有"病"字〕者，先夏至日者为病温〔《伤寒论》"病温"作"温病""病暑"作"暑病"〕，后夏至日者为病暑，暑当与汗皆出，勿止。

"When a patient contracts cold-evil and then the disease turns into seasonal febrile, if it attacks before summer solstice, it is called the seasonal febrile disease; if it attacks after summer solstice, it is called the summer-heat disease. When treating the summer-heat disease, it should apply diaphorasis to let out the heat through sweating; astringent therapy must not be used."

刺热篇第三十二

Chapter 32
Ci Re
(Acupuncture for Treating the Febrile Diseases of the Viscera)

肝热病者，小便先黄〔按“小便”二字与“先”字误倒，应作“先小便黄”〕，腹痛多卧身热，热争〔《太平圣惠方》卷十七《热病论》引“争”作“盛”〕，则狂言及〔《太平圣惠方》“及”作“多”〕惊，胁满〔《太素》卷二十五《五藏热病》“胁”下无“满”字〕痛，手足躁，不得安卧；庚辛甚，甲乙大汗，气逆则庚辛死。刺足厥阴少阳。其逆则头痛员员〔按“其逆”七字，似误窜移〕，脉引冲头也〔此五字疑古注所错，宜删〕。

In the febrile disease from liver, the syndromes of yellow urine, abdominal pain, be fond of sleeping and fever of the patient will occur first. When the heat is excessive, rave, often be startled, hypochondriac pain, restlessness of the hands and feet, uable to sleep of the patient will occur; if the liver energy is reversing upwards, the patient will have dizziness. The disease will become aggravating on the days of Geng and Xin and the patient will be alleviated with plenty perspiration on the days of Jia and Yi. If the energy of the patient has become disorderly already, he will die on the days of Geng and Xin. In treating, it should prick the Foot Jueyin and the Foot Shaoyang channels.

心热病者，先不乐，数日乃热，热争，则卒心痛〔《甲乙》“则”下无“卒痛”二字，“心”字连下“烦闷”读〕，烦闷〔《太平圣惠方》“闷”作“热”〕善呕，头痛面赤，无汗；壬癸甚，丙丁大汗，气逆则壬癸死。刺手少阴太阳。

In the febrile disease from heart, the patient will appear to be unhappy first, and will have fever after a few days. When the heat is excessive, the patient will have feverish sensation accompanied with restlessness, nausea, headache, redish face and anhidrosis. The disease will become aggravating on the Ren and Gui days, and the patient will be alleviated with plenty perspiration on the days of Bing and Ding. If the energy of the patient has become disorderly already, he will die on the days of Ren and Gui. In treating, it should prick the Hand Shaoyin and the Hand Taiyang channels.

脾热病者，先头重颊痛，烦心颜青〔《甲乙》《病论》并无“颜青”二字〕，欲呕身热，热争，则腰痛不可用〔明抄二“不可”下无“用”字〕俛仰，腹满〔《圣济总录》引“满”下无“泄”字〕泄，两颔痛；甲乙甚，戊已大汗，气逆则甲乙死。刺足太阴阳明。

The patient with the febrile disease from spleen will feel heavy of the head, pain between the two eyes and eyebrows, disquieted, feel like to vomit and have fever of the body first. When the heat is excessive, the patient will have lumbago, unable to stoop or elevate,

have abdominal distention and hypochondriac pain. The disease will be aggravating on the days of Jai and Yi, and the patient will have plenty perspiration on the days of Wu and Ji. If the energy of the patient has become disorderly already, he will die on the days of Jia and Yi. In treating, it should prick Foot Taiyin and the Foot Yangming channels.

肺热病者，先淅然厥，起毫毛，恶风寒〔《太素》《病论》“风”下并无“寒”字〕，舌上黄身热，热争，则喘欬，痛走胸膺〔明抄二“膺”作“应”〕背，不得大息，头痛不堪，汗出而〔《伤寒总病论》引“而”下有“恶”字〕寒；丙丁甚，庚辛大汗，气逆则丙丁死。刺手太阴阳明，出血如大豆〔《伤寒总病论》引作“豆大”〕，立〔《伤寒九十论》引“立”作“疼”〕已。

The patient with the febrile disease from lung will feel cold with goose skin, to have an aversion to wind, have yellow tongue and fever in the body first. When the heat is excessive, the patient will cough with rapid respiration. The cough will shake the chest to cause pain and affects the back. The patient can hardly breath deeply, and the unbearable headache will cause him to have cold sweat continuously. The disease will become aggravating on the days of Bing and Ding, and the patient will be alleviated with plenty of perspiration on the days of Geng and Xin. If the energy of the patient has become disorderly already, he will die on the days of Bing and Ding. In treating, it should prick the Hand Taiyin and Hand Yangming channels. The disease will be cured when blood drops of pea size occur after pricking.

肾热病者，先腰痛骱痠〔《病论》“骱”作“胫”〕，苦渴数饮，身热，热争，则项痛而强，骱寒且痠，足下热，不欲言，其逆则项痛员员澹澹〔《甲乙》“员员”下无“澹澹”二字，按“员员”谓病之急〕然；戊已甚，壬癸大汗，气逆则戊已死。刺足少阴太阳。诸汗者，至其所胜日汗出也〔《太素》无“诸汗”以下十一字〕。

The patient with the febrile disease from kidney will feel pain in the loins, soreness of the legs, thirsty, desires to drink and has fever in the body first. When the heat is excessive, the patient will have headache and a rigid neck, his legs are cool and sore, his feet are hot, and he is relunctant to speak. If the kidney energy goes up adversely, the patient will feel pain and stiffness of the neck. The disease will become aggravating on the days of Wu and Ji, and the patient will be alleviated with plenty perspiration on the days of Ren and Gui. If the energy of the patient has become disorderly already, he will die on the days of Wu and Ji. In treating, prick the Foot Shaoyin and Foot Taiyang channels.

肝热病者，左颊先赤；心热病者，颜〔《病论》“颜”作“额”〕先赤；脾热病者，鼻〔《太平圣惠方》“鼻”作“唇”，《病论》“病”上有“凡”字〕先赤；肺热病者，右颊先赤；肾热病者，颐先赤。病虽未发，见赤〔《太素》“见”下有“其”字〕色者刺之，名曰治未病。热病从部所起者，至〔《太素》“至”下有“其”字〕期而已；其刺之反者，三周而已；重逆则死。诸当汗者，至其所胜日，汗大出也。

In febrile disease, when the heat is in the liver, the red colour will appear on the left cheek of the patient first; when the heat is in the heart, the red colour will appear on the forehead first; when the heat is in the spleen, the red colour will appear on the lips first; when the heat is in the lung, the red colour will appear on the right cheek first; when the

heat is in the kidney, the red colour will appear on the cheeks first. Generally, one should treat at the time when the red colour appears on the face before the disease attacks, which is called the treating in advance.

If the red colour in a specific position of the face is seen before the febrile disease attacks, and if the disease is treated in time, it can be cured on the day which is over-coming. If the treating is in an adverse way, the disease will last for three weeks, but if it is maltreated again, the patient will die. In a word, when treating a febrile disease, diaphoresis should be used, if the treating is in time, the disease can be cured on the day when the visceral energy is overcoming by diaphoresis.

诸治热病，以〔《甲乙》"以"作"先"〕饮之寒水，乃刺之；必寒衣之，居止寒处，身寒而止也。

When treating a febrile disease, ask the patient to drink some cool water first, and then begin the acupuncture treatment. The patient should wear thin dresses and stay in a cool place. In this way, when the heat of the body is eliminated, the disease will be cured.

热病先胸胁痛，手足躁，刺足少阳，补足〔《甲乙》"足"作"手"〕太阴，病甚者为五十九刺，热病始手臂痛〔《甲乙》"臂"下无"痛"字〕者，刺手阳明太阴而汗出止〔《甲乙》"出"下并无"止"字〕。热病始于头首者，刺项太阳而汗出止。热病始于足胫者，刺足阳明而汗出止。热病先身重骨痛，耳聋好瞑〔元残二，越本，吴本"瞑"并作"瞑"〕，刺足少阴，病甚为五十九刺。热病先眩冒〔《太素》"冒"作"胃"〕而热，胸胁满，刺足少阴〔张琦说："少阴"二字衍〕少阳。

In febrile disease, if the patient feels oppression and pain over the chest and hypochondria and restlessness of the hands and feet, it should prick the Foot Shaoyang channel and invigorate the Hand Taiyin channel; if the disease is severe, the Fifty-nine Pricking Method should be used.

If the febrile disease is initiated from the arm, prick the Hand Yangming channel (Shangyang point LI. 1) and the Hand Taiyin Channel (Lieque point LU. 7) until sweating.

If the febrile disease is initiated from the head, prick the Foot Taiying Channel (Tianzhu BL. 10) until sweating.

If the febrile disease is initiated from the tibia of foot, prick the Foot Yangming channel until sweating.

If the patient of the febrile disease feels heavy of the body, pain on the joints of the bone, deafness of the ears and sleepiness, prick the Foot Shaoyin Channel, if the disease is rather severe, prick with the Fifty-nine Pricking Method.

If the patient has the febrile disease and he has dizziness, heat in the stomach, and distention over the chest and hypochondria first, prick the Foot Shaoyang Channel.

太阳〔喜多村直宽说"太阳"疑当作"少阳"〕之脉，色荣颧骨〔张文虎说："言颧不必言骨。林引杨上善"骨"字属下读〕，热病也，荣未交〔于鬯说："'交'当从林校作'夭'，'荣'即色，荣未夭即色未夭"〕，曰〔《太素》"曰"作"日"连上读，今作"令"〕今且得汗，待时而已。与厥阴脉争见者，死期不过三日，其热病内连肾〔此六字疑错简〕，少阳之脉色也

〔林校云："旧无此四字"〕。少阳之脉〔喜多村直宽说："少阳疑当作太阳"〕，色荣颊前〔《太素》"前"作"筋"〕，热病也，荣未交，曰今且得汗，待时而已，与少阴脉争见者，死期不过三日。

When the red colour of the Shaoyang disease appears on the two cheekbones, it is the symbol of heat-type bone disease. If the complexion is not deteriorating, the disease can be recovered on the day when the visceral energy is overcoming and if only the patient has perspiration. But if the pulse condition and other manifestations of the Jueyin Channel is seen at the same time, the patient will die within three days.

When the red colour of the Taiyang Channel appears on the cheeks of the face, it is a symbol of febrile disease. If the complexion of the patient is not deteriorating, the disease will come to remission on the day when the visceral energy is overcoming, if only the patient has perspiration. But if the pulse condition and other manifestions of the Shaoyin Channel is seen at the same time, the patient will die within three days.

热病气穴：三椎下间主胸中热，四椎下间主鬲〔《太素》"鬲"下无"中"字〕中热，五椎下间主肝热，六椎下间主脾热，七椎下间主肾热，荣在骶也〔《太素》无"骶也"二字，"荣在"二字属下读〕，项上三椎陷者中也。颊下逆颧为大瘕，下牙车为腹满，颧后为胁痛。颊上者，鬲上也。

When treating the febrile disease with the points where the yang energy passes, regular pricking position should be applied: below the third vertebra is to purge the heat of the lung; below the fourth vertebra is to purge the heat of the heart; below the fifth vertebra is to purge the heat of the liver; below the sixth vertebra is to purge the heat of the spleen; below the seventh vertebra is to purge the heat of the kidney. When measuring the vertebra: The Dazhui (Big Vertebra) point is in the middle of the depression below the third cervical vertebra. When inspecting the complexion of the patient, the disease in the abdomen can be infered, such as, when the red colour moves upwards from the lower part of the cheek to the cheekbone, it shows the disease of dysentery; when the red colour appears in Jiache (Mandibular Joint) point, it shows abdominal distention; when the red colour appears behind the cheekbones, it shows the hypochondriac pain. When the red colours are seen in various parts above, they all show the diseases above the diaphram.

评热病论篇第三十三

Chapter 33
Ping Re Bing Lun
(On Febrile Disease)

黄帝问曰：有病温者，汗出辄〔《伤寒百证歌》引“辄”作“而身”〕复热，而脉躁疾不为汗衰〔《病论》卷十《温病候》“疾”作“病”。“脉躁”应断句，“疾”字属下读〕，狂言不能食，病名为何？岐伯对曰：病名阴阳交，交者〔《病论》“交”上有“阴阳”二字〕死也。帝曰：愿闻其说。岐伯曰：人所以汗出者，皆生于谷，谷生于精。今邪气交争于骨肉而得汗者，是邪却而精胜也。精胜，则当能食〔《太素》卷二十五《热病说》“当”下无“能”字〕而不复热〔《太素》《外台》引“热”上无“复”字〕，复热者邪气也，汗者精气也；今汗出而辄复热者，是邪胜也，不能食者，精无俾〔《太素》作“精母”，精母，瘅也〕也，病而留者〔《脉经》《伤寒补亡论》并作“汗而留热者”〕，其寿可立而倾也。且夫《热论》曰：汗出而脉尚躁盛者死。今脉不与汗相应，此不胜〔《病论》“胜”作“称”〕其病也，其死明矣。狂言者是失志，失志者死。今见三死，不见一生，虽愈必死也。

Yellow Emperor asked: “The patient with febrile disease still has fever and irritating pulse after sweating, his disease is not alleviated after sweating, he also has ravings and he refuses to eat, what is the disease?” Qibo answered: “It is called the Yinyang Complex and it is a fatal disease.”

Yellow Emperor said: “I hope to hear about it.” Qibo said: “The sweat is stemmed from water and cereals which are converted into refined energy for nourishing the whole body, when the refined energy of water and cereals is excreted to the surface of skin, it is sweat. In the combat of evil-energy against the healthy-energy between the bone and muscle, if the refined-energy wins, the evil-energy will be excreted along with the sweat, and the patient will be recovered, as he has no more fever, and the water and cereals can be converted again, he will have appetite to eat. If the patient still has fever after perspiration, it shows the refined-energy has been overcome by the evil-energy, the sweating can no longer let out the evil-energy, but can only consume the essence. When the evil-energy is overabundant and the refined-energy is debilitating, the water and cereals can not be converted, and the patient will refuse to eat. Stop eating will cause the deficiency of the refined fluid and cause the heat-evil to become overabundant even more. When the patient has plenty of sweat but the fever does not come down, the death of the patient is expected at any moment, as it is stated in 《On Heat》: ‘when the patient has perspiration with an irritating and overabundant pulse condition, the patient will die’; presently, the pulse condition is not in conformity with the condition of perspiration, and the refined-energy is unable to overcome the evil-energy, so the

symptom of death is evident; as to the ravings of the patient, it is due to the loss of consciousness, and the loss of consciousness is also the symptom of death. Now, the patient has have three symptoms of death without any lease of life, although there are some conditions turning to the better, the patient will die as well."

帝曰：有病身热汗出烦满，烦满不为汗解，此为何病？岐伯曰：汗出而身热者，风也；汗出而烦满不解者，厥也，病名曰风厥。帝曰：愿卒闻之。岐伯曰：巨阳主气〔《甲乙》作"太阳为诸阳主气"〕，故先受邪；少阴与其为表里也，得热则上从之，从之则厥也。帝曰：治之奈何？岐伯曰：表里刺之，饮之服汤〔《太素》"饮"下无"服"字〕。

Yellow Emperor asked: "Some patients who have fever, have sweat and has the disquieted mood at the same time, that is, the disquieted mood can not be eased up by perspiration, what is the disease?" Qibo said: "When a patient has fever and sweat at the same time, it is due to the wind-evil; when the sweating can not ease up the disquietness, it is due to the reversing up of the vital energy, and the disease is called the wind-jue." Yellow Emperor said: "I hope to hear about it." Qibo said: "The Taiyang Channel dominates all the energies of Yang, and Taiyang Channel is the superficies of the body, so it is easy to be invaded. The Shaoyin Channel and the Taiyang Channel are the superficies and the interior, if the Shaoyin Channel is reversing up under the effect of the fever of Taiyang Channel, it will become the jue-syndrome." Yellow Emperor asked: "How to treat it?" Qibo said: "Prick the points of the Taiyang and Shaoyin channels and take decoctions."

帝曰：劳风为病何如？岐伯曰：劳风法〔《医垒元戎》引作"发"〕在肺下，其为病也，使人强上〔于鬯说："'上'疑'工'之误，强工即强项"〕冥视，唾出若涕，恶风而振寒，此为劳风之病〔按"此为"六字衍，《千金》无此六字〕。帝曰：治之奈何？岐伯曰：以救俛仰。巨阳引。精者三日，中年者五日，不精者七日，咳出青黄涕，其状如〔《太素》"如"下有"稠"字〕脓，大如弹丸，从口中若鼻中出〔"鼻中出"下脱"为善"二字，应据《千金》《医心方》补〕，不出则伤肺〔《千金》"不出"上有"若"字〕，伤肺则死也。

Yellow Emperor asked: "What is lao feng (wind syndrome when being overstrained) disease?" Qibo said: "The initial attack of lao feng disease is under the lung, its syndromes appear to be stiffness of the neck and head, dim of the eyesight, spitting sticky sputum, has an aversion to wind, and chill." Yellow Emperor asked: "How to treat it?" Qibo said: "The patient should pay attention to rest chiefly, and next, Yang energy of the Taiyang Channel should be induced to remove the evil energy of depression with the help of taking medicine. With the treatment, a strong man can be recovered in three days, a middle aged man with weaker energy can be recovered in five days, and an old man with deficient energy can be recovered in seven days. The patient will cough up sputum in greenish-yellow colour, like sticky pus in the size of an ammunition ball. It is the best choice to remove the sticky sputum from the mouth or nose. If it can not be cough out, it will injure the lung, and when the lung is injured, the patient will die."

帝曰：有病肾风者，面胕痝〔《甲乙》卷八第五"然"下有"肿"字〕然壅，害于言，可刺不？岐伯曰：虚不当刺，不当刺而刺，后五日其气必至。帝曰：其至何如？岐伯曰：至必

少气时热〔《甲乙》“时”下无“热”字，“时”字属下读〕，时热从胸背上至头，汗出，手热，口乾苦渴〔吴本无“口乾”二字，滑抄本“苦”作“善”〕，小便黄，目下肿，腹中鸣，身重难以〔《甲乙》“难”下无“以”字〕行，月事不来，烦而不能食〔滑抄本“烦而”下无“不能食”三字〕，不能正偃，正偃则欬〔“欬”下脱“甚”字〕，病名曰风水，论在《刺法》中。

Yellow asked: “The patient who suffers from kidney-wind has edema on the face and dorsum of foot, swelling under the eyes like crouching silkworms, and has alalia, can this kind of patient be pricked?” Qibo said: “As the kidney is asthenic, it must not apply pricking, if pricking is applied, the evil-energy will certainly occur.” Yellow Emperor asked: “What is the condition when the evil-energy occurs?” Qibo said: “When the evil-energy comes, the patient will be short of breath, has fever frequently from the chest and back to the head, sweating, has hotness of hands, being thirsty, has yellow urine, swelling of eyelids, borborygmus, heaviness of the body, and find difficulty in moving. If the patient is a woman, her menstruation will cease. The patient will also have irritable and depressed sensation of the chest, being unable to stoop or lift, and he will cough severely if he stoops or lifts. The disease is called the windy-water, which is expounded minutely in《The Method of Pricking》.”

帝曰：愿闻其说：岐伯曰：邪之所凑，其气必虚，阴虚者、阳必凑之，故少气时热而汗出也〔《甲乙》“也”字作“小便黄”〕。小便黄者，少腹中有热也。不能正偃者，胃中不和也。正偃则欬甚，上迫肺也〔“上”上脱“气”字〕。诸有水气者、微肿先见于目下也。帝曰：何以言？岐伯曰：水者阴也，目下亦阴也，腹者至阴之所居，故水在腹者，必使目下肿也。真〔明抄本“真”作“其”〕气上逆，故口苦舌乾〔《太素》“口”上无“故”字〕，卧〔《太素》“卧”作“故”〕不得正偃，正偃则咳出清水也。诸水病者，故不得卧，卧则惊，惊则咳甚也。腹中鸣者，病本于胃也〔明抄本“病”下无“本”字。张琦说：“‘胃’当作‘脾’”〕。薄脾则烦不能食〔《医垒元戎》卷十引“脾”作“胃”〕，食不下者，胃脘隔也。身重难以行者，胃脉在足也。月事不来者，胞脉闭也，胞脉者属心〔《阴阳别论》“属”下有“于”字〕而络于胞中，今气上迫肺，心气不得下通，故月事不来也。帝曰：善。

Yellow Emperor said: “I hope you can tell me the reason about it.” Qibo said: “The accumulation of the evil-energy is mainly due to the deficiency of the healthy-energy. When the kidney is injured by wind-evil, the essence of the kidney will be asthenic, it is called the asthenia of Yin; when Yin is asthenic, Yang will take advantage to invade, and it is the Yang violates Yin. In this case, it will cause the asthenic of the refined-energy, short of breath, fever and sweating of the patient. When the lower abdomen is hot and the heat is in the lower warmer, yellow urine will occur. When the patient fails to lie on his back, it is because his stomach is not harmonious; when the lying on back aggravates the cough, it is because the reversing up of the fluid to the lung. All patients with the syndrome of retention of fluid have slight swelling under the eyes, it is due to the spleen earth fails to control the kidney water, and the water controls instead.”

Yellow Emperor asked: “Why is it?” Qibo said: “Water belongs to Yin, the position under the eye belongs to Yin as well, the abdomen is the place where the extreme Yin lo-

cates, so there is accumulation of water in the abdomen and slight swelling appears under the eyes. When the heart energy reverses up, the mouth will feel bitter, the tongue will become dry and the patient can not lie on his back, if he lies on his back, he will cough out clear water. Every patient invaded by water-energy can not lie on his back, if he lies on his back he will feel startled and uneasy which will cause the coughing even severe. Borborygmus is caused by asthenia of spleen. When the water-energy coerces the stomach, the patient will feel irritating and refuse to eat. When the patient is unable to swallow any food, it is due to there is some hinderance in the stomach. When the body feels heavy and the patient finds difficulty in moving, it is because of the channel energy of stomach runs to the feet downwards. The ceasing of menstruation of a woman is due to the stagnation of the uterus collaterals. The uterus energy belongs to the heart, and the uterus collaterals connect the uterus, when the water energy reverses up to coerce the lung, the heart energy will be unable to communicate with the lower part of the body and the menstruation will cease." Yellow Emperor said: "Good."

逆调论篇第三十四

Chapter 34
Ni Tiao Lun
(On Maladjustments)

黄帝问曰：人身非常〔于鬯说：“‘常’本‘裳’字”〕温也，非常〔应作裳〕热也，为之热而烦满者何也？岐伯对曰：阴气少而阳气胜，故热而烦满也。

Yellow Emperor asked: "When one has fever and feels oppressed but not owning to the wearing of warm clothes, what is the reason?" Qibo answered: " It is due to the deficiency of Yin energy and the overabundant of Yang energy, in this case, it will cause the patient to have fever and feel disquieted."

帝曰：人身非衣寒也，中非有寒气〔《太素》卷三十《身寒》“寒”下无“气”字〕也，寒从中生〔滑抄本“生”作“出”〕者何？岐伯曰：是人多痹气也〔《甲乙》“痹”下无“气也”二字〕，阳气少，阴气多，故身寒如从水中出。

Yellow Emperor said: " When one is wearing thin dresses to the weather, and has no cold-evil inside, but the cold is like sending from inside, what is the reason?" Qibo said: " It is because of the piatient has contracted bi-syndrome, his yang energy is deficient and his Yin energy is plenty, and his body is cold as if he has just come out from the cool water."

帝曰：人有四支〔按“四支”下似脱“先”字〕热，逢风寒〔《全生指迷方》引无“寒”字。“如火”应作“于火”〕如炙如火者何也？岐伯曰：是人者，阴气虚，阳气盛，四支〔《甲乙》“四支”下有“热”字〕者阳也，两阳相得，而阴气虚少，少水〔《太素》“水”上无“少”字，“灭”作“减”〕不能灭盛火，而阳独治，独治者，不能生长也，独胜而止耳，逢风而如炙如火者，是人当肉烁也。

Yellow Emperor said: " Some people have fever in the extremities first, when he encounters wind, he will be hot as if being scorched by the fire, and why is it?" Qibo said: "This kind of people is asthenic and deficient in Yin energy and is overabundant in Yang energy, since the extremities belong to Yang, and when the two Yangs are combining, it will cause the Yin energy to become asthenic and deficient so as not be able to reduce the overabumdant Yang fire, and the Yang energy will be solely overabundant in the exterior. When the Yang energy is prosperous all by itself in the exterior, it will stop growing. Whenever the wind is encountered, the patient will be hot like being scorched, and his muscle will become emaciated gradually."

帝曰：人有身寒，汤火不能热，厚衣不能温，然不冻栗，是为何病？岐伯曰：是人者，素肾气胜，以水为事；太阳气衰，肾脂枯不长；一水不能胜两火〔高世栻“‘一水’七字以下七字，重于此，衍文”〕，肾者水也，而生于骨，肾不生〔《圣济总录》卷二十引“生”作

"荣"〕，则髓不能满，故寒甚至骨也。所以不能冻〔据王注"能"字衍〕栗者，肝一阳也〔孙鼎宜说："当作'胆一阳也'"〕，心二阳也〔孙鼎宜说"当作'心二阴也'"〕，肾孤藏也，一水不能胜〔《甲乙》"胜"下有"上下"二字〕二火，故不能冻栗，病名曰骨痹，是人当挛节也。

Yellow Emperor said: " There is a kind of people who has cold in the body but are not feeling hot when drawing near to the fire, nor feeling warm when wearing thick clothes, yet they are not shivering with cold, and what is the disease?" Qibo said: " This kind of people always has an overabundant kidney energy, they depend on water and wetness to earn their livings which cause their Taiyang energy to become debilitating, and their kidney-adipose stop growing. Kidney is a viscus of water and takes charge of the bone, when the kidney energy is not prosperous, the bone marrow will not be abundant. The reason of his not shivering with cold is: the gallbladder is the prime minister-fire of the first Yang, and the heart is the monarch-fire of the second Yin, kidney is a solitary viscus, and a single kidney water will not be able to overcome the two fires above and bellow of the heart and gallbladder, so, in spite of the coldness, he is not shivering. The disease is called the bone bi-syndrome, and the patient with this syndrome will suffer from contracture of the joints."

帝曰：人之肉苛者，虽近衣絮、犹尚苛也，是谓何疾？岐伯曰：荣气虚卫气实也〔《素问识》云"此七字不相冒，恐是衍文〕，荣气虚则不仁，卫气虚则不用，荣卫俱虚，则不仁且不用，肉如故也，人身与志不相有，曰死。

Yellow Emperor said: " There is a kind of people whose muscle is numb and tough, he has no sensation even when his muscle touches the clothes or cotton, what is the disease?" Qibo said: " When one's Rong energy is asthenic, his skin and muscle will become numb, when one'e Wei energy is asthenic, his limbs can hardly move; when both the Rong and Wei energies are asthenic and weak, numbness and debility will occur, and the muscle will be tough and numb all the more. If one's physique is not suiting his consciousness, he will die."

帝曰：人有逆气不得卧而息有音者；有不得卧而息无音者；有起居如故而息有音者；有得卧，行而喘者；有不得卧，不能行〔滑寿说："能行"上衍"不"字〕而喘者；有不得卧，卧而喘者；皆何藏使然？愿闻其故。岐伯曰：不得卧而息有音者，是阳明之逆也，足三阳者下行，今逆而上行，故息有音也。阳明者，胃脉也，胃者，六腑之海，其气亦下行，阳明逆不得从其道，故不得卧也。《下经》曰：胃不和则卧不安。此之谓也。夫起居如故而息有音者，此肺〔《太素》卷三十《卧息喘逆》"肺"作"脾"〕之络脉逆也；络脉不得随经上下，故留经而不行，络脉之病人也微，故起居如故而息有音也。夫不得卧，卧则喘者，是水气之客也；夫水者，循津液而流也，肾者，水脏，主津液，主卧与喘也。帝曰：善。

Yellow Emperor said: " When suffering from the adverseness of vital energy, some of the patients can not lie down and has sound in his respiration; some can not lie down without the sound of respiration; some can lead a normal daily life but has sound in respiration; some can lie down but has rapid respiration as soon as he moves about; some can not lie down, but can move about with rapid respiration; some can not lie down and will have rapid respiration as soon as lying down. Among all the cases, which one is due to the visceral disease? I hope

to know the reason about them."

Qibo said: "In the case of unable to lie down and has sound of respiration, it is due to the reversing up of the energy of the Yangming Channel. As the energy of the Foot Yangming Channel should run downwards, its reversing up now makes the respiration not going on very smoothly and causes sound. The Yangming is a stomach channel, and the stomach is the sea of the six bowels, the stomach energy should run downwards also; so, if the Yangming energy is reversing, the stomach energy stomach energy will be unable to follow its tract to run down-wards, and the patient can not lie on his back. That is why it is stated in 《Xia Jing》(Lower Classies): 'When the stomach is in disharmony, one can hardly lie still'.

"When one can lead a normal daily life with the sound of respiration, it is due to the impediment of the lung colatterals, and the collateral energy can not move up and down along with the channel energy, and the energy will be retained in the channel instead of running in the collatteral; as the disease of the collaterals is comparatively slighter, the patient can lead a normal daily life, however, there is sound in respiration.

"If the patient finds difficulty in lying down and has rapid respiration as soon as lying down, it is due to the invasion of the water energy to the lung; the water energy is running along with the track of the body fluid, and kidney is a viscus of water and takes charge of the body fluid, when one has rapid respiration when lying down, it is due to the affection of the kidney." Yellow said: "Good."

疟论篇第三十五

Chapter 35
Nue Lun
(On Malaria)

黄帝问曰：夫痎疟皆生于风，其蓄作有时者何也？岐伯对曰：疟之始发也，先起于毫毛，伸欠乃作，寒慄鼓颔，腰脊俱痛，寒去则内外皆热，头痛如破〔《病论》“头痛”下无“如破”二字〕，渴欲冷饮。

Yellow Emperor asked: “All cases of malaria are affected by wind-evil, and they have a certain period of incubation before the time of attacking, Why is it?” Qibo answered: “In the initial attack of malaria, cold emerges from the soft hair, then, the patient will be feeling fatigue both in body and in spirit, shivering with cold, trembling of the soft parts on both sides under the chin and will have pain of loins and spine; when the cold is over, the patient will have fever on both inside and outside, head-ache, thirst, and the desire for cold drink.

帝曰：何气使然？愿闻其道。岐伯曰：阴阳上下交争，虚实更作，阴阳相移也。阳并于阴，则阴实而阳〔《太素》“阳”下有“明”字〕虚，阳明虚，则寒慄鼓颔也；巨阳虚，则腰背头项痛〔《太素》《太平圣惠方》引“背”并作“脊”〕；三阳俱虚，则阴气胜，阴气胜则骨寒而痛；寒生于内，故中外皆寒；阳盛则外热，阴虚则内热，外内皆热则喘而渴，故欲冷饮也。

Yellow Emperor asked: “What is the evil-energy which cause the disease to such a condition?” Qibo said: “It is due to the contention between Yin and Yang below and above, alternation of asthenia and sthenia, and the transforming into each other of Yin and Yang. When the Yang energy is merged by Yin, the Yin energy will be sthenic and the Yangming energy will be asthenic.

“When the energy of the Yangming Channel is asthenic, cold shiverings will hapen and cause the trembling of the both sides under the chin; when the energy of the Taiyang Channel is asthenic, the pain of loins, spine, head and neck will happen; when all the three Yang energies are asthenic, the Yin energy will become excessive and will cause cold-ness and pain of the joints. As the coldness is produced from inside, the patient will feel cold both inside and outside; when Yang is overabundant, exterior heat will produce, when Yin is asthenic, interior heat will produce, if both the exterior and interior heats are produced, the patient will have rapid respiration, thirst and the desire for cold drink.

此皆得之〔《太素》《病论》《太平圣惠方》“此”下并无“皆”字〕夏伤于暑，热气盛，藏于皮肤之内，肠胃之外，此荣气之所舍也。此令人汗〔《太素》，《甲乙》，《病源》“汗”下有“出”字〕空疏，腠理开，因得秋气，汗出遇风，及得之以浴〔《太素》《病源》“及”作

“乃”〕，水气舍于皮肤之内，与卫气并居。卫气者，昼日行于阳〔《甲乙》“昼”下无“日”字〕，夜行于阴，此气得阳而外出，得阴而内搏，内外相薄〔《太素》《病源》并无“内外相搏”四字〕，是以日作。

“This kind of disease occurs when the patient is injured by the summer-heat in summer. When the heat is overabundant, it will hide in the skin and beyond the stomach and intestine, ie., the evil-energy will reside in the Ying-energy.

“The summer-heat can cause sweating, the flaccidity of the muscle and the openning of the striae of skin, whenever the autumn energy which is chilling is encountered, the sweating patient will be infected by wind-evil, and the disease will turn to the worse after taking a bath. Thus, when the wind-evil and water-energy retained in the skin and join the Wei-energy, malaria will break out. The Wei-energy circulates in the Yang channels in day time and circulates in the Yin channels in night time, when the evil-energy merges into the Yang-energy, it will disperse externally, when it merges into the Yin energy, it will invade internally, in this way, the disease will attack once a day.”

帝曰：其间日而作者何也？岐伯曰：其气之〔《圣济总录》引“之”下有“所”字〕舍深，内薄于阴，阳气独发，阴邪内著，阴与阳争不得出，是以间日而作也。

Yellow Emperor asked: “Some of the malaria disease attack every other day, and why is it?” Qibo said: “It is because the situation of the evil-energy is rather deep for to approach the Yin energy which is inside, so the Yang energy can only operate outside all by itself, and the malarial-evil will still be retained inside. As the evil-energy can not be dispersed after the contention between Yin and Yang, so, the disease can only attack every other day.”

帝曰：善。其作日晏与其日早者，何气使然？岐伯曰：邪气客于风府，循膂而下，卫气一日一夜大会于风府，其明日〔《病源》“日”下不叠“日”字〕日下一节，故其作也晏〔《病源》“作”下无“也晏此先客于脊背也每止于风府”十四字〕，此先客于脊背也。每至于风府，则腠理开，腠理开则邪气入，邪气入则病作，以此日作稍益晏〔《病源》、《外台》“以此所”作“此所以”。孙鼎宜说：“‘稍’字疑衍”〕也。其出于风府〔《病源》作“卫气之行风府”〕，日下一节〔《太素》“节”作“椎”〕，二十五日下至骶骨；二十六日入于脊内，注于伏膂之脉〔周本“注”下无“于”字，《甲乙》“伏膂”作“太冲”〕；其气上行〔《病源》作“伏冲脉其行”〕，九日出于缺盆之中。其气日高〔《病源》“日高”作“即上”〕，故作日益早也〔《病源》作“故其病稍早发”〕。其间日发者，由邪气内薄于五藏，横连募原也。其道远，其气深，其行迟，不能与卫气俱行，不得皆出〔《太平圣惠方》引无“俱行不得”四字作“不能与卫气皆出”〕，故间日乃作也。

Yellow Emperor said: “Good. Some of the malaria diseases attack earlier day after day, and some of them attack later day after day. What is the reason?” Qibo said: “After the invasion of the evil-energy to the Fengfu (Wind Mansion) point, it shifts downwards along the vertebrae one after another; the Wei-energy often meet the evil-energy at the Fengfu point by taking a day and night time, as the Wei-energy shifts a vertebra downwards each day, thus, the meeting of the evil-energy and the Wei-energy will be later day after day, and the time of the disease-attack will be later day after day also. This is the condition when the evil-

energy resides in the spine. Whenever the Wei-energy reaches the Fengfu point, the striae of skin will open, the evil-energy will take advantage to invade and the disease will break out, this is the reason why the disease breaks out later day after day. When the Wei-energy operates in the Fengfu point, the evil-energy will shift down for a vertebra daily, it reaches the sacral bone below on the twenty-fifth day, reaches the inner side of the spine and pour into the Taichong Chennel on the twenty sixth day, and then it goes up along the Taichong Channel and reaches the Tiantu (Sky Prominence) point of the Ren Channel on the ninth day of ascent. As the evil energy is going upwards and drawing nearer and nearer, it will join the Wei-energy earlier day after day, and the attack of the disease is earlier day after day. As to the case of attacking on every other day, it is due to the evil-energy coercing the viscera inside and connecting the membrane of the diaphram, ie., the zone under the navel, since the distance is comparatively far, the penetration is comparatively deep, and its operation is comparatively slow, it can not come out along with the Wei-energy on the same day, thus, it attacks every other day."

帝曰：夫子言卫气每至于风府，腠理乃发，发则邪气入，入则病作。今卫气日下一节，其气之发也〔《病源》无此五字〕，不当风府，其日作者〔《病源》无此四字〕奈何？岐伯曰：此邪气客于头项循膂而下者也〔林校云："按全元起本及《甲乙》、《太素》自'此邪气客于头项'至'则病作故'八十八字并无。按《病源》亦无此八十八字〕，故虚实不同，邪中异所，则不得当其风府也。故邪中于头项者，气至头项而病；中于背者，气至背而病；中于腰脊者，气至腰脊而病；中于手足者，气至手足而病。卫气之所在，与邪气相合〔明抄本《太素》《病源》并作"舍"〕，则病作。故风无常府，卫气之所发，必开其腠理，邪气之所合，则其府也〔《甲乙》《病源》"府也"并作"病作"〕。

Yellow Emperor said: "As you have said when the Wei-energy reaches the Fengfu point, the striae will open, and the evil-energy will take advantage to invade and cause the dissease, now, the Wei-energy shifts down for a vertebra daily, its has not reached the Fengfu point, but the disease attacks every day, what is the reason?" Qibo said: "The above statement is indicating the condition when the evil-energy invades the head and neck and moves down along the vertebrae of the spine. since the conditions of men are different, some are asthenic and some are sthenic, and the location contracting the evil energy are different, so, the disease is not necessary to break out at the time when the evil-energy reaches the Fengfu point. For instance, when the head contracts the evil-energy, if the Wei-energy reaches and combines with the evil-energy on the head and neck, the disease will break out; when the back contracts the evil-energy, if the Wei-energy reaches and combines the evil-energy on the back. the disease will break out; when the lumbas and spine contract the evil-energy, if the Wei-energy reaches and combines with the evil-energy on the lumbas and spine, the disease will break out, if the Wei-energy reaches and combines with the evil-energy on the limbs, the disease will break out. In a word, anywhere the Wei-energy exists and combines with the evil-energy, it will cause the attack of the disease. Therefore, although the invading location of the evil-energy is not certain, yet, whenever the Wei-energy corresponds

to it, the striae will open, the evil-energy will retains and causes disease."

帝曰：善。夫风之与疟也，相似同类，而风独常在，疟得有时而休者何也？岐伯曰：风气留其处，故常在〔《病源》、《外台》无"故常在"三字〕，疟气随经络，沉以内薄〔林校引《甲乙》作"次以内传"〕，故卫气应乃作。

Yellow Emperor said: "Good. It seems that the diseases of wind-evil and malaria are about the same, but what is the reason that the wind-evil usually has no intermittence in attacking and the malaria sometimes attack in regular time?" Qibo said: "The wind-evil often remains in the same place, and the malaria is circulating along with the channels and collaterals and is transmitted internally in sequence, the disease can only break out until the Wei-energy responds with the evil-energy."

帝曰：疟先寒而后热者何也！岐伯曰：夏伤于大暑〔《病源》"于"下无"大"字〕，其汗大出，腠理开发，因遇夏〔《太素》"夏"下无"气"字，于鬯说"水"字是"小"字之误〕气凄沧之水寒，藏于腠理〔按"腠理"二字衍〕皮肤之中，秋伤于风，则病成矣。夫寒者，阴气也，风者，阳气也〔《太平圣惠方》引"阴""阳"下皆无"气"字〕，先伤于寒而后伤于风，故先寒而后热也，病以时作，名曰寒疟。

Yellow Emperor asked: "When the disease of malaria occurs, the patient feels cold first and then feels hot, what is the reason?" Qibo said: "When one is infected by summer-heat in summer and perspires greatly, his striae will be openned and the mild cold of summer will take advantage to invade, and it will be retained in the skin; when one is infected by wind-evil in autumn, it will become malaria. As cold belongs to Yin and wind belongs to Yang, when one is infected by cold first and then infected by wind, he will be feeling cold first and then feeling hot. The time of the disease-attack is regular, and it is called the cold-type malaria."

帝曰：先热而后寒者何也！岐伯曰：此先伤于风，而后伤于寒，故先热而后寒也，亦以时作，名曰温疟。

Yellow Emperor asked: "In a certain kind of malaria, the patient is feeling hot first, and then feeling cold, what is the reason?" Qibo said: "This is due to his being injured by Yang-evil of wind first, and then by Yin-evil of cold. The time of attack of this disease is also regular, and it is called the warm-type malaria.

其但热而不寒者，阴气先〔《太素》"气"下无"先"字〕绝，阳气独发，则少气烦冤，手足热而欲呕，名曰瘅疟。

"If the patient is feeling hot only and not feeling cold, it is because of the Yin energy of the patient is extremely deficient to cause the Yang energy prosperous all by itself, in this case, the patient will be short of breath and become disquieted, feeling hot in the hands and feet, and feeling like to vomit. The disease is called the dan-malaria."

帝曰：夫经言有余者写之，不足者补之。今热为有余，寒为不足。夫疟者之寒，汤火不能温也，及其热，冰水不能寒也，此皆有余不足之类。当此之时，良工不能止，必须其自衰乃刺之，其故何也？愿闻其说。

Yellow Emperor said: "It is stated in the classics of medicine that it should be purged

when there is a surplus and should be invigorated when there is a deficiency. Presently the hotness is having a surplus and coldness is deficient; the coldness of malaria can not be warmed by hot water nor fire, and its hotness can not be cooled even by iced water; since the coldness and hotness are caused by of the surplus and deficiency, so when it is hot or cold, even a good physician can do nothing to stop it, and acupuncture can only be applied after the cold or heat is declined, why is it so? I hpoe you can tell me the reason."

岐伯曰：经言无刺熇熇之热，无刺浑浑之脉，无刺漉漉之汗，故〔明抄本“为”上无“故”字〕为其病逆，未可治也。夫疟之始发也，阳气并于阴〔“阳”下“气”字衍〕，当是之时，阳虚而阴盛〔“盛”应作“实”〕，外无〔《素问玄机原病式》引“外无”下有“阳”字〕气，故先寒栗也；阴气逆极，则复出之阳，阳与阴复并于外〔张琦说：“外”应作“内”〕，则阴〔周本“阴虚”上无“则”字〕虚而阳实，故先热而渴〔《太素》“故”下无“先”字〕。夫疟气者，并于阳则阳胜，并于阴则阴胜，阴胜则寒，阳胜则热。疟〔《甲乙》“疟”下无“气者”二字〕者，风寒之〔林校引《甲乙》“之”下有“暴”字〕气不常也，病极则复，至病之发也，如火之热，如风雨不可当也。故经言曰：方其盛时〔《太素》“盛时”下有“勿敢”二字〕必毁，因其衰也，事必大昌，此之谓也。夫疟之未发也，阴未并阳，阳未并阴，因而调之，真气得安，邪气乃亡〔《太素》“亡”作“已”〕，故工不能治其已发，为其气逆也。

Qibo said: "It is stated in the classics of medicine that it must not prick when the patient's fever is high, must not prick when the pulse condition is disorderly, and must not prick when the patient is perspiring greatly. This is because the treatment must not be carried on when the disease is going on reversely. In the initial attack of malaria, the exterior Yang merges into the interior Yin, by this time, Yang is asthenic and Yin is sthenic, and the asthenic Yang superficies will be unable to guard outside, so the patient will be shivering with cold first. When the Yin energy reverses to the extreme point, it will turn to the opposite and come out from the Yin and merges with Yang at the exterior. By this time, Yin will be asthenic and Yang will be sthenic, and the patient will be hot and thirsty. When the malarial-evil merges into Yang, the Yang energy will become excessive, when it merges into Yin, the Yin energy will become excessive. When the Yin energy is excessive, the patient will be feeling cold; when the Yang energy is excessive, the patient will be feeling hot. The condition of malaria is changable due to the irregular variations of sudden wind-cold evil, when it is hot to the extreme point, the cold-energy of Yin evil will occur; when it is cold to the extreme point, the hotness of Yang evil will occur. When malaria attacks, the patient can be as hot as the burning fire or as cold as the irresistable wind and rain. Therefore, it is stated in the classics of medicine: 'when the evil-energy is prosperous, one must not attack the evil, the treatment can only be effective when the evil-energy is declined'. Before the attack of malaria when the Yin-energy has not yet been merged into Yang or the Yang-energy has not yet been merged into Yin, a treating in time will not injure the healthy energy and the evil-energy can be removed. The reason of a physician does not treat when the disease is attacking is to avoid the confusion of the healthy-energy and the evil-energy."

帝曰：善。攻之奈何？早晏何如？岐伯曰：疟之且发也，阴阳之且移也，必从四末始也。

阳已伤，阴从之，故先其时〔《甲乙》“故”下有“气未并”三字〕坚束其处，令邪气不得入，阴气不得出，审候见之，在孙络盛坚而血者皆取之，此真〔《太素》“真”作“直”〕往而未得并者也。

Yellow Emperor said: “Good. But how to treat malaria? Should it be treated earlier or later?”

Qibo said: “When malaria is about to attack, the Yin energy and Yang energy will be shifting each other, and the shifting will begin from the four extremities. If the Yang energy is injured, the Yin energy will be affected in the wake of it. So, before the emerging of Yin and Yang, the terminal of the extremities of the patient should be bound firmly with strings to hinder the going in of the evil-energy and the coming out of the Yin-energy, then, examine carefully the fully filled minute collaterals and the location where the blood stagnates, prick to let out the blood and thus the genuine evil will be removed so as to avoid its emergence into the body.”

帝曰：疟不发，其应何如？岐伯曰：疟气者，必更盛更虚，当〔《太素》《甲乙》“当”并作“随”〕气之所在也，病在阳，则热而脉躁；在阴，则寒而脉静；极则阴阳俱衰，卫气相离，故病得〔明抄本“得”作“乃”〕休；卫气集，则复病也。

Yellow Emperor asked: “What is the condition of malaria before it attacks?” Qibo said: “The overabundance and debility of malarial energy take place in turn, it attacks along with the presence of the evil-energy: when the disease is in the Yang, the patient will have fever and his pulse condition will be impetuous and rapid; when the disease is in the Yin, the patient will be cold and his pulse condition will be deep and calm; when the attack of the disease is in the extreme condition, both the Yin and Yang energies will be declining, when the Wei-energy is devorced from the evil-energy, the disease will cease; when the Wei-energy merges with the evil-energy again, the disease will reappear.”

帝曰：时有间二日或至数日发，或渴或不渴，其故何也？岐伯曰：其间日者，邪气与卫气客于六府〔《素问识》云“考上文并无客于六府之说，疑是‘风府’之讹”〕，而有时相失，不能相得，故休数日乃作也。疟者，阴阳更胜也，或甚或不甚，故或渴或不渴。

Yellow Emperor said: “In malaria disease, sometimes it attacks in every other two days, and sometimes it attacks in every several other days; some of the patients are thirsty during the attack, and some are not, what is the reason?” Qibo said: Sometimes the meeting of the evil-energy and the Wei-energy at the Fengfu point is staggering, they can not come out at the same time together due to delay, besides, the Yin and Yang abundance in malaria is alternating and the extents of overabundance and deficiency are often different, so, some of the patient is thirsty and some are not.”

帝曰：论言夏伤于暑，秋必病疟。今疟不必应者何也？岐伯曰：此应四时者也。其病异形者，反四时也。其以秋病者寒甚，以冬病者寒不甚，以春病者恶风，以夏病者多汗。

Yellow Emperor said: “It was stated in the classics of medicine: ‘when one is infected by summer-heat in summer, he will certainly contract malaria in autumn’. but nowadays, the condition is not necessarily like this, and why is it?” Qibo said: “The text of ‘when one is in-

fected by summer-heat in summer, he will certainly contract malaria in autumn' is indicating when it is agreeable with the regular patern of the disease attack in the four seasons, but the malaria with different symptoms does not follow the regular pattern. When malaria attacks in autumn, the patient will have severe cold, when it attacks in winter, the patient will have slight cold, when it attacks in spring, the patient will have the syndrome of having an aversion to wind, when it attacks in summer, the patient will have hyperhidrosis."

帝曰：夫病温疟与寒疟而皆安舍〔《太素》"夫"下无"病"字，而皆作"各"〕，舍于何藏？岐伯曰：温疟者，得之冬中于风，寒气藏于骨髓之中，至春则阳气大发，邪气不能自出〔《甲乙》"邪"作"寒"，何梦瑶说'邪'上当有"若"字〕，因遇大暑，脑髓烁，肌肉消，腠理发泄，或有所用力〔《太素》《病源》"或"并作"因"〕，邪气与汗皆出，此病藏于肾〔《千金》"病"下有"邪气先"三字〕，其气先从内出之于外也。如是者，阴虚而阳盛，阳盛则热矣，衰则气复反入，入则阳虚，阳虚则寒矣〔《外台》"则"下有"复"字〕，故先热而后寒，名曰温疟。

Yellow Emperor asked: "Where do the warm-type malaria and the cold-type reside respectively? Which viscus do they retain in?" Qibo said: "The warm-type malaria is due to the infection of wind-evil in winter, as the cold-energy is retained in the bone marrow, when the Yang energy begin to grow in spring, and if the evil-energy can not be let out all by itself, the patient, when encountering the summer-heat, will feel fatigue, dizziness of head, emaciation of muscle, and his striae will open, by this time, if he exert his strength to do some physical labour, the evil-energy will be excreted along with the sweat. In the disease, the evil-energy harbours in the kidney first, when the disease attacks, the evil-energy will come out from inside. In the beginning of the disease, the Yin energy is asthenic and the Yang energy is partial overabundant which causes fever of the body, but when the Yang partial overabundance come to its extreme, the evil-energy will return into Yin again. When the evil-energy enters into the Yin, Yang will become asthenic again and causes cold. The condition of this disease is hot first and then cold, and it is called the warm-type malaria."

帝曰：瘅疟何如？岐伯曰：瘅疟者，肺素有热，气盛于身，厥逆上冲〔《甲乙》、《外台》并作"厥气逆上"〕，中气实而不外泄〔《太平圣惠方》"气"上无"中"字〕，因有所用力，腠理开，风寒舍于皮肤之内，分肉之间而发，发则阳气盛，阳气盛而不衰则病矣，其气不及于阴〔《太素》、《甲乙》并作"不反之阴"〕，故但热而不寒，气内藏于心〔按"气"上脱"邪"字，应据《千金》补〕而外舍于分肉之间，令人消烁脱〔明抄本"脱"作"肌"〕，肉，故命曰瘅疟。帝曰善。

Yellow Emperor asked: "What is the condition of dan-malaria?" Qibo said: "Dan-malaria is due to the heat in lung in advance, when the lung energy is abundant, it will reverse up, and the sthenic energy will not be able to excrete outside; when the patient happens to exert his strength in labour, his striae will be openned and the wind-evil will take chance to invade, retain itself between the skin and the muscle to cause disease, and the disease will cause the Yang-energy to become overabundant, if the abundante condition sustains, the patient will have fever. As the evil-energy does not return into Yin, the patient will be hot but

has no aversion to cold. In this disease. the evil-energy is harbouring internally and is retaining externally between the muscles. It may cause muscle emaciation of the patient, and the discease is called the dan-malaria." Yellow Emperor said: "Good."

刺疟篇第三十六

Chapter 36
Ci Nue
(On Treating Malaria with Acupuncture)

足太阳之疟，令人腰痛头重，寒从背起，先寒后热，熇熇暍暍然，热止汗出〔《甲乙》巢元方“暍暍”作“渴渴”，《太素》“熇熇暍暍然热止汗出”作“渴渴止汗出”〕，难已，刺郄中出血。

The malaria of Foot Taiyang Channel causes the patient to have lumbago, heaviness of head and chill from the back. He feels cold first and then feels hot, and when the fever is over, he perspires severely. This kinds of malaria can hardly be healed. When treating, it should prick the Weizhong (Popliteal Certre BL. 40) point until bleeding.

足少阳之疟，令人身体解㑊〔《病论》“㑊”作“倦”〕，寒不甚，热不甚〔《甲乙》无“热不甚”三字〕，恶见人，见人心惕惕然，热多汗出甚，刺足少阳。

The malaria of Foot Shaoyang Channel causes the patient to have fatigue of the body, a slight cold, has aversion of meeting people and being frightened when meeting people; the duration of the fever is comparatively long, and the patient perspires a lot. When treating, prick the Foot Shaoyang Channel.

足阳明之疟，令人先寒，洒淅〔按此衍“洒淅”二字，所遗“洒淅”二字应下读〕洒淅，寒甚久乃热，热去汗出〔“出”字误，据王注应作“已”〕，喜见日月〔《病源》、《圣济总录》引“日”下无“月”字〕光火气，乃快然，刺足阳明跗上〔《甲乙》“跗上”下有“及调冲阳”四字〕。

The malaria of Foot Yangming Channel causes the patient to have severe cold first; after a period, he will have fever, and when the heat comes down, the perspiration stops along with it. This kind of patient desires for seeing the sunlight and the flame of fire, and will feel comfortable when seeing them. When treating, prick the Chongyang (Rushing Yang ST. 42) point of Foot Yangming Channel on the dorsum of the foot.

足太阴之疟，令人不乐，好太息，不嗜食，多寒热〔《甲乙》作“多寒少热”〕汗出，病至则善呕，呕已乃衰，即取之〔《甲乙》“取之”下有“足太阴”三字〕。

The malaria of Foot Taiyin Channel causes the patient to become depressed, he sighs often, reluctant to eat with much cold and little fever. He has sweat and vomits when the disease attacks, and being relieved after vomitting. When treating, prick the Gongsun (Collateral Point of Spleen Channel SP. 4) point of the Foot Taiyin Channel.

足少阴之疟，令人〔《外台》引“令人”下有“闷”字〕呕吐甚，多寒热，热多寒少，欲闭户牖而处，其病难已。

The malaria of Foot Shaoyin Channel causes the patient to become depressed, he vomits severly, has cold and fever frequently with much fever and little cold, and he desires to close the door and the windows and stay in the room. This kind of malaria can hardly be healed.

足厥阴之疟，令人腰痛少腹满，小便不利，如癃状〔据《图经》卷五《太冲》条应作"淋淋"〕，非癃也〔似系"如癃"之旁记混入正文〕，数便，意恐惧〔林校云："按《甲乙经》"数便意"三字作"数噫"二字〕，气不足，腹〔《太素》"腹"作"肠"〕中悒悒，刺足厥阴。

The malaria of Foot Jueyin Channel causes the patient to have lumbago, distention of the lower abdomen, dysuria like stranguria. He eructates and becomes frightened often, has deficiency of breath and impediment of the intestine. When treating, prick the Taichong (Great Rush LR. 3) point of the Foot Jueyin Channel.

肺疟者，令人心寒，寒甚〔《千金》"甚"下有"则发"二字〕热，热间〔《千金》"间"下有"则"字〕善惊，如有所见者，刺手太阴阳明。

The malaria of lung causes the patient to feel cold from the heart, when the coldness is in the extreme, fever will come in the wake of it. During the fever, the patient is apt to become frightened as if he has seen something. When treating, prick the Lieque (Branching Crevice LU. 7) point of the Hand Taiyin Channel and the Hegu (Connected Valleys LI. 4) point of the Hand Yangming Channel.

心疟者，令人烦心甚，欲得〔《千金》《外台》"得"作"饮"〕清水，反〔《甲乙》无"反"字〕寒多，不甚热，刺手少阴。

The malaria of heart causes the patient to have strong feverish sensation accompanied with restlessness, desire of drinking cold water, and he has much coldness with little fever. When treating, prick the Shenmen (Spiritual Gate HT. 7) point of the Hand Shaoyin Channel.

肝疟者，令人色苍苍然，太息〔《甲乙》无此二字〕，其状若死者。刺足厥阴见血。

The malaria of liver causes the patient to have pale and green complexion like a dead man. When treating, prick the Foot Jueyin Channel until bleeding.

脾疟者，令人寒，腹中痛，热则肠中〔《太素》杨注《医垒元戎》无"中"字〕鸣，鸣已〔《千金》无"鸣已"二字〕汗出，刺足太阴。

The malaria of spleen causes the patient to have cold which he can hardly bear, pain in the abdomen, borborygmus due to the shifting down of the spleen-heat, and perspiration. When treating, prick the Shangqiu (Shang Hill SP. 5) point of the Foot Taiyin Channel.

肾疟者，令人洒洒〔《甲乙》《千金翼方》《外台》"洒"作"悽"〕然，腰脊痛，宛转〔《医垒元戎》引"宛转"上有"不能"二字〕，大便难，目眴眴〔《病源》"目"下有"眩"字〕然，手足寒，刺足太阳少阴。

The malaria of kidney causes the patient to feel cold and pain in the loins and spine that he can hardly turn about, he also has retention of feces, dizziness, and coldness of the hands and feet. When pricking, prick the Foot Taiyang and Shaoyin Channels.

胃疟者，令人且〔《太素》"且"作"疸"〕病也，善饥而不能食，食而〔《千金翼亏》无"食而"二字〕支满腹大，刺足阳明太阴横脉出血。

The malaria of stomach causes heat in the stomach, the patient feels hungry but he is reluctant to eat, he also has swelling and distention of the abdomen. When treating, prick the Foot Yangming and Taiyin Channel and Collaterals until bleeding.

疟发身方热，刺跗上动脉，开其空，出其〔《甲乙》“出”下无“其”字〕血，立寒；疟方欲寒，刺手阳明太阴，足阳明太阴。疟脉满大急，刺背俞，用中针，傍伍胠俞各一，适肥瘦出其〔《甲乙》“出”下无“其”字〕血也。疟脉小实急，灸胫少阴，刺指井。疟脉满大急，刺背俞，用五胠俞背俞各一，适行至于血也〔林校云：“疟脉满”以下二十二字与前文重复，当从删消”〕。

When the body is having a fever after the attack of malaria, prick the artery on the dorsum of foot to open the acupoint, after the blood is let out, the fever will be declined.

If the patient of malaria is about to become cold, it should prick the Hand Yangming and Taiyin Channels, and the Foot Yangming and Taiyin Channels.

If the pulse condition of the patient with malaria is full, large and rapid, it should prick the shu-points at the back with the needle of middle size, prick each from the five shu-points near the lateral chest wall below the axillae and let out some blood according to the stoutness and leanness of the patient.

If the pulse condition of the patient is small, full and rapid, treat the points of Shaoyin Channel on the shank with moxibustion, and prick the Well points at the tips of fingers and toes.

疟脉缓大虚，便宜〔胡本，谈本，赵本“便”下无“宜”字〕用药，不宜用针。凡治疟，先发如食顷，乃可以治，过之则失时也。诸疟而脉不见〔《甲乙》“而”作“如”〕，刺十指间出血，血去必已，先视身之赤如小豆者尽取之。十二疟者，其发各不同时，察其病形，以知其何脉之病也。先其发〔《太素》“先其”下有“病”字〕时如食顷而刺之，一刺则衰，二刺则知，三刺则已；不已，刺舌下两脉出血，不已，刺郄中盛经出血，又刺项已下侠脊者必已。舌下两脉者，廉泉也。

When the pulse condition of the patient with malaria is slow, large and weak, it should be treated with medicine instead of with acupuncture.

In treating malaria, it should be treated before the attack of about the period of taking a meal, if this period of time is passed, the oppotunity will be missed.

To various kinds of malaria of which the pulse condition is hidden, it should prick hastly between the ten fingers until bleeding, when the blood is let out, the evil-energy will be removed. When there is some red points like adzuk beans appear on the skin, it should be prickd to cause them vanish.

The twelve kinds of malaria stated above are different in appearance when attacking, when examining the symptoms, one can distiguish to what channel the disease belongs. If the pricking is carried out in advance of about the period of a meal, the evil-energy can be alleviated after pricking once, to have significant curative effect of the disease after pricking twice; and the patient can be recovered after pricking thrice. If the patient is not recovered, prick the two blood vessels under the tongue until bleeding. If he is not recovered again,

prick the Weizhong (Popliteal Centre BL. 40) point of which the blood is abundant in the channel and collaterals until bleeding, then, prick the Dazhu (Great Axle BL. 11) and the Fengmen (Windy Gate BL. 12) points under the neck, and the disease will sure to be recovered. The two blood vessels under the tongue are the Lianchuan (Tongue Spring RN. 23) points of Ren Channel.

刺疟者，必先问其病之所先发者，先刺之。先头痛及重者，先刺头上及两额两眉间出血。先项背痛者，先刺之。先腰脊痛者，先刺郄中出血。先手臂痛者，先刺手少阴阳明十指间。先足胫痠痛者，先刺足阳明十指〔按“足阳明”疑应作“足阴阳”〕间出血。风疟，疟发则汗出恶风，刺三阳经背俞之血者。骺痠痛甚〔《甲乙》“痛”下无“甚”字〕，按之不可，名曰胕〔吴本“胕”作“附”〕髓病，以镵针针绝骨出血，立已。身体小痛，刺至阴〔《甲乙》无“至阴”二字，“刺”字连下读〕，诸阴之井无出血，间日一刺。疟不渴，间日而作，刺足太阳；渴而间日作，刺足少阳；温疟汗不出，为五十九刺。

When treating malaria by pricking, it must be made clear by asking the patient which part of the body has the pain first, and the part should be pricked first. If the patient has pain and heaviness on the head first, it must prick the head, the two temples and between the two eyebows first until bleeding; when the disease attacks the neck and back first, it should prick the neck and back first; when the loins and spine is painful first, prick the Weizhong (Popliteal Centre BL. 40) point first until bleeding. When it is painful in the arm first, prick the points between the ten fingers of the Hand Yin and Yang Channels.

When it is sore in the shank first, prick the points between the ten fingers of the Foot Yin and Yang Channels.

When the wind-malaria attacks, the patient perspires and has aversion to wind, prick the shu-points of the Taiyang Channel at the back until bleeding.

When the shank is sore and the patient can not withstand pressing, it is called the disease of the marrow in bone, prick the Juegu (ie. Xuanzhoug or Suspended Bell GB. 39) point until bleeding and the pain will be relieved.

If the body is painful slightly, prick the Jing points of the Various Yin Channels every other day without letting out any blood.

If the patient of malaria is not thirsty and the disease attacks every other day, prick the Foot Taiyang Channel. If the patient is thirsty and the disease attacks every other day, prick the Foot Shaoyang Channel.

To the patients of warm-type malaria with no perspiration, apply the Fifty-nine Pricking Therapy.

气厥论篇第三十七

Chanpter 37
Qi Jue Lun
(The Diseases Due to the Inter-transference of Cold and Heat Evils Between Various Organs)

黄帝问曰：五藏六府，寒热相移者何？岐伯曰：肾移寒于肝〔明抄本“肝”作“脾”〕痈〔《医垒元戎》引“痈”上有“发为”二字〕肿少气。脾移寒于肝，痈肿筋挛。肝移寒于心，狂隔〔《太素》“隔”作“鬲”〕中。心移寒于肺，肺消〔《甲乙》、《圣济总论》“肺消”上并有“为”字〕，肺消者饮一溲二，死不治。肺移寒于肾，为涌水，涌水者，按腹不坚〔《甲乙》“按”下有“其”字，《太素》“不”作“下”〕，水气客于大肠，疾行则〔《甲乙》“则”作“肠”〕鸣濯濯，如囊裹浆，水之病也〔《太素》作“治主肺者”〕。

Yellow Emperor asked: "What are the conditions of the inter-transference of cold and heat between the five solid organs and the six hollow organs?"

Qibo said: "When the cold of kidney is transfered into the spleen, the patient will be swelling and short of breath.

"When the cold of spleen is transfered into the liver, the patient will have the disease of carbuncle and the contraction of the tendons.

"When the cold of liver is transfered into the heart, the patient will have mania and the impediment of heart-energy.

"When the cold of heart is transfered into the lung, diabetes involving the lung will occur, the patient's urine will be of two times with that of the water he drinks. It is a fatal disease which can by no means to be cured.

"When the cold of lung is transfered into the kidney, water will be retained in the large intestine and cause failure of lowering the abdomen when being pressed. As the water is invading the large intestine, one can hear the water moving inside when walks rapidly like water in a bag, and, to this diesese, it should mainly treat the lung.

脾移热于肝，则为惊衄。肝移热于心，则死。心移热于肺，传为鬲消。肺移热于肾，传为柔痓。肾移热于脾，传为虚，〔张琦说：“‘虚’字衍”》〕肠澼，死，不可治。胞移热于膀胱，则癃〔四库本“癃”作“必”〕溺血。膀胱移热于小肠，鬲肠〔《伤寒论》引“肠”作“热”〕不便，上为口糜〔《太素》“糜”作“靡”〕。小肠移热于大肠，为虙瘕〔《太素》作“密疝”〕，为沉。大肠移热于胃，善食而瘦入〔按“入”字疑衍〕，谓之食亦。胃移热于胆，亦曰食亦。胆移热于脑，则辛頞〔“頞”音扼“頞”又称“下极”位于左右侧内眦之中内〕鼻渊，鼻渊者〔《圣济总论》引无“鼻渊”以下九字〕，浊涕下不止也，传为衄蔑瞑目，故得之气厥也〔《太素》作“厥气”〕。

"When the heat of spleen is transfered into the liver, the patient will be shocked with terror and has epistaxis.

"When the heat of liver is transfered into the heart, the patient will die.

"When the heat of heart is transfered into the lung, if being protracted and developed, it will become diabetes involving the upper warmer.

"When the heat of lung is transfered into the kidney, if being protracted and developed, it will become soft-type convulsive disease.

"When the heat of the kidney is transfered into the spleen, if being protracted and developed, it will become pi from intestine (bloody stool) which can hardly be healed.

"When the heat of uterus is transfered into the urinary bladder, the patient will have hematuria.

"When the heat of the bladder is transfered into the small intestine, stagnation of heat, retention of faeces and the up-going of heat will occur, and it will cause aphthosis.

"When the heat of the small intestine is transfered into the large intestine, if the stagnated heat is not dispersed, abdominal mass or hemorrhoid will occur.

"When the heat of the large intestine is transfered into the stomach, the patient will eat plenty but being emaciated, and the disease is called the polyphagia-emaciation syndrome.

"When the heat of the stomach is transfered into the gallbladder, it is also called the polyphagia-emaciation syndrome.

"When the heat of the gallbladder is transfered into the brain, one will feel pungent in the nose bridge and will have sinusitis, if being protracted and developed, epistaxis and blur vision of the eyes will occur, and they are caused by the reversing up of the gallbladder energy."

咳论篇第三十八

Chapter 38
Ke Lun
(On Cough)

黄帝问曰：肺之令人咳何也？岐伯对曰：五藏六府皆令人咳，非独肺也。帝曰：愿闻其状。岐伯曰：皮毛者肺之合也，皮毛受邪气〔《伤寒明理论》引“邪”作“寒”〕，邪气以从其合也。其寒饮食入胃，从肺脉上至〔《太素》“至”作“注”〕于肺，则肺寒〔《太素》《伤寒明理论》引并无“则肺寒”三字〕，肺寒则外内合邪，因而客之，则为肺咳。五藏各以其时受病，非其时，各传以与之。人与天地相参，故五藏各以治时，感于寒则受病，微则为咳，甚则为泄为痛。乘秋则〔《太素》林校引全本无“乘秋则”三字〕肺先受邪，乘春则肝先受之，乘夏则心先受之，乘至阴〔《外台》《太平圣惠方》并引作“季夏”〕则脾先受之，乘冬则肾先受之。

Yellow Emperor asked: “The lung can cause one cough, and why is it?” Qibo answered: “Not only the lung but all the five solid and six hollow organs can cause one cough.”

Yellow Emperor said: “I hope you can tell me in detail.” Qibo said: “The skin and hair take charge of the superficies and they are in concert with the lung, when the skin and hair contract the cold-energy, the cold-energy will intrude into the lung. If one has drunken cold water, or has taken cold food, the cold-energy will enter into the stomach and ascend to the lung through the lung vessel and cause the lung to contract cold. In this way, the cold-evil inside and outside will be combined and retained in the lung, and cough will occur.

“As to the cough of the five solid organs and six hollow organs, they are the diseases affected in the season by which the five solid organs dominate respectively, they are not affected in the season by which the lung dominates, but are transfered from the diseases of the five solid organs.

“Man is corresponding to heaven and earth. When the five solid organs being affected by the cold-evil in their respective dominating seasons, one will contract disease. If the affection is slight, cough will occur; if the infection is severe, and the cold-energy has intruded into the interior, it will become diarrhea and abdominal pain.

“Generally speaking, the lung will be affected by evil first in autumn, the liver will be affected by evil first in spring, the heart will be affected by evil first in summer, the spleen will be affected by evil first in late summer, and the kidney will be affected by evil first in winter.”

帝曰：何以异之？岐伯曰：肺咳之状，咳而喘息有音，甚则唾血。心咳之状，咳则心痛，喉中介介如梗〔《太素》、《外台》引“梗”并作“哽”〕状，甚则咽肿喉痹。肝咳之状，咳则

两胁〔《千金》《外台》引"两胁"并作"左胁"〕下痛，甚则不可以转〔《千金》《外台》引并作"甚者不得转侧"〕，转则两胠下满〔《医心方》作"两脚下满"〕。脾咳之状，咳则右胁下〔《外台》引"胁"下无"下"字〕下痛，阴阴引肩背，甚则不可以动，动则咳剧。肾咳之状，咳则腰背相引而痛，甚则咳涎。

Yellow Emperor asked: "Then, how to distinguish the different kinds of coughs?"

Qibo said: "The symptoms of lung cough are: there is sound of respiration when one coughs, and spitting blood when the case is severe.

"The symptoms of heart cough are: one will be feeling heartache when coughs, feeling like something is obstructing in the throat, and the throat is swelling with pain and stagnation when the case is severe.

"The symptoms of liver cough are: pain in the left side of the thorax when one coughs, and he is unable to walk when the case is severe, if he walks, the two feet will be swelling.

"The symptoms of spleen cough are: pain in the right side of the thorax when one coughs, recessive pain attacking the shoulders and back, and he is unable to move when the case is severs, and the patient will cough as soon as he moves about.

"The symptoms of kidney cough are: pains of the loins and the back are affecting each other, and one will cough out mucus when the case is severe."

帝曰：六府之咳奈何？安所受病？岐伯曰：五藏之久咳，乃移于六府。脾咳不已，则胃受之，胃咳之状，咳而呕，呕甚则长虫出。肝咳不已，则胆受之，胆咳之状，咳呕胆汁。肺咳不已，则大肠受之，大肠咳状，咳而遗失。心咳不已，则小肠受之，小肠咳状，咳而失气，气与咳俱失〔《太素》"气"下有"者"字"失"作"出"〕。肾咳不已，则膀胱受之，膀胱咳状，咳而遗溺。久咳不已，则三焦受之，三焦咳状，咳而腹〔《医心方》"腹"作"肠"〕满，不欲食饮〔"饮"字衍〕，此皆〔《太平圣惠方》"此皆"下有"寒气"二字〕聚于胃关于肺，使人多涕唾，而面浮〔《圣济总录》引"面"下有"目"字〕肿气逆也。

Yellow Emperor asked: "What about the symptoms of cough in the six hollow organs, and how are the diseases affected?" Qibo said: "When the cough of the five solid organs is protracted, it will be transmitted into the six hollow organs.

"For instance, when the spleen cough is protracted, the stomach will be affected; the symptom of the stomach cough is cough with vomitting, and roundworms can be vomitted out when the case is severe.

"When the liver cough is protracted, the gallbladder will be affected; the symptom of the gallbladder cough is: the bitter liquid can be vomitted out when coughing.

"When the lung cough is protracted, the large intestine will be affected; the symptom of the large intestine cough is: the fecal incontinence occurs when one coughs.

"When the heart cough is protracted, the small intestine will be affected; the symptom of the small intestine cough is: breaking wind as soon as coughing, and usually, breaking wind and cough occur at the same time.

"When the kidney cough is protracted, the bladder will be affected; the symptom of the bladder cough is: the incontinence of urine when coughing.

"The various kinds of cough stated above, if being protracted, the triple warmer will be affected; the symptoms of the triple warmer cough are: the distention of the intestine, and the patient reluctants to eat.

"No matter from which viscus the affection stems from, it is due to the accumulation of cold-evil in the stomach, and the cold-evil is connecting the lung. It will cause one to have plenty of thick sputum, edema of the face and eyes, and the adverseness of the vital energy."

帝曰：治之奈何！岐伯曰：治藏者治其俞，治府者治其合，浮肿者治其经。帝曰：善。

Yellow Emperor asked: "How to treat it?" Qibo said: "When treating the cough of the five solid organs, prick the Shu-points; when treating the cough of the hollow organs, prick the He-points; to the patient of edema caused by cough, dredge the channel by pricking the points of the related channel." Yellow Emperor said: "Good."

举痛论篇第三十九

Chapter 39
Ju Tong Lun
(On the Pathology of Pain)

黄帝问曰：余闻善言天者，必有验于人；善言古者，必有合于今；善言人者，必有厌于已。如此，则道不惑而要数极，所谓明〔胡本讹本，元残二，赵本吴本“明”并叠“明”字，按“明明”谓明甚〕也。今余问于夫子，令言而可知，视而可见，扪而可得，令验于已而发蒙解惑，可得而闻乎？岐伯再拜稽首对曰：何道之问也？帝曰：愿闻人之五藏卒痛，何气使然？岐伯对曰：经脉流行不止、环周不休，寒气入经而〔《太素》“入”下有“焉”字，“而”作“血”〕稽迟，泣而不行，客于脉外则血少，客于脉中则气不通，故卒然而痛。

Yellow Emperor said: "I am told that when one is good at dicussing the law of heaven, he must be able to verify the law of heaven to man; when one is good at discussing events in the past, he must be able to connect the past with the present; when one is good at commenting on others, he must be able to integrate them with himself, it is only in this way, can one be not in a puzzle in the principles of medicine, and to obtain and know the truth thoroughly.

"Now I want to ask you about the way of diagnosis which can be understood when by speech, visible when by seeing, and tangible when by touching, so that I can have some realization about it. I hope to hear about your advice to enlighten my ignorance and remove my perplexion."

Qibo asked: "What principles do you want to know?" Yellow Emperor said: "I want to hear about what are the evil-energies that cause the sudden pain of the viscera?" Qibo answered: "The blood and energy in the channels are circulating unceasingly in the whole body, when the cold-evil invades the channle, the blood in the channel will become stagnating, and the pain will suddenly occur."

帝曰：其痛或卒然而止者，或痛甚不休者，或痛甚不可按者，或按之而痛止者，或按之无益者，或喘〔按“喘”误，疑应作“揣”，“动”有“痛”义〕动应手者，或心与背相引而痛者，或〔《太素》“或”下有“心”字〕胁肋与少腹相引而痛者，或腹痛引阴股者，或痛宿〔谓抄本“宿”作“夙”〕昔而成积者，或卒然痛死不知人，有少〔《太素》“有”下无“少”字〕间复生者，或痛而呕者，或腹痛而后〔《太素》“后”作“复”〕泄者，或痛而闭〔滑抄本“闭”作“闷”〕不通者，凡此诸痛，各不同形，别之奈何？

Yellow Emperor said: "Some of the pains stop by themselves all of a sudden; some of the acute pains can not be stopped; some of the pains are so severe that can not withstand the massage and pressing; some of the pains can be alleviated by massage and pressing; some

of them can not be alleviated by massage and pressing; some of them occur as soon as the hand touches the abdomen; sometimes the pain of heart and the pain of the back are affecting each other; sometimes the pain of the heart, the pain of the hypochondrium and the pain of the lower abdomen are affecting each other; sometimes the pain of the abdomen is pulling the inner side of the thigh; some of the pains are protracted to become abdominal mass; some acute pains occur suddenly to cause the patient to become unconscious like a dead man but revives after a while; some patients feel pain and vomit at the same time: some of the patients have abdominal pain and diarrhea; some patients feel pain and oppression over the chest. Since all the cases are different, how can they be distinguished?"

岐伯曰：寒气客于脉〔《太素》"脉"作"肠"〕外则脉寒〔《太素》"脉"并作"肠"〕，脉寒则缩踡，缩踡则脉〔《太素》并作"肠"〕绌急，绌急则外引小络，故卒然而痛，得炅〔音窘，热也〕则痛立止；因重中于寒，则痛久矣。

Qibo said: "When cold-evil invades the outside of the intestine and causes the intestine to contract cold, the intestine will be shrinking and winding like being sewed, as it affects the fine collaterals outside, pain will occur suddenly; but the pain can be ceased if only heat is attached. But if it is invaded by cold-evil again, the pain will not be alleviated in a short time.

寒气客于经脉之中，与炅气相薄则脉满，满则痛而不可按〔滑抄本，柯校本并作"甚而不休"〕也。寒气稽留，炅气从上〔"上"误，似应作"之"〕，则脉充大而血气乱，故痛甚不可按也。

"When the cold-evil invades into the channel and persecutes the heat in the channel, the contention between them will cause the channel to become full and substantial, and the channel will become sthenic. Under this condition, severe and unceasing pain will occur.

"When the cold-evil retains, the heat-evil will appear in the wake of it, and the combat between the cold-evil and the heat-evil will cause the channel to become full and substantial. As the energy and blood are confusing inside, the severe pain will not be able to withstand the pressing.

寒气客于肠胃之间，膜原之下，血〔《太素》"血"作"而"〕不得散，小络〔《宣明论方》"络"作"腹"〕急引故痛，按之则血〔据王注所据本"血"字应作"寒"〕气散，故按之痛止。

"When the cold-evil invades the location between the intestine and the stomach, and the membranes connecting the diaphram, intestine and stomach, if it is not dispersed, the fine collaterals nearby will become tightened, and the drawing will cause pain; but when the evil energy and cold is dispersed by massage and pressing, the pain will be alleviated.

寒气客于侠脊之脉，则深〔《史载之方》"则"下无"深"字〕按之不能及，故按之无益也。

"When the cold-evil invades into the Du Channel, even a heavy pressing would not be able to reach the focus of the disease, so, the pressing will be ineffective.

寒气客于冲脉，冲脉起于关元，随腹直上，寒气客〔《太素》无"寒气客"三字〕则脉

不通，脉不通则气因〔《史载之方》引作“脉因之则气不通”〕之，故揣动应手矣。

“When the cold-evil invades the Chong Channel, as the Chong Channel begins from the Guanyuan (Energy Pass) point and traces up along the abdomen, the Chong Channel will be obstructed, and the energy will be stagnated on account of it. Thus, the pain will occur as soon as the hand touches the abdomen.

寒气客于背俞之脉则〔胡本、读本、赵本、吴本“则”下并有“血”字〕脉泣，脉泣则血虚，血虚则痛，其俞注于心〔《史载之方》引“其”作“背”，“注”作“主”〕，故相引而痛，按之则热气至，热气至则痛止矣。

“When the cold-evil invades the channel of the back shu, the blood circulation will become unsmooth to cause athenia of the blood and bring about pain. Since the shu point in the back is connected with the heart, their drawing against each other will cause pain. When one presses the spot of pain with hand, the hand focus will become hot, and as soon as the focus is hot, the pain will be alleviated.

寒气客于厥阴之脉，厥阴之脉者，络阴器系于肝，寒气客于脉中，则血泣脉急，故胁肋与少腹相引痛矣。

“When the cold-evil invades the Jueyin Channel which surrounds the external genitals and connects the liver, when the cold-evil retains, the blood circulation will become unsmooth and the pulse condition will become rapid, the hypochondrium and the lower abdomen will draw against each other and cause pain.

厥〔按“厥气”与下“寒气”误倒〕气客于阴股，寒气上及少腹，血泣在下相引，故腹痛引阴股。

“When the cold-evil invades into the inner side of the thigh, the disharmony of the energy and blood will cause the blood circulation of the lower abdomen and the inner side of the thigh to become unsmooth and affecting each other. In this way, the pain of the abdomen will affect the inner side of the thigh.

寒气客于小肠膜原之间，络血之中，血泣不得注于大经，血气稽留不得行，故宿昔而成积矣。

“When the cold-evil invades the location between the small intestine and the membrane of the diaphram and the collateral-blood, it causes the blood to become unsmooth and fails to enter into the Small-intestine Channel, the energy and blood will become obstructed and retained. When the condition is protracted, hernia will occur.

寒气客于五藏，厥逆上泄〔柯校本“泄”作“壅”〕，阴气竭〔《张琦说：“竭”作法“极“》〕，阳气未入，故卒然痛死不知人，气复反〔“反”字疑衍〕则生矣。

“When the cold-evil invades into the five viscera, the energy of Jueni will be reversing up to cause overabundance of the Yin energy and the impediment of the Yang energy. In this case, the patient will suddenly become unconscious die of pain; If the Yang energy is recovered, the patient can be revived again.

寒气客于肠胃，厥逆上出，故痛而呕也。

“When the cold-evil invades into the stomach and intestine, the energy of Jueni will be

reversing up, and the abdominal pain and vomiting will occur.

寒气客于小肠，小肠不得成聚，故后泄腹痛矣。

"When the cold-evil invades into the small intestine, and the small intestine fails to take charge of the reception, the water and cereals will not be able to retain in the small intestine, diarrhea and abdominal pain will occur.

热气留于小肠，肠中痛，瘅热焦渴，则坚乾〔《儒门事亲》引作"便坚"〕不得出，故痛而闭不通矣。

"When the heat-evil retains in the small intestine, pain will occur in the intestine, and the patient will be hot and thirsty, together with dry stool and retention of feces. These conditions above can be made known by asking the patient."

帝曰：所谓言而可知者也。视而可见奈何？岐伯曰：五藏六府，固〔明抄本"固"作"面"〕尽有部，视其五色，黄赤为热，白为寒，青黑为痛，此所谓视而可见者也。

Yellow Emperor said: "What are the diseases which can be understood by sight seeing?" Qibo said: "The various parts of the face represent the five solid organs and the six hollow organs respectively, when the five colours of the patient's complexion are inspected, the disease can be understood: yellow and red complexions stand for heat, white complexion stands for cold, the green and black complexions stand for pain, and these are the conditions which can be known by sight seeing."

帝曰：扪而可得奈何？岐伯曰：视其主病之脉，坚而血及陷下者，皆可扪而得也。

Yellow Emperor said: "What are the disease conditions that can be made known by palpation?" Qibo said: "It is known mainly according to the pulse condition. When the pulse condition is firm and substantial, it is the overabundance of the evil-energy; when the pulse condition is bogged down, it is deficient of the healthy-energy. All of them can be made known by palpation."

帝曰：善。余知〔《太素》"知"作"闻"〕百病生于气也。怒则气上〔《病源》"上"并作"逆"〕，喜则气缓，悲则气消，恐则气下，寒则气收〔《云笈七签》引"收"作"聚"〕，炅〔《病源》、《太平圣惠方》引"炅"并作"热"〕则气泄，惊〔《太素》《病源》"惊"并作"忧"〕则气乱，劳则气耗，思则气结，九气不同，何病之生？岐伯曰：怒则气逆，甚则呕血及飧泄，故气上矣。喜则气和志达〔《病源》《太平圣惠方》"气和"下并无"志达"二字〕，荣卫通利，故气缓矣。悲则心系急，肺布叶举，而上焦〔《甲乙》"而上焦"作"两焦"〕不通，荣卫不散〔《太平圣惠方》引无"荣卫不散"四字〕，热气在中，故气消矣。恐则精却，却则上焦闭，闭则气还，还则下焦胀，故气不行〔林校云："'不行'当作'下行'"〕矣。寒则腠理闭〔《病源》并作"寒则经络埃涩"〕，气不行，故气收矣。炅则腠理开，荣卫通，汗大泄，故气泄。惊则心无所倚，神无所归，虑无所定，故气乱矣。劳则喘息汗出，外内皆越，故气耗矣。思则心有所存，神有所归，正气留而不行，故气结矣。

Yellow Emperor said: "Good, I am told that many diseases are effected by the energy. Such as, when one is in a fury, the energy will be reversing up; when one is overjoyed, the energy will be relaxed, when one is sorrow-stricken, the energy will be dispersed; when one is in terror, the energy will be bogged down; when one encounters cold, the energy will be

assembled; when one encounters heat, the energy will be discharged; when one is in excessive melancholy, the energy will be confusing; when one is over fatigue, the energy will be consumed; when one is anxious and worrying, the energy will be stagnated. The nine energy changes are different, and what diseases can they bring about?"

Qibo said: "When one is in a fury, the energy will be reversing up, when the case is severe, hematemesis and lienteric diarrhea will occur. So, it is called the 'adverseness of vital energy'.

"When one is in a joyous mood, the energy will be harmonious and both the Ying and Wei energies will be unobstructed. So it is called the 'relaxation of energy'.

"When one is sorrow-stricken greatly, his heart and its tissues connecting the viscera will become strained, the lobes of the lung will become swelling up, the upper and middle warmer will be obstructed, and the heat inside will remain retaining. So, it is called the 'dissipation of energy'.

"When one is in terror, the refined energy will be declined, and the decline of the energy below will cause obstruction of the upper warmer, as the energy can not reach the upper warmer, it will return to the lower warmer, and the energy stagnation will cause fullness and distention of the lower warmer. It is called the 'unstableness and descent of the energy'.

"The cold-evil causes the channel and collaterals to become rough, and the circulation of the Ying and Wei energies to become obstructed. So, it is called the 'collecting of energy'.

"The heat causes the openning of the striae and the excessive excretion of the Ying and Wei energies along with the sweat. So, it is called the 'excretion of the energy'.

"When one is in excessive terror, the beat of heart will cause him to feel like helpless, it seems that his spirit and mind have nowhere to rest, and his misgiving has nowhere to stop. So, it is called the 'confusing of the energy'.

"When one is fatigue with excessive labour, he will have rapid respiration and plenty of sweat, comsumption will occur in both the exterior and the interior. So it is called the 'consumption of the energy'.

"When one is in excessive anxiety, his heart will be injured and his spirit will become dull, the energy will be stagnated and fails to circulate. So it is called the 'stagnation of energy'".

腹中论篇第四十

Chapter 40
Fu Zhong Lun
(On Abdominal Diseases)

黄帝问曰：有病心腹满，旦食则不能暮食，此为何病？岐伯对曰：名为鼓胀。帝曰：治之奈何？岐伯曰：治之以鸡矢醴一剂知，二剂已。帝曰：其时有复发者何也？岐伯曰：此饮食不节，故时有病也。虽然其病且已，时故当病，气聚于腹也。

Yellow Emperor asked: "There is a kind of disease with fullness and distention of epigastrium and abdomen, it the patient takes food in the morning he will be reluctant to eat in the evening. What is the disease?" Qibo said: "It is called distention of grain."

Yellow Emperor asked: "How to treat it?" Qibo said: "It can be treated with the wine of chicken droppings, when one dose is taken, it will be effective, and when two doses are taken, the disease will be cured."

Yellow Emperor said: "Sometimes the disease can be reappeared again, and why is it so?" Qibo said: "When the patient is careless about his food and drink, sometimes the disease may reappear again, sometimes when the patient contracts cold again at the time when he is about to be recovered, and the cold-evil is accumulating in the abdomen, the disease can reappear again."

帝曰：有病胸胁支满者，妨于食，病至则先闻腥臊臭〔《全氏指迷方》引“臭”作“鼻”，“鼻”字疑属下读〕，出清液〔《甲乙》“液”作“涕”〕，先〔于鬯说：“‘先’字衍”〕唾血，四支清，目眩，时时前后血，病名为何？何以得之？岐伯曰：病名血枯，此得之年少时，有所〔“所”字疑衍〕大脱血；若醉入房中，气竭肝伤，故月事衰少不来也。帝曰：治之奈何？复以何术？岐伯曰：以四乌鲗骨一藘茹〔按“藘茹”似应作“茹藘”〕二物并合之，丸以雀卵，大如小豆，以五丸为后饭，饮以鲍鱼汁，利肠〔《太素》“肠”作“胁”〕中及伤肝也。

Yellow Emperor said: "There is a kind of disease with distention and oppression over the chest and the hypochondrium which hinders the taking in of food. Prior to the out burst of the disease, stinking and foul smell are smelt, and the patient has clear nasal discharge, spitting blood, cold in the extremities, dizziness, bloody stool and hematuria. What is the disease, and how is it contracted?"

Qibo said: "It is called blood-exhaustion. When the patient contracted hemorrhage when he was young, and the remnant of the disease took root in the body, or due to the patient's conducting sexual intercourse after drunkenness to exhaust his refined energy, and his liver become injured. For a woman, her menstruation will become decline, less or ceasing."

Yellow Emperor asked: "How to treat it and how can the blood and energy be recovered?" Qibo said: "Combine four portions of cuttle-bone and one portion of rubia root and prepare them with the bird's egg to form pills in the size of a red bean. Take five pills along with the abalone soup before meal. The medicine will be helpful to cure the distention of the hypochondrium and invigorate the liver which is injured."

帝曰：病有少腹盛，上下左右皆有根，此为何病？可治不？岐伯曰：病名曰伏梁。帝曰：伏梁何因而得之？岐伯曰：裹大〔《太素》《千金》"裹"下并无"大"字〕脓血，居肠胃之外，不可治，治之每切，按之致〔《圣济总录》引"致"作"至"〕死。帝曰：何以然？岐伯曰：此下则因〔孙鼎宜说："'因'当作'困'〕阴，必下脓血，上则迫胃脘，生〔孙鼎宜说："'生'当作'至'"〕鬲，侠〔《太素》"侠"作"使"〕胃脘内痈，此久病也，难治。居齐上为逆，居齐下为从〔孙鼎宜说："逆从二字当乙转方与上文'不可治'义合"〕，勿动亟夺，论在《刺法》中。

Yellow Emperor said: "There is a kind of disease with fullness in the lower abdomen and the focuses of disease are on above, below, left and right. What is the disease, and can it be healed?"

Qibo said: "It is called fuliang (ancient name for the disease with epigastric fullness and mass)."

Yellow Emperor asked: "How is the fuliang disease contracted?" Qibo said: "When the purulence and blood are wrapped in the lower abdomen and locate in the outside of the intestine and the stomach, it is hard to treat. When treating, severe pain will occur, if the pressing to the focus is too hard, the patient may die."

Yellow Emperor asked: "Why is it so?" Qibo said: "If the heavy pressing is in the lower part, it will hurt the Yin, if the pressing is in the upper part, it will coerce the area between the stomach and the diaphram to cause carbuncle in the gastric cavity. This is a deep-seated and protracted disease which can hardly be cured. When the disease is above the navel, it is a case with favourable prognosis, when it is under the navel, it is a case with unfavourable prognosis, and the patient must avoid frequent physical labour. The disease is recorded and expounded in detail in the《Pricking Therapy》."

帝曰：人有身体髀股胻皆肿，环齐而痛，是为何病？岐伯曰：病名伏梁，此风根也。其气溢〔《甲乙》校注引《素问》"溢"作"泄"〕于大肠而著于肓，肓之原在齐下，故环齐而痛也，不可动之，动之为水溺涩之病。

Yellow Emperor asked: "When the leg, thigh and hip are all swelling and with pain around the navel, what is the disease?" Qibo said: "It is also called fuliang and it is stemmed from the wind-cold. When the wind-cold is discharged from the large intestine and retains on the membrane outside of the intestine, and as the root of the membrane which is outside of the intestine is on the Qihai point, pain will occur around the navel. This disease must not be treated rashly, if it is treated improperly, dysuria will occur."

帝曰：夫子数言热中消中，不可服高梁芳草石药，石药发瘨〔何校云："《甲乙》'瘨'作'疽'"〕，芳草发狂。夫热中消中者，皆富贵人也，今禁高梁，是不合其心，禁芳草石药，是

病不愈，愿闻其说。岐伯曰：夫芳草之气美，石药之气悍，二者其气急疾坚劲，故非缓心和人，不可以服此二者〔明抄二无“不可”七字〕。帝曰：不可以服此二者，何以然？岐伯曰：夫热气慓悍，药气亦然，二者相遇，恐内伤脾，脾者土也而恶木，服此药者，至甲乙日更论〔《甲乙》作“当愈甚”〕。

Yellow Emperor said："You have said many times that when one contracts the disease of retention of heat-evil in the middle warmer and diabetes involving the middle warmer, he must not take the refined cereals and foods or delicious taste, nor should he use the drugs of fragrant flavour and the medicine of the stone kind, as the medicine of stone kind, when taken, it may cause the subcutaneous ulcer, and the drugs of fragnant flavour may cause mania. As most of the patients who contract the disease of retention of heat-evil in the middle warmer and diabetes involving the middle warmer are rich people or people of the upper class in society, they are not accustomed to abstain from delicious food, but the disease will not be cured if the drugs of fragrant flavour and the medicine of the stone kind are not applied. I hope to hear your opinium about it."

Qibo said："Most drugs of fragrant flavour are hot in property and most medicines of the stone kind are violent, and both of them are urgent, swift, firm and vigorous. They can by no means to relax the body and spirit of a man."

Yellow Emperor asked："Then why are these two kinds of medicine must not be taken?" Qibo said："The heat-evil itself is urgent and vigorous, and so are the energies of medicine, when they join together, the spleen will be injured; as the spleen-energy belongs to earth, and earth detests the subjugation of wood, if the medicine are taken, the disease will become aggravated when encountering the days of Jia or Yi."

帝曰：善。有病膺肿颈痛胸满腹胀，此为何病？何以得之？岐伯曰：名厥逆。帝曰：治之奈何？岐伯曰：灸之则瘖，石之则狂，须其气并，乃可治也。帝曰：何以然？岐伯曰：阳气重上〔“上”字疑涉下衍〕，有余于上，灸之则阳气入阴，入则瘖，石之则阳气虚〔胡本，元残二“气虚”并作“出内”〕，虚〔“虚”字疑误，据王注应作“出”〕则狂；须其气并而治之，可使全〔《甲乙》“全”作“愈”〕也。

Yellow Emperor said："Good. There is a kind of disease with swelling and pain over the chest and neck, fullness of chest and distention of the abdomen. What is the disease and how is it being contracted?" Qibo said："It is called Jueni."

Yellow Emperor asked："How to treat it?"Qibo said："If the disease is treated with moxibustion, the patient will have dysphonia; when it is treated with stone needle, the patient will have mania. It can only be treated at the time when the upper and the lower energies intercourse." Yellow Emperor asked："Why is it so?" Qibo said："The Yang energy is ascending, so, the patient is heavy and has a surplus above, if moxibustion is applied, it will be supporting fire with fire, when Yang is overabundant and Yin is debilitating, Yang energy will take advantage to enter into Yin, and the debilitating Yin energy will not be able to support the root of tongue, and dysphonia will occur; if the disease is treated will stone needle, the blood will be discharged along with the pricking to cause the debility of Yin, and the de-

bility of Yin will cause the overabundance of Yang which will cause mania. When treating, it is neccessary to wait until the intercourse of the upper energy and the lower energy, so as the disease may be cured."

帝曰：善。何以知怀子之且生也？岐伯曰：身有病而无邪脉也。

Yellow Emperor said:"Good. How can one know that a woman is pregnant and will give birth to a bady?" Qibo said: "One can know it by diagnosis, when the woman seems to have disease, but has no signs of disease in the palpation, then she is pregnant."

帝曰：病热而有所痛者何也？岐伯曰：病热者，阳脉也，以三阳之动〔《甲乙》"动"作"盛"〕也，人迎一盛〔《甲乙》"盛"下有"在"字〕少阳，二盛太阳、三盛阳明，入阴也〔《太素》、《甲乙》并无此三字〕。夫阳入于阴，故病在头与腹，乃䐜胀而头痛也。帝曰：善。

Yellow Emperor asked: "There is a kind of disease of having fever and pains in various parts in the body, and what is the reason?" Qibo said: "All diseases with fever appear in the Yang pulse, and when the patient has fever, all the pulse conditions of the three Yang channels are overabundant. When Renying pulse is two times as large as the Cunkou pulse, the disease is in the Shaoyang Channel; when it is three times as targe as the cunkou pulse, the disease is in the Taiyang Channel; when it is four times as as the cunkou pulse, the disease is in the Yangming Channel. When the evil-energy enters into Yin channels from Yang channels, the disease is in head and abdomen, and the headache and abdominal pain will occur." Yellow Emperor said: "Good."

刺腰痛篇第四十一

Chapter 41
Ci Yao Tong
(The Pricking Therapy for Lumbago of Various Channels)

足太阳脉令人腰痛，引项脊尻背如重状，刺其郄中太阳正经出血，春无见血。

When the Foot Taiyang Channel contracts disease, it will cause the patient to have lumbago, and the pain will make the patient to feel like something heavy is on his neck, spine, buttocks and back. When treating, it should prick the Weizhong point (Politeal Centre BL. 40) of the Foot Taiyang Channel until bleeding. If it is in spring the pricking must not cause bleeding.

少阳〔“少阳”下脱“脉”字，下“阳明”“足少阴”亦脱“脉”字〕令人腰痛，如以针刺其皮中〔《圣济总录》引“皮”下无“中”字〕，循循然不可以俯仰，不可以顾〔《甲乙》“可以”下有“左右”二字〕，刺少阳成骨之端出血，成骨在膝外廉之骨独起者〔此句十一字疑为上文“成骨”之释语，传写误入正文〕，夏无见血。

The pain of lumbago caused by the disease of Foot Shaoyang Channel is like the pricking of skin by the needle. If it becomes aggravated gradually, it will cause one unable to face up and down, nor can he look around. When treating, it should prick the starting point of the tibia until bleeding. If it is in summer, the pricking must not cause bleeding.

阳明令人腰痛，不可以顾，顾如有见者，善悲，刺阳明于䯒前三痏，上下和之出血，秋无见血。

The lumbago caused by the disease of Foot Yangming Channel is so painful that the patient can not look back, if he looks back, he seems to have seen something, and besides, the patient is often sorrow-stricken. When treating, prick the Zusanli point (Foot Three Li ST. 36) of the Foot Yangming Channel until bleeding to cause the combination of the upper and the lower energies. If it is in autumn, the pricking must not cause bleeding.

足少阴令人腰痛，痛引脊内廉〔《太素》作“引脊内痛”〕，刺少阴于内踝上二痏，春无见〔《太素》“见”作“出”〕血，出血太多，不可复也。

The lumbago caused by the Foot Shaoyin Channel draws the inner side of the spine to become painful. When treating, it should prick the Fuliu point (Repeating Slip KI. 7) of Shaoyin Channel twice. If it is in spring, the pricking must not cause bleeding; if the bleeding is excessive, the blood will become asthenic and will be hard to recover.

厥阴之脉，令人腰痛，腰中如张弓弩弦，刺厥阴之脉，在腨踵鱼腹之外，循之累累然，乃刺之，其病令人善〔《素问识》云：“其病”以下十五字与前四经腰痛之例不同，恐是衍文〕言，默默然不慧，刺之三痏。

The lumbago which is brought by the disease of Foot Jueyin Channel causes the pain so severe and tight like the string of a bow which is fully drawn. When treating, prick the collatteral of Jueyin. One can seek by touching to locate the location which is like a string of pearls between the calf and the outer flank of the fish belly sticking out in the middle of the heel (the Ligou point LR. 5) and make the pricking.

解脉令人腰痛，痛引肩〔《太素》“引肩”作“引膺”〕目𥆧𥆧〔《太素》“𥆧”作“𥇦”〕然，时遗溲，刺解脉，在膝〔《太素》“膝”作“引”，袁刻《太素》“筋肉”作“筋内”〕筋肉分间郄外廉之横脉出血，血变而止。

The lumbago which is brought by the disease of the horizontal Untied Channel will cause pain of the chest, getting dim of the eyesight and incontinence of urine of the patient. When treating, prick the Untied Channel to cause bleeding, and stop the pricking when the blood in purple turns into red. The Untied Channel is on the horizontal line of the muscular prominence between the two tendons behind the knee (Weiyang point BL. 39).

解脉令人腰痛如引带〔《甲乙》“如引带”作“如裂”〕，常如折腰状，善恐；刺解脉，在郄中结络如黍米，刺之血射以黑，见赤血而已。

The lumbago which is brought about by the Scattered Channel causes the loins feel like cracking when ache, and normally, they are like being broken, besides, the patient is apt to get angry. When treating, prick the Untied Channel to let out the purple blood, and stop the pricking when the blood turns red. The knot of the Untied Channel is on the juncture of collaterals in a size of a glutinous millet.

同阴之脉，令人腰痛，痛如小锤居其中，怫然肿〔四库本“肿”作“痛”〕；刺同阴之脉，在外踝上绝骨之端，为三痏。

The lumbago which is brought about by the disease of the Tongyin Channel which is an extra collateral of the Foot Shaoyang Channel is like a small hammer knocking inside which is very painful. When treating, it should prick the Tongyin Channle for three times. The Tongyin Channel is on the Yangfu point (Yang Support GB. 39) which is on the lower end of the tibia above the external malleolus.

阳维之脉，令人腰痛，痛上怫然〔《太素》“怫然”下有“脉”字〕肿；刺阳维之脉，脉与太阳合腨下间，去地一尺所。

The lumbago which is brought about by the disease of the Yangwei Channel (one of the eight extra channels) causes the site of pain in the channel swelling up abruptly. When treating, it should prick the Yangwei Channel. As the Yangwei Channel joins the Taiyang Channel, the acupoint pricked should be under the calf which is about one foot above the ground.

衡络之脉，令人腰痛，不可以俛仰，仰则恐仆，得之举重伤腰，衡络绝，恶血归〔《铜人图经》卷五《殷门》“归”作“注”〕之，刺之在郄阳筋〔《甲乙》“筋之”作“之筋”〕之间，上郄数寸，衡居为二痏出血。

The lumbago which is brought about by the disease of the Belt Channel causes the patient can not face up and down, if he faces up, he might fall. This disease was caused by lifting weight and the hurting of the loins, and the evil blood poured into the Belt Channel to

cause it became impeded. When treating, prick the Weiyang point (Politeal Yang BL. 39) and the Yinmen point (Big Red Gate BL. 37) twice and let out the blood. The two acupoints are several inches under the horizontal collateral of the buttock.

会阴之脉，令人腰痛，痛上〔明抄二“上”作“止”〕漯漯然汗出，汗干令人欲饮，饮已欲走〔“走”字疑误似应作“溲”〕，刺直阳〔“直阳”应作“会阴”林校谓“直阳之脉即会阴之脉”〕之脉上三痏，在蹻上郄下五寸横居，视其盛者出血。

The disease of the Huiyin Channel (channel passing the perineum) will cause lumbago. When the pain stops, the patient will perspire continuously, when the sweat is dried, the patient will desire for drink, and after drinking, he will desire for urination. When treating, prick the Huiyin Channel three times on the position above the Yangqiao Channel and five inches under the Weizhong point where the blood in the collateral is abundant. Prick until bleeding.

飞阳之脉，令人腰痛，痛上拂拂然，甚则悲以恐，刺飞阳之脉，在内踝上五寸，少阴之前，与阴维之会〔《太素》“维”下无“之”字〕。

The lumbago which is brought about by the disease of Feiyang Channel (an extra collateral of Foot Taiyang) causes the patient feel restless and even go so far as to have the moods of sorrow and terror. When treating, prick the Feiyang Channel. The pricking position is on the intersection of Feiyang Channel and the Yinwei Channel in front of the Shaoyin Channel five inches above the medial malleolus.

昌阳之脉，令人腰痛，痛引膺，目䀮䀮然，甚则反折，舌卷不能言；刺内筋为二痏，在内踝上大筋前，太阴后，上踝二寸所。

When the lumbago which is brought about by the disease of the Fuliu Channel effects the chest, it makes the eyes blur, when the case is serious, the loins and the back will not be able to stoop down, and the tongue will curl and shrink that the patient will not able to speak. When treating, prick the Fuliu point (Repeating Slip KI. 7) for two times, which is in front of the large tendon, behind the Taiyin Channel and above the medial malleolus, ie., two inches above the medial malleolus.

散脉，令人腰痛而热，热甚生烦，腰下如有横木〔明抄二夹注：“木一作脉”〕居其中，甚则遗溲；刺散脉，在膝前骨〔《太素》“膝前”下无“骨”字〕肉分间，络外廉束脉，为三痏。

The lumbago which is brought about by the disease of the Scattered Channel (an extra channel of Foot Taiyin) causes the fever of the patient, when it is serious, the patient will be irritable and restless, like a channel which is running horizontally inside. When the case is severe, incontinence of urine will occur. When treating, prick the Scattered Channel for three times. The Scattered Channel is between the muscular stria in front of the knee connecting the small tendon of the lateral aspect of the leg.

肉里之脉，令人腰痛，不可以咳，咳则筋缩急〔《太素》“缩”作“挛”，《甲乙》“缩”下无“急”字〕，刺肉里之脉为二痏〔此二字有错简，应据《圣济总录》移在“少阳绝骨之后”句下。〕，在太阳之外，少阳绝骨之后〔《甲乙》“后”作“端”〕。

The lumbago which is brought about by the disease of Rouli Channel causes the patient

can hardly bear the coughing, if he coughs, contraction of tendons will occur. When treating, prick the Rouli Channel for two times. The Rouli Channel is at the Xuanzhong point (or Juegu point, Suspended Bell GB. 39) of the Shaoyang Channel of the outer flank of the Taiyang Channel.

腰痛侠脊而痛至头，几几然，目𥆧𥆧〔《太素》作“䀹䀹”：“䀹䀹”惊视貌”〕欲僵仆，刺足太阳郄中出血。腰痛上寒，刺足太阳阳明；上热，刺足厥阴；不可以俛仰，刺足少阳；中热而喘刺足少阴，刺郄中出血〔“出血”应作“血络”〕。

When the lumbago affects the spine and the pain goes up to the top of head, the head will feel heavy and the eyes will be staring and it seems that the patient if going to fall down. When treating, prick the Weizhong point (Popliteal Centre BL. 40) until bleeding.

If there is the feeling of cold during the pain, the Foot Taiyang and Foot Yangming channels should be pricked; if there is the feeling of heat during the pain, the Foot Jueyin Channel should be pricked; if the patient can not face up and down, the Foot Shaoyang Channel should be pricked; if the pain is accompanied with internal heat-syndrome and rapid breathing, the Foot Shaoyin Channel and the blood within the collateral of Weizhong point should be pricked.

腰痛上寒，不可顾，刺足阳明；上热，刺足太阴；中热而喘，刺足少阴。大便难，刺足少阴。少腹满，刺足厥阴。如折，不可以俛仰，不可举，刺足太阳，引脊内廉，刺足少阴。

When the patient is feeling cold during the lumbago and can not look around, it should prick the Foot Yangming Channel; when he is feeling hot during the lumbago with dryness-heat syndrome, it should prick the Foot Taiyin Channel; when the lumbago is accompanied with internal-heat syndrome and rapid breathing, it should prick the Foot Shaoyin Channel.

When the lumbago is accompanied with constipation, it should prick the Foot Shaoyin Channel, When the lumbago is accompanied with the fullness and distention of the lower abdomen, it should prick the Foot Jueyin Channel. When one's loins are painful like being broken, unable to face up and down or to move about, it should prick the Foot Taiyang Channel. When the lumbago is effecting the inner flank of the spine, it should prick the Foot Shaoyin Channel.

腰痛引少腹控䏚，不可以仰。刺腰尻交者，两髁胂上，以月生死为痏数，发针立已。左取右，右取左。

When the lumbago affects the lower abdomen, drawing the hypochondrium to cause uneasiness, and the patient can not stand erect, it should prick the Xialiao point (in between the space of bone) under the buttock on the hard muscle of the hipbone under both sides of the loins. The times of pricking should be calculated according to the wax and wane of the moon to cause the pricking effective. In pricking, when the pain is on the left side, prick the acupoint of the right side, when the pain is on the right side, prick the acupoint on the left side.

风论篇第四十二

Chapter 42
Feng Lun
(On Wind-evil)

黄帝问曰：风之伤人也，或为寒热，或为热中，或为寒中，或为疠〔《甲乙》《千金》“疠”并作“厉”〕风，或为偏枯，或为风也，其病各异，其名不同〔明抄二无“或为”以下十二字〕，或内至五藏六府，不知其解，愿闻其说。

Yellow Emperor asked: “When the wind-evil invades the body, some cause the patient to have chilliness and fever, some cause the retention of heat-evil in the middle warmer, some cause the retention of cold-evil in the middle warmer, some cause leprosy, some cause hemiplegia, and some invade into the interior to reach the viscera. I don't know the reason, and I hope you can tell me.”

岐伯对曰：风气藏于皮肤之间，内不得通〔《千金》《医心方》“通”并作“泄”〕，外不得泄〔《千金》、《医心方》“泄”并作“散”〕；风者善行而数变，腠理开则洒〔《甲乙》“洒”作“凄”〕然寒，闭则热而闷，其寒也则衰食饮，其热也则消肌肉，故使人佚慄而不能食，名曰寒热。

Qibo answered: “When the wind-evil invades into the skin, it can not be dispersed to the interior, nor can it be diffused to the exterior.

“The wind is swift in moving and can be developed into various diseases, when the stria of the skin is open, it will cause one to feel cold, when the stria is closed, it will cause one to have feverish sensation accompanied with restless. When the patient has cold, his food and drink will be reduced, then he has fever, his muscle will become emaciated. Thus, when one has no appetite and reluctant to eat, he has the disease of cold and heat.

风气与阳明入胃，循脉而上至目内眦，其人肥则风气不得外泄〔滑抄本“泄”作“出”〕，则为热中而目黄；人〔《圣济总录》引“人”上有“其”字〕瘦则外泄而寒〔“而寒”二字衍文〕，则为寒中而泣〔《千金》“泣”作“泪”〕出。

“The wind-evil enters into the stomach through the Yangming Channel and goes up along the channel to reach the inner canthus of eyes. If the patient is fat, the wind-evil can hardly be diffused to the exterior, when the retention is protracted, it will become the retention of the heat-evil in the middle warmer, and the eyeballs of the patient will become yellow; if the patient is thin, his Yang energy can easily be dispersed to the exterior, it will become the retention of cold-evil in the middle warmer, and the patient will be falling tears often.

风气与太阳俱入，行诸脉俞，散于分肉〔“分肉”二字误倒，据王注应作“肉分”，谓内

之分理〕之间，与卫〔《病源》“卫”作“血”、《太平圣惠方》“干”作“搏”〕气相干，其道不利，故使肌肉愤䐜〔《太素》“愤”作“贲”，“疡”作“伤”〕而有疡，卫气有所凝而不行，故其肉有不仁也。疠者，有荣气热胕〔“有荣气热胕”应为“荣卫热”〕，其气不清，故使其鼻柱坏而色败，皮肤疡溃，风寒客于脉而不去，名曰疠风，或名曰寒热〔滑抄本无此五字〕。

When the wind-evil invades the body through the Taiyang Channel, it reaches the shu-points of various channels, spreads between the muscle striae and mixes with the blood and energy, in this way, the routs of the energy will become obstructed, and the muscle will be swelling up to become injured. If the Wei-energy is stagnated to effect its circulation, the muscle will become numb and have no sence to the pain and itching.

"Leprosy is caused by the heat of both the Rong and Wei energies, when the energy and blood are not refined and injures the nose bridge, the complexion will be deteriorated and the skin become worn-out. As the protracted retention of the wind-evil in the channel can not be removed, it causes leprosy.

以春甲乙〔《外台》“甲乙”下有“日”字，下丙丁等同〕伤于风者为肝风，以夏丙丁伤于风者为心风，以季夏戊己伤于邪〔《甲乙》《千金》“邪”并作“风”〕者为脾风，以秋庚辛中于邪〔《甲乙》“千金”“中于邪”并作“伤于风”〕者为肺风，以冬壬癸中于邪者为肾风。

"When one is injured by wind-evil on the Jia and Yi days of spring, it is the liver-wind; when one is injured by the evil-wind on the Bing and Ding days in summer, it is the heart-wind; when one is injured by the wind-evil on the Wu and Ji days in late summer (long summer) it is the spleen-wind; when one is injured by the wind-evil on the Geng and Xin days in autumn, it is the lung-wind; when one is injured by the wind-evil on the Ren and Gui days in winter, it is the kidney-wind.

风〔《太素》《甲乙》“风”下并有“气”字〕中五藏六府之俞，亦为藏府之风，各入其门户所〔《太素》“所”作“之”〕中，则为偏风。风气〔《太平圣惠方》“气”作“邪”〕循风府而上，则为脑风。风入系头〔按《甲乙》注云：“一本作‘头系’”。头系是头中的目系、目系，谓目睛人脑之系〕，则为目风，眼〔《太素》“眼”作“眠”，“眠寒”二字属下节〕寒。饮酒中风，则为漏风。入房汗出中风，则为内风。新沐中风，则为首风。久风入中，则为肠风飧〔《千金》“肠风”下无“飧泄”二字〕泄。外在腠理，则为泄风。故〔《千金》“故”下有“曰”字〕风者百病之长也，至其变化，乃为他病也，无常方，然致有风〔吴注本“有”作“自”〕气也。

"When the wind-evil invades into the shu-points of the five solid organs and the six hollow organs, it will become the wind of the five organs and the six hollow organs. Regardless of collateral, channel, viscus or bowel, when any of them is invaded by the wind-evil, it will become the residing of wind-evil on one side of the body.

"After the invasion of the wind-evil, it goes up along the Fengfu Channel to reach the brain, and brain-wind syndrome will occur; when the wind-evil enters into the series of the eye, the eye-wind syndrome will occur.

"When one catches cold during sleep or contracts the wind-evil after drunken, the perforated-wind syndrome will occur.

"When one perspires in sexual intercourse and contracts wind-evil, the endogenous wind syndrome will occur, when one contracts wind evil immediataly after the washing of the hair, the head-wind syndrome will occur.

"When the wind-evil retains in the striae of skin for a long time and injures the spleen and stomach, the fresh blood in stool caused by wind-evil will occur.

"As to the cold-evil retained in between the striae outside, it will become the endogenous wind-evil.

"Thus, the wind-evil is the main factor to induce various diseases, it has many variations, and has no regular patern when it turns to become other diseases. But, in the last analysis, the diseases are stemmed from the invasion of the wind-evil."

帝曰：五藏风之形状不同者何？愿闻其诊及其病能。

Yellow Emperor said: "What are the differences between the appearances of the wind syndromes of the five solid organs? I hope to hear about the essentials about the inspection and the appearances of the diseases."

岐伯曰：肺风之状，多汗恶风，色皏然白，时咳短气，昼日则差，暮则甚，诊在眉上，其色白。

Qibo said: "The symptoms of the lung-wind syndrome are hyperhidrosis, the patient has an aversion to wind, white complexion, cough now and then and short of breath, and the symptoms are comparatively mild in day time and become more acute in the evening. During the inspection, take note of the position above the eyebrow which should be white.

心风之状，多汗恶风，焦绝，善怒吓〔按"善怒"属于心，不合，《医心方》引《小品方》正作"喜悲"〕，赤色，病甚则言不可快〔《千金》、《类编朱氏集验医方》引作"言语不快"〕，诊在口〔高注本引"口"作"舌"，《三因方》引作"舌"〕，其色赤。

"The symptoms of the heart-wind syndrome are hyperhidrosis, the patient has an aversion to wind. The patient is withered and thin, often in sorrow with red complexion. When the infection is severe, disturbance of speech will occur. During the inspection, take note of the colour of the tongue which should be red.

肝风之状，多汗恶风，善悲〔按"善悲"于肝无属，《医心方》引无"善悲"二字〕，色微苍，嗌乾善怒，时憎女子，诊在目下，其色青。

The symptoms of the liver-wind syndrome are hyperhidrosis, the patient has an aversion to wind, slightly green in complexion, dry throat, apt to get angry and detests of woman now and then. During inspection, take note of the position under the eyes which should be green.

脾风之状，多汗恶风，身体怠堕〔《圣济总录》引"堕"作"惰"〕，四支不欲动，色薄〔按"薄"字衍〕微黄，不嗜食，诊在鼻上，其色黄。

"The symptoms of the spleen-wind syndrome are hyperhidrosis, the patient has an aversion to wind, fatigue, reluctant to move the extremities and reluctant to eat. During inspection, take note of the position above the nose which should be yellow.

肾风之状，多汗恶风，面痝然浮肿，脊〔《太素》"脊"上有"腰"字〕痛不能正〔按

“正”字当作“久”，应据《外台》《医心方》改〕立，其色炲，隐曲不利〔《外台》引作“隐曲膀胱不通”〕，诊在肌上，其色黑。

“The symptoms of the kidney-wind syndrome are hyperhidrosis, the patient has an aversion to wind, edema of the face, pain in the loin and spine, unable to stand long, black complexion like the smook from burning coal and has dysuria. During inspection. take note of the two cheeks which should be black.

胃风之状，颈〔《病源》“颈”作“头”〕多汗恶风，食饮不下，鬲〔《病源》、《千金》“鬲”并作“鬲下”〕塞不通，腹善〔《病源》“腹”下无“善”字〕满，失衣则䐜胀，食寒则泄，诊形瘦而腹大。

“The symptoms of the stomach-wind syndrome are hyperhidrosis on the forehead, the patient has an aversion to wind, stagnation and impediment under the diaphram and distention of the abdomen that the patient can hardly take food and drink. If the patient wears too little to the weather, he will have distention of the abdomen, if he takes the cold food, he will have diarrhea. When inspecting, take note of the characteristic of the thin body with a large abdomen of the patient.

首风之状，头〔《甲乙》“头”下有“痛”字〕面多汗恶风，当先风一日，则病甚，头痛不可以出内〔《三因方》引“出”下无“内”字〕，至其风日〔《云笈七签》引“日”作业”〕，则病少愈。

“The symptoms of the head-wind syndrome are headache, hyperhidrosis on the face and has an aversion to wind. On the previous day of the attack of the disease, the patient feels painful in advance, has headache and is reluctant to go outside. The disease will turn to the better on the days when the wind being abundant.

漏风之状，或〔滑抄本无“或”字〕多汗，常不可〔《圣济总录》引“不可”上无“常”字〕单衣，食则汗出，甚则身汗〔《圣济总录》引“汗”作“寒”〕，喘息〔据杨注应无“喘息”二字〕恶风，衣常〔全本“常”作“裳”〕濡，口干善渴，不能劳事。

“The perforated-wind syndrome are: the patient has hyperhidrosis and can not wear thin clothes, he perspires as soon as taking food. When the perspiration is excessive, he will feel cold in the body and has an aversion to wind His clothes are always soaked with sweat, he is thirsty and desires for drink, he also can not tolerate the fatigue.

泄〔林校云：“疑此‘泄’字‘内”之误也”〕风之状，多汗，汗出泄衣上〔《医心方》引“泄衣上”作“沾衣裳”〕，口中干，上渍其风，〔明抄二无“上渍”四字，《素问识》说“上渍其风”四字未详，或恐是衍文〕不能劳事，身体尽痛则寒。帝曰：善。

“The symptom of the endogenous wind are: the patient has hyperhidrosis so as to wet his clothes, dryness in the mouth, pain in the whole body and feeling of cold, he can not tolerate the fatigue also.” Yellow Emperor said: “Good.”

痹论篇第四十三

Chapter 43
Bi Lun
(On Bi-disease)

黄帝问曰：痹之〔《甲乙》“之”作“将”〕安生？岐伯对曰：风寒湿三气杂〔《甲乙》“杂”作“合”〕至，合〔《甲乙》“合”作“杂”〕而为痹也。其风气胜者为行痹，寒气胜者为痛痹，湿气胜者为著痹也。

Yellow Emperor asked: "How does the bi-disease come about?" Qibo answered: "When evil-energies of wind, cold and wetness attack at the same time in mixture, it will combine to become the bi-disease: when it is emphasized on wind, it is called the migratory arthralgia, when it is emphasized on cold, it is called the cold-type arthralgia, when it is emphasized on wetness, it is called the adversive arthralgia."

帝曰：其有五者何也？岐伯曰：以冬遇此者为骨痹，以春遇此者为筋痹，以夏遇此者为脉痹，以至阴〔张琦说：“当作‘季夏’”〕遇此者为肌痹，以秋遇此者为皮痹。

Yellow Emperor asked: "Why are the bi-disease divided into five kinds, and what are they?" Qibo said: "When the disease is contracted in winter, it is called the bone bi-syndrome; when it is contracted in spring, it is called the tendinous bi-syndrome; when it is contracted in summer, it is called the channel bi-syndrome; when it is contracted in late sumer, it is called the myalgia; when it is contracted in autumn, it is called the skin itching."

帝曰：内舍五藏六府，何气使然？岐伯曰：五藏皆有合，病久而不去者，内舍于其合也。故骨痹不已，复感于邪，内舍于肾；筋痹不已，复感于邪，内舍于肝；脉痹不已，复感于邪，内舍于心；肌痹不已，复感于邪，内舍于脾，皮痹不已，复感于邪，内舍于肺。后谓痹者，各以其时重感〔《甲乙》“感”上无“重”字〕于风寒湿之气也。

Yellow Emperor said: "Some evils of the bi-disease retain in the five solid organs and the six hollow organs, what energy makes it so?" Qibo said: "The five solid organs are corresponding with the tendon, channel, muscle, skin and bone. When the evil retains in the bodily position which is corresponding to a certain viscus and not being removed for a long time, it will cause the related viscus to become debilitating. Thus, when the bone bi-syndrome is protracted, and the evils of wind, cold and wetness are contracted again, the evil—energy will retain in the kidney; when the tendinous bi-disease is protracted and the evils are contracted again, it will retain in the liver; when the channel bi-syndrome is protracted, and the evils are contracted again, it will retain in the heart; when the myalgia is protracted and the evils are contractecd again, it will retain in the spleen; when the skin itching is protract-

ed and the evils are contracted again, it will retain in the lung. Therefore, the bi-disease is formed in the dominating season by the repeated invasion of the evil-energies of wind, cold and wetness.

凡痹之客五藏者，肺痹者，〔《圣济总录》引"肺痹者"下有"胸背痛甚上气"六字〕，烦满喘而呕；心痹者，脉不通，烦则心下鼓，暴上气而喘，嗌乾善噫，厥气上则恐；肝痹者，夜卧则惊，多饮数小便，上为引如怀〔"为"字衍，本句应作"上引如怀妊"〕；肾痹者，善胀，尻以代踵，脊以代头；脾痹者，四支解堕，发咳〔《全生指迷方》引"咳"作"渴"〕呕汁〔《三因》卷三《叙论》引"汁"作"沫"〕，上为大〔"大"应作"不"〕塞；肠痹者，数饮而出不得，中气喘争〔《三因方》引"争"作"急"〕，时发飧泄；胞痹者，少腹膀胱，按之内痛〔"内痛"《太素》作"两髀"，"两髀"有太阳脉气所过〕，若沃以汤，涩于小便，上为清涕。

"When the bi-disease invades the five solid organs, their symptoms are different. The symptoms of the lung-bi-syndrome are: acute pain in the chest and back, reversing up of the vital energy, restless and depressive, rapid respiration and vomiting. The symptoms of the cardiac bi-syndrome are: impediment of the channel, irritability, palpitation of the heart, sudden rushing up of the energy to cause rapid respiration, dryness of the throat and frequent eruction, as the adverse energy is up-pressing the heart, it causes the patient to become frightened. The symptoms of the hepatic bi-syndrome are: being frightened. The symptoms of the hepatic bi-syndrome are: being terrified often when sleeping at night, desire for drinking, frequent micturition, distention of the lower abdomen like being pregnant. The symptoms of the kidney bi-syndrome are: swelling of the whole body, can sit only but can not walk due to the swelling, can only lower the head but can not lift it up. The patient feels like his coccyx is touching the ground, his cervical bones are slanting down, and his spinal vertebrae are springing up. The symptoms of the splenic bi-syndrome are: tiredness and weakness of the extremities, thirsty, vomiting foam and has stagnation in the chest. The symptoms of the intestinal bi-syndrome are: frequent drinking, dysuria, insufficient of the middle warmer energy to cause rapid respiration and sometimes has diarrhea. The symptoms of the bladder bi-syndrome are: feeling hot like being sprinkled with hot soup when the thighs are pressed by hands, dysuria and running of clear mucus in the nose.

阴气者，静则神藏，躁则消亡，饮食自倍，肠胃乃伤。淫气喘息，痹聚在肺；淫气忧思，痹聚在心；淫气遗溺〔《太素》作"欧唾"，按《宣明五气篇》"肾为唾"〕，痹聚在肾；淫气乏竭〔《太素》"竭"作"渴"〕，痹聚在肝；淫气肌〔《太素》"肌"作"饥"〕绝，痹聚在脾。

"When the Yin energy of the five solid organs is calm, the spirit will be kept inside, when it is irritating, it will apt to be dispersd outside. If the food and drink are taken excessively, the intestine and the stomach will be injured. When one has rapid respiration at the time of the energy is disharmonious and abnormal, the evil energies of wind, cold and wetness will apt to accumulate in the lung; when one is in melancholy and anxiety at the time of the energy being disharmonious and abnormal, the evil energies of wind, cold and wetness will apt to accumulate in the heart; when one vomits at the time of the energy being dishar-

monious and abnormal, the evil energies of wind, cold and wetness will apt to accumulate in the kidney; when one is tired and thirsty at the time of the energy being disharmonious and abnormal, the evil energies of wind, cold and wetness will apt to accumulate in the liver; when one is extremely hungry to injure the stomach at the time of the energy being disharmonious and abnormal, the evil energies of wind, cold and wetness will apt to accumulate in the spleen.

诸痹不已，亦益内也〔《太素》"内也"作"于内"〕，其风气胜者，其人易已也。

"When the various kinds of the bi-disease are protracted, they will penetrate deeper and deeper into the interior of the body. If wind is prevailing in the bi-disease, the patient can be recovered more easily."

帝曰：痹，其时有死者，或疼久者，或易已者，其故何也？岐伯曰：其入藏者死，其留〔《太素》"留"和"流"〕连筋骨间者疼久，其留皮肤间者易已。

Yellow Emperor asked: "Some of the bi-disease causes death of the patient, some are protracted and can not be cured in a long time, and some can be cured in a short time, what is the reason?" Qibo said: "If the bi-disease has entered into the viscera, the patient will die; if it lingers in the tendon and bone, the pain will be protracted; if it retains in the skin only, the patient can be recovered more easily."

帝曰：其客于六府者何也？岐伯曰：此亦其食饮居处，为其病本也。六府亦各有俞，风寒湿气中其俞，而食饮应之，循俞而入，各舍其府也。

Yellow Emperor asked: "Sometimes the bi-disease invades into the six hollow organs, and why is it?" Qibo said: "When one fails to practise temperance in eating and drinking or does not live in an appropriate environment, it will become the main reason of bringing about the bi-disease. There are shu points in all the six hollow organs, when the evils of wind, cold and wetness invade a certain shu -point outside, and at the same time, the patient is injured by improper food and drink inside, the evil will penetrate through the shu-point and retain in the said hollow organ."

帝曰：以针治之奈何？岐伯曰：五藏有俞，六府有合，循脉之分，各有所发，各随〔《太素》、《甲乙》"随"作"治"〕其过，则病瘳也。

Yellow Emperor asked: "Can it be treated with acupuncture?" Qibo said: "In the five solid organs, there are shu-points, in the six hollow organs, there are corresponding-points (The stomach corresponds to Sanli point, the gallbladder corresponds to the Yangling Quan point, the large intestine corresponds to the Quchi point, the small intestine corresponds to the Xiaohai point, the triple warmer corresponds to the Weiyang point, and the bladder corresponds to the Weizhong point), and the onset of the disease has a definite location on the channel. Thus, when the specific location where the disease abides is treated, the disease will be cured."

帝曰：荣卫之气，亦令人〔《太素》"令"作"合"，本句应作"荣卫之气亦合为痹乎"〕痹乎？岐伯曰：荣者，水谷之精气也，和调于五藏，洒陈于六府，乃能入于脉也。故循脉上下，贯五藏，络六府也。卫者，水谷之悍气也，其气慓疾滑利，不能入于脉也，故循皮肤之

中，分肉之间，熏于肓膜，散〔《甲乙》“散”作“聚”〕于胸腹，逆其气则病，从其气则愈，不与风寒湿气合，故不为痹。

Yellow Emperor asked: " Can the Rong and Wei energies combine with the three evils of wind, cold and wetness to become the bi-disease?" Qibo said: " The Rong energy is a refined energy which is transformed from water and cereals. It harmoizes the five solid organs and spreads to the six hollow organs, it can enter into the channels and can circulate up and down along the channels to link up the five solid organs and contact the six hollow organs. The Wei-energy is the rough energy which is transformed from water and cereals, its property is urgent and slippery, but it can not enter into the channels and can only move about under the skin and between the striae outside of the channels to fumigate the diaphram and assemble itself in the chest and abdomen. In normal condition, the Rong energy moves along within the channel and the Wei energy moves outside of the channel, they both go round the whole body and begin again without ceasing. When the circulation is in an abnormal condition, the patient will be ill; when it is in the normal condition, he will be recovered. Since the Rong and Wei energies are circulating without ceasing, they do not combine with the three evil-energies of wind, cold and wetness, and in this case, the bi-disease can by no means occur."

帝曰：善。痹或痛，或不痛，或不仁，或寒、或热，或燥〔此二字疑衍，因下文未涉及燥〕，或湿，其故何也？岐伯曰：痛者，寒气多也，有寒故〔《太素》“有”下有“衣”字〕痛也。其不痛不仁者，病久入深，荣卫之行涩，经络时疏，故不通〔《甲乙》“通”作“痛”〕，皮肤不营，故为不仁。其寒者，阳气少，阴气多，与病相益，故寒也〔《甲乙》“寒也”作“为寒”〕。其热者，阳气多，阴气少，病气胜〔《圣济总录》引无此三字〕，阳遭阴〔明抄本“遭”作“乘”〕，故为痹热〔《甲乙》“为”下无“痹”字〕。其多汗而濡者，此其逢湿甚〔《太素》“甚”作“胜”〕也，阳气少，阴气盛，两气相感，故汗出而濡也。

Yellow Emperor said: " Good. Some of the bi-diseases are painful and some are not, Some of the patients have numbness and some of them are accompanied with different conditions of chilliness, fever and wetness, what is the reason?" Qibo said: " The pain is due to the excessiveness of the cold-evil, in addition to the wearing thin dress of the patient, the cold both inside and outside will cause pain. If the patient has numbness but has no pain, it is due to the deep penetration of the evil when the disease is protracted which causes the obstruction of the circulations of the Rong and Wei energies. But in the case when the channel is not obstructed occasionally, the pain will not occur. When the skin is malnourished, numbness will occur. If the cold-evil is excessive, the Yang energy will become less and the Yin energy will become more, and the Yin energy will aggravate the evil energies of wind, cold and wetness in the bi-disease, so the patient is cold. When the heat is excessive, the Yang energy will become more and the Yin energy become less, the Yang will override the Yin, so the patient is hot. When the patient has hyperhidrosis and wetness all over his body, it is due to the contraction of excessive wetness, and his Yang energy will be deficient and his Yin energy will have a surplus; When the Yin energy responds the wetness energy, it will cause the hyperhidrosis to wet the whole body."

帝曰：夫痹之为病，不痛何也？岐伯曰：痹在于〔《太素》，《甲乙》引"在"下并无"于"字〕骨则重，在于〔"于"字衍〕脉则血凝〔《甲乙》"则"下无"血"字〕而不流，在于筋则屈不伸，在于肉〔"于"字衍〕则不仁，在于皮则寒，故具此五者则不痛也。凡痹之类，逢寒则虫〔《太素》《甲乙》"虫"作"急"〕，逢热则纵。帝曰：善。

Yellow Emperor asked: " Some of the bi-disease are not painful and why are they?" Qibo said: " When bi-disease is in the bone, the patient will feel heavy of the body; when the bi-dsease is in the channel, the channel will be staganted and impeded; when the bi-disease is in the tendon, the tendon will be crooked and unable to stretch; when the bi-disease is in the muscle, the muscle will become mumb; when the bi-disease is in the skin, the patient will feel cold; if any of the above five symptoms occurs, the patient will not be painful. In most diseases of the bi-kind, constriction and tightness will occur when encountering cold, and relaxation and getting loose will occur when encountering heat." Yellow Emperor said: " Good."

痿论篇第四十四

Chapter 44
Wei Lun
(On Flaccidity)

黄帝问曰：五藏使人痿何也？岐伯对曰：肺主身之皮毛，心主身之血脉，肝主身之筋膜，脾主身之肌肉，肾主身之骨髓，故肺热叶焦，则皮〔《甲乙》“则皮”上有“焦”字〕毛虚弱急薄，著则生痿躄也；心气热，则下脉厥而上，上则下脉虚，虚则生脉痿，枢折挈〔“挈”上疑脱“不”字〕，胫纵而不任地也；肝气热，则胆泄口苦筋膜乾，筋膜乾则筋〔《太素》“则”下无“筋”字〕急而挛，发为筋痿；脾气热，则胃乾而渴，肌肉不仁，发为肉痿；肾气热，则腰脊不举，骨枯而髓〔《难经·十五难》“枯”下无“而”字〕减，发为骨痿。

Yellow Emperor asked："All the five solid organs can cause flaccidity of a man, and why is it?" Qibo answered："The lung takes charge of the skins and hairs of the whole body, the heart takes charge of the channels of the whole body, the liver takes charge of the tendons of the whole body, the spleen takes charge of the muscles of the whole body, and the kidney takes charge of the bone marrows of the whole body.

"Thus, when there is heat in the lung, the lobes of the lung will be withered and the skin and hair will become weak and pressing; when the case is severe. flaccidity of feet will occur.

"When there is heat in the heart, the descending energy in the channel will ascend reversely to cause abundance on the upper part of the body and deficiency in the lower, and the lower deficiency will cause the vascular flaccidity-syndrome; the patient will feel like the broken of the joints which can not contact with each other, and his shank will become flabby to cause inability of walking.

"When there is heat in the liver, the bile will rise up to cause bitterness in the mouth, the aponeurosis will become withered due to malnourishment, and when the aponeurosis are withered, flaccidity-syndrome involving the tendon will occur.

"When there is heat in the spleen, it will cause the dryness of the body fluid in the stomach, the patient will be thirsty and has numbness in the muscle to cause muscular flaccidity-syndrome.

"When there is heat in the kidney, the seminal fluid will be exhausted, the loins and the spine will be unable to move about, the withering of the bone and the reduction of the marrow will cause the occurence of the flaccidity-syndrome involving the bone."

帝曰：何以得之？岐伯曰：肺者，藏之长也，为心之盖也；有所失亡，所求〔滑抄本作“求之”〕不得，则发肺鸣，鸣则肺热叶焦〔《甲乙》无“故曰”以下九字〕，故曰，五藏因肺

热叶焦，发为痿躄，此之谓也。悲哀太甚，则胞〔高世栻说："胞"应作"包"，"包络"心包之络也〕络绝，胞络绝，则阳气内动，发则心下崩〔《圣济总录》"胞络"以下十三字作"阳气动中"〕，数溲血也。故《本病》曰：大经空虚，发为肌〔《太素》"肌"作"脉"〕痹，传为脉痿。思想无穷，所愿不得，意淫〔《素问校伪》引古抄本"淫"作"浮"〕于外，入房太甚，宗筋弛纵，发为筋痿，及为白淫，故《下经》曰：筋痿者，生于肝〔《太素》"于"下无"肝"字〕使内也。有渐于湿，以水为事，若有所留，居处相〔《甲乙》"相"作"伤"〕湿，肌肉濡渍，痹而不仁，发为肉痿。故《下经》曰：肉痿者，得之湿地也。有所远行劳倦，逢大热而渴，渴则阳气内伐〔《三因方》卷九《五痿证例》引"伐"作"乏"〕，内伐则〔明抄二"热"上无"内伐则"三字〕热舍于肾，肾者水藏也，今水不胜火，则骨枯而髓虚〔《甲乙》"虚"作"空"〕，故足不任身，发为骨痿。故《下经》曰：骨痿者，生于大热也。

Yellow Emperor asked: " How does the flaccidity come about?" Qibo said: " Lung is the leader one among various viscera, and it is the canopy of the heart, when one's wish can not be satisfied and he becomes very disapointed, his heart-fire will scorch the lung to cause noise in respiration, and the heat of lung will cause its fluid to become exhausted This is the reason of the occurence of the flaccidity of feet.

"When one is in excessive sorrow, the pericardium will be injured, and the Yang energy will stir inside to cause hematochezia. So, it is stated in the《Chapter of Origin of Disease》when the large channel is deficient, it will cause channel bi-syndrome, and ultimately become the vascular flaccidity-syndrome.

"If one deliberates excessively when his wish is not fulfilling to cause his thought always floating outside, or when one is over-fatigue in sexual activities to cause the flabby of the tendons, tendinous bi-syndrome and go so far as to have nocturnal emission or leucorrhea. So, it is stated in the:《Lower Classics》, 'the tendinous bi-disease is caused by excessive sexual activities'.

"When one contracts the wet-evil and is addicted to drink, the wetness-heat will retain inside; as he resides in a wet place, the wetness will invade from outside and cuase numbness of the muscle. The wetness both inside and outside will cause muscular flaccidity-syndrome. So, it is stated in the《Lower Classics》: 'the muscular flaccidity-syndrome is caused by the protracted living in the wet place'.

"When one is tired after a long jurney in hot weather and become thirsty which is a phenominon of the deficient Yangming energy inside, the asthenic heat will invade into the kidney. As the kidney is an organ pertaining to water, and presently, the water is unable to overcome the heat of fire, the marrow will be emptied, the two feet can no longer support the body, and the flaccidity-syndrome involving the bone will occur. So, it is stated in the《Lower Classics》: 'the flaccidity-syndrome involving the bone is caused by the excessive heat.'"

帝曰：何以别之？岐伯曰：肺热者色白而毛败，心热者色赤而络脉溢，肝热者色苍而爪枯，脾热者色黄而肉蠕动〔《太平御览人事部》引"蠕动"作"软"〕，肾热者色黑而齿槁。

Yellow Emperor asked: " How to distinguish the five flaccidities?" Qibo said: " When

the heat-evil is in the lung, the complexion of the patient is white and his hair is corrupted; when the heat-evil is in the heart, his compexion is red and his minute collaterals are appearing; when the heat-evil is in the liver, his complexion is green and his nails are dry; when the heat-evil is in the spleen, his complexion is yellow and his muscle is soft; when the heat-evil is in the kidney, his complexion is black and his teeth are withered."

帝曰：如夫子言可矣，论言治痿者独取阳明，何也？岐伯曰：阳明者，五藏六府之海，主闰〔吴本，朝本“闰”作“润”〕宗筋，宗筋主束骨〔“宗筋”下有“者”字，“主束骨”作“束骨肉”〕而利机关也。冲脉者，经脉之海也，主渗灌谿谷，与阳明合于宗筋，阴阳揔宗筋之会，会于气街，而阳明为之长，皆属于带脉，而络于督脉。故阳明虚则宗筋纵，带脉不引，故足痿不用也。

Yellow Emperor said: "What you have said is desirable. But, it is stated in the ancient books that when treating the flaccidity, it should treat the Yangming Channel alone, and why is it?"

Qibo said: "Yangming Channel is the source of the five solid and the six hollow organs, it nourishes the convergence of the tendons which control the bone and muscles and smooths the joints. The Chong Channel is the sourse of channels, it permeates and irrigates the striae of muscles. Both the Chong Channel and the Yangming Channel connect the tendons, and both the Yin channels and the Yang channels are assembling with the convergence of tendons and get together again at the Qichong point (Rushing Energy 30). The Yangming Channel is their leader and they all related to the Belt Channel and connecting the Du Channel. Thus, when the Yangming Channel is insufficient, the convergence of the tendons will become flabby and thereby can not be controlled by the Belt Channel. As a result, the feet will become flaccid and unavailable."

帝曰：治之奈何？岐伯曰：各补其荥而通其俞，调其虚实，和其逆顺，筋、脉、骨、肉各以其时受月，则病已矣。帝曰：善。

Yellow Emperor asked: "How to treat it?" Qibo said: "It can be treated with invigorating the Xing-energy and dredging the Shu-energy to adjust the asthenic and sthenic, favourable and unfavourable conditions. Regardless of the tendon, channel, bone, or muscle, when it is treated in the month when the related visceral energy is prosperous, the disease may be cured." Yellow Emperor said: "Good".

厥论篇第四十五

Chapter 45
Jue Lun
(On Jue-syndrome)

黄帝问曰：厥之寒热者何也！岐伯对曰：阳气衰于下，则为寒厥；阴气衰于下，则为热厥。

Yellow Emperor asked："Why are there the cold-type jue-syndromes and the heat-type jue-syndrome?" Qibo answered："When the Yang energy begins to decline in the feet, it is the cold-type jue-syndrome, when the Yin energy begins to decline in the feet, it is heat-type jue-synarome."

帝曰：热厥之为热也〔《甲乙》、《千金》"热厥"下并无"之为热也"四字〕，必起于足下者何也？岐伯曰：阳气起于〔林校引《甲乙》"起"作"走"〕足五指之表，阴脉者〔《太素》、《病沅》、《千金》"集于"上并无"阴脉者"三字〕集于足下，而聚于足心，故阳气〔《太素》、《甲乙》"阳"下并无"气"字〕胜则足下热也。

Yellow Emperor asked："The heat-type jue-syndrome is certain to emerges from the foot, and why is it?" Qibo said："The Yang energy passes through the outer flank of the five toes, concentrates under the foot and assembles on the sole, When Yang is abundant under the foot, it will produce heat."

帝曰：寒厥之为寒〔《甲乙》《千金》并无"之为寒也"四字〕也，必从〔《甲乙》《千金》"从"并作"起"，《太素》《病沅》"而上于膝者"并作"始上于膝下"〕五指而上于膝者何也？岐伯曰：阴气起于五指之里，集于膝下〔《千金》无"下"字〕而聚于膝上，故阴气胜，则从五指至膝上寒，其寒也，不从外，皆从内也〔《太素》、《病沅》并作"内寒"〕。

Yellow Emperor asked："The cold-type jue-syndrome initiates regularly from the five toes and then go up to the location under the knee, and what is the reason?" Qibo said："The Yin energy emerges from the inside of the five toes, and accumulates on the knee. When the Yin energy is abundant, it can cause the cold to emerge from the toes and then goes up to the knee; the cold is not the kind of cold which invades the body from outside, but is the cold due to the asthenic Yang from inside."

帝曰：寒厥何失〔"失"字误，疑应作"如"〕而然也？岐伯曰：前阴者，宗〔《甲乙》"宗"作"众"〕筋之所聚，太阴阳明之所合也。春夏则阳气多而阴气少，秋冬则阴气盛而阳气衰。此人者质壮，以秋冬夺于所用，下气上争不能复，精气溢下，邪气因从之而上也；气因〔《太素》"因"作"居"〕于中，阳气衰，不能渗营其经络，阳气日损，阴气独在，故手足为之寒也。

Yellow Emperor asked："How does the cold-type jue-syndrome come about?" Qibo

said: " The anterior yin (external genitals) is the place where the various tendons assemble and it is also the juncture of the Taiyang Channel of spleen and the Yangming Channel of stomach. Generally, in spring and summer, the Yang energy is plenty and the Yin energy is little, in autumn and winter, the Yin energy is prosperous and the Yang energy is deficient. Mostly, the patient of the cold-type jue-syndrome is self-assured that he is having a strong body, neglects to practise temperance to the sexual activities in autumn and winter when the Yang energy is declined, it causes the Yin energy below to float up and contend with the Yang energy, As the Yang energy can not be stored inside, the Yin energy which is cold will be reversed up to become the cold-type jue-syndrome. Since the cold-evil is harbouring inside, the Yang energy will decline in the wake of it, and it will not be able to permeat and operate in the channels and collaterals. In this way, the Yang energy is injured every day, and finally, the Yin energy will be existing solely, and as a result, the patient will have cold extremities."

帝曰：热厥何如而然也？岐伯曰：酒入于胃，则络脉满而经脉虚；脾主为胃行其津液者也，阴气虚则阳气入〔孙鼎宜说："入"当作"实"〕，阳气入则胃不和，胃不和则精气竭，精气竭则不营其四支也。此人必数醉，若饱以入房，气聚于脾中不得散，酒气与谷气相薄〔《太素》"薄"当作"搏"〕，热盛于中〔《病沅》"盛于中"作"起于内"〕，故热偏于身内热而溺赤也。夫酒气盛而慓悍，肾气有〔胡本，元残二，吴本，朝本，"有"并作"曰"〕衰，阳气独胜，故手足为之热也。

Yellow Emperor asked: " How does the heat-jue-syndrome come about?" Qibo said: " When alcohol is taken, it will cause the collaterals to fill with blood, and the channels, on the contrary, become empty. As the spleen is to help the stomach for transporting the essence of water and cereals, if alcohol is excessively taken, the spleen will have nothing to transport and cause the Yin energy to become asthenic; when the Yin energy is asthenic, the Yang energy will be sthenic, and the stomach energy will become disharmonious, and thus, the refined energy of water and cereals will be reduced, and the extremities can hardly be nourished. The patient of this kind must be drunken frequently and conducting sexual intercourse after being well-fed, his kidney energy is so asthenic that his gate of life has no more energy to support the spleen, and the energy in the spleen will be stagnated without being dispersed. When the energy of alcohol and the energy of cereals are combating, heat will emerge from inside, and fever all over the body and the deep-coloured urine will occur. As the energy of alcohol is abundant and violent, and the kidney energy is declining day after day, the Yang energy will become solely abundant inside and both the hands and feet will be hot."

帝曰：厥或令人腹满，或令人暴不知人，或至〔《病沅》"或"下无"至"字〕半日远至一日乃知人者何也？岐伯曰：阴气盛于上则下虚，下虚则腹胀满；阳气盛于上，则下气重上，而邪气逆，逆则阳气乱，阳气乱则不知人也。

Yellow Emperor asked: " Some jue-syndromes cause one to have distention of the abdomen, some cause one to become unconscious all of a sudden and can not regain consciousness until half a day or even one whole day, and what is the reason?" Qibo said: " When the

Yin energy is abundant partially on the upper part of the body, one will be deficient in the lower and the abdomen will apt to have distention; when the Yang energy is abundant partially on the upper part, the Yin energy will join and go along with it. As the evil-energy is going in the adverse direction, the adverse evil-energy will cause confusion of the Yang energy, and when the Yang energy is confused, one will lost consciousness all of a sudden."

帝曰：善。愿闻六经脉之厥状病能〔王注所据本无“病能”二字，疑衍〕也。岐伯曰：巨阳之厥，则肿〔《太素》“肿”作“踵”，据《太素》杨注“头”应作“皆”〕首头重，足不能行，发为眴仆；阳明之厥，则癫疾欲走呼，腹满不得卧，面〔“面”上有“卧则”二字〕赤而热，妄见而妄言；少阳之厥，则暴聋颊肿而〔《病源》“而”作“胸”〕热，胁痛，骭不可以运；太阴之厥，则腹满䐜胀，后不利，不欲食，食则呕，不得卧；少阴之厥，则口乾〔《太素》《病沅》《千金》“口”并作“舌”〕溺赤，腹满心痛；厥阴之厥，则少腹肿痛，腹〔《太素》“腹”作“䐜”〕胀，泾溲不利，好卧屈膝，阴缩肿〔《甲乙》“缩”下无“肿”字〕，骱〔《太素》、《病沅》“骱”并作“胫”〕内热。盛则写之、虚则补之，不盛不虚，以经取之。

Yellow Emperor said: "Good. I hope to hear about the syndromes of the jue-disease in the six channels." Qibo said: "The jue-disease of the Taiyang Channel causes one to feel heavy on the head and heel, to become dim-sighted which causes one to fall down. The patient is unable to walk due to the weakness of legs.

"The jue-disease of Yangming Channel causes one to have mania, running while shouting, distention of the abdomen and inability of lying down. When the patient lies down, his complexion will be come red and will have fever; what he has seen are peculiar things, and what he has spoken are nonsense.

"The jue-disease of Shaoyang Channel causes one to become deaf suddenly, to have swelling in the cheeks, hotness in the chest, pain on the lateral sides of the thorax, and the thighs can not move.

"The jue-disease of the Taiyin Channel causes one to have distention of the abdomen, constipation, reluntance of eating and vomits after eating, the patient is unable to lie quietly.

"The jue-disease of the Shaoyin Channel causes one to have dry tongue, deep-coloured urine, distention of the abdomen and heartache.

"The jue-disease of the Jueyin Channel causes one to have swelling and pain of the lower abdomen, fullness and distention of the abdomen, dysurla, the desire of curlling up when lying, atrophy of the external genitals and hotness on the inner side of the shanks.

"When treating the jue-disease, apply the purgation therapy when the body of the patient is strong, and apply the invigorating therapy when the body of the patient is weak. To patients of ordinary body which is not strong nor weak, aply acupuncture therapy to prick the main points of the related channel.

太阴厥逆〔《太素》作“足太阴脉厥逆”，下“少阳”等类推〕，骭急挛，心痛引腹，治主病者；少阴厥逆，虚满呕变，下泄清〔《太素》“清”作“青”，柯校云：“‘清’疑‘青水’二字”〕，治主病者；厥阴厥逆，挛、腰痛，虚满前闭，谵言，治主病者；三阴俱逆，不

得前后，使人手足寒，三日死。太阳厥逆，僵仆，呕血善衄，治主病者；少阳厥逆，机关不利，机关不利者，腰不可以行，项不可以顾，发肠痈不可〔“不可”应作“犹可”〕治，惊者死；阳明厥逆，喘咳身热，善惊，衄呕〔《甲乙》“衄”下有“血”字〕血。

“When the Jueni disease of Foot Taiyin Channel is contracted, the convulsion of shanks and heartache which effects the abdomen will occur. When treating, prick the points on the channel which are associated to the disease. When the Jueni disease of the Foot Shaoyin Channel is contracted, distention and fullness of the abdomen, vomiting and green watery diarrhea will occur. When treating, prick the points on the channel which are associated to the disease. When the Jueni disease of the Foot Jueyin Channel is contracted, convulsion, lumbago, dysuria and speaking nonsense will occur. When treating, prick the points on the channel which are associated to the disease. If the Jueni of Taiyin, shaoyin and Jueyin channels are all contracted siumltaneously, and the patient will have retention of feces and urine, cold extremities from the tips to the elbows or knees, and he will die in three days.

“When the Jueni disease of the Foot Taiyang Channel is contracted, the patient will have coma to fall down frequently and has nasal hemorrhage often. When treating, prick the points on the channel which are associated to the disease.

“When the Jueni disease of Foot Shaoyang Channel is contracted, the tendons, bones and the joints will not be nimble, the loins can hardly move about, and the neck can hardly look back; if the pyogenic infection of intestine occurs at the same time, the disease will have chance to be cured but if the patient is terrified again, he will die.

“When the Jueni disease of the Foot Yangming Channel is contracted, rapid respiration, cough, fever of the body, being frightened often, nasal hemorrhage and hematemesis will occur.

手太阴厥逆，虚满而咳，善呕沫，治主病者，手心主、少阴厥逆，心痛引喉，身热死，不（《甲乙》“不”下有“热”字）可治；手太阳厥逆，耳聋泣出，项不可以顾，腰不可以俯仰〔王冰说：“项不可二句，脉不相应，疑古错简文”〕，治主病者；手阳明、少阳厥逆、发喉痹、嗌肿，痓〔林校全本引“痓”作“痉”，谓颈项强急〕，治主病者。

“When the Jueni disease of the Hand Taiyin Channel is contracted, asthenic-fullness of the chest and abdomen, cough, vomiting of the phlegm and water frequently will occur. When treating, prick the points on the channel which are associated to the disease.

“When the Jueni disease of the Pericardium Channel of Hand Jueyin or the Heart channel of Hand Shaoyin is contracted, heartache which affects the throat will occur, if the patient has fever, he will die, if he has no fever, the disease can be cured.

“When the Jueni disease of the Hand Taiyang Channel is contracted, one will become deaf and will have falling tears in the eyes. When treating, prick the points on the channel which are associated to the disease.

“When the Jueni disease of the Hand Yangming and Shaoyang Channel is contracted, it can develope into sorethroat, pharynx swelling, and stiffness of the neck, When treating, prick the points on the channel which are associated to the disease.”

病能论篇第四十六

Chapter 46
Bing Neng Lun
(On Various Diseases)

黄帝问曰：人病胃脘痈者，诊当何如？岐伯对曰：诊此者当候胃脉，其脉当〔《圣济总录》"脉"下并无"当"字〕沉细〔《甲乙》"细"作"濇"，下"细"字同〕，沉细者气逆，逆者人迎甚盛，甚盛则热；人迎者胃脉也，逆而盛，则热聚于胃口而不行，故胃脘为痈也。

Yellow Emperor asked: "How can one diagnose the carbuncle of the gastric cavity?" Qibo answered: "In diagnosing this kind of disease, the stomach pulse should be inspected first, In this disease, the fuyang pulse (also called Chongyang pulse, located over the anterior at the dorsum of foot, reflecting the disorders of the spleen and stomach of the patient) must be sunken and rough, which reflects the reversing up of the stomach energy; when the stomach enery is rsversing up, the Renying (pulse of the cervical arteries lateral to the thyroid cartilage) will pulsate severely, which shows there is fever in the patient. As the Renying pulse is the artery of the stomach, and the sunken and rough fuyang pulse is the unfavourable condition of the energy, when the pulsation of the Renying pulse is florishing, it shows the heat is accumulating in the stomach without dispersing, thus, the carbuncle will occur in the gastric cavity."

帝曰：善。人有卧而有所不安者何也？岐伯曰：藏有所伤，及精有所之寄则安〔《甲乙》作"情有所倚，则卧不安"〕，故人不能悬其病也。

Yellow Emperor said: "Good. Some people can not sleep calmly and what is the reason?" Qibo said: "This is because there is injury in his viscera, or his sentiment is rather radical. If the two reasons are not removed, he can not sleep calmly."

帝曰：人之不得偃仰者何也？岐伯曰：肺者藏之盖也，肺气盛则脉大，脉大则不得偃卧，论在《奇恒阴阳》中。

Yellow Emperor asked: "Some people can not lie on his back, and why is it?" Qibo said: "The lung situates on the highest position and covers all the other organs, when the evil-energy is filling abundantly in the lung, the collaterals of the lung will be swelling, and when it is swelling, one can not lie on his back. There was such a discussion in the《Extraordinary and Normal Yin and Yang》of ancient times."

帝曰：有病厥者，诊右脉沈而紧，左脉浮而迟，不然病主安在？岐伯曰：冬诊之，右脉固当沉紧，此应四时，左脉浮而迟，此逆四时，在左当主病在肾，颇关在肺，当腰痛也。帝曰：何以言之？岐伯曰：少阴脉贯肾络肺，今得肺脉，肾为之病，故肾为腰痛之病也。

Yellow Emperor asked: "Some people become ill due to the adverseness of the vital en-

ergy, according to palpation, the pulse of his right hand is sunken and tight, and the pulse of his left hand is floating and slow, and where is the disease?" Qibo said: "In winter, if the right pulse is sunken and tight, it is normal as it is accordance with the four seasons; if the left pulse is floating and slow in winter, it is abnormal as it is against the four seasons, and there is disease in the kidney. As the floating pulse condition is about similar to the lung pulse which is floating, the patient will have lumbago."

Yellow Emperor asked: "Why is it so?" Qibo said: "The Shaoyin Channel runs through the kidney and connects the lung, since, at present, the floating and slow pulse occur in winter, it shows the deficiency of the kidney energy. When there is disease in the kidney, the patient will suffer from lumbago."

帝曰：善。有病颈痈者，或石治之，或针灸〔《甲乙》"或"下并有"以"字，柯校云："依下文，'灸'字疑衍"〕治之，而皆已，其真〔《甲乙》"真"作"治"〕安在？岐伯曰：此同名异等者也。夫痈气之息者，宜以针开除〔"除"字疑衍〕去之，夫气盛血聚者，宜石而写之，此所谓同病异治也。

Yellow Emperor said: "Good. To the patient of the carbuncle on neck, sometimes it is treated with stone needle, some-times it is treated with metal needle, and they can all be cured, and why it is so?" Qibo said: "This due to the diseases are having the same name but belong to different types. If the carbuncle is formed by the accumulation of the stagnated energy, it should be pricked by the metal needle to open the acupoint and clear away the evil-energy; if the carbuncle is matured with pus together with abundant stagnated energy and blood, they should be let out with the stone needle. It is the so called treating the same disease in different ways."

帝曰：有病怒狂者，此病安生？岐伯曰：生于阳也。帝曰：阳何以使人狂？岐伯曰：阳气者〔《千金》"气"下无"者"字〕，因暴折而难决，故善怒也，病名曰阳厥。帝曰：何以知之？岐伯曰：阳明者常动，巨阳少阳不动，不动而动大疾，此其候也。帝曰：治之奈何？岐伯曰：夺〔《太素》、《甲乙》"夺"并作"衰"〕其食即已，夫食入于阴，长气于阳，故夺其食即已。使之服以生铁洛〔《太素》"洛"作"落"〕为饮，夫生铁洛〔作"落"〕者，下气疾也。

Yellow Emperor asked: "There is a disease which causes one apt to be raved with fury, and how does it come about?" Qibo said: "It is due to the overabundance of the Yang energy." Yellow Emperor asked: "Why can the Yang energy cause one to become mad?" Qibo said: "When the Yang energy meets with the setback suddenly and can not be dredged, it will cause one to get angry, and the disease is called the Yang-type Jue." Yellow Emperor asked: "How can one know the disease is about to come about?" Qibo said: "For a normal man, some points (such as Renying point) on the Yangming Channel pulsate prominantly, but some points on the Taiyang Channel (such as Tianchuang point S. I. 16) and on the Shaoyang Channel (such as Tianrong point S, I. 17) only pulsate faintly. If the pulse which should pulsate faintly becomes very rapidly all of a sudden, it is the syndrome of Yang type syncope and the patient is apt to get angry and become mad." Yellow Emperor asked: "How

to treat it?" Qibo said: "When his meals and food are reduced the disease can be revovered. When the food enters into the stomach, it will promote the Yang energy, so, when the food is reduced, the Yang energy will become declined, and the disease will be recovered. Besides, the patient can also take some soup of iron filings which has curable effect to the disease of the mania kind."

帝曰：善。有病身热解堕〔《政和经史证备用草本》引“身热”下有“者”字，“解堕”二字自为句〕，汗出如浴，恶风少气，此为何病？岐伯曰：病名曰酒风。帝曰：治之奈何？岐伯曰：以泽泻、术各十分，麋衔五分，合，以三指撮，为后饭。

Yellow Emperor said: "Good. Some people has fever all over the body, feeling tired in the extremities, sweating all over like taking a bath, has an aversion to wind and is short of breath, what is the disease?" Qibo said: "It is called the wind-evil syndrome due to drinking." Yellow Emperor asked: "How to treat it?" Qibo said: "Take the oriental water plantain (Rhi-zoma Alismatis) and large-headed atractylodes (Rhizoma Atractylodis Macrocephalae) ten portions each, pyrola (Herba Pyrolae) five portions, mix and grind them into powder, and take the quantity which can be picked up with three fingers for each time before meal.

所谓深之细者，其中手如针也，摩之切之，聚者坚也，博〔“博”疑误，似应作“搏”〕者大也。《上经》者，言气之通天也；《下经》者言病之变化也；《金匮》者，决死生也；《揆度》者，切度之也；《奇恒》者，言奇病也。所谓奇者，使奇病不得以四时死也；恒者，得以四时死也，所谓揆者，方切求之也，言切求其脉理也〔《太素》无“言切”以下七字〕；度者，得其病处，以四时度之也。

"The so called sunken and fine pulse is like needle when it responds to the fingers in palpation; when the pulse is concentrating and not dispersing after being pushed and pressed, it is the firm pulse; when the Yin and Yang are combating, it is the gigantic pulse.

"The《Upper Classics》is the book discussing the relation between the nature and the activities of human body; the《Lower Classics》is the book discussing the variations of diseases; the《Golden Chamber》is the book discussing the diagnosis of diseases and the determinations of the survival and death of the patient; the《Observing and Judging》is the book discussing the determination of diseases according to the pulse condition from palpation; the《Extraordinary and Ordinary Diseases》is the book discussing and analysizing the abnormal diseases. The extraordinary diseases indicate the fatal diseases which are not effected by the four seasons; the ordinary diseases indicate the fatal diseases which are effected by the weather change of the four seasons. 'Judge' indicates integrating the favourable and infavourable conditions of the four seasons to analyse the treating methods of the disease and determine the death or survival of the patient according to the result of the diagnosis."

奇病论篇第四十七

Chapter 47
Qi Bing Lun
(On Extraordinary Diseases)

黄帝问曰：人有重身，九月而瘖，此为何也？岐伯对曰：胞之络〔“之络”二字误倒，应据《太平御览》乙正〕脉绝也。帝曰：何以言之？岐伯曰：胞络者系于肾，少阴〔《太平御览》引“阴”下，无“之”字〕之脉，贯肾〔按《灵枢经脉篇》“贯”作“属”〕系舌本，故不能言。帝曰：治之奈何？岐伯曰：无治也，当十月复。《刺法》曰：无损不足，益有余，以成其疹〔《甲乙》“疹”作“辜”〕。然后调之〔《太素》，《甲乙》并无“然后”四字〕，所谓无损不足者，身羸瘦，无用鑱石也；无益其〔“其”字衍〕有余者，腹中有形而泄〔孙鼎宜说：“‘泄’当作‘补’”，下同〕之，泄之则精出而病独擅中，故曰疹成〔《甲乙》“疹成”作“成辜”〕也。

Yellow Emperor asked: “In the ninth months of a woman's pregnancy, there is no vioce when she speaks, what is the reason?” Qibo answered: “it is because of the collaterals in her uterus are obstructed.”

Yellow Emperor asked: “Why is it so?” Qibo said: “The collaterals of the uterus are connecting the kidney, and the Kidney Channel of Shaoyin belongs to the kidney and the root of tongue, so, when the collaterals of the uterus are obstructed, she will speak without voice.”

Yellow Emperor asked: “How to treat it?” Qibo said: “it is not necessary to treat at all, when the pregnancy is completed after ten months, it will be recovered naturally.

“It was stated in the《Acupuncture》of ancient times; ‘one must not injure when there is an insufficiency, nor invigorate when there is a surplus so that it may not cause the evil-energy to become a solid tumor’.

“The so-called not to injure when there is an insufficiency means when the patient is thin, it must not treat with the stone needle. The so-called not to invigorate when there is a surplus means, although after invigoration, the spirit of the patient may turn to the better, but something solid like abdominal mass may occur.”

帝曰：病胁下满气逆〔《甲乙》“气逆”下并有“行”字，按“行”字应属下读，《国语·晋语》书注：“‘行’，历也”〕，二三岁不已，是为何病？岐伯曰：病名曰息积〔《甲乙》“积”作“贲”〕，此不妨于食，不可灸刺，积为导引服药〔《圣济经》无“服药”二字〕，药不能独治也。

Yellow Emperor asked: “Some people has fullness and distention over the hypochondrium and adverseness of the vital energy lasting for two or three years, and what is the dis-

ease?" Qibo siad: " It is called lump located at right hypochondrium, the patient can eat and drink as usual without doing him any harm. When treating, it must not apply moxibustion and acupuncture, but should dredge the energy and blood with a long-term physical exercise, and the disease can not be cured solely by medicine."

帝曰：人有身体髀股䯒皆肿，环齐而痛，是为何病？岐伯曰：病名曰伏梁。此风根也，其气溢于大肠，而著于肓，肓之原在齐下，故环齐而痛也。不可动之，动之为水溺濇之病也。

Yellow Emperor asked: " Some people is swelling in his hips, thighs and legs and has pain around his navel, what is the disease?" Qibo said: " It is called fuliang (ancient name for the disease with epigastric fullness and mass) which is mainly caused by the wind-evil. As the evil-energy is spreading all over the outside of the large intestine and retains in the adipose membrane, and the source of the adipose membrane is under the navel, so there is pain around the navel. To this kind of disease, it should not apply medicine for purgating, if the purgation therapy is applied, dysuria will occur."

帝曰：人有尺脉数甚〔《甲乙》"脉数"作"肤缓"〕，筋急而见，此为何病：岐伯曰：此所谓疹〔《甲乙》"疹"作"狐"〕筋，是人腹必急〔《太素·疹筋》"是"下无"人"字〕，白色黑色见，则病甚。

Yellow Emperor asked: " Somebody whose Chi pulse (the proximal throbbing of the radial pulse) pulsates slowly, what is the disease?" Qibo said: " It is called hujin (abdominal pain and convulsion of extremities). When it is contracted, abdominal pain will occur. If there is white or black colour occur on the skin, the disease will be more serious."

帝曰：人有病头痛以数岁〔《甲乙》"痛"下无"以"字〕不已，此安得之？名为何病？岐伯曰：当有所犯大寒，内至骨髓，髓者〔《甲乙》"髓"上有"骨"字〕以脑为主，脑逆故令头痛〔《太素》"令"下有"人"字〕，齿亦痛〔《太素》"亦"下有"当"字〕，病名曰厥逆〔《针灸资生经》卷六《头痛》引"厥逆"下有"头痛"二字〕。帝曰：善。

Yellow Emperor asked: " Somebody has headache lasting for many years, how is it contracted?" Qibo siad: " Some part of the body must have been invaded by the cold-evil. When the cold-evil invades the bone marrow, the brain will be invaded as the brain is a main part of the bone marrow, and the syndrome of headache and toothache will occur. The disease is called the head-ache due to attack of cold-evil." Yellow Emperor said: " Good."

帝曰：有病口甘者，病名为何？何以得之？岐伯曰：此五气〔《医说》引"五"作"土"〕之溢也，名曰脾瘅。夫五味入口，藏于胃，脾为之行其精气，津液在脾〔《外治》作"溢在于脾"〕，故令人口甘也；此肥美之所发也，此人必数食甘美而多肥也，肥者令人内热，甘者令人中满，故其气上溢，转为消渴。治之以兰，除陈气也。

Yellow Emperor asked: " Some people have sweet taste in the mouth, what is the disease, and how does it come about?" Qibo said: " It is due to the overflowing of the earth-energy, and the disease is called pidan (heat and wetness in spleen). Generally, the food enters through the mouth, stores in the stomach, be converted into the refined substance by the spleen and being transported to various organs. At present, however, the spleen fails to operate normally, and the up-flowing of the body fluid will cause sweetness in the mouth. This

disease is seduced by the fine and delicious food, and most of the patients with this disease usually have nice and delicious food. The fatty and delicious food can cause the inner heat of a man, and the sweet taste can cause one to have fullness and distention of the chest, and the up-flowing of the spleen energy may be transferred into diabetes. It should be treated with stem the of orchid which can remove the staleness heat."

帝曰：有病口苦取阳陵泉〔明抄本“有病”下并无“口苦取阳陵泉”六字〕，口苦者病名为何？何以得之？岐伯曰：病名曰胆瘅。夫肝者中之将也〔林校云：“按《甲乙》曰：胆者中精之府，五藏取决于胆，咽为之使，疑“肝者中之将也”文误〕，取决于胆，咽为之使。此人者，数谋虑不决，故胆虚气上溢〔《甲乙》“胆”下无“虚”字，按“溢”误，应作“嗌”〕，而口为之苦。治之以胆募俞，治在《阴阳十二官相使》中。

Yellow Emperor asked: "Some patients have bitterness in the mouth, what is the disease and how does it come about?" Qibo said: "The disease is called Dandan (heat and wetness in gallbladder). The gallbladder is a clean hollow organ, it determins the conditions of all the five viscera and also controls the pharynx and larynx. The patient with Dandan disease is always gloomy with continuous worry, so that the gallbladder can not bring its normal functions into full play, and the bile will be overflowing upwards and cause bitterness in the mouth. When treating, prick the front Mu-point of gallbladder (Riyue point GB. 24) and Danshu point (BL. 19). The principle of treating is written in the《Mutual-assistance of the Twelve Organs of Yin and Yang》."

帝曰：有癃者，一日数十溲，此不足也。身热如炭〔《太素》“炭”下有“火”字〕，颈膺如格，人迎躁盛，喘息气逆，此有余也。太阴脉微细如发者〔明抄本“细”上无“微”字〕，此不足也，其病安在？名为何病？岐伯曰：病在太阴，其盛在胃，颇在肺，病名曰厥，死不治，此所谓得五有余二不足也。帝曰：何谓五有余二不足？岐伯曰：所谓五有余者〔张琦说：“‘五’字衍，下‘五病’之‘五’字亦衍”〕，五病之气有余也，二不足者〔张琦说：“‘二’字衍”〕，亦病气之不足也。今外得五有余，内得二不足，此其身不表不里，亦正死〔《甲乙》“正死”作“死证”〕明矣。

Yellow Emperor asked: "Some one has frequent micturition with several decades of times in a day which is the case of insufficiency; his body is hot like charcoal, seems to have something blocking between the neck and the chest, his Renying pulse is irritating, he has rapid breathing and adverseness of vital energy, which show the cases of having a surplus; his Cunkou pulse is thin like hair, and it is the symbol of insufficiency. Now, where is the disease located and what is the disease?" Qibo said: "The origin of the disease is in the Taiyin Channel, it is caused by the excessive heat of the stomach, and its syndrome is manifested on the lung. The disease is called jue-syndrome, and it is a fatal disease. The disease is caused by the five cases of having a surplus and the two cases of being insufficient."

Yellow Emperor asked: "What are the five cases of having a surplus and the two cases of being insufficient?" Qibo said: "The so-called having a surplus is indicating there is a surpuls in the evil-energy, and the so-called being insufficient indicates the insufficiency of the evil-energy. Since, at present, there are five kinds of pulse conditions and other manifesta-

tions showing surplus in the exterior (five cases of surplus: hot like charcoal in the body, obstruction between neck and chest, irritation of the Renying pulse, rapid breathing, and adverseness of the vital energy) and there are two kinds of pulse conditions and other manifestations showing insufficient in the interior (two cases of insufficient: the pulse is thin like hair, several decades times of urination in a day), the patient can not be treated from the superfices, nor can be treated from the interior, so, he is having a fatal disease"

帝曰：人生而有病癫疾者〔《太平御览》《医说》引“而”下无“有”字〕，病名曰何？安所得之？岐伯曰：病名为胎病。此得之在母腹中时，其母有所大惊〔《千金》《圣济总录》“所”下并有“数”字〕，气上而不下，精气并居，故令子发为巅疾〔《太平御览》引“发”下无“为”字〕也。

Yellow Emperor asked: " Some people have epilepsy since he was born, what is the disease, and how does it come about?" Qibo said: " It is called the infantile epilepsy. It is because the mother was frightended severely several times when the baby was in her womb, her vital energy reversed upwards and failed to come down, and the assembling of the energy of fright caused the baby to have epilepsy when he was born. "

帝曰：有病痝然如有水状〔《甲乙》“水”下并有“气”字〕，切其脉大紧，身无痛者，形不瘦，不能食，食少，名为何病？岐伯曰：病生在肾〔《甲乙》“生”作“主”〕，名为肾风，肾风而不能食，善惊〔《甲乙》“惊”作“不”〕，惊已，心气〔《太素》“心”下无“气”字〕痿者死。帝曰：善。

Yellow Emperor asked: " Someone is swelling like edema in his face, his pulse condition is gigantic and tight, he has no pain in the body and is not emaciated, but he can not eat or can eat only a little, what is the disease?" Qibo said: " The root of this disease is in the kidney, and it is called the wind-evil syndrome of kidney. When the patient of wind-evil syndrome come to the stage of failing to take food or can eat only very little, if he often being frightened or being firghtened continuously, he will have heart faliurs and die. " Yellow Emperor said: " Good. "

大奇论篇第四十八

Chapter 48
Da Qi Lun
(On Strange Diseases)

肝满〔“满”应作“脉”，以后“心脉”“肝脉”均同〕肾满肺满皆实，即〔《太素》“即”作“皆”〕为肿。肺为雍〔《太素》《甲乙》“雍”并作“痈”，按“肺”下“之”字衍〕，喘而两胠满：肝雍，两胠〔《太素》“胠”作“胁”〕满，卧则惊，不得小便；肾雍，脚〔《太素》《甲乙》“脚”并作“胠”《脉经》“少”并作“小”〕下至少腹满，胫有大小，髀骱大〔《甲乙》“骱”作“胫”，无“大”字〕跛，易偏枯。

When the pulse conditions of the liver, kindey and lung are all substantial, abundant and full, they can all cause swelling.

When one contracts the lung abscess, rapid respiration and distention of the two lateral sides of the thoraxes will occur; when one contracts the liver abscess, distention of the two lateral sides of the thoraxes, fright during sleep and dysuria will occur; when one contracts the kidney abscess, distention over the hypochondrium and the lower abdomen, swelling of the two lateral sides of the tibia now and then, deformation of the thighs and legs will occur, the patient can not keep his body in balance when walking, and he is apt to have hemiplegia.

心脉满大，痫瘛筋挛；肝脉小急，痫瘛筋挛；肝脉骛，暴有所惊骇，脉不至若瘖，不治自已。

When the heart pulse is full and gigantic, it shows the internal heat is excessive, epilepsy, cramp of hands and feet, and the stiffness of tendons will occur. If the liver pulse is small and tight, which shows asthenic-cold of the liver, epilepsy, cramp of hands and feet and the stiffness of tendons will also occur. If the liver pulse is rapid, or the pulse can not be felt due to the fright of the patient and he also has dysphonia, it is the phenomenum of the adverseness of vital energy due to fright. It is not necessary to treat at all as it will be recovered when the patient is calmed down.

肾脉小急，肝脉小急，心脉小急〔《太素》“心脉”下无“小急”二字，“心脉”二字连下读〕不鼓皆为瘕。

When the kidney pulse is small and tight, the liver pulse is also small and tight, and the heart pulse is not hitting under the fingers, it shows the stagnation of the blood which may become abdominal mass.

肾肝并沉〔王注“肾肝”下并有“脉”字〕为石水，并浮为风水，并虚为死，并小弦欲〔《全生指迷方》引作“为”〕惊。

When both the kidney pulse and the liver pulse are sunken, indurative edema will occur.

When both the pulse conditions of kidney and liver are floating, it is edema caused by wind-evil and it is a fatal disease. If they are small and wiry like a bow string, the disease of terror will occur.

肾脉大急沉，肝脉大急沉，皆为疝。

When the pulse condition of kidney is gigantic, rapid and sunken, or the pulse condition of the liver is gigantic, rapid and sunken, hernia will occur.

心脉搏滑急〔《太素》"搏"作"揣"、《广推·释诂》"揣"动也，"心脉搏，谓心脉之动，"滑急"即谓滑紧〕为心疝，肺脉沉搏〔准上文例，"搏"亦应作"揣"》〕为肺疝。

When the condition of the heart pulse is slippery and tight, it is the heart-channel colic; when the condition of the lung pulse is sunken, it is the lung-channel colic.

三阳急为瘕，三阴急为疝〔《太素》《甲乙》并无"三阴急为疝"五字〕，二阴急为痫厥，二阳急为惊。

When the coming of the bladder pulse and the small intestine pulse are urgent, it is the abdominal mass; when the coming of both the heart and kidney pulses are urgent, it is the disease of epileptic syncope, when the coming of both the stomach and large intestine pulses are urgent, it is the disease of terror.

脾脉外鼓，沉为肠澼，久自已。肝脉小缓为肠澼，易治。肾脉小搏沉，为肠澼下血，血温身〔《尤怡说："温"当作"溢"》〕热者死。心肝澼亦下血〔"澼亦下血"误衍，《全生指迷方》引正作"心肝脉小，沈濇为肠澼"〕，二藏同病者可治，其脉小沉濇为肠澼，其身热者死，热见〔《甲乙》"见"作"甚"〕七日死。

When the pulse condition of spleen is stirring and sunken, it is diarrhea which can can be recovered in a certain period. The patient with diarrhea whose liver pulse is small and slow, it can be cured easily. When the patient of diarrhea with bloody stool whose kidney pulse is small and sunken, if his blood is overflowing and he has a fever, he will die. When the patient of diarrhea whose heart pulse and liver pulse are both small, sunken and choppy, as both the two viscera are sick and wood produces fire, the disease can be cured. If the patient has a fever, he may die, when the fever is severe, he will die in seven days.

胃脉沉鼓〔"鼓"字涉下衍，此当作"胃脉沈濇"〕濇，胃外鼓大，心脉小坚急〔《全生指迷方》引"小"下无"坚"字〕，皆鬲〔"鬲"字误，似应作"为"〕偏枯，男子发左，女子发右，不瘖舌转，可治，三十日起，其从者，瘖，三岁起，年不满二十者，三岁死。

When the pulse condition of the stomach is sunken and choppy, or floatting and gigantic together with a rapid and small heart pulse, it shows the energy and blood is stagnated which can cause hemiplegia. If the disease of a man is on the left side, or of a woman is on the right side, speaking without dysphonia and the tougue can operate freely, the disease can be cured in about thirty days. If the disease if a man is on the right side or of a woman is on the left side, having dyaphonia when speaking, the disease can be recovered in about three years. If the patient is less than twenty years old and his body is developing, he will die in three years.

脉至而搏，血衄〔《甲乙》作"衄血"〕身热者死，脉来悬钩浮为常脉。

When the coming of the pulse is gigantic and strong in responding the fingers, and the patient has hemorrhage and fever, he will die. When the coming of the pulse is suspending without root, and is somewhat hooked and floating, it is the proper pulse for hemorrhage.

脉至如喘，名曰暴厥。暴厥者，不知与人言。脉至如〔《甲乙》“如”作“而”〕数，使人暴惊，三四日自已。

When the coming of the pulse is urgent like rushing currents, it is the syncope with sudden onset. The patient of syncope with sudden onset becomes unconscious and can not talk only for the time being. When the coming of the pulse is rapid, it is the heat-evil rushing the heart and causes one to become frightened suddenly. When the heat has come down, the patient will be quiet natrually, and the disease will be recovered in about three or four days.

脉至〔“至”下脱“如”字〕浮合，浮合如数〔张琦以“浮合如数”四字为衍文〕，一息十至以上，是经气予不足也，微见九十日死；脉见如火薪〔明抄本，《太素》“薪”并作“新”〕然，是心精之予夺〔《甲乙》“精”下无“之”字，“予夺”即“之夺”，“夺”古“脱”也〕也，草乾而死；脉至如散叶〔《甲乙》作“丛棘”，张琦说：“丛棘，弦硬杂乱之象”〕，是肝气予虚也，木叶落而死；脉至如省客，省客者，脉塞而鼓，是肾气予不足也，悬去枣华而死；脉至如丸泥，是胃精予不足也，榆荚落而死；脉至如横格，是胆气予不足也，禾熟而死；脉至如弦缕，是胞精予不足也，病善言，下霜而死，不言可治；脉至如交漆〔《太素》“漆”作“荚”〕，交漆者，左右傍至也，微见三十日死；脉至如涌泉〔《太素》“如”下无“涌”字〕，浮鼓肌〔《太素》“肌”作“胞”〕中，太阳气予不足也，少气味〔张琦说：“此二字衍”〕，韭英而死；脉至如颓土〔《太素》《脉经》“颓”并作“委”，按“委”有“弃”义〕之状，按之不得〔《甲乙》“不得”作“不足”〕，是肌气予不足也，五色先见〔《甲乙》“五色”下无“先”字〕，黑白垒发死；脉至如悬雍，悬雍者，浮揣切之益大，是十二俞之予不足也，水凝而死；脉至如偃刀，偃刀者，浮之〔《甲乙》“之”下有“气”字〕小急，按之坚大急〔《甲乙》“大”下无“急”字〕，五藏菀熟，寒热独并于肾也，如此其人不得坐，立春而死；脉至如丸，滑不直〔《甲乙》“直”作“著”〕手，不直手者，按之不可得也，是大肠气予不足也，枣叶生而死；脉至如华〔《甲乙》“华”并作“春”〕者，令人善恐，不欲坐卧，行立常听，是小肠气予不足也，季秋而死。

When the coming of the pulse is like the assembly of floating waves, ie., the very frequent coming of the waves, the pulsation is more than ten times in a respiration, it shows the insufficiency of the energies of the twelve channel in human body. The patient will die whithin ninety days from the occurance of the said pulse condition. When the coming of the pulse is like the beginning of the burning fire, it shows the refined energy of the heart is exhausting, the patient will die at the beginnibg of winter when the grasses are withered.

When the coming of the pulse is like overgrowing thorns, it is the pulse condition of extreme asthenic of the liver energy, the patient will die at the time when the leaves are falling.

When the coming of the pulse is very substantial like being blocked yet bouncing up to hit th fingers, it shows the refined energy of the kidney has become extremely insuffcient, and the patient will die in the period between the jujube tree comes into flower and the falling

of the petal.

When the coming of the pulse is like a clay ball which is firm, short and choppy, it shows the energy of the stomach has become insufficient, the patient will die in the beginning of summer when the elm leaves fall.

When the coming of the pulse is like something blocking horizontally under the fingers, it shows the energy of the gallbladder has become insufficient, the patient will die in late autumn when the crops become mature.

When the coming of the pulse is like string or thread, it shows the energy of the collaterals in the uterus has become insufficient. If the patient has polylogia, he will die in the season when the frost descends; if he does not talk much, the disease can be cured.

When the coming of the pulse is like the intersection in left and right of the beanpods, the patient will die within thirty days from the occurance of the pulse.

When the coming of the pulse is like the spring water stirring in the uterus, it shows the energy of the Taiyang Channel has become insufficient, the patient will die in long summer when the flowers of the Chinese chives occur.

When the coming of the pulse is like waste dust which is inadequate when by hard pressing, it shows the energy of the muscle has become insufficient. When the black and white complexions of the patient occur frequently, the patient will die.

When the coming of the pulse is like a hanging jar which seems to become larger and larger when being felt lightly, it shows the insufficiency of the retained energies of the twelve shu-points, and the patient will die in winter when the water is frozen.

When the coming of the pulse is like the blade facing up, small and rapid when being felt lightly, gigantic and firm when being felt heavily, it is the stagnated heat storing in the five viscera, and the cold-syndrome associated with the heat-syndrome is retaining in the kidney, the patient with this disease can not sit up and he will die on the Beginning of Spring.

When the coming of the pulse is like a shot, can hardly be touched due to slippery, and can not be held when being pressed, it shows the refined energy of the large intestine has become insufficient, and the patient will die in early summer when the leaves of the jujube tree begin to grow.

When the coming of the pulse is like pounding of rice which causes one to become frightened frequently, unable to sit down or to sleep at ease, hearing sounds often when standing or walking, it shows the refined energy of the small intestine has become insufficient, and the patient will die in late autumn.

脉解篇第四十九

Chapter 49
Mai Jie
(On Channels)

太阳所谓肿腰〔柯校云：“‘肿腰’当云‘腰肿’”〕肿痛者，正月太阳〔于鬯说：“‘太阳’二字疑涉下衍”〕寅，寅太阳也，正月阳气出在〔明抄本“在”作“于”〕上，而阴气盛，阳未得自次也，故肿腰脽痛也。病偏虚为跛〔《太素》卷八《经脉病解》“偏”上无“病”字〕者，正月阳气冻〔读本，赵本，吴本“冻”并作“东”〕解地气而出也，所谓偏虚者，冬寒颇有不足者，故偏虚为跛也。所谓强上引背〔《太素》无“引背”二字〕者，阳气大上而争，故强上也。所谓耳鸣者，阳气万物〔张文虎说：“‘万物’二字衍”〕盛上而跃，故耳鸣也。所谓甚则狂巅疾者〔《图经》注引无“甚则”二字〕，阳尽在上，而阴气从下，下虚上实，故狂巅疾也，所谓浮为聋者，皆在气也。所谓入中为瘖者，阳盛已衰，故为瘖也。内夺而厥，则为瘖俳，此肾虚也。少阴不至〔《太素》“不至”下重“少阴不至”四字〕者，厥也。

In Taiyang channel, there is the disease of swelling and distention of the loins and pain of the buttock. This is because the first (lunar) month of the year is Yin, and the month of Yin belongs to Taiyang. In the first month, the Yang energy begins to emerge from above, while the cold energy of Yin is still prosperous, and the Yang energy can not expand itself freely without impediment yet, so, it causes pain in the loins and the buttock.

The condition of lameness due to the partial asthenic of Yang energy in the body is: when the Yang energy come from the east in the first month, it thaws the energy of the frozen earth and ascends, as the weather is still cold, the Yang energy in the body is still insufficient, so, the asthenic Yang energy can only reside in the body slanting to one side, and the syndrome of lameness will occur.

The condition of headache and stiffness of the neck is due to the contention of Yang energies when rising.

The condition of tinnitus is due to the overabundance and the activity of the Yang energy above.

The condition of mania is: the Yang energy is staying above exclusively, unable to combine the Yin energy below, the Yin energy asthenia below and the Yang energy sthenia above will caues mania.

The deafness caused by the Yang energy floating above is due to the up-flaming of the Yang energy and the failure of fire to come down.

The condition of dysphonia is the Yang energy enters into the interior and the Yang energy has already become asthenic.

When one's sexual activities is excessive, the disease of Jueni (coldness of limbs) will occur, it can develope into dysphonia, aphasia and paralysis of limbs. The disease is due to the declination of the kidney which can not be reached by the energy of Shaoyin Channel. When the energy of the Shaoyin Channel is not approaching, the disease of Jueni will occur.

少阳所谓心胁痛者，言少阳盛也〔《太素》“盛”作“戌”，下“盛者”同，孙鼎宜说“‘言’字衍”〕，盛者心之所表也，九月阳气尽而阴气盛，故心胁痛也。所谓不可反侧者，阴气藏物也〔《太素》杨注《图经》“阴气”上有“九月”二字〕，物藏〔四库本“物藏”作“藏物”〕则不动，故不可反侧也。所谓甚则跃者，九月万物尽衰，草木毕落而堕，则气去阳而之阴，气盛而阳之下长，故谓跃。

The condition of pain in the heart and hypochondrium of Shaoyang Channel is: the Shaoyang belongs to the ninth lunar month of the year which is the month of Xu. Xu belongs to Shaoyang Channel which is connecting the pericardium, and the onset of the disease will affect the heart channel. In the ninth month, the Yang energy is about to become exhausting, and the Yin energy is becoming more and more prosperous, so, it causes the pains of the heart and the hypochondrium.

The condition of unable to toss and turn when lying of the patient is: the Yin energy become prosperous gradually from the ninth month, all things on earth are going to hide, and they all appear to be calm and motionless, since the energy of the Shaoyang Channel in human body is also affected, so, the patient can not toss and turn.

The condition of the disease of Yao is: in the ninth lunar month, all things begin to decline, the grasses and trees are withered and bare, and the energy of man is turning from Yang to Yin, if the Yang energy is prosperous, it will be active below as well, so it is called the disease of Yao (being active).

阳明所谓洒洒振寒者，阳明者午也，五月盛阳之阴也，阳盛而阴气加之，故洒洒振寒也。所谓胫肿而股不收者，是五月盛阳之阴也，阳者衰于五月，而一阴气上，与阳始争。故胫肿而股不收也。所谓上喘而为水者，阴气下而复上，上则邪客于藏府间，故为水也。所谓胸痛少气者，水气在藏府也〔《太素》“水”下无“气”字〕，水者阴气也，阴气在中，故胸痛少气也。所谓甚则厥，恶人与火，闻木音则惕然而惊者，阳气与阴气相薄，水火相恶，故惕然而惊也。所谓欲独闭户牖而处者，阴阳相薄也，阳尽而阴盛，故欲独闭户牖而居。所谓病至则欲乘高而歌，弃衣而走者，阴阳复〔林校引本句无“复”字，疑衍〕争，而外并于阳，故使之弃衣而走也。所谓客孙脉则头痛鼻鼽腹肿者，阳明并于上，上者则其孙络太阴也〔《太素》“络”作“脉”〕，故头痛鼻鼽腹肿也。

The condition of shivering all over the body with cold is: the Yangming Channel is prosperous in the fifth lunar month of the year. It is the time when Yang is extreme and Yin begins to emerge. The disease of the Yangming Channel is like the season of which the Yang is extreme with Yin is adding gradually, when Yangming is invaded by Yin which is associated with cold, the syndrome of shivering with cold all over the body will occur.

The condition of the swelling of the legs of the patient and the inability of stretching and bending his thighs is due to the making mischief of the Yin energy in the abundant Yang. In

the fifth lunar month, The Yang energy begins to decline and the energy of the first Yin begins to ascend and contend with the Yang energy. When the energy of the Yangming Channel becomes disharmonious, the syndrome of swelling of the legs and inability of bending and stretching the thighs will occur.

The condition of adverse rising of lung-energy to become edema is due to the reversing up of the Yin energy and the invasion of the Yin evil to the spleen and stomach, When the wetness is excessive it will transform into watar and reverse up to invade the lung to cause dyspnea.

The condition of chest pain and short of breath is due to the retaining of water in the viscera, as the fluid belongs to the Yin energy when it retains in the body, the syndrome of chest pain and short of breath will occur.

The condition of becoming to the disease of Jueni when the disease is severe is: the patient detests fire and light, becomes frightened when hearing the sound of hitting wood. It is due the friction between the Yin and Yang energies, and the disharmony of water and fire that cause the fright of the patient.

The condition of desiring to shut the doors and windows and live in solitued of the patient is due to the conflict between the Yin energy and Yang energy, when the Yang energy is declined, the Yin energy will become prosperous to make the patient prefer calmness, so, he desires to close the doors and windows and live in solitule.

The coldition of desiring to mount to a high place and sing aloud, running here and there with the clothes taken off of the patient during the onset of the disease is: the Yang energy becomes overabuudant after its contention with the Yin energy and the evil energy has combined into the Yang channel, causing the patient to have coma, becomes unconcious, and desires to run here and there with his clothes taken off.

The condition of headache, stuffy nose, running nose and abdominal distention when the evil-energy invades the minute collaterals of the upper part of the body is: due to the evil-energy of Yangming Channle has combined with the fine collaterals of the upper part of the body and the Taiyin Channel. When the evil-energy enters into the fine collaterals of the upper part of the body, it will cause the headache, stuffy nose and running nose of the patient, when the evil-energy enters into the Taiyin Channel, it will cause abdominal distention.

太阴所谓有病胀者，太阴子也〔《太素》“太阴”下有“者”字〕，十一月万物气皆藏于中，故曰病胀；所谓上走心为噫者，阴盛而上走于阳明，阳明络属心，故曰上走心为噫也；所谓食则呕者，物盛满而上溢，故呕也；所谓得后与气则快然如衰者，十二月〔胡本，诶本，赵本，吴本“二”并作“一”〕阴气下衰，而阳气且〔《图经》卷二《足大阴脾经》注引“且”作“自”〕出，故曰得后与气则快然如衰也。

The condition of the distention on the Taiyin Channel is due to the Taiyin Channel being prosperous in the eleventh lunar month of the year which is the month of Zi, and the eleventh lunar month is the month of storing and hiding of all things. By this time, the Yang energy of a man is also hiding and storing, if the evil-energy is stored inside also, the syn-

drome of abdominal fullness and distention will occur.

The condition of the rising up of the Yin energy to the heart to cause eructation is: due to the overabundance of the Yin energy which rises up to invade the stomach Channel of Foot Yangming, as the collaterals of the Yangming Channel is connecting the heart, so, when the heart channel is invaded by the Yin energy, the syndrome of eructation will occur.

The condition of vomiting after taking food of the patient is due to the food fails to be digested, and when the stomach is fully filled and the food is overflowing upwards, the patient will vomit.

The condition of feeling very comfortable of the patient when he has no detention of feces or to break wind is due to the Yin energy is extremely overabundant in the eleventh lunar month, and from then on, the Yin energy will decline gradually and the Yang energy will turn up natually. So, the patient will feel very comfortable when losing bowels and breaking wind.

少阴所谓腰痛者，少阴者肾〔“肾”字误，应作“申”〕也，十〔《太素》“十”作“七”〕月万物阳气皆伤，故腰痛也。所谓呕咳上气喘者，阴气在下，阳气在上，诸阳气浮，无所依从，故呕咳上气喘也。所谓色色〔《太素》“色色”作“邑邑”，“坐”上无“久”字，连下读，“邑邑”忧貌〕不能久立久坐，起则目䀮䀮无所见者，万物阴阳不定未有主也〔《图经》卷一《足少阴肾经》注引“主”作“生”〕，秋气始至，微霜始下，而方杀万物，阴阳内夺，故目䀮䀮无所见也。所谓少气善怒者，阳气不治，阳气不治，则阳气不得出，肝气当治而未得，故善怒，善怒者，名曰煎厥。所谓恐如人将捕之者，秋气万物未有毕去〔《太素》“有”作“得”〕，阴气少，阳气入，阴阳相薄，故恐也。所谓恶闻食臭者，胃无气，故恶闻食臭也。所谓面黑如地色〔孙鼎宜产：“‘地’当作‘炧’炧即炭也”〕者，秋气内夺，故变于色也。所谓咳则有血者，阳脉伤也，阳气未盛于上〔孙鼎宜说：“‘未’字疑衍，阳气盛于上即上文阳气在上之义，‘满’谓邪满也”〕而脉满，满则咳，故血见于鼻也。

The condition of lumbago in the Shaoyin Channel is due to the shaoyin begins at the seventh lunar month of the year which is the month of Shen. In the seventh lunar month, all the three Ying have risen up, and the Yang energy in human body becomes declined together with that of the season. So, lumbago will occur.

In the condition of vomiting, adverseness of the vital energy and rapid breathing of the patient is due to the Yin energy is overabundant below, and the Yang energy is floating above, as the Yang energy can adhere to nothing, the syndromes of vomiting, cough, adverseness of vital energy and rapid breathing will occur.

The condition of the prolonged worry and disapointment of the patient, unable to stand, being dazzled and can see nothing when sitting up is due to the Yin energy and Yang energy are both unstable. When the season of the chilly energy of autumn has arrived, the frost begins to descended slightly, and all things are withered and bare due to it. The case of the Yin and Yang contention in the human body is exactly the same, so, the patient's eyes are blur and can see nothing.

The condition of short of breath and often gets angry of the patient is due to the Yang

energy can no more play its normal role, the energy of the Shaoyang Channel can not come out, and the stagnated liver energy can not be dispersed, so, the patient is apt to get angry, and the disease is called 'scorching syncope'.

The condition of the patient is often frightened as if someone is going to arrest him is due to the autumn energy has just descended, the Yang energies in all things have not yet been removed thoroughly, the weather is still not cold and some of the Yang energy is still remaining inside as the weather is still hot, the frequent conflict of Yin and Yang energies cause the patient to become frightened often.

The condition of having an aversion to the odour of food of the patient is due to the stomach fails to digest the food, so, he detest the odour of food.

The condition of black complexion like charcoal of the patient is due to his quintessence has been exhausted by the autumn energy, and his complexion turns to black.

The condition of hemoptysis is due to the injury of collaterals in the upper part of the body. As the Yang energy is overabundant above, and the blood is filling the vessels, the blood-filling of vessels in the upper part will cause cough, and the syndrome of cough and epistaxis will occur.

厥阴所谓㿗疝，妇人少腹肿者，厥阴者辰也，三月阳中之阴，邪在中，故曰㿗疝少腹肿也。所谓腰脊〔"脊"字疑衍，《灵枢·经脉》肝足厥阴之脉，是动则病腰痛，并未言"脊"〕痛不可以俯仰者，三月一振荣华，万物一俯而不仰也〔《太素》"万物"上有"而"字〕。所谓㿗癃疝〔《太素》作"钉癃"，小便难也〕肤胀者，曰阴亦盛而脉胀不通〔《太素》作"曰阴一盛，而胀阴胀不通"〕，故曰㿗癃疝也〔《太素》无"疝"字〕。所谓甚则嗌干热中者，阴阳相薄而热，故嗌干也。

The disease of swelling of scrotum of male or distention of the lower abdomen of female in Jueyin Channel is: the starting month of Jueyin is Chen which is the third lunar month of the year. The third lunar month is the time when the Yang energy is just asthenic and the Yin energy is about to exhaust, and it is the season of Yin in the Yang. When the evil energy is accumulated inside, the swelling of the scrotum of male or distention of the lower abdomen of female will occur.

The condition of lumbago which causes one can not face up and down is: due to the Yang energy is stirring in the third lunar month of the year, the grasses and trees then are flourishing, all branches and leaves are bowing down, showing the tendency of bending without lifting. The disease of a man is in accordance with it, and the disease of lumbago will cause one unable to face up and down.

The condition of swelling of the external genitals, skin and muscle of the patient is due to the over-abundance of the Jueyin energy to cause distention and impediment of Yin, the swelling of the external genitals and dysuria.

The condition of dryness of the laryngopharynx and retention of heat-evil in the middle warmer is due to the internal heat produced from the conflict between Yin and Yang. It can cause dryness of the laryngopharynx.

刺要论篇第五十

Chapter 50
Ci Yao Lun
(The Essentials of Acupuncture)

黄帝问曰：愿闻刺要。岐伯对曰：病有浮沈，刺有浅深，各至其理，无过其道，过之则内伤，不及则生外壅〔《按“生”字衍〕，壅则邪从之，浅深不得，反为大贼，内动〔《甲乙》“动”作“伤”〕五藏，后生大病。故曰：病有在毫毛腠理者，有在皮肤者，有在肌肉者，有在脉者，有在筋者，有在骨者，有在髓者。

Yellow Emperor asked: “ What are the essentials of acupuncture?” Qibo answered: “ The extents of severeness of diseases are different, and in treating, the depth of pricking should also be different. In treating, the pricking should reach the depth where it ought to be, and must not exceed the proper criterion. If the pricking is too deep, the viscus will be hurt, if the pricking is too shallow, it will unable to reach the focus and will cause stagnation of the energy and blood outside, in this case, the evil-energy may take advantage to invade. Therefore, if the depth of the pricking is improper, it can, on the contrary, cause great damage. If the viscus inside is hurt, the patient will contract serious disease.

“The fact is some diseases are in the fine hair and striae, some are in the skin, some are in the muscle, some are in the channel, some are in the tendon, some are in the bone and some are in the marrow.

是故刺毫毛腠理无伤皮，皮伤则内动肺，肺动则秋病温疟〔《甲乙》“温疟”下有“热厥”二字〕，泝泝〔《甲乙》作“淅淅”《广雅·释诂二》：“淅，洒也”“洒然”寒貌〕然寒慄。

“Thus when pricking the fine hair and striae, the skin must not be hurt, if the skin is injured, it will affect the lung inside. When the lung can not bring its functions into full play, the patient will have warm-type malaria and cold extremities due to heat-evil in autumn will occur, and can develope into the syndrome of rigor and cold.

刺皮无伤肉，肉伤则内动脾，脾动则七十二日四季之月，病腹胀烦〔《甲乙》“烦”下有“满”字〕，不嗜食。

“When pricking the skin, the muscle must not be hurt, if the muscle is injured, it will affect the spleen inside. When the spleen can not bring its functions into full play, the patient will have the syndromes of restlessness, distention of abdomen and will be reluctant to eat in the last eighteen days of every season when the spleen energy is abundant.

刺肉无伤脉，脉伤则内动心，心动则夏病心痛。

“When pricking the muscle, the vessel must not be hurt, if the vessel is injured, it will affect the heart. When the heart can not bring its functions into full play, heartache will oc-

cur in summer.

刺脉无伤筋，筋伤则内动肝，肝动则春病热而筋驰。

"When pricking the vessel, the tendon must not be hurt, if the tendon is injured, if will affect the liver inside. When the liver can not bring its functions into full play, the disease of heart will occur in spring, and the tendons of the patient will also become flaccid.

刺筋无伤骨，骨伤则内动肾，肾动则冬病胀、腰痛。

"When pricking the tendon, the bone must not be hurt, if the bone is injured, it will affect the kidney inside. When the kidney can not bring its functions into full play, the syndromes of abdominal distention and lumbago will occur in winter.

刺骨无伤髓，髓伤则销铄胻酸，体解㑊然不去矣。

"When pricking the bone, the marrow must not be hurt, if the marrow is affected, the marrow will be withered gradually to cause aching pain of the legs and thighs, the patient will be tired and weak and reluctant to move."

刺齐论篇第五十一

Chapter 51
Ci Qi Lun
(The Proper Depth of Pricking)

黄帝问曰：愿闻刺浅深之分。岐伯对曰：刺骨者无伤筋，刺筋者无伤肉，刺肉者无伤脉，刺脉者无伤皮；刺皮者无伤肉，刺肉者无伤筋，刺筋者无伤骨。

Yellow Emperor asked: "What are the differences of the depth of pricking in acupuncture therapy?" Qibo answered: "In deep pricking; when pricking the bone, one must not prick shallowly to hurt the tendon, when pricking the tendon, one must not prick shallowly to hurt the muscle, when pricking the muscle, one must not prick shallowly to hurt the vessel, when pricking the vessel, one must not prick shallowly to hurt the skin; in shallow pricking; when pricking the skin, one must not prick deeply to hurt the muscle, when pricking the muscle, one must not prick deeply to hurt the tendon, when pricking the tendon, one must not prick deeply to hurt the bone."

帝曰：余未知其所谓，愿闻其解。岐伯曰：刺骨无伤筋者，针至筋而去，不及骨也；刺筋无伤肉者，至肉而去，不及筋也；刺肉无伤脉者，至脉而去，不及肉也；刺脉无伤皮者，至皮而去，不及脉也。

Yellow Emperor said: "I do not quite understand what you mean, please explain it to me." Qibo said: "The so called when pricking the bone, one must not prick shallowly to hurt the tendon means; when pricking the bone, it must not reach the tendon only which has not yet reached the bone, and stops the pricking or pulls off the needle; the so called when pricking the tendon, one must not prick shallowly to hurt the muscle means: when pricking the tendon, one must not prick shallowly to reach the muscle only which has not yet reached the tendon and stops the pricking or pulls off the needle; the so called when pricking the vessel, one must not prick shallowly to hurt the skin means: do not prick shalllowly to reach the skin only which has not yet reached the vessel, and stops the pricking or pulls off the needle.

所谓刺皮无伤肉者，病中皮中，针入皮中，无伤肉也；刺肉无伤筋者，过肉中筋也；刺筋无伤骨者，过筋中骨也，此之谓反也。

"The so called when pricking the skin, do not hurt the muscle means: when the disease is in the skin, only the skin should be pricked, one must not prick excessively to hurt the muscle. The so called when pricking the muscle, do not hurt the tendon means: the pricking should only reach the muscle where the disease resides, if the pricking is excessive, it will hurt the tendon. The so called when pricking the tendon, do not hurt the bone means: the

pricking should only reach the tendon where the dieease resides, if the pricking is excessive, it is the irregular handling of acupuncture."

刺禁论篇第五十二

Chapter 52
Ci Jin Lun
(The Forbiden Positions in Pricking)

黄帝问曰：愿闻禁数，岐伯对曰：藏有要害，不可不察，肝生于左，肺藏于右，心部于表，肾治〔《云笈七签》“治”作“位”〕于里，脾为〔赵本，吴本“为”并作“谓”〕之使，胃为之市，鬲肓之上，中有父母，七节之傍，中有小〔《太素》《甲乙》“小”并作“志”〕心，从之有福，逆之有咎。

Yellow Emperor said: “ I hope you can tell me the forbiden positions in pricking. ” Qibo said: “ In the five viscera, they all have vital parts which one must pay attention to. The liver is on the left side; the lung is on the right side; the heart takes charge of the exterior of the body; the kidney controls the interior of the body; the spleen transports the refined substances of water and cereasls to various viscera like a servant; the stomach accommodates water and cereals like a market; above the diaphram, there is the sea of energy which maintains the life, and by the side of the seventh vertebra is the refined substance of kidney. When pricking, one must adhere to the rules of acupuncture so as to obtain the curative effect. If the rules are violated, the pricking will be erroneous.

刺〔《太平圣惠方》“刺”下有“若”字〕中心，一日死，其动为噫。刺中肝，五日死，其动为语〔《甲乙》“语”作“欠”〕。刺中肾，六〔《诊要经终论》“六”作“七”〕日死，其动为嚏。刺中肺，三日〔《诊要经终论》“三”作“五”〕死，其动为咳。刺中脾，十〔《诊要经终论》“十”作“五”〕日死，其动为吞。刺中胆，一日半死，其动为呕。

“If the heart is hurt by pricking erroneously, the patient will die in one day, and its allergic reaction os eructation.

“If the liver is hurt erroneously, the patient will die in five days, and its allergic reaction is yawning.

“If the kidney is hurt erroneously, the patient will die in seven days, and the allergic reaction is sneezing.

“If the lung is hurt erroneously, the patient will die in five days, and its allergic reaction is coughing.

“If the spleen is hurt erroneously, the patient will die in five days, and its allergic reaction is swallowing.

“If the gallbladder is hurt erroneously, the patient will die in one and half days, and its allergic reaction is vomiting.

刺跗上，中大脉，血出不止死。刺面，中溜脉，不幸为盲。刺头，中脑户，入脑〔《圣

济总录》引无“入脑”二字〕立死。刺舌下，中脉太过，血出不止为瘖。刺足下布络中脉，血不出为肿。刺郄中〔《“郄中”下脱“中”字》〕大脉，令人仆脱色。刺气街中脉，血不出为肿，鼠仆〔《千金》《圣济总录》“仆”并作“鼷”，模骨尽处去中行五寸，有肉核名鼠鼷〕。刺脊间中髓，为伛。刺乳上，中乳房，为肿，根蚀。刺缺盆中内陷，气泄，令人喘〔《医心方》引“喘”下无“咳”字〕咳逆。刺手鱼腹内陷，为肿。

"When pricking the dorsum of the foot, if the artery of the eminent head of the radius is hurt erroneously, the patient will bleed continuously and die.

"When pricking the face, if the vessels connecting the eyes are pricked erreneously, it will cause the patient to become blind.

"When pricking the head, if the Naohu point (Brain Window DU 17) is hurt erroneously, the patient will die immediately.

"When pricking the Lianquan point (Tongue Spring CV (RN) 23) under the tongue, if the channel is pricked too deeply, the continuous bleeding will cause dysphonia of the patient.

"When the spreading collaterals under the foot are hurt by pricking, the blood will be unable to come out and swelling will occur.

"When pricking the Weizhong point (Popliteal Centre BL. 41) too deeply and hurt the large vessel erroneously, it may cause the patient to faint with white complexion.

"When pricking the Qichong point (Rushing Energy ST. 30), if the channel is hurt erroneously, and the blood can not come out, the stagnated blood will cause swelling and pain of the muscle kernel by the pubic bone.

"When the spine marrow is hurt erroneously by pricking the spinal pace, hunchback of the patient will occur.

"When pricking the Ruzhong point (Breast Centre ST. 17), if the breast is hurt erroneously, it will swell and cause corrosive trauma.

When pricking the Quepen point (Supraclavicular Fossa ST. 12)too deeply to excrete the energy, it will cause dyspnea.

"When pricking the muscle above the Yuji point (Thenar Prominence LU. 10) too deeply, it will cause swelling in a certain part of the body.

无刺大醉，令人气〔“气”疑应作“脉”，王注所据本原作“脉乱”〕乱。无刺大怒，令人气逆。无刺大劳人，无刺新〔《太平圣惠方》引“新”作“大”〕饱人，无刺大饥人，无刺大渴人，无刺大惊人。

"Do not prick the one who is in the state of drunkenness, if he is pricked, his pulse will be confusing. Do not prick the one who is in great anger, if he is pricked, he will have adverseness of vital energy. Do not prick the one who is over-fatigue, one who is exceedingly full up, one who is exceedingly hungry, one who is exceedingly thirsty nor the one who is exceedingly frightened.

刺阴股中大脉，血出不止死。刺客主人内陷中脉，为内漏、为聋。刺膝髌出液，为跛。刺臂太阴脉，出血多立死。刺足少阴脉，重虚出血，为舌难以言。刺膺中陷，中肺〔《圣济总

录》引“肺”作“脉”〕，为喘逆仰息。刺肘中内陷，气归之，为不屈伸。刺阴股下三寸内陷，令人遗弱。刺腋下胁间内陷，令人咳。刺少腹中膀胱，溺出，令人少腹满。刺腨肠内陷为肿。刺〔《千金》“刺”下有“目”字〕匡上陷骨中脉，为漏为盲。刺关节中液出不得屈伸。

“When pricking the acupoints in the inner flank of the thigh, if the large pulse is hurt erroneously, the patient will bleed continuously and die.

“When pricking the cave-in above the eye of Shangguan point (Upper Pass GB. 3), if the collaterals are hurt erroneously, pus will occur in the ears to cause deafness of the patient.

“When pricking the knee-cap, if liquid comes out, the patient will become lame.

“When pricking the Tianfu point (Heaven Mansion LU. 3), if the Hand Taiyin Channel is hurt erroneously, and if the bleeding is plenty, the patient will die very soon.

“When pricking the Foot Shaoying Channel into bleeding, it will cause the kidney to become more asthenic, the syndrome of inability to speak of the patient due to his tongue becoming not so nimble will occur.

“When pricking the chest too deeply and hurt the channel, dyspnea, cough and the syndrome of rapid breathing of the patient when facing up will occur.

“When pricking the Chize point (One foot Marsh Lu. 5) and the Quze point (Crooked Marsh P. 3) too deeply, the energy will stagnate in a certain locality, and the inability of bending and stretching of the arms of the patient will occur.

“When pricking the position at the three inches below the inner flank of the thigh too deeply, it will cause incontinence of urine.

“When pricking between the armpit and the lateral side of the thorax too deeply, it will cause cough of the patient.

“When pricking the abdomen too deeply and hurt the bladder, the urine will flow into the abdominal cavity and cause abdominal distention of the patient.

“When pricking the calf too deeply, it will cause swelling in a certain part of the body.

“When pricking the bone of the orbit and hurt the collaterals, it will cause continuous lacrimation and even blindness of the patient.

“When pricking the lumbar vertebra or the joints of the four limbs, if there is liquid flowing out, the patient will lose the ability of bending, stretching and moving.”

刺志论篇第五十三

Chapter 53
Ci Zhi Lun
(On Treating Asthenia and Sthenia with Acupuncture)

黄帝问曰：愿闻虚实之要，岐伯对曰：气实形实，气虚形虚，此其常也，反此者病；谷盛气盛，谷虚气虚，此其常也，反此者病；脉实血实，脉虚血虚，此其常也，反此者病。

Yellow Emperor said："I hope you can tell me the essentials about asthenia and sthenia." Qibo said："When the energy is substantial and the body is also substantial or when the energy is deficient and the body is also deficient, it is the normal condition; when the condition is on the contrary, it is the diseased condition. When one takes plenty of food and he has a overabundant energy, or when he can take only a little food and his energy is insufficient, it is the normal condition; when the condition is on the contrary, it is the diseased condition. When the pulse is substantial and the blood is also substantial, or when the pulse is deficient and the blood is also deficient, it is the normal condition; when the condition is on the contrary, it is the diseased condition."

帝曰：如何而反？岐伯曰〔林校云："据《甲乙》"曰"下当补"气盛身寒"四字〕：气虚身热，此谓反也，谷入多而气少，此谓反也；谷不入〔"不入"误，应作"入少"〕而气多，此谓反也；脉盛血少，此谓反也；脉少〔"少"误，应作"小"〕血多，此谓反也。

Yellow Emperor asked："What is the condition when it is abnormal?" Qibo said：When the healthy energy is overabundant but the body is cold, or when the energy is deficient but the body is hot, they are both the abnormal conditions, When one can eat plenty but his energy is insufficient, it is an abnormal condition; when one can eat only a little but has an overabundant energy, it is also the abnormal condition. When the pulse is substantial, but the blood is insufficient, it is an abnormal condition; When the pulse is deficient but the blood is plenty, it is also an abnormal condition.

气盛身寒，得之伤寒。气虚身热，得之伤暑。谷入多而气少者，得之有所脱血，湿居下也，谷入少而气多者，邪在胃及与肺也。脉小血多者，饮中热也。脉大血少者，脉有风气，水浆不入，此之谓〔张琦说"此之谓"三字衍〕也。

"When the energy is overabundant but the body is cold, it is due to the injury by the cold-evil. When the energy is insufficient but the body is hot, it is due to the injury by the summer-heat.

"When one can eat a lot but has few energy is due to the wetness-evil accumulating below after the loss of blood.

"When one can eat only a little but his energy has a surplus shows the evil-energy re-

tains in the stomach and has reached the lung.

"When the pulse is small but the blood is plenty and the patient has a red complexion, it is caused by the heat in the middle warmer due to excessive drinking of wine. When the pulse is large but the blood is few, it is due to the patient has contracted wind-evil without drinking any water and soup.

夫实者，气入也，虚者，气出也；气实者，热也，气虚者，寒也。入实者，左手开针空也；入虚〔《素问识》云："当是'出虚'"〕者，左手闭针空也。

"The so-called sthenia indicates the evil-energy has entered the body. The so-called asthenia indicates the healthy energy has exhausted inside. When the evil-energy is sthenic, heat will produce; when the healthy energy is asthenic, cold will occur.

"When treating the sthenia-syndrome with acupuncture, it should open the needle hole with the left hand so as to purge; when treating the asthenia-syndrome with acupuncture, it should close the needle hole which is pricked with the left hand so as to invigorate."

针解篇第五十四

Chapter 54
Zhen Jie
(Explaination on Needles)

黄帝问曰：愿闻九针之解，虚实之道。岐伯对曰：刺虚则实之者，针下热也，气实乃热也〔《太素》无“气实”五字〕；满而泄之者，针下寒也，气虚乃寒也〔《太素》无“气虚”五字〕；菀陈则除之者，出恶血也。邪胜则虚之者，出针勿按；徐而疾则实者，徐出针而疾按之；疾而徐则虚者，疾出针而徐按之；言实与虚者，寒温气多少也。若无若有者，疾不可知也。察后与先者，知病先后也。为虚与实者，工〔《太素》“工”下有“守”字〕勿失其法。若得若失者，离其法也。虚实之要，九针最妙者，为其各有所宜也。补写之时〔林校据《甲乙经》“补写之时”下脱“以针为之”四字〕者，与气开阖相合也。九针之名，各不同形者，针穷其所当补写也。

Yellow Emperor said: “I hope you can explain to me about the nine needles and the different methods in treating asthenia and sthenia.” Qibo said: “When treating asthenia with acupuncture, it should apply the invigorating method, when there is hotness under the needle, it shows the healthy energy has been aroused to cause normality; when treating sthenia with acupuncture, it should apply the purging method, when there is coolness under the needle, it shows the evil-energy has been purged to cause normality. The blood in which the long stagnated evil-energy resides should be let out. When pricking the patient whose evil-energy is overabundant, do not close the needle hole by pressing so as to let out the evil energy. The so-called ‘slow first and then swift to cause sthenia’ indicates after pulling the needle slowly, press and close the needle hole swiftly so that the healthy energy may not be excreted. The so-called ‘swift first and then slow to cause asthenia’ indicates after pulling the needle swiftly, leave the needle hole openned without pressing it so that the evil-energy can be dispersed. The so-called asthenia and sthenia here indicates that in asthenia, the energy is few and cold, and in sthenia, the energy is plenty and warm; if the hot or cold feeling is not obvious, then the asthenia or sthenia of the disease will be hard to be distinguished. When one inspects the condition of the early and later stage of the disease, it is for to make sure of the branch and root of the disease. A physician can only avoid error when he knows the asthenia or sthenia of the disease and adhere to the rules of acupuncture. If the physician does not know for certain the way of treating (such as applying purgation when it should be invigorated, or applying invigoration when it should be purged), his treating will divorce from the rule.

“When treating asthenia or sthenia, one must apply the nine kinds of needle flexibly.

The nine kinds of needle can suit the various kinds of disease.

"When applying the invigorating method or the purging method, the needle used should be in concert with the openning and closing for the energy.

"The so called nine needles means there are nine kinds of needle in various form and have different names, and each kind of them has a specific role for invigorating and purging.

刺〔《太素》"刺"下有"其"字，下"刺虚"同〕实须其虚者，留针阴气隆至〔明抄本"隆至"下有"针下寒"三字〕，乃去针也；刺虚须其实者，阳气隆至，针下热乃去针也。经气已至，慎守勿失者，勿变更也。深浅在志者，知病之内外也；近远如一者，深浅其候等也。如临深渊者，不敢堕也；手如握虎者，欲其壮也；神无营于众物者，静志观病人，无左右视也；义无邪下者，欲端以正也；必正其神者，欲瞻病人目制其神，令气易行也。所谓三里者，下膝三寸也；所谓跗之者〔林校云："'跗之'上作'跗上'"〕，举膝〔"膝"是"脉"之误字〕分易见也；巨虚者，蹻足骱独陷者；下廉者，陷下者也。

"When treating the sthenia-syndrome by pricking, purge therepy should be used, the needle should be retained in the body and wait for the coming of the abundant Yin energy, pull the needle after there is a cold feeling under the needle. When treating the asthenia-syndrome by pricking, the invigorating method should be used, after pricking, wait for the coming of the abundant Yang enery, and pull the needle after there is a hot feeling under the needle.

"The so-called one must wait carefully until getting the acupuncture feeling means: do not change the pricking method rashly.

"The so-called one must be certain about the depth of the pricking means: one must know clearly the exterior and the interior of the disease.

"The so-called both the distance-pricking and the nearby-pricking should be in the same way means: the methods of waiting the acupuncture feeling in both the severe or slight diseases are the same.

"The so-called one should feel like standing upon edge of abyss in pricking means: one must not be indolent and careless in pricking.

"The so-called holding the needle like holding a tiger means: the pricking must be firm and forceful.

"The so-called concentrating the mind without paying attention to things outside means: inspect the patient calmly without looking around.

"The so-called the pricking must not be slanting means: the needle inserted must be upright.

"The so-called set right the spirit of the patient means: watch attentively the eyes of the patient to control his spiritual activities, so as the channel energy can flow easily.

"The Zusanli point (Foot Three Li ST. 36) is the name of the acupoint three inches under the knee at the lateral side. The Chongyang point (Rushing Yang ST. 42) is on the dorsum, it can be easily seen when pricking the artery. The Shangjuxu point (Upper Huge Passage ST. 37) is in the bogging position on the lateral side of the tibia, it can be pricked when

the leg is lifting up. The Xiajuxu point (Lower Huge Passage ST. 35) is below the bogging position stated above."

帝曰：余闻九针，上应天地四时〔《类说》引“天地”下并无“四时”二字〕阴阳，愿闻其方，令可传于后世〔《太素》“世”下有“而”字〕以为常也。岐伯曰：；夫一天、二地、三人、四时、五音、六律、七星、八风、九野，身〔《太素》“身”作“人”〕形亦应之，针各有所宜，故曰九针。人皮应天，人肉应地，人脉应人，人筋应时，人声应音，人阴阳合气〔柯逢时说：“依《九针论》‘合气’二字衍”〕应律，人齿面目应星，人出入气〔《太素》“气”下有“口”字〕应风，人九窍三百六十五络应〔《太平圣惠方》引“应”下有“九”字〕野，故一针皮，二针肉，三针脉，四针筋，五针骨，六针调阴阳，七针益精，八针除风，九针通九窍，除〔据《太素》杨注“除”字当作“应”〕三百六十五节气，此之谓各有所主也〔《太平圣惠方》引“主”作“立”〕。人心意应八风，人气应天，人发齿耳目五声应五音六律，人阴阳脉血气应地，人肝目应之九。

Yellow Emperor said: "I am told that the nine needles are corresponding with the heaven, earth, Yin and Yang, I hope you can tell me the causal relation about it, so that it may be handed down to the later generations and become the routine in treating." Qibo said: "The various parts of the human body is corresponding with the followings: one corresponds with heaven, two corresponds with earth, three corresponds with man, four corresponds with the four seasons, five corresponds with the five notes, six corresponds with the six rules in poem prescribing rhymes and syllables which regulate each other, seven corresponds to the sveen stars, eight corresponds to the eight kinds of wind, and nine corresponds to the nine open fields. The various kinds of needle suit different diseases respectively, and they are called the nine needles.

"The skin of a man is like the sky that covers all things; the muscle of a man is like the earth which is thick and solid; the flourishing and decline of the channel is like the robustness and senility of a man; the functions of tendons in various parts of the body are like the different weathers in the four seasons; the vioce of a man is corresponding with the five notes in the nature; the solid and hollow organs, Yin and Yang are like the six rules in poem in which the rhymes and syllables are coordinating each other; the arrangement of teeth and the five sense organs of man are like that of the constellation in the sky; the respiration of man is like the wind in the nature; the nine orifices and the three hundred and sixty five collaterals which are spreading all over the body are like the nine open fields.

"So, the first kind of needle is used to prick the skin, the second kind of needle is used to prick the muscle, the third kind of needle is used to prick the vessel, the fourth kind of needle is used to prick the tendon, the fifth kind of needle is used to prick the bone, the sixth kind of needle is used to adjust the Yin and Yang, the seventh kind of needle is used to invigorate the refined energy, the eighth kind of needle is used to expel the wind-evil, the ninth kind of needle is used to dredge the energies of the nine orifices to respond to the energies of the three hundred and sixty five acupoints, so each kind of the nine needles has the specific function.

"The thoughts and ideas of a man is changing without regular pattern like the eight kinds of winds; the healthy energy of a man is like the continuous operation of heaven; the hairs, teeth, ears and eyes of man are coordinative perfectly like the five notes and the six prescribed rules in the poem; the blood, energy, Yin and Yang channel are like the earth that promote the birth and growth of all things; the liver-energy of man which communicates with the eyes is corresponding to the number of nine."

长刺节论篇第五十五

Chapter 55
Chang Ci Jie Lun
(Supplemental Commentary On Pricking)

刺家不诊〔孙鼎宜说："按'不诊'或为'来诊'"〕，听病者言，在头，头疾痛，为藏〔林校据全元起本无"藏"字〕针之，刺至骨，病已上〔朝本，明抄本"上"并作"止"〕，无伤骨肉及皮，皮者道也。

When a physician who is keen in acupuncture to treat the disease, he always hears the auto-anamnesis of the patient. When the headache of the patient is severe, the acupoint on the head should be pricked, and stop the pricking when the head-ache is relieved. In pricking, the bone, muscle and skin must not be hurt. The passage of the needle should be limited in the skin so that the bone and muscle may not be hurt.

阴〔《太素》"阴"作"阳"〕刺，入一傍四处〔《太素》"四"下无"处"字〕，治寒热。深专者，刺大藏；迫藏刺背，背〔《太素》"刺背"下不重"背"字〕俞也。刺之迫藏，藏会，腹中寒热〔《太素》"寒热"下有"气"字〕去而止。与刺之要，发针而浅出血。

It pricking the Yang, prick straightly in the middle once, and prick slantingly in the left and right sides for four times with which to cure the disease of cold and heat.

If the evil-energy has penetrated inside to attack the viscera specifically, the five viscera should be pricked. When the evil-energy is approaching the five viscera, the back-shu points should be pricked as the shu-points are the locations where the viceral-energy assembles. The pricking should be stopped when the abdominal cold and heat has been dispersed. Generally, there should be a slight bleeding when pulling the needle.

治腐〔《太素》"腐"作"痈"〕肿者刺腐上，视痈小大深浅〔《太素》"深浅"下无"刺"字〕刺，刺大者多血，小者深之〔楼英说："'大者多血，小者深之'衍文也"〕，必端内针为故止。

When treating the carbuncle, the carbuncle should be pricked. One should inspect the size and the depth of the carbuncle first and prick properly to let out the pus; the pricking must be straight.

病在少腹有积，刺皮髓〔《太素》"皮髓"作"腹齐"〕以下，至少腹而止；刺侠脊两傍四椎间，刺两髂髎季胁肋间，导腹中气热〔全本作"热气"〕下已。

When there is a mass in the lower abdomen, it should prick the positions from the abdomen down to the lower abdomen, then prick the points on the two sides of the fourth vertebra, the Femur-Juliao (Squatting Crevice GB. 29) on the lateral sides of the hip bone and the acupoints on the hypochondrium to cause the heat of the abdomen moving downwards,

and the disease will be cured.

病在少〔“少”作“小”〕腹，腹痛不得大小便，病名曰疝，得之寒；刺少腹两股间〔《甲乙》作“得寒则少腹胀，两股间冷”〕，刺腰髁骨间，刺而多〔“多”疑当作灸〕之，尽炅病已。

When the disease is in the lower abdomen, and the pain causes one unable to move bowels and to pass urine, it is called hernia. When the cold is contracted, it will cause one to have abdminal distention and coldness between the thighs. In treating, it should prick the loins and locations between the hip bones and treat with moxibustion after pricking. The disease will be cured when the lower abdomen becomes hot thoroughly.

病在筋，筋挛〔《太素》“挛”下有“诸”字〕节痛，不可以行，名曰筋痹。刺筋上为故，刺分肉〔《太素》“分”下无“肉”字，按王注：“分谓肉分间有筋维络处也”〕间，不可中骨也；病起〔“病起”二字衍〕筋炅，病已止。

When the disease is in the tendon and the patient is seized with cramp, has pain in the jionts and unable to walk, it is called the tendinous bi-syndrome. When treating, it should prick the tendon as the tendon is in the juncture of the muscles. The pricking must reach the tendon in the juncture of the muscles, but the bone must not be hurt. When the sensation of hotness in the tendon is felt, it shows the disease has been cured and the pricking sbould be stopped.

病在肌肤，肌肤尽痛，名曰肌痹，伤于寒湿。刺大分、小分，多发针而深之，以热为故；无伤筋骨，伤筋骨，痈〔《甲乙》“痈”作“寒”〕发若变；诸分尽热，病已止。

When the disease is in the skin and both the skin and muscle are painful, it is called the myalgia and it is caused by the invasion of the cold-wetness. When treating, it should prick the acupoints in the large and small junctures of the muscles. The pricking should be deep and in various locations until the hotness is felt. In pricking, it must not hurt the tendon and bone, if the tendon and bone are hurt, the cold-evil will attack and cause disease. When the hot feelingis felt in the large and small junctures of muscles after pricking, it shows the disease has been cured and the pricking should be stopped.

病在骨，骨重不可举，骨髓酸痛，寒气至〔孙鼎宜说：“‘至’下疑有‘骨’字”〕，名曰骨痹，深者刺，无伤脉肉为故，其道〔《太素》“其道”作“至其”〕大分小分，骨热病已止。

When the disease is in the bone, the patient will feel heavy of the bone and can hardly move, if the marrow is sore and the bone is extremly cold, it is the bone bi-syndrome. In treating, the pricking should be deep, but the vessel and muscle must not be hurt. When the needle reaches the bone between the large and small junctures of muscles and the hot feeling of the bone is felt, the disease will soon be recovered, and the pricking should be stopped.

病在诸阳脉，且寒且热〔按“且寒”四字，涉下误衍〕，诸分且寒且热，名曰狂。刺之虚脉，视分尽热，病已止。病初发，岁一发，不治，月一发，不治，月四五发，名曰癫病。刺诸分诸脉〔《甲乙》作“其脉”，连下读〕，其无寒者以针调〔《甲乙》无“其”字，“无”作“尤”，“调”作“补”〕之，病〔金本，胡本，讹本，赵本，吴本“病”下并有“已”字〕止。

When the disease is in various Yang channels (Hand and Foot Taiyang, Shaoyang and

Yangming channels) and there is hot and cold feelins now and then in the junctures of muscles, it is the disease of mania. When treating, it should apply the purging therapy to disperse the evil-energies of the Yang channels; when the hot feeling is felt in all the junctures of muscle, the disease will be recovered very soon, and the pricking should be stopped.

When mania is newly contracted, it will attack once a year, if the treating is delayed, it will attack once a month, if it is not treated again, it will attack four or five times in a month which is called epilepsy.

When treating, it should prick the large and small junctures of the muscle, If the channel is extremely cold frequently, the invigorating therapy should be applied. When the disease turns to the better, the pricking should be stopped.

病风且寒且热，炅汗出，一日数过〔《甲乙》“过”作“欠”按“欠”疑是“次”之坏字〕，先刺诸分理络脉；汗出且寒且热，三日一刺，百日而已。

When the disease of the patieat is caused by wind-evil, the syndrome of hot and cold at times will occur, the patient perspires when he is hot and the disease comes on several times a day. When treating, the junctures of muscle, skin and the collaterals should be prick first. If the patient remains to perspire and feels hot and cold at times, he should be pricked in every other three days, and after treating for one hundred days, the disease will be cured.

病大风，骨节重，鬚眉堕，名曰大风，刺肌肉为故，汗出百日，刺骨髓，汗出百日，凡二百日，鬚眉生而止针。

When one contracts leprosy, the patient will feel heavy in the joints all over his body, and his beards and eyebrows are falling, it is called the disease of leprosy. When treating, it should prick the muscle to cause sweating, and after the one-hundred-day-pricking, prick again the bone morrow for another one hundred days to cause sweating. The whole process should last for two hundred days before ceasing the pricking.

皮部论篇第五十六

Chapter 56
Pi Bu Lun
(On the Parts of Skin)

黄帝问曰：余闻皮有分部，脉有经纪，筋有结络，骨有度量。其所生病各异，别其分部，左右上下，阴阳所在，病之始终，愿闻其道。

Yellow Emperor said: "I am told that the various parts of skin are belonging to the twelve channels respectively, in the distribution of vessels, some are vertical and some are horizontal, in the distribution of tendons, there are knots and collaterals; in the distribution of bones, some of them are large and long and some of them are small and short. The diseases stemmed from various organs are different, and they can only be distinguished by the parts of skin which belong to various channels respectively, and besides, one must also take into account of the upper and lower, left and right positions, the attribute of Yin or Yang and the process of developement of the disease. I hope you can tell me further about it."

岐伯对曰：欲知皮部以经脉为纪者〔《太素》"纪"下无"者"字〕，诸经皆然。阳明之阳，名曰害蜚，上下同法。视其部中有浮络者，皆阳明之络也。其色多青则痛，多黑则痹，黄〔据《太素》"黄赤"上脱"多"字〕赤则热，多白则寒，五色皆见，则寒热也。络盛则入客于经，阳主外，阴主内。

Qibo asid: "When one wants to determine to which channel the part of skin belongs, it should base on the locations where the channel reaches and passes. The conditions of all the twelve channels are the same.

"The Yang-collaterals of Yangming Channel which reaches and passes the part of skin is called 'Haifei' (the killing energy which hinders birth and growth). The conditions of Hand Yangming Channel and Foot Yangming Channel are the same. The floating collaterals seen in the part of skin are all the floating collaterals of the Yangming Channel, if the collaterals are mostly green, it shows there is pain; if they are mostly black, it shows there is bi (the disease of blocking of extremities, meridians and viscera by evils); if they are mostly yellowish-red, it shows there is heat; if they are mostly white, it shows there is cold; if all the five colour are existing it shows there is the disease of alternating heat and cold. When the evil-energy of the collaterals is over-abundant, it will invade into its channel. The collaterals belong to the Yang and they take charge of the exterior, and the channels belong to Yin take charge of the interior.

少阳之阳，名曰枢持，上下同法。视其部中有浮络者，皆少阳之络也。络盛则入客于经。故在阳者主内，在阴者主出，以渗于内，诸经皆然〔"故在阳"以下十九字，张琦以为伪误，

孙鼎宜以为衍文，吴注本册此十九字〕。

“The Yang-collaterals of shaoyang Channel which reach and pass the part of skin are called ‘shuchi’ (the axle of pivot), and the conditions of the Hand Shaoyang Channel and Foot Shaoyang Channel are the same. The floating collaterals seen in the part of skin are all the collaterals of Shaoyang Channel. When the evil-energy in the collaterals is overabundant, it will penetrate into its channel.

太阳之阳，名曰关枢，上下同法。视其部中有浮络者，皆太阳之络也。络盛则入客于经。

“The Yang collaterals of Taiyang Channel which reach and pass the part of skin is called ‘Guanshu’ (the controlling pivot). The conditions of both the Hand Taiyang and Foot Taiyang are the same. The floating collaterals seen on the part of skin are all the collaterals of Taiyang Channel. When the evil-energy in the collaterals is overabundant, it will penetrate into its channel.

少阴之阴，名曰枢儒，上下同法。视其部中有浮络者，皆少阴之络也。络盛则入客于经，其入经也，从阳部注于经〔“经”蒙上误，似应作“筋”〕；其〔《太素》“其”下有“经”字，按“经”字应在“出”字下，为“其经出者”〕出者，从阴内〔《太素》“阴”下无“内”字，按“阴内”应作“阴部”《甲乙》作“阴部”“阴部”谓脉也〕注于骨。

“The Yin-collaterals in Shaoyin Channel which reach and pass the part of skin is called ‘shuru’ (the axle sleeve of pivot). The conditions of the Hand Shaoyin Channel and the Foot Shaoyin channel are the same. The flooting collaterals seen on the part of skin are all the collaterals on the shaoyin Channel. When the evil-energy in the collateral is over-abundant, it will penetrate into its channel. When the evil-energy invades into the channel, it will pour into the tendon through the collaterals; if it does not invade the channel, it will pour into the bone through the vessel.

心主〔张琦说：“‘心主’当作‘厥阴’”〕之阴，名曰害肩，上下同法。视其部中有浮络者，皆心主〔当作“厥阴”〕之络也。络盛则入客于经。

“The Yin-collaterals in the Jueyin Channel which reach and pass the part of skin is called ‘Haijian’ (harming the shoulder). The conditions of the Hand Jueyin channel and the Foot Jueyin channel are the same. The floating collaterals seen are all the collaterals of the Jueyin Channel. When the evil-energy in the collateral is overabundant, it will penetrate into its channel.

太阴之阴，名曰关蛰，上下同法。视其部中有浮络者，皆太阴之络也，络盛则入客于经。凡十二经络〔《太素》“经”下无“络”字〕脉者，皮之部也。

“The Yin-collaterals in the Taiyin Channel which reach and pass the part of skin is called ‘Guanzhe’ (the sealed hibernant). The conditions of the Hand Taiyin Channel and the Foot Taiyin Channel are the same. The floating collaterals seen in the part of skin are all the floating collaterals of the Taiyin Channel. When the evil-energy in the collaterals is overabundant, it will penetrate into its channel. In a word, all the twelve channels belong to various parts of skin respectively.

是故百病之始生也，必先于皮毛〔吴注本“毛”作“也”，《太素》《甲乙》“先”下有

"客"字〕，邪中之则腠理开，开则入客于络脉，留而不去，传入于经，留而不去，传入于府，廪于〔《类说》"入手"下无"府廪于"三字〕肠胃。邪之始入于皮也，泝〔《甲乙》"泝"作"淅"，"淅然"寒貌〕然起毫毛，开腠理；其入于络也，则络脉盛色变；其入客于经也，则感虚乃陷下。其留于筋骨之间，寒多则筋挛骨痛；热多则筋弛骨消，肉烁䐃破，毛直而败。

"So, all diseases start definitely from the part of skin first When the evil attacks the skin, the striae will be kept openned and the evil-energy will invade the collaterals, when the evil retains long, it will be transmited into the channel inside, when it retains in the channel long, it will be transmited into the intestine and stomach. When the evil invades the skin, One will shiver with cold with the fine hairs of the skin standing up and the striae openning. When the evil-energy invades the collaterals, the collaterals will be fully filled, and the colour of the patient's complexion will be changed. When the evil invades the channel, the patient will have the syndrome of bogging down and weak pulse and deficient breath. If the evil retains in between the tendon and bone, and when the cold-energy is overabundant, the patient will have spasm of the muscle and pain in the bone; when the heat-energy is overabundant, the patient will have muscular flaccidity, and he will be weak in the bone, his muscle in the shoulder and elbows will be deteriorative and his skin and hair will become withered."

帝曰：夫子言皮之十二部，其生病皆何如？岐伯曰：皮者脉之部也，邪客于皮则腠理开，开则邪入客于络脉，络脉满则注于经脉，经脉满则入舍于府藏也，故皮者〔《甲乙》"皮"下无"者"字〕有分部，不与而生大病也。帝曰：善！

Yellow Emperor asked: "What are the conditions of the infections of the twelve parts of skin you said?" Qibo said: "The skin is the place where the collaterals spread, when the evil-energy invades the skin, the striae will be openned; when the striae are openned, the evil-energy will invade into the collaterals; when the collateral is fully filled with evil-energy, it will be poured into the channel; when the channel is fully filled, it will go further and retain in the viscera. Thus, when the evil-energy invades the skin, if the treating is in time, the disease can be recovered soon, if the treatment is delayed, the evil-energy will penetrate into the viscera and cause serious disease."

经络论篇第五十七

Chapter 57
Jing Luo Lun
(On Collaterals)

黄帝问曰：夫络脉之见也，其五色各异，青黄赤白黑不同，其故何也？岐伯对曰：经有常色而络无常变也。

Yellow Emperor asked："When the collaterals appear outside，they have five different colours of green，yellow，red，white and black，and what is the reason?"

Qibo answered："The colour of the channel is not changing，but the colour of the collateral is changable."

帝曰：经之常色何如？岐伯曰：心赤、肺白、肝青、脾黄、肾黑，皆亦应其经脉之色也。

Yellow Emperor asked："What are the regular colours of the twelve channels?"Qibo answered："The twelve channels are connecting the five viscera，and the colours of the five viscera are different：the heart is red，the lung is white，the liver is green，the spleen is yellow and the kidney is black. In the twelve channels，the colour of the channel is the same with that of the viscus it connects."

帝曰：络之阴阳，亦应其经乎？岐伯曰：阴络之色应其经，阳络之色变无常，随四〔《太素》"随"下无."四"字〕时而行也。寒多则凝泣，凝泣则青黑；热多则淖泽，淖泽则黄赤；此皆常色，谓之无病〔明抄二夹注云："'此皆'八字，当在'随时而行'之下"〕，五色具〔《太素》"具"作"俱"〕见者，谓之寒热。帝曰：善。

Yellow Emperor asked："Are the Yin (deep) collateral and the Yang (shallow) collaterals correspond with the regular colour of the channel to which they belong?"

Qibo answered："The colour of the Yin collateral corresponds with the colour of its related channel，but the colour of the Yang collateral is changable，and the colour changes along with the change of the weather.

"When the weather is extremely cold，the blood will be tardy and stagnated，and its colour will be greenish-black；when the weather is extremely wet and hot，the blood will be moist and smooth，and its colour will be yellowish-red. These colours are normal which show a good health of the body. If the five colours are appearing at the same time，it is caused by the extreme cold or extreme heat of the body. Yellow Emperor said："Good."

气穴论篇第五十八

Chapter 58
Qi Xue Lun
(On Acupoints)

黄帝问曰：余闻气穴三百六十五，以应一岁，未知其所〔《太素》“所”下有“谓”字〕，愿卒闻之。岐伯稽首再拜对曰：窘乎哉问也！其非圣帝，孰能穷其道焉！因〔《太素》“因”作“固”〕请溢意尽言其处。帝捧手逡巡而却曰：夫子之开余道也，目未见其处，耳未闻其数，而目以明，耳以聪矣。岐伯曰：此所谓圣人易语，良马易御也。帝曰：余非圣人之易语也，世言真数开人意，今余所访问者真数，发蒙解惑，未足以论也。然余愿闻夫子溢志尽言其处，令解其意，请藏之金匮，不敢复出。

Yellow Emperor said: "I am told that a man has three hundred and sixty five acupoints which correspond with the day-number of a year, but I don't know their positions, I hope you can tell me about it."

Qibo bowed twice and said: "This is an embarrassing problem. How can one infer its principle save a sagacious emperor. Since you have mentioned it, I will try my best to explain it."

Yellow Emperor cupped one of his hand in the other before his chest and said modestly: "If you can tell me the essentials and inspire me to understand the acupoints which I have not seen and heard before, it will be just like causing me to have bright eyes and keen eares". Qibo said: "Your excellent ability of comprehension is just like the so-called 'a sage is always clever enough to understand things well, and a good horse can easily be reined'"

Yellow Emperor said: "I am not the kind of sage you said who is so brilliant. But even an ordinary person, his thought will be openned up when he knows the number of the acupoints in the meridians (this is what I want to know). What I am asking you is to enlighten me on my ignorance and remove my perplexity only, and I am not asking you to discuss its subtle theory. Since you have said that you want to try your best to explain the positions of the acupoints and make the essentials known to me, I will keep the record or your explaination in a golden chest saftly and never lose it."

岐伯再拜而起曰：臣请言之，背与心相控而痛，所治天突与十椎及上纪〔《太素》“上纪”下有“下纪”二字〕，上纪者，胃脘也，下纪者关元也。背胸邪系〔《太素》“邪上无“胸背”二字，“系”作“主”〕阴阳左右，如此其病前后痛濇，胸胁痛而不得息，不得卧，上气短气偏〔林校云：“按别本‘偏’作‘满’”〕痛，脉满起，斜出尻脉，络胸胁〔《太素》“胸”下无“胁”字〕支心贯鬲、上肩加天突，斜下肩交十椎下〔《太素》“下”者“藏”字，杨上善说：“下藏者，下络肾藏也”〕

Qibo bowed deeply once again, then he rose up and said: "In that case, I will try to explain it. When one's back and chest are drawing each other with pain, it should be treated by pricking the Tiantu point (CV (RN) 22) of the Ren Channel, the Zhongshu point (DU. 7) of the Du Channel, the Zhongwan point (CV (RN) 12) and the Guanyuan point (CV (RN) 4).

"When the evil-energy attacks the left and right sides and Yin and Yang, the pain of the chest and the hypochondrium will cause the patient to respire difficulty, be unable to lie on his back. The adverse rising of the lung-enargy causes the rapid respiration, short of breath, distention, fullness and pain. When the evil energy is filled in the channel it will rise up and shift to the large collateral, then, slanting to the buttock, chest, heart, diaphram, scapula and intersects with the Ren Channel at Tiantu point, then slanting downwards to the shoulder and join the kidney below the tenth vertebra of the back.

藏俞五十穴，府俞七十二穴，热俞五十九穴，水俞五十七穴，头上五行，行五，五五二十五穴，中胎两傍各五，凡十穴，大椎〔《太素》"大椎"作"大杼"，按"上"疑是"下"〕上两傍各一，凡二穴，目瞳子浮白二〔"浮白"下脱"各"字，王注"左右言之，各二为四也"〕穴，两髀厌分〔《太素》"厌"下无"分"字〕中二穴，犊鼻二穴，耳中多所闻二穴，眉本二穴，完骨二穴，项中央一穴，枕骨二穴，上关二穴，大迎二穴，下关二穴，天柱二穴，巨虚上下廉四穴，曲牙二穴，天突一穴，天府二穴，天牖二穴，扶突二穴，天窗二穴，肩解二穴，关元一穴，委阳二穴，肩贞二穴，瘖门一穴，齐一穴，胸俞十二穴，背俞二穴，膺俞十二穴，分肉二穴，踝上横二穴，阴阳跻四穴，水俞在诸分，热俞在气穴，寒热俞在两骸厌中二穴，大禁二十五，在天府下五寸，凡三百六十五穴，针之所由行也。

"In the five solid organs, each of them has five kinds of of shu-point which are Jing, Xing, shu, Jing and He, and each kind of shu-points has five acupoints, five times five makes twenty five, and they amount to fifty points in the left and right sides as following:

Acupoints in five solid organs	Liver	Heart	Spleen	Lung	Kidney
Jing (wood)	Dadun (LR. 1)	Shaochong (HT. 9)	Yinbai (SP. 1)	Shaoshang (LU. 11)	Yong-Quan (KI. 1)
Xing (Fire)	Xingjian (LR. 2)	Shaofu (HT. 8)	Dadu (SP. 2)	Yuji (LU. 10)	Rangu (KI. 2)
Shu (Earth)	Taichong (LR. 3)	Shenmen (HT. 7)	Taibai (SP. 3)	Taiyuan (LU. 9)	Taixi (KI. 3)
Jing (Metal)	Zhongfeng (LR. 4)	Lingdao (HT. 4)	Shangqiu (SP. 5)	Jingqu (LU. 8)	Fuliu (KI. 7)

He (Water)	Quchuan (LR. 8)	Shaohai (HT. 3)	Yinling-quan (SP. 9)	Chize)LU. 5)	Yingu (KI. 10

"In the six hollow orsans, each of them has six kinds of shupoint which are Jing, Xing, shu, Yuan, Jing and He, and each kind of shu-points has six acupoints, six times six makes thirty six. They amount to seventy two points in the left and right sides as following:

Shu in six Hollow organs	Gall-bladder	Stomach	Large intestine	Small intestine	Triple warmer	Bladder
Jing (Metal)	Qiaoyin (GB. 44)	Lidui (ST. 45)	Shangyang (II.1)	Shaoze (SI. 1)	Guan-chong (SJ1)	zhiyin (BL. 67)
Xing (water)	Xiaxi (GB. 43)	Neiting (ST. 44)	Erjian (LI. 2)	Qiangu (SI. 2)	Yemen (SJ. 2)	Tonggu (BL. 66)
Shu(wood)	Linqi (GB. 41)	Xiangu (ST. 43)	Sanjian (LI. 3)	Houxi (SI. 3)	Zhongzhu (SJ. 3)	Shugu (BL. 65)
Yuan	Qiuxu (GB. 40)	Chong-yang (ST. 42)	Hegu (LI. 4)	Wangu (SI. 4)	Yangchi (SJ. 4)	Jinggu (BL. 64)
Jing(fire)	Yangfu (GB. 38)	Jiexi (ST. 41)	Yangxi (LI. 5)	Yanggu (SI. 5)	Zhigou (SJ. 6)	Kunlun (BL. 60)
He(Earth)	Yangling-quan(GB.34)	Sanli (ST. 36)	Quchi (LI. 11)	Xiaohai (SI. 8)	Tianjing (SJ. 10)	Weizhong (BL. 40)

"The acupoints for treating the heat-syndrome are fifty nine. In the section of head, there are five rows and each row has five acupoints. In the middle row, there are the five points of Shangxing (DU23), Xinhui (DU. 22), Qianding (DU. 21), Baihui (DU. 20) and Houding (DU. 19); on each of the two sides are Wuchu (BL. 5), Chengguang (BL. 6), Tongtian (BL. 7), Luoque (BL. 8) and Yuzhen (BL. 9) points, and they amount to ten points on the left and right sides; on each of the further two sides are Head-Linqi (GB. 15), Muchuang (GB. 16), Zhengying (GB. 17), Chengling (GB. 18) and Naokong (GB. 19) points, they amount to ten points in the left and right sides. The total of the above acupoints are twenty five. Besides, there are the Dashu (BL. 11), Yingzhu, Quepen (ST. 12), Fengmen (BL. 12) points on each side, they amount to eight points on the left and right sides; Qichong (ST. 30)Sanli (ST. 36), Shangjuxu (ST. 37) and Xiajuxu (ST. 39) points on each

side, they amount to eight points in the left and right sides; Yunmen (LU. 2), Yugu (Jianyu LI. 15), Weizhong (BL. 40) and Yaoshu (DU. 2) points on each side, they amount to eight points in the left and right sides; Pohu (BL. 42), Shentang (BL. 44), pomen (Hunmen BL. 47), Yishe (BL. 49) and Zhishi (BL. 52) points on each sides, they amount to ten points in the left and right sides. The total acupoints for treating the heat-syndrome are fifty nine points.

"The acupoints for treating the syndrome of fluid retention are fifty seven. There are five rows above the buttock, and each row has five acupoints. Along the middle of the spine where the Du Channel pases are the five points of Jizhong (DU. 6), Xuanshu (DU. 5), Mingmen (DU. 4) Yaoshu (DU. 2) and Chang-qiang (DU. 1) points. One and half inches beside the spine where the Foot Taiyang Channel passes are the Dachangshu (BL. 25) Xiaochangshu (BL. 27), Pangguangshu (BL. 28), Zhonglushu (BL. 29), Baihuanshu (BL. 30) points, they amount to ten points in the left and right sides. Three inches by the two sides of the spine where the Foot Taiyang Channel passes are Weicang (BL. 50), Huangmen (BL. 51), Zhishi BL. 52), Baohuang (BL. 53) and Zhibian (BL. 54) points, they amount to ten points in the left and right sides. The total points above are twenty five. Besides, above the musculus rectus femoris, there are two rows, and each of them where the Foot Shaoyang passes has five acupoints. They are Zhongzhu (KI. 15), Siman (KI. 14), Qixue (KI. 13), Dahe (KI. 12), and Henggu (KI. 11) points, and they amount to ten points in the left and right sides. By the sides of Chong Channel and Foot Shaoyin Channel where the Foot Yangming Channel passes are Wailing (ST. 26), Daju (ST. 27), Shuidao (ST. 28), Guilai (ST. 29) and Qichong (ST. 30) points, they amount to ten points in the left and right sides. Above each ankle, there is a row, and each row where the Foot Shaoyin Channel and the Yinjiao Channel pass has six acupoints. They are Taichong (LR. 3), Fuliu (KI. 7), Yingu (KI. 10), Zhaohai (KI. 6), Jiaoxin (KI. 8) and Zhubin (KI. 9) points, and they amount to twelve points in the left and right sides. The total acupoints for treating the syndrome of fluid retention are fifty seven points.

"In the section of head, there are five rows, and each row has five acupoints, and five times five makes twenty five points (the twenty five points in the five rows on head above for treating the heat-syndrome).

"One and half inches by the two sides of the spine, there are five acupoints on each side. By the side of the third vertebra is Feishu (BL. 13), by the side of the fifth vertebra is Xinshu (BL. 15), by the side of the ninth vertebra is the Ganshu (BL. 18), by the side of the eleventh vertabra is Pishu (BL. 20), By the side of the fourteen vertebra is the Shenshu (BL. 23) and they amount to ten points on the left and right sides.

"On the two sides below tre Dazhui point are the two Dazhu points (BL. 11).

"Half inch by each side of the outer canthus are the two Mutong points (Tongziliao GB. 1), on the upper part behind each otomastoid are the two Fubai points (GB. 10). They amount to four points on the left and right sides.

"In the joint of the greater trochanter (uppermost part of the lateral aspect of the thigh where exists the prominence of femur) is the Huantiao point (GB. 30). They amount to two points on the left and right sides.

"The Dubi point (ST. 35) is between the knee cap and the tibia. They amount to two points in the left and right sides.

"The Duosowen point (Tinggong SI. 19) is in the cave-in in the corner of the ear lobe. They amount to two points on the left and right sides.

"The Meiben point (Cuanzhu BL. 2) is in the cave-in of the eyebrow, and they amount to two points on the left and right sides.

"The Wangu point (GB. 12) is inside of the hairline behind the ear. They amount to two points on the left and right sides.

"The Fengfu point (DU. 16) is on the neck one inch inside the hairline. It has only one point.

"The Zhengu point (Touqiaoyin GB. 11) is under the occipital bone seven fen above the wangu point. They amount to two points on the left and right sides.

"The shangguan point (Kezhuren GB. 3) is in front of the ear. They amount to two points in the left and right sides.

"The Daying point (ST. 5) is in the artery one inch and three fen of the cave-in in front of the curve of chin. They amount to two points on the left and right sides.

"The Xiaguan point (ST. 7) is three inches below the Shangguan point, and they amount to two points on the left and right sides.

"The Tianzhu point (BL. 10) is behind the head five inches inside of the hairline, they amount to two points on the left and right sides.

"The Shangjuxu point (ST. 37) is three inches below the Foot Sanli point, the Xiajuxu point (ST. 39) is three inches below the Shangjuxu point. They amount to four points on the left and right sides.

"The Quya point (Jiache ST. 6) is in the cave-in of the cheek terminal eight fen below the ear. They amount to two points on the left and right sides.

"The Tiantu point (RN. 22) is four inches under the Adam's apple, there is only one point.

"The Tianfu point (LU. 3) is three inches under the armpit, they amount to two points on the left and right sides.

"The Tianyou point (SJ. 16) is beside the large tendon behind the Tianrong point and in front of the Tianzhu point under the Wangu point and above the hairline. They amount to two point on the left and right sides.

"The Futu point (LI. 18) is one and half inches beside the Renying point and one inch above the Tianding point between the large tendons of the neck. They amount to two points on the left and right sides.

"The Tianchuang point (SI. 16) is one inch behind the Futu point between the large ten-

dons of the neck under the curved chin. They amount to two points on the left and right sides.

"The Jianjie point (Jianjing GB. 21) is in the cave-in of the shoulder one inch beside the neck and one inch above the Jianliao point. They amount to two points on the left and right sides.

"The Guanyuan point (RN. 4) is three inches under the navel on the white line of the abdomen. There is only one point.

"The Weiyang point (BL. 39) is on the outer side of the Weizhong point on the external terminal of the popliteal fosse. They amount to two points on the left and right sides.

"The Jianzhen point (SI. 9) is under the scapula, and they amount to two points on the left and right sides.

"The Yinmen point (Yamen DU 15) is on the top of neek, five fen inside the hairline. There is only one point.

"In the middle of the navel is the Shenque point (RN. 8) which must not be pricked. It has only one point.

"On each side of the two sides of the Ren Channel on the chest, there are the six acupoints of shufu (KI. 27), Yuzhong (KI. 26), Shen-cang (KI. 25), Lingxu (KI. 24), Shengfeng (KI. 23) and Buguo (Bulang KI. 22). The vertical distance of every point is one inch and six fen, They amount to twelve points on the left and right sides.

"The Dazhu point (BL. 11) is on the back, it is one and half inches beside the first thoracic vertebra. They amount to two points on the left and right sides.

"On each side of the chest, there are the Yunmen (LU. 2), Zhongfu (LU. 1), Zhourong (SP. 20), Xiongxiang (SP. 19), Tianxi (SP. 18) and Shidou (SP. 17) points. They amount to twelve points on the left and right sides, and they are all six inches beside the Ren Channel.

"The Fenrou point (Yangfu GB. 38) is four inches above the outer ankle of the foot in the pace between the strips of muscles at the lower end of os fibula. They amount to two points on the left and right sides.

"Above the inner and the outer ankle, each of them has an acupoint: the Jiaoxin point (KI. 8) is two inches above the inner ankle, and the Fuyang point (BL. 59) is two inches above the outer ankle. They amount to four points in the left and right sides.

"The Yinqiao point (Zhaohai KI. 6) is under the inner ankle, the Yangqiao point (Shenmai BL. 62) is five fen under the outer ankle. They amount to four points on the left and the right sides.

"The fifty seven points for treating the syndromes of retention of fluid are on the spaces between the strips of muscles and the fifty nine points for treating the syndromes of heat-evils are on the intersections of various channels. The points for treating the syndromes of cold-evil is the Xiyang-guan point (GB. 33) on the narrow place on the outer flank under the knee. They amount to two points on the left and right sides.

"The Dajin point (Wuli LI. 13) is five inches under the Tianfu point. This acupoint must not be pricked more than twenty five times: when it is pricked for twenty five times, the shu-energy will be exhausted and the patient will die. This is the reason the point is called Dajin (great prohibition).

"The three hundred and fifty five acupoints are all the importont positions for applying the needles."

帝曰：余已知气穴之处，游针之居，愿闻孙络谿谷，亦有所应乎？岐伯曰：孙络三百六十五穴会，亦以应一岁，以溢奇邪，以通荣卫〔按"以通"四字涉下误衍〕，荣卫稽留，卫散荣溢〔按"卫散"四字，疑为"气竭血著"之旁注，误入正文〕，气竭〔《太素》"竭"作"浊"〕血著，外为发热，内为少气，疾写无怠，以通荣卫，见而写之，无问所会。

Yellow Emperor said: "Now I know the positions of the acupoints for applying the needles, I want to know further to what the minute collaterals, joints and the valleys and grooves between the strips of muscles are corresponding."

Qibo said: "The three hundred and sixty-five points which join the minute collaterals and grooves of muscle are corresponding to the number of days of a year. The function of the minute collaterals is to remove the evil-energy. When the evil energy invades the body, it will cause the stagnation of the Rong and Wei energies, crude and turbid of the breathing, coagulation of the blood, fever in the exterior and short of breath in the interior, if the minute collateral is pricked by needle immediately without delay to discharge the evil-energy, the Rong and Wei energies will become unimpeded. so, whenever the above condition is seen, it should apply the purging therapy by pricking, regardless of the acupoint's position."

帝曰"善。愿闻溪谷之会也。岐伯曰〔胡本，读本，赵本"曰"下并无"善"字〕：肉之大会为谷，肉之小会为谿，肉分之间，谿谷之会，以行荣卫，以会〔《甲乙》"会"作"舍"〕大气，邪溢气壅，脉热肉败，荣卫不行，必将为脓，内销骨髓，外破大腘，留于节凑，必将为败。积寒留舍，荣卫不居，卷肉缩筋，肋肘不得伸，内为骨痹，外为不仁，命曰不足，大寒留于谿谷也。谿谷三百六十五穴会，亦应一岁，其小痹淫溢，循脉往来，微针所及，与法相同。

Yellow Emperor said: "I want to know further about the convergence of valleys and groves." Qibo said: "The larger space between the strips of muscles is called the "valley", the smaller space between the strips of muscles is called the "grove". Thus, in between the strips and groves of muscles, the Rong and Wei energies can pass through, and the evil energy can reside. When the evil-energy invadcs and resides in the valley and groove, the healthy-energy will become stagnated to cause the blood-heat and the deterioration of the muscle, the Rong and Wei energies will be unable to pass through and the muscle will become swelling, in this case, the marrow will be destroyed inside and the larger protruding part of the muscle will be broken outside. If the evil-energy retains in between the bone and muscle, the disease of corruption will occur. When the cold-evil is retaining long, the Rong and Wei energies will not be able to circulate normally and the tendon will shrink and unable to be stretched due to the excessive coldness inside, in this case, it can cause bone bi-syn-

drome inside and numbness outside. The above syndromes are stemmed from the retention of the excessive cold in the valleys and the grooves. The valleys and groves join the three hundred sixty five acupoints are also corresponding with the day-number of a year. If a slight cold is retaining long, it may be accumulated to become more, and it can also circulate along the vessel to cause disease. The evil-energy can be purged by using the small needle like in common pricking treatment."

帝乃辟左右而起，再拜曰：今日发蒙解惑，藏之金匮，不敢复出，乃藏之金兰之室，署曰气穴所在。岐伯曰：孙络之脉别经者，其血盛而当写者，亦三百六十五脉，并注于络，传注十二络脉、非独十四络脉也，内解写于中者十脉。

Yellow Emperor sent away the people who attended beside, rose up and bowed again and again, saying: "Your speech today enlightens my ignorance and relieve my perplexity. I will keep the record of your words in a golden chest, and will by no means lose it, I will store the golden chest in the royal library and name the record as "The Positions of the Acupoints."

Qibo said: "The difference of the vessel of the minute collateral and that of the channel is that the vessel of the minute collateral can discharge the blood when it is abundant. As the three hundred and sixty five vessels are all connecting the collaterals, the overabundant blood can be poured to the collaterals and then to the channels. The pouring is not limited in the fourteen channels (the twelve channels and the Du and Ren channels), even when the meridian in the bone is invaded by the evil, the blood can also pour into the channels of the five solid organs (ten channels in left and right)."

气府论篇第五十九

Chapter 59
Qi Fu Lun
(The Acupoints Associate with Various Channels)

足太阳脉气所发者七十八〔《太素》"八"作"三"〕穴：两眉头各一，入发至顶〔林校云："'项'当作'顶'"〕三寸半，傍五，相去寸，其浮气在皮中者凡五行，行五，五五二十五，项中大筋两傍各一，风府两傍各一，侠背〔《太素》"背"作"脊"〕以下至尻尾二十一节，十五间各一，五藏之俞各五，六府之俞各六，委中以下至足小指傍各六俞。

The Acupoints issued from the Foot Taiyin channel's energy are seventy three。

The Cuanzhu point (BL. 2) is in the cave-in of the brow. They amount to two points in the left and right sides.

From the Cuanzhu point up to the hairline and from the middle point of the hairline up to the Qianding point (DU. 21), the distance is three and half inches, on the line are the Shen-ting point (DU. 24), Shangxing point (DU. 23) and Xinhui point (DU. 22). The row with the Qianding point is the middle row, one and half inches beside the middle row are the two side rows, and one and half inches beside the two side rows are the two further side rows. The distance from the middle row to the further side row is three inches.

There are five rows of the channel energy floating on the top of head. In the middle row, there are the five points of Xinhui (DU. 22), Qianding (DU. 21, Baihui (DU. 20), Houding (DU. 19) and Qiangjian (DU. 18) which belongs to the Du Channel. On each of the two side rows are the Wuchu (BL. 5), Chengguang (BL. 6), Tongtian (BL. 7), Luoque (BL. 8) and Yuzhen (BL. 9) points which belong to the Taiyang channel. They amount to ten points in the left and right sides. On each of the further rows are the Head-linqi (GB. 15), Muchuang (GB. 16), Zhengying (GB. 17), Chengling (GB. 18), and Naokong (GB. 19) points which are pertaining to the Shaoyang Channel, They amount to ten points in the left and right sides. The total points in the five rows are twenty five.

On the left and right sides of the large tendon of the neck are the two Tianzhu points (BL. 10).

By the sides of the Fengfu point are the two Fengchi points (GB. 20).

Among the twenty one vertebrae from the thoracic vertebrae to the coccyx, there are fifteen points of which each of them is one and half inches beside the interspinal space on each of the left and right sides including the five shu-points of the five solid organs and the six hollow organs. They are Feishu (BL. 13) which is one and half inches beside the third vertebra, Jueyin-shu (BL. 14) which is one and half inches beside the fourth vertebra, Xinshu

(BL. 15) which is one and half inches beside the fifth vertebra, Geshu (BL. 17) which is one and half inches beside the seventh vertebra, Ganshu (BL. 18) which is one and half inches beside the ninth vertebra, Danshu (BL. 19) which is one and half inches beside the tenth vertebra, Pishu (BL. 20) which is one and half inches beside the eleventh vertebra. Weishu (BL. 21) which is one and half inches beside the twelfth vertebra, Sanjiaoshu (GB. 22) which is one and half inches beside the thirteenth vertebra, Shenshu (BL. 23) which is one and half inches beside the fourteenth vertebra, Dachangshu (BL. 25) which is one and half inches beside the sixteenth vertebra, Xiaochangshu (BL. 27) which is one and half inches beside the eighteenth vertebra, Pangguangshu (BL. 28) which is one and half inches beside the nineteenth vertebra, Zhonglushu (BL. 29) which is one and half inches beside the twentieth vertebra and Baihuanshu (BL. 30) which is one and half inches beside the twenty first vertebra. They amount to thirty points in the left and right sides.

From the Weizhong point down to the left and right sides of the little toe are six points on each side, they are Weizhong (BL. 40) which is in the cave-in in the artery of the indistinct line in the middle of the fossa poplitea, kunlun (BL. 60) which is five fen behind the outer ankle of the foot, Jinggu (BL. 64) which is in the cave-in of the dorso-ventral boundary under the large bone of the ouuter flank of the foot, Shugu (BL. 65) which is in the cave-in of the dorso-ventral boundary behind the basic joint on the outer flank of the little toe, Tonggu (BL. 66) which is in the cave-in of the dorso-ventral boundary in front of the basic joint on the outer flank of the little toe and Zhiyin (BL. 67) which is about one fen beside the corner of the toe nail on the outer flank of the little toe. They amount to twelve points on the left and right sides.

足少阳脉气所发者六十二穴：两角上各二，直目上发际内各五，耳前角上各一，耳前角下各一，锐发下各一，客主人各一，耳后陷中各一，下关各一，耳下牙车之后各一，缺盆各一掖下三寸，胁下至胠，八间各一，髀枢中傍各一，膝以下至足小指次指各六俞。

The acupoints issued from the Foot Shaoyang channel's energy are sixty two. On the forehead angle are the Tianchong point (GB. 9) which is two inches in the hairline behind the ear, and the Qubin point (GB. 7) which is in the cave-in of the hairline above the ear. They amount to four points on the left and right sides.

From the pupil up into the hairline are the five points of Head-linqi (GB. 15) which is five fen in the hairline above the eye, Muchuang (GB. 16) which is one inch behind the Head-linqi point, Zhengying (GB. 17) which is one inch behind the Muchuang point, Chengling (GB. 18) which is one and half inches behind the Zhengying point and Naokong (GB. 19) which is one and half inches behind the Chengling point. They amount to ten points in the left and right sides.

Above the temple is the Hanyan point (GB. 4). They amount to two points on the left and right sides.

Under the temple is the Xuanli point (GB. 6). They amount to two points on the left and right sides.

In the acute angle of the hairline in front of the auricle is the Heliao point (SJ. 22). They amount to two points on the left and right sides.

Under the Heliao point is the Kezhuren point (Shangguan GB. 3). They amount to two points on the left and right sides.

In the cave-in under the earlope is the Yifeng point (SJ. 17). They amount to two points in the left and right sides.

Under the Kezhuren point is the Xiaguan point (ST. 7). They amount to two points on the left and right sides.

On the terminal of the curved jaw under the ear is the Jiache point (ST. 6). They amount to two points on the left and right sides.

In the cave-in of the transverse under the shoulder is the Quepen point (ST. 12). They amount to two points on the left and right sides.

Three inches under the axilla are the three points of Yuanye (GB. 22), Zhejin (GB. 23) and Tianchi (PC. 1). In the spaces of ribs on the hypochondrium on each side are the six points of Riyue (GB. 24), Zhangmen (LR. 13), Daimai (GB. 26), Wushu (GB. 27), Weidao (GB. 28) and Juliao (GB. 29). They amount to eighteen points on the left and right sides.

By the side of the uppermost part of the lateral aspect of the thigh where exists the prominence of femur is the Huantiao point (GB. 30) which is above the greater trochanter of the outer flank of the thigh. They amount to two points on the left and right sides.

From the knee to the sides of the little toe and the forth toe are the six points of Yanglingsquan (GB. 34) which is one inch under the knee, Yangfu (GB. 38) which is four inches above the outer ankle, Qiuxu (GB. 40) which is before and under the outer ankle, Linqi (GB. 15) which is in the cave-in behind the basic joint between the fourth and the little toes, Xiaxi (GB. 43) which is in the cave-in in front of the basic joint in the juncture of the little toe and the fourth toe, and Qiaoyin (GB. 44) which is one fen beside the nail of the fourth toe. They amount to twelve points on the left and right sides.

足阳明脉气所发者六十八穴：额颅发际傍各三，面鼽骨空各一，大迎之骨空各一，人迎各一，缺盆外骨空各一，膺中骨间各一，侠鸠尾之外，当乳下三寸，侠胃脘各五，侠齐广三寸〔高注本“三寸”作“二寸”〕各三，下齐二寸，侠之各三，气街动脉各一，伏菟上各一，三里以下至足中指各八俞，分之所在穴空。

The acupoints issued from the Foot Yangming channel are sixty eight. By the side of the brow, skull and the hairline is Xuanlu point (GB. 5) which is in the temple, Yangbai point (GB. 14) which is one inch above the eyebow, and Touwei point (ST. 8) which is in the hairline on the frontal corner one and half inches beside the Benshen point. They amount to six points on the left and right sides.

In front of the cheekbone under the eye is the Sibai point (ST. 2). They amount to two points on the left and right sides.

In the cave-in one inch and three fen in front of the curved jaw is the Daying point (ST. 5). They amount to two points on the left and right sides.

Beside the Adam's apple is the Renying point (ST. 9). They amount to two points in the left and right sides.

In the cave-in above the Quepen point is the Tianliao point (SJ. 15). They amount to two points on the left and right sides.

Under the clavicle along the line of mamma, there is an acupoint between each space of the ribs. They are the six points of Qihu (ST. 13) which is under the clavicle, Kufang (ST. 14) which is in the first space of the ribs, Wuyi (ST. 15) which is in the second space of the ribs, Yingchuang (ST. 16) which is in the third space of the ribs, Ruzhong (ST. 17) which is in the fourth space of the ribs, and Rugen (ST. 18) which is in the fifth space of the ribs. They amount to twelve points on the left and right sides.

Outside of the dovetail which is three inches under the mamma and beside the gastric cavity, there are on each side the five points of Burong (ST. 19), Chengman (ST. 20), Liangmen (ST. 21), Guanmen (ST. 22) and Taiyi (ST. 23). The Burong point is under the terminal of the fourth rib, and from Burong point to Taiyi point, the distance of each point between the other is one inch, and their distances from the middle line are two inches. They amount to ten points on the left and right sides.

Two inches by each side of the navel are the three points of Huaroumen (ST. 24) which is one inch under the Taiyi point, Tianshu (ST. 25) which is one inch under the Huaroumen point, and Wailing (ST. 26) which is one inch under the Tianshu point. They amount to six points on the left and right sides.

Two inches under the navel on each side are the three points of Daju (ST. 27), Shuidao (ST. 28) and Guilai (ST. 29). The distances between them are all one inch. They amount to six points on the left and right sides.

The Qijie point (Qichong ST. 30) is one inch under the Guilai point. They amount to two points on the left and right sides.

Six inches above the musculus rectus femoris is the Biguan point (ST. 31). They amount to two points on the left and right sides.

On each side from the Zusanli point down to the middle toe of the foot are the eight points of Zusanli (ST. 36) which is three inches under the Xiyan point and outside of the tibia and fibula between the two tendons, Shanglian (Shangjuxu ST. 37) which is three inches below the Zusanli point, Xialian (Xiajuxu ST. 30) which is three inches below the Shanglian point, Jiexi (ST. 41) which is on the cave-in of the foot dorsum where tieing the shoe lace, Chongyang (ST. 42) which is just before the second and third joints of the metatarsal bone, Xiangu (ST. 43) which is in the cave in behind the basic joint outside of the second toe, Neiting (ST. 44) which is in the front cave-in of the basic joint outside of the second toe, and Lidui (ST. 45) which is one fen beside the corner of the nail outside of the second toe. They amount to sixteen points on the left and right sides.

手太阳脉气所发者三十六穴：目内眦各一，目外〔明抄本“外”下有“眦”字〕各一，鼽骨下各一，耳郭〔《甲乙》“郭”作“廓”〕上各一，耳中各一，巨骨穴各一，曲掖上骨穴各一，柱骨上陷者各

一，上天窗四寸各一，肩解各一，肩解下三寸各一，肘以下至手小指本各六俞。

The acupoints issued from the Hand Taiyang channel's energy are thirty six. One fen beside the inner canthus is the Jingming point (BL. 1). They amount to two points on the left and right sides.

Five fen beside the outer canthus is the Tongziliao point (GB. 1). They amount to two points on the left and right sides.

Under the cheek bone on the face in the cave-in of the sharp bone is the Quanliao point (SI. 18). They amount to two points on the left and right sides.

Under the hairline above the auricle is the Jiaosun point (SJ. 20). They amount to two points on the left and right sides.

Below and in front of the external auditory meatus, behind the condylian process of the lower palatine bone is the Tinggong point (SI. 19). They amount to two points on the left and right sides.

In the cave in of the terminal of the shoulder where the two bones join is the Jugu point (L. I. 16). They amount to two points on the left and right sides.

In the cave in above the axilla in the back, above the Jianzhen point and below the Jugu point is the Naoshu point (SJ. 10). They amount to two points on the left and right sides.

In the upper cave-in of the spinous process of the seventh cervical vertebra above the Quepen point is the Jianjing point (GB. 21). They amount to two points on the left and tight sides.

Four inches above the Tianchuang point behind the ear and one inch under the Fubai point is the Qiaoyin point (GB. 11). They amount to two points in the left and right sides.

At the shoulder joint behind the small protruding bone of the shoulder is the Bingfeng point (SI. 12). They amount to two points on the left and right sides.

In the cave-in of the large bone behind the Bingfeng point, three inches under the shoulder joint is the Tianzong point (SI. 11). They amount to two points on the left and right sides.

From the elbow down to the small finger's tip are the six points of Xiaohai (SI. 8) which is in the cave-in five fen beside the elbow terminal outside of the large bone in-side of the elbow, Yanggu (SI. 5) which is in the wrist under the sharp bone on the outer flank of the hand, Wangu (GB. 12) which is in front of the wrist on the outer flank of the hand, Houxi (SI. 3) which is in the cave-in of the basic joint behind the outer flank of the small finger, Qiangu (SI. 2) which is in the cave in in front of the basic joint on the outer flank of the small finger, and Shaoze (SI. 1) which is one fen beside the corner of the nail on the outer flank of the tip of the small finger. They amount to twelve points on the left and the right sides.

手阳明脉气所发者二十二穴：鼻空外廉、项上各二；大迎骨空各一；柱骨之会各一，髃骨之会各一，肘以下至手大指次指各六俞。

The acupoints issued from the Hand Yangming channel's energy are twenty two. Five

fen outside of the nostril is the Yingxiang point (LI. 20), in the sternocleidomastoid muscle beside the neck is the Futu point (LI. 18). They amount to four points on the left and right sides.

One inch and three fen in front of the curved jaw is the Daying point (ST. 5). They amount to two points on the left and right sides.

Above the Ouepen point on the neck, one inch behind the Futu point in the spinous process of the seventh cervical vertebra where the neck joins the shoulder is the Tianding point (LI. 17). They amount to two points on the left and right sides.

In the cave-in of the split in the terminal of the upper limb and the shoulder, in the joint of acromion scapulae is the Jianyu point (LI. 15). They amount to two points in the left and right sides.

On each side of the line from the elbow down to the thumb and forefinger are the six points of Shousanli (LI. 10) which is in the cave-in between the two tendons on the wrist, Hegu (LI. 4) which is in the cave-in of the bone juncture of the thumb and forefinger, Sanjian (LI. 3) which is in the cave-in benind the inner flank of the basic joint of the forefinger, Erjian (LI. 2) which is in the cave-in in front of the inner flank of the basic joint of the forefinger, and Shangyang (LI. 1) which is one fen beside the corner of nail of the inner flank of the forefinger. They amount to twelve points on the left and right sides.

手少阳脉气所发者三十二穴；鼽骨下各一，眉后各一，角上各一，下完骨后各一，项中足太阳之前各一，侠〔《太素》“扶”上无“侠”字〕扶突各一，肩贞各一，肩贞下三寸分间各一，肘以下至手小指次指本各六俞。

The acupoints issued from the Hand Shaoyang Channel's energy are thirty two. Below the cheek bone is the Quanliao point (SI. 18). They amount to two points on the left and right sides.

In the cave-in behind the eyebrow is the Sizhukong point (SJ. 23). They amount to two points on the left and right sides.

In the cave-in in the hairline below the Xuanlu point is the Xuanli point (GB. 6). They amount to two points on the left and right sides.

Below the Wangu point is the Tianyou point (SJ. 16). They amount to two points on the left and right sides.

In the cave-in the hairline under the Naokong point in front of the Foot Taiyang Channel on the neck is the Fengchi point (GB. 20). They amount to two points on the left and right sides.

In the space of the large tendon of the neck beside the Futu point is the Tianchuang point (SI. 16). They amount to two points on the left and right sides.

One inch below the Naoshu point behind and below the shoulder joint is the Jianzhen point (SI. 9). They amount to two points on the left and right sides.

Three inches below the Jianzhen point in the upper arm by the terminal of the shoulder is the Jianliao point (SJ. 14), on the outside behind the arm, three inches below the Jianliao

point is the Naohui point (SJ. 13), outside of the upper arm, two and half inches below the Naohui point is the Xiaoluo point (SJ. 12). They amount to six points on the left and right sides.

On each side of the line from the elbow to the tips of the small finger and the forefinger are the six points of Tianjing (SJ. 10) which is on the split of the two tendons of the fibula behind the large bone one inch above the elbow, Zhigou (SJ. 6) which is in the cave-in between the two bones three inches behind the wrist on the outer flank of the forearm, Yangchi (SJ. 4) which is in the middle behind the wrist joint, Zhongzhu (SJ. 3) which is in the cave-in behind the basic joint between the small and fourth fingers, Yemen (SJ. 2) which is in the cave in between the basic joints of the small and the fourth fingers, and Guanchong (SJ. 1) which is one fen beside the fourth finger nail. The above points amount to twelve points on the left and right sides.

督脉气所发者二十八穴：项中央二，发际后中八，面中三，大椎以下至尻尾及傍十五穴，至骶下凡二十一节，脊椎法也。

The acupoints issued from the Du channle's energy are twenty eight.

In the middle of the neck are the two points of Fengfu (DU. 16) which is one inch in the hairline in the middle of the neck and Yamen (DU. 15) which is five fen in the hairline in the middle of the neck.

From the middle point of the front hairline straight to the rear are the eight points of Shengting (DU. 24) which is five fens in the hairline, Shangxing (DU. 23) which is one inch in the hairline, Xinhui (DU. 22) which is one inch behind the Shangxing point, Qianding (DU. 21) which is one and half inches behing the Xinhui point, Baihui (DU. 20) which is one and half inches behind the Qianding point, Houding (DU. 19) which is one and half inches behind the Baihui point and Qiangjian (DU. 18) which is one and half inches benind the Houding point, and Naohu (DU. 17) which is one and half inches behind the Qiangjian point.

On the central part of the face are the three points of Suliao (DU. 25) which is on the apex nasi, Shuigou (DU. 26) which is in the nasolabial groove, and Yinjiao (DU. 28) which is in the upper lip above the incisor teeth.

From the Dazhui point down to and beside the sacral bone are fifteen points. They are the Dazhui point (DU. 14) which is in the upper space of the first vertebra, Taodao point (DU. 13) which is in the lower space of the first vertebra, Shenzhu point (DU. 12) which is in the lower space of the third vertebra, Shendao point (DU. 11) which is in the lower space of the fifth vertebra, Lingtai point (DU. 10) which is in the lower space of the six vertebra, Zhiyang point (DU. 9) which is in the lower space of the seventh vertebra, Jinsuo point (DU. 8) which is in the lower space of the ninth vertebra, Zhongshu point (DU. 7) which is in the lower space of the tenth vertebra, Jizhong point (DU. 6) which is in the lower space of the eleventh vertebra, Xuanshu point (DU. 5) which is in the lower space of the thirteenth vertebra, Mingmen point (DU. 4) which is in the lower space of the fourteenth verte-

bra, Yangguan point (DU. 3) which is in the lower space of the sixteenth vertebra, Yaoshu point (DU. 2) which is in the lower space of the twentieth vertebra, Changqiang point (DU. 1) which is under the sacrum and coccyx, and Huiyang point (BL. 35) which is five fen beside the coccyx.

From the first vertebra (the first thoracic vertebra) down to the sacrum and coccyx (the Yaoshu point) are twenty one vertebrae which are the standards for seeking the acupoints by counting the vertebrae.

任脉之气所发者二十八穴：喉中央二，膺中骨陷中各一，鸠尾下三寸，胃脘五寸，胃脘以下至横骨六寸半一〔顾观光说：" '一' 上当脱 '寸' 字，'大' 谓每寸一穴也"〕，腹脉法也。下阴别一，目下各一，下唇〔"下唇" 应之作 "唇下"〕一，龈交一。

The acupoints issued from the Ren Channel's energy are twenty eight. In the middle of the throat are two points, They are the Lianquan point (RN. 23) which is in the cave-in under the chin and above the Adam's apple, and the Tiantu point (RN. 22) which is in the cave-in on the upper terminal of the sternum.

In each cave-in between the sterna is an acupoint, and they amount to six points. They are the Xuanji point (RN. 21) which is one inch below the Tiantu point, Huagai point (RN. 20) which is in the cave-in one inch below the Xuanji point, Chest-Zigong point (RN. 19) which is in the cave-in, one inch and six fen below the Huagai point, Yutang point (RN. 18) which is one inch and six fen below the Chest-Zigong point, Tanzhong point (RN. 17) which is in the cave-in between the two breast, one inch and six fen below the Yutang point, and Zhongting point (RN. 16) which is in the cave-in one inch and six fen below the Tanzhong point.

In the three inches length from the dovetail (the xiphoid process of the sternum) are the three points of Jiuwei (RN. 15) which is five fen below the dovetail, Juque (RN. 14) which is one inch below the Jiuwei point, and Shangwan (RN. 13) which is one inch below the Juque point. In the five inches length of the gastric cavity which is from the Zhongwan point to the Qizhong point are the five points of Zhongwan (RN. 12) which is one inch below the Shangwan point, Jianli (RN. 11) which is one inch below the Zhongwan point, Xiawan (RN. 10) which is one inch below the Jianli point. Shuifen (RN. 9) which is one inch below the Xiawan point, and Shenque (RN. 8) which is one inch below the Shuifen point in the middle of the navel. In the six and half inches length from the gastric cavity to the pubic bone which is one inch below the navel, are the six points of Abdomen-Yinjiao (RN. 7) which is one inch below the navel, Qihai (RN. 6) which is one and half inches below the navel, Shimen (RN. 5) which is two inches below the navel, Guanyuan (RN. 4) which is three inches below the navel, Zhongji (RN. 3) which is one inch below the Guanyuan point, and Qugu (RN. 2) which is one inch below the Zhongji point on the pubic bone. These are the rules for pricking the acupoints in the abdomen from the dovetail to the pubic bone.

In the perineum, there is the Huiyin point (RN. 1).

Seven fen below the eyes are the Chengqi points (ST. 1). They amount to two points on

the left and right sides.

Below the lower lip in front of the chin is the Chengjiang point (RN. 24).

In the seam of the upper teeth and the middle of the upper incisor is the Yinjiao point (DU. 28).

冲脉气所发者二十二穴：侠鸠尾外各半寸至齐寸一，侠齐下傍各五分至横骨寸一，腹脉法也。

The acupoints issued from the Chong Channel are twenty two. Five fen by each side of the middle line are the six points of Youmen (KI. 21) which is five fen beside the Juque point, Tonggu (KI. 20) which is one inch below the Youmen point, Yindu (Shigong KI. 19) which is one inch below the Tonggu point, Shiguan (KI. 18) which is one inch below the Yindu point, Shangqu (KI. 17) which is one inch below the Shiguan point and Huangshu (KI. 16) which is five fen beside the navel one inch below the shangqu point. They amount to twelve points on the left and right sides from the Youmen point to the navel, and the distances from one point to the other are all one inch.

Five fen of each side of the middle line from the navel to the pubic bone are five points which are one inch from one to the other. They are the Zhongzhu point (KI. 15) which is one inch below the Huangshu point, Suifu point (Siman, KI. 14) which is one inch below the Zhongzhu point, Baomen point (Qixue, KI. 13) which is one inch below the Suifu point, Dahe point (Yinwei, KI. 12) which is one inch below the Baomen point, and Henggu point (Xiaji, KI. 11) which is one inch below the Dahe point. They amount to ten points on the left and right sides.

足少阴舌下，厥阴毛中急脉各一，手少阴各一，阴阳跻各一，手足诸鱼际脉气所发者〔孙鼎宜说：“‘者’下脱‘各一’二字，手足共四，故曰诸”。手鱼际，肺经穴名，足鱼际，谓足太阴大都穴〕，凡三百六十五穴也。

The acupoints issued from the Foot Shaoyin Channel are the two Lianquan points of kidney Channel on each side under the tongue.

The acupoints associate to the Jueyin Channel are the two Jimai points (LR. 12) on the left and right sides. They are in the suprapubic mangin.

The Xi-point of the Hand Shaoyin Channel is the Yinxi point (HT. 6) which is five inches behind the wrist. They amount to two points on the left and right sides.

The acupoints of the Yinjiao Channel are the two Jiaoxin points (KI. 8) which are two inches above the inner ankles; The acupoints of the Yangjiao Channel are the two Fuyang points (BL. 59) which are three inches above the outer ankles. They amount to four points on the left and right sides.

Each of the Hand-Yuji point (LU. 10) and the Foot-Yuji point (Dadu SP. 2) which belong to the Taiyin Channel has two points on the left and right sides. They amount to four points.

The total points above amount to three hundred and sixty five (some of the points occur repeatedly of allernately due to their associations to different channels).

骨空论篇第六十

Chapter 60
Gu Kong Lun
(On the Cavity of the Bone)

黄帝问曰：余闻风者百病之始也，以针治之奈何？岐伯对曰：风从外入，令人振寒，汗出头痛，身重恶〔《太素》《骨空》“恶”下有“风”字〕寒，治在风府，调其阴阳，不足则补，有余则写。

Yellow Emperor asked: "I am told that the wind-evil is the source of all diseases, what method should be applied when treating with acupuncture?"

Qibo answered: "When the wind-evil invades the body, it causes the patient to have cold shiverings, perspiration, headache, the feeling of heaviness in the body and have the aversion to wind. When treating, the Fengfu point (DU. 16) should be pricked to adjust the Yin and Yang. If the patient's healthy energy is insufficient, the invigorating method should be applied, if the evil-energy is having a surplus, the purging method should be applied.

大风颈项痛，刺风府，风府在上椎；大风汗出，灸譩譆，譩譆在背下俠脊傍三寸所，厌之，令病者呼譩譆，譩譆应手。

"If a greater wind-evil is contracted and the neck is painful, the Fengfu point which is on the first cervical vertebra should be pricked. If a greater wind-evil is contracted and the patient is sweating, prick the Yixi point (BL. 45) which is three inches beside the sixth vertebra of the spine on the back, when the point is pressed by fingers, the patient will feel painful and cry out the sound of Yixi, and by this time, the physician will feel the bouncing of pulse under the fingers.

从风憎风，刺眉头。失枕，在肩上〔《太素》“上”下有“之”字，按“在”上疑脱“治”字〕横骨间。折，使榆〔“榆”《太素》吴本作“揄”〕臂，齐肘正，灸脊中。

"To the patient who has aversion to the braving of wind, the Chanzhu point (BL. 2) in the brow should be pricked.

"To the syndrome of pain in the neck, the points on the transverse of the shoulder should be pricked. When the arm is painful like being broken, ask the patient to stretch his hands by the two sides first, and then apply moxibustion to the central part in the middle of the connecting line on the back between the two elbows.

𦙶络季胁引少腹而痛胀，刺譩譆。

"When the lower abdomen is drawn by the insubstantial and soft part under the hypochondrium with pain, the Yixi point should be pricked.

腰痛不可以转摇，急引阴卵，刺八髎与痛上，八髎在腰髎分间。

"When the lumbago causes the patient unable to turn aside or sway, and his testes become uncomfortable when the pain is severe, the four liao-points and the site of pain should be pricked. The shangliao point (BL. 31) is the first sacral foramen which is one inch beside the eighteenth vertebra, the Ciliao point (BL. 32) is the second sacral foramen which is eight fen beside the nineteenth vertebra, the Zhongliao point (BL. 33) is the third sacral foramen which is seven fen beside the twentieth vertebra, and Xialiao point (BL. 34) is the fourth sacral foramen which is six fen beside the twenty-first vertebra. The liao-points amount to eight points on the left and right sides.

鼠瘘，寒热，还刺寒府，寒府在〔《太素》“在”下无“附”字〕附膝外解营，取膝上外者使之拜，取足心者使之跪。

"When scrofula is contracted, the patient will have chillness and fever, the Hanfu point (Xiyangguan GB. 33) which is in the seam of the bone beside the knee cap should be pricked. When pricking the points in the outer flank of the knee, the patient should make the posture of bowing; when pricking the Yongquan point (KI. 1) which is on the sole of foot, the patient should make the posture of kneeling.

任脉者，起于中极之下，以上毛际，循腹里上关元，至咽喉，上颐循面入目。冲脉者，起于气街，并少阴〔《甲乙》“少阴”作“阳明”〕之经，侠齐上行，至胸中而散。任脉为病，男子内结七疝，妇子带下〔《难经·二十九难》“带下”作“为”〕瘕聚。冲脉为病，逆气里急。

"The Ren Channel starts from the Huiyin point (RN. 1) between the external genitals and the anus and ascends to the suprapubic hair margin and then ascends along the middle line of the abdomen (the white line of the abdomen) to the Guanyuan point (one inch above the Zhongji point), upper part of the abdomen, the chest, throat and cheek to the lower gum by passing the Chengjiang point, and finally reaches the Chengqi point (ST. 1) below the eye.

"The Chong Channel starts from the Qijie point (Qichong ST. 30) which is parallel to the Yangming Channel, advancing along the left and right sides of the navel, and scatters when reaching the middle of the chest.

"When there is pathologic change in the Ren Channel, a man will contract the seven kinds of hernia in the abdomen, a woman will contract the abdominal mass. When there is pathologic change in the Chong Channel, the vital energy will reverse up and cause pain of the abdomen.

督脉为病，脊强反折〔滑抄本“折”作“张”〕。督脉者，起于少腹以下骨中央。女子入系廷孔，其孔，溺孔之端也。其络循阴器合篡〔《太素》《甲乙》“篡”作“纂”〕间，绕篡后，别绕臀，至少阴与巨阳中络者〔王注无“者”字凝衍〕合，少阴上股内后廉，贯脊属肾，与太阳起于目内眦，上额交巅，上入络脑，还出别下项，循肩髆，内侠脊抵腰中，入循膂络肾〔《太素》“络肾”下有“而止”二字〕；其男子循茎下至篡，与女子等，其少腹直上者，贯齐中央，上贯心入喉，上颐还唇，上系两目之下中央。此生病，从少腹上冲心而痛，不得前后，为冲疝；其女子不孕，癃痔〔《太素·督脉》杨注：“有本无‘痔’字”〕遗溺嗌乾。督脉生病治督脉，治在骨上，甚者在齐下营。

“When there is a pathologic change in the Du Channel, it will cause stiffness of the spine and the patient will be unable to face up and down.

“The Du Channel starts from the middle of the hip bone under the lower abdomen. For a woman, it starts from inside of the external urethral orifice, its collaterals branch off along the vaginal orifice, join the perineum and surround the outside of the anus; another branch of Du Channel surrouds the buttock to the Shaoyin channel and then join the middle collaterals of the Taiyang Channel. The Shaoyin Channel ascends from the back of the inner thigh, penetrates through the spine and connects the kidney.

“The Du Channel also starts with the Foot Taiyang Channel from the inner canthus of the eye, they ascend to the forehead, and join the top of the head, their collaterals reach the brain, and from the brain, a branch of collateral descends to the neck, shoulder, arm, and loin, and finally to the kidney.

“For a man, the Du Channel descends to the perineum along the penis which is the same like that of a woman The difference is that the Du Channel ascends straight from the lower abdomen, penetrates through the centre of the navel, passing the heart and throat, surrounds the lips and reach the location below the two eyes.

“When there is pathologic change in the Du Channel, the energy will rush up from the lower abdomen to the heart and causes pain, the patient will be unable to pass urine nor to move bowels and contracts the disease which is called the hernia by impact; for a woman, it will cause her to have the syndromes of sterility, dysuria, enuresis and dryness of the laryngopharynx, etc. In a word, when the Du Channel contracts disease, the Du Channel should be treated, when the disease is light, treat the points in the spine or in the transverse by pricking, if the disease is severe, prick the Yinjiao point (RN. 7) under the navel.

其上气有音者，治其喉中央，在缺盆中者，其病〔孙鼎宜说：“‘上’字衍”〕上冲喉者治其渐，渐者，上侠颐也。

“To the patient who has the syndrome of rapid breathing with sound, prick the Lianquan point (RN. 23) and the Tiantu point (RN. 22) when treating. If the vital energy reverses up to impact the throat, prick the Daying point (ST. 5) by the curved bone of jaw.

蹇，膝伸不屈，治其楗。坐而膝痛，治其机。立而暑解〔尤怡说：“‘暑’当是‘骨’字，骨解言骨散堕如解也”〕，治其骸关。膝痛，痛及拇指治其腘。坐而膝痛如物隐者，治其关。膝痛不可屈伸，治其背内，连骺若折，治阳明中俞髎。若别，治巨阳少阴荥。淫泺胫痠〔《太素》“泾泺”下无“胫痠”二字〕，不能久立，治少阳之维〔“维”误，应作“络”，核王注原作“络”〕，在外上五寸。

“To the patient who has difficulty in walking and can not bend his knee, prick the Biguan point (ST. 31) in his thigh when treating; to the patient whose knee is painful when sitting down, prick the Huantiao point (GB. 30) when treating; to the patient whose bones are scatter and falling like being separated, prick the Yangguan point (GB. 33) in the knee joint when treating; when the pain on the knee drawing the thumb and the great toe, prick the Weizhong point (BL. 40) in the poplitea. When the knee is painful like something hiding

inside when sitting down, prick the greater trochanter; when the knee is painful that can not be stretched or bent, prick the shu-points of the Foot Taiyang Channel on the back; when the pain affecting the leg like being broken, prick the Xiangu point (ST. 43) which is the Shu-point of the Foot Yangming Channel; when the knee is painful as if its sections are parting, prick the Xing-points of the Taiyang and Shaoyin channels; when the knee is sore and weak, and the patient can not stand long, prick the point five inches above the outer ankle which is on the collateral of the Shaoyang Channel.

辅骨上，横骨下为楗，侠髋为机膝解为骸关，侠膝之骨为连骸，骸下为辅，辅上为腘，腘上为关，头〔《太素》“头”作“项”杨上善说：项横骨，项上头后王、枕也〕横骨为枕。

"Above the fibula and below the pubic bone is the femur bone, between the hip point is the pivot, the juncture of the knee is called the knee joint, the prominent bone beside the knee is the knee cap, below the knee cap is the fibula, above the fibula is the popliteal fossa, the moving joint above the popliteal fossa is called the clue, the horizontal bone behind the neck is the occipital bone.

水俞五十七穴者，尻上五行，行五；伏菟上两行，行五，左右各一行，行五；踝上各一行，行六穴，髓空在脑后三分，在颅际锐骨之下，一在龈基下，一在项后中复骨下，一在脊骨上空在风府上；脊骨下空，在尻骨下空，数髓空在面侠鼻，或骨空在口下当两肩；两髆骨空，在髆中之阳，臂骨空在臂阳〔《太素》“骨”下无“空”字〕，去踝四寸两骨空之间；股骨上空在股阳〔孙鼎宜说：“出上”二字恐误倒〕，出上膝四寸；骺骨空在辅骨之上端，股际骨空在毛中动〔《太素》“动”下有“脉”字〕下；尻骨空在髀骨之后，相去四寸。扁骨有渗理凑〔《太素》“理”下无“凑”字〕，无髓孔，易髓〔顾观光说：“‘易髓’二字当乙转”。“易”作“亦”解》〕无孔。

"The Shu-points for treating the water-syndrome are fifty seven: there are five rows above the sacral bone, and in each row, there are five points. In the middle row which is the Du Channel, there are the five points of Jizhong (DU. 6), Xuanshu (DU. 5), Mingmen (DU. 4), Yaoshu (DU. 2) and Changqiang (DU. 1). On each side-row beside the Du Channel is the Foot Taiyang Channel, and on each side, there are the five points of Dachangshu (BL. 25), Xiaochangshu (BL. 27), Pangguangshu (BL. 28), Zhonglushu (BL. 29) and Baihuanshu (BL. 30) and they amount to ten points on the left and right sides. On each further side-row which is also the Taiyang Channel are the five points of Weishu (BL. 21), Huangmen (BL. 51), Zhishi (BL. 52), Baohuang (BL. 53) and Zhibian (BL. 54), and they amount to ten points in the left and right sides. Above the Futu point beside the Ren Channel there are two rows, on each row are the five points of Zhongzhu (KI. 15), Siman (KI. 14), Qixue (KI. 13), Dahe (KI. 12) and Henggu (KI. 11), and they amount to ten points on the left and right sides. On each of the further side beside the Foot Shaoyin Channel which is on the Foot Yangming Channel are the five points of Wailing (ST. 26), Daju (ST. 27), Shuidao (ST. 28), Guilai (ST. 29) and Qichong (ST. 30), and they amount to ten points on the left and right sides. Above each inner ankle there is a row, and on each row are the six points of Taichong (LR. 3), Zhaohai (KI. 6), Fuliu (KI. 7), Jiaoxin (KI. 8), Zhubin

(KI. 9) and Yingu (KI. 10), and they amount to twelve points on the left and right sides.

"The cavity of bone which leads to the bone marrow is also called the cavity of marrow. The cavity of bone of the Fengfu point (DU. 16) is five fen behind the brain under the sharp bone of the skull; the cavity of bone of the Chengjiang point (RN. 24) is in the cave-in of the lower gum; the cavity of bone of Yinmen point (Yamen point DU 15) is in the middle behind the neck under the Fugu point; the cavity of bone of the Naohu point (DU. 17) is above the Fengfu point in the upper cavity of the spine; the cavity of bone of Changqiang point (DU. 1) is below the spine in the lower cavity of the sacral bone. Besides the nose of the face, there are also some cavities of bone, some of them lead to the brain which are the Chengqi (ST. 1), Juliao (ST. 3), Quanliao (SI. 18), Jingming (BL. 1), Sizhukong (SJ. 23), Tongziliao (GB. 1), Tinghui (GB. 2) and Yingxiang (LI 20) points, some of the bone cavities are below the mouth, or on the two shoulders like the two Daying points (ST. 5).

"The cavity of bone of the shoulder is on the outer flank of the shoulder. The cavity of bone of the arm is on the outer flank of the arm, four inches above the wrist between the two bones which are the Sanyangluo points (SJ. 8) of the Hand Shaoyang Channel.

"The cavity of bone on the thigh is in the outer flank of the thigh, four inches above the knee, which is the Futu point (ST. 32).

"The cavity of tibia and fibula is on the upper terminal of the fibula which is the Dubi point (ST. 35).

"The cavity of bone of the upper thigh is in the artery of the suprapubic hair margin on the two terminals of the pubic bone below the lower abdomen. The cavity of the sacral bone is four inches behind the femur which are the eight Liao-points.

"Each piece of bone in the body which is round has marrow in it, and each bone with marrow has a passway for the marrow which is the cavity of marrow, but the bone in flat shape whose striae is irrigated by blood instead of by marrow, it has no cavity for the marrow.

灸寒热之法，先灸项大椎，以年为壮数，次灸橛〔《太素》作“厥”〕骨，以年为壮数，视背俞陷者灸之，举〔《太素》“举”作“与”〕臂肩上陷者灸之，两季胁之间灸之，外踝上绝骨之端灸之，足小指次指间灸之，腨下陷脉灸之，外踝后灸之，缺盆骨上切之坚痛如筋者灸之，膺中陷骨间灸之，掌束骨下灸之，齐下关元三寸灸之，毛际动脉灸之，膝下三寸〔《甲乙》“膝”作“脐”，“三”作“二”〕分间灸之，足阳明跗上动脉灸之，巅上一灸之 。犬所啮〔《太素》作“齧”，《说文》“齧”，噬也”〕之处灸之三壮，即以犬伤病法灸之。凡当灸二十九处〔《太素》“九”作“七”〕，伤食灸之，不已者，必视其经之过於阳者，数刺其俞而药之。

"When treating the cold and fever, apply moxibustion to the Dazhui point first, and determine the number of moxa cones used in one treatment according to the age of the patient, then, apply moxibustion to the points in the sacral bone and use the number of the cones according to the age of the patient.

"When treating, inspect first the back of the patient, and treat with moxibustion where

there is a cave-in. The patient should lift his arm horizontally so as the location of the cave-in may treated on the shoulder (the Jianyu point LI. 15) may be treated. Treat with moxibustion to the point between the two hypochondria (Jingmen point GB. 25). Treat with moxibustion to the lower end of the fibula above the outer ankle (Yangfu GB. 38). Treat with moxibustion to the point in front of the basic joint of the little toe and the fourth toe (Xiaxi point GB. 43). Treat with moxibustion to the cave-in below the calf (Chengjin point BL. 56). Treat with moxibustion to the Kunlun point (BL. 60). behind the outer ankle Kunlun point (BL. 60).

"Treat with moxibustion to the location which is hard and painful like that of the tendon when being pressed by hand above the supraclavicular fossa. Treat with moxibustion to the Guanyuan point (RN. 4) which is three inches below the navel. Treat with moxibustion to the Qichong point (ST. 30) in the artery of the suprapubic hair margin. Treat with moxibustion to the Zusanli point (ST. 36) between two tendons two inches under the knee. Treat with moxibustion to the Chongyang point (ST. 42) where there is artery on the dorsum. Treat with moxibustion to the Baihui point (DU. 20) which is at the centre on top of the head.

"When one is bitten by a dog, the injured part should be treated with moxibustion by applying three moxa-cones in a treatment in accordance with the method of treating the dog's bite, as the dog's bite can also cause cold and fever.

"The above points for treating the syndrome of cold and fever amount to twenty seven.

"The syndrome of dyspepsia should be treated with moxibustion as dyspepsia can also cause cold and fever. If the disease can not be cured by moxibustion, the patient's channel should be inspected, if his Yang-evil is overabundant, his Shu-points should be pricked repeatedly, and at the same time, medicine should be taken."

水热穴论篇第六十一

Chapter 61
Shui Re Xue Lun
(On the Shu-points for Treating the Fluid-retention Syndrome and Fever)

黄帝问曰：少阴何以主肾？肾何以主水？岐伯对曰：肾者，至〔《太素》“阴”上无“至”字〕阴也，至阴者，盛水也；肺者，太阴也〔《太素》作“肾者少阴”〕，少阴者，冬脉也，故其本在肾，其末在肺，皆积水也。帝曰：肾何以能聚水而生病？岐伯曰：肾者，胃之关也〔《太素》“也”作“闭”〕，关门〔赵本“门”作“阀”〕不利，故聚水而从其类也。上下溢于皮肤，故为胕肿，胕肿者，聚水而生病也。

Yellow Emperor asked："Why is it that the Shaoyin determines the condition of the kidney, and the kidney determines the condition of the water?" Qibo answered："Kidney is the location to store the extreme Yin, and Yin belongs to the water, so, the kidney is the viscus which determines the condition of water. Kidney belongs to Shaoyin, and Shaoyin is most prosperous in winter, and winter is the season which corresponds with water, therefore, the root of edema is in the kidney, and its symptom is manifested in the lung. If the viscus of lung or kidney is not sound, the accumulation of fluid will occur."

Yellow Emperor asked："How can the kidney acumulate the fluid and cause disease?"Qibo answered："The kidney is like the sluice gate of the stomach, when the sluice gate does not work, the fluid will be accumulated and the evil-energy will run wild, when the fluid overflows about the skin, peritoneal fluid will occur. The come about of the peritoneal fluid is due to the continuous accumulation of the fluid."

帝曰：诸水皆生〔《甲乙》“生”作“主”〕于肾乎？岐伯曰：肾者，牝藏也，地气〔《医垒元戎》引“地气”下无“上者”二字〕上者属于肾，而生水液也，故曰至阴。勇而劳甚则肾〔《圣济总录》引“勇”上有“故人”二字，孙鼎宜说：“‘肾’字业上‘甚’字声衍”〕汗出，肾汗〔《太素》“汗”上无“肾”字〕出逢于风，内不得入于藏府〔《太素》作“入其藏”〕，外不得越于皮肤，客于玄〔《太素》“玄”作“六”〕府，行于皮里〔四库本“里”作“肤”，按《太素》作“肤”〕，传为胕肿，本之于肾，名曰风水。所谓玄府者，汗空也〔《太素》无“也”字〕。

Yellow Emperor asked："Are all the fluid-retention syndromes originated from kidney?" Qibo answered："Kidney is a Yin viscus, when the earth-energy communicates with kidney, fluid will produce, so the kidney is called the viscus of extreme Yin. If anyone is self-assured for his courage to conduct excessive sex intercourse or take part in excessive labour, he will be sweating, and when the wind-evil invades the body during the sweating, his sweat pores

will close all of a sudden, as the perspiration has not completed, the sweat can not return to its viscus inside, neither can it be discharged to the skin outside, the fluid will fill the skin and cause edema.

"The disease is caused by the affection of the kidney, and is also caused by the wind-evil, so it is called the edema caused by wind-evil."

帝曰：水俞五十七处者，是何〔《太素》"何"下有"所"字〕主也？岐伯曰：肾俞五十七穴，积阴之所聚也，水所从出入也。尻上五行行五者，此〔《太素》"此"下有"皆"字〕肾俞，故水病下为胕肿大腹，上为喘呼，不得卧者，标本俱病，故肺为喘呼，肾为水肿，肺为逆〔《太素》"逆"下有"故"字〕不得卧，分为相输俱受者，水气之所留也。伏菟上各二行行五者，此肾之街〔"街"作"所冲"〕也，三阴之所交结于脚也。踝上各一行行六者，此肾脉之下行也，名曰太冲。凡五十七穴者，皆藏之阴络，水之所客也。

Yellow Emperor asked: "The number of the Shu-points for treating the fluid-retention syndrome are fifty seven, by which viscus are they related?" Qibo answered: "The fifty seven Shu-points of the kidney are the locations where the Yin energy accumulates and they are also the locations where the fluid comes in and goes out. There are five rows above the buttock, and each row has five points, they amount to twenty five points and they are all the Shu-points of kidney, and they are the Shu-points dominated by the Du Channel and the Foot Taiyang Channel. When the fluid-retention is in the lower part, edema of the dorsum and swelling of the abdomen will occur; if the fluid-retention is in the upper part, rapid breathing and failure of lying on the back of the patient will occur. This is the case of disease in both the root and the branch: the rapid breathing associates with the lung and edema associates with the kidney, when the lung is coerced by the up-reversing flow of the water-energy, the patient will not be able to lie on his back. As the spreading of the kidney-energy and the lung-energy are correlated with each other, the retention of fluid will cause both the viscera to suffer disease.

"Above the Futu point beside the Ren Channel are two rows on which each rows are the five points of Zhongzhu (KI. 15), Siman (KI. 14), Qixue (KI. 13), Dahe (KI. 12) and Henggu (KI. 11); on each of the two further sides are the five points of Wailing (ST. 26), Daju (ST. 27), Shuidao (ST. 28), Guilai (ST. 29) amd Qichong (ST. 30). They amount to twenty points on the left and right sides, and they are all the passways of the kidney energy and the three Yin Channels of Foot. Above each inner ankle, there is the row for the kidney energy to descend to the Yongquan point which is called the Taichong line. On each line of the left and the right there are the six points of Taichong (LR. 3), Fuliu (KI. 7), Yingu (KI. 10), Zhaohai (KI. 6), Jiaoxin (KI. 8) and Zhubin (KI. 9), and they amount to twelve points on the left and right sides. The above fifty seven points are all the Yin collaterals of the viscera and they are also the locations where the water-energy retains. They should be pricked when treating the fluid-retention syndrome."

帝曰：春取络脉分肉何也？岐伯曰：春者木始〔《太素》"木"下无"始"字〕治，肝气始生，肝气急，其风疾，经脉常深，其气少，不能深入，故取络脉分肉〔《甲乙》"肉"下有

"之"字〕间。

Yellow Emperor asked: "When treating in spring, it should prick the shallow position where the collateral and muscular layer locate, and what is the reason?" Qibo answered: "Spring is the season when the grasses and trees begin to grow and the liver which corresponds to spring will manifest vigor and vitality also. The property of the liver is rather urgent and it changes swiftly like the wind. The channel-energy of a man resides deeply inside in winter, and it begins to send off in spring, thus in spring, the channel-energy is still little outside and abundant inside. So, when the evil-energy invades, it can only reach the shallow position where the collateral and muscle locate instead of reaching deeply inside where the channel-energy is abundant. Therefore, when treating, it should only prick the shallow position where the collateral and muscular layer locate."

帝曰：夏取盛经分腠，何也？岐伯曰：夏者火始治，心气始长，脉瘦气弱，阳气留〔《太素》《甲乙》"留"作"流"〕溢，热熏分腠〔《甲乙》作"血温于腠"〕，内至于经，故取盛经分腠，绝肤而病去者，邪居浅也。所谓盛经者，阳脉也。

Yellow Emperor asked: "When treating in summer, it should prick the Yang collaterals which are prosperous and floating between the skin and the muscle, and what is the reason?" Qibo answered: "The fire-energy dominates in summer and the heart-energy begins to become prosperous in correspondence by this time, although the of fire-energy is still weak in its initial stage, yet it fills with Yang energy, when it becomes prosperous gradually and spreads into the whole body, the heat will fumigate the floating and prosperous collaterals between the muscle and the striae and reach the channel inside. As the Yang energy is abundant in the channel, the evil-energy can by no means invade, so, when the pricking reaches only the shallow position which is the collateral between the muscle and striae, it will extinguish the evil-energy in the skin. The floating collaterals between the muscle and the striae are that of the Yang Channels."

帝曰：秋取经俞何也？岐伯曰：秋者金始治，肺将收杀〔按"杀"疑误，似应作"敛"〕，金将胜火，阳气在合，阴气初胜，湿气及体，阴气未盛，未能深入，故取俞以写阴邪，取合以虚阳邪，阳气始衰，故取于合。

Yellow Emperor asked: "When treating in autumn, it should prick the Shu-points of the channels, and what is the reason?" Qibo answered: "The metal dominates in autumn, the lung in the body which corresponds to it also manifests the appearance of chilliness and restraint like autumn. When the metal-energy is prosperous and the fire-energy is becoming declined, metal will overcome the fire and the Yang energy will penetrate inside to enter into the He-points of the channel. As the Yin energy is only in its initial stage of being prosperous, its wetness is not strong enough to penetrate deeply into the body. So, when treating, it should prick the Shu-points to purge the Yin evil. Since the Yang energy then only begins to decline and enters into the He-points, so the He-points should be pricked to excrete the Yin evil."

帝曰：冬取井荥〔全本，胡本，吴本"荣"作"荥"〕何也？岐伯曰：冬者水始治，肾方

闭，阳气衰少，阴气坚盛〔《太素》“坚盛”作“紧”〕，巨阳伏沈，阳脉〔赵本，朝本，“脉”作“气”〕乃去，故取井以下阴逆，取荣〔应作荥〕以实阳气。故曰冬取井荥，春不鼽衄，此之谓也。

Yellow Emperor asked: "When treating in winter, it should prick the Jing-points and the Xing-points, and what is the reason? Qibo answered: "The water dominates in winter, the kidney in the body which corresponds to it also manifests the appearance of the declining Yang when the Yin becomes abundant in winter. As the energy of the Foot Taiyang Channel is sinking on the bone, and the Yang energy descends in the wake of it, so, it should prick the Jing-points to restrain the excessive and up-reversing Yin energy and prick the Xing-points to enrich the Yang energy which is insufficient. That is why the saying goes: 'When the Jing-points and the Xing-points are pricked in winter, one will not contract allergic rhinitis and epistaxis in spring'。"

帝曰：夫子言治热病五十九俞，余论〔“论”疑误〕其意，未能领〔《太素》“能”下无“领”字〕别其处，愿闻其处，因闻其意。岐伯曰：头上五行行五者，以越诸阳之热逆也；大杼、膺俞、缺盆、背俞，此八者，以写胸中之热也；气街、三里、巨虚上下廉，此八者，以写胃中之热也；云门、髃骨、委中、髓空，此八者，以写四支之热也；五藏俞傍五，此十者，以写五藏之热也，凡此五十九穴者，皆热之左右也。

Yellow Emperor said: "Now I understand the general idea of the fifty nine Shu-points for treating the fever, but I do not know clearly their positions. I hope you can tell me their positions and how can they excrete the heat." Qibo answered: "On the head, there are five rows and each row has five points, they amount to twenty five points. As all the Yang energies are ascending to the head, the heat can be excreted when pricking the twenty five points. On the middle row which is the Du Channel, are the five points of Shangxing (DU. 23), Xinhui (DU. 22), Qianding (DU. 21), Baihui (DU. 20) and Houding (DU. 19). On each of the side-row which is the Foot Taiyang Channel are the five points of Wuchu (BL. 5), Chengguang (BL. 6), Tongtian (BL. 7), Luoque (BL. 8) and Yuzhen (BL. 9), and they amount to ten points on the left and right sides. On each of the further side-row which is the Foot Shaoyang Channel are the five points of Linqi (GB. 15), Muchuang (GB. 16), Zhengying (GB. 17), Chengling (GB. 18) and Naokong (GB. 19) and they amount to ten points on the left and right sides.

"The Dazhu point (BL. 11) of the Foot Taiyang Channel is beside the Dazhui point on the neck. The Yingshu point (Zhongfu, LU. 1) of the Taiyang Channel is six inches beside the middle of the chest; the Quepen point (ST. 12) of the Foot Yangming Channel is in the cave-in of the clavicle on the shoulder; the Beishu point (Fengmen, BL. 12) of the Foot Taiyang Channel is one and half inches beside the second vertebra. They amount to eight points on the left and right sides. As they are all on the chest or back, the heat of chest can be excreted by pricking them.

"The Qijie point (Qichong, ST. 30) is on the terminal of the pubic bone under the lower abdomen where there is artery and it can be felt when touching with hand, the Sanli point

(Zusanli, ST. 36) is in the muscle between the two tendons on the outside of the tibia and fibula three inches below the knee; the Shangjuxu point (ST. 37) is three inches below the Sanli point; the Xiajuxu point (ST. 39) is three inches below the Shangjuxu point. They amount to eight points on the left and right sides. All the eight points belong to the Foot Yangming Channel, the heat in the stomach can be excreted by pricking them.

"The Yunmen point (LU. 2) of the Hand Taiyin Channel is below the clavicle six inches beside the middle of the chest; The Yugu point (Jianyu LI. 15) on the acromion scapula of the Hand Yangming Channel is beside the terminal of the shoulder; the Weizhong point (BL. 40) of the Foot Taiyang Channel is in the middle of the poplitea in the artery on the indistinct line behind the knee; the Suikong point (Henggu, KI. 11) of the Foot Shaoyin Channel is on the suprapubic hair margin five fen beside the middle of the upper margin of the pubic bone. They amount to eight points on the left and right sides. The channels with the eight points are passing the four limbs and the heat of the four limbs can be excreted by pricking them.

"The Shu-points of the five viscera are on the back, and they all located on one and half inch beside the spine: the Feishu point (BL. 13) is in the space of the third vertebra; the Xinshu point (BL. 15) is in the space of the fifth vertebra; the Ganshu point (BL. 18) is in the space of the ninth vertebra; the Pishu point (BL. 20) is in the space of the eleventh vertebra,; the Shenshu point (BL. 23) is in the space of the fourteenth vertebra. They amount to ten points on the left and right sides. The ten points all belong to the Foot Taiyang Channel, and the heat of the five viscera can be excreted by pricking them.

"The fifty nine points above are all the points for treating the fever."

帝曰：人伤于寒而传〔《太平御览》引“传”下“转”〕为热，何也？岐伯曰：夫寒盛〔《太素》“盛”作“甚”〕则生热也。

Yellow Emperor asked: "When one contracts the cold-evil, it transforms into fever, and what is the reason?" Qibo said: "It is because the cold-evil is abundant outside, and the Yang-energy is shut inside, when the energy and blood become stagnated, it produces fever."

调经论篇第六十二

Chapter 62
Tiao Jing Lun
(On Adjusting the Channels by Pricking)

黄帝问曰：余闻刺法言，有余写之，不足补之，何谓有余？何谓不足？岐伯对曰：有余有五，不足亦有五，帝欲何问？帝曰：愿尽闻之。岐伯曰：神有〔《甲乙》"神有"下叠"有"字，下气，血，形，志同〕余有不足，气有余有不足，血有余有不足，形有余有不足，志有余有不足，凡此十者，其气不等也。

Yellow Emperor asked："I am told that when the disease is in the state of having a surplus，the purge therapy should be applied，when the disease is in the state of being insufficient，the therapy of invigoration should be applied，but what is the condition of having a surplus or being insufficient?" Qibo answered："There are five conditions of having a surplus and five conditions of being insufficient. Which one do you want to know?" Yellow Emperor said："I like to hear all about them." Qibo said："In spirit，in energy，in blood，in shape and in will，they all have the conditions of having a surplus or being insufficient. These ten conditions develope along with different situations and they are changeful."

帝曰：人有精气津液，四支、九窍、五藏、十六部，三百六十五节，乃生百病，百病之生，皆有虚实。今夫子乃言有余有五，不足亦有五，何以生之乎？岐伯曰：皆生于五藏〔林校云：按《甲乙经》无"五藏"二字〕也。夫心藏神，肺藏气，肝藏血，脾藏肉，肾藏志，而此成形。志意通，〔《甲乙》"通"下有"达"字〕内连骨髓，而成身形五藏。五藏之道，皆出于经隧，以行血气，血气不和，百病乃变化而生，是故守经隧焉。

Yellow Emperor said："In the refined energy，fluid，the four extremities，five viscera，nine orifices，sixteen channels and three hundred and sixty five bone joints of a man，all of them can contract disease，and all the diseases contracted are of asthenic or sthenic. Now you only mention five conditions of having a surplus and five conditions of being insufficient，and how do they come about?"

Qibo said："They are all stemmed from the five viscera. The heart controls the spirit，the lung controls the energy，the liver controls the blood，the spleen controls the muscle，and the kidney controls the will，with these functions，the five viscera are formed. when the spirit and will are unimpeded，the bone marrows inside are mutual connecting and the whole body is formed. The communication between the five viscera depends on the channel tunnel which enables the circulation of the energy and blood. If the energy and blood are not in harmony，various diseases will occur. Thus，the channel tunnel must be unimpeded."

帝曰：神有余不足何如？岐伯曰：神有余则笑不休，神不足则悲，血气未并，五藏安定，

邪客於形，洒淅起於毫毛，未入於经络也，故命曰神之微。帝曰：补写奈何？岐伯曰：神有余，则写其小络之血〔守校本“血”作脉〕，出血勿之深斥，无中其大经，神气乃平。神不足者，视其虚络，按〔《甲乙》《太素》“按”本作“切”〕而致之，刺而利〔《甲乙》“利”作“和”〕之，无出其血，无泄其气，以通其经，神气乃平。帝曰：刺微奈何？岐伯曰：按摩勿释，著针勿斥，移气于不足〔林校云：“按《甲乙》及《太素》作‘移气于足’，无‘不’字”〕，神气乃得复。

Yellow Emperor asked："What will happen when the spirit is having a surplus or being insufficient?" Qibo sad："When there is a surplus in the spirit，one will laugh at the top of his voice continuously，when the spirit is insufficient，one will be melancholic. If the evil-energy has not yet mingled with the blood and energy，the five viscera can remain their stablity. By this time，the evil-energy retains shallowly in the body，the cold-evil is only on the skin and the soft hair instead of reaching the channel and it is called the slight disease of the spirit."

Yellow Emperor asked："How to apply invigoration and purge in treating?" Qibo said："When one's spirit is having a surplus，prick the small collateral until bleeding to purge but must not insert the needle deeply to hurt the large channel in this way，the spirit can be adjusted to become normal. When the spirit is insufficient，the invigorating therapy should be applied. Seek along the asthenic collateral to reach the focus and prick with needle，guard against bleeding nor the letting out of the energy，when the channel and collaterals are dredged，the spirit will be a ajusted to become normal."

Yellow Emperor asked："How to treat the slight disease of the spirit with pricking?" Qibo said："Do not lift up the hand when massaging，the insertion of needle must not be deep，when the energy and blood are led to the location which is insufficient and becomes substantial，the spirit will be recovered."

帝曰：善！有余〔《太素》“有余”上并有“气”字〕不足奈何？岐伯曰：气有余则喘咳上气，不足则息〔“息”下脱“不”字〕利少气。血气未并，五藏安定皮肤微病，命曰白气微泄。帝曰：补写奈何？岐伯曰：气有余，则写其经隧，无伤其经，无出其血，无泄其气；不足，则补其经隧，无出其气。帝曰：刺微奈何？岐伯曰：按摩勿释，出针视之，曰我〔《甲乙》“我”作“故”〕将深之，适人〔《太系》萧校引《甲乙》“人”作“入”〕必革，精气自伏，邪气散乱，无所休〔《太素》“休”作“优”〕息，气泄腠理，真气乃相得。

Yellow Emperor said："Good，What will happen when the energy is having a surplus or being insufficient?" Qibo said："When the energy is having a surplus，rapid breathing，cough and up-reversing of the energy of the patient will occur；when the energy is insufficient，difficult respiration and short of breath will occur. If the evil-energy has not yet mingled with the energy and blood，the five viscera can remain its stability. By this time，the evil-energy can only invade the skin and injure the lung-energy slightly and the disease is called the slight discharge of the white-energy. The lung-energy is also called the white-energy as the colour of metal is white."

Yellow Emperor asked："How to treat the disease with invigoration and purgation?" Qibo

said: "When the energy is having a surplus, the channel should be purged by pricking, but it must not cause bleeding to excrete the energy, and the channel must not be injured. If the energy is insufficient, the channel should be invigorated, but the energy must not be discharged."

Yellow Emperor asked: "How to treat the slight disease of energy by pricking?" Qibo said: "When treating, massage the focus without loosening the hand, show the needle to the patient and tell him that you are going to prick deeply so as to cause the refined-energy of the patient to conceal inside, and change into shallow pricking when inserting, in this way, the evil-energy can not but disperse to outside as it can retain nowhere. When the evil-energy is excreted through the striae, the healthy-energy will be restored."

帝曰：善！血有余不足奈何？岐伯曰：血有余则怒，不足则恐〔《太素》"恐"作"悲"〕；血气未并，五藏安定，孙络水〔金本，赵本，明抄本"水"并作"外"〕溢，则经〔《甲乙》"经"作"络"〕有留血。帝曰：补写奈何？岐伯曰：血有余，则写其盛经出其血；不足，则视〔《太素》"视"作"补"〕其虚经内针其脉中，久留而视；脉大，疾出其针，无令血泄。帝曰：刺留血奈何？岐伯曰：视其血络，刺出其血，无令恶血得入于经，以成其疾。

Yellow Emperor said: "Good. What are the conditions when the blood is having a surplus and being insufficient?" Qibo said: "Liver controls the blood, when the blood is having a surplus, the liver-energy will be over-abundant, angry associates with the liver, when the liver-energy is over-abundant, one will apt to get angry. The liver and the gallbladder are connecting, when the blood in the liver is insufficient, the energy of gallbladder will become timid and cause the patient to have sorrow. If the evil-energy has not yet mingled with the energy and blood, the five viscera can remain the stability, but the over-abundant evil-energy in the minute collaterals may become overflowed and cause the retention of blood in the collaterals."

Yellow Emperor asked: "How to treat it with invigoration and purge?" Qibe said: "When the blood is having a surplus, purge the collateral which is filled with abundant evil-energy, and prick until bleeding. If the blood is insufficient, prick and invigorate the collateral of which the energy is insufficient. If the pulse of the patient is normal in magnitude, the period of the needle retention should be longer and should watch the eyes of the patient to inspect the response, if the pulse is full and gigantic, the needle should be pulled off instantly to avoid bleeding."

Yellow Emperor asked: "How to prick the collateral which is retained with blood?" Qibo said: "Prick the collateral in which there is the blood retention until bleeding, but take note of the malicious blood not to flow into the channel and cause other diseases."

帝曰"善！形有余不足奈何？岐伯曰：形有余则腹胀，泾溲不利，不足则四支不用。血气未并，五藏安定，肌肉蠕动，命曰微风。帝曰：补写奈何？岐伯曰：形有余则写其阳经，不足则补其阳络。帝曰：刺微奈何？岐伯曰：取分肉间，无中其经，无伤其络，卫气得复，邪气乃索。

Yellow Emperor said: "Good. What are the conditions when the shape is having a sur-

plus and being insufficient?" Qibo said: "When the shape (physique) is having a surplus, swelling of the abdomen and dysuria will occur. When the shape is insufficient, the limbs will not be nimble. If the evil-energy has not yet mingled with the energy and blood, the five viscera can remain the stability, as the wind-evil can only reach the muscle, there will be only the feeling of wriggling in the muscle. The disease is called the slight wind."

Yellow Emperor asked: "How to invigorate or purge when treating?" Qibo said: "Purge the energy of the Stomach channel of Foot Yangming when the shape is having a surplus, and invigorate the energy of Stomach collateral of Foot Yangming when the shape is insuficient."

Yellow Emperor asked: "How to prick the disease of slight wind?" Qibo said: "Prick the muscle under the skin to disperse the evil-energy, but the channel must not be pricked and the collateral must not be hurt. In this way, the Wei-energy can be recovered, and the evil-energy can be dissipated."

帝曰：善！志有余不足奈何？岐伯曰：志有余则腹胀飧泄，不足则厥，血气未并，五藏安定，骨节有动。帝曰：补写奈何？岐伯曰：志有余则写然筋〔林校云："详诸处引然各者多云'然骨之前血者'疑少"骨之"二字，'前'字误作'筋'字〕血者，不足则补其复溜。帝曰：刺未并奈何！岐伯曰：即取之，无中其经，邪所〔《甲乙》作"以去其邪"〕乃能立虚。

Yellow Emperor said: "Good. What are the conditions when the will is having a surplus and being insufficient?" Qibo said: "Will belongs to kidney, when the will is diseased by having a surplus, it is caused by the evil-energy which is having a surplus in the kidney. Kidney is a viscus of cold and water, when its evil-energy is having a surplus, the cold-energy will become over-abundant and causes distention of the abdomen and lienteric diarrhea. When the will is insufficient, it is due to the insufficiency of the primodial Yang energy in the kidney which will cause cold limbs. When the evil-energy has not yet mingled with the energy and blood, the five viscera can remain the stability, but there is the feeling of slight trembling in the bone joint as the kidney has been affected by the evil-energy and the bone associates with the kidney."

Yellow Emperor asked: "How to invigorate and purge when treating?" Qibo said: "When the will is having a surplus, prick the Rangu point (KI. 2) until bleeding to purge, when the will is insufficient, prick the Fuliu point (KI. 7) for invigoration."

Yellow Emperor asked: "How to prick when the evil-energy has not yet mingled with the energy and blood?" Qibo said: "Prick the trembling bone joint. Do not prick the channel but only prick the location where the evil-energy retains and the evil-energy can be eliminated right away."

帝曰：善！余已闻虚实之形，不知其何以生！岐伯曰：气血以〔赵本"以"作"已"〕并，阴阳相倾，气乱于卫，血逆于经，血气离居，一实一虚。血并于阴，气并于阳，故为惊狂；血并于阳，气并于阴，乃为炅中；血并于上，气并于下，心烦惋〔《甲乙》"惋"作"闷"〕善怒；血并于下，气并于上，乱〔《太素》"乱"上有"气"字〕而喜忘。帝曰：血并于阴，气并于阳，如〔《太素》"如"作"于"字〕是血气离居，何者为实？何者为虚？岐伯曰：血气

者，喜温而恶寒，寒则泣不能流，温则消而去之，是故气之所并为血虚，血之所并为气虚。

Yellow Emperor said: "Good. Now I have heard the various appearances of asthenia and sthenia, but I do not know how do they come about." Qibo said: "The asthenia and sthenia are caused by the imbalance of the Yin and Yang due to the mingling of the evil-energy with the energy and blood. When the evil-energy runs wild to disturb the Wei-energy, and the blood runs reversely along the channels and collaterals, they all leave their proper positions, and the conditions of being asthenic and sthenic will occur. If the blood mingles with the Yin-evil, and the energy mingles with the Yang-evil, the syndrome of terror and mania will occur. If the blood mingles with the Yang-evil, and the energy mingles with the Yin evil, the syndrome of internal heat will occur. If the blood mingles with the evil-energy in the upper part of the body, and the energy mingles with the evil-energy in the lower part of the body, it will cause one to become irritable, distressed and apt to get angry. If the blood mingles with the evil energy in the lower part of the body, and the energy mingles with the evil-energy in the upper part of the body, it will cause one to have disorder of the vital energy and amnesia."

Yellow Emperor asked: "When the blood mingles with the Yin-evil, and the energy mingles with the Yang-energy, they all leave their proper positions, how can we know whether it is asthenic or sthenic?" Qibo said: "Both the energy and blood are fond of warmness and detest coldness, the coldness can cause the energy and blood to become stagnated and impeded, while the warmness can cause the energy and blood to circulate more easily. Thus, when the energy is partialy over-abundant, the blood will be asthenic, when the blood is partialy over-abundant, the energy will be asthenic."

帝曰：人之所有者、血与气耳。今夫子乃言〔四库本"言"作"曰"〕血并为虚，气并为虚，是无实乎？岐伯曰：有者为实，无者为虚，故气并则无血，血并则无气，今血与气相失，故为虚焉。络之与孙脉〔明抄本"孙脉"作"孙络"〕俱输〔《甲乙》"输"作"注"〕于经，血与气并，则为实焉。血之与气并走于上，则为大厥，厥则暴死，气〔《太素》"复反"上无"气"字〕复反则生，不反则死。

Yellow Emperor said: "The energy and blood are most important in human body, now you have said that both the partial over-abundance of blood and the partial over-abundance of energy are the conditions of being asthenic, then is there any condition of being sthenic?" Qibo said: "When there is a surplus, it is sthenia, when there is an insufficiency, it is asthenia, thus, when the energy combines with the Yang, the blood will be insufficient, when the blood combines with Yin, the energy will be insufficient, since both the energy and blood have left their proper positions and are out of balance, they are in the condition of asthenia. Both the energy and blood in the collaterals and minute collaterals are flowing to the channels, if the energy and blood mingle in the collateral, it will become sthenic. If the energy and blood mingle and ascend along the channels and collaterals to his head, coma will occur, and coma can cause one to die suddenly. If one's blood can descend and return again, his head will be relieved, and the patient may come to life again, if it fails to return, he will

die."

帝曰：实者何道从来？虚者何道从去？虚实之要，愿闻其故。岐伯曰：夫阴与阳，皆有俞会，阳注于阴，阴满之外，阴阳匀平，以充其形，九候若一，命曰平人。夫邪之生〔《甲乙》"之"下有"所"字〕也，或生于阴，或生于阳，其生于阳者，得之风雨寒暑〔"暑"字误应作"湿"〕；其生于阴者，得之饮食居处〔《太素》《甲乙》"居处"作"起居"〕，阴阳喜怒。

Yellow Emperor asked: "Where does the sthenic-evil come from and where does the asthenic-evil go to, and what are the essentials of asthenia and sthenia?" Qibo said: "Both the Yin channels and the Yang channels are having the shu-points for infusing and joining each other. When the energy and blood of the Yang channel is transfused into the Yin channel, the energy and blood in the Yin channel will be filled up and flow to else-where of the body, in this way, the Yin and Yang can be kept in balance and permeating the body so as the pulse conditions of the nine sub-parts may be identical and normal. Some of the infections caused by the evil-energy are from the internal injuries of Yin and some are from the external cause of Yan. The infections from Yang are due to the invasion of wind, rain, cold and wetness, and those from Yin are due to the intemperance of taking food and drink, abnormal daily life, excessive sexual activities and moodiness."

帝曰：风雨之伤人奈何？岐伯曰：风雨之伤人也，先客于皮肤，传入于孙脉，孙脉满则传入于络脉，络脉满则输于大〔《甲乙》"则输"作"乃注"，孙鼎宜说："'大'字疑衍"〕经脉，血气与邪并客于分腠之间，其脉坚大，故曰实。实者外坚充满，不可按之〔《甲乙》"按"下并无"之"〕，按之则痛。帝曰：寒湿之伤人奈何？岐伯曰：寒湿之中人也，皮肤不〔《太素》《甲乙》"肤"下并无"不"字〕收，肌肉坚紧〔《太素》"坚"下无"紧"字〕，荣血泣，卫气去，故曰虚。虚者聂〔《太素》"聂"作"慑"〕辟，气不足〔《太素》《甲乙》"不足"下并有"血泣"二字〕，按之则气足以温之，故快然而不痛。

Yellow Emperor asked: "What are the conditions when people is injured by the wind and rain?" Qibo said: "When the wind and rain hurt the body, it invades into the skin first, then enters into the minute collateral, when the minute collateral is filled, the evil-energy will be transmitted into the collateral, when the collateral is filled, it will be transmitted into the channel, when the evil-energy mingles with the energy and blood and invades the location between the muscle and striae under the skin, the gigantic pulse condition will occur, and it is the syndrome of sthenia. In sthenic syndrome, it seems firm and substantial in the exterior, but the skin and muscle can not tolerate touching and pressing which will cause pain."

Yellow Emperor asked: "What are the conditions when the cold-wetness injures the people?" Qibo said: "When the cold-wetness injures the people, it will cause sudden shrink of the skin, hardness of the muscle, stagnation of the Ying-blood and exhaustion of the wei-energy, and it is the syndrome of asthenia. The patient with asthenic syndrome is often nervous and short of breath, but when being pressed and massaged with hands, the flow of blood will become fluent, the breath will become sufficient, and the patient will feel warm comfortable and painless."

帝曰：善！阴之生实奈何？岐伯曰：喜怒不节，则阴气上逆，上逆则下虚，下虚则阳气走之，故曰实矣。帝曰：阴之生虚奈何？岐伯曰：喜〔“喜”字误，似应作“恐”，《举痛论》“恐则气下”〕则气下，悲则气消，消则脉虚空〔《太素》“虚”下无“空”字〕，因寒饮食，寒气熏满〔《甲乙》作“动藏”〕，则血泣气去，故曰虚矣。

Yellow Emperor said: “Good. What are the conditions of the sthenic syndrome stem from Yin?” Qibo said: “When one is often getting angry without temperance, the Yin energy will reverse upward, which will cause the deficiency of the Yin energy in the lower part, and the Yang energy will take the place, so it is the sthenic syndrome.”

帝曰：经言阳虚则外寒，阴虚则内热，阳盛则外热、阴盛则内寒，余已闻之矣，不知其所由然也。岐伯曰：阳受气于上焦，以温皮肤分肉之间，令〔全本、读本、赵本，“令”并作“今”，《太素》《甲乙》“不通”上并不叠“上焦”二字〕寒气在外，则上焦不通，上焦不通，则寒气〔《太素》《甲乙》“寒”下并无“气”字〕独留于外，故寒慄。帝曰：阴虚生内热奈何？岐伯曰：有所劳倦，形气衰少，谷气不盛，上焦不行，下脘（《甲乙》“下焦”）不通，胃气热、热气〔《甲乙》《病沅》并无“热气”二字〕熏胸中，故内热。帝曰：阳盛生外热奈何？岐伯曰：上焦不通利，则皮肤致密，腠理闭塞，玄府不通〔《太素》《甲乙》并无“玄府”二字〕，卫气不得泄越，故外热。帝曰：阴盛生内寒奈何？岐伯曰：厥气上逆、寒气积于胸中而不写，不写则温气去，寒独留，则血凝泣，凝则脉不通，其脉盛大以濇，故中寒〔“中寒”据杨注应作“寒中”〕。

Yellow Emperor said: “It was said in the ancient classics: ‘When Yang is deficient, external cold will produce; when Yin is deficient, internal heat will produce: when the Yang is overabundant, external heat will produce, when Yin is overabundant, internal cold will produce’. I have heard about the saying, but I do not know its reason.” Qibo said: “All Yangs receive the energy from the upper warmer, they are for warming the location between the skin and the muscle. Now, as the cold energy invades from outside, the energy of the upper warmer can not reach the location between the skin and muscle, as the cold remains on the surface alone, the syndrome of shivering with cold will occur.”

Yellow Emperor asked: “What is the condition when the asthenic Yin produces the internal heat?” Qibo said: “When one is fatigue excessively, his strength in the body will become insufficient. As a result, the upper warmer will not be able to channel out the tastes of the five cereals, the lower part of the gastric cavity will not be able to transform the cereals into essence, and the stagnated stomach energy will produce heat to fumigate the chest. This is the condition when the asthenic Yin produces the internal heat.”

Yellow Emperor asked: “What is the condition when the over-abundant Yang produces the external heat?” Qibo said: when the upper warmer is ineffective, the skin will become tight and the striae impeded, causing the Wei-energy can not be excreted outside and the external heat will occur.”

Yellow Emperor asked: “What is the condition when the over-abundant Yin produces the internal cold?” Qibo said: “As the energy of Jueni (coldness of limbs) is up-reversing, the cold-energy accumulated in the chest and can not be excreted downward, it will cause the

Yang-energy to disperse and leave the cold-energy in the chest alone. As a result, the blood will be stagnated, the channel will be impeded, and the pulse condition will be gigantic and choppy to become the syndrome of the middle warmer."

帝曰：阴与阳并〔《太素》作“阴之与阳”〕，血气以并，病形以成，刺之奈何？岐伯曰：刺此者，取之经隧，取血于营，取气于卫，用形哉，因四时多少高下。帝曰：血气以并，病形以成，阴阳相倾，补写奈何？岐伯曰：写实者气盛乃内针，针与气俱内〔《素问校伪》引古抄本“俱”下无“内”字〕，以开其门，如利其户；针与气俱出，精气不伤，邪气乃下，外门不闭，以出其疾；摇大其道，如利其路，是谓大写，必切而出，大气乃屈。帝曰：补虚奈何？岐伯曰；持针勿置，以定其意，候呼内针，气出针入，针空四塞，精无从去，方实而疾出针，气入针出，热不得还，闭塞其门，邪气布散，精气乃得存，动气候时〔《太素》作“动勿候时”，谓及时入针出针〕，近气不失，远气乃来，是谓追之。

Yellow Emperor asked: "When Yin mingles with Yang, and at the same time mingles with the energy and blood to cause disease, how to treat it by pricking?" Qibo said: "When treating, prick the channel and also prick the Ying-blood inside of the channel and the Wei-energy outside of the channel, at the same time, inspect the tall or short, fat or thin type of build of the patient, and refer to the different weather of the season to determine the times of pricking and the upper or lower pricking position of the body."

Yellow Emperor asked: "When the evil-energy has mingled with the energy and blood, and the Yin and Yang become imbalanced, how to apply the therapy of invigoration and purgation?"Qibo said:"The way of purging the sthenia is to insert the needle when the evil-energy is over-abundant, and cause both the needle and the energy enter into the body together so as to open the gate for discharging the evil-energy. When pulling the needle, cause the needle and the energy to come out together, and keep the refined energy uninjured, in this way the evil-energy will be extinguished. The needle hole must not be closed but should sway the needle heavily to enlarge the exit and cause the evil-energy to come out thoroughly, and it is called the therapy of great purgation. When pulling the needle, it should be swift so as the evil energy can be quitted."

Yellow Emperor asked:"How to invigorate the syndrome of asthenia?"Qibo said:"Keep a calm mood before pricking, prick when the patient exhales and insert the needle when the inhalation ends. In this way, it will be tight around the needle hole and the refined-energy will not be excreted. Pull the needle swiftly when the energy is in the state of sthenic to let in the energy. In this way, the heat under the needle will not come out along with the needle, its exit of dispersing will be blocked. Thus, the evil-energy will soon be dispersed, and the refined energy will be retained. In a word, in pricking both the insertion and the pulling of the needle should lose no opportunity so as that the energy obtained may not be missing through the needle, and the energy which has not yet come can be induced. This is called the therapy of invigortion."

帝曰：夫子言虚实者有十，生于五藏，五藏〔《甲乙》“五藏”上不叠“五藏”二字〕五脉耳，夫十二经脉皆生其〔《太素》《甲乙》“其病”上并有“视”字〕病，今夫子独言五藏，

夫十二经脉者，皆络三百六十五节，节有病必被经脉，经脉之病，皆有虚实，何以合之？岐伯曰：五藏者，故得六府与为表里，经络支节，各生虚实，其病所居，随而调之。病在脉、调之血；病在血、调之络；病在气，调之卫；病在肉，调之分肉；病在筋，调之筋；病在骨，调之骨〔《太素》无“病在”六字〕；燔针劫刺其下及与急者；病在骨，焠〔《太素》“焠”作“卒”〕针药熨；病不知所痛，两跻为上；身形有痛，九候莫病，则缪刺之；痛在于左而右脉病者，巨刺之。必谨察其九候，针道备〔《甲乙》作“毕”〕矣。

Yellow Emperor said: "You have said the ten kinds of asthenia and sthenia are produced from the five channels of the five viscera, but in fact, the twelve channels in the body can all contract diseases; you have mentioned the five viscera only, but the twelve channels are connecting the three hundred and fifty five acupoints, when the acupoint contracts disease, it will affect the channel, and the diseases of the channel are of sthenic and asthenis, and how do they correspond to the asthenia and sthenia of the five viscera?" Qibo said: "The five solid organs and the six hollow organs are related and they are the superficies and interior. All the diseases in the channels collaterals and their related points are having the conditions of asthenia and sthenia, and they should be adjusted according to the location of the focus by inspecting.

"If the disease is in the channel, adjust the blood; if the disease is in the blood, adjust the collateral; if the disease is in the energy, adjust the Wei-energy; if the disease is in the muscle, adjust the muscle under the skin; if the disease is in the tendon, adjust the tendon and prick the focus of the disease and the location of contracture with the heated needle, if the disease is in the bone, prick deeply and then warm the focus with medicine after pulling the needle. If the patient is unaware of his pain, prick the Yangqiao and the Yinqiao channels; if the patient is feeling pain and the pulse conditions of the nine sub-parts are normal, apply the contralateral collateral pricking therapy (prick the right side when the pain is in the left and vice versa); if the pain is on the left side and the diseased pulse is on the right side, apply the contralateral channel pricking therapy. In a word, inspect the pulse condition of the nine sub-parts of the pulse carefully before pricking so as a complete way of pricking may be engaged."

缪刺论篇第六十三

Chapter 63
Miu Ci Lun
(On Contralateral Pricking)

黄帝问曰：余闻缪刺，未得其意，何谓缪刺？岐伯对曰：夫邪之客于形也，必先舍于皮毛，留而不去，入舍于孙脉〔明抄本“脉”作“络”〕，留而不去，入舍于络脉，留而不去入舍于经脉，内连五藏，散于肠胃，阴阳俱感〔《太素》“俱感”作“更盛”〕，五藏乃伤，此邪之从皮毛而入，极于五藏之次也，如此则治其经焉。今邪客于皮毛，入舍于孙络，留而不去，闭塞不通、不得入于经，流溢〔《甲乙》《外台》“溢”上并无“流”字〕于大络，而生奇病也。夫邪客大络者，左注右，右注左，上下左右〔《太素》“上下”下无“左右”二字〕，与经相干，而布于四末。其气无常处，不入于经俞，命曰缪刺。

Yellow Emperor asked："I am told there is a kind of contralateral pricking，but I do not know its meaning，after all，what is the contralateral pricking？"

Oibo answered："When the evil-energy invades the body，it begins on the skin and soft hair，if it retains there and not leaving，it will enter into the collateral；if it retains again，it will enter into the channel to join the five viscera and then disperses to the intestine and the stomach. In this way，the Yin and Yang will become even more overabundant alternately and the five viscera will be injured. This is the sequence of the evil-energy transmission from the skin and soft hair to the viscera. Therefore，when treating. it should prick the channel with the ordinary pricking. If the evil-energy invades the skin and the soft hair and then retains in the minute collateral，but can not reach the channel due to the impediment of the collateral branch of the channel，it will flow into the large collateral，and the infection will appear on one side，ie.，the disease on the left side appears on the right side and vice versa. When the evil-energy enters into the large collateral，it flows from left to right and then from right to left，up and down along the large collateral which joins the channel and spreads to the four extremities. As the evil-energy runs in all directions not staying in a proper place，nor flowing into the shu-points in the channel，thus，the contralateral pricking is necessary."

帝曰：愿闻缪刺以左取右以右取左奈何〔《甲乙》无此二字〕？其与巨刺何以别之？岐伯曰：邪客于经，左盛则右病，右盛则左病，亦有移易者，左痛未已而右脉先病，如此者，必巨刺之，必中其经，非络脉也。故络病者，其痛与经脉缪处，故命日缪刺。

Yellow Emperor said："I like to hear the reason of when the disease is on the left side，prick the right side，and when the disease is on the right side，prick the left side in contralateral pricking，and how is it distinguished from the opposing needling？" Qibo said："As the

evil-energy of the left side and the right side are connecting, so, when the channel is invaded by the evil-energy, if the evil-energy is over-abundant on the left side, it often causes the disease on the right side, if the evil-energy is over-abundant on the right side, it often causes the disease on the left side. But sometimes, the condition is different: when the pain of the left side has not yet recovered, the vessels on the right side begin to contract disease. In this case, the evil-energy is not in the collateral, but in the channel. So, the opposing needling which will be reaching the channel should be applied. If the evil-energy is in the collateral of which the depth of the pain is different from that of the channel, the contralateral pricking should be applied."

帝曰：愿闻缪刺奈何？取之何如？岐伯曰：邪客于足少阴之络，令人卒心痛，暴胀，胸胁支满，无积者，刺然骨之前出血，如食顷而已。不已〔《甲乙》《太素》并无此二字〕，左取右，右取左。病新发者，取五日〔《太素》《甲乙》"五日"上并无"取"字，按"取"误应作"刺"〕，已。

Yellow emperor said: "I like to know what is contralateral pricking and how to apply it?" Qibo said: "when the evil energy invades the collateral of Foot Shaoyin, it will cause one to have heartache, distention of abdomen and fullness of the chest and hypochondrium suddenly. If the patient has no abdominal mass, prick the Rangu point (KI. 2) until bleeding, and the disease will be recovered in the period of a meal. Prick the left side when the disease is on the right side, and prick the right side when the disease is on the left side. If the disease is the case of recurrence, it can only be recovered five days after the pricking.

邪客于手少阳之络，令人喉痹舌卷，口干心烦，臂外〔《太素》"外"作"内"〕廉痛，手不及头，刺手中指〔《太素》作小指〕次指爪甲上，去端如韭叶各一痏，壮者立已，老者有顷已，左取右，右取左。此新病数日已。

"When the evil-energy invades the collateral branch of the Hand Shaoyang Channel, the syndromes of sorethroat, curled tongue, dryness of the mouth, feeling disquieted, and pain in the outer flank of the arm so as unable to lift it up to the head will occur. When treating prick the Guanchong point (SJ. 1) which is in the distance of the Chinese chive leaves beside the nail on the tip of the finger next to the small finger, prick once each on the left and right side.

For a man who is in his prime of life, the disease will be recovered immediately, for an old man, the disease will be recovered after a short time. Prick the right side when the disease is on the left side, and prick the left side when the disease is on the right side. If the disease is newly contracted, it will be recovered a few days after the pricking.

邪客于足厥阴之络，令人卒疝暴痛，刺足大指爪甲上，与肉交者各一痏，男子立已，女子有顷已，左取右，右取左。

"When the evil-energy invades the collateral branch of the Foot Jueyin Channel, it will cause one to have hernia with sudden pain, prick the Dadun point (LR. 1) which is on the connection of the nail and the skin on the toe once on each of the left and right side. For a man, the disease will be recovered immediately, for a woman, it will be recovered after a

while. Prick the right side when the disease is on the left side, and prick the left side when the disease is on the right side.

邪客于足太阳之络，令人头项〔《太素》《甲乙》“项”下并有“痛”字〕肩痛，刺足小指爪甲上，与肉交者各一痏，立已，不已，刺外踝下三痏，左取右，右取左，如食顷已〔《太素》无“如食”四字〕。

"When the evil-energy invades the collateral branch of the Foot Taiyang Channel it will cause one to have headache and pain on the neck and shoulder. When treating, prick the Zhiyin point (BL. 67) which is on the connection between the nail and the muscle above the tip of the little toe. Prick once on each of the left and right side, and the disease will be recovered immediately. If it is not recovered, prick the Jinmen point (BL. 63) below the outer ankle for three times. If the disease is on the left side, prick the right side, if the disease is on the right side, prick the left side.

邪客于手阳明之络，令人气满胸中，喘息〔《甲乙》“息”作“急”〕而支胠，胸中热，刺手大指、次指爪甲上，去端如韭叶，各一痏，左取右，右取左，如食顷已。

"When the evil-energy invades the collateral branch of the Hand Yangming Channel, it will cause one to have distention of vital energy in the chest, rapid breathing and heat in the chest. When treating, prick the Shangyang point (LI. 1) which is in the distance of the Chinese chive leaf width beside the tip of the nail of the forefinger next to the thumb. Prick once each on the left and right side. Prick the right side when the disease is on the left side, and prick the left side when the disease is on the right side. The disease will be recovered in the period of a meal.

邪客于臂掌之间，不可〔《甲乙》“不”下无“可”字〕得屈，刺其踝后，先以指按之痛，乃刺之，以月死生为〔《明抄本“为”下有“痏”字〕数，月生一日一痏，二日二痏〔按“二痏”下脱“渐多之”三字，应据《刺腰痛篇》王注引补〕，十五日十五痏，十六日十四痏〔按“十四痏”下脱“渐少之”三字，应据《刺腰痛篇》王注引补〕。

"When the evil-energy invades the collateral of the palm and the joint of wrist fail to bend, the basic joint of the wrist should be pricked. Press the focus which is painful first and then insert the needle. The number of times of pricking should be determined by the wax and wane of the moon: when the moon is waxing, prick once on the first day of the lunar month, prick twice on the second day of the lunar month, and add one pricking day after day. When the moon is waning in the second half of the month, prick fifteen times on the fifteenth day of the lunar month, prick fourteen times on the sixteenth day of the lunar month, and minus one pricking day after day.

邪气客于足〔《太素·量缪刺篇》“于”下无“足”字〕阳跻之脉，令人目痛从内眦始，刺外踝之下半寸所各二痏，左刺右，右刺左，如行十里顷而已。

"When the evil-energy invades the Yangqiao Channel, it will cause pain starting from the inner canthus. When treating, prick twice the Shenmai point (BL. 62) which is half inch below the outer ankle. Prick twice each on the left and right side. When the disease is on the left side, prick the right side, and when the disease is on the right side, prick the left side,

the disease will be recovered in the period of a ten li walk (an hour).

人有所堕坠，恶血留内，腹中满〔《卫生宝鉴》"满"作"痛"〕胀，不得前后，先饮利药，此上伤厥阴之脉，下伤少阴之络，刺足内踝之下，然骨之前，血脉〔林校云："脉"疑是"络"字〕出血，刺足跗上动脉，不已，刺三毛上各一痏，见血立已，左刺右，右刺左。善悲惊〔《太素》"悲"下有"善"字〕不乐，刺如右方。

"When one is injured from tumbling and the stagnated blood retains in the body, it will cause abdominal pain, the retention of feces and dysuria. When treating, the medicine for dispersing the stagnation should be taken first. Since the Jueyin Channel on the upper part and the Shaoyin Collateral of the lower part have been hurt, it should prick the superficial venulus in front of the Rangu point (KI. 2) below the inner ankle until bleeding, and also prick the Chongyang point (ST. 42) on the artery of the dorsum. If the pricking is ineffective, prick the Dadun point (LR. 1) on the toe once each on the left and right side, the disease will be recovered immediately after bleeding. Prick the right side when the disease is on the left side, and prick the left side when the disease is on the right side. If the patient is apt to become melancholic, frightened and unhappy, the way of pricking should be the same as above.

邪客于手阳明之络，令人耳聋，时不闻音〔《太素》"闻"下无"音"字〕，刺手大指次指爪甲上去端如韭叶各一痏，立闻，不已，刺中指爪甲上与肉交者立闻，其不时闻者，不可刺也。耳中生风者，亦刺之如此数，左刺右，左刺左。

"When the evil-energy invades the collateral branch of the Hand Yangming Channel, it will cause one to become deaf and often can hear nothing. When treating, prick the Shaoshang point (LU. 11) which is on the tip of the thumb, and the Shangyang point (LI. 1) which is on the tip of the forefinger in a dislance of the chinese chive leaf width beside the nail. Prick once on each of them of the left and right side and the sense of hearing can be restored immediately. If the pricking is ineffective, prick the Zhongchong point (PC. 9) which is on the connection between the muscle and the nail of the middle finger, and the patient can hear immediately; if he still can not hear, it shows that the energy of the collateral has been severed and will be ineffective by pricking. When the patient has tinnitus as if hearing the sound of the wind, the method and the times of pricking should be the same as above. Prick the right side when the disease is on the left side, and prick the left side when the disease is on the right side.

凡痹往来行无常处者，在分肉间痛而刺之，以月死生为数，用针者〔《明抄本无"用针"十一字〕随气盛衰，以为痏数，针过其日〔《太素》"日"作"月"〕数则脱气，不及日数则气不写，左刺右，右刺左，病已止，不已，复刺之如法，月生一日一痏，二日二痏，渐多之；十五日十五痏，十六日十四痏，渐少之。

"To the patient with bi-syndrome, as the pain of the bi-syndrome has no definite location, it should prick the site where the muscle is painful, The times of pricking should be based on the date of wax and wane of the moon, if the times of pricking are less then it should be, the evil-energy will not be removed. If the disease is on the left side, prick the

right side, and if the disease is on the right side, prick the left side. When the disease is recovered, the pricking should be stopped. If the disease is not recovered, the same method above should be applied again. When the moon is waxing prick once on the first day of the lunar month, prick twice on the second day of the lunar month, and add one pricking day after day; when the moon is waning, prick fifteen times on the fifteenth day of the lunar month, prick fourteen times on the sixteenth day of the lunar month, and minus one pricking day after day.

邪客于足阳明之经〔《太素》、《甲乙》"经"并作"络"〕，令人鼽衄上齿寒，刺足中指次指〔《甲乙》、《太素》"中指"下并无"次指。二字〕爪甲上，与肉交者各一痏，左刺右，右刺左。

"When the evil-energy invades the collateral Foot Yangming Channel, it will cause one to have rhinorrhea, epistaxis and chillness of the upper teeth. If should prick the Lidui point (ST. 45) which is on the connection between the nail and the muscle of the middle toe once on each of the left and right side. Prick the right side when the disease is on the left side, and prick the left side when the disease is on the left side.

邪客于足少阳之络，令人胁痛不得息，咳而汗出，刺足小指次〔《甲乙》"小指"下无"次指"二字〕指爪甲上，与肉交者各一痏，不得息立已，汗出立止，咳者温衣饮食，一日已。左刺右，右刺左，病立已。不已，复刺如法。

"When the evil-energy invades the collateral branch of the Foot Shaoyang Channel, it will cause one to have syndromes of hypochondriac pain, difficult respiration, cough and sweating. When treating, prick the Qiaoyin point (GB. 44) which is on the connection between the skin and the nail on the tip of the fourth toe once on each of the left and right side. In this way, the difficult respiration will be relieved and the sweating will stop. If the patient coughs, take note to keep warm of the dress and the food, and it will be recovered in one day, Prick the right side when the disease is on the left side, and prick the left side when the disease is on the right side, the disease can be removed immediately. If it is not recovered, prick again according to the method above.

邪客于足少阴之络，令人嗌痛〔《甲乙》"嗌""咽"〕，不可内食，无故善怒，气上走贲〔四库本"贲"下无"上"字〕上，刺足下中央之脉，各三痏，凡六刺，立已，左刺右，右刺左。

"When the evil-energy invades the collateral branch of the Foot Shaoyin Channel, it will cause one to have the syndromes of pain in the pharynx, unable to eat, angry without cause and the up-reversing of vital energy against the diaphram. When treating prick the Yongquan point (KI. 1) on the sole, and prick three times each on the left and right side which amount to six times, and the disease will be recovered immediately. Prick the right side when the disease is on the left side and prick the left side when the disease is on the right side.

嗌中肿，不能内唾，时不能出唾者，刺然骨之前，出血立已，左刺右，右刺左。

"When the pharynx and larynx become swelling so as the patient is unable to swallow

the saliva, and the saliva in the mouth can not be spitted out, it should prick the Rangu point (KI. 2) in front of the navicular bone anterior to the medial malleolus until bleeding, and it will have curative effect immediately. Prick the right side when the disease is on the left side, and prick the left side when the disease in on the right side.

邪客于足太阴之络，令人腰痛，引少腹控胁，不可以仰息，刺腰尻之解，两胂之上，是腰俞〔《太素》无此三字〕，以月死生为痏数，发针立已，左刺右，右刺左。

"When the evil-energy invades the collateral branch of the Foot Taiyin channel, it will cause one to have lumbago which affects the lower part of the hypochondrium, and one can not breath with the chest sticking out. When treating, prick the Xialiao point (BL. 34) which is on the muscle beside the spine in the seam of bones between the loin and the buttock. The times of pricking are determined by the days of the waxing and waning of the moon. After pricking, it will be effective immediately. Prick the right side when the disease is on the left side, and prick the left side when the disease is on the right side.

邪客于足太阳之络，令人拘挛背急，引胁而痛，刺之从项始，数脊椎侠脊，疾按之应手如痛，刺之傍三痏，立已。

"When the evil-energy invades the collateral branch of the Foot Taiyang Channel, it will cause one to have contracture in the back which affects the hypochondrium to become painful. When treating, count the vertebra behind the neck and press along the sides of the spine where the patient is painful. Prick three times beside the spine and it will be effective.

邪客于足少阳之络，令人留于〔"留于"二字衍〕枢中痛，髀不可举，刺枢中以毫针，寒则久留针，以月死生为〔"为"下脱"痏"字，应据《太素》《甲乙》补〕数，立已。

"When the evil-energy invades the collateral branch of the Foot Shaoyang Channel, it will cause pain around the site of the Huantiao point causing the thigh fails to lift. When treating, prick the Huantiao point (GB. 30) with a fine needle, if the cold is severe, the needle retention should be longer. Determine the times of the pricking according to the date of waxing and waning of the moon, and the disease will be recovered immediately.

治诸经刺之，所过者不病，则缪刺之。

"In treating the diseases in various channels with pricking, when the location where the channel passes is not painful, it shows that the focus is on the collateral, and the contralateral pricking should be applied.

耳聋，刺手阳明，刺其通〔《甲乙》"通"作"过"〕脉出耳前者。

"When treating the syndrome of deafness, prick the Shangyang point (LI. 1) of the Hand Yangming Channel. If it is not effective, prick the Tinggong point (SI. 19) of the Hand Yangming Channel which leads to the front of the ear.

齿龋，刺手阳明〔《甲乙》"阳明"下有"立已"二字〕，不已，刺其脉入齿中〔金刻本，读本，赵本"中"下并有"者"字〕，立已。

"In treating the dental caries, prick the Shangyang point (LI. 1) of the Hand Yangming Channel, and it will be effective immediately. If it is ineffective, prick the channel between the teeth to let out the malicious blood, and it will be effective immediately.

邪客于五藏之间，其病也，脉引而痛，时来时止，视其病〔《太素》《甲乙》病下并有“脉”字〕，缪刺之于手足爪甲上，视其脉，出其血，间日一刺，一刺不已，五刺已。

“When the evil-energy invades into the five viscera, the pain of the channel and the collateral are affecting each other. Sometimes the pain stems from the collateral, sometimes, it terminates in the channel. The disease channel must be ascertained first, and then, prick until bleeding. Prick every other day. If the disease is not recovered after one pricking, it will be recovered after five continuous prickings.

缪传引上齿，齿唇寒痛〔《甲乙》“寒”下无“痛”字〕，视其手背脉〔按“脉血”疑作“血络”〕血者去之，足阳明〔“足阳明”上有“刺”字〕中指爪甲上一痏，手大指次指爪甲上各一痏，立已，左取右，右取左。

“When the Hand Yangming Channel is diseased and the evil-energy being transmitted erroneously to the upper teeth, which causes the pain of the teeth and the lips, inspect the back of the hand of the patient and seek the collateral with blood retention and prick until bleeding, then prick the Neiting point (ST. 44) of the Foot Yangming Channel above the nail of the middle finger and the Shangyang point (LI. 1) of the Hand Yangming channel above the nail of the forefinger. Prick each point once and the disease will be recovered immediately. Prick the right side when the disease is on the left side and prick the left side when the disease is on the right side.

邪客于手足少阴太阴足阳明之络，此五络，皆会于耳中，上络左角，五络俱竭，令人身脉皆动，而形无知也，其状若尸，或曰尸厥，刺其〔《甲乙》“络”下有“者”字〕足大指内侧爪甲上，去端如韭叶，后刺足心，后刺足中指〔“中指”应作“大指次指。〕爪甲上各一痏，后刺手大指内侧，去端如韭叶，后刺手心主〔《太素》无“后刺”五字〕，少阴锐骨之端各一痏，立已。不已，以竹管吹其两耳〔《甲乙》“耳”下有“中”字，按“两耳”下脱“立已不已”四字〕，鬄〔《甲乙》作“剔”，剔又同“剃”〕其左角之发方一寸，燔治，饮以美酒一杯，不能饮者灌之，立已。

“As the five channels of Hand Shaoyin, Foot Shaoyin, Hand Taiyin, Foot Taiyin and Foot Yangming are all assembling in the ear, and they ascend to surround the frontal angle above the left ear, if the channel-energy of all the five kinds of collateral are exhausted when the evil energy invades, it will cause one to lose consciousness, in spite of the operations of the channels in the whole body are normal, the patient will appear like a corpse, and it is called the syncope. When treating, prick the Yinbai point (SP. 1) which is in a distance of Chinese chive leaf width from the tip beside the nail of the inner flank of the toe, then prick the Yongquan point (KI. 1) on the sole, prick each of the Lidui point (ST. 45) on the second toe once, and then, prick each of the Shaoshang point (LU. 11) which is in the distance of a Chinese chive leaf width from the tip of the inner flank on the thumb, and the Shenmen point (HT. 7) of the Shaoyin Channel which is on the terminal of the sharp bone behind the palm once, and the disease will be recovered immediately. if the pricking is ineffective, blow the two ears of the patient with a bamboo tube and the disease can be recovered immediately. If the blowing is ineffective, shave one square inch of the hair on the left frontal angle of the

patient and burn it with fire, grind the residue into powder, mix with wine of good quality and drink. If the patient can not drink due to loss of consciousness, it should be poured into the patient's mouth, and the patient will be recovered immediately.

凡刺之数，先〔《太素》"先"上有"必"字〕视其经脉，切而从〔《甲乙》"从"作"循"〕之，审其虚实而调之，不调者，经刺之，有痛而经不病者缪刺之，因视其皮部有血络者尽取之，此缪刺之数也。

"Generally, in pricking, inspect the pulse condition of the patient first, touch and press his pulse carefully with the hand to know whether the disease is of sthenic or of asthenic, and adjust the energy and blood of the patient. If the condition is partially sthenic or partially asthenic, prick the channel with opposing needling. If the patient is painful but the channels are not affected, apply the contralateral pricking. Besides, the skin must be inspected, if there is superficial venules, the stagnated blood should be let out. This is the principle of the contralateral pricking."

四时刺逆从论篇第六十四

Chapter 64
Si Shi Ci Ni Cong Lun
(The Regular and Adverse Treatments of Acupuncture in the Four Seasons)

厥阴有余，病阴痹；不足，病生〔明抄本，明抄二“病”。下并无“生”字〕热痹；滑则病狐疝风；涩则病少腹积气。

When the energy of the Jueyin Channel is excessive, the yin-type bi-syndrome will occur; when it is insufficient, the heat-type arthralgia will occur; when the pulse condition is slippery, the inguinal hernia due to wind-evil will occur, when the pulse condition is choppy, it shows there is retention of energy in the lower abdomen.

少阴有余，病皮痹隐轸〔《永乐大典》卷一万三千八百七十七引“轸”作“疹”按“隐轸”即“瘾胗”〕；不足，病肺痹；滑则病肺风疝，涩则病积溲血。

When the energy of the Shaoyin Channel is excessive, skin itching and urticaria will occur; when it is insufficient, the lung-bi-syndrome will occur; when the pulse condition is slippery, lung hernia due to wind-evil will occur, when the pulse condition is choppy, abdominal mass and hematuria will occur.

太阴有余，病肉痹寒中；不足，病脾痹；滑则病脾风疝；涩则病积心腹时满。

When the energy of the Taiyin Channel is excessive, myalgia and cold in the middle warmer will occur; when it is insufficient, splenic bi-syndrome will occur; when the pulse condition is slippery, splenic hernia due to wind-evil will occur; when the pulse condition is choppy, abdominal mass and distention of the heart and abdomen will often occur.

阳明有余，病脉痹，身时热；不足，病心痹；滑则病心风疝；涩则病积时善惊。

When the energy of the Yangming Channel is excessive, the channel bi-syndrome will occur, and the patient will often have fever; when it is insufficient, the cardiac bi-syndrome will occur; when the pulse condition is slippery, heart-channel colic due to wind-evil will occur, when the pulse condition is choppy, the patient will have abdominal mass and panic.

太阳有余，病骨痹身重；不足病肾痹；滑则病肾风疝；涩则病积善时〔明抄二“积”下无“善时”三字〕巅疾。

When the energy of the Taiyang Channel is excessive, bone bi-syndrome will occur, and the patient will feel heavy of the body; when it is insufficient, kidney bi-syndrome will occur; when the pulse condition is slippery, kidney hernia due to wind-evil will occur, when the pulse condition is choppy, it shows the patient will have the abdominal mass or the disease on head often.

少阳有余，病筋痹胁满；不足病肝痹；滑则病肝风疝；濇则病积时筋急目痛。

When the energy of the Shaoyang Channel is excessive, tendinous bi-syndrome will occur, and the patient will feel fullness of the hypochondrium; when it is insufficient, hepatic bi-syndrome will occur: when the pulse condition is slippery, hepatic hernia due to cold-evil will occur, when the pulse condition is choppy, it shows abdominal mass, and the patient will have contracture of tendon and sore eyes.

是故春气在经脉，夏气在孙络，长夏气在肌肉，秋气在皮肤，冬气在骨髓中。帝曰：余愿闻其故。岐伯曰：春者、天气始开，地气始泄，冻解冰释，水行经通，故人气在脉。夏者、经满气溢、入〔“入字衍，应据姚止庵说删〕孙络受血，皮肤充实。长夏者、经络皆盛，内溢肌中。秋者、天气始收，腠理闭塞，皮肤引急。冬者盖藏，血气在中，内著骨髓，通于五藏。是故邪气者，常随四时之气血而入客也，至其变化不可为〔明抄二“为”作“以”〕度，然必从其经气，辟除其邪，除其邪〔明抄二无此三字〕，则乱气不生。

Thus in spring, the energy is in the channel; in summer, the energy is in the minute collateral; in long summer, the energy of wetness and earth is in the muscle; in autumn, the energy of dryness and metal is in the skin: in winter, the energy is in the bone marrow.

Yellow Emperor said: “ I like to hear the reason of why the spring energy is in the channel, the energy of summer is in the minute collateral, the energy of long summer is in the muscle, the energy of autumn is in the skin, and the energy of winter is in the bone marrow?” Qibo said: “ In spring, the Yang energy begins to rise, and the earth energy has just revealed, the frozen earth has thawed out, the ice has been melted, the water can flow in the river, and all things come to life again. Thus the energy of man which is corresponding with the spring energy is located in the channel. In summer, all things are growing, the energy in the channel is full and over-abundant, the minute collateral can be nourished fully by the blood, and the skin becomes ruddy and substantial. Thus the energy of man which is corresponding with the summer energy is located in the minute collateral. In long summer, both the channel and the collateral are prosperous and they can moist the muscle completely, as the long summer associates with the spleen ,and the spleen associates with the muscle so the energy of man which is corresponding to the long summer energy is located in the muscle. In autumn, the weather begings to restrain itself, the striae of human body becomes closed and the skin becomes shrinking in the wake of it, so, the energy of man which is corresponding to the autumn energy is located in the skin. In winter which is the season of shutting and hiding, the energy and blood store in the body, the refined energy is attaching the bone marrow and communicating with the five viscera, so, the energy of man which is corresponding to the winter energy is located in the bone marrow. Therefore, the evil-energy often invades into the body along with the various conditions of the energy and blood in different season, and its specific variations can hardly be inferred. But in treating, the evil-energy must be removed according to the different locations where the energy resided in various seasons. In this way, the disease may not occur. ”

帝曰：逆四时而生乱气奈何？岐伯曰：春刺络脉，血气外溢，令人少气；春刺肌肉，血

气环逆，令人上气；春刺筋骨，血气内著，令人腹胀。夏刺经脉，血气乃竭，令人解㑊〔《诊要经络论》林校引本句“㑊”作“堕”，“堕”系“惰”之借字，“解㑊”即“解隋”〕；夏刺肌肉，血气内却，令人善恐；夏刺筋骨，血气上逆，令人善怒。秋刺经脉，血气上逆，令人善忘；秋刺络脉，气不外行〔林校引全元起本作“气不卫外”〕，令人卧不欲动；秋刺筋骨，血气内散，令人寒慄。冬刺经脉，血气皆脱，令人目不明；冬刺络脉，内〔“内”是“血”之误字〕气外泄，留为大痹；冬刺肌肉，阳气竭绝，令人善忘〔林校引作“善渴”〕。凡此四时刺者，大逆之病〔林校引全元起本作“六经之病”〕，不可不从也，反之，则生乱气相淫病焉。故刺不知四时之经，病之所生，以从为逆，正气内乱，与精相薄。必审九候。正气不乱，精气不转。

Yellow Emperor said: "What is the conditon when the blood and energy become disorderly and when violating the law of the seasonal weather change in treating?" Qibo said: "The energy of spring is in the channel, if the collateral is pricked in spring, the blood and the energy will be overflowing outside to cause short of breath of the patient; if the muscle is pricked in spring, the blood and energy will circulate disorderly to cause rapid breathing of the patient; if the tendon and bone are pricked in spring, the blood and energy will be retained inside to cause abdominal distention of the patient. The energy of summer is in the minute collaterals. if the channel is pricked in summer, the blood and energy will be exhausted to cause fatigue of the patient; if the muscle is pricked in summer, the blood and energy will be shut inside, the Yang energy will be obstructed to cause one apt to become terrified; if the tendon and bone are pricked in summer, the blood and energy will be reversing up to cause one apt to get angry. The energy of autumn is in the skin, if the channel is pricked in autumn, the blood and energy will be reversing up causing one to have amnesia; if the collateral is pricked in autumm, the energy will become deficient and fail to guard outside, the patient will have lethargy and reluctant to move about; if the tendon and bone are pricked in autumm, the energy and blood will become disorderly inside to cause shivering with cold of the patient. The energy of winter is in the bone marrow, if the channel is pricked in winter, the patient will have blurred vision and prostration due to the debility of energy and blood; if the collateral is pricked in winter, the blood and energy will be excreted outside to cause the deficiency of visceral energy and the evil-energy stagnated in the five viscera; if the muscle is pricked in winter the Yang energy will be exhausted to cause thirsty of the patient. These various contraindications in pricking related to the four seasons must be followed when treating the diseases of all the six channels. If they are violated, the disorderly energy will produce, and the unchecked disorderly energy will cause the disease to turn to the worse. Thus, when one knows not the location of the channel energy of the four seasons and the condition of the disease's incidence, taking the agreeable condition as the adverse condition, it will cause the healthy energy to become confused inside, and the evil-energy to combat with the healthy energy. Therefore, in diagnosis, one must inspect the pulse condition of the three parts and the nine sub-parts of the pulse condition so that the healthy energy may not be confused, and the healthy energy may not combat with the evil-energy."

帝曰：善。刺五藏，中心一日死，其动为噫；中肝五日死，其动为语〔林校引《甲乙》"语"作"欠"〕；中肺三日死，其动为咳；中肾六日死，其动为嚏欠〔林校引《甲乙》无"欠"字〕；中脾十日死，其动为吞。刺伤人五藏必死，其动则依其藏之所变候知其死也。

Yellow Emperor said："Good. In pricking the five viscera，when the heart is hit，the patient will die in one day，its syndrome of the affection is eructation；when the liver is hit，the patient will die in five days，its syndrome of the affection is yawning；if the lung is hit，the patient will die in three days，its syndrome of the affecton is coughing；if the kidney is hit，the patient will die in six days，its syndrome of the affection is frequent sneezing；when the spleen is hit the patient will die in ten days，its syndrome of the affection is swallowing. In a word，when one of the five viscera is injured by pricking，the patieet will surely die. The syndrome of afection indicates which viscus is injured，and the date of the patient's death can be known also."

标本病传论篇第六十五

Chapter 65
Biao Ben Bing Chuan Lun
(The Branch and Root and the Transfering Sequence of the Disease)

黄帝问曰：病有标本，刺有逆从奈何？岐伯对曰：凡刺之方，必别阴阳，前后相应，逆从得施，标本相移，故曰：有其在标而求之于标，有其在本而求之于本，有其在本而求之于标，有其在标而求之于本，故治有取标而得者，有取本而得者，有逆取而得者，有从取而得者，故知逆与从，正行无问〔吴注本"问"作"间"〕，知标本者，万举万当，不知标本、是谓妄行。

Yellow Emperor asked: "In diseases, some belong to the branch and some belong to the root; in pricking, sometimes, the regular treating is applied, and sometimes, the adverse treating is applied, and what is the reason?"

Qibo said: " Generally, in pricking, one must distinguish whether the disease belongs to Yin or Yang, and integrate the early stage and the latter stage of the disease first, and then determine whether the agreeable or adverse treating should be applied, Thus, to some of the diseases of branch, their branches are treated, to some of the diseases of root, their roots are treated; to some of the diseases of root, its branches are treated and to some of the diseases of branch, their roots are treated. Among the treatings, some are effective when treating the branch, some are effective when treating the root; some are effective when applying the agreeable treating, and some are effective when applying the adverse treating. Therefore, when one knows the principle of the agreeable and adverse treating, he can set his mind at ease in treating without misgiving, when one knows the principle of treating the diseases of branch and root, he will be sure to succeed and can cure the patient repeatedly. If one knows not the principle of branch and root of the disease. he can only treat wantonly.

夫阴阳，逆从，标本之为道也，小而大，言一而知百病之害。少而多，浅而博，可以言一而知百也。以浅而知深，察近而知远，言标与本，易而勿及。

"The principle of Yin and Yang, regular and adverse treating, and branch and root of the disease enables one to understand whether the disease is slight or severe, causes one to know the harms of various diseases by commencing from a certain point, besides, it enables one to know more about the disease from knowing only a little, to inspect the disease in an extensive scope instead of from a limited scope, to comprehend various diseases by inferring one disease, from the grasping the superficial knowledge to the profound knowledge, and to know what is afar by inspecting the near. The principle of branch and root can be understood easily, but it is hard to be carried out.

治反为逆，治得为从。先病而后逆者治其本；先逆而后病者治其本；先寒而后生病者治其本；先病而后生寒者治其本；先热而后生病者治其本；先热而后生中满者治其标〔《灵枢·病本》“热”作“病”，滑寿说：“此句当作‘先病而后生热者治其标’”〕先病而后生寒者治其本；先病而后泄者治其本；先泄而后生他病者治其本；必且调之，乃治其他病；先病而后先中满〔金本，胡本，赵本吴本“先中满”并作“生中满”，明抄二“而后”下无“先”字〕者治其标；先中满而后烦心者治其本。人有客气，有同〔林校引全本“同”作“固”〕气。小大不利治其标；小大利治其本；病发而有余，本而标之，先治其本，后治其标；病发而不足，标而本之，先治其标，后治其本。谨察间甚，以意调之，间者并行，甚者独行。先小大不利而后生病者治其本〔明抄本，明抄二“先小大不利”十三字移上“小大利治其本”句下〕。

“When treating adversely, it is the reverse treating, when the treating is in an routine way, it is the agreeable treating.

When the disharmony of energy and blood is caused by a certain disease, the disease is the root, and the disease should be treated first; when the disease is caused by the disharmony of energy and blood, the disharmony of energy and blood is the root, and the energy and blood should be treated first.

“When the cold-evil is contracted first, and then other disease occurs, then the cold-evil is the root which should be treated first, when other disease is contracted first, and then the cold-evil occurs, then the other disease is the root which should be treated first.

“When the patient contracts heat-evil first, and then other disease occurs, then the heat-evil is the root which should be treated first; when the other disease is contracted first and then the heat-evil occurs, the branch which is the heat-evil should be treated first.

“When the patient contracts other disease first and then the diarrhea occurs, treat the root which is the other disease first; when the patient has diarrhea first and then other disease occurs, treat the root which is the diarrhea and adjust the stomach first, and then treat the other disease.

“When other disease is contracted first and then the abdominal flatulence occurs, the branch which is the abdominal flatulence should be treated first: when the abdominal flatulence is contracted first, and then the irritation of heart occurs, treat the root which is the abdominal flatulence first.

In the human body, there exists the evil-energy and the healthy energy.

“When other disease is contracted first and then the retention of feces and urine occur, the branch which is the retention of feces and urine should he treated first; if there is no retention of feces and dysuria, the root which is the disease contracted first should be treated first.

“When the disease is sthenic, it shows the evil-energy is having a surplus, the root which is the evil-energy should be treated first, and then adjust the healthy energy. when the disease is asthenic, it shows the healthy energy is insufficient, the branch which is the healthy energy should be supported first, and then treat the evil-energy.

Before treating, inspect carefully whether the disease is a slight one or a severe one, and

then adjust it accordingly. when the disease is a slight one. the therapy of supporting the healthy energy and the therapy of eliminating the evil energy can be carried on at the same time; when the disease is a severe one, treat first the branch or the root according to its specific condition. If the retension of feces and urine occurs first and then the other disease occurs, treat the retension of feces and urine which is the root first.

夫病传者〔沈祖 说“传“当作”转”〕，心病先心痛，一日而咳；三日胁支痛；五日闭塞不通，身痛体重；三日不已，死。冬夜半，夏日中。

“The transfering sequence of the disease is as following: when the heart disease is contracted, the patient will have heartache; in about one day, the disease will transfer to the lung, and cough will occur; on the third day, the disease will transfer to the liver, fullness and pain in the hypochondrium of the patient will occur; on the fifth day , the disease will transfer to the spleen, retention of feces and the pain and heaviness of the body will occur; if the disease lasts for another three days, the patient will die. In winter, he will die at midnight, in summer, he will die at noon.

肺病喘咳，三日而胁支满痛；一日身重体痛；五日而胀；十日不已，死。冬日入，夏日出。

“When the lung disorder is contracted, rapid breathing and cough of the patient will occur: in about three days, the disease will transfer to the liver and the fullness and pain in the hypochondrium will occur: in about one day, the disease will transfer to the spleen, and the feeling of heaviness and pain of the body will occur: on the fifth day, the disease will transfer to the kidney , and swelling of the body will occur; if the disease lasts for another ten days, the patient will die. In winter, he will die when the sun sets, in summer, he will die when the sun rises.

肝病头目眩，肋支满，三日体重身痛；五日而胀；三日腰脊少腹痛，胫酸；三日不已，死。冬日入〔林校引《甲乙〕作“日中”〕，夏早食。

“When the liver disorder is contracted, the patient will feel distention in the hypochondrium, in about three days, the disease will transfer to the spleen, and the patient will feel heavy and painful of the body; on the fifth day the disease will transfer to the stomach, and abdominal distention will occur; in another three days, the disease will transfer to the kidney, and pain of the spinal column and the lower abdomen, and the soreness of the legs will occur; if the disease lasts for another three days, the patient will die. In winter, he will die at noon, in summer, he will die at the breakfast time.

脾病身痛体重，一日而胀；二日少腹腰脊痛胫酸；三日背胆筋痛，小便闭；十日不已，死。冬人定，夏晏食。

“When the spleen disorder is contracted, the patient will feel pain and heaviness of the body; in about one day, the disease will transfer to the stomach and the distention of the stomach will occur; on the second day the disease will transfer to the kidney, and the pain of the spinal column and the lower abdomen and the soreness of the legs will occur; on the third day, the disease will transfer to the bladder, the pain of the tendon of the back bone and dy-

suria will occur; if the dsease lasts for another ten days, the patient will die. In winter, he will die at the hour when people rests (7:00—9:00pm), in summer, he will die at the supper time.

肾病少腹腰脊痛，胻酸，三日背胆筋痛，小便闭；三日腹胀；三日两胁支痛，三日不已、死。冬大晨，夏晏晡。

"When the kidney disorder is contracted, the patient will have pain in the lower abdomen, spinal column and the legs; on the third day, the disease will transfer to the bladder, and pain in the tendon of the back and dysuria will occur: in another three days, the disease will transfer to the small intestine, and the distention of the lower abdomen will occur; in another three days, the disease will transfer to the heart, and fullness and pain of the hypochondrium will occur; if the disease lasts for another three days, the patient will die. In winter, he will die at dawn, in summer, he will die at the supper time.

胃病胀满，五日少腹腰脊痛，胻酸；三日背胆筋痛，小便闭；五日身体重；六日不已，死。冬夜半后，夏日昳。

"When the stomach disorder is contracted, the patient will feel fullness and distention of the stomach: on the fifth day, the disease will transfer to the kidney, and the pain in the lower abdomen and the spinal column, and soreness of the legs will occur; in another three days, the disease will transfer to the bladder, and pain of the tendon of the back bone and dysuria will occur; in another five days, the disease will transfer to the spleen, and the patient will feel heavy of the body; if the disease lasts for another six days, the patient will die. In winter, he will die after midnight, in summer, he will die in the afternoon.

膀胱病小便闭，五日少腹胀，腰脊痛，胻酸；一日腹胀；一日身体痛；二日不已，死。冬鸡鸣，夏下晡。

"When the bladder disorder is contracted, the patient will have dysuria; on the fifth day, the disease will transfer to the kidney, distention of the lower abdomen and pain in the back bone and soreness of the legs will occur; in about one day, the disease will transfer to the small intestine, and abdominal distention will occur; in about one day, the disease will transfer to the heart, and the feeling of heaviness and pain of the body will occur; if the disease lasts for another two days, the patient will die. In winter, he will die after midnight, in summer, he will die in the afternoon.

诸病以次是〔金本"次"下无"是"字〕相传，如是者，皆有死期，不可刺，间一藏止〔林校引《甲乙》无"止"字〕，及至三四藏者，乃可刺也。

"If the disease transfers from viscus to viscus one by one in the above sequence, the patient will die on the estimated date stated above, and pricking must not be applied. If it transmits in every other viscus or in every three or four viscus, the pricking is permissible."

天元纪大论篇第六十六

Chapter 66
Tian Yuan Ji Da Lun
(The Yin and Yang of the Five Elements Motion and the Six Kinds of Weather as the Guiding Principles of the Universe)

黄帝问曰：天有五行，御五位，以生寒、暑、燥、湿、风。人有五藏，化五气，以生喜、怒、思、忧、恐。论言五行相袭而皆治之，终期之日，周而复始，余已知之矣，愿闻其与三阴三阳之候奈何合之？

Yellow Emperor asked: "The five elements of the nature associate with the five orientations of east, west, south, north and the centrality to produce the weathers of cold, heat, dryness, wetness and wind. The five viscera of man activate the vital energy to produce the five emotions of overjoy, anger, melancholy, anxiety and terror. In the chapter of the《Six Cycles of Sixty Days and the States of Viscera》states that the energy of the element's motion which dominates the days of the year one after another is in a definite sequence, it completes its cycle on the last day of the year and then begins to start again. I have known the contents, but I hope to know how the five elements motion coincide with the six energies, ie., the three energies of Yin and the three energies of Yang?"

鬼臾区稽首再拜对曰：昭乎哉问也。夫五运阴阳者，天地之道也，万物之纲纪，变化之父母，生杀之本始，神用之府也，可不通乎！故物生谓之化，物极谓之变，阴阳不测谓之神，神用无方谓之圣。夫变化之为用也，在天为玄，在人为道，在地为化，化生五味，道生智，玄生神。神在天为风，在地为木；在天为热，在地为火；在天为湿，在地为土；在天为燥，在地为金；在天为寒，在地为水。故在天为气，在地成形，形气相感而化生万物矣。然天地者，万物之上下也，左右者，阴阳之道路也，水火者，阴阳之徵兆也，金木者，生成之终始也。气有多少，形有盛衰，上下相召，而损益彰矣。

Gui Yuqu cupped his hands, bowed again and again and said: "What an explicit question you have asked. The Yin and Yang of the five elements motion is the law of the universe, the guiding principle of all things, the source of various variations, the base of growth and injury, and the supreme headquater of the spiritual activities, could it be said that it should not be understood thoroughly?

"The growth of all things is called the Transformation, when the growth developes into its extreme stage, it is called the change, when the change of Yin and Yang becomes unanticipated, it is called Divinity, when the property of the divinity is changing constantly, it is sacred. As to the functioning of the changeful divinity, in heaven, it is the universe which is profound and can hardly be inferred, in man, it is the penetrating principle, and on earth, it

is the growth and developement of all things. As the earth promotes growth and developement, it produces the five tastes for nourishing all things; when a man understands the penetrating principle, it produces the wisdom; when the heaven is elusive, it produces divinity.

"In the variation of the divinity, in heaven, it is wind, on earth, it is wood; in heaven it is heat, on earth it is fire; in heaven it is wetness, on earth it is earth; in heaven it is dryness, on earth it is metal; in heaven it is cold, on earth it is water. In a word, in heaven, they are the shapeless six kinds of weather, and on earth, they are the shaped five elements. when the elements and the weathers responding with each other, it causes the growth and developement of all things.

"Therefore, the heaven and earth are the limits for all things to rise and fall, the left and right are the routes for Yin and Yang to ascend and descend, the water and fire are the manifestations of Yin and Yang, and the spring and autumn are the beginning and the terminal of growth and harvesting. There is differential in plenty and few of the energy, and there is diversity in overabundance and deficiency of the five elements, when the shaped elements and the shapeless energies inspiring each other, the phenomenon of having a surplus and insufficiency will become apparent."

帝曰：愿闻五运之主时也何如？鬼臾区曰：五气运行，各终期日，非独主时也。帝曰：请闻〔守校本"闻"作"问"〕其所谓也。鬼臾区曰：臣积〔"积。疑作"稽"〕考《太始天元册》文曰：太虚廖廓，肇基化元，万物资始，五运终天，布气真灵，总统坤元，九星悬朗，七曜周旋，曰阴曰阳，曰柔曰刚，幽显既位，寒暑驰张，生生化化，品物咸章。臣斯十世，此之谓也。

Yellow Emperor said: " I hope to know how the five elements motion control the condition of the four seasons". Gui Yuqu said: " The five elements motion take turns to control the year's seasons and days, they are not controlling the four seasons merely."

Yellow Emperor said: " I hope you can tell me the reason about it." Gui Yuqu said: " I have read the ancient book of the《Primordial Universe》in which stated: 'The primordial energy in the spacious sky is the foundation of generation, and the growth and developement of all things depend on it. As the five elements motion are having their regular patterns, the four seasons of spring, summer, autumn and winter are formed. The refined energy of heaven and earth spreads extensively and controls all things in the universe, so, the nine stars illuminate above and the seven celestial bodies (sun, moon and the five planets) are revolving around, through which the distinction of Yin and Yang and the different properties of firmness and mildness can be distinguished. Due to the proper operation of Yin and Yang, the coming and going of the four seasons and the shifting of day and night, all things can grow and develope and become prosperous. This proposition has heen handed down in my family for ten generations."

帝曰：善。何谓气有多少，形有盛衰？鬼臾区曰：阴阳之气各有多少，故曰三阴三阳也。形有盛衰，谓五行之治，各有太过不及也。故其始也，有余而往，不足随之，不足而往，有余从之，知迎知随，气可与期。应天为天符，承岁为岁直，三合为治。

fire."

帝曰：其于三阴三阳，合之奈何？鬼臾区曰：子午之岁，上见少阴；丑未之岁，上见太阴；寅申之岁，上见少阳；卯酉之岁，上见阳明；辰戌之岁，上见太阳；巳亥之岁，上见厥阴，少阴所谓标也。厥阴所谓终也。厥阴之上，风气主之；少阴之上，热气主之；太阳之上，湿气主之；少阳之上，相火主之；阳明之上，燥气主之；太阳之上，寒气主之。所谓本也，是谓六元。

Yellow Emperor asked: "How do the five-element motions and the six kinds of weather integrate with the three Yins and the three Yangs?" Gui Yuqu said: "In both the Zi year and the Wu year, the Shaoyin controls the heaven; in both the Chou and Wei year, the Taiyin controls the heaven, in both the Yin and Shen year, the Shaoyang controls the heaven, in both the Mao year and the You year, the Yangming controls the heaven, in both the Chen year and the Xu year, the Taiyang controls the heaven ,in both the Si year and the Hai year, the Jueyin controls the heaven. In the sequence of the duodecimal cycle, the Yin and Yang begin from the Zi year and end in the Hai year. The Jueyin is dominated by the wind-energy, the Shaoyin is dominated by the heat-energy, the Taiyin is dominated by the wetness-energy, the Shaoyang is dominated by the prime minister fire energy, the Yangming is dominated by the dryness-energy, the Taiyang is dominated by the cold-energy. As the wind, heat, wetness, fire, dryness and cold are the proper energies of the three Yins and the three Yangs themselves, so they are called the Primordial Energy of Heaven."

帝曰：光乎哉道！明乎哉论，请著之玉版，藏之金匮，署曰《天元纪》。

Yellow Emperor said: "You have made a very explicit explanation. Please write it down in a jade tablet, I will keep it in a golden cabinet, and name it as the《Record of the Primordil Energy of Universe》."

of weather, on earth, there are five elements. The six kinds of weather which associate with heaven take six years to complete a cycle, and the five elements which associate with the earth take five years to complete a cycle. When the five elements' motion combine with the six kinds of weather, it is thirty years or an era which comprises seven hundred and twenty solar terms. After one thousand four hundred and fourty solar terms in a cycle of sixty years, all the cases of having a surplus or insufficiency can be revealed."

帝曰：夫子之言，上终天气，下毕地纪，可谓悉矣。余愿闻而藏之，上以治民，下以治身，使百姓昭著〔明抄本无"使百姓昭著，上下和亲，德泽下流，子孙无忧"十七字〕，上下和亲，德泽下流，子孙无忧，传之后世，无有终时，可得闻乎？鬼臾区曰：至数之机，迫迮以微，其来可见，其往可追，敬之者昌，慢之者亡。无道行私，必得天殃，谨奉天道，请言真要。

Yellow Emperor said: "You have explained the weather of heaven up above and the era on earth down below exhaustively. I will keep what you said in mind so as the distresses of the people can be removed and the health of myself can be maintained. I want to hand it down to the later generations perpetually, but can you tell me more about it?"

Gui Yuqu said: "The law of the five elements motion and the six kinds of weather combination is rather subtle, yet its future can be inspected and its past can be traced. when one pays good attention to the law of change, he can avoid diseases, when one neglects it, he will contract diseases or even die. When one violates the natural law and behaves in his own way, disaster will occur. so, one must be careful in adapting the natural law of the element's motion and the six kinds of weather. Now, let me tell you the true essential."

帝曰：善言始者，必会于终。善言近者，必知其远，是则至数极而道不惑，所谓明矣。愿夫子推而次之，令有条理，简而不匮，久而不绝，易用难忘，为之纲纪。至数之要，愿尽闻之。鬼臾区曰：昭乎哉问！明乎哉道！如鼓之应桴，响之应声也。臣闻之：甲己之岁，土运统之；乙庚之岁，金运统之；丙辛之岁，水运统之；丁壬之岁，木运统之，戊癸之岁，火运统之。

Yellow Emperor said: "when one is good in explaining the beginning, he must know well the result, when one is sagacious in commenting the simple, he must understand what is profound. It is only in this case can the principle of the five element motion and the six kinds of weather be made explicit without misgiving, I hope you can push ahead a further step to make its contents more systematic, concise yet not lacking, easy to be applied, easy to be remembered in outline, so that it may be handed down for a long time. I hope to know the principle about the five-element motions and the six kinds of weather thoroughly."

Gui Yuqu said: "what a brillant question you have asked. The principle of the five elements motion and the six kinds of weather is quite evident, it is as sure as the sound when the drumsticks hit the drum, and the echo of a sound. I was told that the entire years of Jia and Ji are dominated by the earth, the entire years of Yi and Geng are dominated by the metal, the entire years of Bing and Xin are dominated by the water, the entire years of Ding and Ren are dominated by the wood, and the entire years of Wu and Gui are dominated by the

called the Due Year, such as when the Wood motion encounters the Mao year; when the fire motion encounters the wu year; when the metal motion encounters the You year; when the water motion encounters the Zi year. when the element's motion, the controlling energy of heaven, and the duodecimal order of the year are all agreeing, it is called the tripple agreement of the year of heaven tally and convergence, in which its energy is not having a surplus or being insufficient."

帝曰：上下相召奈何？鬼臾区曰：寒暑燥湿风火，天之阴阳也，三阴三阳上奉之。木火土金水火，地之阴阳也，生长化收藏下应之。天以阳生阴长，地以阳杀阴藏。天有阴阳，地亦有阴阳。木火土金水火，地之阴阳也，生长化收藏。下应之。天以阳生阴长，地以阳杀阴藏。天有阴阳，地亦有阴阳，木火土金水火（《困学纪闻》卷九《天道》引无“木火土金水火，地之阴阳也，生长化收藏”十六字）地之阴阳也，生长化收藏。故阳中有阴，阴中有阳。所以欲知天地之阴阳者。应天之气，动而不息，故五岁而右迁，应地之气，静而守位，故六期而环会，动静相召，上下相临，阴阳相错，而变由生也。

Yellow Emperor asked: "What is the condition when the heaven and earth inspiring each other?" Gui Yuqu said: "The cold, heat, dryness, wetness, wind and fire are the Yin and Yang of heaven, and the three Ying and the three Yangs of a man correspond with them. The wood, monarch-fire, earth, metal, water and prime minister-fire are the Yin and Yang of earth and the generation, growth, developement, harvesting and storing are corresponding to them.

"In heaven, the Yang generates and the Yin promotes growing, on earth, the Yang restrains and the Yin stores.

"There are Yin and Yang in the six kinds of weather in heaven, and there are Yin and Yang in the five elements of earth. when the Yin and Yang of heaven and that of earth combine, it causes the natural changes of generation, growth, developement, harvesting and storing of all things. The heavenly energy will not be able to descend when there is no Yin, and the earthly energy will not be able to ascend when there is no Yang. Thus, there must be Yin in Yang, and there must be Yang in Yin. When one wants to know the Yin and Yang of heaven and earth, he must know their operations. The five-element motions of earth which correspond with the six kinds of weather in heaven are moving continuously, it moves rightward for five years to complete a cycle and then begins again; the six kinds of weather of heaven which correspond with the five-element motions on earth complete a cycle every six years. Under the interaction of heaven and earth, motion and motionless, up above and down below and the interlacement of Yin and Yang, changes will occur."

帝曰：上下周纪，其有数乎？鬼臾区曰：天以六为节，地以五为制，周天气者，六期为一备；终地纪者，五岁为一周。君火以明，相火以位〔明抄本无“君火”以下八字〕，五六相合，字七百二十气为一纪，凡三十岁；千四百四十气，凡六十岁而为一周，不及太过，斯皆见矣。

Yellow Emperor asked: "Is there any numerical limit in the operations of heaven and earth which goes round and begins again?" Gui Yuqu said: "In heaven, there are six kinds

Yellow Emperor said: " Good. But what is the meaning of there is differentia of plenty and few in energy, and there is diversity of overabundance and deficiency in the five elements?" Gui Yuqu said: " In the Yin and Yang erergies, there are the differentia of plenty and few, and hence there are the distinctions of three Yins and three Yangs. The Yin is divided into three Yins according to the more or less content of Yin in it: when the Yin is more, it is Taiyin, when it is less, it is Shaoyin, when it is even less, it is Jueyin (the first Yin is Jueyin, the second Yin is Shaoyin, the third Yin is Taiyin). The Yang is divided into three Yangs according to the more or less content of Yang in it: when the Yang is more, it is Taiyang, when it is less, it is Yangming, when it is even less, it is Shaoyang (the first Yang is Shaoyang, the second Yang is Yangming, the third Yang is Taiyang).

"The over abundance and deficieny of the five elements motion means their excessive or insufficient domination of the year. If an element's motion is excessive in dominating the year, then its domination next year will be insufficient such as when the domination of wood motion of the Ren year is excessive, then the domination of wood motion in Ding year (five years after Ren year) will be insufficient, when the domination of the fire motion in Wu year is excessive, then the domination of the fire motion in the Gui year (five years after Wu year) will be insufficient, when the domination of earth motion in the Jia year is excessive, then the domination of earth motion in Ji year (five years after Jia year) will be insufficient, when the domination of the metal motion in the Geng year is excessive, the domination of the metal motion in the Yi year (five years after Geng year) will be insufficient, when the domination of the water motion in the Bing year is excessive, then the domination of the water motion in the Xin year (five years after Bing year) will be insufficient. when the domination begins with a condition of having a surplus, the insufficient condition of domination will come in the wake of it; such as: when the Jia year of earth motion is excessive, the succeeding Yi year of metal motion will be insufficient; when the Zi year of Shaoyin is having a surplus, the succeeding Chou year of Taiyin will be insufficient. When the domination begins with a condition of insufficiency, the dominating condtition of having a surplus will come in the wake of it, such as: when the Yi year of metal motion is insufficient, the succeeding Bing year of water motion will have a surplus; when the Chou year of Taiyin is insufficient, the succeeding Yin year of Shaoyang will have a surplus.

"When one understands the principle of having a surplus and insufficiency, he will be able to know which year will be having a surplus and which year will be insufficient. When the element's motion corresponds and tallies with the controlling energy of heaven it is called the Heaven Tally, such as when the earth motion dominates the year and the controlling energy of heaven is Taiyin; When the fire dominatos the year, and the controlling energv of heaven is Shaoyang and Shaoyin; when the metal dominates the year, and the controlling energy of heaven is Yangming; when the wood dominates the year, and the controlling energy of heaven is Jueyin; when the water dominates the year, and the controlling energy of heaven is Taiyang. When the element's motion agrees with the duodecimal order of the year, it is

五运行大论篇第六十七

Chapter 67
Wu Yun Xing Da Lun
(On the Five Elements' Motion)

黄帝坐明堂，始正天纲，临观八极，考建五常，请天师而问之曰：论言天地之动静，神明为之纪；阴阳之升降，寒暑彰其兆。余闻五运之数于夫子，夫子之所言，正五气之各主岁尔，首甲定运，余因论之。鬼臾区曰：土主甲己、金主乙庚，水主丙辛，木主丁壬，火主戊癸。子午之上，少阴主之；丑未之上，太阴主之；寅申之上，少阳主之；卯酉之上，阳明主之；辰戌之上，太阳主之；巳亥之上，厥阴主之。不合阴阳，其故何也？

Sitting in the bright hall (the Policy Proclaiming Hall), Yellow Emperor began to check the stars in the zodiac of heaven and surveyed the terrain of the eight orientations on earth to study the reasons of the Yin and Yang variations of the five elements' motion.

He sent Qibo to him and asked him: "In some books, it is stated that the motion and the motionless of heaven and earth are regulated by the moving degree of the sun and moon, and the symptoms of the moving up and down of the Yin and Yang are manifested by the cold and heat of the seasons.

"I have heard the law of the five elements' motion you explained, as you have said: the energies of the five-element motions dominate the year respectively, and it begins in the Jia year. I discussed what you said with Gui Yuqu, but he said: the earth motion dominates the years of Jia and Ji, the metal motion dominates the year of Yi and Geng, the water motion dominates the years of Bing and Xin, the wood motion dominates the years of Ding and Ren, the fire motion dominates the years of Wu and Gui; in the two years of Zi and Wu, the Shaoyin controls the heaven, in the two years of Chou and Wei, the Taiyin controls the heaven, in the two years of Yin and Shen, the Shaoyang controls the heaven, in the two years of Mao and You, the Yangming controls the heaven, in the two years of Chen and Xu, the Taiyang controls the heaven, in the two years of Si and Hai, the Jueyin controls the heaven. What he said was not in comformity with the Yin and Yang you said, and what is the reason?"

岐伯曰：是明道也，此天地之阴阳也。夫数之可数者，人中之阴阳也，然所合，数之可得者也，夫阴阳者，数之可十，推之可百，数之可千，推之可万。天地阴阳者，不以数推，以象之谓也。

Qibo said: "The reason is evident, it is because the Yin and Yang. Gui Yuqu said are the Yin and Yang of the five elements' motion on earth and the six kinds of weather in heav-

en. The Yin and Yang in human body are countable, such as blood is Yin and energy is Yang; solid organs are Yin and hollow organs are Yang, the interior is Yin and the superficies is Yang. When the Yin and Yang of human body combine with that of the heaven and earth, it can be calculated by analogy, such as, it can be inferred from ten to one hundred or from one thousand to ten thousand, but the number of Yin and Yang in heaven and earth can not be counted with number, but can only be obtained by estimation."

帝曰：愿闻其所始也。岐伯曰：昭乎哉问也！臣览《太始天元册》文，丹天之气，经于牛女戊分；黅天之气，经于心尾己分；苍天之气，经于危室柳鬼；素天之气，经于亢氐昴毕；玄天之气，经于张翼娄胃。所谓戊己分者，奎壁角轸，则天地之门户也。夫候之所始，道之所生，不可不通也。

Yellow Emperor said: "I hope to know how it begins." Qibo said: "What a brilliant question you have put forward. I have read the ancient book of the《Primordial Universe》in which it was stated: 'In ancient times, people saw there was in the sky the red energy lying in between the two stars of Niu and Nu position and the Wu position of northwest; there was yellow energy lying in between the two stars of Xin and Wei position and the position of Ji of southeast; there was green energy lying in between the two stars of Wei and Shi position and the two stars of Liu and Gui position; there was white energy lying in between the two stars of Kang and Di position and the two stars of Mao and Bi position; and there was black energy lying in between the two stars of Zhang and Yi position and the two stars of Lou and Wei Position'. The so-called Wu position is where the two stars of Kui and Bi locate, and the Ji position is where the two stars of Jiao and Zhen locate. The two stars of Kui and Bi locate in between the solar terms of Beginning of Autumn and Beginning of Winter; the two stars of Jiao and Zhen locate in between the solar terms of Beginning of Spring and Beginning of Summer. So, they are the gates of the heaven and earth, and they are also the beginning of the solar terms which is the starting point of Yin and Yang of heaven and earth, and one must not be ignorant of it."

帝曰：善。论言天地者，万物之上下，左右者，阴阳之道路，未知其所谓也。岐伯曰：所谓上下者，岁上下见阴阳之所在也。左右者，诸上见厥阴，左少阴，右太阳；见少阴，左太阴，右厥阴；见太阴，左少阳，右少阴；见少阳，左阳明，右太阴；见阳明，左太阳，右少阳；见太阳，左厥阴，右阳明。所谓面北而命其位，言其见也。

Yellow Emperor said: "Good, It was stated in the《Primordial Universe》: 'The heaven and earth are the upper and lower ranges for all things to rise and fall, and the left and right are the routes for Yin and Yang to ascend and descend'. But I do not understand its meaning."

Qibo said: "To rise means the Yin or Yang position of the six kinds of weather controlling the heaven above, to fall means the Yin or Yang position of the five elements' motion affecting the earth below. Left and right are the left or right positions of the controlling of the heaven. When the Jueyin appears on the position of controlling the heaven, the left will be Shaoyin and the right will he Taiyang; when the Shaoyin appears on the position of control-

ling the heaven, the left will be Taiyin and the right will be Jueyin; when the Taiyin appears on the position of controlling the heaven, the left will be the Shaoyang and the right will be the Shaoyin; when the Shaoyang appears on the position of controlling the heaven, the left will be the Yangming and the right will be the Taiyin: when the Yangming appears on the position of controlling the heaven, the left will be the Taiyang and the right will be the Shaoyang; when the Taiyang appears on the position of controlling the heaven, the left will be the Jueyin and the right will be the Yangming. This is the case of the facing north to determine the position of Yin and Yang in indicating the various appearances of Yin and Yang in controlling the heaven."

帝曰：何谓下？岐伯曰：厥阴在上，则少阳在下，左阳明，右太阴；少阴在上，则阳明在下，左太阳，右少阳；太阴在上，则太阳在下，左厥阴，右阳明；少阳在上，则厥阴在下，左少阴，右太阳；阳明在上，则少阴在下，左太阴，右厥阴；太阳在上，则太阴在下，左少阳，右少阴；所谓面南而命其位，言其见也。上下相遘、寒暑相临，气相得则和，不相得则病。

Yellow Emperor asked: "What is the meaning of affecting the earth below?" Qibo said: "When the Jueyin is on the position of controlling the heaven, then the Shaoyang will be on the position of affecting the earth, the Yangming will be on the left and Taiyin will be on the right; when the Shaoyin is on the position of controlling the heaven, then Yangming will be on the position of affecting the earth, and Taiyang will be on the left and Shaoyang will be on the right; when the Taiyin is on the position of controlling the heaven, then Taiyang will be on the position of affecting the earth, and Jueyin will be on the left and Yangming will be on the rignt; when the Shaoyang is on the position of controlling the heaven, then Jueyin will be on the position of affecting the earth, and Shaoyin will be on the left and Taiyang will be on the right; when the Yangming is on the position of controlling the heaven, then the Shaoyin will be on the position of affecting the earth, and Taiyin will be on the left and Jueyin on the right; when the Taiyang is on the position of controlling the heaven, then, the Taiyin will be on the position of affecting the earth, and Shaoyang will be on the left and Shaoyin will be on the right. Here, I am talking about the positions of Yin and Yang when one is facing south, and the different appearances of Yin and Yang positions in controlling the heaven and affecting the earth.

"In the intercourses of energies above and below, and the effects of different weathers, if the energies are promoting each other, it will cause harmony, if they are subjugating each other, it will cause disease."

帝曰：气相得而病者何也？岐伯曰：以下临上不当位也。

Yellow Emperor asked: "Sometimes the disease occurs when the six kinds of weather are in harmony, and what is the reason?" Qibo said: "The controlling heaven should happen in the first half of the year, and the affecting earth should happen in the second half of the year. When the controlling heaven is in the second half of it or the affecting earth is in the first half of it, they are in the wrong positions and disease will occur."

帝曰：动静何如？岐伯曰：上者右行，下者左行，左右周天，余而复会也。帝曰：余闻鬼臾区曰，应地者静。今夫子乃言下者左行，不知其所谓也，愿闻何以生之乎？岐伯曰：天地动静，五行迁复，虽鬼臾区其上候而已，犹不能遍明。夫变化之用，天垂象，地成形，七曜纬虚五行丽地；地者，所以载生成之形类也。虚者，所以列应天之精气也。形精之动，犹根本之与枝叶也。仰观其象，虽远可知也。

Yellow Emperor asked: "What are the conditions when the energies control the heaven and affecting the earth?" Qibo said: "The energy that controls the heaven is turning rightward, and energy that affects the earth is turning leftward, they return to their original position after turning right or left for one year."

Yellow Emperor said: "Gui Yuqu told me that the energies which correspond to the earth are motionless, now you say that the energy of the elements' motion affecting the earth is turning leftward, I do not know the reason. I hope you can tell me how can it move?"

Qibo said: "The motion and motionless of heaven and earth are changing, and the five elements' motion are turning in cycle. Although Gui Yuqu knows the pattern of movement of heaven, but he does not know thoroughly the details of the left and right.

"In the process of natural changes, the heaven creates the constellations, the earth shapes up all things, the sun, moon and the five planets are abiding by their orbits in the interstellar space, and the five elements are attaching the earth. The earth is loading all the visible things. The sun, moon and the five stars are spreading in heaven. All things on earth and the movements of sun, moon and the five stars in the sky are related with each other closely like the trunk of a tree connecting its branches and leaves. when we lift up our heads and watch the celestial phenomena, we can know the celestial body even it is far away."

帝曰：地之为下否乎？岐伯曰：地为人之下，太虚之中者也。帝曰：冯乎？岐伯曰：大气举之也。燥以干之，暑以蒸之，风以动之，湿以润之，寒以坚之，火以温之。故风寒在下，燥热在上湿气在中，火游行其间，寒暑六入，故令虚而生化也。故燥胜则地干，暑生则地热，风胜则地动，湿胜是地泥，寒胜则地裂，火胜则地固矣。

Yellow Emperor asked: "The earth is on below, isn't it?" Qibo said: "The earth is under the human being, and it is in the interstellar space."

Yellow Emperor asked: "Is the earth supported by something?" Qibo said: It is supported by the atmosphere (containing the six energies of wind, cold, heat, wetness, dryness and fire) in the interstellar space.

"The dryness energy causes the earth to become dry, the heat energy causes it to evaporate, the wind energy causes it to move, the wetness energy causes it to become moist, the cold energy causes it to become firm and substantial, and the fire energy causes it to become warm.

"The wind and cold situate below, the dryness and heat situate above, the wetness is in the middle, and the fire energy is moving up and down. The six energies invade the earth respectively within the year, and the earth can grow and breed all things under their effect.

"When the dryness energy is excessive, the earth will become dry, when the heat energy

is excessive, the earth will become hot, when the wind energy is excessive, all things on earth will be moving, when the wetness energy is excessive, the earth will become moist, when the cold energy is excessive the earth will be frozen with crackings, when the fire energy is excessive, the earth will become substantial and firm."

帝曰：天地之气，何以候之？岐伯曰：天地之气，胜复之作，不形于诊也。《脉法》曰：天地之变，无以脉诊，此之谓也。

Yellow Emperor asked: "As the universe and men are having the same energy, how to detect the energies which is controlling the heaven and affecting the earth by palpation?" Qibo said: "The six kinds of weather in heaven and the five elements' motion on earth are changeful in invading and retaliating which do not appear in the pulse of man. That is why in 《The Pulsation》 stated: The changes of heaven and earth can not be inspected by pulsation."

帝曰：间气何如？岐伯曰：随气所在，期于左右。帝曰：期之奈何？岐旧曰：从其气则和，违其气则病，不当其位者病，迭移其位者病，失守其位者危，尺寸反者死，阴阳交者死。先立其年，以知其气，左右应见，然后乃可以言死生之逆顺。

Yellow Emperor asked: "How to inspect the intermediate energy (the energy between the controlling the heaven and that affecting the earth) by palpation?" Qibo said: "One can detect the position of the intermediate energy by inspecting the left and right pulse. When the energy is on the left, the left pulse will be responding, when the energy is on the right, the right pulse will be responding."

Yellow Emperor asked: "what is the condition when the pulse corresponds with the energy?" Qibo said: "When the energy arrives and the pulse also arrives, the energy and pulse are in harmony, when the pulse arrives but the energy fails to arrive, the energy and pulse are disharmonious, in this case, the disease will occur.

"When the energy is on the left and the pulse is on the right, it is the diseased pulse in the wrong position, when the corresponding pulse often shifts its position, it is also the diseased pulse; when the subjugating pulse appears while its fundamental pulse is missing, the patient will be in danger, when the Cun pulse and the Chi pulse appear reversedly in the due year, the patient will die; when the pulse apears on the left in the year of Yin in which its corresponding pulse should be on the right, or it appears on the right in the year of Yang in which its corresponding pulse should be on the left, it is the alteration of the pulse, the patient will also die.

"One must ascertain first which energy is controlling the heaven and which energy is affecting the earth in the year, from which to sort out the intermediate energies on the left and on the right, then can the patient's death, survival, unfavourable or favourable prognosis can be inferred."

帝曰：寒暑燥湿风火，在人合之奈何？其于万物何以生化？岐伯曰：东方生风，风生木，木生酸，酸生肝、肝生筋、筋生心。其在天为玄，在人为道，在地为化。化生五味，道生智，玄生神，化生气。神在天为风，在地为木，在体为筋，在气为柔，在藏为肝。其性为暄，其德为和，其用为动，其色为苍，其化为荣，其虫毛，其政为散，其令宣发，其变摧拉，其眚

为陨，其味为酸，其志为怒。怒伤肝，悲胜怒；风伤肝，燥胜风；酸伤筋，辛胜酸。

Yellow Emperor asked: "How do the six kinds of weather of cold, heat, dryness, wetness, wind and fire coincide with the human body, and how can they promote the growth of all things?"

Qibo said: "For the variations of the six kinds of weather, in heaven, it is the mysterious phenomenon, in man; it is the way of adapting the change, and on earth, it is the influence of generating and growing of all things. The influence of earth produces the five tastes of various things, the adapting way of man produces the wisdom, and the mysterious phenomenon of heaven produces the divinity. As the earth can promote the generation and growth of all things, the six kinds of weather are produced from it.

"The east produces the wind, the wind can cause the energy of wood to grow, the wood energy can produce the sour taste, the sour taste can nourish the liver, the blood in liver can nourish the tendon. As the tendon is produced from the liver, the liver associstes with the wood, and wood can produce fire, so, the liver can also nourish the heart. In heaven , it is the wind; in the five elements, it is the wood; in human body, it is the tendon; in its influence to things, it is softness; in the five viscera, it is the liver; in attribution, it is warmness; in essence, it is modest; its function is movement; its colour is dark-green; in variation, it is glory; in animal, it is beast; in affect, it is dispersing; in season, it is the harmonic and scattering energy; in alteration, it is apt to be broken; its jeopardy is falling, its taste is sour: in mood, it is anger. The anger can injure the liver, and melancholy can restrain anger; the wind energy can injure the liver, and the dryness energy can restrict the wind energy; when the sour taste is excessive, it will injure the tendon, and the acrid taste can restrict the sourness.

南方生热，热生火，火生苦，苦生心，心生血，血生脾。其在天为热，在地为火，在体为脉，在气为息，在藏为心，其性为暑，其德为显，其用为躁，其色为赤，其化为茂，其虫羽，其政为明，其令郁蒸，其变炎烁，其眚燔焫，其味为苦，其志为喜。喜伤心，恐胜喜；热伤气，寒胜热；苦伤气，咸胜苦。

"The south produces the heat, the heat can cause the fire energy to become prosperous, the fire energy can produce the bitter taste, the bitter taste can nourish the heart, the heart can produce the blood, when the blood is abundant, it can nourish the spleen. In the six kinds of weather of heaven, it is heat; in the five elements on earth, it is fire; in man, it is the channel; in function, it can promote the growth of all things; in viscera, it is the heart; in attribute, it is the summer heat; in essence, it is displaying; in function, it is irritability: in animal, it is bird; in function, it is reasonable; in season, it is the extreme heat and vaporization; in alteration, it is apt to be burned; its jeopardy is the fire accident; in taste, it is bitterness; in moods, it is overjoy. When the overjoy is excessive, it will injure the heart, and terror can overcome overjoy. When the heat is excessive, it will injure the energy, and the cold energy can restrain the heat energy; when excessive bitter taste is addicted, it can also injure the energy, and the salty taste can restrain the bitterness.

中央生湿，湿生土，土生甘，甘生脾，脾生肉、肉生肺。其在天为湿，在地为土，在体为肉，在气为充，在脏为脾。其性静兼，其德为濡，其用为化，其色为黄，其化为盈，其虫倮，其政为谧，其令云雨，其变动注，其眚淫溃，其味为甘，其志为思，思伤脾，怒胜思；湿伤肉，风胜湿，甘伤脾，酸胜甘。

"The centrality produces wetness, the wetness energy can promote the earth energy, the earth energy can produce the sweet taste of the crops, the sweet taste can nourish the spleen energy, and the spleen energy can nourish the muscle when the muscle is strong, the lung energy will be abundant. In the six kinds of weather, it is the wetness; in the five elements, it is earth; in man, it is the muscle; in function, it is the substantiality of the body; in viscera it is the spleen; its property is the tranquility and the compatibility of cold energy and heat energy; in essence, it is smoothness; in function, it can generate and promote the growth of all things: in colour, it is yellow; in alteration, it is fullness; in animal, it belongs to the animal without hair, shell and scale kind; in affect, it is tranquility; in season, it is overcast and rain; in its variation, it is apt to have torrential rain or excessive and continuous rain and its disaster is like the dam burst after enduring rain; in taste, it belongs to the sweet kind; in moods, it belongs to anxiety. when one has excessive anxiety, it will injure the spleen, and anger can restrain the anxiety. The wetness can injure the muscle, and the wind energy can restrain the wetness. When excessive sweet taste is addicted, it can also injure the spleen, and sour taste can restrain the sweetness.

西方生燥，燥生金，金生辛，辛生肺，肺生皮毛，皮毛生肾。其在天为燥，在地为金，在体为皮毛，在气为成，在脏为肺。其性为凉，其德为清，其用为固，其色为白，其化为敛，其虫介，其政为劲，其令雾露，其变肃杀，其眚苍落，其味为辛，其志为忧。忧伤肺，喜胜忧；热伤皮毛，寒胜热；辛伤皮毛，苦胜辛。

"The west produces the dryness, the dryness energy can promote the metal energy, the metal energy can produce the acrid taste, the acrid taste can nourish the lung energy, the lung energy can nourish the skin and soft hairs, when the skin and soft hair are moistened, they can produce the kidney-fluid. In the six kinds of weather, it is dryness; in the five elements, it is the metal; in man, it is the skin and the soft hair; in function, it can accomplish things; in viscera, it is the lung. In property, it is coolness; in essence, it is the quietness; in variation, it is reinforcement; its colour is white; its alteration is restraining; in animal, it belongs to the cyprid kind; in affect, it belongs to being vigorous; in season, it belongs to the season of emerging mists and falling dew; in alteration, it is the chilling life and the restraint of all things; its disaster is causing the grasses and woods to become dry and withered away; in tastes, it is acrid; in moods, it is melancholy. The excessive melancholy can injure the lung, the mood of overjoy can restrain the melancholy. when the heat is excessive, it will injure the skin and the soft hair, the cold energy can restrain the heat. when the acrid taste is excessive, it can also injure the skin and the soft hair, and the bitter taste can restrain the acridness.

北方生寒，寒生水，水生咸，咸生肾，肾生骨髓，髓生肝。其在天为寒，在地为水，在

体为骨，在气为坚，在脏为肾。其性为凛，其德为寒，其用为〔明抄本“为”下补“藏”字〕，其色为黑，其化为肃，其虫鳞，其政为静，其令〔明抄本“令”下补“霰雪”二字〕，其变凝冽、其眚冰雹，其味为咸，其志为恐。恐伤肾，思胜恐；寒伤血，燥胜寒，咸伤血，甘胜咸。五气更立，各有所先，非其位则邪，当其位则正。

“The north produces the cold, the cold energy can promote the water energy to become prosperous, the water energy can produce the salty taste, the salty taste can nourish the kidney energy, the kidney energy can nourish the bone marrow, when the bone marrow is substantial, it can nourish the liver. In the six kinds of weather, it is cold; in the five elements, it is water; in the human body, it is the bone. Its affect is reinforcing the substance; in viscera, it is the kidney. Its property belongs to coolness, its essence belongs to coldness, its function is storing, its colour is black; in alteration, it is the solemnity and silence of all things; in animals, it belongs to the scaled animal kind; in affect, it is motionless; in seasons, it is the season of falling snow; in variation, it is the frozen ice in bitter cold; in disaster, it is the hailstone in the wrong time; in the five tastes, it is the salty taste; in mood, it is terror. When one has excessive terror, it will injure the kidney, the anxiety can restrain the terror; when the cold is excessive, it will injure the channel, the dryness energy can restrain the cold; the salty taste can injure the channel; the sweet taste can restrain the salty taste.

“The energies from the five orientation are taken place alternately in definite sequence. When the weather is not in conformity with the four seasons of the orientation, such as cold in summer and hot in winter, it is the evil energy; when it is in conformity with the four seasons of the orientation, it is the healthy energy.”

帝曰：病生之〔读本，赵本，吴本“生之”并乙作“之生”〕变何如？岐伯曰：气相得则微，不相得则甚。帝曰：主岁何如？岐伯曰：气有余，则制己所胜而侮所不胜；其不及，则己所不胜侮而乘之，己所胜轻而侮之。侮反受邪〔滑本无“侮而受邪”四字〕，侮而受邪，寡于畏也。帝曰：善。

Yellow Emperor asked: “ what is the condition when one contracts the disease?” Qibo said: “ when the weather is on their proper position according to the five orientations, the disease will be slight, when they are not on their proper position, the disease will be severe.”

Yellow Emperor said: ‘ what is the condition of the element’s motion in dominating the year?” Qibo said: ‘ When the element’s motion arrives at the time when it should not arrive, it shows the energy is excessive, not only it will invade the element’s energy which it can subjugate (such as wood subjugates earth), but will also subjugate reversely the element which can overcome itself (such as wood subjugates metal reversely). When the element’s motion is not arriving when it should arrive, it shows the energy is insufficient, when it is insufficient, it will not only be subjugated by the element which can overcome itself (such as wood being subjugated by the metal), but also will be subjugated reversely by the element which can not overcome itself (such as earth subjugates wood reversely). In the principle of

the five elements' motion, there is overcoming and also retaliating, when an element invades other element, it will be invaded by the evil energy, and the invasion is brought about by the running riot of itself." Yellow Emperor said: "Good."

六微旨大论篇第六十八

Chapter 68
Liu Wei Zhi Da Lun
(The Exquisite Meaning of Six Energies)

黄帝问曰：呜呼！远哉，天之道也，如迎浮云，若视深渊，视深渊尚可测，迎浮云莫知其极，夫子数言谨奉天道，余闻而藏之，心私异之，不知其所谓也。愿夫子溢志尽言其事，令终不灭，久而不绝，天之道可得闻乎？岐伯稽首再拜对曰：明乎哉问，天之道也！此因天之序，盛衰之时也。

Yellow Emperor asked: "Alas! How profound is the principle of heaven: It is like the floating cloud above, and the deep abyss below. One can measure the abyss but can by no means to know the extent of the floating cloud. You have said many times that one should abide by the principle of heaven carefully, and I have kept what you said in mind, but I am still doubtful as I do not know its reason. I hope you can tell me in detail, so that it may not be lost and can be handed down for a long time. Now, can I hear the details about the principle of heaven from you?" Qibo bowed again and again and said: "What a brilliaint question you have asked! This is the so called the principle of heaven is the prosperity and decline displayed in time sequence by the natural changes."

帝曰：愿闻天道六六之节盛衰何也？岐伯曰：上下有位，左右有纪。故少阳之右，阳明治之；阳明之右，太阳治之；太阳之右，厥阴治之；厥阴之右，少阴治之；少阴之右，太阴治之；太阴之右，少阳治之。此所谓气之标，盖南面而待也。故曰：因天之序，盛衰之时，移光定位，正立而待之，此之谓也。

Yellow Emperor said: "I hope to hear the reasons of the prosperity and decline in time sequence of the six sixty days (a year)."

Qibo said: "There are the regular positions for the six dominating energies above and below, and there are certain rule in situating in the right and left. So, on the right side of Shaoyang, Yangming is taking charge; on the right side of Yangming, Taiyang is taking charge; on the right side of Taiyang, Jueyin is taking charge; on the right side of Jueyin, Shaoyin is taking charge; on the right side of Shaoyin, Taiyin is taking charge; on the right side of Taiyin, Shaoyang is taking charge. These are the branches of the three Yins and the three Yangs, and one should observe it when facing south. The prosperity and decline of the time sequence of the nature can be determined by surveying the shifting of the sun's shadow."

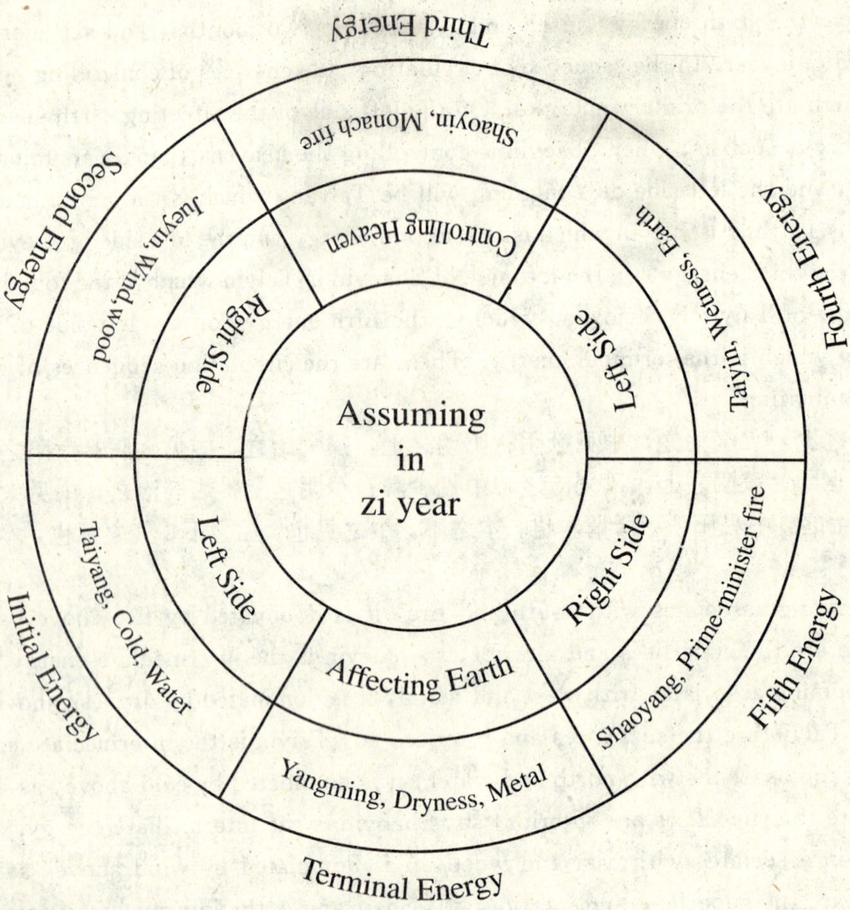

The diagrame of the energies of controlling the heaven, affecting the earth, on the left side and on the right side.

Diagram Illustration:

Controlling heaven, affecting earth, left side and right side are the proper terms in the theory of the five elements' motion and the six kinds of weather variations which indicate the six energies dominationg upwards, downwards, left and right. The meaning of upwards and downwards is the heaven and earth, the meaning of left and right is the time. Controlling heaven indicates dominating the heaven energy. and affecting earth indicates dominating the earth energy. In a year, the energy of controlling heaven dominates in the first half of the year, and the energy of affecting earth dominates in the second half of the year. Besides the energies of controlling heaven and affecting earth, the other four energies are the intermediate energies which are on the left and right sides. The six steps which are turning left step by tep show each one of the six energies dominates alternately the seasons of the year. The ini-

tial energy (the first energy) begins from the solar term of Great cold and ends in the terminal energy (the sixth energy), each energy takes up two months, and six energies take up the period of a year. In the sequence of circulating, the energies of controlling heaven and affecting earth are the primary energies. On the left side of the affecting earth energy, it is the initial energy. such as, when Shaoyin is controlling the heaven, then, Yangming is affecting the earth, and the left side of Yangming will be Taiyang which is the initial energy. On the left side of Taiyang is Jueyin which is the second energy: on the left side of Jueyin is Shaoyin which is the third energy: on the left side of Shaoyin is Taiyin which is the fourth energy, on the left side of Taiyin is Shaoyang which is the fifth energy; on the left side of Shaoyang is Yangming which is the terminal energy. These are the circulating sequences of the six energies in dominating.

少阳之上，火气治之，中见厥阴；阳明之上，燥气治之，中见太阴；太阳之上，寒气治之，中见少阴；厥阴之上，风气治之，中见少阳；少阴之上，热气治之，中见太阳；太阴之上，湿气治之，中见阳明。所谓本也，本之下，中之见也，见之下，气之标也，本标不同，气应异象。

"Shaoyang associates with south and fire, it is dominated by fire above, as Shaoyang and Jueyin are the superfices and interior, so, Jueyin is the intermediate energy.

"Yangming associates with west and metal, it is dominated by dryness above, as Yangming and Taiyin are the superfices and interior, so, Taiyin is the intermediate energy.

"Taiyang associtès with north and water, it is dominated by cold above, as Taiyang and Shaoyin are the superfices and interior, so, Shaoyin is the intermediate energy.

"Jueyin associates with east and wood, it is dominated by wind above, as Jueyin and Shaoyang are the superfices and interior, so, Shaoyang is the intermediate energy.

"Shaoyin associates with south and the monarch fire, it is dominated by heat above, as Shaoyin and Taiyang are the superfices and interior, so, Taiyang is the intermediate energy.

"Taiyin associates with southwest and earth, it is dominated by wetness above, as Taiyin and Yangming are the superfices and interior, so Yangming is the intermediate energy.

The energies dominating above are the root-energies of the three Yangs. The energies being dominated by the root-energies are the branch-energies. Between the root-energies and branch-energies and above the root-energies are the intermediate energies.

(Root)

Cold	Dryness	Fire		Wetness	Heat	Wind
Shaoyin	Taiyin	Jueyin	Inter mediate energy)	Yangming	Taiyang	Shaoyang
Taiyang	Yangming	Shaoyang		Taiyin	Shaoyin	Jueyin

(Branch)

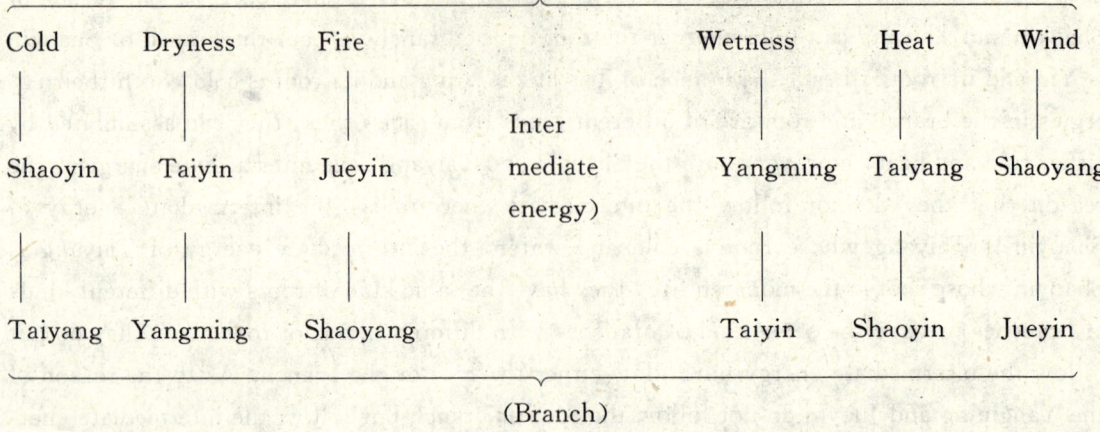

Diagram of the root, branch and intermediate energies of the six channels.

The energies dominating above are the root-energies of the three Yangs. The energies being dominated by the root-energies are the branch-energies. Between the root-energies and branch-energies and above the root-energies are the intermediate energies.

Diagram illustration:

The energies of the six channels take the wind, cold, heat. wetness, dryness and fire as the roots, and take the three Yangs and the three Yins as the branches. Between the roots and branches, there are the intermediate energies, such as, the Shaoyang and Jueyin are the superfices and interior (gallbladder and liver are the superfices and interior), the triple warmer and the pericardium are superfices and interior, Yangming and Taiyin are the superfices and interior (stomach and spleen are the superfices and interior, large intestine and the lung are the superfices and interior), Taiyang and Shaoyin are the superfices and interior (the bladder and the kidney are the superfices and interior. and small intestine and the heart are the superfices and interior). As the superfices and the interior are connecting, they are the intermediate energies to each other.

As the dominating six energies are different in following the root, branch and intermediate energy, their effects in response are different. Such as, the Shaoyang and Taiyin are following the root, the Shaoyin and Taiyang are following the root or the branch, the Yangming and Jueyin do not follow the root nor branch, but follow the intermediate energy. The root of Shaoyang is fire and its branch is Yang; the root of Taiyin is wetness and its branch is Yin, both their root-and branch-energies are of the same kind, so, they follow the root; as to the reason of that both the Shaoyang and Taiyin are having their intermediate energies, but they do not follow them is that: the intermediate energy of Shaoyang (fire) is the wind wood of Jueyin, as the wood and fire energies are of the similar kind, the wood assimilates with fire, so, it does not follow the intermediate energy. The intermediate energy of Taiyin

(Wetness earth) is the dryness metal of Yangming, as the earth generates metal, the dryness assimilates with wetness, so, it does not follow the intermediate energy. The reason of Shaoyin and Taiyang can follow either the root or the branch is that: the branch of Shaoyin is Yin and its root is heat, the branch of Taiyang is Yang and its root is cold, both their energies in the branch and root are of different kinds from each other, they can assimilated by either cold and heat, however, both the Shaoyin and Taiyang have intermediate energies, the reason that they do not follow the intermediate energies is: the intermediate energy of Shaoyin is Taiyang whose root is cold and water, the intermediate energy of Taiyang is Shaoyin whose root is the monarch fire, they have the same kind of roots with different kinds of branches or have the same kind of branches with different kinds of roots, so, they do not follow the intermediate energy but follow either the root or the branch. As to the reason of the Yangming and Jueyin do not follow the root or branch but follow the intermediate energy, it is because the intermediate energy of Yangming (dryness) is Taiyin whose root energy is wetness and earth, and dryness will assimilate with wetness; the intermediate energy of Jueyin (wind) is Shaoyang whose root energy is the prime minister-fire, and the wind will assimilate with fire. Thus, both the Yangming and Jueyin do not follow the root nor the branch, but follow the intermediate energies. At the same time, when the Yangming (dryness) encounters its intermediate energy which is Taiyin (wetness), it will become non-dryness, when the Jueyin (wind and wood) encounters its intermediate energy which is Shaoyang (fire), the wood will be burnt away; so, when the Yangming and Jueyin encounter their intermediate energies they will follow the intermediate energies. In a word, in the assimilation of the root and branch, when the wind encounters fire, wood will be assimilated by fire, when the dryness encounters wetness, dryness will be assimilated by wetness. As the targets of which to follow are various, the responses are different. In treating, sometimes the disease can be cured when following the root, sometimes it can be cured when following the branch, sometimes it can be cured by following either the root or branch, and sometimes it can be cured when following the intermediate energy.

Diagram Illustration:

The solid organs and the hollow organs are the roots which are the interiors; the twelve channels are the branches which are the superfices, The energies which are the superfices and interior with the solid and hollow organs are the intermediate energies. The intermediate energies situate in between the roots and branches for liaison, they are also called the links. Such as the Bladder channel of Foot Taiyang links the kidney, the kidney channel of Foot Shaoyin links the bladder, etc.

帝曰：其有至而至，有至而不至，有至而太过，何也？岐伯曰：至而至者和；至而不至，来气不及也；未至而至，来气有余也。帝曰：至而不至，未至而至如何？岐伯曰：应则顺，否则逆，逆则变生，变则病。帝曰善。请言其应。岐伯曰：物，生其应也，气，脉其应也。

Yellow Emperor said: " Sometimes the dominating energy of the six energies arrives when the season arrives, sometimes it arrives lagging behind the season, sometimes, it ar-

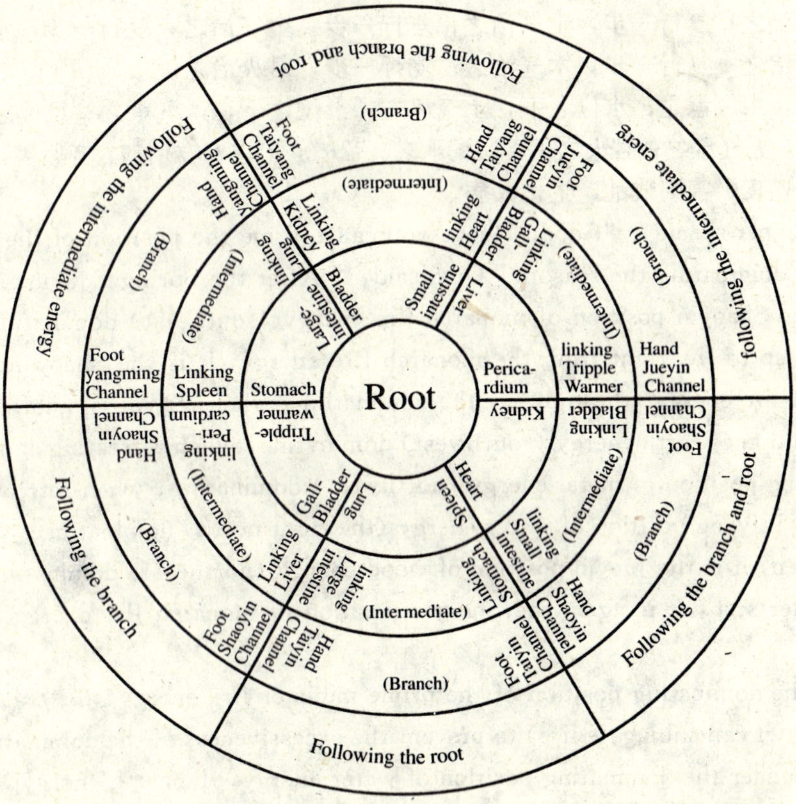

Diagram of the root, branch and intermediate energy of the viscera

rives prior to the season, and what is the reason?" Qibo said: " when the dominating energy arrives in the right season, it is the moderate energy; when the energy has not yet arrived and the season has arrived already, it is the condition of short of energy; when the energy arrives in advance and the season has not arrived yet, it is the energy which is having a surplus."

Yellow Emperor asked: " What are the conditions when the dominating energy has not yet arrived and the season has already arrived and the condition of the energy comes in advance when the season has not yet arrived?" Qibo said: " When the arriving of the energy corresponds with the season, it is the agreeable condition, when the coming of the energy fails to correspond with the season, it is the adverse condition, when the adverse condition appears, change will happen, and the change will cause disease."

Yellow Emperor said: "Good. I hope you can tell me the meaning of corresponding." Qibo said: "The conditions of all things corrospond to the different stages of their growth, and the various pulse conditions corrospond to the diferent kinds of the six-weather."

帝曰：善。愿闻地理之应六节气位何如？岐伯曰：显明之右，君火之位也；君火之右，退行一步，相火治之；复行一步，士气治之；复行一步，金气治之；复行一步，水气治之；复行一步，水气治之；复行一步，木气治之；复行一步，君火治之。

相火之下，水气承之；水位之下，土气承之；土位之下，风气承之；风位之下，金气承之；金位之下，火气承之；君火之下，阴精承之。帝曰：何也？岐伯曰：亢则害，承乃制，制则生化，外列盛衰，害则败乱，生化大病。

Yellow Emperor said: "Good. I hope you can tell me the position of the six kinds of weather when dominating the season." Qibo said: "After the Spring Equinox (in the right east), it is the Shaoyin position of monarch fire energy (southeast) dominating: when retreating one step to the right from the monarch fire energy, it is the Shaoyang position of prime minister fire energy (the right south) dominating: when retreating another step, it is the Taiyin position of earth energy (southwest) dominating; when retreating another step, it is the Yangming position of metal energy (northwest) dominating; when retreating another step, it is the Taiyang position of water energy (the right north) dominating; when retreating another step, it is the Jueyin position of wood energy (northeast) dominating; when retreating another step, it is again the Shaoyin position of monarch fire energy (southeast) dominating.

"Under the dominating position of the prime minister fire energy, the water energy is restricting (water can subjugate fire) to prevent the excessiveness of the dominating of prime minister fire, under the dominating position of water energy, the earth energy is restricting (earth can subjuget water), under the dominating position of the earth energy, the wind energy is restricting (wood can subujgate earth), under the dominating position of the wind energy, the metal energy is restricting (metal can subjugate wood), under the dominating position of the metal energy, the fire energy is restricting (fire can subjugate metal), under the dominating position of the monarch-energy, the Yin essence is restricting (water can subjugate fire)."

Yellow Emperor asked: "Why is it so?" Qibo said: "When the six energies are hyperactive in dominating, they will do harm, so, they must be restricted in certain extent. It is only in this way can the growth and transformation of all things be carried on. When the six energies are excessive or insufficient, they will do harm to the mechanism of growth and transformation and cause severe affection."

帝曰：盛衰何如？岐伯曰：非其位则邪，当其位则正，邪则变甚，正则微。帝曰：何谓当位？岐伯曰：木运临卯，火运临午，土运临四季，金运临酉，水运临子，所谓岁会，气之平也。帝曰：非位何如？岐伯曰：岁不与会也。

Yellow Emperor asked: "What are the conditions of the prosperity and decline in the nature?" Qibo said: "When the energy is not in its proper position, it is the evil energy; when

it is in its proper position, it is the healthy energy. When the evil energy causes disease, the disease will be changeful, when the healthy energy causes disease, it will be a slight one."

Yellow Emperor asked again: "What is the meaning of the proper position?" Qibo said: "When the wood motion encounters the year of Mao which is the Ding Mao year; When the fire motion encounters the Wu year which is the Wu Wu year; When the earth motion encounters the Chen, Xu, Chou and Wei years which are the Jia Chen year, the Jia Xu year, the Ji Chou year and the Ji Wei year when the metal motion encounters the year of You which is the Yi You year, when the water motion encounters the Zi year which is the Bing Zi year, they are all the years of which the decimal cycle converges with the duodecimal cycle. They are called the convergent year in which their energies are in the proper positions. In the convergent year. the energy will be normal and moderate without the condition of being excessive or defficient." Yellow Emperor asked: "What is the condition when the energy is not in its proper position?" Qibo said: "In the year of non-convergence of which the energy has the condition of excessiveness or defficiency, it is the year of which the energy is not in its proper position."

帝曰：土运之岁，上见太阴；火运之岁，上见少阳、少阴；金运之岁，上见阳明；木运之岁，上见厥阴；水运之岁，上见太阳，奈何？岐伯曰：天之与会也。故《天元册》曰天符。

Yellow Emperor asked: "What are the conditions when the earth motion is dominating the year and Taiyin is controlling the heaven; when the fire motion is dominating the year and Shaoyang or Shaoyin is controlling the heaven; when the metal motion is dominating the year and Yangming is controlling the heaven; when the wood motion is dominating the year and Jueyin is controlling the heaven; when the water motion is dominating the year and Taiyang is controlling the heaven?" Qibo said: "They are the conditions of the energy controlling the heaven converges with the energy of the element's motion. This condition is called Heaven Tally in the ancient book of《Origin of the Universe》."

天符岁会何如？岐伯曰：太乙天府之会也。

Yellow Emperor asked: "What is the condition when the heaven tally occurs simultaneously with the convergent year?" Qibo said: "It is the case of the coincidence of the weather that controls heaven, the year's motion, the orientation of the duodecimal cycle and the attribute of the five-element. which is called the heaven tally in the primordial unity of Yin and Yang."

帝曰：其贵贱何如？岐伯曰：天符为执法，岁位为行令，太乙天符为贵人。帝曰：邪之中也奈何？岐伯曰：中执法者，其病速而危；中行令者，其病除而特〔赵本，吴本"特"并作"持"〕中贵人者，其病暴而死。帝曰：位之易也何如？岐伯曰：君位臣则顺，臣位君则逆，逆则其病近，其害速；顺则其病远，其害微。所谓二火也。

Yellow Emperor asked: "Are there any difference in nobility and humbleness between them?" Qibo said: "The Heaven Tally is like the official that enforces the law, the Convergent Year is like the officer that executes the order, and the Heaven Tally in the Primordial Unity of Yin and Yang is like a noble man."

Yellow Emperor asked: " What is the difference in the three cases when one is affected by evil energy and contracts disease?" Qibo said: " When one is affected by the evil energy of the official that enforces the law, the disease will be acute and dangerous, when one is affected by the evil energy of the officer that excecute the order, the disease will be moderate, and the evil energy and the healthy energy will be at a stalemate, when one is affected by the evil energy of the noble man, the disease will occur all of a sudden and the patient will die instantly. "

Yellow Emperor asked: " What is the condition when the six energies exchange their positions?" Qibo said: " When the monarch situates in the position of the courtier, it is the agreeable condition, when the courtier situates in the position of the monarch, it is the adverse condition, In the adverse condition, the disease will be acute and dangerous, The so called the exchanging of energies' position is indicating the monarch fire and the prime minister fire. "

帝曰：善。愿闻其步何如？岐伯曰：所谓步者，六十度而有奇，故二十四步积盈百刻而成日也。

Yellow Emperor said: " Good I like to hear what is the meaning of a step. " Qibo said: " One day is a degree, 60 days and 87.5 notches make a step. In a year, it is 365.25 degrees, and 24 steps make 4 years. The remainder one fourth degree (25 notches) in each year will be accumulated in four years into 100 notches which is one day. "

帝曰：六气应五行之变何如？岐伯曰：位有终始，气有初中，上下不同，求之亦异也。帝曰：求之奈何？岐伯曰：天气始于甲，地气始于子，子甲相合，命曰岁立，谨候其时，气可与期。帝曰：愿闻其岁，六气始终，早晏何如？岐伯曰：明乎哉问也！甲子之岁，初之气，天数始于水下一刻，终于八十七刻半；二之气，始于八十七刻六分，终于七十五刻；三之气，始于七十六刻，终于六十二刻半；四之气，始于六十二刻六分，终于五十刻；五之气，始于五十一刻，终于三十七刻半；六之气，始于三十七刻六分，终于二十五刻，所谓初六，天之数也

Yellow Emperor asked: " What is the condition of variation when the six energies correspond with the five elements?" Qibo said: " The position of every energy in the six energies that dominating the season has its beginning time and its terminal time. In energies, there are the difference of the initial energy, intermediate energy, energy of heaven and energy of earth, and they should not be calculated in the same all way. "

Yellow Emperor asked: " How to calculate them?" Qibo said: " The decimal cycle of heaven starts from Jia, and the duodecimal cycle of earth starts from Zi, when Jia encounters Zi, it is the beginning of the year. When one calculates the changes from the beginning of the year carefully, the convergent time of the starting point and the terminal in the six energies can be obtained. "

Yellow Emperor asked: " Can I hear about the early or late, beginning and terminal conditions of the six energies in the year?" qibo said: " What a brilliant Question you have asked. In the year of Jia Zi. the initial energy starts at the first notch under the water level

of the clepsydra and ends at the 87. 5th notch, the second energy starts from the 87. 6th notch and ends at the 75th notch, the third energy starts from the 76th notch and ends at the 62. 5th notch, the fourth energy starts from the 62. 6th notch and ends at the 50th notch, the fifth energy starts from the 51st notch and ends at the 37. 5 notch, the sixth energy starts from the 37. 6 notch and ends at the 25th notch. There are the notches' number of the beginning and terminal of the first cycle of the six energies.

乙丑岁，初之气，天数始于二十六刻，终于一十二刻半；二之气，始于一十二刻六分，终于水下百刻；三之气，始于一刻，终于八十七刻半；四之气，始于八十七刻六分，终于七十五刻；五之气，始于七十六刻，终于六十二刻半；六之气，始于六十二刻六分，终于五十刻；所谓六二，天之数也。

"In the year of Yi Chou, the initial energy starts from the 26th notch and ends at the 12. 5 notch, the second energy starts from the 12. 6th notch and ends at the 100th notch under the water level of the clepsydra the third energy starts from the lst notch and ends at the 87. 5th notch, the fourth energy starts from the 87. 6 notch and ends at the 75th notch, the fifth energy starts from the 76th notch and ends at the 62. 5th notch, the sixth energy starts from the 62. 6th notch and ends at the 50th notch. There are the notches' number of the beginning and terminal of the second cycle of the six energies.

丙寅岁，初之气，天数始于五十一刻，终于三十七刻半；二之气，始于三十七刻六分，终于二十五刻；三之气，始于二十六刻，终于一十二刻半；四之气，始于一十二刻六分，终于水下百刻；五之气，始于一刻，终于八十七刻半；六之气，始于八十七刻六分，终于七十五刻，所谓六三，天之数也。

"In the year of Bing Yin, the initial energy starts from the 51st notch and ends at the 37. 5th notch, the second energy starts from the 37. 6th notch and ends at the 25th notch, the third energy starts from the 26th notch and ends at the 12. 5th notch, the fourth energh starts from the 12. 6th notch and ends at the 100th notch under the water level of the clepsydra, the fifth energy starts from the lst notch and ends at the 87. 5th notch, the sixth energy starts from the 87. 6th notch and ends at the 75th notch. These are the notches' number of the beginning and terminal of the third cycle of the six energies.

丁卯岁，初之气，天数始于七十六刻，终于六十二刻半；二之气，始于六十二刻六分，终于五十刻；三之气，始于五十一刻，终于三十七刻半；四之气，始于三十七刻六分，终于二十五刻；五之气，始于二十六刻，终于一十二刻半；六之气，始于一十二刻六分，终于水下百刻，所谓六四，天之数也。次戊辰岁，初之气复始于一刻，常如是无已，周而复始。

"In the year of Ding Mao, the initial energy starts from the 76th notch and ends at the 62. 5 notch; the second energy starts from the 62. 6th notch and ends at the 50th notch, the third energy starts from the 51st notch and ends at the 37. 5th notch; the fourth energy starts from the 37. 6th notch and ends at the 25th notch; the fifth energy starts from the 26th notch and ends at the 12. 5th notch, the six energy starts from the 12. 6th notch and ends at the 100th notch under the water level of the clepsydra. These are the notches' number of the beginning and terminal of the fourth cycle of the six energies. Nextly, the initial

energy in the Wu Chen year starts again from the lst notch of the clepsydra to move continuously according to the sequence stated above which goes round and begin again."

帝曰：愿闻其岁候何如？岐伯曰：悉乎哉问也！日行一周，天气始于一刻，日行再周，天气始于二十六刻，日行三周，天气始于五十一刻，日行四周，天气始于七十六刻，日行五周，天气复始于一刻，所谓一纪也。是故寅午戌岁气会同，卯未亥岁气会同，辰申子岁气会同，巳酉丑岁气会同，终而复始。

Yellow Emperor asked: "What is the condition in counting the year?" Qibo said: "How thoroughly you have asked. In the first cycle of the sun's circulation, the six-energy starts from the first notch, in the second cycle of its circulation, the six-energy starts from the 26th notch, in the third cycle of its circulation, the six-energy starts from the 51st notch, in the fourth cycle of its circulation, the six-energy starts from the 76th notch, in the fifth cycle of its circulation, the six-energy starts again from the lst notch. There are the four cycles of the six energies which is called the period of four years.

"Thus, the starting and the terminal notches of the six energies in the years of Yin, Wu and Xu are the same; the starting and the terminal notches in the years of Mao, Wei and Hai are the same; the starting and the terminal notches in the years of Chen, Shen and Zi are the same; and the starting and terminal notches in the year of Si, You and Chou are the same. In a word, the six energies are circulating continuously, they go round and to the end begin again."

帝曰：愿闻其用也。岐伯曰：言天者求之本，言地者求之位，言人者求之气交。帝曰：何谓气交？岐伯曰：上下之位，气交之中，人之居也。故曰天枢之上，天气主之；天枢之下，地气主之；气交之分，人气从之，万物由之。此之谓也。帝曰：何谓初中？岐伯曰：初凡三十度而有奇，中气同法。帝曰：初中何也？岐伯曰：所以分天地也。帝曰：愿卒闻之。岐伯曰：初者地气也，中者天气也。

Yellow Emperor said: "What are the functions of the six energies?" Qibo said: "Referring heaven, it should search after the dominating six energies of cold, heat, dryness, wetness, wind and fire; referring earth, it should search after the six positions of metal, wood, water, prime minister fire, earth and monarch fire in dominating the seasons; referring man, it should search after the intersection of the heaven energy and the earth energy."

Yellow Emperor asked: "What is the intersection of heaven energy and earth energy?" Qibo said: "The heaven energy descends from above, and the earth energy ascends from below, and the intersection of heaven energy and earth energy is in the zone where the human being lives. So, above the middle zone (the space between heaven and earth), it is dominated by heaven, below the middle zone, it is dominated by earth and in the section where the heaven energy and the earth energy intersect exists the human energy, and all things generate from this section."

Yellow Emperor asked: "What are the initial energy and the intermediate energy?" Qibo said: "The initial energy has thirty days odd (30.4375 days), and the intermediate energy has the same number of days."

Yellow Emperor asked: "Why there is the intermediate energy besides the initial energy?" Qibo said: "They are the grounds for to distinguish the heaven and earth."

Yellow Emperor said: "I like to know the details of it." Qibo said: "The initial energy is the earth energy and the intermediate energy is the heaven energy."

帝曰：其升降何如？岐伯曰：气之升降，天地之更用也：帝曰：愿闻其用何如？岐伯曰：升已而降，降者谓天；降已而升，升者谓地。天气下降，气流于地；地气上升，气腾于天。故高下相召，升降相因，而变作矣。帝曰：善。寒湿相遘，燥热相临，风火相值，其有闻〔读本，吴本，朝本"闻"并作"间"〕乎？岐伯曰：气有胜复，胜复之作，有德有化，有用 有变，变则邪气居之。

Yellow Emperor asked: "What is the condition of the ascent and descent of the energies?" Qibo said: "The ascent of the earth energy and the descent of the heaven energy are the mutual functions of the heaven energy and the earth energy."

Yellow Emperor asked: "What are their functions?" Qibo said: "The function of heaven is to ascend first and then descends, the function of earth is to descend first and then ascends. When the heaven energy descends, it will spread on the earth, when the earth energy ascends, it will be transpired into heaven. When the upper and lower energies are working in coordination with each other and the ascending and descending energies promoting each other, changes will occur."

Yellow Emperor said: "Good. Is there any variation when cold is encountering wetness when dryness is abiding by the heat and when the wind is bounding up with the fire?" Qibo said: "In the six energies, there are the energies of overcoming and retaliating, some are pertaining to the essence, some are pertaining to the promotion of growth and some are causing the change. When the change occurs, it will bring about the retention of the evil energy."

帝曰：何谓邪乎？岐伯曰：夫物之生从于化，物之极由乎变，变化之相薄，成败之所由也。故气有往复，用有迟速，四者之有，而化而变，风之来也。帝曰：迟速往复，风所由生，而化而变，故因盛衰之变耳。成败倚伏游乎中何也？岐伯曰：成败倚伏生乎动，动而不已，则变作矣。

Yellow Emperor asked: "what is the evil energy?" Qibo said: "The growth of all things depends on transformations, and the matures of all things are due to the changes. The combate between the change and the transformation is the source of growth and ruin. So, there are the energies of going and returning which can be swift or slow. The different conditions in the going, returning, swift and slow will cause the transformation and change, and they are the source of the wind energy."

Yellow Emperor said: "The different conditions of going, returning, swift and slow of the energy cause the wind energy to generate, and the process from the transformation to the change is formed by the variations of prosperity and decline. But, no matter in the promotion or ruin, their incubative factors are all stemmed from the change, and why is it?" Qibo said: "Due to the motions of the six energies, the factors of promotion and ruin are incubating in each other, and the continuous moving will cause the change."

帝曰：有期乎？岐伯曰：不生不化，静之期也。帝曰：不生化乎？岐伯曰：出入废则神机化灭，升降息则气立孤危，故非出入，则无以生长壮老已；非升降，则无以生长化收藏。是以升降出入，无器不有。故器者生化之宇，器散则分之，生化息矣。故无不出入，无不升降，化有小大，期有近远，四者之有，而贵常守，反常则灾害至矣。故曰：无形无患。此之谓也。帝曰：善。有不生不化乎。岐伯曰：悉乎哉问也！与道合同，惟真人也。帝曰：善。

Yellow Emperor asked："Is there any case of ceasing after the occurence of change? Qibo siad："When there is no growth and no transformation, it is the time of ceasing."

Yellow Emperor asked："Is there any case of the stopping of generating and transforming?" Qibo said："In animal kind, if the respiration is ceased, its life will be perished at once; in the plant and mineral kind, when its Yin and Yang fail to ascend and descend, its vitality will be withered away. Thus, if there is no going out and coming in, there will be no process of birth, growth, robustness, senility and death; if there is no ascent and descent, there will be no process of generating, growth, blooming, yieling fruit or crop and finally storing. So, in all visible things, they are having the energies of going out, coming in, ascent and descent . Therefore, the existance of growth and transformation depends upon the existance of the visible things. If the visible body disappeared, the growth and transformation will be extinguished. So, none of the visible things are without the energies of going out, coming in, ascent and descent, only there are the differences in extent and the earlier or later in time. In ascent and descent, it is important to remain normality, and disaster will occur when the abnormal condition happens, and it is only in the invisible thing can the disaster be avoided."

Yellow Emperor sakd："Good. Is there any human being that goes beyond the scope of growth and transformation?" Qibo said："what an exhaustive question you have asked. It is only a perfect man who can merge himself with the natural law, and changes along with the nature can do it." Yellow Emperor said："Good."

气交变大论篇第六十九

Chapter 69
Qi Jiao Bian Da Lun
(Changes in the Intersection of Energies)

黄帝问曰：五运更治，上应天期，阴阳往复，寒暑迎随，真邪相薄，内外分离，六经波荡，五气倾移，太过不及，专胜兼并，愿言其始，而有常名，可得闻乎？岐伯稽首再拜对曰：昭乎哉问也！是明道也。此上帝所贵，先师传之，臣虽不敏，往闻其旨。帝曰：余闻得其人不教，是谓失道，传非其人，慢泄天宝。余诚菲德，未足以受至道；然而众子哀其不终，愿夫子保於无穷，流於无极，余司其事，则而行之奈何？岐伯曰：请遂言之也。《上经》曰：夫道者上知天文，下知地理，中知人事，可以长久，此之谓也。帝曰：何谓也？岐伯曰：本气位也，位天者，天文也，位地者，地理也，通于人气之变化者，人事也。故太过者先天，不及者后天，所谓治化而人应之也。

Yellow Emperor asked: "The alternations of the five-element motions correspond with the six kinds of weather of heaven, the coming and going of Yin and Yang follow the sequential changes of cold and heat seasons, The combat of the healthy energy and the evil energy causes the divorce of the superfices and the interior in human body, the fluctuation of blood and energy of the six channels and the shifting and the imbalance of the energies of the five viscera cause the excessiveness or insufficiency of the human visceral energy and that of the domination of the five element-motion to the year.

I hope to hear the principle about its beginning and the syndromes reflected to the human body. Can you tell me?" Qibo bowed and answered: "What an explicit question you have asked. It is an important principle that should be explained clearly, and it is a valuable principle handed down by the preceeding physicians. Although I am not clever enough to understand it thoroughly, but I had heard about its meaning in the past."

Yellow Emperor said: "I am told that when one fails to teach when meeting the proper person, he will miss the chance of imparting the principle, when one passes the principle to an unworthy person, it will be the same as neglecting the valuable principle. Although I am wanting in ability and shallow in knowledge that I may not be capable to push ahead with the principle of medicine, yet I have the compassion for the people who died of diseases. I hope you can impart the knowledge to me so that many lives of the people may be saved, and the medical principle may be handed down for a long time. I will take charge of the matter abiding with the rules. What do you think about it?"

Qibo said: "I will try my best to explain it. It was stated in the《Upper Classics》: When one knows the principle, he will know the astronomy in heaven above, the geography

on earth below, the human affairs in the middle, and he will live long."

Yellow Emperor asked: "What is the meaning of it?" Qibo said: "The fundamental thing here is to infer the energy-positions of heaven, earth and man. When the energy situates in heaven, it is the energy that controls the weather; when the energy situates on the earth, it is the six steps that affecting the earth; when the energy communicates with man, it is taking charge of the variations of human affairs. So, the excessive energy arrives prior to the season, the insufficient energy arrives behind the season, and the abnormal condition confuses Yin and Yang and causes the regular and irregular changes of the weather, and the human body is also changing along with is."

帝曰：五运之化，太过何如？岐伯曰：岁木太过，风气流行，脾土受邪。民病飧泄，食减体重，烦冤，肠鸣腹支满，上应岁星。甚则忽忽善怒，眩冒巅疾。化气不政，生气独治，云物飞动，草木不宁，甚而摇落，反胁痛而吐甚，冲阳绝者死不治，上应太白星。

Yellow Emperor asked: "What is the condition when the activity of energy of the five elements' motion are excessive?"

Qibo said: "When the activity of energy of wood motion is excessive, it will cause the wind energy to prevail and the spleen earth will be injured by it. When the spleen fails to convey, one will contract diarrhea, he will have the symptoms of reducing food, feeling heavy of the limbs, feeling distressed, gurgling of the intestine and abdominal distention. As the wood energy is excessive, the corresponding Jupiter in the sky will be bright. If the wind energy is exceedingly prosperous, one will apt to get angry all of a sudden, having the symtoms of dizziness, sudden black out and grow dim of the eyes, diseases on head, etc. These are the phenomena when the earth energy fails to implement its decree and the wood energy is overabundant solely. So, the wind energy will be running wildly, causing the clouds flying in the sky, the grasses and woods on earth swaying, and the leaves and branches falling down. In man, he will have hypochondriac pain and continuous vomiting. If the subjugation of the wood energy to the earth energy causes the severance of the Chongyang pulse, the patient will by on means to be cured and die. When the wood energy tends to become weak after reaching its extreme, Venus in the sky will be unusually bright (metal overcomes wood).

岁火太过，炎暑流行，金肺受邪。民病疟，少气咳喘，血溢血泄注下，嗌燥耳聋，中热肩背热，上应荧惑星。甚则胸中痛〔《三因方》卷五引无“胁痛”二字〕，胁支满胁痛，膺背肩胛间痛，两臂内痛，身热骨痛〔林校“骨”字是“肤”字之误〕而为浸淫。收气不行，长气独明，雨水霜寒，上应辰星。上临少阴少阳，火燔焫，冰〔读本，赵本，明抄本“冰”并作“水”〕泉涸，物焦槁，病反谵妄狂越，咳喘息鸣，下甚血溢泄不已，太渊绝者死不治，上应荧惑星。

"When the energy of fire motion is excessive, the energy of summer-heat will be pervailing, and the lung metal will be injured by it, people will contract malaria, have the symtoms of short of breath, cough, rapid breathing, spitting blood, epistaxis, hematochezia, watery diarrhea, dry throat, deafness, hot in the chest, hot in the shoulders and back, etc. As the fire energy is excessive, the corresponding Mars in the sky will be bright. If the fire energy

is exceedingly prosperous, people will have the symptoms of pain in chest, fullness under the hypochondria, pain between the chest, back and scapula, pain in the inner side of the arms, fever in the body, pain in the skin to cause sores of infestation, etc. These are the phenomena when the metal energy fails to implement its decree and the fire energy becomes overabundant solely. After the fire energy reaches its extreme, it turns conversely to become week, so, the water energy takes advantage to invade and causes the coming of the rain, ice, frost and cold. The corresponding Mercury in the sky will be bright (water overcomes fire). In the period of when the fire energy is prosperous solely, the condition of the Shaoyin (heat energy is dominating above) or the Shaoyang (fire is dominating above) controlling the weather is encountered, the energy of fire and heat will be hyperactive like the burning of the fire. It will cause the spring to become dry up, the plants to become withered and man will suffer, continuous hematuria and hematochezia. If the subjugating of the fire energy to the metal energy is too much, causing the severance of the Taiyuan pulse, most of the patients can by no means be cured and die. As the fire energy is excessive, the corresponding Mars in the sky will be bright.

岁土太过，雨湿流行，肾水受邪。民病腹痛，清厥意不乐，体重烦冤，上应镇星。甚则肌肉萎，足痿不收，行善瘈，脚下痛，饮发中满食减，四支不举。变生得位，藏气伏，化气独治之，泉涌河衍，涸泽生鱼，风雨大至，土崩溃，鳞见于陆，病腹满溏泄肠鸣，反下甚而太谿绝者，死不治，上应岁星。

"When the energy of the earth motion is excessive, the energy of rain and wetness will be prevailing, and the energy of kidney water will be injured by it. The patient will have abdominal pain, cold extremities, depression of the spirit, heaviness of the body and be boring. As the earth energy is excessive, the corresponding Saturn in the sky will be bright. If the earth energy is exceedingly prosperous, the wetness energy will be partial overabundant and the spleen energy will be injured due to overabundance. As a result, the muscle in human body will become withered, the flaccidity of feet causes one unable to walk, the patient will often have contraction, pain in the heel, abdominal distention due to the retention of the water-evil and reduction of food so as he can not move his extremities. These are the conditions when the water energy fails to play its role and the earth energy is dominating the season and become prosperous solely. When the wetness earth turns weak after excessive abundance, the water energy will control the earth energy reversely, the spring water will become overflowing, the rivers will be filling with water and the fish will breed in the dried ponds. It may go so far as to have violent storm causing the dykes to collapse, the water in the river becomes flooded and the fishes appear on the dry land. Man will contract abdominal fullness and distention, diarrhea with loose stool, borborygmus, continuous diarrhea, etc. If the kidney water energy is excessively damaged to cause the severance of the Taixi pulse, the patient can by no means to be cured and die. When the water energy is injured, its son energy which is the wood energy (water generates wood) will retaliate for its mother, the corresponding Jupiter in the sky will be bright.

岁金太过，燥气流行，肝木受邪。民病两胁下少腹痛，目赤痛眦疡〔《三因方》引“疡”作“痒”〕，耳无所闻。肃杀而甚，则体重烦冤，胸痛引背，两胁满且痛引少腹，上应太白星。甚则喘咳逆气，肩背痛，尻阴〔《圣济总录》卷一中引作：“下连”〕股膝髀腨胻足皆病，上应荧惑星。收气峻，生气下，草木敛，苍干凋陨，病反暴痛，胠胁不可反侧，咳逆甚而血溢，太冲绝者死不治，上应太白星。

“When the energy of metal motion is excessive, the energy of dryness will be prevailing and the liver wood will be injured by it. A man will suffer from pain under the hypochondriac region and the lower abdomen, has red eyes, pain in the eyes, itching in the canthus, deafness, etc. When the energy of dryness metal is exceedingly prosperous, it will cause heaviness of the body, feeling of disquieted and unhappy, chest pain drawing the back, fullness and distention of the two hypochondria which affect the lower abdomen. As the metal energy is excessive, the corresponding Venus in the sky will both be bright. when the metal energy is prosperous to its extreme, it will turn weak gradually, the son energy of wood energy (fire energy) will take advantage to retaliate for its mother. When the fire energy subjugates the lung metal, man will have the symptoms of rapid breathing, cough, adverseness of vital energy, pain in the shoulders and back, etc. As the metal energy is too weak to produce the kidney water, the diseases of thigh, knee, calf and leg will occur. As the fire energy is prosperous, the corresponding Mars in the sky will be bright. If the metal energy is exceedingly severe, the wood energy (energy for generating) will be restricted and the grasses, and woods will become less prosperous, or even cause the green leaves to become withered and falling down. In a man, when the liver energy is restricted, the syndromes of acute headache, pain in the hypochondria causing inability to turn around, cough, adverseness of vital energy, spitting blood, and hemorrhage will occur. If the lung metal subjugating the liver wood so hard to cause the severance of the Taichong pulse, most of the patients will die. As the metal energy is prosperous, the corresponding Venus in the sky will be bright.

岁水太过，寒气流行，邪害心火。民病身热烦心，躁悸，阴厥上下中寒，谵妄心痛，寒气早至，上应辰星。甚则腹大胫肿，喘咳，寝汗出憎风，大雨至，埃雾朦郁，上应镇星。上临太阳，雨冰雪，霜不时降，湿气变物，病反腹满肠鸣，溏泄食不化，渴而妄冒，神门绝者死不治，上应荧惑辰星。

“When the energy of the water motion is excessive, the cold energy will be prevailing, and the heart fire will be injured by it. Man will contract bodily fever, oppression over the chest, feeling of anxiety, palpitation, asthenic-cold due to the attack of cold evil, chillness over the whole body, delirium, and cardialgia. As to the climate, the cold energy will arrive in advance. Since the water energy is in excess, the corresponding Mercury in the sky will be bright. If the water energy is exceedingly prosperous to which the spleen earth can no more restrict it, man will contract the syndromes of hydroperitoneum, edema of the shank, rapid breathing, cough, night sweat and have an aversion to wind. As the water energy is prosperous, the heavy rain will fall, and the dust and mist will cause haziness. When the water energy reaches its extreme and begins to turn weak gradually, the earth energy (son energy of

fire energy) will take advantage to retaliate for its mother, and the corresponding Saturn in the sky will be bright. When the cold water energy is partial abundant and the condition of Taiyang cold energy controlling the weather is encountered, the combination of the two cold energies will cause the falling of hail, frost and snow, and the excessiveness of wetness will cause things to become deformed. In a man, the syndromes of abdominal distention, borborygmus, diarrhea with loose stools, indigestion of food, thirsty and dizziness will occur. If the water energy subjugates the fire energy too hard to cause the severance of Shenmen pulse, the patient can by no means to be cured and die. As the fire can not overcome water, the corresponding Mars in the sky will be dark, and the Mercury will be bright."

帝曰：善。其不及何如？岐伯曰：悉乎哉问也！岁木不及，燥廼大行，生气失应，草木晚荣，肃杀而甚，则刚木辟著，悉萎苍干，上应太白星，民病中清，胠胁痛，少腹痛，肠鸣溏泄，凉雨时至，上应太白星，其谷苍。上临阳明，生气失政，草木再荣，化气乃急，上应太白、镇星，其主苍早〔沈祖丝说："'主'上脱'谷'字，'早'为'曰'之讹"〕。复则炎暑流火，湿性燥，柔脆草木焦槁，下体再生，华实齐化，病寒热疮疡痱胗痈痤，上应荧惑、太白，其谷白坚。白露早降，收杀气行，寒雨害物，虫食甘黄，脾土受邪，赤气后化，心气晚治，上胜肺金，白气乃屈，其谷不成，咳而鼽，上应荧惑、太白星。

Yellow Emperor said: "Good. Then, what is the condition when the energy of the five elements' motion is insufficient?" Qibo said: "What an exhaustive question you have asked. When the energy of the wood motion is insufficient, the energy of dryness metal will be prevailing (metal subjugating the wood even more hardly), the energy for generating which is the liver wood will not be able to arrive in time, and the grasses and woods will postpone their flourishing. When the metal energy is hyperactive, the strong and sturdy trees will be broken like being split, the tender branches and leaves will become withered. As the energy of dryness metal is excessive, the corresponding Venus in the sky will be bright. In man, the syndromes of asthenia cold of the middle warmer energy, pain in the hypochondria and lower abdomen, borborygmus and diarrhea with loose stool will occur. In weather, the cold rain will fall now and then. As the metal energy is abundant, the corresponding Venus in the sky will be bright. As the wood energy is restricted, the energy for generating will be insufficient, the crops will be immature with green and grey colour. When the dryness energy is overabundant, and the condition of Yangming controllng the weather is encountered, the wood energy will not be able to implement its decree and fails to restrict the earth, the earth energy will arise and the grasses and woods will be flourishing again. As the energy of generation and transformation is urgent, the crops can hardly become mature. Since both of the dryness energy and the earth energy are prosperous, so, both the Venus and Saturn in the sky will be bright. As the wood energy is restricted causing the crops to become grey and white, its son energy (fire energy) will be retaliating for its mother, the weather will become as hot as fire, all the wet things will become dry, the soft and tender branches and leaves of plants will be born anew from the root and finally reach the stage of appearing flowers and fruits. In man, the syndromes of cold and heat, sores and furuncle will occur. In

corresponding, both the Mars and Venus in the sky will be bright. But due to the restriction of the fire energy to the metal energy (harvest energy), the crops can hardly become mature, the white dew descends in advance between the summer and autumn and the severe and restraining energy will be prevailing. The cold rain in the wrong time injures all things and the sweet and yellow crops are bitten by bugs. When the metal energy is prosperous, the wood energy will be restricted, the fire energy (son of the wood enegy) will be retaliating to become active, but due to water energy (the son energy of the metal energy) can restrict the fire, the fire energy can only become active later and the heart energy will postpone its effect. When the fire is capable to overcome the metal energy, the metal energy will be subdued, the energy of harvest will not be prevailing and the crops will not be able to become mature. In man, the syndromes of cough and running nose will occur. As the fire energy and the metal energy are combating, both the Mars and Venus in the sky will be bright.

岁火不及，寒乃大行，长政不用，物荣而下，凝惨而甚，则阳气不化，乃折荣美，上应辰星，民病胸中痛〔《三因方》引作“胃”〕，胁支满，两胁痛，膺背肩胛间及两臂内痛，郁冒朦昧，心痛暴瘖，胸腹大，胁下与腰背相引而痛，甚则屈不能伸，髋髀如别，上应荧惑、辰星，其谷丹。复则埃郁，大雨且至，黑气乃辱，病鹜溏腹满，食饮不下，寒中肠鸣，泄注腹痛，暴挛痿痹，足不任身，上应镇星、辰星，玄谷不成。

“When the energy of the fire motion is insufficient, the cold energy of water will be prevailing a large scale (water subjugates fire), the erergy of growth which is of summer will not be able to implement its decree, the plants will turn to desolation from prosperity. when the cold energy of water is excessive, the Yang energy will not be able to promote growth and transformation, and the flourishing of all things will be destroyed. The corresponding Mercury in the sky will be bright. In man, the syndromes of stomachache, fullness and pain in the hypochondriac region, pain in the chest, pain between the back and the scapula and pain in the inside flank of the arm, stagnation and up-rising of vital energy, blur sight, heartache, sudden dysphonia, enlargement of chest and abdomen will occur. The back and loins under the hypochondria drawing each other with pain, when the condition is severe, the patient will be unable to face up and down and is painful as if his hip bone and the thigh bone are being split. As the fire energy is restricted by water energy, the corresponding Mars in the sky will be dark, the Mercury will be bright, and the five crops will be immature with red colour. When the water energy retricts the heart fire, the earth energy (the son energy of fire energy) will come to retaliate for it mother, the energy of wetness earth will be evaporated to become clouds, and the pouring rain will soon be falling. As the earth energy is capable to overcome the water energy, the water energy will be subdued. But when the earth energy becomes partial abundant, the spleen will fail to convey and transform, a man will have diarrhea with loose stool, abdominal fullness, failing to take in food, cold in the abdomen, borborgymus, continuous diarrhea, abdominal pain, sudden contracture of the limb, flaccidity and numbness of feet that he can not support his body. As the water energy is restricted by the earth energy, the corresponding Saturn in the sky will be bright, the Mercury

will be dark and the crops in black colour will not mature.

岁土不及，风乃大行，化气不令，草木茂荣。飘扬而甚，秀而不实，上应岁星。民病飧泄霍乱，体重腹痛，筋骨繇复，肌肉瞤酸，善怒，藏气举事，蛰虫早附，咸病寒中，上应岁星、镇星，其谷黅。复则收政严峻，名木苍凋，胸胁暴痛，下引少腹，善太息，虫食甘黄，气客于脾，黅谷乃减，民食少失味，苍谷乃损，上应太白，岁星。上临厥阴，流水不冰，蛰早来见，藏气不用，白乃不复，上应岁星，民乃康。

"When the energy of earth motion is insufficient, the wind energy will be prevailing in a large scale (wood subjugates earth), and the earth energy which is transformation will not be able to implement its decree. As the wood wind energy can promote the growth of all things, the grasses and woods will be flourishing. Nevertheless, due to the excessive floating of wind, the crops and fruits can hardly be yielded although their appearances are graceful. The corresponding Jupiter in the sky will be bright. In a man, the syndromes of lienteric diarrhea, cholera, heaviness of the body. abdominal pain, loose and rigidity of the extremities, bouncing of muscle with aches will occur, and the patient will apt to get angry often. As the wood energy subjugates the spleen earth causing the earth unable to subjugate water, the water energy will take advantage to become active, and the hibernants will hibernate early. In a man, the syndrome of asthenic cold of the middle-warmer energy will occur. In corresponding, the Jupiter in the sky will be bright, and the Saturn will be dark. In crops, they will become yellow and can hardly be mature. As the earth energy is restricted by the wood energy, the metal energy (son energy of the earth energy) will retaliate for its mother, so, the autumn energy (metal) will be prosperous, and the energy of clearing and descending, restraining and severing will be prevailing, thus, the big trees will become withered and bare. In man, the sudden pain in the chest and hypochondrium affecting the lower abdomen will occur, and the patient will sigh often. When the metal energy is overabundant, its son energy (water energy) will also be prosperous. When the water energy is prosperous, the sweet crops in yellow colour being bitten by the bugs, and the crops in yellow will reduce their production. As the metal energy is overcoming the wood, the green crops are injured, The corresponding Venus in the sky is bright and the Jupiter is dark. By this time, if the condition of Jueyin controlling the weather and the Shaoyang affecting the earth are encountered, the flowing water will not be able to get frozen and the hibernated worms will appear again. As the energy of cold water fails to play its role, the metal energy will not be abundant again. So, the Jupiter in the sky will be bright, and the people will be healthy.

岁金不及，炎火乃行，生气乃用，长气专胜，庶物以茂，燥烁以行，上应荧惑星，民病肩背瞀重，鼽嚏血便注下，收气乃后，上应太白星，其谷坚芒。复则寒雨暴至，乃零冰雹霜雪杀物，阴厥且格，阳反上行，头脑户痛，延及囟顶发热，上应辰星，丹谷不成，民病口疮，甚则心痛。

"When the energy of the metal motion is insufficient, the fire energy will be prevailing (fire subjugates metal). As the metal energy is not strong enough to subjugate the wood, the generating energy which is of wood will be able to implement its decree, and the growth

energy which is of fire will also be abundant, and all things will become flourishing. When the fire energy is prosperous, the weather will become harmful with dryness and scorching heat and the corresponding Mars in the sky will be bright. As the lung metal is subjugated by the heart fire, man will have the syndromes of heaviness of shoulder and back, running nose, sneezing, hemotochezia, continuous diarrhea etc. As the metal energy is restricted, the harvest energy of autumn will come later. The corresponding Venus in the sky will be dark, the crops of white colour will not be able to become mature. When the metal energy is brought under control, its son energy (water energy) will retaliate for its mother, thus, the cold rain will come all of a sudden and the hail, frost and snow will fall in the wake of it, and all things will be injured. When a man is disturbed by the cold evil, the Yang energy will arise to cause headache, the pain of the brain and fever of the body. The corresponding Mercury in the sky will be bright. The crops in red colour will not become mature, and a man will often contract aphthosis or even heartache.

岁水不及，湿乃大行，长气反用，其化乃速，暑雨数至，上应镇星，民病腹〔《三因方》“腹”作“肿”〕满身重，濡泄寒疡流水，腰股痛发，腘腨股膝不便，烦冤，足痿，清厥，脚下痛，甚则胕肿，藏气不政，肾气不衡，上应辰星，其谷秬。上临太阴，则大寒数举，蛰虫早藏，地积坚冰，阳光不治，民病寒疾于下，甚则腹满浮肿，上应镇星，其主黅谷。复则大风暴发，草偃木零，生长不鲜，面色时变，筋骨并辟，肉瞤瘛，目视𥆨𥆨，物疏璺，肌肉胗发，气并鬲中，痛于心腹，黄气乃损，其谷不登，上应岁星。

"When the energy of the water motion is insufficient, the energy of wetness will be prevailing in a large scale (earth subjugates water). As the water energy is not strong enough to control the fire, the growth energy which is of fire, on the contrary, will be able to implement its decree. When the growth energy is playing its role. the energy of transformation will act swiftly and speed up the growth and the transformation of all things. Due to the evaporations of all things, the summer rain will fall frequently. The corresponding Saturn in the sky will be bright. In man, the syndromes of abdominal fullness, heaviness of the body, diarrhea due to wetness-evil, sore with dilute pus, pain in the loins and thigh, feeling uneasy of the poplitea, calf, thigh and knee, feeling disquieted and unhappy, flaccidity of the feet, cold extremities, pain in the foot and even edema will occur. These are the conditiong when the hiding energy of winter can not implement its decree and the kidney energy becomes imbalanced. The corresponding Mercury in the sky will be dark, and the crops in black colour will not become mature. By this time, if the condition of Taiyin controlling the weather and the cold water affecting the earth is encountered, the great cold energy will invade often and the worms will be hiding early. On earth, there will be thick frozen ice, and the sunlight in the sky will not be able to bring its warmness into play. People will contract cold syndrome in the lower part, and the abdominal fullness and edema will occur when the case is severe. The corresponding Saturn in the sky will be bright and the crops of yellow colour will be mature. As the earth energy is restricted by the water energy, the son energy of the water energy (wood energy) will be retaliating for its mother, the strong squall will come suddenly,

the grasses will be bending over, the woods will be withered and lose its lustre due to the dryness and being cracked by the blowing of wind. As the wood wind subjugates the spleen earth, the complexion of man will lose its lustre, the tendons and bones become contracted and painful, the muscle bouncing with spasm, the two eyes can not see things clearly and seems to have faint cracks on the things seen and rubella will grow in the muscle. If the wind energy invades the diaphram, the heartache and abdominal pain will occur. As the wood energy is exceedingly prosperous and the earth energy (yellow energy) is injured, the crops of yellow colour can hardly become mature. The corresponding Jupiter in the sky will be bright."

帝曰：善。愿闻其时也。岐伯曰：悉哉问也！木不及，春有鸣条律畅之化，则秋有雾露清凉之政，春有惨凄残贼之胜，则夏有炎暑燔烁之复，其眚东，其藏肝，其病内舍胠胁，外在关节。

Yellow Emperor said: "Good. I hope you can tell me about the relation between the energy of the five motions and the four seasons." Qibo said: "What an exhaustive question you have asked. When the energy of the wood motion is insufficient, and the metal energy is not subjugating, there will be moderate energy like gentle breeze in spring and there will be clear and cool normal weather with mist and dew in autumn; if the metal energy is subjugating the insufficient wood, there will be cold and destitude metal energy in spring and the son energy of the wood (fire energy) will retaliate to cause hot weather like burning fire in summer. The calamity often occurs in the east, in a man, the disease often occurs in the liver. The attacking position of the disease is in the hypochondrium inside and joints outside.

火不及，夏有炳明光显之化，则冬有严肃霜寒之政，夏有惨凄凝冽之胜，则不时有埃昏大雨之复，春眚南，其藏心，其病内舍膺胁，外在经络。

"When the energy of the fire motion is insufficient in summer and the water energy is not subjugating, there will be moderate energy in summer and a severe and cold normal weather with frost in winter: if the water energy is subjugating the insufficient fire then. there will be desolate and cold weather in summer and the gloomy sky with dust and pouring rain occur frequently. Its calamity often occur in the south, and in human body, it often occurs in the heart. The attacking position of the disease is in the chest and hypochondrium inside and channels and collaterals outside.

土不及，四维有埃云润泽之化，则春有鸣条鼓拆之政，四维发振拉飘腾之变，则秋有肃杀霖霪之复，其眚四维，其藏脾，其病内舍心腹，外在肌肉四支。

"When the energy of the earth motion is insufficient and the wood energy is not subjugating, there will be moderate energy moistening with dusts and clouds in the four corners (southwest, northeast, southeast and northeast), and there will be normal weather with wind, bird's warblings and sprouting of grasses and woods in spring: if the wood energy is subjugating the insufficlent earth, there will be the abnormal conditions of rising squall in the air, swaying and breaking of the grasses and woods in the four corner months (southeast, northwest, southwest and northwest on the third, ninth, twelfth and sixth months),

and there will be the shady cool weather with continuous rain in autumn. Its calamity often occurs in the four corners, in human body, it often occurs in the spleen. The attacking position of the disease is in the heart and abdomen inside and in the muscles and the extremities outside.

金不及，夏有光显郁蒸之令，则冬有严凝整肃之应，夏有炎烁燔燎之变，则秋有冰雹霜雪之复，其眚西，其藏肺，其病内舍膺胁肩背，外在皮毛。

"When the energy of the metal motion is insufficient and the fire energy is not subjugating, there will be moderate energy with apparent wetness and vapour in summer, and there will be the corresponding normal bitter cold, frozen and severe weather in winter; if the fire energy is subjugating the insufficient metal, then , there will be summer heat like burning fire in summer, and there will be the corresponding weather of ice, hail, frost and snow in autumn. Its calamity often occur in the west, in human body, it often occurs in the lung. The attacking position is in the chest, hypochondrium, shoulder and back inside, and the skin and soft hair outside.

水不及，四维有湍润埃云之化，则不时有和风生发之应，四维发埃昏骤注之变，则不时有飘荡振拉之复，其眚北，其藏肾，其病内舍腰脊骨髓，外在谿谷踹膝。夫五运之政，犹权衡也，高者抑之，下者举之，化者应之，变者复之，此生长化成收藏之理。气之常也，失常则天地四塞矣。故曰：天地之动静，神明为之纪，阴阳之往复，寒暑彰其兆，此之谓也。

"When the energy of the water motion is insufficient, and the earth energy is not subjugating, there will be normal energy with moisture dusts and clouds in the four corner months, and there is the response of generating gentle breeze often; if the earth energy is subjugating the insufficient water, then, there will be the gloomy sky with mists, dusts and pouring rain in the corner months. There will be often the conditions of squall rising in the air to cause the swaying and breaking of the grasses and woods. Its calamity often occurs in the north, in human body it often occurs in the kidney. The attacking position of the disease is in the spine and bone marrow inside, the intermuscular septum, heel and knee outside.

"The function of the five-motion energies is to keep balance in each other. It restricts the motion energy which is excessive, and assists the one which is insufficient, to the normal activity of energy. It will have normal response, to the abnormal ones, it restores it to become normal. This is the natural law of all things in their process of birth, growth, transformation, harvesting and storing and the routine sequence of the four seasons. If the law is violated, the energy of heaven and earth will be obstructed in all directions and become impeded. Thus, the activity of heaven and earth can be refered by the movements of the sun, moon and stars, and the coming and going symptoms of Yin and Yang are displayed by the alternations of the cold and hot seasons."

帝曰：夫子之言五气之变，四时之应，可谓悉矣。夫气之动乱，触遇而作，发无常会，卒然灾合，何以期之？岐伯曰：夫气之动变，固不常在，而德化政令灾变，不同其候也。帝曰：何谓也？岐伯曰：东方生风，风生木，其德敷和，其化生荣，其政舒启，其令风，其变振发，其灾散落。南方生热，热生火，其德彰显，其化蕃茂，其政明曜，其令热，其变销烁，其灾

燔焫。中央生湿，湿生土。其德溽蒸，其化丰备，其政安静，其令湿，其变骤注，其灾霖溃。西方生燥，燥生金，其德清洁，其化紧敛，其政劲切，其令燥，其变肃杀，其灾苍陨。北方生寒，寒生水，其德凄沧，其化清谧，其政凝肃，其令寒，其变凓冽，其灾冰雪霜雹。是以察其动也，有德有化，有政有令，有变有灾，而物由之，而人应之也。

Yellow Emperor said："You have explained quite exhaustively the changes of the five-motion energies correspond with the four seasons，but the running wild of the energy is aroused only when being offended，since the out burst of the running wild has no regular pattern，how can we anticipate its sudden occurrence in advance?" Qibo said："Although the running wild and changes of the five energies have no regular pattern，but they can be inferred by their different functions，abilities of transforming and their variations."

Yellow Emperor asked："Why is it so?" Qibo said："The east produces the wind，and the wind can promote the prosperity of the wood energy. Its characteristic is to spread the moderate energy，its ability is to promote growth and transformation and cause the breeding and flourishing of all things，its authority of office is to cause all things to unfold and bloom，its appearance is the wind，its variation is the howling of the squall，its calamity is to blow off all things and cause desolation.

"The south produces the heat，and heat can promote the prosperity of the fire energy. Its characteristic is brightness and prominence，its ability is to promote growth and transformation so as to cause all things to become numerous and prosperous，its authority of office is to illuminate all things with light，its appearance is heat，its variation is the burning heat of fire，its calamity is to melt all things.

"The centrality produces the wetness，and the energy of wetness can promote the prosperity of the earth energy. Its characteristic is wetness-heat，its ability is to promote growth and transfromation and cause all things to become plump and comprehensive，its authority of office is to causes all things to become calm，its appearance is wetness，its variation is the continuous pouring rain，its calamity is the unceasing rain，collapse of the earth and spoil of the mud.

"The west produces the dryness，the energy of dryness can produce the prosperity of the metal energy. Its characteristic is cleanliness，its ability is to promote growth and transformation and causes all things to become retrenched and restrained，its authority of office is to cause all things to become strong and sharp by drying，its appearance is dryness，its variation is causing all things to become severe and descending，its function is to cause all things to become severe and descending，its calamity is to cause all things to become grey，withered and falling.

"The north produces cold，and the cold can promote the prosperity of the water energy. its characteristic is cold，it ability of promoting growth and transformation is to cause all things to become peaceful and quiet，its authority of office is to cause all things to become solidified and in an orderly manner，its appearance is cold，its variation is bitter cold，its calamity is the ice，snow，frost and hail.

"So, when observing their activities, one can see there are characteristic ability of promoting growth and transformation, authority of office, appearance, variation and calamity, and all things and men are corresponding with it."

帝曰：夫子之言岁候，不及其太过，而上应五星。今夫德化政令，灾眚变易，非常而有也，卒然而动，其亦为之变乎。岐伯曰：承天而行之，故无妄动，无不应也。卒然而动者，气之交变也；其不应焉。故曰：应常不应卒。此之谓也。帝曰：其应奈何？岐伯曰：各从其气化也。

Yellow Emperor said: "You have explained the excessive and the insufficient conditions of the five motions and the changes corresponding with the five stars. Now, when the characteristic, promotion of growth and transformation, authority of office, appearance, calamity and variation are not appearing in a routine pattern, but in an unexpected way, will the five-motion be changing along with it?" Qibo said: "If the five-motion is following the way of heaven, then, it will be sure to correspond with the five stars. The unexpected change of the overcoming and retaliating is due to the change in the intersection of the weather, which has no relation with the five stars. This is the condition of the so called: 'The five stars are corresponding to the regular rule, not to the sudden change.'"

Yellow Emperor asked: "In what way the five stars correspond with the elements' motion?" Qibo said: "The five stars are following the activity of the energy of weather respectively, such as the Saturn corresponds with the activity of wetness energy, the Jupiter corresponds with the activity of the wind energy. the Venus corresponds with the activity of the dryness energy, and Mercury corresponds with the activity of the cold energy.

帝曰：其行之徐疾逆顺何如？岐伯曰：以道留久，逆守而小，是谓省下；以道而去，去而速来，曲而过之，是谓省遗过也；久留而环，或离或附，是谓议灾与其德也；应近则小，应远则大，芒而大倍常之一，其化甚；大常之二，其眚即也；小常之一，其化减；小常之二，是谓临视，省下之过与其德也。德者福之，过者伐之。是以象之见也，高而远则小，下而近则大，故大则喜怒迩，小则祸福远。岁运太过，则运星北越，运气相得，则各行以道。故岁运太过，畏星失色而兼其母，不及则色兼其所不胜。肖者瞿瞿，莫知其妙，闵闵之当，孰者为良，妄行无征，示畏侯王。

Yellow Emperor asked: "In the movements of the five stars, there are swift and slow in speed, adverse and agreeable in direction. and what do they illustrate?: Qibl said: "If the five-star lingers in the course of the agreeable direction, or stays on the same degree with faint light, it is like inspecting the good and evil behavior of the people under its jurisdiction; if the five-star passes along its track and returns quickly or passes in twists and turns, it is like to know whether there is any people under its jurisdiction whose good or bad behavior have been neglcted or being slipped away; if the five-star stays long, turning around or staying on and off, it is like deliberating to release calamities or blessings to the people under its jurisdiction. If the time for the delivery of calamities or blessings to the people is drawing near, the light of the five-star will be faint, if the delivery is remote, the light of the star will be bright. If the star-light is two times as big as usual, it is the hyperaction of the activ-

ity of energy; when the star-light is three times as big as usual, calamities will occur instantly; when the star-light is only half as big as usual, it shows the reduction of the activity of energy; when, the star-light is only one fourth as big as usual, it is called the estimating which means inspecting the faults and merits of the people below, and will bestow blessing to those who have merrits and release calamities to those who have faults.

"Thus, when the five-star appears to be high and far away, the level of its overcoming and relatiating will be light, if the five-star appears to be low and near, the degree of its overcoming and retaliating will be heavy. when the star-light is bright, it shows the time of the releasing calamities or blessing will be close, when the star-light is faint, it shows the time of releasing calamities or blessings will be remote.

"When the energy of the element's motion is excessive, the corresponding star will leave its track and move northward, such as, when the energy of wood motion is excessive, the Jupiter which dominates the year will leave its track and move northward. It is only when the energy of the five-motion is on the proper position and proper time, can the corresponding star which dominating the year moves along within its track.

"Therefore, when the energy of the element-motion is excessive, the star it restricts will not be bright, and at the same time, it has also the colour of it's motion star, such as, when the energy of the wood motion is excessive, the Saturn which it overcomes will be dark, and at the same time, Saturn will also have the red colour of its mother star (Mars). When the energy of the element's motion is insufficient, not only the corresponding star itself is dark, but also the light of the star of which the coresponding element is being restricted, the Jupiter will not be bright and the Venus to which the Jupiter can not overcome (metal restricts wood) will be bright also.

"In a word, the principle of the change in heaven is subtle and is hard to be understood, but it is suitable and beneficial. As to the people casting horoscope who are ignorant and unwilling to learn, they do not really understand the astronomy, they can only use it to puzzle and threaten the lords and kings."

帝曰：其灾应何如？岐伯曰：亦各从其化也。故时至有盛衰，凌犯有逆顺，留守有多少，形见有善恶，宿属有胜负，征应有吉凶矣。

Yellow Emperor asked: "In what way the five-star corresponds with the calamities?" Qibo said: "The corresponding change of the five-star to the calamities varies in different activities of the energy of the element's motion respectively. Thus, when they arrive in accordance with different seasons there are the conditions of overabundance and decline; in the invasions of the motion star, there are the adverse and agreeable conditions; in the periods of their retention, there are the conditions of long and short time; in the appearances, there are the good and evil conditions; in subordinations, there are different conditions of victory and defeat in each other; in their corresponding symptoms to all things and men, there are blessings and calamities."

帝曰：其善恶何谓也？岐伯曰：有喜有怒，有忧有丧，有泽有燥，此象之常也，必谨察

之。帝曰：六者高下异乎？岐伯曰：象见高下，其应一也，故人亦应之。

Yellow Emperor asked: "What kind of appearance stands for blessing or calamity?" Qibo said: "In the appearances of the five-star, there are the difference of over-joy, anger melancholy, depression, moist and dryness which are the common appearances of the stars, and one should observe them carefully."

Yellow Emperor asked: "In the different attitudes of the star's location with the six appearances of overjoy, anger, etc., are there any differences when affecting men?" Qibo said: "Although the high and low attitudes of the stars are different, their influencs to the world are the same, so, there is no difference when affecting men."

帝曰：善。其德化政令之动静损益皆何如？岐伯曰：夫德化政令灾变，不能相加也。胜复盛衰，不能相多也。往来小大，不能相过也。用之升降，不能相无也。各从其动而复之耳。

Yellow Emperor said: "Good. What are the affects, damages and benefits of their charateristics, transforming ability, jurisdiction and enforcing decree to man?" Qibo said: "Their characteristics, ability of transformation, jurisdiction and enforcing decree are determined by the good or bad behaviours of men which are regular and can not be increased or decreased wantonly; when the energy of overcoming is excessive, the energy of retaliating will be excessive, when the energy of overcoming is deficient, the energy of retaliating will also be deficient. They are of direct proportion which can not be increased one sidely; the period of days of overcoming and retaliating are also the same, and they can not surpass one another. The ascent and the descent of Yin and Yang of the five elements are integrating with each other and they will not diminish in one side only. Their corresponding conditions are related with the energy of the five motions."

帝曰：其病生何如？岐伯曰：德化者气之祥，政令者气之章，变易者复之纪，灾眚者伤之始，气相胜者和，不相胜者病，更感于邪则甚也。

Yellow Emperor asked: "What are their affects to the disease." Qibo said: "the characteristic of its ability of generation and transformation is the amicability and harmonization of the year's energy; the appearance of its authority of office is the prominent evidence of the year's energy; the variation is the outline for its repeatition; and the calamity is the source of injuries of all things. When the energy of men suits the energy of the year, there will be calm and peace, when the energy of men fails to suit the energy of the year, disease will occur, if the evil-energy is affected again, the disease will become even more severe."

帝曰：善。所谓精光之论，大圣之业，宣明大道，通于无穷，究于无极也。余闻之，善言天者，必应于人，善言古者，必验于今，善言气者，必章于物，善言应者，同天地之化，善言化言变者，通神明之理，非夫子孰能言至道欤！乃择良兆而藏之灵室，每旦读之，命曰《气交变》，非斋戒不敢发，慎传也。

Yellow Emperor said: "Good. Your brilliant and profound theory has reached the standard of the cause of the sages and your knowledge of good comment has reached an inexhaustible realm. I am told that he who is good in explaining the principle of heaven can adapt it to men; he who is good in relating the ancient things can apply them to the present: he

who is good in expounding the activity of energy can display the activity of energy on all things explicitly, he who is good in explaining the response can integrate it with the creation of heaven and earth, he who is good in in interpreting the growth, transformation and change knows the principle of the nature, and who can deliver such a refined and marvelous principle except you? I will keep your words in the room of excellent orchid room and read it every morning. I will name it as the 'Changes in the Intersection of Energies'. I will be careful not to open the book when I am not sincere enough, and I will hand it down to the later generations."

五常政大论篇第七十

Chapter 70
Wu Chang Zheng Da Lun
(On the Energies of the Five Elements' Motion)

黄帝问曰：太虚寥廓，五运迴薄，衰盛不同，损益相从，愿闻平气何如而名？何如而纪也？岐伯对曰：岐伯对曰：昭乎哉问也！木曰敷和，火曰升明，土曰备化，金曰审平，水曰静顺。

Yellow Emperpr asked: 'The sky is spacious and boundless, and the five elements' motion circulates swiftly and unceasingly. As there are the different conditions of prosperity and declination, its injury and benefit to human body are varied. I hope to hear how to nominate and distinguish the moderate energies of the five elements' motion。" Qibo said: " What an explicit question you have asked. When the wood energy is moderate, it spread harmony and softness, and it is called the 'Spreading Harmony'; when the fire energy is moderate, it ascends and becomes bright, and it is called the 'Ascending Brightness'; when the earth energy is moderate, it spreads the energies of growth and transformation extensively to all things, and it is called the 'Extensive Activation of Energy'; when the metal energy is moderate, it is refreshing but not restraining hard and it is called the 'Cautious Punishment'; when the water energy is moderate, it is calm and fluent, and it is called the 'Calm and Agreeable'。"

帝曰：其不及奈何？岐伯曰：木曰委和，火曰伏明，土曰卑监，金曰从革，水曰涸流。帝曰：太过何谓？岐伯曰：木曰发生，火曰赫曦，土曰敦阜，金曰坚成，水曰流衍。

Yellow Emperor asked: "What are the conditions when they are insufficient?" Qibo said: " when the wood energy is insufficient, it is tortuous without the harmonious energy of Yang, and it is called 'Disharmony'; when the fire energy is insufficient, it hides without illuminating, and it is called 'Hiding Light'; when the earth energy is insufficient, it lies low whithout promoting growth and transformation, and it is called 'Descending Low'; when the energy of metal is insufficient, it is like leather without the energy of firmness, and it is called 'Leather-like'; when the energy of water is insufficient, it is dry without the energy of moisture, and it is called 'Drying Flow'。"

Yellow Emperor asked: " What are conditions when they are excessive?? Qibo said: "when the wood energy is excessive, the growth and transformation of all things will come in advance, and it is called 'Early Generation'; when the energy of fire is excessive, the flaming of fire will be very strong, and it is called the 'Conspicious Flame'; when the energy of earth is excessive, it is high and thick, and it is called 'High and Thick'; when the energy of

metal is excessive, it will be very hard, and it is called 'Firm and Blocked'; when the energy of water is excessive, it will be overflowing, and it is called the 'Flooding'。"

帝曰：三气之纪，愿闻其候。岐伯曰：悉乎哉问也！敷和之纪，木德周行，阳舒阴布，五化宣乎，其气端，其性随，其用曲直，其化生荣，其类草木，其政发散，其候温和，其令风，其藏肝，肝其畏清，其主目，其谷麻，其果李，其实核，其应春，其虫毛，其畜犬，其色苍，其养筋，其病里急支满，其味酸，其音角，其物中坚，其数八。

Yellow Emperor asked: "what are the symbols of the moderate, insufficient and excessive energies and how to distinguish them?" Qibo said: "How exhaustive your question is. The symbol of 'spreading Harmony' which is the moderate energy of wood is prevailing all around causing the Yang energy to relax, the Yin energy to spread and cause the activities of energy of the five elements' motion to become unimpeded and moderate. The moderate energy of wood is upright: its property is agreeable to the transformation of all things; its variation is crooked or straight: its ability of promoting growth and transformation is to cause all things to become prosperous; it subordinates to the grass and wood kind; its function is difussion, its symptom is mildness; its manifestation is the wind; its corresponding viscus of a man is the liver. The liver wood is afraid of the lung metal and the liver associates to the eyes. In crops, it is the fiber crops; in kinds of fruit, it is the plum; in the parts of fruit, it is the kernel; in seasons, it is spring; in worms, it is the caterpillar; in animals, it is the dog; in colours, it is dark-green; its refined energy nourishes the tendon; in diseases, they are the tenesmus and the abdominal distention; in the five tastes, it is sourness; in the five tones, it is the Jue; in substances, it is of the firm kind; in the accomplishing number in the mystic diagram, it is eight.

升明之纪，正阳而治，德施周普，五化均衡，其气高，其性速，其用燔灼，其化蕃茂，其类火，其政明曜，其候炎暑，其令热，其藏心，心其畏寒，其主舌，其谷麦，其果杏，其实络，其应夏，其虫羽，其畜马，其色赤，其养血，其病瞤瘛，其味苦，其音徵，其物脉，其数七。

"The symbol of 'Ascending Brightness' which is the moderate energy of fire is the universal implementing of the decree of fire causing the activities of the five-element energy to develope in a balanced way. The moderate energy of fire is ascending; its property is swift in moving; its affect is scorching and burning heat; its ability of promoting growth is to cause all things to become flourishing; in categories, it belongs to fire; its function is to illuminate light; in weathers, it is the hot summer; its authority of office is to implement the decree of heat; in viscus, it is the heart, and the heart is afraid of the kidney water; in human body, it associates with the tongue; in the five crops, it is the wheat; in the kinds of fruit, it is the apricot; in the parts of fruit, it is the sponge; in seasons, it is the summer; in worms, it is the flying insect; in animals, it is the horse; in colours, it is red; its refined energy nourishes the blood; in diseases, it is the bouncing and spasm of the muscle; in the five tastes, it is the bitterness; in the five tones, it is Zhi; in substances, it belongs to the channel and collateral kind; its accomplishing number in the mystic diagram is seven.

备化之纪，气协天休，德流四政，五化齐修。其气平，其性顺，其用高下，其化丰满，其类土，其政安静，其候溽蒸，其令湿，其藏脾，脾其畏风，其主口，其谷稷，其果枣，其实肉，其应长夏，其虫倮，其畜牛，其色黄，其养肉，其病否，其味甘，其音宫，其物肤，其数五。

"The symbol of 'Extensive Activation of Energy' which is the moderate energy of earth is the coordination of the thickness of the earth energy with the harmonious energy of heaven. The energy spreads in all directions causing the activities of the five elements to become prosperous simultaneously. The moderate energy of earth is mild; its property is agreeable; in variations, it is either high or low; its ability is to promote growth, to cause all things to become abundant and full; in categories, it belongs to earth; in functions, it is causing all things to become calm and silence; in weathers, it is the weather of vapourizing wetness and heat; in the manifestations, it is the wetness; its corresponding internal organ of a man is the spleen, the spleen is afraid of the liver wood, and the spleen associates with the mouth; in crops, it is the millet; in kinds of fruit, it is the jujube; in the parts of fruit, it is the pulp of fruit: in seasons, it is the long summer; in worms, it is the naked worm; in animals, it is the cow; in colours, it is yellow; its refined energy nourishes the muscle; in diseases, it is the feeling of stagnation and oppression; in the five tastes, it is sweetness; in the five tones, it is Gong: in substances, it belongs to the skin kind: its accomplishing number in the mystic diagram is five.

审平之纪，收而不争，杀而无犯，五化宣明，其气洁，其性刚，其用散落，其化坚敛，其类金，其政劲肃，其候清切，其令燥，其藏肺，肺其畏热，其主鼻，其谷稻，其果桃，其实壳，其应秋，其虫介，其畜鸡，其色白，其养皮毛，其病咳，其味辛，其音商，其物外坚，其数九。

"The symbol of 'Caustious Punishment' which is the moderate energy of metal is restraining yet without conflicting, chillness yet without persecution, so as the activities of the energy of the five elements' motion may become smooth and clarified. The moderate energy of metal is clean; its property is firm and straight forwards; in variation, it is scattering; its ability of promoting growth and transformation is to cause all things to yield fruit and restrained; in categories, it belongs to the metal; its function is to cause all things to become clean and solemn; its symptoms are coolness and urgency; its manifestation is dryness; its corresponding internal organ of a man is the lung, the lung is afraid of the heart fire, and the lung associates with the nose; in crops, it is rice; in kinds of fruit, it is the peach; in the parts of fruit, it is the shell; its corresponding season is autumn; in worms, it is the cyprid: in livestocks, it is the chicken; in colours, it is white: its refined energy nourishes the skin and hair: in diseases, it is the cough: in the five tastes, it is acridness; in the five tones, it is Shang: in substances, it is of the hard shell outside, its accomplishing number in the mystic diagram is nine.

静顺之纪，藏而勿害，治而善下，五化咸整，其气明，其性下，其用沃衍，其化凝坚，其类水，其政流演，其候凝肃，其令寒，其藏肾，肾其畏湿，其主二阴，其谷豆，其果栗，其

实濡，其应冬，其虫鳞，其畜彘，其色黑，其养骨髓〔吴本"骨"下无"髓"字〕，其病厥，其味咸，其音羽，其物濡，其数六。

"The symbol of 'Calm and Agreeable' which is the moderate energy of water is the storing of all things without doing any harm. It promotes the growth and transformation and is good at flowing lowly to cause the energies of the five elements' motion to become completed. The moderate energy of water is calm and bright; its property is tending to descend; in variation, it is irrigating and overflowing; its ability of promoting growth is solidifying; in categories, it belongs to the liquid; its function is to cause the inexhaustibility of water in the spring, well and river; its symptoms are coldness and calmness; its manifestation is coldness; its corresponding internal organ of a man is the kidney, the kidney is afraid of the spleen earth, and the kidney relates to the posterior yin (anus) and the anterior yin (external gentals and urethral orifice); in crops, it is pea; in the kinds of fruit, it is the chestnut, in the parts of fruit, it is the juice; its corresponding season is winter; in worms, it is the scaled worm: in livestock, it is the pig; in colours, it is black; its refined energy nourishes the bone; in diseases, it is the adversness of vital energy; in the five tastes, it is salty; in the five tones, it is Yu; in substances, it belongs to the liquid kind; in the accomplishing number of the mystic diagram, it is six.

故生而勿杀，长而勿罚，化而勿制，收而勿害，藏而勿抑，是谓平气。

"When the energy is in the condition of promoting generation yet not persecuting, promoting growth yet not punishing, promoting transformation yet not preventing, restraining yet not interfering, storing yet not suppressing, it is called the moderate energy.

委和之纪，是谓胜生。生气不政，化气乃扬，长气自平，收令乃早。凉雨时降，风云并兴，草木晚荣，苍乾凋落，物秀而实，肤肉内充。其气敛，其用聚，其动緛戾拘缓，其发惊骇，其藏肝，其果枣李，其实核壳，其谷稷稻，其味酸辛，其色白苍，其畜犬鸡，其虫毛介，其主雾露凄沧，其声角商。其病摇动注恐，从金化也，少角与判商同，上角与正角同，上商与正商同；其病支废痈肿疮疡，其甘虫，邪伤肝也，上宫与正宫同。萧飋肃杀，则炎赫沸腾，眚于三，所谓复也。其主飞蠹蛆雉，乃为雷霆。

"The symbol of 'Disharmony' which is the insufficient energy of wood motion is the obstruction of the generating energy. When the generating energy of wood can not play its role, the transforming energy of earth will be spreading, the growth energy of fire will become calm and the harvesting energy of metal will come in advance, thus, the cool rain falling now and then, the wind and clouds will arise, the growth of the grasses and woods pospones and they apt to become withered. But when the crops are yielding, the husks and grains are substantial. The property of the insufficient energy of wood is restraining; its function is collecting; its variation in human body is the contraction and relaxation of the tendon; in disease, it is liable to fright; its corresponding internal organ of a man is the liver; in the kinds of fruit, they are the jujube and the plums; in the parts of the fruit, they are the kernel and the shell; in the crops, they are the millet and the rice; in the five tastes, they are the sourness and acridness; in colours, they are white and green; in animals, they are the

dog and the chicken; in worms, they are the caterpillar and the cyprid; in the weathers they are the weathers of mist, dew and cold; in the five tones, they are Jue and Shang; in the attacks of diseases, they are the shaking and the frightening due to the insufficiency of the wood motion, and the wood assimilates with the metal. By this time, the tone of Lesser Jue (insufficient energy of wood) is similar with the tone of Lesser Shang (insufficient energy of metal). When Jueyin is controlling the weather, it is the tone of Upper Jue (when wood wind is dominating the weather), when the insufficient energy of wood motion receives the help of the dominating energy which is the wood wind, it makes the tone of Upper Jue to become similar with the tune of Right Jue (the moderate energy of wood). when the Yangming is controlling the weather, it is the tone of Upper Shang (Dryness dominating the weather), as the insulficient energy of the wood motion is subjugated by the dominating energy which is the dryness metal, it causes the tone of Upper Shang to become similar with the tone of Right Shang (moderate energy of metal). In the diseases, they are the swelling of the extremities, sores, parasitic infestation due to the injury of the liver energy by the metal energy. By this time, the tone of Upper Gong (wetness dominating the weather) is similar with the tone of Right Gong (moderate energy of earth). When the wood is restricted by the metal, the autumn energy will be chilly and restraining, but the flaming heat will come in the wake of it. Its calamity is from the east, and it is called the retaliation. When the wood is restricted by the metal, the fire-related flying insects, moth, maggot and pheasant will appear. when the wood energy is extremely weak, the thunderbolt will occur. Thus, when the wood energy is insufficient, it associates with the appearance of the flying insect, moth, maggot, pheasant and thunder.

伏明之纪，是谓胜长。长气不宣，藏气反布，收气自政，化令乃衡；寒清数举，暑令乃薄。承化物生，生而不长，成实而稚，遇化已老。阳气屈伏，蛰虫早藏。其气郁，其用暴，其动彰伏变易。其发痛，其藏心，其果栗桃，其实络濡，其谷豆稻，其味苦咸，其色玄丹，其畜马彘，其虫羽鳞，其主冰雪霜寒，其声徵羽。其病昏惑悲忘，从水化也，少徵与少羽同，上商与正商同。邪伤心也，凝惨凓冽则暴雨霖霪，眚于九〔胡本、读本、吴本“九”作“七”〕。其主骤注雷霆震惊，沈黔淫雨。

“The symbol of ‘Hiding Light’ which is the insufficient energy of the fire motion is the obstruction of the growth energy. When the fire can not play its role, the water energy will take chance to spread widely, the harvest energy will play its role, the earth energy will be calm, the energy of cold will appear now and then, and the energy of summer heat will become weak. Although all things are generated by the influence of the transforming energy of earth, yet, due to the insufficiency of the energy of the fire motion, the crops can hardly grow after generation; although it can yield, yet its grain will be small and thin, when the transforming energy of long summer is met, it will become decrepit in advance. Due to the hiding of Yang energy, the worms will hibernate prior to the regular season. The insufficient energy of the fire is stagnant; its function is urgency; its variation is either revealing or hiding without certainty; in the attacks of disease, it is pain; in the corresponding internal organ

of a man is the heart, in the kinds of fruit, they are the chestnut and peach; in the parts of fruit, they are the sponge and the juice; in crops, they are the pea and the rice; in the five tastes, they are the bitterness and the saltness; in colours, they are black and red; in animals, they are horse and pig; in worms, they are the flying insect and the scaled worm; it dominates the weathers of ice, snow, frost and cold; in the five tones, they are Zhi and Yu; in the diseases of a man, they are the falling into stupor and muddle, feeling sorrow and has amnesia due to the assimilation of fire to the water. By this time, the tone of Lesser Zhi (insufficient energy of fire) will be similar with the tone of Lesser Yu (ingufficient energy of water), When Yangming is controlling the weather, it is the tone of Upper Shang (dryness dominating the weather), as the fire can not control the metal, the tone of Upper Shang is similar with the tone of Right Shang (moderate energy of metal). As the energy of the fire motion is deficient, the heart energy (fire) will be injured by the water energy, the weather will become overcast and cloudy, and the pouring rain will fall in the wake of it. The calamities are from the four directions. Since fire is restricted, the torrential rain and the claps of thunder will occur. When the fire is restricted extremely by water, the weather will turn to cloudy and rainy, so, the insufficient energy of the fire motion associates with the appearance of the torrential rain, thunderbolt and unceasing rain.

卑监之纪，是谓减化。化气不令，生政独彰，长气整，雨乃愆，收气平，风寒并兴，草木荣美，秀而不实，成而粃也。其气散，其用静定，其动疡涌分溃痈肿，其发濡滞，其藏脾，其果李栗，其实濡核，其谷豆麻，其味酸甘，其色苍黄，其畜牛犬，其虫倮毛，其主飘怒振发，其声宫角，其病留满否塞，从木化也，少宫与少角同，上宫与正宫同，上角与正角同，其病飧泄，邪伤脾也。振拉飘扬，则苍乾散落，其眚四维，其主败折虎狼，清气乃用，生政乃辱。

"The symbol of 'Descending Low' which is the insufficient energy of earth motion, is the reduction of the transforming energy. When the transforming energy of earth can not play its role, the generation energy of wood will be prevailing solely, although the growth energy of fire can be kept intact, yet the rain will not fall on due time; although the harvesting energy is stable, yet the wind and cold will appear simultaneously; although the grasses and woods are flourishing, yet they can hardly yield seeds, and the yields of crops are only of the blighted grain kind. The insufficient energy of the earth motion is slackness; its function is to cause sedateness and stabilization; in variation, it is the festering and swelling of the ulcer; the attack of disease is the wetnss and stagnation; its corresponding internal organ of a man is the spleen; in the kinds of fruit, they are the plum and chesnut; in the parts of fruit, they are the nut and the kernel; in the crops, they are the pea and the fibre crops; in five tastes, they are the sourness and sweetness; in five colours, they are dark green and yellow; in live-stocks, they are the cow and the dog; in worms, they are the naked worm and the caterpillar; the weather it dominates is the blowing of gale and the swaying of trees; in five tones, they are Gong and Jue; in diseases, they are the feelings of distention and stagnation and the dissimilation of earth to wood. By this time, the tone of Lesser Gong (insufficient en-

ergy of earth) is similar with the tone of Lesser Jue (insufficient energy of wood). when Taiyin is controlling the weather, it is the tone of Upper Gong (wetness dominating the weather), since the insufficient energy of the earth motion receives the help of the dominating wetness, the tone of Upper Gong is similar with the tone of Right Gong (moderate energy of earth). When Jueyin is controlling the weather, it is the tone of Upper Jue (wind dominating the weather), as the energy of the earth motion is insufficient, together with the subjugation of the wind energy that is controlling the weather, the tone of Upper Jue is similar with the tone of Right Jue (moderate energy of wood). In diseases, it is the lienteric diarrhea due to the injury of the spleen by the wood energy. As the earth energy is deficient, and the wood energy is prosperous, the gale will blow all of a sudden, the grasses and woods will be swaying and broken to become withered and falling. Its calamities are from the four corners (southeast, northwest, southwest and northeast), and its corruption and injury are like the ferocious damage of the wild beasts of tiger and wolf. As the cool and clear weather is prevailing, the functions of the energy of generation will be subdued.

从革之纪，是谓折收，收气乃后，生气乃扬，长化合德，火政乃宣，庶类以蕃。其气扬，其用躁切，其动铿禁瞀厥，其发咳喘，其藏肺，其果李杏，其实壳络，其谷麻麦，其味苦辛，其色白丹，其畜鸡羊，其虫介羽，其主明曜炎烁，其声商徵，其病嚏咳鼽衄，从火化也，少商与少徵同，上商与正商同，上角与正角同。邪伤肺也。炎光赫烈，则冰雪霜雹，眚生七，〔胡本，读本、吴本、"七"并作"九"〕其主鳞伏彘鼠，岁气早至，乃生大寒。

"The symbol of 'Leather-like' which is the insufficient energy of the metal motion is the reduction of the harvest energy. When the harvest energy of metal postpones, the generating energy of wood will be blazing. When the fire energy combines with the earth energy, the function of fire energy will be fully played and all kinds of plant will be flourishing. The insufficient energy of the metal motion is ascending; its function is impetuousness; its variations are the rapid breathing, cough, aphonia, opperssion over the chest and the adverseness of vital energy; in the attacks of disease, they are cough and rapid breathing. Its corresponding internal organ of man is the lung; in kinds of fruit, they are the plum and apricot; in the parts of fruit, they are the shell and the sponge; in crops, they are the fibre crop and glutinous millet; in five tastes, they are the bitterness and the acridness; in colours, they are white and red; in live-stocks, they are the chicken and the sheep; in worms, they are the flying insect and the cyprid; the weathers it dominates are the fine and hot weathers; in the five tones, they are the tones of Shang and Zhi; in attacks of disease, they are the sneezing, coughing, running nose and hemorrhage due to the insufficient energy of the metal motion and the assimilation of metal with fire. By this time, the tone of Lesser Shang (insufficient energy of metal) is similar with the tone of Lesser Zhi (insufficient energy of fire). When Yangming is controlling the weather, it is the tone of Upper Shang (dryness dominating the weather), since the insufficient energy of metal motion receives the help of the dominating dryness, the tone of Upper Shang is similar with the tone of Right Shang (moderate energy of metal). When Jueyin is controlling the weather, it is the tone of Upper Jue (wood domi-

nating the weather), Since the metal is unable to control the wood, so, the tone of Upper Jue is similar with the tone of Right Jue (moderate energy of wood). This is due to the lung benig injured by the fire energy. As the metal is declining and the fire is prosperous, the flame will be bright and vigorous, but when the fire is extremely prosperous, the water will come to retaliate, and the ice, snow, frost and hail will come in the wake of it. The calamity is in the south, and the scaled worms, small reptiles will come out. The storing energy of winter will arrive in advance, and the weather will become very cold.

涸流之纪，是谓反阳，藏令不举，化气乃昌，长气宣布，蛰虫不藏，土润水泉减，草木条茂，荣秀满盛。其气滞，其用渗泄，其动坚止，其发燥槁，其藏肾，其果枣杏，其实濡肉，其谷黍稷，其味甘咸，其色黅玄，其畜彘牛，其虫鳞倮，其主埃郁昏翳，其声羽宫，其病痿厥坚下，从土化也，少羽与少宫同，上宫与正宫同，其病癃闷，邪伤肾也，埃昏骤雨，则振拉摧拔，眚于一，其主毛显狐狢，变化不藏。

"The symbol of 'Drying Flow' which is the insufficient energy of the water motion is the condition of substitution of the Yin energy by the Yang energy. As the storing energy of water can not play its role, the transforming energy of earth will become prosperous, the growth energy will be spreading as well, and the hibernants will not be hiding in time. The earth will be moist, the water in the spring will become less, the grasses and woods will be flourishing and all things will be graceful, plump and prosperous. The insufficient energy of water motion is stagnation, its function is the slow seeping; its variation is firm and fullness; its attack in disease is the dried up of body fluid; its corresponding internal organ of a man is the kidney; in kinds of fruit, they are the jujube and apricot; in the parts of fruit, they are the juice and the pulp; in crops, they are the glutinous millet and millet; in the five tastes, they are the sweetness and the saltiness; in colours, they are the yellow and black; in live-stocks, they are the pig and the cow; in worms, they are the scaled worm and the nacked worm; it dominates the weathers with rising clouds of dust and the gloomy sky; in the five tones, they are the tones of Yu and Gong; in diseases, they are the muscular flaccidity, coldness of the extremities and hard tumor in the lower part of the body due to the insufficient energy of the water motion and the assimilation of water with the earth. When the energy of the water motion is insufficient, the tone of Lesser Yu (insufficient energy of water) is similar with the tone of Lesser Gong (insufficient energy of earth). When Taiyin is controlling the weather, it is the tone of Upper Gong (wetness dominating the weather); since the energy of water motion is insufficient, and at the same time, it is subjugated by wetness that is dominating the weather, the tone of Upper Gong is similar with the tone of Right Gong (moderate energy of earth). In diseases, it is urodialysis or dysuria due to the injury of the kidney energy by the earth energy. As the energy of water motion is insufficient, the sky will be gloomy with dust and the rain will fall suddenly. when the water energy is subjugated by the earth energy excessively, the wood energy (son energy of water) will come to retaliate for its mother, so, the strong gale will rise and the trees will be pulled out and destroyed. The calamity occurs in the north, the caterpillar and the beast of the fox kind will

appear, and the variation will not be concealing.

故乘危而行，不速而至，暴虐无德，灾反及之，微者复微，甚者复甚，气之常也。

"Thus, When the energies of the five element's motion is insufficient, its overcoming energy will take chance to invade rudely, but the son energy of the energy which is being subjugated will come to retaliate, if the injury of the mother energy is slight, the retaliating will be slight also, if the injury of the mother energy is severe, the retaliation will be severe also, and this is the regular rule of the activity of energy.

发生之纪，是谓启敕，土疏泄，苍气达，阳和布化，阴气乃随，生气淳化，万物以荣。其化生，其气美，其政散，其令条舒，其动掉眩巅疾，其德鸣靡启坼，其变振拉摧拔，其谷麻稻，其畜鸡犬，其果李桃，其色青黄白，其味酸甘辛，其象春，其经足厥阴少阳，其藏肝脾，其虫毛介，其物中坚外坚，其病怒。太角与上商同。上徵则其气逆，其病吐利。不务其德，则收气复，秋气劲切，甚则肃杀，清气大至，草木凋零，邪乃伤肝。

"The symbol of 'Early Generation' which is the excessive energy of the wood motion is the spreading of the gentle Yang energy to promote the growth of all things. Due to the excessiveness of the wood energy, the earth energy becomes loose and diffusing, the serene energy of grasses and woods are unimpeded, the Yang energy spreads in all directions and the yin energy retreats. The energy of generation promotes the growth and transformation of all things, and causes them to become flourishing. The excessive energy of the wood motion is fine; its authority of office is spreading outwards; its manifestations are the smoothness and the extension; in the affections of the body, they are shaking, dizziness and the diseases on the top of head; its characteristics are the scattering of the breeze and the making of renovations; in variation, it is the destroying and breaking of the trees by the violent gale; in crops, they are the fibre crop and the rice; in live-stocks, they are the chicken and the dog; in the kinds of fruit, they are the plum and the peach; in colours, they are green, yellow and white; in the five tastes, they are the sourness, sweetness and acridness; its correspoding season is spring; in the channels of man, they are the foot Jueyin and shaoyang; in the internal organs of a man, they are the spleen and the liver; in worms, they are the caterpillar and the cyprid; in substances, it is the substance of firm and hard both inside and outside; in diseases, it is the getting angry; when the wood energy is excessive, it can resist the overcoming metal energy, so the tone of Greater Jue (excessive energy of wood) is similar with the tone of Upper Shang (dryness dominating the weather). when the monarch-fire of Shaoyin or the minister-fire of Shaoyang is controlling the weather, it is the tone of Upper Zhi. (heat or fire is dominating the weather), since the son enegy of wood (fire energy) is controlling its mother energy (wood energy) reversely, in a man, there will be the adverseness of vital energy to cause vomiting and diarrhea. If the wood energy is self-assured of its ability and invade the earth too maliciously, then, the metal energy (son energy of earth) will come to retaliate causing the implementing of the autumn decree, the energies of chillness and restraint will occur; the weather will become cool suddenly, and the grasses and woods will become withered and falling. As the energy of the wood motion is debilitating, the evil energy will in-

jure the liver of man.

赫曦之纪，是谓蕃茂，阴气内化，阳气外荣，炎暑施化，物得以昌。其化长，其气高，其政动，其令鸣〔明抄本"鸣"作"明"〕显，其动炎灼妄扰，其德暄 暑郁蒸，其变炎烈沸腾，其谷麦豆，其畜羊彘，其果杏栗，其色赤白玄，其味苦辛咸，其象夏，其经手少阴太阳，手厥阴少阳，其藏心肺，其虫羽鳞，其物脉濡，其病笑疟疮疡血流狂妄目赤。上羽与正徵同，其收齐，其病痓〔张琦说："其收"六字疑衍'痓'为大阳病，与火运无与〕，上徵而收气后也。暴烈其政，藏气乃复，时见凝惨，甚则雨水霜雹切寒，邪伤心也。

"The symbol of 'Conspicious Flame' which is the excessive energy of the fire motion is in prosperity. When things encounter Taiyang energy, the Yin energy will retreat from inside and the Yang energy will be flourishing outside, the summer-heat will play its role of vapourizing and the grasses and woods will be flourishing. The excessive energy of the fire motion is the promotion of growth; its energy is ascending; its authority of office is to promote; its manifestation is obviousness; its affection to human body are the high fever and the uneasiness; its charateristics are summer-heat, wetness and vapourizing; its variation is the extreme heat like boiling; in crops, they are the wheat and the pea; in live-stocks, they are the sheep and the pig; in the kinds of fruit, they are the apricot and the chestnut; in colours, they are the white and the black; in the five tastes, they are the bitterness, acridness and the sourness; its corresponding season is summer; in the six channels of the body, they are the Hand Shaoyin, Taiyang, Hand Jueyin and Shaoyang; in the internal organs of a man, they are the heart and the lung; in worms, they are the flying insects and the scaled worms; in substances , they are the channel, collateral, juice and fluid; in affections of disease, they are the laughing, malaria, sores, bleeding, mania and red eyes. As the excessive fire energy can be restricted by the cold water which controls the weather, so, the tone of Greater Yu (excessive energy of water) is similar with the tone of Right Zhi (moderate energy of fire). When the fire energy is excessive and the fire energy is controlling the weather at the same time, the combining of the two fires will injure the metal energy, and the role of harvest energy will be postponed. If the energy of the fire motion is extremely violent, the water energy (son energy of metal energy) will come to retaliate for its mother, the scene of condensation and destitude will occur, the rain, frost and hail will fall and the weather will become extremely cold. When the energy of the fire motion falls into a decline, the evil energy will injure the heart of human body.

敦阜之纪，是谓广化，厚德清静，顺长以盈，至阴内实，物化充成，烟埃朦郁，见于厚土，大雨时行，湿气乃用，燥政乃辟，其化圆，其气丰，其政静，其令周备，其动濡积并稸，其德柔润重淖，其变震惊飘骤崩溃，其谷稷麻，其畜牛犬，其果枣李，其色黅玄苍，其味甘咸酸，其象长夏，其经足太阴阳明，其藏脾肾，其虫倮毛，其物肌核，其病腹满，四支不举，大风迅至，邪伤脾也。

"The symbol of 'High and Thick' which is the excessive energy of the earth motion is the excessive energy of transformation. The characteristc of earth is thick and calm, it causes all things to suit the season to grow and become full and abundant. As the refined energy

of earth can substantialize things internally, it makes all things to be transformed and being shaped. When the earth energy is excessive, it will vapourize like smokes and dusts that occur above the hill, the pouring rain will appear, the wetness energy will run amuck and the power of dryness will keep out of the way. The ability of the excessive energy of the earth motion is satisfactoriness; its energy is abundant; its authority of office is to keep calm; its manifestation is comprehensiveness; its affection to human body is the accumulation of wetness; its characteristics are smoothness and gloss; its variations are the shock of the thunderbolt, sudden fall of torential rain and the landslide: in crops, they are the millet and the fibre crop; in live-stocks, they are the cow and the dog; in the kinds of fruit, they are the jujube and the plum; in colours, they are yellow, black and green; in five tastes, they are the sweetness, saltness and the sourness; its corresponding season is the long summer; in the six channels of a man, they are the Foot Taiyin and Yangming; in the internal organs of a man, they are the spleen and the kidney; in worms, they are the naked worm and the caterpillar; in substances, they belong to the meat and the kernal kind; in the attacks of diseases they are the abdominal fullness and the failing of lifting up the extremities. When the energy of earth motion is excessive to injure the water, the wood energy (son energy of water energy) will come to retaliate for its mother, so, the strong gale will occur instantly. Since the energy of earth falls into a decline, in the course of combate with the wood, the evil energy will injure the spleen of man.

坚成之纪，是为收引，天气洁，地气明，阳气随，阴治化，燥行其政，物以司成，收气繁布，化洽不终。其化成，其气削，其政肃，其令锐切，其动暴折疡疰，其德雾露萧飋，其变肃杀雕零，其谷稻黍，其畜鸡马，其果桃杏，其色白青丹，其味辛酸苦，其象秋，其经手太阴阳明，其脏肺肝，其虫介羽，其物壳络，其病喘喝，胸凭仰息，上徵与正商同，其生齐，其病咳。政暴变，则名木不荣，柔脆焦首，长气斯救，大火流，炎烁且至，蔓将槁，邪伤肺也。

"The symbol of 'Firm and Blocked' which is the excessive energy of the metal motion is the restraining of Yang. As the energy of heaven is clean and the energy of earth is smooth and unimpeded and the energy of dryness metal is able to play its role causing all things to yield fruits. But since the harvest energy is spreading frequently, the transforming energy will not be able to play its role thorougthly. The excessive energy of the metal motion reduces the growth, its functions are cutting and weakening; its authorities of office are the excessive chilliness and restraint; its manifestations are sharpness and urgency; in the affections to human body, they are the bone fracture and the sore in skin; its charateristics are the sough of mists and dew; its variations are chilliness and desolation; in crops, they are the rice and the glutinous millet; in live-stocks, they are the chicken and horse; in the kinds of fruit, they are the peach and the apricot; in colours, they are white, green and red; in the five tastes, they are the acridness, sourness and the bitterness; its corresponding season is autumn; in channels of a man, they are the Hand Taiyin and Yangming; in internal organs of a man, they are the lung and the liver: in worms, they are the flying insects and the cater-

pillars; in substance, they belong to the shell and the sponge kind; in diseases, they are the rapid breathing and expiratory dyspnea which cause the patient fall to lie down. As the excessive metal energy can be restricted by the fire energy, so, the tone of Upper Zhi (fire dominating the weather) is similar with the tone of Right Shang (moderate energy of metal). As the metal energy is restricted, it can no longer subjugate the wood, so, the energy of generation will be able to keep balance with the energies of growth, transforming, harvesting and storing, and the disease occurred will be cough only. If the excessive energy of the metal motion implements its decree despotically, then, the big trees will not be flourishing, the tender and weak grasses and woods will be withered and die, the growth energy of summer will be resumed, the heat will be prevailing and the creeping weed will be withered. When the energy of the metal falls into a decline, the evil energy will injure the lung of a man.

流衍之纪，是谓封藏。寒司物化，天地严凝，藏政以布，长令不扬。其化凛，其气坚，其政谧，其令流注，其动漂泄沃涌，其德凝惨寒雰，其变冰雪霜雹，其谷豆稷，其畜彘牛，其果栗枣，其色黑丹黅，其味咸苦甘，其象冬，其经足少阴大阳，其脏肾心，其虫鳞倮，其物濡满，其病胀，上羽而长气不化也。政过则化气大举，而埃昏气交，大雨时降，邪伤肾也。故曰：不恒其德，则所胜来复，政恒其理，则所胜同化。此之谓也。

"The symbol of 'Flooding' which is the excessive energy of the water motion is shutting and hiding. By this time, the hiding energy is dominating, the weather is cold, the things on earth are frozen, and the growth energy can not play its role. The activating ability of the excessive energy of the water motion is to cause cold; its energies are the firmness and solidification; its authority of office is calmness; its manifestations are the wetness and the pouring of water; as the effects to man, they are diarrhea with pain and salivation; its characteristic is the cold energy of gloominess; its variations are the weathers of ice, snow, frost, and hail; in crops, they are the pea and the millet; in live-stocks, they are the pig and the cow; in the kinds of fruit, they are the chestnut and the jujube; in colours, they are black, red and yellow; in five tastes, they are the saltiness, bitterness and the sweetness; its sign is winter; in the six channels of a man, they are the Foot Shaoyin and Taiyang; in the internal organs of a man, they are the kidney and the heart; in worms, they are the scaled worm and the naked worm; in substance, it belongs to the liquid which is full; in disease, it is the abdominal distention due to the inability of the spreading of the growth energy of fire. If the excessive energy of the water motion injures the fire energy too much, the earth energy (son enercy of fire) will come to retaliate for its mother, the combat of water and earth will cause the pouring rain. When the energy of water motion falls into a decline, the evil energy will injure the kidney of a man.

"Thus, when the element's energy fails to remain its normal function, and relying its ability to bully the weak one excessively, another element's energy which can overcome it will come to retaliate. If the element's energy implements its function normally, even though it is invaded by a strong element's energy, the strong element's energy may also be assimilated。"

帝曰：天不足西北，左寒而右凉；地不满东南，右热而左温；其故何也？岐伯曰：阴阳

之气，高下之理，太少之异也。东南方，阳也，阳者其精降于下，故右热而左温。西北方，阴也，阴者其精奉于上，故左寒而右凉。是以地有高下，气有温凉，高者气寒，下者气热，故适寒凉者胀，之〔按“之”应作“适”〕温热者疮，下之则胀已，汗之则疮已，此腠理开闭之常，太少之异耳。

Yellow Emperor asked: "The heaven energy is insufficient in the northwest to cause coldness in the north and coolness in the west; the earth energy is not full in the southeast to cause hotness in the south and warmness in the east, what is the reason?" Qibo said: "It is because the Yin and Yang energie in heaven and earth and in the high and low altitudes of the terrain are different in extent. The southeast belongs to Yang, and the refined energy of Yang descends from up above, so the south is hot and the east is warm; the north-west belongs to Yin, and the refined energy of Yin ascends from below, so, the west is cool and the north is cold. Thus, in terrain, there are the alttitudes of high and low; in weather, there are the weathers of warm and cold. When the altitude is high, the weather is cold, when the altitude is low, the weather is hot. When one goes to the cold and cool place in northwest, he is apt to contract abdominal distention, when he goes to the warm and hot place in southeast, he is apt to contract sores. The patient who suffers from abdominal distention can be cured by applying the drugs of purgation, to the patient who suffers from sores can be cured by applying the diaphoretic drugs, and these are the common condition concerning the weather, terrain and the openning and shutting of the striae of human body, when treating, it can be varied according to the different extents of the disease's condition。"

帝曰：其余寿夭何如？岐伯曰：阴精所奉其人寿，阳精所降其人夭。帝曰：善。其病也，治之奈何？岐伯曰：西北之气散而寒之，东南之气收而温之，所谓同病异治也。故曰：气寒气凉，治以寒凉，行水渍之；气温气热。治以温热，强其内守，必同其气，可使平也，假者反之。帝曰：善。一州之气，生化寿夭不同，其故何也？岐伯曰：高下之理，地势使然也。崇高则阴气治之，污下则阳气治之，阳胜者先天，阴胜者后天，此地理之常，生化之道也。帝曰：其有寿夭乎？岐伯曰：高者其气寿，下者其气夭。地之小大异也，小者小异，大者大异。故治病者，必明天道地理，阴阳更胜，气之先后，人之寿夭，生化之期，乃可以知人之形气矣。

Yellow Emperor asked: "How do the refined energies of Yin and Yang affect the life span of a man?" Qibo said: "The people staying in the place where the refined energy of Yin is ascending, their striae will be dense, and they will live long. The people living in the place where the refined energy of Yang is descending, their striae will be loose and they will die early。"

Yellow Emperor said: "Good. But how to treat the disease?"

Qibo said: As the weather in the northwest is cold, one must disperse the external coldness and clear away the internal heat; the weather in the southwest is warm and hot, one must collect and restrain the excreted Yang energy and warm the internal coldness, and these are the ways in treating the same disease with different ways. Therefore, the people living in the place of cold weather often have internal heat, and it can be treated with the

drugs of cold nature or soak with decoction; the people living in the place of hot weather often have endogenous cold-syndrome, and it can be treated with the warming therapy to expel the cold, besides, one must guard against the excretion of the true Yang of the patient. In treating, it must be in accordance with the local weather and make the energy to become agreeable and moderate. To the cold disease of pseudo heat syndrome of the fever of pseudo cold syndrome, it should be treated in the reverse way。"

Yellow Emperor said: "Good. But in the same place and in the same weather, the growth conditions and the life spans of men are different, and what is the reason?" Qibo said: "It is due to the different altitude of the terrain. In the terrain with high altitude, the weather is dominated by the Yin energy and it is cold; in the place with low altitude, the weather is dominated by the Yang energy and it is hot. When the Yang energy is excessive, the weather will come prior to the season, when the Yin energy is excessive, the weather will lag behind the season, and this is the common law between the high and low altitude and the early or late generation and growth of all things。"

Yellow Emperor asked: "Is it related to the life span of a man?" Qibo said: "In the terrain of high altitude, the primordial energy of a man is stable due to the cold weather, so, he will live long; in the terrain of low altitude, the primordial energy of a man is excretive due to the hot weather, and he will die early. The difference of life spans are also related with the size of the region: the life span of a man in a small region will be shorter and the life span of a man is longer in a large region. Thus, in treating, one must know the law of heaven and the terrain, the condition of overcoming of Yin and Yang, the early or late coming of the weather, the life span of man, and the time of generation and transformation, then can one know the physique and the mechanism of energy of man。"

帝曰：善。其岁有不病，而藏气不应不用者何也？岐伯曰：天气制之，气有所从也。帝曰：愿卒闻之。岐伯曰：少阳司天，火气下临，肺气上从，白起金用，草木眚，火见燔焫，革金且耗，大暑以行，咳嚏鼽衄鼻窒，口疡，寒热胕肿，风行于地，尘沙飞扬，心痛胃脘痛，厥逆鬲不通，其主暴速。

Yellow Emperor said。" Good. Sometimes, when according to the dominating energy of the year, one should have contracted the disease, but the disease does not occur; or when the related visceral energy should be corresponding, but fails to correspond and what is the reason?" Qibo said: "It is due to the visceral energy of a man must follow a certain energy which controls the weather。"

Yellow Emperor said: "I hope to hear the details about it。" Qibo said: "when the prime minister-fire of Shaoyang is controlling the weather, the fire energy will be spreading, the lung will be subjugated by the fire energy first, and the metal will follow the weather which is dominated by fire above, the metal will assimilated with the fire and will play the role of fire, so, the grasses and woods on earth will be injured, the scorching fire will injure the metal and the summer-heat will be prevailing. In a man, the diseases of coughing, sneezing, hemorrhage, stuffy nose, sores, malaria and edema will occur.

"When the liver wood of Jueyin is affecting the earth energy, the wind will rise on earth, the dust and sand will be flying. In a man, the diseases of heartache, stomachache, coldness of limbs, obstruction between the chest and the diaphram will occur instantly.

阳明司天，燥气下临，肝气上从，苍起木用而立，土乃眚，凄沧数至，木伐草萎，胁痛目赤，掉振鼓慄，筋痿不能久立。暴热至，土乃暑，阳气郁发，小便变，寒热如疟，甚则心痛，火行于槁，流水不冰，蛰虫乃见。

"When the dryness metal of Yangming is controlling the weather, the dryness energy will descend to the earth, and the liver energy will be subjugated first, the wood liver will follow the weather which is dominated by dryness above, and the wood will assimilate with metal and play the role of metal, so, the earth energy will be injured, the cool energy will come now and then, the wood will be destroyed and the grasses withered. In a man, the diseases of pain on the lateral sides of the thorax, red eyes, shaking, shivering, flaccidity syndrome involing the muscle and inability to stand long will occur. As Yangming is controlling the weather, the monarch-fire of Shaoyin will be affecting the earth energy, so, the summer-heat will arrive and the earth energy will become hot and vaporized. In a man, the Yang energy will be stagnated inside to cause diseases; the urine will turn yellow, the alternating episodes of chilliness and fever like malaria will occur, and the patient may go so far as to have heartache. During the time when the fire energy is prevailing, the grasses and woods become withered, the flowing water will not freeze and the hibernants will be seen outside.

太阳司天，寒气下临，心气上从，而火且明，丹起金乃眚，寒清时举，胜则水冰，火气高明，心热烦，嗌乾善渴，鼽嚏，喜悲数欠，热气妄行，寒乃复，霜不时降，善忘，甚则心痛。土乃润，水丰衍，寒客至，沉阴化，湿气变物，水饮内稸，中满不食，皮痹肉苛，筋脉不利，甚则胕肿，身后痈。

"When the cold water of Taiyang is controlling the weather, the cold energy will descend on the earth and the heart fire will be restricted. The fire energy will follow the weather which is dominated by the cold above, and fire will assimilate with water and play the role of water. As fire is invaded by water, the fire will turn to subjugate the metal, and the metal will be injured. As a result, the cold and cool energies will occur and the water will freeze. As the fire energy is compelled to flame up, the diseases of heart-heat, oppression over the chest, dry throat, running nose, sneezing, melancholy, frequent yawn will occur: the heat energy will run wantonly above, the cold energy will come to retaliate below, the cold frost will descend now and then, and the spirit and energy of man will be injured. As the heart fire energy is invaded by the water energy, the patient will be forgetful, he even goes so far as to have heartache. As Taiyang is controlling the weather, the wetness earth energy of Taiyin will be affecting the earth energy. Since earth can control water, so, the earth energy will be moistened, and the water will be abundant. When the guest energy of cold water occurs, the fire will assimilate with the wetnss earth, and all things will be deformed due to the cold-wetness energy. In a man, the diseases of fluid retention, inability to take in food due to abdominal fullness, numbness of the skin and numbness of the muscle will occur. The

patient may even go so far as to contract edema and can hardly turn his body.

厥阳司天，风气下临，脾气上从，而土且隆，黄起，水乃眚，土用革，体重，肌肉萎，食减口爽，风行太虚，云物摇动，目转耳鸣。火纵其暴，地乃暑，大热消烁，赤沃下，蛰虫数见，流水不冰，其发机速。

"When the wind wood of Jueyin is controlling the weathar, the wind energy will descend on the earth, and the spleen energy will be restricted, the earth energy will assimilate with the wood energy and play the role of wood. When the earth is invaded by the wood, the earth will turn to restrict the water, the water will be injured and the functions of earth will be altered as well. In a man, the diseases of heaviness of the body, muscular atrophy, reduction of taking in food, flat taste in the mouth will occur. As the wind energy is moving in the sky, the clouds, grasses and woods will be swaying, and man will suffer dizziness and tinnitus. As the Jueyin is controlling the weather, the prime minister-fire Shaoyang will affect the earth energy, the fire energy will be prevailing, and the earth will have scorching heat like summer. In a man, the diarrhea with bloody stool will occur. By this time, the hibernants can often be seen outside, the flowing water is not frozen, and the attacks of the disease is very rapid.

少阴司天，热气下临，肺气上从，白起金用，草木眚，喘呕寒热，嚏鼽衄鼻窒，大暑流行，甚则疮疡燔灼，金烁石流。地乃燥清〔读本，赵本，吴本"燥"下并无"清"字〕，凄沧数至，胁痛善太息，肃杀行，草木变。

"When the monach-fire of Shaoyin is controlling the weather, the heat energy will descend on the earth, and the lung engery will be restricted and it will follow the weather which is dominated by the heat above. The metal will assimilate with fire and play the role of fire, so, the grasses and woods will be injured. In a man, the diseases of rapid breathing, vomiting, cold and heat, sneezing, running nose, hemorrhage and stuffy nose will occur. As the fire energy is in power, the great heat of summer will be prevailing, the diseases of sores and high fever may even occur. The sweltering summer heat seems capable to melt the metal and stone. As Shaoyin is controlling the weather, the dryness metal of Yangming will affect the earth energy, the dryness energy will move on earth and the cold and cool energies will come now and then. In a man, the pain in the lateral sides of the thorax will occur, and the patient will sigh often. As the chilly and restraining energies are prevailing, the appearance and the build of grasses and woods will be altered.

太阴司天，湿气下临，肾气上从，黑起水变〔林校云："详前后文，'变'下少'火乃青'三字"〕，埃冒云雨，胸中不利，阴痿，气大衰，而不起不用。当其时，反腰脽痛，动转不便也，厥逆。地乃藏阴，大寒且至，蛰虫早附，心下否痛，地裂冰坚，少腹痛，时害于食，乘金则止水增，味乃咸，行水减也。

When the wetness earth of Taiyin is controlling the weather, the wetness energy will descend on the earth, the kidney energy will be restricted and it will follow the weather which is dominated by wetness above. The water will assimilate with the earth and play the role of earth, and the clouds and rains will occur. In man, the diseases of unquietness of the

chest, impotence, extreme debility of Yang energy, fails to erect and inability of conducting sexual action will occur. By this time, the loins and the buttocks of the patient will be painful, and he will have difficulty to turn around. As Taiyin is controlling the weather, the cold water energy of Taiyang will affect the earth energy, the cold water energy will attach the earth, the great cold will come and the hibernants will hide press close to the earth in advance. In the attack of the disease, the epigastric fullness with pain will occur. If the cold energy is excessive, the earth will be frozen to cracks, the water will be frozen, and in man, the syndrome of pain in the lower abdomen affecting the food intake will occur. When the water energy invades the lung metal energy, the water will be active, When it encounters the metal, the cold energy will be even prominent (metal produces water), as a result, the water in the spring and the well will be increased, its taste will become salty due to the reduction of water poured from the river。"

帝曰：岁有胎不孕不育，治之不全，何气使然？岐伯曰：六气五类，有相胜制也，同者盛之，异者衰之，此天地之道，生化之常也。故厥阴司天，毛虫静，羽虫育，介虫不成；在泉，毛虫育，倮虫耗，羽虫不育。少阴司天，羽虫静，介虫育，毛虫不成；在泉，羽虫育，介虫耗不育。太阴司天，倮虫静，鳞虫育，羽虫不成；在泉，倮虫育，鳞虫〔林校云："详'鳞虫'下少一'耗'字"〕不成。少阳司天，羽虫静，毛虫育，倮虫不成；在泉，羽虫育，介虫耗，毛虫不育。阳明司天，介虫静，羽虫育，介虫不成；在泉，介虫育，毛虫耗，羽虫不成。太阳司天鳞虫静，倮虫育；在泉，鳞虫耗〔林校云："详此当作'鳞虫育，羽虫耗'"〕，倮虫不育。诸乘所不成之运，则甚也。故气主有所制，岁立有所生，地气制已胜，天气制胜已，天制色，地制形，五类衰盛，各随其气之所宜也。故有胎孕不育，治之不全，此气之常也，所谓中根也。根于外者亦五，故生化之别，有五气五味五色五类五宜也。帝曰：何谓也？岐伯曰：根于中者，命曰神机，神去则机息。根于外者，命曰气立，气止则化绝。故各有制，各有胜，各有生，各有成。故曰：不知年之所加，气之同异，不足以言生化，此之谓也。

Yellow Emperor asked: "Some of the worms can be pregnant and multiply each year and some can not, their conditions of generation are different, and what is the reason?" Qibo Said: "The, five kinds of worm (caterpillar, flying insect, naked worm, cyprid and scaled worm) which are bred by the six-weather and the five-element are overcoming and subjugating each other. If the six-weather is similar with the energy of the five-element's motion, the living things will be exuberant, if they are different with each other, the living things will fall into a decline. This is the rule of breeding in the universe and the natural law of growth and transformation. Thus, when Jueyin is controlling the weather, the caterpillar will be kept intact and remained calm, the flying insect will be able to multiply, and the cyprid will not grow up. When Jueyin is affecting the earth energy, the caterpillar will be able to multiply, the naked worm will be injured and the flying insect will not be able to multiply.

When Shaoyin is controlling the weather, the flying insect will be kept intact and remained calm, the cyprid will be able to multiply, and the caterpillar will not grow up. When Shaoyin is affecting the earth energy, the flying insect will be able to multiply, the cyprid will be injured and will not be able to multiply.

"When Taiyin is controlling the weather, the naked worm will be kept intact and remained calm, the scaled worm will be able to multiply and the flying insect will not grow up. When Taiyin is affecting the earth energy, the naked worm will be able to multiply, but the scaled worm will be injured and will not grow up.

"When Shaoyang is controlling the weather, the flying insect will be kept intact and remained calm, the caterpillar will be able to multiply and the naked worm will not grow up. When the Shaoyang is affecting the earth energy, the flying insect will be able to multiply, the cyprid will be injured and the caterpillar will not be able to multiply.

"When Shaoyang is controlling the weather, the cyprid will be kept intact and remained calm, the flying insect will be able to multiply, and the cyprid will not grow up. When Yangming is affecting the earth energy, the cyprid will be able to multiply, the caterpillar will be injured and the flying insect will not grow up.

"When Taiyang is controlling the weather, the scaled worm will be kept intact and remained calm, and the naked worm will be able to multiply. When the Taiyang is affecting the earth energy, the scaled worm will be able to multiply, the flying insect will be injured, and the naked worm will not able be to multiply.

"If the energy of the element's motion being subjugated by the six-weather to hinder the growth, the condition will be even more serious. Thus, each of the six energies has its targets of dominating and overcoming, and each year's energy motion has its function of promoting growth and transformation to certain thing, the energy that affects the earth energy often controls the enegry which it can overcome, and the energy that controls the weather often restricts the energy which can overcome itself; the energy that controls the weather determines the colour, and the energy that affects the earth energy determines the shape. The prosperity and declination of the five kinds of worm in propagation depend on the conditions of the six weathers, and thus, there are the different conditions of pregnacy and sterility. It is not due to the imcompleteness of generating and transforming energies, but it is the normal condition in the energy of element's motion, which is called the 'Internal source of Vitality'.

"As to the living things without consciousness (like trees and crops), their source of vitality is outside, and they have different extent of generation and transformation according to the different conditions of the element's motion. As a result, they are of the five odours of the foul, scorched, fragrant, stink and rancid, the five tastes of sourness, bitterness, acridness, saltness, and sweetness, the five colours of green, yellow, red, white and black, and the five kinds of worm of caterpillar, flying insect, naked worm, scaled worm and cyprid, and they each plays its proper role to suit each other。"

Yellow Emperor asked: "Why is it so?" Qibo said: "when the source of vitality of the living thing hides inside, it is called the mechanism of the spirit, if the spirit moves away, the mechanism of generation and transformation will be severed. When the source of vitality stays outside, it is called the 'Establishment of Engrgy', when the outside energy stops, the

generation and transformation will be stopped. Thus, each of the element's motion has something to control, to overcome, to generate and to accomplish. If one does not know the arriving time of the energy of the year and the six weathers, the similarity and difference of the six weather, he will not understand the conditions of generation and transformation。"

帝曰：气始而生化，气散而有形，气布而蕃育，气终而象变，其致一也。然而五味所资，生化有薄厚，成熟有少多，终始不同，其故何也？岐伯曰：地气制之也，非天不生地不长也，帝曰：愿闻其道。岐伯曰：寒热燥湿，不同其化也。故少阳在泉，寒毒不生，其味辛，其治苦酸，其谷苍丹。阳明在泉，湿毒不生，其味酸，其气湿，其治辛苦甘，其谷丹素。太阳在泉，热毒不生，其味苦，其治淡咸，其谷黅秬。厥阴在泉，清毒不生，其味甘，其治酸苦，其谷苍赤。其气专，其味正。少阴在泉，寒毒不生，其味辛，其治辛苦甘，其谷白丹。太阴在泉，燥毒不生，其味咸，其气热，其治甘咸，其谷黅秬。化淳则咸守，气专则辛化而俱治。

Yellow Emperor asked: "Since when the energy is formed, there will be generation and transformation, when the energy moves, it will accomplish the substance of thing, when the energy spreads, there will be multiplication, when the energy ends, the shape of thing will be changing, and all their substances are alike. But in the conditions of receiving the energies of the five tastes, there are the different conditions of heavy and slight in generation and transformation, different extents in promoting the maturity, and the different affections at the beginning and the end and what is the reason?" Qibo said: "It is due to the different energy that affects the earth energy causing the different conditions of promoting the generation and transformation, and it is not due to the failure of the heaven energy to produce life and earth energy to promote growth。"

Yellow Emperor said: " I hope to know the reason about it。" Qibo said: " The activities of energy of the cold, heat, dryness and wetness are different, so, when the prime-minister-fire of Shaoyang is affecting the earth energy, the cold toxicant will not produce. As fire restricts metal, metal assimilates with the fire, so, the taste is acrid: as the Shaoyang associates with the fire and its intermediate energy Jueyin associates with wood, so, the main tastes for treating are the bitterness and sourness. In the colours of the crops they are green and red.

"When the dryness metal of Yangming is affecting the earth energy, the wet toxicant will not produce. As metal restricts wood, it assimilates with the metal, so, its taste is sourness, and its energy is the wetness; as the Yangming metal is acrid, the prime minister-fire which controls heaven energy is bitter, and the wetness is sweet, so, the main tastes for treating are acridness, bitterness and sweetness. In the colours of the crops, they are red and white.

"When the cold water of Taiyang is affecting the earth energy, the hot toxicant will not produce. As water restricts the fire and the fire assimilates with the water, so, its taste is bitterness; the main tastes for treating are mildness and saltness. In the colours of the crops, they are yellow and black。"

"When the wind wood of Jueyin is affecting the earth energy, the cool toxicant will not

produce. As the wood restricts the earth and earth is assimilated with the wood, so, its taste is sweet; the taste of wood is sour, when prime minister-fire is controlling the weather, its taste is bitter, so, the main tastes for treating are sourness and bitterness. In the colours of the crops, they are green and red. Since the Jueyin is affecting the earth, and Shaoyang is controlling the weather, as wood produces fire, the activity of energy will be concentrating and its taste will be pure.

"When the monarch-fire of Shaoyin is affecting the earth energy, the cold toxicant will not produce. As the fire restricts the metal and the metal is assimilated with the fire, so, its taste is acrid. As the taste of metal energy which controls the weather is acridness, the taste of fire which is affecting the earth energy is bitterness, and the taste of intermediate energy is sweetness, so, the main tastes for treating are acridness, bitterness and sweetness. In the colours of the crops, they are white and red.

"When the wetness earth of Taiyin is affecting the earth energy, the dry toxicant will not produce. As the earth restricts the water and the water assimilates with the earth, so, its taste is saltiness and its energy is hot. As the taste of wetness earth is sweet, the taste of the cold water which controls the weather is salty, so, the main tastes for treating are sweetness and saltness. Its colours in the crops are yellow and black. As Taiyin is affecting the earth energy, its activating of energy will be pure and thick, as the earth can ristrict the water, so, its saltness can be kept inside, since the earth produces the metal, so, the energy produced will be unified and pure. As a result, the acridness can also become active and dominates with the wetness earth jointly.

故曰：补上下者从之，治上下者逆之，以所在寒热盛衰而调之。故曰：上取下取，内取外取，以求其过。能毒者以厚药，不胜毒者以薄药，此之谓也。气反者，病在上，取之下；病在下，取之上；病在中，傍取之。治热以寒，温而行之；治寒以热，凉而行之；治温以清，冷而行之；治清以温，热而行之。故消之削之，吐之下之，补之写之，久新同法。

"Therefore, to the disease induced by the insufficient energy that controls the heaven energy or the insufficient energy that affects the earth energy, the invigorating therapy should be applied, and the invigoration should be carried on favourably with the energy; to the disease induces by the excessive energy that controls the heaven energy or the excessive energy that affects the earth energy, the therapeutic method should be applied, and the treatment should be carried on reversely to the energy, and all treatments should be aimed to adjust the cold, heat, overabundance and decline. So, no mater when treating the excessive energy with medicine, eliminating the indigestive food with purgative drugs, applying internal management or treat with external measures, one must find out first the reason of insufficiency or the excessiveness of the energy. Apply the medicine with violent property and rich flavour to the patient which has a strong body which is capable to withstand toxin, and give the medicine with mild property and light flavour to the patient who has a weak body and can not withstand toxin. If the condition of the disease is abnormal, treat the upper part of the body, When the disease is in the lower part, and treat the left or right side when the disease

is in the middle. When treating the fever, apply the drugs with cold property, and the decoction should be taken when it is warm; when treating the cold disease, apply the drugs with hot property, and take the decoction when it is cold; when treating the seasonal febrile disease, apply the drugs with cool property, and the decoction should be taken when it is cold; when treating the cool disease, apply the drugs with warm property, and the decoction should be taken when it is hot. As the patient's body has the different conditions of being sthenic and asthenic, the ways in treating must not be the same. According to the different conditions of the patient, use the dispelling therapy, whittling therapy, vomiting therapy, purgative therapy and the invigorative therpy respectively. This rule must be observed in treating both the protracted and the newly contracted diseases。"

帝曰：病在中而不实不坚，且聚且散，奈何？岐伯曰：悉乎哉问也！无积者求其藏，虚则补之，药以祛之，食以随之，行水渍之，和其中外，可使毕已。

Yellow Emperor asked: "In the case of inside disease which is not substantial nor firm, sometimes it concentrates to become shaped, sometimeg it disperses to become shapless, and how to treat it?" Qibo said: "what an exhaustive question you have asked. If there is no stagnation, the reason of the disease should be seeked from the internal organs. If the disease is of asthenic, the invigorating therapy should be applied first, then, nourish the patient with food and drink, soak and bathe the affected part with hot decoction to adjust the interior and the exterior of the patient, so as the disease may be cured。"

帝曰：有毒无毒，服有约乎？岐伯曰：病有久新，方有大小，有毒无毒，固宜常制矣。大毒治病，十去其六；常〔《素问玄机原病式·火》引"常"作"小"〕毒治病，十去其七；小〔《原病式》引"小"作"常"〕毒治病，十去其八；无毒治病，十去其九；谷肉果菜，食养尽之，无使过之，伤其正也。不尽，行复如法，必先岁气，无伐天和，无盛盛，无虚虚，而遗人夭殃，无致邪，无失正，绝人长命。帝曰：其久病者，有气从不康，病去而瘠，奈何？岐伯曰：昭乎哉圣人之问也！化不可代，时不可违。夫经络以通，血气以从，复其不足，与众齐同，养之和之，静以待时，谨守其气，无使倾移，其形乃彰，生气以长，命曰圣王。故《大要》曰：无代化，无违时，必养必和，待其来复。此之谓也。帝曰：善。

Yellow Emperor asked: "Is there any restriction when taking the poisonous and poisonless drugs: "Qibo said: "In diseases, some are protracted and some are newly contracted; in prescriptions, some of the quantities are large and some are small: in decoctions, some drugs are of toxicant and some are not; and there are certain rules in taking them. The drugs with great toxicity should be ceased when the disease is removed by 60%; the drugs with small toxicity should be ceased when the disease is removed by 70%; the common drug should be ceased when the discase is removed by 80%; the drug without any toxicity should be ceased when the disease is removed by 90%. After the ceasing of drug, the patient should take the cereals, meats, fruits and vegetables to eliminate all the remaining evil energy. If some of the evil energy is still remaining, the patient may take the drug again according to the way stated above. Thus, one must be sure to know in advance the partial overabundance of the year's energy, avoid to attack the harmonized primordial energy, nor to cause the sthenic en-

ergy becoming even more sthenic and the asthenic energy becoming even more asthenic, so as not to leave the patient with future trouble. In a word, not to make the evil energy to become more abundant and not to forfeit the patient's healthy energy to ruin his life.

Yellow Emperor asked: "Sometimes, the healthy energy of the patient with protracted disease can not be recovered, although the disease has been removed, yet he is still having an emaciated and weak body, can we do anything with it?" Qibo said: "what a brilliant question you have asked. The ability of promoting the generation and transformation energy of the heaven and earth to all things can not be substituted by man, and the sequence of the four seasons must not be violated by man. One can only suit the activity of the energies of the four seasons to maintain the unimpediness of the channels and the collaterals, and the fluent circulation of the energy and blood, so as to resume its normal condition from insufficiency gradually. when invigorating or adjusting the energy, one must observe carefully and guard the healthy energy prudently against waste and comsumption. By this way, the physique of the patient can be recovered and the vital energy may be increased day after day, and this is the so called 'The Method of the Holy King'. In the《Essentials》, it was stated: 'Do not substitude the activity of energy with the power of man, and do not violate the movements of the four seasons, one must keep calm and be patient to wait for the restoration of the healthy energy'。" Yellow Emperor said: "Good。"

六元正纪大论篇第七十一

Chapter 71
Liu Yuan Zheng Ji Da Lun
(On the Changes and Symbols of the Five Elements' Motion and the Six Kinds of Weather in the Cycle of Sixty Years)

黄帝问曰：六化六变，胜复淫治，甘苦辛咸酸淡先后，余知之矣。夫五运之化，或从五气，或逆天气，或从天气而逆地气，或从地气而逆天气，或相得，或不相得，余未能明其事。欲通天之纪，从地之理，和其运，调其化，使上下合德，无相夺伦，天地升降，不失其宜，五运宣行，勿乖其政，调之正味，从逆奈何？岐伯稽首再拜对曰：昭乎哉问也，此天地之纲纪，变化之渊源，非圣帝孰能穷其至理欤！臣虽不敏，请陈其道，令终不灭，久而不易。

Yellow Emperor said: "Now I understand the normal and abnormal conditions about the six energies, the relations between the overcoming energy and the retaliating energy, the treatment for balancing Yin and Yang and the reasons of the early or late generation and transformation caused by the tastes of sweetness, bitterness, acridness, sourness and mildness. But sometimes, the activity of the energy of the five-element is agreeable with the energy that controls the heaven energy, sometimes, it violates it, sometimes it agrees with the energy that affects the earth energy, but goes against the energy that controls the heaven energy; sometimes it agrees with the energy that controls the heaven energy but goes against the energy that affects the earth energy; sometimes they are fit with each other, sometimes they are not, I do not understand the reason. I want to follow the law of the six energies of heaven, obey the rule of the five elements of earth, regulate the energy activity of the five elements' motion, so that the energies up above and down below may not violate each other, the rise and fall of the heaven and earth energies may in their routine patterns, the five elements being unimpeded without deviating from their authorities of office, and to adjust the agreeable or reverse activity of energy with the five tastes. How should I do it?"

Qibo bowed again and again and said: "What an explicit question you have asked! This is the guiding principle of generation and transformation of heaven and earth, and it is the origin of the changes of the six-energy and the five-motion. who can make a thorough inquiry to its quintessence save a wise sage? Although I am not talented, yet I like to illustrate its principle to you, so that it may be last long without changing."

帝曰：愿夫子推而次之，从其类序，分其部主，别其宗司，昭其气数，明其正化，可得闻乎？岐伯曰：先立其年以明其气，金木水火土运行之数，寒暑燥湿风火临御之化，则天道可见，民气可调，阴阳卷舒，近而无惑，数之可数者，请遂言之。

Yellow Emperor said: "I hope you can distinguish the host energy, the guest energy, the dominating energy and the subordinate energy in the six kinds of weater according to the categories and sequences, and clarify the symbols and the rules of the activity of the energy of the five-motion for me。"

Qibo said: "One must set the decimal cycle and the duodecimal cycle of the year first to ascertain the dominate energy of the year, to know the conditions of the metal, wood, water, fire and earth energies of the five-element motion that dominating the year and the principal and subordinate changes of the six weather of cold, heat, dryness, wetness, fire and wind. In this way, the law of nature can be understood. the energy mechanism of man can be adjusted and the reasons of victory and defeat of Yin and Yang can be known without perplexity. The symbols of the weather and the element's motion can be traced by calculation, and I like to try my best to explain it。"

帝曰：太阳之政奈何？岐伯曰：辰戌之纪也。

Yellow Emperor asked: "what are the conditions of the five elements' motion and the six kinds of weather when Taiyang is controlling the heaven energy?" Qibo soid: "They are the two years which are marked by the symbols of Chen and Xu of the duodecimal cycle.

太阳　太角　太阴　壬辰　壬戌　其运风，其化鸣紊启拆，其变振拉摧拔，其病眩掉目瞑。

太角初正　少徵　太宫　少商　太羽终

"In the Chen year and the Xu year, the cold water of Taiyang controls the heaven energy, and the wetness earth Taiyin affects the earth energy, if the excessive energy of wood motion is encountered, they are the two years of Ren Chen and Ren Xu, The energy of the year's motion dominates the wind, when the domination is normal, the wood will sound gentlely in the blowing of wind. and all things will begin to awake. when the dominatin is abnormal, the gale will shake the grasses and trees, and they will be broken and destroyed. As the wind energy is excessive, people will contract the diseases of dizziness and dim-sighted of eyes. As the year's motion is wood, and Ren is a year of Yang, so, the guest motion starts from the Greater Jue and terminates in the Greater Yu (the sequence is Greater Jue, Lesser Zhi, Greater Gong, Lesser Shang and Greater Yu). The start and the terminal of the host motion are similar with that of the guest motion.

太阳　太徵　太阴　戊辰　戊戌同正徵。　其运热，其化暄暑郁燠，其变炎烈沸腾，其病热郁。

太徵　少宫　太商　少羽终　少角初

"When Taiyang controls the heaven energy and Taiyin affects the earth energy, if the excessive energy of the fire motion is encountered, they are the two years of Wu Chen and Wu Xu. Although the fire energies in these two years are excessive, yet they are restricted by the dominating cold water of Taiyang which controls the heaven energy, so, the year's motion is similar with the Right Zhi (year of moderate fire motion). The energy of the year's motion dominates the heat, when the domination is normal, the weather will be warm and

gradually turn into summer-heat and vapouration, if the domination is abnormal, the fire energy will be flaming strongly and the water will be boiling and evapourating. In a man, most of the diseases due to the excessiveness of the fire energy are the stagnation of heat evil. As the year's motion is fire and Wu is a year of Yang, so, the guest motion. starts from the Greater Zhi and terminates on the Lesser Jue (the sequence is Greater Zhi, Lesser Gong, Greater Shang, Lesser Yu and Lesser Jue). The host motion starts from the Lesser Jue and terminates on the Lesser Yu (the sequence is Lesser Jue, Greater Zhi, Lesser Gong, Greater Shang and Lesser Yu).

太阳　太宫　太阴　甲辰岁会同天符　甲戌岁会同天符其运阴埃，其化柔润重泽，其变震惊飘骤，其病湿下重。

太宫　少商　太羽终　太角初　少徵

"When Taiyang controls the heaven energy and Taiyin affects the earth energy, if the excessive earth motion is encountered, they are the two years of Jia Chen (year of convergence and same with the year of heaven tally) and Jia Xu (year of convergence and same with the year of heaven tally). The year's motion dominates the cloudy and rainy weather. When the domination is normal, the earth energy will be soft and moist, the rain and dew will moisten the earth properly; when the dominaion is abnormal, the thunder, lightning and tempest will occur. In a man, the disease caused by the excessive energy of the earth motion is the heaviness of the lower body. As the year's motion is earth, and Jia is a year of Yang, so, the guest motion starts from the Greater Gong and terminates on the Lesser Zhi (the seguence is Greater Gong, Lesser Shang, Greater Yu, Greater Jue and lesser Zhil, The host motion starts form the Greaten Jue and Lesser Zhi), and the host motion starts from the Greater Jue and terminates on the Greater Yu (the sequence is Greater Jue, Lesser Zhi, Greater Gong, Lesser Shang and Greater Yu).

太阳　太商　太阴　庚辰　庚戌　其运凉，　其化雾露萧飋，其变肃杀凋零，其病燥背瞀胸满。

太商　少羽终少角初　太徵　少宫

When Taiyang is controlling the heaven energy and Taiyin energy is affecting the earth energy, if the excessive metal energy is encountered, they are the two years of Geng chen and Gen Xu and the years'motions are similar with that of the Righ Shang which is dominating the coldness. If the domination is normal, it will be of mist and dew, if the domination is abnormal, it will be of restraint and desolation. As the metal energy is excessive people will contract the pain of shoulder, back and the chest. As the motion of the year is metal and Geng is a year of Yang, so the guest motion starts from Greater Shang and terminates on the Lesser Gong (the sequence is Greater Shang, Lesser Yu, Lesser Jue, Greater Zhi and Lesser Gong). The host motion starts from the Lesser Jue and terminates on Lesser Yu (the sequence is Lesser Jue, Greater Zhi, Lesser Gong, Greater Shang and Lesser Yu).

太阳　太羽　太阴　丙辰天符　丙戌天符　其运寒，其化凝惨凓冽，其变冰雪霜雹，其病大寒留於谿谷。

太羽^终 太角^初 少徵 太宫 少商

"When Taiyang is controlling the heaven energy and Taiyin is affecting the earthy energy, if the excessive energy of the water motion is encountered, they are the two years of Bing Chen (heaven tally) and Bing Xu (heaven tally). The motion's energy of the year dominates the coolness. When the domination is normal, there will be the cool weather with ice, snow, frost and hail, when the domination is abnormal, there will be the chilly weather with desolation. People will contract the disease of retention of the cold-energy in the groove. As the year's motion is water and Bing is a year of Yang, so, the guest motion starts from the Greater Yu and terminates on the Lesser Shang (the sequence is Greater Yu Greater Jue, Lesser Zhi and Greater Gong and Lesser Shang), and the host motion starts from the Greater Jue and terminates on the Greater Yu (the sequence is Greater Jue, Lesser Zhi, Greater Gong, Lesser Shang and Greater Yu).

凡此太阳司天之政，气化运行先天，天气肃，地气静，寒临太虚，阳气不令，水土合德，上应辰星镇星。其谷玄黅，其政肃，其令徐。寒政大举，泽无阳焰，则火发待时。少阳〔吴本注"阳"作"阴"〕中治，时雨乃涯，止极雨散，还于太阴，云朝北极，湿化乃布，泽流万物，寒敷于上，雷动于下，寒湿之气，持于气交。民病寒湿，发肌肉萎，足萎不收，濡写血溢。初之气，地气迁，气乃大温，草乃早荣，民乃厉，温病乃作，身热头痛呕吐，肌腠疮疡。二之气，大凉反至，民乃惨，草乃遇寒，火气遂抑，民病气郁中满，寒乃始。三之气，天政布，寒气行，雨乃降，民病寒反热中，痈疽注下，心热瞀闷，不治者死。四之气，风湿交争，风化为雨，乃长乃化乃成，民病大热少气，肌肉痿，足痿，注下赤白。五之气，阳复化，草乃长，乃化乃成，民乃舒。终之气，地气正，湿令行，阴凝太虚，埃昏郊野，民乃乃惨凄，寒风以至，反者孕乃死。故岁宜苦以燥之温之〔林校云："详'故岁'九字，当在'避虚邪以安其正'下，错简在此"〕，必折其郁气，先资其化源，抑其运气，扶其不胜，无使暴过而生其疾，食岁谷以全其真，避虚邪以安其正。适气同异，多少制之，同寒湿者燥热化，异寒湿者燥湿化，故同者多之，异者少之，用寒远寒，用凉远凉，用温远温，用热远热，食宜同法。有假者反常，反是者病，所谓时也。

"Whenever Taiying is controlling the weather and implementing its role, the activity of energy will come prior to the normal weather of the season. The heaven energy will be cold and clear and the earth energy will be calm. As the cold energy is occupying the sky, the Yang energy can not play its role, the cold water (black) and the wetness earth (yellow) promote each other. Their corresponding stars are Mercury and Saturn. The crops that grow are of black and yellow colours. Its phenomenon is solemnness, its function is slowliness. If the function of the cold energy is expanding extremely, the Yang in Yin will be restricted, there will be no evaporating Yang energy on the rivers and lakes, and the suppressed fire energy will watch a chance to burst out. When the fire energy of Shaoyin controls the weather, the rain in proper time will be ceasing. But when the condition developes to the extreme, the rain will be very rare and Taiyin will be dominating again. Then, the earth energy will ascend and turn into clouds which moves north to carry rain, the energy of wetness will be spreading in all directions, and the moistening of rain will reach all things. As the energy of

cold water spreading above, the monarch-fire energy of Shaoyin is acting below, the cold energy and the wetness energy stalemate in the intersection of the heaven and earth energies. By this time, people's diseases of flaccidity of muscles and feet due to the cold-wetnss evil, diarrhea due to wetnss-evil and blood loss will occur.

"In the stage of the initial energy, the prime minister-fire Shaoyin is playing its role. the energy affects the earth energy is shifting, the weather will be very warm and the various kinds of grasses will be flourishing early. In this period, People are apt to contract epidemic and seasonal febrile disease, of which the syndromes are bodily fever, headache, vomiting and red spots on the skin.

"In the stage of the second energy, the dryness metal energy of Yangming is playing its role, the weather of great coolness will occur. People will suffer the gloomy weather, the various kinds of grasses will be suffered in the cold energy, and the fire energy will be restricted. People will suffer the diseases of stagnated energy in the middle warmer and the distention of the chest and abdomen. The energy of cold water of Taiyang will commence from then on.

"In the stage of the third energy when the cold water energy of Taiyang is playing its role, the cold energy will be prevailing and the rain will be falling. People will often contract the cold disease with fever inside so as to have carbuncle, diarrhea, feverish sensation accompanied with restlessness in the chest, coma and depression of the chest. If the disease is not treated in time, the patient will die.

"In the stage of the fourth energy when the wood wind energy of Jueyin is playing its role and the wetness earth of Taiyin is the host motion. In the combat of the wind energy and the wetness energy, the wind can not surpass the wetness and turns into rain which causes all things to grow, transform and become matured. By this time, people often contract high fever, deficiency of vital energy, flaccidity of muscles and feet, diarrhea with whitish and bloody stool.

"In the stage of the fifth energy when the monarch-fire energy of Shaoyin is in the dominating position, due to the presence of the guest energy, the monarch-fire energy can hardly operate. However, due to the combination of the Monarch-fire of Shaoyin and the wetness earth of Taiyin, the grasses will be growing, transforming and getting into shape, and people will be at ease without disease.

"In the stage of the terminal energy, the wetness earth energy of Taiyin is playing its role, the earth energy will be prosperous and the wetness energy will be prevailing. The Yin energy will be clotting in the sky, the dust and sand will be flying to cover the outskirts, and people will feel unhappy and distressful under this kind of weather. If the cold wind which overcomes the wetness arrives, it will affect the human body, the pregnant woman may be hurt and has abortion. If one wants to weaken the excessive energy which causes stagnation, he must cultivate the source of generation and transformation to restrict the excessive energy of the element's motion, and support the energy of the element's motion which is not over-

coming. In this way, it may avoid the partial overabundant or partial deficient energy which causes disease. Besides, the patient should take the crops of the year in green and yellow colours which are in accordance with the energy of the year's motion to preserve the true energy, to keep away from the debilitating evil and thief evil energy to maintain the healthy energy. Thus, in this year, the patient should take more food of bitter taste to dispel the wetness, more medicine of bitter taste and warm nature to dispel the cold. Set the quantity of medicine according to the similarity of differance of the motion's energies. If the motion and energy are both cold and wet, the medicine of dry and hot nature should be applied; if the motion and energy are different with cold and wetness, the medicine for drying the wetness-evil should be applied; when the motion and energy are similar, apply more medicine of the appropriate taste; when the motion and energy are different, the dosage of the medicine should be small. Avoid the cold weather when applying the medicine of cold nature. Avoid warm weather when applying the medicine of warm nature, and aviod the hot weather when applying the medicine of hot nature. When taking food or drink, the same rules stated above should also be observed. If the substitutionary energy is playing its role and the weather is abnormal, such as hot in winter and cold in summer, and the evil energy, on the contrary, is overabundant, it must not follow the rule of avoiding the hot or cold weather stated above rigidly to cause disease, but treat the disease in some other way. This is the so called treat differently according to different conditions。"

帝曰：善。阳明之政奈何？岐伯曰：卯酉之纪也。

Yellow Emperor said: "Good. what is the condition of the five elements' motion and the six kinds of weather when Yangming is controlling the heaven energy?" Qibo said: "They are the years which are marked by the symbols of Mao and You of the duodecimal cycle.

阳明　少角　少阴　清热胜复同，同正商。丁卯岁会　丁酉　其运风清热

少角初正太徵　少宫　太商　少羽终

"When the dryness metal energy of Yangming is controlling the heaven energy and the monarch-fire energy of Shaoyin is affecting the earth energy, if the insufficient energy of wood motion is encountered, the overcoming cool energy and the retaliating fire energy will occur simultaniously. As the wood energy is insufficient this year, and Yangming is controlling the heaven energy (metal subjugates wood), so, the Upper Shang is similar with the Right Shang (moderate energy of metal). They are the years of Ding Mao (the year of convergence) and Ding You. The motion's energy of the year is wind, the overcoming energy is coolness and the retaliating energy is heat of monarch-fire. As the year's motion is wood, and Ding is a year of Yin, so, the guest motion starts from the Lesser Jue and terminates on the Lesser Jue, (The sequence is Lesser Jue, Greater Zhi, Lesser Gong, Greater Shang and Lesser Yu). The start and the terminal of the host motion are similar with that of the guest motion.

阳明　少徵　少阴　寒雨胜复同　同正商。癸卯同岁会癸酉同岁会其运热寒雨。

少徵　太宫　少商　太羽终　太角初

"When Yangming is controlling the heaven energy and Shaoyin is affecting the earth energy, if the insufficient energy of the fire motion is encountered, the overcoming cold energy and the retaliating rain (wetness) energy will occur simutaneously. As the fire energy is insufficient, and Yangming is controlling the heaven energy, so, the upper Shang is similar with the Right Shang. They are the two years of Gui Mao (same with the year of convergence) and Gui You (same with the year of convergence). The motion's energy of the year is heat, the overcoming energy is cold and the retaliating energy is rain. As the year's motion is fire and Gui is a year of Yin, so, the guest motion starts from the Lesser Zhi and terminates on the Greater Jue (the sequence is Lesser Zhi, Greater Gong, Lesser Shang, Greater Yu and Greater Jue), and the host motion starts from the Greater Jue and terminates on the Greater Yu (the sequence is Greater Jue, Lesser Zhi, Greater Gong, Lesser shang and Greater Yu).

阳明　少宫　少阴　风凉胜复同。已卯　已酉　其运雨风凉

少宫　太商　少羽[终]少角[初]　太徵

"When Yangming is controlling the heaven energy and Shaoyin is affecting the earth energy, if the insufficient energy of the earth energy is encountered, the overcoming wind energy and the retaliating cool energy will occur simultaneously. They are the two years of Ji Mao and Ji You. The motion's energy of the year is rain, the overcoming energy is wind and the retaliating energy is coolness. As the year's motion is earth and Ji is a year of Yin, so the guest motion starts from the Lesser Gong and terminates on the Greater Zhi (the sequence is Lesser Gong, Greater Shang, Lesser Yu, Lesser Jue and Greater Zhi), and the host motion starts from the Lesser Jue and terminates on the Lesser Yu (the sequence is Lesser Jue, Greater Zhi, Lesser Gong, Greater Shang and Lesser Yu).

阳明　少商　少阴　热寒胜复同，同正商。乙卯天符，乙酉岁会，太乙天符。其运凉热寒。

少商　太羽[终]　太角[初]　少徵　太宫

"When Yangming is controlling the heaven energy and Shaoyin is affecting the earth energy, if the insufficient energy of the metal motion is encountered, the overcoming heat energy and the retaliating cold energy will occur simultaneously. The upper Shang will be similar with the Right Shang. They are the two years of Yi Mao (year of heaven tally) and Yi You (year of convergence and heaven tally). The motion's energy of the Year is coolness, the overcoming energy is heat and the retaliating energy is cold. As the year's motion is metal and Yi is a year of Yin, so, the guest motion starts from the Lesser Shang and terminates on the Greater Gong (the sequence is Lesser Shang, Greater Yu, Greater Jue, Lesser Zhi and Greater Gong), and the host motion starts from the Greater Jue and terminates on the Greater Yu (the sequence is Greater Jue, Lesser Zhi, Greater Gong, Lesser Shang and Greater Yu).

阳明　少羽　少阴　雨风胜复同，辛卯少宫同。辛酉　辛卯　其运寒雨风。

少羽[终]　少角[初]　太徵　太宫　太商

"When Yangming is controlling the heaven energy and Shaoyin is affecting the earth energy, if the insufficient energy of water motion is encountered, the overcoming rain (wetness energy) and the retaliating wind energy will occur simultaneously. As the water energy is insufficient and the earth energy subjugates it excessively, the Lesser Yu is similar with the Lesser Gong. They are the two years of Xin Chou and Xin Mao. The motion's energy of the year is cold, the overcoming energy is rain, and the retaliating energy is wind. As the year's motion is water and Xin is a year of Yin, so, the guest motion starts from the Lesser Yu and terminates on the Greater Shang (the sequence is Lesser Yu, Lesser Jue, Greater Zhi, Greater Gong and Greater Shang), and the host motion starts from the Lesser Jue and terminates on the Lesser Yu (the sequence is Lesser Jue, Greater Zhi, Greater Gong, Greater Shang and Lesser Yu).

凡此阳明司天之政，气化运行后天，天气急，地气明，阳专其令，炎暑大行，物燥以坚，淳风乃治，风燥横运，流于气交，多阳少阴，云趋雨府，湿化乃敷。燥极而泽，其谷白丹，间谷命太者，其耗白甲品羽，金火合德，上应太白荧惑。其政切，其令暴，蛰虫乃见，流水不冰，民病咳嗌塞，寒热发，暴振溧癃闷，清先而劲，毛虫乃死，热后而暴，介虫乃殃，其发躁，胜复之作，扰而大乱，清热之气，持于气交。初之气，地气迁，阴始凝，气始肃，水乃冰，寒雨化。其病中热胀，而目浮肿，善眠，鼽衄，嚏欠，呕，小便黄赤，甚则淋。二之气，阳乃布，民乃舒，物乃生荣。厉大至，民善暴死。三之气，天政布，凉乃行，燥热交合，燥极而泽，民病寒热，四之气，寒雨降，病暴仆，振慄谵妄，少气，嗌乾引饮，及为心痛痈肿疮疡虐寒之疾，骨痿血便。五之气，春令反行，草乃生荣，民气和，终之气，阳气布，候反温，蛰虫来见，流水不冰，民乃康平，其病温。故食岁谷以安其气，食间谷以去其邪，岁宜以咸以苦以辛，汗之、清之、散之，安其运气，无使受邪，折其郁气，资其化源。以寒热轻重少多其制，同热者多天化，同清者多地化，用凉远凉，用热远热，用寒远寒，用温远温，食宜同法。有假者反之，此其道也。反是者，乱天地之经，扰阴阳之纪也。

"Whenever the dryness metal energy of Yangming is controlling the heaven energy and play its role, the activity of energy will lag behind the normal weather of the season, and the weather will be pressing. As the monarch-fire energy of Shaoyin is affecting the earth energy, the earth energy will be bright. As the Yang energy is dominating the season, the scorching heat will be prevailing, and the grasses and woods will become dry and hard which can only be recovered by the blowing of the warm breezes. As the wind and dryness energies lie across the year and run into the intersection of the heaven and earth energies, it causes more Yang energy and less Yin energy. The clouds and rains occur often and the wetness energy of earth spreads. But when the extreme dryness turns into wetness, the rain will fall. The crops of the year activated by the healthy energy are of red and white colours, and the maturity of the intermediate crops are promoted by the excessive intermediate energy. The beetle and the flying insect kind will be injured and can not multiply. The metal and fire energies combine to play their roles, their corresponding stars above are Venus and Mars. The energy of metal is pressing and the energy of fire is rash and violent, so, the hibernants will appear, the water will be flowing without freezing, people will contract the diseases of

cough, disphagia, sudden cold and heat, shivering and retention of urine and feces. As Yangming is controlling the heaven energy, it determines the weather of the first half of the year, so, the weather is cool and pressing in the first half of the year, and the caterpillar will die; as Shaoyin is affecting the earth energy, it determines the weather of the second half of the year, so the weather is hot and urgent in the second half of the year and the cyprid will be injured. Since the attacks of the metal energy and the fire energy are both urgent, the changing of the overcoming and retaliating energies are often disorderly and the cool and heat energies stalemate in the intersection of the heaven and earth energies.

"In the stage of the initial energy, the wetness earth energy of Taiyin is playing its role, the earth energy is shifting, and the Yin energy begins to condense, as a result, the weather becomes chilly and restraining, the water freezes, and the cold rain is in the making. When man is invaded by the weather, he will contract the diseases of internal heat-syndrome, fullness of the chest, edema of the face and eyes, somnolence, rhinorrhea, epistaxis, sneezing, yawning, vomiting, yellowish. red urine, frequency of urination, urgency of micturition, dysuria and dripping of urine etc.

"In the stage of the second energy, the prime minister-fire energy of Shaoyang is playing its role. The Yang energy is spreading, people will feel comfortable and the grasses and woods are flourishing. But the epidemic will run wild for a while and will cause death of the people.

"In the stage of the third energy, the dryness metal of Yangming is playing its role. The cool energy operates and the dryness energy and the heat energy are coordinating. When the dryness energy reaches its extreme, it turns into moisture. People will often contract malaria.

"In the stage of the fourth energy, the cold water Taiyang energy is playing its role. The cold rain falls. People will contract the diseases of falling down suddenly, shivering with cold, speaking nonsense, short of breath, dry throat, thirsty, heartache, carbuncle, cold-type malaria, flaccidity-syndrome involing the bone, bloody stool and hematochezia.

"In the stage of the fifth energy, the wind wood energy of Jueyin is playing its role, and autumn will implement spring's decree instead. The grasses are growing gracefully again and people are also comfortable.

"In the stage of the terminal energy, the monarch-fire heat energy of Shaoyin is playing its role, the Yang energy is spreading all around, and the weather, on the contrary, is warm. The hibernants can be seen outside, and the flowing water can not freeze. People are quiet and healthy but they are easy to contract seasonal febrile disease.

"In the year like this, one should take crops of the year which are of white or red colour to stablize the healthy energy, take the intermediate crop of which its maturity is promoted by the intermediate energy to expel the evil energy. Apply the medicine with the tastes of saltiness, bitterness and acridness, besides, apply the therapies of diaphoresis, heat-clearing and dispersing to suit the energy of the element's motion, Protect the patient against the evil energy, weaken the stagnated energy and assist the source of generation and transformation,

Apply different medicine according to the extent of cold and heat: when the energy that controls the heaven energy and the motion that affects the earth energy are both hot, treat with the medicine of cool nature, when both the energy and the motion are not cool, treat with the medicine of hot nature. Do not apply the medicine of cool nature in cool weather, do not apply the medicine of hot nature in hot weather, do not apply the medicine of cold nature in cold weather, and do not apply the medicine of warm nature in warm weather, When taking the food and drink, the same rule stated above should be observed. When the substitutionary energy is dominating and the weather is abnormal, the disease should be treated in some other way. These are the methods of adapting the natural law, if they are violated, it will up set the rule of the natural changes and the law of Yin and Yang。"

帝曰：善。少阳之政奈何？岐伯曰：寅申之纪也。

Yellow Emperor said: "Good. What is the condition when Shaoyang is controlling the heaven energy?" Qibo said: "They are the two years which are marked by symbols of Yin and Shen of the duodecimal cycle.

少阳　太角　厥阴　壬寅同天符　壬申同天符　其运风鼓，其化鸣紊启坼，其变振拉摧拔，其病掉眩，支胁，惊骇。

太角初正　少徵　太宫　少商　太羽终

"When Shaoyang is controlling the heaven energy and Jueyin is affecting the earth energy, if the excessive energy of the wood motion is encountered, they are the two years of Ren Yin (same with the year of heaven tally) and Ren Shen (same with the year of heaven tally). The motion's energy of the year dominates the wind and the moving, When the domination is normal, the woods will sound gently in the blowing of wind, and all things will begin to awake, when the domination is abnormal, the gale will blow to shake and destroy the grasses and trees. As the wind energy is excessive, peopel will contract the diseases of dizziness, pain in the hypochondria and frightening. As the year's motion is wood and Ren is a year of Yang, so, the guest motion starts from the Greater Jue and terminates on the Greater Yu. (the sequence is Greater Jue, Lesser Zhi, Greater Gong, Lesser Shang and Greater Yu). The start and the terminal of the host motion are similar with that of the guest energy.

少阳　太徵　厥阴　戊寅天符　戊申天符。其运暑，其化暄嚣郁燠，其变炎烈沸腾，其病上热郁，血溢血泄心痛。

太徵　少宫　太商　少羽终　少角初

"When Shaoyang is controlling the heaven energy and Jueyin is affecting the earth energy, if the excessive energy of the fire motion is encountered, they are the two years of Wu Yin (year of heaven tally) and Wu Shen (year of heaven tally). The motion's energy of the year dominates the summer-heat. When the domination is normal, it is the hot summer, when the domination is abnormal, it is the scorching heat and the boiling temperature. As the fire energy is excessive in a man, the diseases of fever in the upper part of the body, overflowing of blood, hematochezia and epigastric pain due to blood stasis will occur. As the

year's motion is fire and Wu is a year of Yang, so, the guest motion starts from the Greater Zhi and terminates on the Lesser Jue (the sequence is Greater Zhi, Lesser Gong, Greater Shang, Lesser Yu and Lesser Jue), and the host motion starts from the Lesser Jue and terminates on the Lesser Yu (the sequence is Lesser Jue, Greater Zhi, Lesser Gong, Greater Shang and Lesser Yu.)

少阳　太宫　厥阴　甲寅　甲申　其运阴雨，其化柔润重泽，其变震惊飘骤，其病体重，胕肿痞饮。

太宫　少商　太羽终　太角初　少徵

"When Shaoyang is controlling the heaven energy and Jueyin is affecting the earth energy, if the excessive energy of the earth motion is encountered, they are the two years of Jia Yin and Jia Shen. The motion's energy dominates the cloudy and rainy weather. When the domination is normal, the weather will be soft and moist, when the domination is abnormal, there will be shocking and the sudden blowing of the wind. As the earth energy is excessive, people will contract the diseases of heaviness of the body, edema and retention of fluid in the body causing the feeling of fullness and oppression. As the year's motion is earth and Jia is a year of Yang, so, the guest motion starts from the Greater Gong and terminates on the Lesser Zhi (the sequence is Greater Gong, Lesser Shang, Greater Yu, Greater Jue and Lesser Zhi), and the host energy starts from Greater Jue and terminates on the Greater Yu (the sequence is Greater Jue, Lesser Zhi, Greater Gong, Lessonr Shang and Greater Yu).

少阳　太商　厥阴　庚寅　庚申同正商　其运凉，其化雾露清切，其变肃杀凋零，其病肩背胸中。

太商　少羽终　少角初　太徵　少宫

When Shaoyang is controlling the heaven energy and Jueyin energy is affecting the earth energy, if the excessive metal energy is encountered, they are the two years of Geng Yin and Gen Shen and the year's motions are similar with that of the Right Shang which is dominating the coolness. If the domination is normal, it will be of restraint and desolation. As the metal energy is excessive, people will contract the pain of shoulder, back and the chest. As the motion of the year is metal and Geng is a year of Yang, so, the guest motion starts from Greater Shang and terminates on Lesser Gong (the sequence is Greater Shang, Lesser Yu, Lesser Jue, Greater Zhi and Lesser Gong). The host motion starts from the Lesser Jue and terminates on Lesser Yu (the sequence is Lesser Jue, Greater Zhi, Lesser Gong, Greater Shang and Lesser Yu).

少阳　太羽　厥阴　丙寅　丙申　其运寒肃，其化凝惨凓冽，其变冰雪霜雹，其病寒浮肿。

太羽终　太角初　少徵　太宫　少商

"When Shaoyang is controlling the heaven energy and Jueyin is affecting the earth energy, if the excessive energy of the water motion is encountered, they are the two years of Bing Yin and Bing Shen. The motion's energy of the year dominates the cold and chillness. When the domination is normal, there will be the weather of condensation, desolation and

coldness, when the domination is abnormal, there will be the weather of ice, snow, frost and hail. People will contract the diseases of cold and edema. As the year's motion is water and Bing is a year of Yang, so, the guest motion starts from the Greater yu and terminates on the Lesser Shang (the sequence is Greater Yu, Greater Jue, Lesser Zhi, Greater Gong and Lesser Shang), and the host motion starts from the Greater Jue and terminates on the Greater Yu (the sequence is Greater Jue, Lesser Zhi, Greater Gong, Lesser Shang and Greater Yu).

凡此少阳司天之政，气化运行先天，天气正，地气扰，风乃暴举，木偃沙飞，炎火乃流，阴行阳化，雨乃时应，火木同德，上应荧惑岁星，其谷丹苍，其政严，其令扰，故风热参布，云物沸腾，太阴横流，寒乃时至，凉雨并起。民病寒中，外发疮疡，内为泄满。故圣人遇之，和而不争，往复之作，民病寒热疟泄，聋瞑呕吐，上怫肿色变。初之气，地气迁，风胜乃摇，寒乃去，候乃大温，草木早荣。寒来不杀，温病乃起，其病气怫于上，血溢目赤，咳逆头痛，血崩胁满，肤腠中疮。二之气，火反郁，白埃四起，云趋雨府，风不胜湿，雨乃零，民乃康，其病热郁于上，咳逆呕吐，疮发于中，胸嗌〔《三因方》引“嗌”作“臆”〕不利，头痛身热，昏愦脓疮。三之气，天政布，炎暑至，少阳临上，雨乃涯，民病热中，聋瞑血溢，脓疮咳呕，鼽衄渴嚏欠，喉痹目赤，善暴死。四之气，凉乃至，炎暑闲化，白露降，民气和平，其病满身重。五之气，阳乃去，寒乃来，雨乃降，气门乃闭，刚木早凋，民避寒邪，君子周密。终之气，地气正，风乃至，万物反生，霿雾以行，其病关闭不禁，心痛，阳气不藏而咳。抑其运气，赞所不胜，必折其郁气，先取化源，暴过不生，苛疾不起。故岁宜咸辛宜酸，渗之泄之，渍之发之，观气寒温以调其过，同风热者多寒化，异风热者少寒化，用热远热，用温远温，用寒远寒，用凉远凉，食宜同法，此其道也。有假者反之，反是者病之阶也。

"Whenever Shaoyang is controlling the heaven energy and is playing its role, the activity of energy comes prior to the normal weather of the season, the heaven energy is normal, but the earth energy is stirring. The wind will rise all of a sudden, the trees will be blown down, the sand and dust will be flying and the scorching fire energy will be prevailing. When the wind energy of Jueyin combines with the prime minister-fire energy of Shaoyang, the rain will fall in time. The fire and wood energies coordinate to play their roles, the corresponding stars above are Mars and Jupiter, and the corresponding crops are of red and dark-green colours. As the prime minister-fire Shaoyang is controlling the heaven energy and the character of fire is urgent, so, its authority of office is strict; as the wind wood energy is affecting the earth energy, and the character of wind is mobile, so, its appearance is stirring. When the wind energy and the heat energy mix in the intersection of the heaven and earth energies, the evaporation will like clouds flying above. Once the energy of wetness earth runs amuck, the cold energy will come often, and the cold rain will fall in the wake of it. Under this condition, people will contract the syndrome of internal stagnation of cold which causes sores outside and diarrhea and abdominal fullness inside. When a wise man encounters the condition, he will be able to adjust the cold and heat energies to stop their contention. If the cold and heat energies contend time and again, the diseases of malaria, diarrhea, deafness, closing of eyes, vomiting, stagnation of the heart and lung energies, swelling and changing

colour of the skin will occur.

"In the stage of the initial energy, the monarch-fire energy of Shaoyin is playing its role. The earth energy is shifting, the wind energy is hyperactive, the wind is waving, the cold energy is retreating, the weather is becoming warm and the grasses and trees are flourishing, as the remainder cold can not cut their lustre thoroughly. By this time the seasonal febrile disease will occur, and people will often contract the depressive syndrome due to disorder of vital energy in the upper part or the body, bleeding, red eyes, cough, adverseness of vital energy , headache, metrorrhagia, fullness and distention over the hypochondria and sore on the skin.

"In the stage of the second energy, the wetness earth energy of Taiyin is playing its role, and the monarch-fire energy of Shaoyin, on the contrary is being restricted. So, the white energy is rising everywhere and the weather becomes cloudy and rainy; as the wind energy can not surpass the wetness energy, the drizzles will fall now and then, people will be very comfortable and healthy. If there is any disease, they will be the stagnation of heat in the upper part of the body, cough, adverseness of vital energy, vomiting, internal ulcer, pain in the muscle of chest, headache, fever over the body, unquietness and sore with pus.

"In the stage of the third energy, the heat energy of Shaoyang is playing its role, the weather is scorching hot. As both the host and guest energies are playing the role of prime minister-fire of Shaoyang, the rain will be ceased. By this time, people will often contract the internal heat-syndrome, deafness, closing of eyes, hemorrhage, cough, vomiting, stuffy nose, running nose, nasal hemorrhage, yawning, obstruction and pain in the throat, red eyes. Sometimes, the patient may die all of a sudden.

"In the stage of the fourth energy, the cool guest energy of Yangming adds on the wetness energy of Taiyin which is dominating the season, the weather will be hot and cool alternately. The white dew will fall and people will feel ease and calm. If there are any diseases, they will be the fullness of chest and the heaviness of the body.

"In the stage of the fifth energy, the cold water energy of Taiyang is playing its role, the heat of the Yang energy is dispersed and the cold energy comes in the wake of it. The rain falls and the striae and orifices of man are shrinking, and the trees of the hard wood become withered in advance. People will keep away from the cold and live causually.

"In the stage of the terminal enery, the wind energy of Jueyin is playing its role. As the wind energy is moving, all things become growing and transforming, and the gloomy frost occurs frequently. Under this condition, people will often contract the diseases of incontinence of feces and urine, heartache and cough due to inability of shutting the Yang energy. When treating, it should suppress the excessive motion energy, assist the insufficent motion's energy, weaken the stagnated energy and treat the source of generation and transformation first. If the excessive motion's energy is not happening, then, no serious disease will occur. when treating, one should apply the medicine of salty, acrid and sour tastes, and apply the therapies of excreting, purgative, soaking and diaphoresis within the year. Ob-

serve the coldness and the warmness of the motion's energy of the year and adjust it not to become excessive, when the energy of the year's motion is similar with the assimilating wind energy that affects the earth energy, or similar with the assimilating heat energy that controls the heaven energy, treat with more medicine of cold and cool nature to clear the heat; when they are not similar, treat with less medicine of cold and cool nature. Do not apply the medicine of hot nature in hot weather, do not apply the medicine of warm nature in warm weather, do not apply the medicine of cold nature in cold weather, and do not apply the medicine of cool nature in cool weather. when taking food and drink, the rules stated above should be observed as well. If a substitutionary energy is dominating and the weather is abnormal, the disease should be treated in some other way. These are the fundamental rules which must not be violated, so as not to cause other disease。"

帝曰：善。太阴之政奈何？岐伯曰：丑未之纪也。

Yellow Emperor said:"Good. What is the condition when Taiyin is controlling the heaven energy? Qibo said: "They are the two years which are marked the symbols of Chou and Wei of the duodecimal cycle.

太阴　少角　太阳　清热胜复同，同正宫。丁丑　丁未　其运风清热。

少角初正　太徵　少宫　太商　少羽终

"When Taiyin is controlling the heaven energy and Taiyang is affecting the earth energy, if the insufficient energy of the wood motion is encountered, the overcoming cool energy and the retaliating heat energy will occur simultaneously. As the wood energy is insuffcient and earth energy is playing its role, the upper Gong is similar with the Right Gong. They are the two years of Ding Chou and Ding Wei. The motion's energy of the year is wind, the overcoming energy is cool and the retaliating energy is heat. As the year's motion is wood and Ding is a year of Yin, so, the guest motion starts from the Lesser Jue and terminates on the Lesser Yu (the sequence is Lesser Jue, Greater Zhi, Lesser Gong, Greater Shang and Lesser Yu). The start and the terminal of the host motion are similar with that of the guest energy.

太阴　少徵　太阳　寒雨胜复同。　癸丑　癸未　其运热寒雨。

少徵　太宫　少商　太羽终太角初

"When Taiyin is controlling the heaven energy and Taiyang is affecting the earth energy, if the insufficient energy of fire motion is encountered, the overcoming cold energy and the retaliating rain(wetness)energy will occur simultaneously. They are the two years of Gui Chou and Gui Wei. The motion's energy of the year is heat, the overcoming energy is cold and the retaliating energy is rain. As the year's motion is fire and Gui is a year of Yin, so, the guest motion starts from the Lesser Zhi and terminates on the Greater Jue (the sequence is Lesser Zhi, Greater Gong, Lesser Shang, Greater Yu and Greater Jue), and the host motion starts from the Greater Jue terminates on the Greater Yu (the sequence is Greater Jue, Lesser Zhi, Greater Gong. Lesser Shang and Greater Yu).

太阴　少宫　太阳　风清胜复同，同正宫。己丑太乙天符　己未太乙天符，其运雨风清。

少宫　太商　少羽[终]　少角[初]　太徵

"When Taiyin is controlling the heaven energy and Taiyang is affecting the earth energy, if the insufficient energy of the earth motion is encountered, the overcoming wind energy and the retaliating cool energy will occur simultaneously. Although the earth energy is insufficient in the year, yet it receives the help of wetness earth energy which is controlling the heaven energy, so, the Upper Gong is similar with the Right Gong. They are the two years of Ji Chou (year of convergence and heaven tally) and Ji Wei (year of convergence and heaven tally). The motion's energy of the year is rain, the overcoming energy is wind and the retaliating energy is coolness. As the year's motion is earth and Ji is a year of Yin, so, the guest motion starts from the Lesser Gong and terminates on the Greater Zhi (the sequence is Lesser Gong, Greater Shang, Lesser Yu, Lesser Jue and Greater Zhi), and the host motion starts from the Lesser Jue and terminates on the Lesser Yu (the sequence is Lesser Jue, Greater Zhi, Lesser Gong, Greater Shang and Lesser Yu).

太阴　少商　太阳　热寒胜复同，乙丑　乙未　其运凉热寒。

少商　太羽[终]　太角[初]　少徵　太宫

"When Taiyin is controlling the heaven energy and Taiyang is affecting the earth energy, if the insufficient energy of metal is encountered, the overcoming heat energy and the retaliating cold energy will occur simultaneously. They are the two years of Yi Chou and Yi Wei. The motion's energy of the year is coolness, the overcoming energy is heat and the retaliating energy is cold. As the year's motion is metal and Yi is a year of Yin, so, the guest motion starts from the Lesser Shang and terminates on the Greater Gong (the sequence is Lesser Shang, Greater Yu, Greater Jue, Lesser Zhi and Greater Gong), and the host motion starts from the Greater Jue and terminates on the Greater Yu (the sequence is Greater Jue, Lesser Zhi, Greater Gong, Lesser Shang, Greater Yu).

太阴　少羽　太阳　雨风胜复同，同正宫。辛丑[同岁会]　辛未[同岁会]　其运寒雨风。

少羽[终]　少角[初]　太徵　少宫　太商

"When Taiyin is controlling the heaven energy and Taiyang is affecting the earth energy, if the insufficient energy of water motion is encountered, the overcoming rain energy and energy of the retaliating wind energy will occur simultaneously. As the water energy is insufficient in the year and it is excessively overcome by the wetness earth energy that controls the heaven, the upper Gong is similar with the Right Gong. They are the two years of Xin Chou (same with the year of convergence) and Xin Wei (same with the year of convergence). The motion's energy of the year is cold, the overcoming energy is rain and the retaliating energy is wind. As the year's motion is water and Xin is a year of Yin, so, the guest motion starts from the Lesser Yu and terminates on the Greater Shang (the sequence is Lesser Yu, Lesser Jue, Greater Zhi, Lesser Gong and Greater Shang), and the host motion starts from the Lesser Jue and terminates on the Lesser Yu (the sequence is Lesser Jue, Greater Zhi, Lesser Gong, Greater Shang and Lesser Yu).

凡此太阴司天之政，气化运行后天，阴专其政，阳气退辟，大风时起，天气下降，地气

上腾，原野昏霿，白埃四起，云奔南极，寒雨数至，物成于差夏。民病寒湿，腹满，身䐜愤，胕肿，痞逆寒厥拘急。湿寒合德，黄黑埃昏，流行气交，上应镇星辰星。其政肃，其令寂，其谷黅玄。故阴凝于上，寒积于下，寒水胜火，则为冰雹，阳光不治，杀气乃行。故有余宜高，不及宜下，有余宜晚，不及宜早，土之利，气之化也，民气亦从之，间谷命其太也。初之气，地气迁，寒乃去，春气正，风乃来，生布万物以荣，民气条舒，风湿相薄，雨乃后。民病血溢，筋络拘强，关节不利，身重筋痿。二之气，大火正，物承化，民乃和，其病温厉大行，远近咸若，湿蒸相薄，雨乃时降。三之气，天政布，湿气降，地气腾，雨乃时降，寒乃随之。感于寒湿，则民病身重胕肿，胸腹满。四之气，畏火临，溽蒸化，地气腾，天气否隔，寒风晓暮，蒸热相薄，草木凝烟，湿化不流，则白露阴布，以成秋令。民病腠理热，血暴溢疟，心腹满热，胪胀，甚则胕肿。五之气，惨令已行，寒露下，霜乃早降，草木黄落，寒气及体，君子周密，民病皮腠。终之气，寒大举，湿大化，霜乃积，阴乃凝，水坚冰，阳光不治。感于寒，则病人关节禁固，腰脽痛，寒湿推于气交而为疾也。必折其郁气，而取化源，益其岁气，无使邪胜，食岁谷以全其真，食间谷以保其精。故岁宜以苦燥之温之，甚者发之泄之。不发不泄，则湿气外溢，肉溃皮拆而水血交流。必赞其阳火，令御甚寒，从气异同，少多其判也，同寒者以热化，同湿者以燥化，异者少之，同者多之，用凉远凉，用寒远寒，用温远温，用热远热，食宜同法。假者反之，此其道也，反是者病也。

"Whenver Taiyin is controlling the heaven energy and play its role, the activity of energy comes lagging behind the normal weather of the season. As the Yin energy is dominating, the Yang energy retreats, the gale blows frequently, the heaven energy descends, the earth energy ascends, the open wild country is indistinct and gloomy, the white clouds rise and move south, the cold rain falls often, and the crops can only become matured after the Beginning of Autumn. People will contract the diseases of cold-wetness, abdominal distension, fullness of the body, edema, obstruction and oppression of the chest, adverseness of vital energy, cold extremities due to asthenia of Yang energy and stiffness of muscles and limbs. The wetness energy coordinates with the cold energy causing the sky gloomy with yellow and black dusts floating in the intersection of the heaven and earth energies. The corresponding stars above are Saturn and Mercury, its authority of office is solemnity, its appearance is calm, and the corresponding crops are of yellow and black colours. As the energy of wetness earth condenses above, the energy of cold water retains below, and the water can overcome the fire, so, the hail will occur. when the Yang energy can no more play its role, the Yin energy will be prevailing. In the year with excessive motion's energy, the crops should be planted on highland, in the year with insufficient motion's energy, it should be planted on lowland; in the year with excessive motion's energy, the crops should be planted late, and in the year with insufficient motion's energy, the crops should be planted early. The ability of promoting growth of the earth stems from the breeding of nature, and the human bodily energy is of the same. The maturity of the intermediate crops is due to the receiving of the excessive intermediate energy.

"In the stage of the initial energy, the wind energy of Jueyin is playing its role. The earth energy and the cold energy shift away, the spring arrives, the gentle breezes come, the

vital energy spreads everywhere, and things become flourishing and men feel comfortable. As the wetness earth of Taiyin is controlling the heaven energy, the wind energy and the wetness energy are combating, the rain will not fall in time. Under the influence of the weather, people will contract the diseases of hemorrhage in mouth and nose, stiffnss and contraction of muscles, joint disease, heaviness of the body and flaccidity syndrome involving the muscle.

"In the stage of the second energy, the monarch-fire Shaoyin energy is playing its role, all things are being bred, and people are stable and calm. As the fire is abundant, the pestilence will be prevailing far and near. It is only when the wetness energy vaporizes and combats with the heat energy, can the timely rain fall.

"In the stage of the third energy, Taiyin controls the heaven energy and plays its role, the wetness energy descends and the earth energy ascends, the rain will fall in time and the cold energy will come in the wake of it. If a man contracts the cold-wetness, he will have the diseases of heaviness of the body, edema and distention of the chest and abdomen.

"In the stage of the fourth energy, the vigorous prime minister-fire of Shaoyang is playing its role. The wetness energy vaporizes, the earth energy rises, the heaven energy being obstructed, the cold wind blows in the mornings and in the evenings, the vaporized wetness and the heat energy are combating each other and there seems to have a thin cloud spreading between the grasses and woods. As the wetness energy is stagnant and the white dew falls, it appears to be the harvest season of autumn. By this time, people will contract the diseases of hot skin, bleeding all of a sudden, malaria, heat and distention in heart and abdomen, or even to have edema.

"In the stage of the fifth energy, the dryness metal energy of Yangming is playing its role. The cold dew descends, the heavy frost falls early, the grasses and woods become yellow and withered, and the human body is invaded by the cold energy. People who are good at preserving health are living cautiously to guard against contracting disease. By this time, the disease of striae of skin will occur often.

"In the stage of the terminal energy, the cold water energy of Taiyang is playing its role. The cold energy is very strong, the wetness energy operates, the cold frost assembles, the water is frozen into hard ice and the Yang energy can hardly play its role. People will contract the diseases of stiffness of the joints, pain in the loins and legs due to the stalemate of the cold energy and the wetness energy in the intersection of the heaven and the earth energies.

"When treating, the stagnated energy must be weakened to enforce the source of transformation, restrict the excessive motion's energy of the year to avoid the injury of the abundant evil energy. Take the crop of the year which is the same colour of the year's motion to maintain the healthy energy, and take the intermediate crop whose maturity is promoted by the excessive intermediate energy to preserve the refined energy.

"In this year, the medicine of bitter taste and the therapies of drying and warming

should be applied; to the diseases which are severe, the inducing diaphoresis and purgative therapies should be applied. If the wetness energy is not dispelled, it will be overflowing outside to cause the decay of muscle, the crack of skin and the bleeding of blood. Assist the Yang fire to resist the bitter cold and determine the way of treating and the quantity of applying the medicine according to the similarity or difference of the energy and motion. When the motion's energy of the year and the energy that controls the heaven energy are both of coolness, adjust them with the medicine of hot nature; when they are both of wetness, adjust them with the medicine of dry nature; apply smaller dosage of medicine when they are different, and apply larger dosage when they are similar. Do not apply medicine of cool nature in the cool weather, do not apply the medicine of cold nature in the cold weather, do not apply medicine of warm nature in the warm weather, and do not apply the medicine of hot nature in the hot weather. when taking food and drink, the rule stated above should be observed as well. If a substitutionary energy is dominating and the weather is abnormal, the disease should be treated in some other way. These are the fundamental rules which must not be violated to cause disease。"

帝曰：善。少阴之政奈何？岐伯曰：子午之纪也。

Yellow Emperor said: "Good. What is the condition when Shaoyin is controlling the heaven energy?" Qibo said: "They are the years which are marked by symbols of Zi and Wu of the duodecimal cycle.

少阴　太角　阳明　壬子　壬午　其运 风鼓，其化鸣紊启折，其变振拉摧拔，其病支满。

太角[初正]　少徵　太宫　少商　太羽[终]

"When Shaoyin is controlling the heaven energy and Yangming is affecting the earth energy, if the excessive energy of wood motion is encountered, they will be the two years of Ren Zi and Ren Wu. The motion's energy of the year dominates the wind and the moving. when the domination is normal, the wood will sound gentlly in the blowing of wind and the earth energy begins to awake, when the domination is abnormal, the gale will be blowing to break and destroy the grasses and trees. People will contract the disease of epigastric fullness. As the year's motion is wood and Ren is a year of Yang, so, the guest motion starts from the Greater Jue and terminates on the Greater Yu (the sequence is Greater Jue, Lesser Zhi, Greater Gong, Lesser Shang and Greater Yu). The start and the terminal of the host motion are similar with that of the guest motion.

少阴　太徵　阳明　戊子天符　戊午太乙天符　其运炎暑，其化暄曜郁燠，其变炎烈沸腾，其病上热血溢。

太徵　少宫　太商　少羽[终]少角[初]

"When Shaoyin is controlling the heaven energy and Yangming is affecting the earth energy, if the excessive energy of the fire motion is encountered, they are two years of Wu Zi (year of heaven tally) and Wu Wu (year of heaven tally and convergence). The motion's energy of the year dominates the summer heat: when the domination is normal, the weather is warm, hot and evaporating, moist weather with heavy rain will occur, when the domination

is abnormal, the weather will be scorching hot like boiling. In a man, the disease of heat-syndrome in the upper part of the body and hemorrhage will occur. As the year's motion is fire and Wu is a year of Yang, so the guest motion starts from the Greater Zhi and terminates on the Lesser Jue (the sequence is Greater Zhi, Lesser Gong, Greater Shang, Lesser Yu and Lesser Jue), and the host motion starts from the Lesser Jue and terminates on the Lesser Yu (the sequence is Lesser Jue, Greater Zhi, Lesser Gong, Greater Shang and Lesser Yu).

少阴　太宫　阳明　甲子　甲午　其运阴雨，其化柔润时雨，其变震惊飘骤，其病中满身重。

太宫　少商　太羽终　太角初少徵

"When Shaoyin is controlling the heaven energy and Yangming is affecting the earth energy, if the excessive energy of the earth motion is encountered, they are the two years of Jia Zi and Jia Wu. The year's motion dominates the cloudy and rainy weather. When the domination is normal, the weather will be soft and moist, when the domination is abnormal, there will be shocking and sudden blowing of the wind, and people will contract the diseases of abdominal flatulence and heaviness of the body. As the year's motion is earth and Jia is a year of Yang, so the guest motion starts from the Greater Gong and terminates on the Lesser Zhi (the sequence is Greater Gong, Lesser Shang, Greater Yu, Greater Jue and Lesser Zhi), and the host motion starts from the Greater Jue and terminates on the Greater Yu (the sequence is Greater Jue, Lesser Zhi, Greater Gong, Lesser Shang and Greaterr Yu).

少阴　太商　阳明　庚子同天符庚午同天符　同正商　其运凉劲，其化雾露萧飋，其变肃杀凋零，其病下清。

太商　少羽终　少角初　太徵　少宫

"When Shaoyin is controlling the heaven energy and Yangming is affecting the earth energy, if the excessive energy of metal motion is encountered, they are the two years of Gen Zi (same with the year of heaven tally) and Geng Wu (same with the year of heaven tally). As the monach-fire energy of Shaoyin is Controlling the heaven energy and the year's motion is the excessive metal. So the upper Zhi is similar with the Right Shang. The year's motion dominates the cold and pressing weather. When the domination is normal, the weather of frost, dew and desolateness will ocour, when the domination is abnormal, the chilly weather and the withering of trees will occur. People will contract the diseases of diarrhea and coolness of the lower body. As the year's motion is metal and Geng is a year of Yang, so, the guest motion starts from the Greater Shang and terminates on the Lesser Gong (the sequence is Greater Shang, Lesser Yu, Lesser Jue, Greater Zhi and Lesser Gong), and the host motion starts from the Lesser Jue and terminates on the Lesser Yu (the sequence is Lesser Jue, Greater Zhi, Lesser Gong, Greater Shang and Lesser Yu).

少阴　太羽　阳明　丙子岁会　丙午　其运寒，其化凝惨凓冽，其变冰雪霜雹，其病寒下。

太羽终　太角初　少徵　太宫　少商

"When Shaoyin is controlling the heaven energy and Yangming is affecting the earth energy, if the excessive energy of water motion is encountered, they are the two years of Bing Zi (year of convergence) and Bing Wu. The motion's energy dominates the coldness. When the domination is normal, the weather will be cold, when the domination is abnormal, the weather will be of ice, snow, frost and hail. People will contract the asthenia-cold of the middle warmer and cold in abdomen and feet. As the year's motion is water and Bing is a year of Yang, so, the guest motion starts from the Greater Yu and terminates on the Lesser Shang (the sequence is Greater Yu, Greater Jue, Lesser Zhi, Greater Gong and Lesser Shang), and the host motion starts from the Greater Jue and terminates on the Greater Yu (the sequence is Greater Jue, Lesser Zhi, Greater Gong, Lesser Shang and Greater Yu).

凡此少阴司天之政，气化运行先天，地气肃，天气明，寒交暑，热加燥，云驰雨府〔张琦说"上热下燥无湿化流行之理，'云驰'十二字必误衍〕，湿化乃行，时雨乃降，金火合德，上应荧惑太白。其政明，其令切，其谷丹白。水火寒热持于气交而为病始也。热病生于上，清病生于下，寒热凌犯而争于中，民病咳喘，血溢血泄，鼽嚏，目赤，眦疡，寒厥入胃，心痛，腰痛，腹大，嗌乾肿上。初之气，地气迁，燥将去，寒乃始，蛰复藏，水乃冰，霜复降，风乃至，阳气郁，民反周密，关节禁固，腰脽痛，炎暑〔张琦说："'炎暑'二句不伦，必误衍"〕将起，中外疮疡。二之气，阳气布，风乃行，春气以正，万物应荣，寒气时至，民乃和，其病淋，目瞑目赤，气郁于上而热。三之气，天政布，大火行，庶类蕃鲜，寒气时至。民病气厥心病，寒热更作，咳喘目赤。四之气，溽暑至，大雨时行，寒热互至。民病寒热，嗌乾，黄瘅，鼽衄，饮发。五之气，畏火临，暑反至，阳乃化，万物乃生乃长荣，民乃康，其病温。终之气，燥令行，余火内格，肿于上，咳喘，甚则血溢。寒气数举，则霿雾翳，病生皮腠，内舍於胁，下连少腹而作寒中，地将易也，必抑其运气，资其岁胜，折其郁发，先取化源，无使暴过而生其病也，食岁谷以全真气，食间谷以辟虚邪。岁宜咸以软之，而调其上，甚则以苦发之，以酸收之，而安其下，甚则以苦泄之，适气同异而多少之，同天气者以寒清化，同地气者以温热化，用热远热，用凉远凉，用温远温，用寒远寒，食宜同法。有假则反，此其道也，反是者病作矣。

"Whenever Shaoyin is controlling the heaven energy and playing its role, the activity of energy comes prior to the normal weather of the season. The earth energy shrinks and the heaven energy is bright and clear. The cold energy ascends to intersect with the summer energy, and the heat energy descends to mix with the dryness energy, the metal energy and the fire energy are coordinating to play their roles. The corresponding stars above are Mars and Venus. The government of heaven energy is bright, and the manifestation of earth energy is urgent, the colour of the corps is red and white, the cold and heat energies stalemate against each other in the intersection of heaven and earth energies to cause the diseases of men. The disease of heat-evil appears in the upper part of the body, the disease of cold-evil appears in the lower part of the body, and the disease of mutual contending of cold and heat appears in the middle part of the body. Under these conditions, people will often contract the diseases of cough, rapid breathing, bleeding of the mouth and nose, bloody stool, stuffy nose, running nose, sneezing, red eyes, sore in the canthus, cold-jue type syndrome in the stomach,

heartache, lumbago, abdominal distention, dry throat, swelling in head and face, etc.

"In the stage of the initial energy, the cold water of Taiyang is playing its role. The earth energy shifts away, the dryness energy removes, the cold energy begins to become active, the insects hibernate, the water in the river freezes, the cold frost falls again, the cold wind blows frequently and the Yang energy is restricted by the cold energy. By this time, a man should be careful about his living. If one fails to take care of himself, he will contract the diseases of inconvenience in moving the joints and pain in the loins and buttocks. In the period before the scorching weather, one may contract internal or external sores.

"In the stage of the second energy, The wood wind of Jueyin is playing its role. The Yang energy spreads, the wind energy moves about, the spring energy is very comfortable to men, and all things are flourishing. But due to the monarch-fire that controls the heaven energy is not yet abundant, the cold energy comes still quite offen. As the motion's energies of wind and fire are harmonized with the season, people will feel calm and comfortable. Due to the heat energy, people will contract the diseases of dysuria, red eyes, stagnated qifen in the upper warmer and fever of the body.

"In the stage of the third energy, the monarch-fire energy of Shaoyin that controls the heaven energy and the motion's energy of minister-fire are combining to play their roles. The fire energy will be abundant and all things will be flourishing and bright, but due to the frequent invasion of the cold energy, people will often contract the diseases of cold extremities due to heat-evil, heartache, alternative attacks of heat and cold, cough, rapid breathing and red eyes.

"In the stage of the fourth energy, the wetness earth energy of Taiyin is playing its role. The wet weather of hot summer arrives and the big rain falls frequently. The cold and heat occur alternately and people will contract the diseases of cold and heat, dry throat, jaundice, stuffy nose, running nose, epistaxis, accumulation of excessive fluid in the body, etc.

"In the stage of the fifth energy the minister-fire of Shaoyang is playing its role, the weather is scorching hot although it is autumn, yet the Yang energy operates and spreads, so all things become flourishing and people are in good health. If there is any disease, it will be the common seasonal febrile disease.

"In the stage of the terminal energy, the dryness metal of Yangming is playing its role, but the remaining fire-evil causes trouble inside of the body and people will often contract sewelling of head and face, cough and rapid breathing. When it is severe, the hemorrhage of mouth and nose will occur. As the cold energy flows frequently, the scene of hazy sky and dense mist will occur. In a man, the external disease will appear on the striae of skin, the internal disease will retain in the hypochondria, and the disease of cold may tie down to the lower abdomen. By this time, the earth energy will be shifting away.

"In treating, one must restrict the motion's energy which is excessive, assist the energy which is overcome by the motion's energy of the year, and weaken the stagnated energy.

Adjust the source of generation and transformation, and prevent it to become excessive to cause disease. Take the year's crops of which their colours are corresponding to that of the element's motion of the year, and take the intermediate crops of which their growth are promoted by the excessive intermediate energy so as to prevent evil energy. In the year, the medicine or food of salty taste and cold nature should be applied to soften the firmness and adjust the upper part of the body, and take the medicine or food of bitter taste for purgation further; besides. the medicine or food of sour taste should be taken to restrain and stable the lower part of the body. Determine the large or small quantity of the medicine according to the similarity or difference of the motion with the energy. when both the year's motion and the energy that controls the heaven energy are hot, treat with the medicine of cool or cold nature, when the year's motion and the energy that affects the earth energy are both cool, treat with the medicine of hot or warm nature. Do not apply the medicine of hot nature in hot weather, do not apply medicine of cool nature in cool weather, do not apply the medicine of warm nature in warm weather, and do not apply the medicine of cold nature in cold weather. When taking food and drink, the rule stated above should be observed as well. If a substitutionary energy is dominating and the weather is abnormal, the disease should be treated in some other way. These are the fundamental rules which must not be violated to cause disease。"

帝曰：善。厥阴之政奈何？岐伯曰：巳亥之纪也。

Yellow Emperor said:"Good. What is the condition when Jueyin is controlling the heaven energy?" Qibo said: "They are the years marked by the symbols of Si and Hai of the duodecimal cycle.

厥阴　少角　少阳　清热胜复同，同正角。丁巳天符　丁亥天符　其运风清热。

少角[初正]　太徵　少宫　太商　少羽[终]

"When Jueyin is controlling the heaven energy and Shaoyang is affecting the earth energy, if the insufficient energy of wood is encountered, the overocoming energy of coolness and the retaliating energy of heat will occur simultaneously. As the insufficient wood energy receives the help of Jueyin which controls the heaven energy, so, the Upper Jue is similar with the Right Jue(moderate wood energy). They are the two years of Ding Si(year of heaven tally) and Ding Hai (year of heaven tally). The motion's energy of the year is wind, the overcoming energy is coolness and the retaliating energy is heat. As the year's motion is wood and Ding is a year of Yin, so, the guest motion starts from the Lesser Jue and terminates on the Lesser Yu (the sequence is Lesser Jue, Greater Zhi, Lesser Gong, Greater Shang and Lesser Yu). The start and the terminal of the host motion are the same.

厥阴　少徵　少阳　寒雨胜复同。癸巳[同岁会]　癸亥[同岁会]　其运热寒雨。

少徵　太宫　少商　太羽[终]太角[初]

"When Jueyin is controlling the heaven energy and Shaoyang is affecting the earth energy, if the insufficient energy of fire is encountered, the overcoming energy of cold and the retaliating energy of rain will occur simultaneously. They are the two years of Gui Si (same

with the year of convergence) and Gui Hai (same with the year of convergence). The motion's energy of the year is heat, the overcoming energy is cold, and the retaliating energy is rain. As the year's motion is fire and Gui is a year of Yin, so, the guest starts from the Lesser Zhi and terminates on the Greater Jue (the sequence is Lesser Zhi. Greater Gong, Lesser Shang, Greater Yu and Greater Jue, and the host motion starts from the Greater Jue and terminates on the Greater Yu (the sequence is Greater Jue, Lesser Zhi, Greater Gong, Lesser Shang and Greater Yu).

厥阴　少宫　少阳　风清胜复同，同正角。己巳　己亥　其运雨风清。

少宫　太商　少羽[终]　少角[初]　太徵

"When Jueyin is controlling the heaven energy and Shaoyang is affecting the earth energy, if the insufficient energy of the earth motion is encountered, the overcoming energy of wind and the retaliating energy of coolness will occur simultaneously. As the insufficient energy of earth motion is overcome by wood wind energy which controls the heaven energy, and earth energy assimilates with the wood energy, so, the Upper Jue is similar with the Right Jue. They are the two years of Ji Si and Ji Hai. The motion's energy of the year is rain, the overcoming energy is wind and the retaliating energy is coolness. As the year's motion is earth, and Ji is a year of Yin, so, the guest motion starts from the Lesser Gong and terminates on the Greater Zhi (the sequence is Lesser Gong, Greater Shang, Lesser Yu, Lesser Jue and Greater Zhi), and the host motion starts from the Lesser Jue and terminates on the Lesser Yu (the sequence is Lesser Jue, Greater Zhi, Lesser Gong, Greater Shang and Lesser Yu).

厥阴　少商　少阳　热寒胜复同　同正角。乙巳　乙亥　其运凉热寒。

少商　太羽[终]　太角[初]　少徵　太宫

"When Jueyin is controlling the heaven energy and Shaoyang is affecting the earth energy, if the insufficient energy of metal motion is encountered , the overcoming energy of heat and the retaliating energy of coldness will occur simultaneously. As the energy of metal motion is insufficient, and wood wind of Jueyin is controlling the heaven energy, the metal can no more control the wood, and wood plays its role, so, the Upper Jue is similar with the Right Jue. They are the two years of Yi Si and Yi Hai. The motion's energy of the year is coolness, the overcoming energy is heat, and the retaliating energy is coldness. As the year's motion is metal and Yi is a year of Yin, so, the guest motion starts from the Lesser Shang and terminates on the Greater Gong (the sequence is Lesser Shang, Greater Yu, Greater Jue, Lesser Zhi and Greater Gong), and the host motion starts from the Greater Jue and terminates on the Greater Yu (the sequence is Greater Jue, Lesser Zhi, Greater Gong, Lesser Shang and Greater Yu).

厥阴　少羽　少阳　雨风胜复同。辛巳　辛亥　其运寒雨风。

少羽[终]　少角[初]　太徵　少宫　太商

"When Jueyin is controlling the heaven energy and Shaoyang is affecting the earth energy, if the insufficient energy of water motion is encountered, the overcoming energy of rain

and the retaliating energy of wind will occur simultaneously. They are the two years of Xin Si and Xin Hai. The motion's energy of the year is coldness, the overcoming energy is rain and the retaliating energy is wind. As the year's motion is water and Xin is a year of Yin, So, the guest motion starts from the Lesser Yu and terminates on the Greater Shang (the sequence is Lesser Yu, Lesser Jue, Greater Zhi, Lesser Gong and Greater Shang), and the host motion starts from the Lesser Jue and terminates on the Lesser Yu (the sequence is Lesser Jue, Greater Zhi, Lesser Gong, Greater Shang and Lesser Yu).

凡此厥阴司天之政，气化运行后天，诸同正岁，气化运行同天，天气扰，地气正，风生高远，炎热从之，云趋雨府，湿化乃行，风火同德，上应岁星荧惑。其政挠，其令速，其谷苍丹，间谷言太者，其耗文角品羽。风燥火热，胜复更作，蛰见来见，流水不冰，热病行于下，风病行于上，风燥胜复形于中。初之气，寒始肃，杀气方至，民病寒于右之下。二之气，寒不去，华雪水冰，杀气施化，霜乃降，名草上焦，寒雨数至，阳复化，民病热于中。三之气，天政布，风乃时举，民病泣出耳鸣掉眩。四之气溽暑湿热相薄，争于左之上，民病黄乃而为胕肿。五之气，燥湿更胜，沉阴乃布，寒气及体，风雨乃行。终之气，畏火司令，阳乃大化，蛰虫出见，流水不冰，地气大发，草乃生，人乃舒，其病温厉，必折其郁气，资其化源，赞其运气，无使邪胜。岁宜以辛调上，以咸调下，畏火之气，无妄犯之。用温远温，用热远热，用凉远凉，用寒远寒，食宜同法。有假反常，此之道也，反是者病。

"Whenever Jueyin is controlling the heaven energy and playing its role, the activity of the energy comes lagging behind the normal weather of the season, if the year's moderate energy is encountered, the activation of energy will come in conformity with the normal weather of the season. As the wood wind energy is controlling the heaven energy, so the heaven energy will be stirring, and as monarch-fire energy of Shaoyin is affecting the earth energy, the earth energy will be normal. As the wood energy is above, the wind will be blowing high and far, as the fire energy is below, the scorching heat will be pursuing. The carrying of rain by the clouds is the symbol of the spreading of the wetness earth energy, and it is the effect of the coordination of the wind energy and the fire energy. The corresponding stars above are Jupiter and Mars. Its authority of office is wind and stirring, and the decree of fire is urgent. The corresponding crops are those of dark-green and red colours, and the maturity of the intermediate crops are promoted by the excessive intermediate energy. As the dryness wind and the hot fire energies are combating, the hibernants occur again outside, and the flowing water can not be frozen. In a man, the diseases of heat-evil are apt to appear in the lower part of the body, the diseases of wind-evil are apt to appear in the upper part of the body, and the diseases of the contention of wind and dryness energies are apt to appear in the middle part of the body.

"In the stage of the initial energy, the dryness energy of Yangming is playing its role, The cold energy is urgent, the energies of chillness and restraint have just arrived, and people will often contract the disease of cold under the right hypochondrium.

"In the stage of the second energy, the cold water energy of Taiyang is playing its role. The cold energy is retaining, the snow is flying and the water in the river freezes, the ener-

gies of chilliness and restraint are playing their roles, the falling of the cold frost causes the tips of the grasses become withered and the cold rain falls frequently. As the monarch-fire of Shaoyin is dominating the season, the Yang energy will be dispersing again, and people will contract the disease of retention of heat-evil in the middle warmer.

"In the stage of the third energy, the wind energy of Jueyin is playing its role and the wind blowe frequently. People will often contract the diseases of tears in eyes, tinnitus and dizziness.

"In the stage of the fourth energy, the monarch-fire energy of Shaoyin is playing its role. The wet summer arrives, and the wetness energy (host energy) and the heat energy (guest energy) are combating in the left side of the upper body. People will contract the diseases of jaundice and edema often.

"In the stage of the fifth energy, the dryness host energy of Yangming and the guest energy of wetness Taiyin are becoming even more abundant, the weather is usually cloudy, the cold energy invades men and the storm will occur.

"In the stage of the terminal energy, the guest energy of the minister-fire Shaoyang is playing its role. The Yang energy is overabundant, the hibernants come out often, the flowing water can not be frozen, The earth energy is developing, the various kinds of grasses are growing again, and people will feel comfortable, but the seasonal febrile disease is apt to be contracted.

"When treating, one must weaken the overcoming energy that causes the retained energy, assist the source of generation and transformation, enhance the motion's energy and prevent the evil energy from being excessive. In the year, apply the acrid taste to adjust the wind energy above, and apply the salty taste to adjust the fire energy below, and the prime minister-fire should be pacified and must not be offended rashly. Do not apply the medicine of warm nature in warm weather, do not apply the medicine of hot nature in hot weather, do not apply the medicine of cold nature in cold weather, and do not apply the medicine of cool nature in cool weather. When taking food and drink, the rules stated above should be observed as well. When the substitutionary energy is dominating and the weather is abnormal, the disease should be treated in some other way. These are the fundamental rules for treating, and they must not be violated to cause disease。"

帝曰：善。夫子言可谓悉矣，然何以明其应乎？岐伯曰：昭乎哉问也！夫六气者，行有次，止有位，故常以正月朔日平旦视之，睹其位而知其所在矣。运有余，其至先，运不及，其至后，此天之道，气之常也。运非有余非不足，是谓正岁，其至当其时也。帝曰：胜复之气，其常在也。灾眚时至，候他奈何？岐伯曰：非气化者，是谓灾也。

Yellow Emperor said; Good. Your words are exhaustive enough but how to know its respond?" Qibo said: "What an evident question you have asked. The movement of the six weathers are all having their regular sequences and definite orientations. One should observe it in the dawn on the first day of the first lunar month. According to its position, one can know whether it is corresponding or not. When the energy of the year's motion is excessive,

the activity of energy will come prior to the normal weather of the season, when the energy of the year's motion is insufficient, the activity of energy will come lagging behind the normal weather of the season. This is the principle of heaven and the law of the six weathers. If the energy of the year's motion is neither excessive nor insufficient, it is the so called the 'normal year', and the activity of energy comes with the normal weather of the season together。"

Yellow Emperor asked:"There often occurs the overcoming energy, the retaliating energy and the calamities, how to examine them?" Qibo said: "When the activity of energy is not in its proper position, it may be considered to be the calamity。"

帝曰：天地之数，终始奈何？岐伯曰：悉乎哉问也！是明道也。数之始，起于上而终于下，岁半之前，天气主之，岁半之后，地气主之，上下交互，气交主之，岁纪毕矣。故曰位明，气月可知乎，所谓气也。帝曰：余司其事，则而行之，不合其数何也？岐伯曰：气用有多少，化洽有盛衰，衰盛多少，同其化也。帝曰：愿闻同化何如？岐伯曰：风温春化同，热曛昏火夏化同，胜与复同，燥清烟露秋化同，云雨昏暝埃长夏化同，寒气霜雪冰冬化同，此天地五运六气之化，更用盛衰之常也。

Yellow Emperor asked: "What are the orders of the initial and terminal symbols and periodical change of the energies that controls the heaven energy and affects the earth energy?" Qibo said: "What an exhaustive question you have asked. Surely you are keen in researching the medicine. It starts from the heaven energy and ends in the earth energy, the heaven energy dominates in the first half of the year, the earth energy dominates in the second half of the year, and the intersecting energy of heaven and earth dominates the mutual actions of the heaven and earth energies. This is the entire condition of the law of the activity of energy in the year. Thus, when one knows the upper, lower, left and right positions of the energy, he can know which energy is dominating the month respectively. It is the so called knowing the orders of the initial and terminal domination of the heaven and earth energies。"

Yellow Emperor said: " I have examined the matter and have behaved as what you said, but sometimes, the domination of the heaven and earth energies does not agree with the corresponding weather of the year, and what is the reasen?" Qibo said: " The affect of the six kinds of weather are sometimes excessive and sometimes insufficient, when they combine with the five elements' motion, the energy may be prosperous or declining. Since the cases are different, there exists the assimilation。"

Yellow Emperor asked: " What is assimilation?" Qibo said: " The windy and warm energy assimilates with the wood energy of spring, the depressing hot energy assimilates with the fire energy of summer. There are also assimilations in the overcoming energy and the retaliatins energy, the energies of dryness, coolness, smoke and dew assimilate with the metal energy of autumn, and the energies of frost and snow assimilate with the water energy of winter. These are the assimilations of the Six kinds of weather in heaven and the five elements motion on earth and it is the regular law of the interaction of prosperity and decline。"

帝曰：五运行同天化者，命曰，天符，余知之矣。愿闻同地化者何谓也？岐伯曰：太过

而同天化者三，不及而同天化者亦三，太过而同地化者三，不及而同地化者亦三。此凡二十四岁也。帝曰：愿闻其所谓也。岐伯曰：甲辰甲戌太宫下加太阴，壬寅壬申太角下加厥阴，庚子庚午太商下加阳明，如是者三。癸巳癸亥少徵下加少阳，辛丑辛未少羽下加太阳，癸卯癸酉少徵下加少阴，如是者三。戊子戊午太徵上临少阴，戊寅戊申太徵上临少阳，丙辰丙戌太羽上临太阳，如是者三。丁巳丁亥少角上临厥阴，乙卯乙酉少商上临阳明，己丑己未少宫上临太阴，如是者三。除此二十四岁，则不加不临也。帝曰：加者何谓？岐伯曰：太过而加同天符，不及而加同岁会也。帝曰：临者何谓？岐伯曰：太过不及，皆曰天符，而变行有多少，病形有微甚，生死有早晨晏耳。

Yellow Emperor said："I have known already that when the motion's energy of the year agrees with the energy that controls the heaven energy is called the heaven tally. I hope to know further the condition when the energy of the year's motion agrees with the energy that affects the earth energy。" Qibo said："There are three cases when the excessive energy of the year's motion agrees with the energy that controls the heaven energy and there are three cases when the insufficient energy of the year's motion agrees with the energy that controls the heaven energy, and there are three cases when the excessive energy of the year's motion agrees with the energy that affects the earth energy, there are therr cases when the insufficient energy of the year's motion agrees with the energy that affects the earth energy. They are all together twenty four years with different cases."

Yellow Emperor said："I hope to know the meaning of three。" Qibo said："In the two years of Jia Chen and the Jia Xu the excessive energy of the earth motion assimilates with Taiyin that affects the earth energy; in the years of Ren Yin and Ren Shen, the excessive energy of wood motion assimilates with Jueyin that affects the earth energy; in the years of Geng Zi and Geng Wu, the excessive energy of metal motion assimilates with Yangming that affects the earth energy. These are the three cases when the excessive enegy agrees with the energy that affects the earth energy.

"In the two years of Gui Si and Gui Hai, the insufficient energy of the fire motion assimilates with Shaoyang that affects the earth energy; in the years of Xin Chou and Xin Wei, the insufficient energy of water motion assimilates with Taiyang that affects the earth energy; in the years of Gui Mao and Gui You, the insufficient energy of the fire motion assimilates with Shaoyin that affects the earth energy. These are the three cases when the insufficient energy agrees with the energy that affects the earth energy.

"In the two years of Wu Zi and Wu Wu , tne excessive energy of the five motion assimilates with Shaoyin that controls the heaven energy; in the years of Wu Yin and Wu Shen, the excessive energy of the fire motion assimilates with Shaoyang that controls the heaven energy; in the years of Bing Chen and Bing Xu, the excessive energy of the water motion assimilates with Taiyang that controls the heaven energy. These are the three cases when the excessive energy agrees with the energy that controls the heaven energy.

"In the two years of Ding Si and Ding Hai, the insufficient energy of the wood motion assimilates with Jueyin that controls the heaven energy; in the years of Yi Mao and Yi You,

the insufficient energy of the metal motion assimilates with Yangming that controls the heaven energy; in the years of Ji Chou and Ji Wei, the insufficient energy of the earth motion assimilates with Taiyin that controls the heaven energy. These are the three cases when the insufficient energy agrees with the energy that controls the heaven energy.

"Besides the twenty four years, there is no other energy of the year's motion agrees with the energy that controls the heaven energy or affects the earth energy。"

Yellow Emperor asked: "What is the condition when the year's motion agrees with the energy that affects the earth energy?"Qibo said: " When the excessive energy agrees with the energy that affects the earth energy, it is called 'same with the year of heaven tally', when the insufficient energy agrees with the energy that affects the earth energy, it is called 'same with the year of convergence'。" Yellow Emperor asked: " What is the condition when the year's motion agrees with the energy that controls the heaven energy?" Qibo said: " when the cxcessive energy or the insufficient energy agrees with the year's motion, they are both called the heaven tally, only the extents of operation of the energy may be large or may be small, the condition of diseases may be severe or slight, and the time of the patient's survival or death may be early or late。"

帝曰：夫子言用寒远寒，用热远热，余未知其然也，愿闻何谓远？岐伯曰：热无犯热，寒无犯寒，从者和，逆者病，不可不敬畏而远之，所谓时兴〔《素问校讹》引古抄本"兴"作"与"〕六位也。帝曰：温凉何如？岐伯曰：司气以热，用热无犯，司气以寒，用寒无犯，司气以凉，用凉无犯，司气以温，用温无犯，闲气同其主无犯，异其主则小犯之，是谓四畏，必谨察之。帝曰：善。其犯者何如？岐伯曰：天气反时，则可依及胜其主则可犯，以平为期，而不可过，是谓邪气反胜者。故曰：无失天信，无逆气宜，无翼其胜，无赞其复，是谓至治。

Yellow Emperor said: " As you have said, do not apply the medicine of cold nature in cold weather and do not apply the medicine of hot nature in hot weather, I do not know the exact way of doing it, I hope you can tell me specifically。" Qibo said: " When applyng the medicine of hot nature, it must not be contradictory with the heat of the weather. When applying the medicine of cold nature, it must not be contradictory with the cold of the weather. When following this law, the patient will be easy and calm, otherwise, the disease will become more severe, and one must take good care of not violating it. This is indieating the host energy (which dominates the four seasons)and the guest energy (the six-energy that cooperates with the four seasons)。"

Yellow Emperor asked: " since warmness and coolness are inferior to heat and coldness, can the warmness and coolness be violated?" Qibo said: " When the motion's energy is hot , the applying medicine of hot nature should be avoided. When the motion's energy is cold, the applying medicine of cold nature should be avoided, when the motion's energy is cool, the applying medicine of cool nature should be avoided, when the motion's energy is warm, the applying medicine of warm nature should be avoided. When the intermediate energy is similar with the host energy, such as both are hot or both are cold, the energy will be strong and it must not be violated, if the intermediate enegy is different with the host energy, it can be

violated slightly. The coldness, hotness, warmness and the coolness are called the four fears, and they must be observed carefully and pay good attention in avoiding them。"

Yellow Emperor said: " Good. But under the condition when one can not but to violate it, what should one do?" Qibo said: " When the guest energy disagrees with the host energy, the host energy should be followed, when the guest energy is stronger than the host energy, the guest energy may also be violated, but the violation should be limited under the level of balance, and must not be surpassed. This is because the evil-energy, on the contrary, is overcoming the energy that dominates the season. Therefore, when the treating is not violating the arriving time of the guest energy and the host energy, not violating the proper weather of cold, hot, warm and cool and enhancing neither the overcoming energy or the retaliating energy, it is the best way of treating。"

帝曰：善。五运气行主岁之纪，其有常数乎？岐伯曰：臣请次之。

甲子甲午岁

上少阴火　中太宫土运，下阳明金　热化二，雨化五，燥化四，所谓正化日也。其化上咸寒，中苦热，下酸热，所谓药食宜也。

Yellow Emperor said: " Good. Is there any regular number in the activity of energy of the element's motion that dominates the year?" Qibo said: Let me tell you in sequence:

In the years of Jia Zi and Jia Wu, Shaoyin is controlling the heaven energy and Yangming is affecting the earth energy, so, the upper motion is the monarch-fire of Shaoyin, the lower motion is dryness metal of Yangming, and the middle motion of the year is the excessive energy of the earth motion greater Gong. The producing number of the monarch-fire which controls the heaven energy above is two, the producing number of the excessive earth energy of the motion of the year in the middle is five, and the producing number of the dryness energy which affects the earth energy below is four. In the year, there is no overcoming and retaliating energies. As the upper, middle and the lower motions are all assimilated with the healthy energy, it is called the normal activity of energy. When treating the disease caused by the heat energy that controls the heaven energy, the medicine of salty taste and cold nature should be applied, when treating the disease caused by the rain wetness energy of the middle motion, the medicine of bitter taste and hot nature should be applied, when treating the disease caused by the dryness energy that affects the earth energy, the medicine of sour taste and hot nature should be applied. These are the proper ways of applying medicine in these two years.

乙丑乙未岁

上太阴土　中少商金运　下太阳水　热化寒化胜复同，所谓邪气化日也。灾七宫。湿化五，清化四，寒化六，所谓正化日也。其化上苦热，中酸和，下甘热，所谓药食宜也。

"In the years of Yi Chow and Yi Wei, Taiyin is controlling the heaven energy above and Taiyang is affecting the earth energy below, so, the upper motion is the wetness earth of Taiyin and the lower motion is the cold water of Taiyang, and the middle motion is the Lesser Shang which is the insufficient energy of the metal motion. The overcoming energy of as-

similating heat and the retaliating energy of the assimilating cold will occur simultaneously. As the assimilating of both the overcoming and the retaliating energies are abnormal energies, they are called the assimilating of the evil-energy. The calamity caused is in the west, the producing number of the assimilating wetness energy that controls the heaven energy is five, the producing number of the assimilating cool energy of the middle motion is four, the accomplishing number of the assimilating cold energy that affects the earth energy is six. As all the assimilating energies are healthy energies, they are called the assimilating energies are healthy energies, When treating the disease caused by the wetness energy that controls the heaven energy, the medicine of bitter taste and hot nature should be applied, when treating the disease caused by the cool energy of the middle motion of the year, the medicine of sour taste and mild nature should be applied, when treating the disease caused by the cold energy which affects the earth energy, the medicine of sweet taste and hot nature should be applied. These are the proper ways of applying medicine in these two years.

丙寅　丙申岁

上少阳相火，中太羽水运，下厥阴木，火化二，寒化六、风化三，所谓正化日也。其化上咸寒，中咸温，下辛温，所谓药食宜也。

"In the years of Bing Yin and Bing Shen, Shaoyang is controlling the heaven energy above, and Jueyin is affecting the earth energy below, so, the upper motion is the prime minister-fire of Shaoyang, the lower motion is the wood wind of Jueyin, and the middle motion is the Greater Yu which is the excessive energy of the water motion. The producing number of the assimilating prime minister-fire which controls the heaven energy is two, the accomplishing number of the assimilating water energy of the middle motion is six, the producing number of the assimilating wind energy that affects the earth energy is three. As all of the assimilating energies are healthy energies, they are called the assimilation of the healthy energies. When treating the disease caused by the fire energy which controls the heaven energy, the medicine of salty taste and cold nature should be applied, when treating the disease caused by the excessive water energy of the middle motion, the medicine of salty taste and warm nature should be applied , when treating the disease caused by the wind energy that affects the earth energy, the medicine of acrid taste and warm nature should be applied. These are the proper ways of applying medicine in these two years.

丁卯岁会　丁酉岁

上阳明金，中少角木运，下少阴火，清化热化胜复同，所谓邪气化日也，灾三宫。燥化九，风化三，热化七，所谓正化日也。其化上苦小温，中辛和，下咸寒，所谓药食宜也。

"In the years of Ding Mao (year of convergence) and Ding You, Yangming is controlling the heaven energy above and Shaoyin is affecting the earth energy below, so, the upper motion is the dryness metal of Yangming, the lower motion is the heat monarch-fire of Shaoyin and the middle motion is the lesser Jue which is the insufficient energy of the wood motion. The overcoming energy of the assimilating coolness and the retaliating energy of assimilating heat will occur simultaneously. As the assimilating energies are all evil energies, they are

called the assimilation of evil energies. The calamity caused is in the east. The accomplishing number of the assimilating dryness energy which controls the heaven energy is nine, the producing number of the assimilating wind energy of the middle motion is three, and the accomplishing number of the assimilating heat energy which affects the earth energy is seven. As all the assimilating energies are healthy, they are called the assimilation of healthy energies. When treating the disease caused by the dryness energy which controls the heaven energy, the medicine of bitter taste and slight-warm nature should be applied, when treating the disease caused by the insufficient wind energy of the middle motion, the medicine of acrid taste and mild nature should be applied, when treating the disease caused by the heat energy which affects the earth energy, the medicine of salty taste and cold nature should be applied. These are the proper ways of applying medicine in these two years.

戊辰　戊戌岁

上太阳水，中太徵火运，下太阴土，寒化六，热化七，湿化五，所谓正化日也。其化上苦温，中甘和，下甘温，所谓药食宜也。

"In the years of Wu Chen and Wu Xu, Taiyang is controlling the heaven energy above and Taiyin is affecting the earth energy below, so, the upper motion is the cold water of Taiyang, the lower motion is the wetness earth of Taiyin and the middle motion is the greater Zhi which is the excessive energy of the fire motion. The accomplishing number of the assimilating cold energy which controls the heaven energy is six, the accomplishing number of the assimilating fire energy of the middle motion is seven, the producing number of the assimilating wetness energy which affects the earth energy is five. As all the assimilating energies are healthy, they are called the assimilating of healthy energies. When treating the disease caused by the cold energy that controls the heaven energy, the medicine of bitter taste and warm nature should be applied, when treating the disease caused by the fire energy of the middle motion, the medicine of sweet taste and mild nature should be applied, when treating the disease caused by the wetness energy which affects the earth energy, the medicine of sweet taste and warm nature should be applied. These are the proper ways of applying medicine in these two years.

己巳　己亥岁

上厥阴木，中少宫土运，下少阳相火，风化清化胜复同，所谓邪气化日也。灾五宫。风化三，湿化五，火化七，所谓正化日也。其化上辛凉，中甘和，下咸寒，所谓药食宜也。

In the years of Ji Si and Ji Hai, Jueyin is controlling the heaven energy above and Shaoyang is affecting the earth energy below, so, the upper motion is the wind wood energy of Jueyin, the lower motion is prime minister fire of Shaoyang and the middle motion is the lesser Gong which is the insufficient energy of the earth motion. The overcoming energy of the assimilating wind and the retaliating energy of coolness will occur simultaneously. As the assimilating energies of both overcoming and retaliating are abnormal energies the year, they are called the assimilation of evil energies. The calamity caused is in the centre. The producing number of the assimilating wind energy that controls the heaven energy is three, the pro-

ducing number of the assimilating wetness energy of the middle motion is five, and the accomplishing number of the assimilating fire energy which affects the earth energy is seven. As all the assimiating energies are healthy, they are called the assimilation of healthy energies. When treating the disease caused by the wind energy which controls the heaven energy, the medicine of acrid taste and cool nature should be applied, When treating the disease caused by the insufficient earth energy of the middle motion, the medicine of sweet taste and mild nature should be applied, when treating the disease caused by the prime minister-fire energy which affects the earth energy, the medicine of salty taste and cold nature should be applied. These are the proper ways of applying medicine in these two years.

庚午同天符　庚子岁同天符

上少阴火，中太商金运，下阳明金，热化七，清化九，燥化九，所谓正化日也。其化上咸寒，中辛温，下酸温，所谓药食宜也。

In the years of Geng Wu (same with the year of heaven tally) and Geng Zi (same with the year of heaven tally), Shaoyin is controlling the heaven energy above and Yangming is affecting the earth energy below, so, the upper motion is the heat monarch fire of Shaoyin, the lower motion is dryness metal of Yangming, and the middle motion is the greater Shang which is the excessive energy of the metal motion. The accomplishing number of the assimilating heat energy which controls the heaven energy is seven, the accomplishing number of the assimilating cool energy of the middle motion is nine, the accomplishing number of the assimilating dryness energy that affects the earth energy is nine. As all the assimilating energies are healthy, they are called the assimilation of healthy energies. When treating the disease caused by the heat energy which controls the heaven energy, the medicine of salty taste and cold nature should be applied. when treating the disease caused by the coolness energy of the middle motion, the medicine of acrid taste and warm mature should be applied. When treating the disease caused by the dryness energy which affects the earth energy, the medicine of sour taste and warm nature should be applied. These are the proper ways of applying medicine in these two years.

辛未同岁会辛丑岁同岁会

上太阴土，中少羽水运，下太阳水，雨化风化胜复同，所谓邪气化日也。灾一宫。雨化五，寒化一，所谓正化日也。其化上苦热，中苦和，下苦热，所谓药食宜也。

"In the years of Xin Wei (same with the year of convergence) and Xin Chou (same with the year of convergence), Taiyin is controlling the heaven energy above, and Taiyang is affecting the earth energy below, so, the upper motion is the wetness earth of Taiyin, the lower motion is the cold water of Taiyang, and the middle motion is the Lesser Yu which is the insufficient energy of the water motion. The overcoming energy of the assimilating rain and the retaliating energy of the assimilating wind will occur simultaneously. As both the assimilating energies of overcoming and retaliating are the abnormal energies of the year, they are called the assimilation of evil energies. The calamity caused is in the north. The producing number of the assimilating rain energy which controls the heaven energy is five, the produc-

ing number of the assimilating cold energy which affects the earth energy is one, As the assimilating energies are all healthy, they are called the assimilation of healthy energies. When treating the disease caused by the wetness energy which controls the heaven energy, the medicine of bitter taste and hot nature should be applied, when treating the disease caused by the insufficient water energy of the middle motion, the medicine of bitter taste and mild nature should be applied, when treating the disease caused by the cold energy which affects the earth energy, the medicine of bitter taste and hot nature should be applied. These are the proper ways of applying medicine in these two years.

壬申[同天符]　壬寅岁[天同符]

上少阳相火，中太角木运，下厥阴木，火化二，风化八，所谓正化日也。其化上咸寒，中酸和，下辛凉，所谓药食宜也。

In the years of Ren Shen (same with the year of heaven tally) and Ren Yin (same with the year of heaven tally), Shaoyang is controlling the heaven energy above and Jueyin is affecting the earth energy below. So, the upper motion is the prime minister-fire of Shaoyang, the lower motion is the wind wood of Jueyin and the middle motion is greater Jue which is the excessive energy of the wood motion. The producing number of the assimilating fire energy which controls the heaven energy is two, the accomplishing number of the assimilating wind energy which affects the earth energy is eight. As both the assimilating energies are healthy, they are called the assimilation of the healthy energies. When treating the disease caused by the prime minister-fire energy that controls the heaven energy, the medicine of salty taste and cold nature should be applied, When treating the disease causead by the excessive wood energy of the middle motion, the medicine of sour taste and mild nature should be applied. when treating the disease caused by the wind energy which affecting the earth energy, the medicine of acrid taste and cool nature should be applied. These are the proper ways of applying medicine in these two years.

癸酉[同岁会]　癸卯岁[同岁会]

上阳明金，中少徵火运，下少阴火，寒化雨化胜复同，所谓邪气化日也。灾九宫。燥化九，热化二，所谓正化日也。其化上苦小温，中咸温，下咸寒，所谓药食宜也。

"In the years of Gui You (same with the year of convergence) and Gui Mao (same with the year of convergence), Yangming is controlling the heaven energy above and Shaoyin is affecting the earth energy below. So, the upper motion is coolness metal of Yangming, the lower motion is heat monarch-fire of Shaoyin, and the middle motion is the Lesser Zhi which is the insufficient energy of the fire motion. The overcoming energy of assimilating cold and the retaliating energy of rain will appear simultaneously. As the assimilating energies of overcoming and retaliating of the year are both abnormal energies, they are called the assimilating of the evil energies. The calamity caused is in the south. The accomplishing number of the assimilating dryness energy which controls the heaven energy is nine, the producing number of the assimilating heat energy which affects the earth energy is two, As the assimilating energies are both healthy, they are called the assimilation of healthy energies. When

treating the disease caused by the dryness energy which controls the heaven energy, the medicine of bitter taste and slight warm nature should be applied, when treating the disease caused by insufficient fire energy of the middle motion, the medicine of salty taste and warm nature should be applied, when treating the disease caused by the heat energy that affects the earth energy, the medicine of salty taste and cold nature should be applied. These are the proper ways of applying medicine in these two years.

甲戌岁会同天符　甲辰岁岁会同天符

上太阳水，中太宫土运，下太阴土，寒化六，湿化五，正化日也。其化上苦热，中苦温，下苦温，药食宜也。

In the years of Jia Xu (year of convergence and same with heaven tally) and Jia Chen (year of convergence and same with heaven tally). Taiyang is controlling the heaven energy above, Taiyin is affecting the earth energy below. So, the upper motion is the cold water of Taiyang, the lower motion is the wetness earth of Taiyin, and the middle motion is the greater Gong which is the excessive energy of the earth motion. The accomplishing number of the assimilating cold energy which controls the heaven energy is six, and the producing number of the assimilating wetness energy which affects the earth energy is five. As the assimilating energies are both healthy, they are called the assimilation of healthy energies. When treating the disease caused by the cold energy which controls the heaven energy, the medicine of bitter taste and hot nature should be applied, when treating the disease caused by the excessive earth energy of the middle motion, the medicine of bitter taste and warm nature should be applied, when treating the disease caused by the wetness energy which affects the earth energy, the medicine of bitter taste and warm nature should be applied. These are the proper ways of applying medicine in these two years.

乙亥　乙巳岁

上厥阴木，中少商金运，下少阳相火，热化寒化胜复同，邪气化日也。灾七宫。风化八，清化四，火化二，正化度也。其化上辛凉，中酸和，下咸寒，药食宜也。

"In the years of Yi Hai and Yi Si, Jueyen is controlling the heaven energy above and Shaoyang is affecting the earth energy below. So, the upper motion is the wind wood of Jueyin, the lower motion is the prime minister-fire of Shaoyang, and the middle motion is lesser Shang which is the insufficient energy of the metal motion. The overcoming energy of assimilating heat and the retaliating energy of assimilating cold will occur simultaneously. As both the assimilating energies of overcoming and retaliating are the abnormal energies of the year, they are called the assimilation of evil energy. The calamity caused is in the west. The accomplishing numeber of the assimilating wind energy which controls the heaven energy is eight, the producing number of the assimilating cool energy which is the middle motion is four, and the producing number of the prime minister-fire energy that affects the earth energy is two. As the assimilating energies are all healthy, they are called the assimilation of healthy energies. When treating the disease caused by the wind energy which controls the heaven energy, the medicine of acrid tastes and cool nature should be applied, when treating

the disease caused by the dryness energy of the middle motion, the medicine of sour taste and mild nature should be applied, when treating the disease caused by the prime minster-fire energy which affects the earth energy, the medicine of salty taste and cold nature should be applied. These are the proper ways of applying medicine in these two years.

丙子岁会　丙午岁

上少阴火，中太羽水运，下阳明金，热化二，寒化六，清化四，正化度也。其化上咸寒，中咸热，下酸温，药食宜也。

"In the years of Bing Zi (year of convergence) and Bing Wu, Shaoyin is controlling the heaven energy above and Yangming is affecting the earth energy below. So, the upper motion monarch fire is the Shaoyin, the lower motion is the dryness metal of Yangming, and the middle motion greater Yu which is the excessive energy of the water motion. The producing number of the assimilating heat energy which controls the heaven energy is two, the accomplishing number of the assimilating cold energy of the middle motion is six, and the producing number of the assimilating cool energy which affects the earth energy is four. As they are all healthy energies. they are called the assimilation of healthy energies, When treating the disease caused by the heat energy which controls the heaven energy, the medicine of salty taste and cold nature should be applied, when treating the disease caused by the excessive cold energy of the middle motion, the medicine of salty taste and hot nature should be applied, when treating the disease caused by the dryness energy which affects the earth energy, the medicine of sour taste and warm nature should be applied. These are the proper ways of applying medicine in these two years.

丁丑　丁未岁

上太阴土，中少角木运，下太阳水，清化热化胜复同，邪气化度也。灾三宫。雨化五，风化三，寒化一，正化度也。其化上苦温，中辛温，下甘热，药食宜也。

"In the years of Ding Chou and Ding Wei, Taiyin is controlling the heaven energy above, and Taiyang is affecting the earth energy below. So, the upper motion is the vetness earth of Taiyin, the lower motion is the cold water of Taiyang, and the middle motion is the Lesser Jue which is the insufficient energy of the wood motion. The overcoming energy of the assimilating coolness and the retaliating energy of assimilating heat will occur simultaneously. As the assimilating energies of overcoming and retaliating are both abnormal energies of the year, they are called the assimilation of evil energies. The calamity caused is in the east. The producing number of the assimilating wetness energy which controls the heaven energy is five, the producing number of the assimilating wind energy of the middle motion is three, the puoducing number of the assimlating cold energy which affects the earth energy is one, and they are all healthy energies. When treating the disease caused by the wetness energy which controls the heaven energy, the medicine of bitter taste and warm nature should be applied, when treating the disease caused by the insufficient wood energy of the middle motion, the medicine of acrid taste and warm nature should be applied, when treating the disease caused by the cold energy which affects the earth energy, the medicine of sweet taste

and hot nature should be applied. These are the proper ways of aplying medicine in these two years.

戊寅　戊申岁天符

上少阳相火，中太徵火运，下厥阴木，火化七，风化三，正化度也。其化上咸寒，中甘和，下辛凉，药食宜也。

In the years of Wu Yin and Wu Shen (year of heaven tally), Shaoyang is controlling the heaven energy above and Jueyin is affecting the earth energy below. So, the upper motion is the heat prime minister-fire of Shaoyang, the lower motion is the wind wood of Jueyin, and the middle motion is the greater Zhi which is the excessive energy of the fire motion. The accomplishing number of the assimilating fire energy which controls the heaven energy is seven, the producing number of the assimilating wind energy which affects the earth energy is three, and they are all healthy energies. When treating the disease caused by the fire energy which controls the heaven energy, the medicine of salty taste and cold nature should, be applied, when treating the disease caused by the excessive fire energy of the middle motion, the medicine of sweet taste and mild nature should be applied, when treating the disease caused by the wind energy which affects the earth energy, the medicine of acrid taste and cool nature should be applied. These are the proper ways of applying medicine in these two years.

己卯　己酉岁

上阳明金，中少宫土运，下少阴火，风化清化胜复同，邪气化度也。灾五宫。清化九，雨化五，热化七，正化度也。其化上苦小温，中甘和，下咸寒，药食宜也。

"In the years of Ji Mao and Ji You, Yangming is controlling the heaven energy and Shaoyin is affecting the earth energy. So, the upper motion is the dryness metal of Yangming, the lower motion is the monarch-fire of Shaoyin, and the middle motion is the Lesser Gong which is the insufficient energy of the earth motion. The overcoming energy of the assimilating wind and the retaliating energy of the assimilating coolness will occur simultaneously. As the assimilating energies of overcoming and retaliating are both the abnormal energies of the year, they are the assimilation of evil energies. The calamity caused is in the centre. The accomplishing number of the assimilating coolness energy is nine, the producing number of the assimilating rain energy is five, the accomplishing number of the assimilating heat energy is seven, and they are all healthy energies. When treating the disease caused by the dryness energy which controls the heaven energy, the medicine of bitter taste and slight warm nature should be applied, when treating the disease caused by the insufficient earth energy of the middle motion, the medicine of sweet taste and mild nature should be applied, when treating the disease caused by the monarch fire energy which affects the earth energy, the medicine of salty taste and cold nature should be applied, these are the proper ways of applying medicine is these two years.

庚辰　庚戌岁

上太阳水，中太商金运，下太阴土，寒化一，清化九，雨化五，正化度也。其化上苦热，中辛温，下甘热药食宜也。

"In the years of Geng Chen and Geng Xu, Taiyang is controlling the heaven energy above and Taiyin is affecting the earth energy below. so, the upper motion is the cold water of Taiyang, the lower motion is the wetness earth of Taiyin, and the middle motion is the greater Shang which is the excessive energy of the metal motion. The producing number of the assimilating cold energy is one, the accomplishing number of the assimilating coolness energy is nine, the producing number of the assimilating rain energy is five, and they are all healthy energies. When treating the disease caused by the cold energy which controls the heaven energy, the medicing of bitter taste and hot nature should be applied, when treating the disease caused by the excessive metal energy of the middle motion, the medicine of acrid taste and warm nature should be applied, when treating the disease caused by the wetness energy which affects the earth energy, the medicine of sweet taste and hot nature should be applied. These are the proper ways of applying medicine in these two years.

辛巳　辛亥岁

上厥阴木，中少羽水运，下少阳相火，雨化风化胜复同，邪气化度也。灾一宫。风化三，寒化一，火化七，正化度也。其化上辛凉，中苦和，下咸寒，药食宜也。

"In the years of Xin Si and Xin Hai, Jueyin is controlling the heaven energy and Shaoyang is affecting the earth energy. So, the upper motion is the wind wood of Jueyin, the lower motion is the prime minister- fire of Shaoyang, and the middle motion is lesser Yu which is the insufficient energy of water motion. The overcoming energy of assimilating rain and the retaliating energy of wind will occur simultaneously. The assimilating energies of overcoming and retaliating are both abnormal energies of the year, they are called the assimilation of evil energies. The calamity caused is in the north. The producing number of the wind energy which controls the heaven energy is three, the producing number of the assimilating cold energy of the middle motion is one, the accomplishing number of the fire energy which affects the earth energy is seven, and they are all healthy energies. When treating the disease caused by the wind energy which controls the heaven energy, the medicine of acrid taste and cool nature should be applied, when treating the disease caused by the insufficient water energy of the middle motion, the medicine of bitter taste and mild nature should be applied, when treating the disease caused by the prime minister-fire energy which affects the earth energy, the medicine of salty taste and cold nature should be applied. These are the proper ways of applying medicine in these two years.

壬午　壬子岁

上少阴火，中太角木运，下阳明金，热化二，风化八，清化四，正化度也。其化上咸寒，中酸凉，下酸温，药食宜也。

In the years of Ren Wu and Ren Zi, Shaoyin is controlling the heaven energy above and Yangming is affecting the earth energy below. So, the upper motion is the heat monarch-fire of Shaoyin, the lower motion is the dryness metal of Yangming, and the middle motion is the greater Jue Which is the excessive energy of the wood motion. The producing number of the assimilating heat energy which controls the heaven energy is two, the accomplishing number

of the assimilating wind energy of the middle motion is eight, the producing number of the assimilating cool energy which affects the earth energy is four, and they are all healthy energies. When treating the disease caused by the monarch fire energy which controls the heaven energy, the medicine of salty taste and cold nature should be applied, when treating the disease caused by the excessive wind energy of the middle motion, the medicine of sour taste and cool nature should be applied, when treating the desease caused by the dryness energy which affects the earth energy, the medicine of sour taste and warm nature should be applied. These are the proper ways of applying medicine in these two years.

癸未　癸丑岁

上太阴土，中少徵火运，下太阳水，寒化雨化胜复同，邪气化度也。灾九宫。雨化五，火化二，寒化一，正化度也。其化上苦温，中咸温，下甘热，药食宜也。

"In the years of Gui Wei and Gui Chou, Taiyin is controlling the heaven energy and Taiyang is affecting the earth energy. So, the upper motion is the wetness earth of Taiyin, the lower motion is the cold water of Taiyang, and the middle motion is the Lesser Zhi which is the insufficient energy of the fire motion. The overcoming energy of the assimilating cold and the retaliating energy of the assimilating rain will occur simultaneously. Both the assimilating energies of overcoming and retaliating are abnormal energies of the year, they are called the assimilation of evil energies. The calamity is in the south. The producing number of the assimilating rain energy which controls the heaven energy is five, the producing number of the assimilating fire energy of the middle motion is two, the producing number of the assimilating water cold energy which affects the earth energy is one, and they are all healthy energies. When treating the disease caused by the wetness energy which controls the heaven energy, the medicine of bitter taste and warm nature should be applied, when treating the disease caused by the insufficient fire energy of the middle motion, the medicine of salty taste and warm nature should be applied, when treating the disease caused by the cold energy which affects the earth energy, the medicine of sweet taste and hot nature should be applied. These are the proper ways of applying medicine in these two years.

甲申　甲寅岁

上少阳相火，中太宫土运，下厥阴木，火化二。雨化五，风化八，正化度也。其化上咸寒，中咸和，下辛凉，药食宜也。

In the year of Jia Shen and Jia Yin, Shaoyang is controlling the heaven energy, the Jueyin is affecting the earth energy. So, the upper motion is the prime minister-fire of Shaoyang, the lower motion is the wind wood of Jueyin and the middle motion is greater Gong which is the excessive energy of the earth motion. The producing number of the assimilating fire energy which controls the heaven energy is two, the producing number of the assimilating rain energy of the middle motion is five, the accomplishing number of the assimilating wind energy which affects the earth energy is eight, and they are all healthy energies. When treating the disease caused by the fire energy which controls the heaven energy, the medicine of salty taste and cold nature should be applied, when treating the disease caused

by the wetness energy of the middle motion, the medicine of salty taste and mild nature should be applied, when treating the disease caused by the wind energy which affects the earth energy, the medicine of acrid taste and cool nature should be applied. These are the proper ways of applying medicine in these two years.

乙酉太乙天符　乙卯岁天符

上阳明金，中少商金运，下少阴火，热化寒化胜复同，邪气化度也。灾七宫。燥化四，清化四，热化二，正化度也。其化上苦小温，中苦和，下咸寒，药食宜也。

"In the years of Yi You (the year of heaven tally and convergence) and Yi Mao (year of heaven tally), Yangming is controlling the heaven energy and Shaoyin is affecting the earth energy. So, the upper motion is the dryness metal of Yangming, the lower motion is the heat monarch-fire of Shaoyin, and the middle motion is the lesser Shang which is the insufficient energy of the metal motion. The overcoming energy of the assimilating heat and the retaliating energy of the assimilating cold will occur simultaneously. The assimilating energies of overcoming and retaliating are both abnormal and they are the assimilation of evil energies. The calamity is caused in the west. The producing number of the assimilating dryness energy which controls the heaven energy is four, the producing number of the assimilating coolness energy is four, the producing number of the assimilating heat energy which affects the earth energy is two, and they are all healthy energies. When treating the disease caused by the dryness energy which controls the heaven energy, the medicine of bitter taste and slight warm nature should be applied, when treating the disease caused by the insufficient dryness energy of the middle motion, the medicine of bitter taste and mild nature should be applied, when treating the disease caused by the fire energy which affects the earth energy, the medicine of salty taste and cold nature should be applied. These are the proper ways of applying medicine in these two years.

丙戌天符　丙辰岁天符

上太阳水，中太羽水运，下太阴土，寒化六，雨化五，正化度也。其化上苦热，中咸温，下甘热，药食宜也。

"In the years of Bing Xu (year of heaven tally) and Bing Chen (year of heaven tally), Taiyang is controlling the heaven energy above and Taiyin is affecting the earth energy below. So, the upper motion is the cold water of Taiyang, the lower motion is wetness earth of Taiyin, and the middle motion is the Greater Yu which is the excessive energy of water motion. The accomplishing number of the assimilating cold energy which controls the heaven energy is six, the producing number of the assimilating rain energy which affects the earth energy is five, and they are all healthy energies. When treating the disease caused by the cold energy which controls the heaven energy, the medicine of bitter taste and hot nature should be applied, when treating the disease caused by the excessive water energy of the middle motion, the medicine of salty taste and warm nature should be applied, when treating the disease caused by the wetness energy which affects the earth energy, the medicine of sweet taste and hot nature should be applied. These are the proper ways of applying medicine in

these two years.

丁亥[天符]　丁巳岁[天符]

上厥阴木，中少角木运，下少阳相火，清化热化胜复同，邪气化度也。灾三宫。风化三，火化七，正化度也。其化上辛凉，中辛和，下咸寒，药食宜也。

"In the years of the Ding Hai (year of heaven tally) and Ding Si (year of heaven tally), Jueyin is controlling the heaven energy and Shaoyang is affecting the earth energy. So, the upper motion is the wood wind of Jueyin, the lower motion is the prime minister-fire of Shaoyang, and the middle motion is the lesser Jue which is the insufficient energy of the wood motion. The overcoming energy of coolness and the retaliating energy of heat will occur simultaneously. As the energies are the abnormal energies of the year, they are the assimilation of the evil energies. The calamity caused is in the east. The production number of the assimilating wind energy that controls the heaven energy is three, the accomplishing number of the assimilating fire energy that affects the earth energy is seven, and they are all healthy energies. When treating the disease caused by the wind energy which controls the heaven energy, the medicine of acrid taste and cool nature should be applied, when treating the disease caused by the insufficient wood energy of the middle motion, the medicine of acrid taste and mild nature should be applied, when treating the disease caused by the fire energy which affects the earth energy, the medicine of salty taste and cold nature should be applied. These are the proper ways of applying medicine in these two years.

戊子[天符]　戊午岁[太乙天符]

上少阴火，中太徵火运，下阳明金，热化七，清化九，正化度也。其化上咸寒，中甘寒，下酸温，药食宜也。

"In the years of Wu Zi (year of heaven tally) and Wu Wu (year of heaven tally and convergence), Shaoyin is controlling the heaven energy above and Yangming is affecting the earth energy below. So, the upper motion is the monarch-fire of Shaoyin, the lower motion is the dryness metal of Yangming, and the middle motion is the greater Zhi which is the excessive energy of the fire motion. The accomplishing number of the assimilating heat energy which controls the heaven energy is seven, the accompsishing number of the assimilating cool energy which affects the earth energy is nine, and they are both healthy energies. When treating the disease, the medicine of salty taste and cold nature should be applied, when treating the disease caused by the excessive fire energy of the middle motion, the medicine of sweet taste and cold nature should be applied, when treating the disease caused by the cool energy which affects the earth energy, the medicine of sour taste and warm nature should be applied. These are the proper ways of applying medicine in these two years.

己丑[太乙天符]　己未岁[太乙天符]

上太阴土，中少宫土运，下太阳水，风化清化胜复同，邪气化度也。灾五宫。雨化五，寒化一，正化度也。其化上苦热，中甘和，下甘热，药食宜也。

"In the years of Ji Chou (the year of heaven tally and convergence) and Ji Wei (the year of heaven tally and convergence), Taiyin is controlling the heaven energy and Taiyang is af-

fecting the earth energy. So, the upper motion is the wetness earth of Taiyin, the lower motion is the cold water of Taiyang, and the middle motion is the lesser Gong which is the insufficient energy of the earth motion. The overcoming energy of the assimilating wind and the retaliating energy of the assimilating coolness will occur simulaneously. Both the assimilating energies of overcoming and retaliating are the abnormal energies of the year, they are the assimilation of evil energies. The calamity caused is in the centre. The producing number of the assimilating rain energy which controls the heaven energy is five, the producing number of the assimilating cold energy is one, and they are both healthy energies. When treating the disease caused by the rain energy which controls the heaven energy, the medicine of bitter taste and hot nature should be applied, when treating the disease caused by the insufficient earth energy of the middle motion, the medicine of sweet taste and mild nature should be applied, when treating the disease caused by the cold energy which affects the earth energy, the medicine of sweet taste and hot nature should be applied. These are the proper ways of applying medicine in these two years.

庚寅　庚申岁

上少阳相火，中太商金运，下厥阴木，火化七，清化九，风化三，正化度也。其化上咸寒，中辛温，下辛凉，药食宜也。

"In the years of Geng Yin and Geng Shen, Shaoyang is controlling the heaven energy and Jueyin is affecting the earth energy. So, the upper motion is the prime minister-fire of Shaoyang, the lower motion is the wind wood of Jueyin, and the middle motion is the greater Shang which is the excessive energy of the metal motion. the accomplishing number of the assimilating fire energy which controls the heaven energy is seven, the accomplishing number of the assimilating cool energy of the middle motion is nine, the producing number of the assimilating wind energy which affects the earth energy is three, and they are all healthy energies. When treating the disease caused by the fire energy which controls the heaven energy, the medicine of salty taste and cold nature should be applied, when treating the disease caused by the coolness energy of the middle motion, the medicine of acrid taste and warm nature should be applied, when treating the disease caused by the coolness energy of the middle motion, the medicine of acrid taste and warm nature should be applied, when treating the disease caused by the wind energy that affects the earth energy, the medicine of acrid taste and cool nature should be applied. These are the proper ways of applying the medicine in these two years.

辛卯　辛酉岁

上阳明金，中少羽水运，下少阴火，雨化风化胜复同，邪气化度也。灾一宫。清化九，寒化一，热化七，正化度也。其化上苦小温，中苦和，下咸寒，药食宜也。

"In the years of Xin Mao and Xin You, Yangming is controlling the heaven energy and Shaoying is affecting the earth energy. So, the upper motion is the dryness metal of Yangming, the lower motion is the monarch-fire of Shaoyin, and the middle motion is the lesser Yu which is the insufficient energy of the water motion. The overcoming energy of the as-

similating rain and the retaliating energy of wind will occur simultaneously. Both the assimilating energies of overcoming and retaliating are the abnormal energies of the year. The calamity caused is in the north. The accomplishing number of the assimilating coolness energy which controls the heaven energy is nine, the producing number of the assimilating cold energy of the middle motion is one, the accomplishing number of the assimilating heat energy which affects the earth energy is seven, and they are all healthy energies. When treating the disease caused by the dryness energy that controls the heaven energy, the medicine of bitter taste and slight warm nature should be applied, when treating the disease caused by the insufficient water energy of the middle motion, the medicine of bitter taste and mild nature shoul be applied, when treating the disease caused by the monarch-fire energy which affects the earth energy, the medicine of salty taste and cold nature should be applied. These are the proper ways of applying medicine in these two years.

壬辰　壬戌岁

上太阳水，中太角木运，下太阴土，寒化六，风化八，雨化五，正化度也。其化上苦温，中酸和，下甘温，药食宜也。

In the years of Ren Chen and Ren Xu, Taiyang is controlling the heaven energy and Taiyin is affecting the earth energy. So, the upper motion is the cold water of Taiyang, the lower motion is the wetness earth of Taiyin, and the middle motion is the greater Jue, which is the excessive energy of the wood motion. The accomplishing number of the assimilating cold energy which controls the heaven energy is six, the accomplishing number of the assimilating wind energy of the middle motion is eight, the producing number of the assimilating rain energy which affects the earth energy is five, and they are all healthy energies. When treating the disease caused by the cold energy which controls the heaven energy, the medicine of bitter taste and warm nature should be applied, when treating the disease caused by the excessive wind energy of the middle motion, the medicine of sour taste and mild nature should be applied, when treating the disease caused by the wetness energy which affects the earth energy, the medicine of sweet taste and warm nature should be applied. These are the proper ways of applying medicine in these two years.

癸巳同岁会　癸亥岁同岁会

上厥阴木，中少徵火运，下少阳相火，寒化雨化胜复同，邪气化度也。灾九宫。风化八，火化二，正化度也。其化上辛凉，中咸和，下咸寒，药食宜也。

In the years of Gui Si (same with the year of convergence) and Gui Hai (same with the year of convergence), Jueyin is controlling the heaven energy above and Shaoyang is affecting the earth energy below, so, the upper motion is the wood wind of Jueyin, the lower motion is the prime minister-fire of Shaoyang and the middle motion is the lesser Zheng which is the insufficient energy of the fire motion. The overcoming energy of the assimilating cold and the retaliating energy of the assimilating rain will occur simultaneously. Both the assimilating energies of overcoming and retaliating are the abnormal energies of the year. The calamity caused is in the south. The accomplishing number of the assimilating wind energy which

controls the heaven energy is eight, the producing number of the assimilating fire energy which affects the earth energy is two, and they are both healthy energies. When treating the disease caused by the wind energy which controls the heaven energy, the medicine of acrid taste and cool nature should be applied, when treating the disease caused by the insufficient fire energy of the middle motion, the medicine of salty taste and mild nature should be applied, when treating the disease caused by the fire energy which affects the earth energy, the medicine of salty taste and cold nature should be applied. These are the proper ways of applying medicine in these two years.

凡此定期之纪，胜复正化，皆有常数，不可不察。故知其要者，一言而终，不知其要，流散无穷，此之谓也。

"In the cycle of the sixty years period of the combination of the decimal cycle and the duodecimal cycle stated above, the overcoming energy, retaliating energy, and the assimilation of the healthy energy are in regular order which must be inspected carefully. Thus, when one knows the essential points of it, he will understand it by only a few words, if he knows not the essential points, he will be utterly ignorant about it。"

帝曰：善。五运之气，亦复岁乎？岐伯曰：郁极乃发，待时而作也。帝曰：请问其所谓也？岐伯曰：五常之气，太过不及，其发异也。帝曰：愿卒闻之。岐伯曰：太过者暴，不及者徐，暴者为病甚，徐者为病持。帝曰：太过不及，其数何如？岐伯曰：太过者其数成，不及者其数生，土常以生也。

Yellow Emperor said:"Good. Do the overcoming and the retaliating energies of the five-motion energy occur each year like that of the six-energy?" Qibo said: "When the energy of the five-motion is suppressed excessively by the overcoming energy, the retaliating energy will produce and will burst out in a certain time。"Yellow Emperor asked:"Why is it so?" Qibo said:" there are the different conditions of excessive and insufficient in the energies of the five-motion, so the conditions of the bursting out of the retaliating energies are different。"

Yellow Emperor said: " I hope to know it thoroughly。" Qibo said: " The bursting out of the excessive energy is rapid, and that of the insufficent energy is slow, when the rapid energy injures man, the disease will be severe, when the slow energy injures man, the disease will be enduring。" Yellow Emperor asked: " What are the conditions of the number when the energy is excessive or insufficient?" Qibo said: " When the energy is excessive, it is the accomplishing number, when the energy is insufficient, is is the producing number, and earth often applies the producing number。"

帝曰：其发也何如？岐伯曰：土郁之发，岩谷震惊，雷殷气交，埃昏黄黑，化为白气，飘骤高深，击石飞空，洪水乃从，川流漫衍，田牧土驹。化气乃敷，善为时雨，始生始长，始化始成。故民病心腹胀，肠鸣而为数后，甚则心痛胁䐜，呕吐霍乱，饮发注下，胕肿身重。云奔雨府，霞拥朝阳，山泽埃昏，其乃发也，以其四气。云横天山，浮游生灭，怫之先兆。

Yellow Emperor asked:" what is the condition of bursting out when the energy is being suppressed excessively?" Qibo said: " In the bursting out of the suppressed earth energy, it shakes the rocks and the valleys, the thunder sounds in the intersecting energy of heaven and

earth, the sky is covered with hazy dust like evening, the moisture rises and turns into clouds and rain, the storm breaks out from the high mountain and the deep valley to impact the sands and stones to cause floods, and the water in the river rushes on in a torrent. After the retreat of the waters, the remaining earth and stones on ground appear like horses on the pasture. Then, the wetness energy begins to spread, the rain falls in proper time causing the growing and transforming of all things. By this time, people often contract the diseases of distention of the chest and the abdomen, tinnitus and diarrhea, even go so far as to have heartache, distention of the hypochondria, vomiting, cholera, phlegm-retention syndrome, watery diarrhea, edema, heaviness of the body, etc. When the dark clouds cover densely, the rosy rays surround the rising sun, the misty dusts appear in the mountains and rivers, it shows the suppressed earth energy will soon be bursting. The bursting out is in the period of the fourth energy. When the wetness energy is evaporating, the cloud of large size lies across the sky and mountains, the cloud of small size floating, moving about, producing and diminishing, they are the omens of the bursting out of the suppressed earth energy.

金郁之发，天洁地明，风清气切，大凉乃举，草树浮烟，燥气以行，霧雾数起，杀气来至，草木苍乾，金乃有声。故民病咳逆，心胁满，引少腹，善暴痛，不可反侧，嗌乾面尘色恶。山泽焦枯，土凝霜卤，怫乃发也，其气五。夜零白露，林莽声凄，怫之兆也。

"In the bursting out of the suppressed metal energy, the heaven energy is clear and the earth energy is bright, the weather is cool and pressing, and the cool season of autumn arrives. It seems to have floating smoks between the grasses and the trees, the dryness energy prevails, the frost and mists occur frequently, the grasses and woods become grey and withered, and the metal energy begins to give off the sound of autumn. When a man is affected by the dry weather, he will have cough and adverse of vital energy, fullness of the chest and hypochondria affecting the lower abdomen, sudden pain, inability of turning over, dry throat, disgraceful complexion like covering with dust. When the springs dry up, the white bitterns crystalize on the ground like frost, it shows the suppressed metal energy will soon be bursting. The bursting out is in the period of the fifth energy. When the white dew falls at night, the woeful and shrill sounds are heard from the grasses and trees, they are the omens of the bursting of the suppressed metal energy.

水郁之发，阳气乃辟，阴气暴举，大寒乃至，川泽严凝，寒雾结为霜雪，甚则黄黑昏翳，流行气交，乃为霜杀，水乃见祥，故民病寒客心痛，腰脽痛，大关节不利，屈伸不便，善厥逆，痞坚腹满。阳光不治，空积沉阴，白埃昏瞑，而乃发也。其气二火前后。太虚深玄，气犹麻散，微见而隐，色黑微黄，怫之先兆也。

In the bursting out of the suppressed water energy, the Yang energy retreats, the Yin energy sets into motion all of a sudden, the energy of bitter cold arrives, the water in rivers and lakes become frozen, the vapour becomes gloomy, yellow and dark, lingering in the intersecting energy or heaven and earth, the falling of frost injures the grasses and woods, and the water begins to become frozen. By this time, people will often contract the diseases of cold-evil, heartache, pain in the loins, lumbago, difficult in stretching and bending the large

joints, cold extremities, abdominal mass, distention and fullness of the abdomen, etc. When the Ying energy can no more play its role, the gloomy scene appears in the sky, the energy of the white dust becomes dark, it shows that the suppressed water energy will soon be bursting. The time of the bursting out of the suppressed water energy is around the domination of the two fires (the second energy of the monarch fire is in the Spring Equinox of the second lunar month, the third energy of the prime minister-fire is in the Grain Rain of the fourth lunar month. There are about sixty days between the two fires dominaton, in which period the suppressed water bursts out). When the sky is high and far with yellowish-dark energy like disorderly fibre which can be dimly seen, they are the omens of the bursting of the suppressed water energy.

木郁之发，太虚埃昏，云物以扰，大风乃至，屋发折木，木有变。故民病胃脘当心而痛，上支两胁，鬲咽不通，食饮不下，甚则耳鸣眩转，目不识人，善暴僵仆。太虚苍埃，天山一色，或气浊色，黄黑郁若，横云不起，雨而乃发也，其气无常。长川草偃，柔叶呈阴，松吟高山，虎啸岩岫，怫之先兆也。

In the bursting out of the suppressed wood energy, the sky is gloomy with dust, the clouds are stirring, the gale bale blows, the decorations in the corners of the roots are being blown down by the gale, and the trees are broken and destroyed by the breaking forth of the wood energy. By this time, people often contract the diseases of stomachache over the epigastrium, fullness of the arms and the hypochondria, obstruction in the throat, inability of swallowing the food and drink, tinnitus, dizziness, blur of eyes and fail to identify man, hardly distinguish the sky and mountains. sometimes, the turpid energy in yellowish-black colour assembles like clouds lying across the sky without rain, they are the phenomena before the bursting. The rising of the wind energy has no regular time, but one can test it by the following appearances: When the wild grasses beside the river is flattened by the wind blow, the soft leaves turn up side down to manifest their backs, the pine trees whistle in the high mountain, the roars of tigers in the cave are heard, they are the omens of the bursting of the suppressed wood energy.

火郁之发，太虚肿翳，大明不彰，炎火行，大暑至，山泽燔燎，材木流津，广厦腾烟，土浮霜卤，止水乃减，蔓草焦黄，风行惑言，湿化乃后。故民病少气，疮疡痈肿，胁腹胸背，面首四支䐜愤，胪胀，疡痱，呕逆，瘛疭骨痛，节乃有动，注下温虐，腹中暴痛，血溢流注，精液乃少，目赤心热，甚则瞀闷懊憹，善暴死。刻终大温，汗濡玄府，其乃发也，其气四。动复则静，阳极反阴，湿令乃化乃成。华发水凝，山川冰雪，焰阳午泽，怫之先兆也。有怫之应而后报也，皆观其极而乃发也，木发无时，水随火也。谨候其时，病可与期，失时反岁，五气不行，生化收藏，政无恒也。

In the bursting out of the suppressed fire energy, the sun is covered and the sky is gloomy, the scorching heat is prevailing and the summer-heat arrives. The climate among the mountains and rivers is scorching hot, the fluid of the timber is flowing out and the smoke is rising from the big buildings. The frost like bitterns adhere to the surface of the ground, the water in the well reduces day after day, and the thin and long creeping weeds

are turning yellow. As the extreme heat produces the wind, the wind and heat interweaving, people will have alalia, and the spreading of the wetness energy can not arrive on time. In this case, people will often contract the diseases of short of breath, carbuncle, swelling of the hypochondrium, swelling of the chest, back, face, head and the four extremities, tightening of muscle and skin, miliaria vomiting, convulsion of the extremities, ostealgia as if something is wriggling in the joint of bone, water diarrhea, acute abdominal pain, running rashly of blood due to blood-heat, bleeding like streaming, reduction of saliva, red eyes, feverish sensation accompanied with restlessness, even go so far as to become stupid with boredom and oppression, restlessness and sudden death. By the time of the last graduation of the day (end of the Chou double-hours when the energy of the day is most cool), the expected cool weather, on the contrary, is extremely hot, and the sweat poles are moistened by the sweat, it shows the great summer heat will soon be attacking. The attack is in the period of the fourth energy. As motionless comes after motion, the extreme Yang will turn into Yin, the extreme heat will produce wetness, and the spreading of wetness will cause the transformation and the maturity of all things. When the flowers are blooming, but the water in the river is frozen, and the frost and snow are covering the earth, it shows the fire energy is being suppressed. If there is Yang energy rising in the ponds which are facing south, it is the omens of the bursting out of the suppressed fire energy.

" Before the appearance of the retaliating energy, there must be omens, According to observation, all the retaliating energies are being acculmulated to the extreme livel. The retaliating of wood energy has no definite time in bursting, the retaliating of water energy comes around the occurrences of the two fires. When one inspects the season carefully, he can know the cause of the disease. If one does not know the season and violates the motion's energy of the year, then, the understanding of the energies of the five-motion, ie. , the energies of generation, growth, transformation, harvesting, and storing will be all in disorder. Under this case, how can he know the abnormal change of the energies of overcoming and retaliating?"

帝曰：水发而雹雪，土发而飘骤，木发而毁折，金发而清明，火发而曛昧，何气使然？岐伯曰：气有多少，发有微甚，微者当其气，甚者兼其下，征其下气而见可知也。

Yellow Emperor said: " In the bursting out of the suppressed water energy, the hail and snow appear, in the bursting out of the suppressed earth energy, the storm appears, in the bursting out of the suppressed wood energy, the destruction appears, in the bursting out of the suppressed metal-energy, the clear and bright scene appears, in the bursting out of the suppressed fire energy, the scene of muddling appears, and why is it so?" Qibo said: " There are the different conditions of the excessive and insufficient energies of the five elements, and there are the different extents of severeness and slightness in the bursting. When the bursting is slight, it is of the proper energy of its own, when it is severe, it is the bursting of its proper energy along with its supporting energy below. When inspecting the severe or slight extent of the supporting energy below, the extent of attacking condition of the disease can be

known。”

帝曰：善。五气之发，不当位者何也？岐伯曰：命其差。帝曰：差有数乎？岐伯曰：后皆三十度而有奇也。

Yellow Emperor said: “ Good. What is the reason when the attack of the five-energy sometimes do not come in accordance with the proper season?” Qibo said: “ The energy's different condition of being prosperous and deficient causes the early or late arrival of the energy, so there is a time difference。” Yellow Emperor asked: “ Are there any regular difference in days?” Qibo said: “ The differences are all thirty days odds。”

帝曰：气至而先后者何？岐伯曰：运太过则其至先，运不及则其至后，此候之常也。帝曰：当时而至者何也？岐伯曰：非太过非不及，则至当时，非是者眚也。

Yellow Emperor asked: “ Sometimes the arrival of the energy is early, sometimes it is late, what is the reason?” Qibo said: “ when the energy of the year's motion is excessive, the energy will come earlier, when it is insufficient, the energy will come later. and this is the regular pattern of the weather。” Yellow Emperor asked: “ Sometimes the energy comes just in time, and what is the reason?” Qibo said: “ It is because the energy is neither excessive nor insufficient, and it will come on proper time, or else, calamities will occur。”

帝曰：善。气有非时而化者何也？岐伯曰：太过者当其时，不及者归其已胜也。

Yellow Emperor said: “ Good. Sometimes the energy plays its role in the weather which it does not dominate, such as cool in spring instead of in autumn, and what is the reason?” Qibo said: “ The excessive energy plays the role when it dominates the heaven energy, the insufficient energy appears to have the role of its overcoming energy, thus, it plays the role deviate from the corresponding weather。”

帝曰；四时之气，至有早晏高下左右，其候何如？岐伯曰：行有逆顺，至有迟速，故太过者化先天，不及者化后天。

Yellow Emperor asked: “ How to inspect the different conditions of the energy's arrival which may be early or late, high or low, from left or right?” Qibo said: “ The directions of the energy's moving can be agreeable or reversing, the arrivals of the energy can be fast or slow, and the excessive energy will arrive prior to the normol weather of the season, the insufficient energy will arrive lagging behind the normal weather of the season。”

帝曰：愿闻其行何谓也？岐伯曰：春气西行，夏气北行，秋气东行，冬气南行，故春气始于下，秋气始于上，夏气始于中，冬气始于标。春气始于左，秋气始于右，冬气始于后，夏气始于前。此四时正化之常。故至高之地，冬气常在，至下之地，春气常在。必谨察之。帝曰：善。

Yellow Emperor said: “ I hope to know the different conditions of the agreeable or adverse, fast or slow of the activity of the energy。” Qibo said: “ The spring energy moves from east to west, the summer energy moves from south to north, the autumn energy moves from west to east and the winter energy moves from north to south. So, the spring energy commences from below, the autumn energy commences from above, the summer energy commences from the middle to reach outside, the winter energy commences from outside to reach

inside, the spring energy commences from the left (east), the autumn energy commences from the right (west), the winter energy commences from the rear (north), and the summer energy commences from the front (south). These are the normal activities of the energies of the four seasons. Thus, in the very high place, the winter energy often exists. in the very low place, the spring energy often exists, and they should be observed carefully。" Yellow Emperor said: " Good。"

黄帝问曰：五运六气之应见，六化之正，六变之纪何如？岐伯对曰：夫六气正纪，有化有变，有胜有复，有用有病，不同其候，帝欲何乎？帝曰：愿尽闻之。岐伯曰：请遂言之。夫气之所至也。厥阴所至为和平，少阴所至为暄，太阴所至为埃溽，少阳所至为炎暑，阳明所至为清劲，太阳所至为寒雾，时化之常也。

Yellow Emperor asked: " Since the motions of the five elements and the six kinds of weather can be seen outside, then, what are the essentials of the regular and irregular conditions of the six kinds of weather?" Qibo said: " In the normal assimilations of the six kinds of weather, there are the regular assimilation, variation, overcoming energy, retaliating energy, benefits and calamities, and their appearances are all different, which one do you want to know?" Yellow Emperor said: " I hope to know them all。"

Qibo said:" Let me tell you in details. On the arrival of the six-energy, the Jueyin energy is genial, the Shaoyang energy is warm, the Taiyin energy is wet and moist, the Shaoyang energy is hot, the Yangming energy is cool and pressing, and the Taiyang energy is cold. These are the normal phenomena of the activities of energies in the four seasons.

厥阴所至为风府，为璺启，少阴所至为火府，为舒荣；太阴所至为雨府，为员盈；少阳所至为热府，为行出；阳明所至为司杀府，为庚苍；太阳所至为寒府，为归藏；司化之常也。

"On the arrival of the Jueyin energy, the wind assembles which symbolizes the germination of the grasses and woods; on the arrival of the Shaoyin energy, the fire assembles, which symbolizes the gracefulness of all things; on the arrival of the Taiyin energy, the rain assembles, which symbolizes the completeness and plentifulness of all things; on the arrival of the Shaoyang energy, the heat assembles which symbolizes the activity of energy outside; on the arrival of the Yangming energy, the chilly and restraining energies assemble, which symbolizes the condition the getting old of all things; on the arrival of the Taiyang energy, the cold assembles, which symbolizes the hiding of all things. These are the normal phenomena by which the six-energy controls and the changes of all things.

厥阴所至为生，为风摇；少阴所至为荣，为形见；太阴所至为化，为云雨；少阳所至为长，为蕃鲜；阳明所至为收，为雾露；太阳所至为藏，为周密；气化之常也。

On the arrival of the Jueyin energy, all things begin to generate and they are shaken by the winds; on the arrival of the Shaoyin energy, all things become graceful and their shapes are manifesting; on the arrival of the Taiyin energy, all things are growing and transforming, and they are moistened by the clouds and rains; on the arrival of the Shaoyang energy, all things grow and being nourished, and they become flourishing and bright; on the arrival of the Yangming energy, all things become restraining and the mists and dew are falling; on

the arrival of the Taiyang energy, all things are shut and hiding, and the Yang energy is stable. These are the phenomena of the normal changes in the six energies.

厥阴所至为风生，终为肃；少阴所至为热生，中为寒；太阴所至为湿生，终为注雨；少阳所至为火生，终为蒸溽；阳明所至为燥生，终为凉；太阳所至为寒生，中为温；德化之常也。

"On the arrival of the Jueyin energy, the wind produces, but at the end, it is calmness; on the arrival of the Shaoyin energy, heat produces, but its intermediate energy is cold; on the arrival of the Taiyin energy, wetness produces, but at the end, it is the torrential rain; on the arrival of the Shaoyang energy, fire produces, but at the end, it is the wetness-heat; on the arrival of the Yangming energy, coolness produces, but at the end, it is the dryness; on the arrival of the Taiyang energy, cold produces, but its intermediate energy is warm. These are the phenomena of the natural changes in the six energies.

厥阴所至为毛化，少阴所至为羽化，太阴所至为倮化，少阳所至为羽化，阳明所至为介化，太阳所至为鳞化，德化之常也。

"On the arrival of the Jueying energy, the animals with fur can multiply; on the arrival of the Shaoyin energy, the animals with wings can multiply; on the arrival of the Taiyin energy, the animals in naked bodies can multiply, on the arrival of the Shaoyang energy, the insects with wings can multiply; on the arrival of the Yangming energy, the animals with shell can multiply; on the arrival of the Taiyang energy, the animals with scales can multiply. These are the normal phenomena of the six energies in breeding all things.

厥阴所至为生化，少阴所至为荣化，太阴所至为濡化，少阳所至为茂化，阳明所至为坚化，太阳所至为藏化，布政之常也。

"On the arrival of the Jueyin energy, it causes the generation of all things; on the arrival of the Shaoyin energy, it causes the prosperity of all things; on the arrival of the Taiyin energy, it causes the moistening of all things; on the arrival of the Shaoyang energy, it causes the flourishing of all things; on the arrival of the Yangming energy, it causes the substantialness of all things; on the arrival of the Taiyang energy, it causes all things to shut and hide. These are the common laws of the spreading of the six energies and all things are adapting to the changes.

厥阴所至为飘怒太凉，少阴所至为太暄寒，太阴所至为雷霆骤注烈风，少阳所至为飘风燔燎霜凝，阳明所至为散落温，太阳所至为寒雪冰雹白埃，气变之常也。

"On the arrival of the Jueyin energy, the gale roars and the weather becomes cool; on the arrival of the Shaoyin energy, the weather is very hot and very cold alternately; on the arrival of the Taiyin energy, the thunderbolt, torrential rain and violent gale occur; on the arrival of the Shaoyang energy, the whirl wind occurs, the weather is hot in day time and the dew turns into frost at night; on the arrival of the Yangming energy, the grasses and woods become scattering and falling, but the weather, on the contrary, turns warm; on the arrival of the Taiyang energy, the cold snow, ice and hail occur and the white energy on the ground can be seen. These are the common laws of the variation of the six-weather when being hy-

peractive.

厥阴所至为挠动，为迎随；少阴所至为高明，焰为曛；太阴所至为沉阴，为白埃，为晦暝；少阳所至为光显，为彤云，为曛；阳明所至为烟埃，为霜，为劲切，为凄鸣；太阳所至为刚固，为坚芒，为立；令行之常也。

On the arrival of the Jueyin energy, all things are stirring and swaying; on the arrival of the Shaoyin enrgy, there are the high and bright blaze in yellow colour appearing; on the arrival of the Taiyin energy, there are the dismal weather, white dusts and the evaporating energy of wetness earth which cause the haziness of the sky; on the arrival of the Shaoyang energy, there occurs the rainbow, red clouds and scorching heat; on the arrival of the Yangming energy there occurs the smoke, dust, frost, vigorous west wind and the chirp of the insects; on the arrival of the Taiyang energy, there are the hard ice, hitting wind and the maturity of crops. These are the common laws of the six energies when they are playing their roles.

厥阴所至为里急；少阴所至为疡胗身热；太阴所至为积饮否隔；少阳所至为嚏呕，为疮疡；阳明所至为浮虚；太阳所至为屈伸不利；病之常也。

厥阴所至为支痛；少阴所至为惊惑，恶寒，战慄，谵妄；太阴所至为穑满；少阳所至为惊躁，瞀昧，暴病；阳明所至为鼽，尻阴股膝髀腨䯒足病；太阳所至为腰痛；病之常也。

"On the arrival of the Jueyin energy, the disease of muscle contraction will occur; on the arrival of the Shaoyin energy, the diseases of ulceration of skin, papule and fever will occur; on the arrival of the Taiyin energy, the diseases of retention of body fluid and the sensation of oppression of the chest will occur; on the arrival or the Shaoyang energy, the diseases of sneezing, vomiting and sores will occur; on the arrival of the Yangming energy, the diseases of edema of the skin will occur; on the arrival of the Taiyang energy, the diseases of difficulty in stretching and bending the joints will occur. These are the common diseases caused by the six energies.

"On the arrival of the Jueyin energy, the propping pain of the hypochondria will occur; on the arrival of the Shaoyin energy, the diseases of suspicion, shivering with cold, talking nonsence and acting rashly will occur; on the arrival of the Taiyin energy, the disease of abdominal distention will occur; on the arrival of the Shaoyang energy, the diseases of frightening, restlessness, feeling of oppression and mental confusion will occur; on the arrival of the Yangming energy, the diseases of stuffy nose, sneezing, and the disease on the buttock, pubis groove, knee, thigh, fibula and leg will occur; on the arrival of the Taiyang energy, the disease of lumbago will occur. These are the common diseases caused by the six energies.

厥阴所至为緛戾；少阴所至为悲妄衄衊；太阴所至为中满霍乱吐下；少阳所至为喉痹，耳鸣呕涌；阳明所至皴揭；太阳所至为寝汗，痉；病之常也。

"On the arrival of the Jueyin energy, the disease of weakening and contraction of extremities causing the difficulty of turning around will occur; on the arrival of the Shaoyin energy, the diseases of laughing and sorrow without reason, hemorrhage and blood pollution

will occur; on the arrival of the Taiyin energy, the diseases of cholera, vomiting and diarrhea will occur; on the arrival of the Shaoyang energy, the diseases of sore throat, tinnitus and vomiting will occur; on the arrival of the Yangming energy, the disease of coarse skin will occur; on the arrival of the Taiyang energy, the diseases of night sweat, and convulsion of muscle will occur. These are the diseases caused by the six energies.

厥阴所至为胁痛呕泄；少阴所至为语笑；太阴所至为重胕肿；少阳所至为暴注，瞤瘛，暴死；阳明所至为鼽嚏，太阳所至为流泄禁止；病之常也。

"On the arrival of the Jueyin energy, the diseases of pain in the hypochondria, vomiting and diarrhea will occur; on the arrival of the Shaoyin energy, the disease of uuceasing talking and laughing will occur; on the arrival of the Taiyin energy, the diseases of heaviness of the body and edema will occur; on the arrival of the Shaoyang energy, the disease of sudden onset of diarrhea, bouncing of the muscle, and convulstion of the muscle and tendon will occur, and the patient may die all of a sudden; on the arrival of the Yangming energy, the diseases of stuffy nose and sneezing will occur; on the arrival of the Taiyang energy, the disease of incontinence of feces and urine will occur. These are the general rules of causing diseases under the effects of the six energies

凡此十二变者，报德以德，报化以化，报政以政，报令以令，气高则高，气下则下，气后则后，气前则前，气中则中，气外则外，位之常也。故风胜则动，热胜则肿，燥胜则干，寒胜则浮，湿胜则濡泄，甚则水闭胕肿，随气所在，以言其变耳。

In sumarizing the twelve changes stated above, one can see all things are responding to the effects that come from the six energies. The positions of the six energies' arrival are different in high and low, front and rear, inside and outside which will also cause diseases in different positions in high and low, front and rear, inside and outside of the body. When the wind energy is abundant, there will be pain, when the heat energy is abundant, there will be swelling, when the dryness energy is abundant there will be wrinkle of skin, when the cold energy is abundant, there will be watery diarrhea or even go so far as to have retention of urine and edema. In a word, when studying the changes, it must be according to the different locations of the evil energy。"

帝曰：愿闻其用也。岐伯曰：夫六气之用，各归不胜而为化，故太阴雨化，〔张琦说："雨化"应作"湿化"〕施于太阳；太阳寒化，施于少阴；少阴热化，施于阳明；阳明燥化，施于厥阴；厥阴风化，施于太阴。各命其所在以征之也。帝曰：自得其位何如？岐伯曰：自得其位，常化也。帝曰：愿闻所在也。岐伯曰：命其位而方月可知也。

Yellow Emperor said: "I like to hear about the effects of the activity of energy。" Qibo said: "The activity of the six-energy produces when the energy encounters the energy which it overcomes, such as: when the wetness earth energy of Taiyin encounters the cold water energy of Taiyang as earth overcomes water, the water energy of Taiyang will be assimilated by the wetness earth energy of Taiyin; when the cold water energy of Taiyang encounters the heat monarch-fire of Shaoyin as water overcomes fire, the heat energy of Shaoyin will be assimilated by cold energy of Taiyang; when heat energy of Shaoyin encounters the dryness

metal energy of Yangming, as fire overcomes metal, the dryness metal energy of Yangming will be assimilated by the heat energy of Shaoyin; when the dryness metal energy of Yangming encounters the wind wood energy of Jueyin, as metal overcomes wood, the wind energy of Jueyin will be assimilated by the dryness energy of Yangming; when the wind wood energy of Jueyin encounters the wetness, earth energy of Taiyin will be assimilated by the wind energy of Jueyin. One must forecast according to the situated orientations of the six-energy respectively。"

Yellow Emperor asked: " what is the condition when the six-energy dominates in the proper orientation and in the proper month?" Qibo said: " When the six-energy is dominating in one proper orientation of its own and in the proper month, it is the normal condition of the activity of energy". Yellow Emperor said: " I like to know the orientation of situation。" Qibo said: " When the sequence and the position of the six-energy is ascertained, the situating orientation and the dominating month can be known。"

帝曰：六位之气〔明抄本作“六气之位”〕盈虚何如？岐伯曰：太少异也，太者之至徐而常，少者暴而亡。帝曰：天地之气盈虚何如？岐伯曰：天气不足，地气随之，地气不足，天气从之，运居其中而常先也，恶所不胜，归所同和，随运归从而生其病也。故上胜则天气降而下，下胜则地气迁而上，多少而差其分，微者小差，甚者大差，甚则位易气交易，则大变生而病作矣。《大要》曰：甚纪五分，微纪七分，其差可见。此之谓也。

Yellow Emperor asked: " What is the condition when the six-energy is abundant or deficient?" Qibo said: " In energies, there are different conditions of being excessive or insufficient. In the coming of the excessive energy, it is vigorous and rapid, but it will be diminished soon, in the coming of the insufficient energy, it is slow but it can last long。"

Yellow Emperor asked: " what is the condition when the energy is having a surplus or being deficient in controlling the heaven energy and affecting the earth energy?" Qibo said: " When the energy that controls the heaven enrgy is insufficient, the energy that affects the earth energy will ascend in the wake of it; when the energy that affects the earth energy is insufficient. the energy that controls the heaven energy will descend in the wake of it; the energy of the year's motion situates in the intersecting-energy of heaven and earth, and it often ascends or descends prior to that of the heaven energy or the earth energy. The energy detests the energy that controls the heaven energy or affects the earth energy which it can not overcome it, and combines or assimilates with the energy that controls the heaven energy or affects the earth energy which is similar with itself. As assimilation means assisting and combining, the disease will occur in the wake of it. Thus, when the energy that controls the heaven energy is abundant, the heaven energy will descend, when the energy that affects the earth energy is abundant, the earth energy will ascend, and the extent of overcoming determines the different extent of the ascent and descent. When the overcoming energy is slight, the difference of ascent and descent will be small; when the overcoming energy is vigorous, the difference of ascent and descent will be large. If the difference is very large, then, the position of the energy-intersection will be shifted to produce change and disease. It is stated

in the《Essentials》: 'In the year of excessive overcoming, the different of extent is seventy pen cent, in the year of slight overcoming. the difference of extent is fifty per cent, and the differences are perceivable。'"

帝曰：善。论言热无犯热，寒无犯寒。余欲不远寒，不远热奈何？岐伯曰：悉乎哉问也！发表不远热，攻里不远寒。帝曰：不发不攻而犯寒犯热何如？岐伯曰：寒热内贼，其病益甚。帝曰：愿闻无病者何如？岐伯曰：无者生之，有者甚之。帝曰：生者何如？岐伯曰：不远热则热至，不远寒则寒至，寒至则坚否腹满，痛急下利之病生矣，热至则身热，吐下霍乱，痈疽疮疡，瞀郁注下，瞤瘛肿胀，呕，鼽衄头痛，骨节变，肉痛，血溢血泄，淋闷之病生矣。帝曰：治之奈何？岐伯曰：时必顺之，犯者治以胜也。

Yellow Emperor said: " Good. It was stated in the treatise: 'When applying the medicine of hot nature, do not violate the dominating heat energy; when applying the medicine of cold nature, do not violate the dominating cold energy'. I do not want to avoid the heat nor the cold energy, how should I do it?" Qibo said: " How exhaustive your question is. When dispelling the superficial evils, the medicine of hot nature should not be omitted, when dispelling the evils in the interior, the medicine of cold nature should not be omitted。" Yellow Emperor asked: " When one is dispelling neither the superficial evils nor the evils in the interior, but breaks the taboos of applying medicine of hot nature in hot weather and medicine of cold nature in cold weather, what would be the condition?" Qibo said: "In this case, the cold and heat evils will injure the viscera internally, and the disease will become worse。" Yellow Emperor asked: " What will happen to a man who has no disease?" Qibo said: " The man who has no disease will become ill, and the man with disease will become worse。"

Yellow Emperor asked: " What is the condition when the disease is contracted?" Qibo said: " When the hot weather is not avoided, the patient will contract heat evil; when the cold weather is not avoided, the patient will contract cold evil. If the cold evil is extreme, the disease of mass in the chest, abdominal fullness, acute pain and diarrhea will occur. When the heat evil is extreme, the diseases of fever, vomiting, cholera, ulceration, carbuncle, mental confuslon, oppression, diarrhea, convulsion of the body, swelling, running nose, epistaxis, headache, deformation of the joints, pain in the muscle, spitting blood, bloody stool, strangury and dysuria will occur。"

Yellow Emperor asked: " How to treat them?" Qibo said: " It must follow the sequence of the four seasons, if the contraindication has been violated, it should be treated by applying the medicine of cold nature to fever, and applying the medicine of hot nature to the disease of cold。"

黄帝问曰：妇人重身，毒之何如？岐伯曰：有故无殒，亦无殒也。帝曰：愿闻其故何谓也？岐伯曰：大积大聚，其可犯也，衰其太半而止，过者死。

Yellow Emperor asked: " What about applying the violent medicine to a pregnant woman?" Qibo said: If the patient has abdominal mass, the violent medicine will suit the disease, both the mother and the foetus will be unharmed。" Yellow Emperor asked: " What is the

reason?" Qibo said： " To the diseases of great stagnation and accumulation, the violent medicine can be used as it can remove the disease, but when the disease is removed by a good half already, the applying of medicine should be ceased, if the medicine applied is more than enough, it may cause death of the patient。"

帝曰：善。郁之甚者治之奈何？岐伯曰：木郁达之，火郁发之，土郁夺之，金郁泄之，水郁折之，然调其气，过者折之，以其畏也，所谓写之。帝曰：假者何如？岐伯曰：有假其气则无禁也。所谓主气不足，客气胜也。帝曰：至哉圣人之道！天地大化运行之节，临御之纪，阴阳之政，寒暑之今〔赵本，吴本"今"并作"令"〕，非夫子孰能通之！请藏之灵兰之室，署曰《六元正纪》非斋戒不敢示，慎传也。

Yellow Emperor said：" Good. How to treat the disease caused by the extreme suppression of the five elements' energy?" Qibo said： " When the wood energy is suppressed, it should be adjusted to become smooth, when the fire energy is suppressed, it should be dispersed, when the earth energy is suppressed, it should be attacked hastly, when the metal energy is suppressed, it should be dredged, when the water energy is suppressed, it should be restrained, and these are the ways of adjusting the energies. To the excessive energy, it should be subdued by applying purging medicine。" Yellow Emperor asked： " what about treating the disease when a substitutionary energy is dominating?" Qibo said：" when treating the disease during the domination of a substitutionary energy, as the host energy is insufficient and the guest energy is abundant, one may not follow the contraindication of avoiding cold and hot weather。"

Yellow Emperor said：" How profound the theory of the sages is! The principle of the energy activity of heaven and earth, the rules of the operation of the five motions, the essential points of the encountering of the six energies, the functions of Yin and Yang and the influence of the cold and hot weather of the seasons are so recondite, who can understand them save you. Now, let me keep the papers of your words in the royal orchid chamber, and named it as《 On the Changes and Symbols of the Five Elements' Motion and the Six kinds of Weather in the Cycle of Sixty Years》. It will not be allowed to read without fasting and taking a bath previously, and it may be handed down to the later generations cautiously。"

刺法论篇第七十二（亡）

Chapter 72

Ci Fa Lun

(On Pricking Therapy)

(Lost)

本病论篇第七十三（亡）

Chapter 73

Ben Bing Lun

(On the Source of Diseases)

(Lost)

至真要大论篇第七十四

Chapter 74
Zhi Zhen Yao Da Lun
(The Various Changes in the Dominations of the Six Energies and their Relations with the Diseases)

黄帝问曰：五气交合，盈虚更作，余知之矣。六气分治，司天地者，其至何如？岐伯再拜对曰：明乎哉问也！天地之大纪，人神之通应也。帝曰：愿闻上合昭昭，下合冥冥奈何？岐伯曰：此道之所主，工之所疑也。

Yellow Emperor asked："I have understood the principles about the mutual coordination of the five-motion's energies and their mutual alternations when they are excessive or insufficient. But what about the changes induced by the arrivals of the energy that controls the heaven or by that of the energy that effects the earth energy in the seasonal domination of the six energies respectively?" Qibo bowed and said："What an explicit question you have asked. It is the fundamental law of the changes of heaven and earth, and the law for the human body to suit the changes of heaven and earth."

Yellow Emperor said："I hope to know how can one suit the evident principle of heaven above and fit the profound truth of the earth below?" Qibo said："This is the principal part in the medical theory which is unclear to many physicians."

帝曰：愿闻其道也。岐伯曰：厥阴司天，其化以风；少阴司天，其化以热；太阴司天，其化以湿；少阳司天，其化以火；阳明司天，其化以燥；太阳司天，其化以寒。以所临藏位，命其病者也。

Yellow Emperor said："I hope to hear about it." Qibo said："When Jueyin is controlling the heaven energy, the energy is assimilated by the wind; when Shaoyin is controlling the heaven energy, the energy is assimilated by the heat; when Taiyin is controlling by the heaven energy, the energy is assimilated by the wetness; when Shaoyang is controlling the heaven energy, the energy is assimilated by the fire; when Yangming is controlling the heaven energy, the energy is asimilated by the dryness; when Taiyang is controlling the heaven energy, the energy is assimilated by the cold. The names or the diseases are determined by the viscus to which the guest energy befalls."

帝曰：地化奈何？岐伯曰：司天同候，间气皆然。帝曰：间气何谓？岐伯曰：司左右者，是谓间气也。帝曰：何以异之？岐伯曰：主岁者纪岁，间气者纪步也。帝曰：善。岁主奈何？岐伯曰：厥阴司天为风化，在泉为酸化，司气为苍化，间气为动化。少阴司天为热化，在泉为苦化，不司气化，居气为灼化。太阴司天为湿化，在泉为甘化，司气为黅化，间气为柔化。少阳司天为火化，在泉为苦化，司气为丹化，间气为明化。阳明司天为燥化，在泉为辛化，司

气为素化，间气为清化。太阳司天为寒化，在泉为咸化，司气为玄化，间气为藏化。故治病者，必明六化分治，五味五色所生，五藏所宜，乃可以言盈虚病生之绪也。

Yellow Emperor said: “What is the assimilating condition when the energy is affecting the earth energy?” Qibo said: “It is similar with the energy that controls the heaven energy, and the condition of the intermediate energy is also the same.”

Yellow Emperor asked: “What is the intermediate energy?” Qibo said: “It is the energy that takes charge in the left or right side of the energy that controls the heaven energy and that effects the earth energy.”

Yellow Emperor asked: “What is the difference of the energy that controls the heaven energy, the energy that affects the earth energy and the intermediate energy?” Qibo said: “The energy that controls heaven energy and that affects the earth energy dominates the energy activity of the whole year, and the intermediate energy dominates the energy activity for sixty days (one pace).”

Yellow Emperor said: “Good. What is the condition of the energy that dominates the year?” Qibo said: “When Jueyin is controlling the heaven energy, it is assimilated by the wind, when it is affecting the earth energy, it is assimilated by the sourness, when it dominates the year's motion, it is assimilated by the green colour. When it is the intermediate energy, it is assimilated by the mobility. When Shaoyin is controlling the heaven energy, it is assimilated by the heat, when it is affecting the earth energy, it is assimilated by the bitterness, as a monarch, when Shaoyin does not dominate the year's motion, it is the intermediate energy, and is assimilated by the scorching heat. When Taiyin is controlling the heaven energy, it is assimilated by the wetness. When it is affecting the earth energy, it is assimilated by the sweetness, when it dominates the year's motion, it is assimilated by the yellow colour, when it is the intermediate energy, it is assimilated by the softness, when Shaoyang is controlling the heaven energy, it is assimilated by the fire, when it is affecting the earth energy, it is assimilated by the bitterness, when it dominates the year's motion, it is assimilated by the red colour, when it is the intermediate energy, it is assimilated by the brightness, when Yangming is controlling the heaven energy, it is assimilated by the dryness. When it is affecting the earth energy, it is asimilated by the acridness, when it is dominating the year's motion, it is assimilated by the plainness, when it is the intermediate energy, it is assimilated by the coolness. When Taiyang is controlling the heaven energy, it is assimilated by the cold, when it is affecting the earth energy, it is assimilated by the saltiness, when it is dominating the year's motion, it is assimilated by the black colour, when it is the intermediate energy, it is assimilated by the energy of storing.

“Thus, when treating, one must understand the different functions of the energy activities of the six energies, the functions produced by the five tastes and the five colours and what the five viscera like and dislike, then can one know the threads of the surplus and the deficiency of the energy activity and the diseaes.”

帝曰：厥阴在泉而酸化，先余知之矣。风化之行也何如？岐伯曰：风行于地，所谓本也，

余气同法。本乎天者，天之气也，本乎地者，地之气也，天地合气，六节分而万物化生矣。故曰：谨候气宜，无失病机，此之谓也。

Yellow Emperor said: "I have known when Jueyin is affecting the earth energy, it will be assimilated by the sourness, but what is the condition when it is assimilated by wind?" Qibo said: "When Jueyin is affecting the earth energy, the wind moves about earth and the earth energy is assimilated by the wind, and the other five energies are likewise. When the six energies are controlling the heaven energy, they belong to the heaven energy, when the six energies are affecting the earth energy, they belong to the earth energy, when the heaven energy and the earth energy join together, there occur the delimitations of the six stages of the energies, and, in this way, can all things be growing and transforming. Thus, one must pay good attention to the observation of the weather change, and must not let slip the change of treating the diseaes."

帝曰：其主病何如？岐伯曰：司岁备物，则无遗主矣。帝曰：先岁物何也？岐伯曰：天地之专精也。帝曰：司气者何如？岐伯曰：司气者主岁同，然有余不足也。帝曰：非司岁物何谓也？岐伯曰：散也，故质同而异等也，气味有薄厚，性用有躁静，治保有多少，力化有浅深，此之谓也。

Yellow Emperor asked: "What are the main medicines for treating the disease?" Qibo said: "When one prepares properly the medicines of which its energy is similar with the energy that dominates the year, then, no medicine neccessary will be lacking."

Yellow Emperor asked: "What is the reason that one must prepare the medicine of which its energy is similar with the energy that dominates the year?" Qibo said: "It is because such medicine has the specific quintessence of heaven and earth and has better curative effect."

Yellow Emperor asked: "What about the medicines which are similar with the energy of the element's motion that dominates the year?" Qibo said: "They are the same with the energy that controls the heaven energy or affects the earth energy, but they have difference in surplus and deficiency."

Yellow Emperor asked: "What about the medicine of which its energy is not similar with the energy that controls the heaven energy or affects the earth energy?" Qibo said: "The taste of the medicine is impure, it has the essential character but with lower grade. When comparing the medicine with that of the similar energy, they are different in heavy and light taste, different in calm and rash property, different in more of less of curative effect and different in profound and shallow of medical effect."

帝曰：岁主藏害何谓？岐伯曰：以所不胜命之，则其要也。帝曰：治之奈何？岐伯曰：上淫于下，所胜平之，外淫于内〔张琦说："按地气不可云外理于内，疑是'内淫于外'在泉之气，当可云协矣〕，所胜治之。帝曰：善。平气何如？岐伯曰：谨察阴阳所在而调之，以平为期，正者正治，反者反治。

Yellow Emperor asked: "Sometimes the weather of the six energies that domimates the year can injure the five viscera and what is the reason?" Qibo said: "There are the cases of

overcoming and retaliating in all the six energies and the five viscera. Excessive overcoming or retaliating will hurt the five viscera. and this is the crux of the matter."

Yellow Emperor asked: "How to treat it?" Qibo said: " When the energy that controls the heaven energy is partial overabundant to injure the lower part of the body, apply the medicine of proper taste and nature of cold, cool, hot or warm which is overcoming to calm it; when the energy that affects the earth energy is overabundant to injure the external body, apply the medicine of proper taste and nature of cold, hot, cool or warm which is overcoming to treat it."

Yellow Emperor asked: "Good. But sometimes one contracts the disease when the year's energy is moderate, how to treat it?" Qibo said: " One must observe carefully the positions of the three Yin energies and the three Yang energies that control the heaven energy and affect the earth energy, and treat properly until the energy is balanced. When heat syndrome is seen in fever, or cold syndrome is seen in the cold disease, it is the diseaes of normal case which should be treated positively, ie., apply the medicine of cold nature when treating the heat sydrome and apply the medicine of hot nature when treating the cold syndrome; when the heat disease or when the heat syndrome is seen or the cold syndrome is seen in the cold disease, it is the abnormal disease which should be treated reversely, ie., apply the medicine of hot nature when treating the fever and apply the medicine of cold nature when treating the cold disease."

帝曰：夫子言察阴阳所在而调之，论言人迎与寸口相应，若引绳小大齐等，命曰平，阴之所在寸口何如？岐伯曰：视岁南北，可知之矣。帝曰：愿卒闻之。岐伯曰：北政之岁，少阴在泉，则寸口不应；厥阴在泉，则右不应；太阴在泉，则左不应。南政之岁，少阴司天，则寸口不应；厥阴司天，则右不应；太阴司天，则左不应。诸不应者，反其诊则见矣。帝曰：尺候何如？岐伯曰：北政之岁，三阴在下，则寸不应；三阴在上，则尺不应。南政之岁，三阴在天，则寸不应；三阴在泉，则尺不应。左右同。故曰：知其要者，一言而终，不知其要，流散无穷，此之谓也。

Yellow Emperor said: " As you have said that one must treat according to the position of Yin and Yang, but in some medical books, it is stated that the Renying pulse (pulse of the cervical arteries lateral to the thyroid cartilage) condition must be coincide with that of the Cunkou pulse (the pules located along the radial artery proximal to the wrist), like pulling threads which must be of the same length to become even, what about the condition of the cunkou pulse when the pulse of the three Ying is seen?" Qibo said: "There are the different cases of south administration and North administration, it will be clear when inspecting whether it is the south administration (in the Jia and Ji year when the monarch earth is playing its role, it implements its decree facing south) or the north administration (in the eight years of Yi, Geng, Bing, Xin, Ding, Ren, Wu and Gui when the wood, fire, metal and water is playing their roles respectively, as they are all courtiers, they implement their decree facing north)." Yellow Emperor said: " I hope to know it thoroughly." Qibo said: " In the north administration, when Shaoyin is affecting the earth energy, the Cunkou pulse will be

fine, sunken, hidden and can hardly respond the palpating fingers; when Jueyin is affecting the earth energy, the Cunkou pulse of the right hand will be fine, sunken, hidden and can hardly respond the finger; when Taiyin is affecting the earth energy, the Cunkou pulse of the left hand will be fine, sunken, hidden and can hardly respond the finger. In the south administration, when Shaoyin is controlling the heaven energy, the Cunkou pulse will be fine and sunken which will hardly respond the finger; when Jueyin is controlling the heaven energy, the Cunkou pulse in the right hand will be fine and sunken which will hardly respond the finger; when Taiyin is controlling the heaven energy, the Cunkou pulse of the left hand will be fine and sunken which will hardly respond the finger. Whenever the Cunkou pulse is sunken and can hardly be felt, turn the patient's palm up-side-down and a floating and gigantic pulse can be felt."

Yellow Emperor said: "What is the condition of the Chi pulse (the proximal throbbing of the radial pulse)?" Qibo said: "In the north administration, when the three Yins energies affect the earth energy, the Cunkou pulse will not respond; when the three Yins energies control the heaven energy, the Chi pulse will not respond. In the south administration, when the three Yins energies control the heaven energy, the Cunkou pulse will not respond; when the three Yins energies affect the earth energy, the Chi pulse will not respond. The failing respond of the left pulse and the right pulse are the same as above. Thus, the saying goes: 'when one knows the main principle, he can understand it by a single word, if he knows not the main principle, he will go astray.'

帝曰：善。天地之气，内淫而病何如？岐伯曰：岁厥阴在泉，风淫所胜，则地气不明，平野昧，草乃早秀。民病洒洒振寒，善伸数欠，心痛支满，两胁里急，饮食不下，鬲咽不通，食则呕，腹胀善噫，得后与气，则快然如衰，身体皆重。

Yellow Emperor said: "Good. what is the condition when the energies of heaven and earth invade the internal body and cause disease?" Qibo said: "In the year when Jueyin is affecting the earth energy, the wind energy is partial over-abundant, the earth energy will be dim, the wildness will become gloomy and the grasses will form ears early, People will contract cold disease like malaria, frequent groaning, unceasing yawning, heartache, distention in the chest, convulsion and uneasiness of the hypochondria, detest taking food and drink, dysphagia, feel like to vomit after taking food, abdominal distention, eructation, feeling relaxed after moving the bowels or breaking wind, and have the feeling of fatigue.

岁少阴在泉，热淫所胜，则焰浮川泽，阴处反明。民病腹中常鸣，气上冲胸，喘不能久立，寒热皮肤痛，目瞑齿痛颛肿，恶寒发热如疟，少腹中痛，腹大，蛰虫不藏。

"In the year when Shaoyin is affecting the earth energy, the heat energy is partial over-abundant. The energy will be floating above the rivers and lakes, The shady places will become bright and the hibernants will not be hiding. People will contract the disease of gurgling sound in the abdomen, rushing up of the adversed energy to attack the chest, rapid breathing causing the inability of standing long, chillness and fever, pain of the skin, dizzy sight, toothache, swelling of the top, contention of heat and cold like in malaria, pain in the

lower abdomen and swelling of the abdomen.

岁太阴在泉，草乃早荣〔林校云："详'草乃早荣'四字疑衍"〕，湿淫所胜，则埃昏岩谷，黄反见黑，至阴之交。民病饮积，心痛耳聋，浑浑焞焞，嗌肿喉痹，阴病血见。少腹痛肿，不得小便，病冲头痛，目似脱，项似拔，腰似折，髀不可以回。腘如结，腨如别。

"In the year when Taiyin is affecting the earth energy, the wetness energy is partial overabundant. The valley will be gloomy and turbid, the yellow earth turns into black when the wetness earth energy is extreme, and it is the phenomenon of the wetness energy mixing with the earth energy. People will often contract fluid retention, abdominal mass, heartache, deafness, hearing nothing, swelling of the pharynx, sore throat, yin-type disease with bleeding such as stranguria with blood, hematochezia, pain and swelling of the lower abdomen, dysuria, up-attacking of the evil energy to cause headache feeling like the eye balls are going to fall off, the neck is like being pulled up, the loin is like being broken, the thigh can hardly turn back, the knee fossa seems to become solid and the calf seems to become rigid.

岁少阳在泉，火淫所胜，则焰明郊野，寒热更至。民病注泄赤白，少腹痛溺赤，甚则血便，少阴同候。

"In the year when Shaoyang is affecting the earth energy, the fire energy is overabundant. The outskirts will be illuminated with light and the weather will be cold and hot alternately. People will contract watery diarrhea, dysentery with purulent and bloody stools, pain in the lower abdomen, red urine, even go so far as to have hemetochezia, the other syndromes contracted will be similar with that of when Shaoyin is affecting the earth energy.

岁阳明在泉，燥淫所胜，则霿雾清暝。民病喜呕，呕有苦，善太息，心胁痛不能反侧，甚则嗌乾面尘，身无膏泽，足外反热。

" In the year when Yangming is affecting the earth energy, the dryness energy is partial abundant. The mists will cause hazziness and one can hardly see anything. The weather will be cold. People will often contract vomiting, bilious vomiting, frequent sighing, pain in the heart and the hypochondria causing the patient unable to turn around. When the disease becomes worse, the pharynx will be dry, the complexion will become dusty, the skin of the whole body will become withered without lustre, and the outer flank of the foot will be feeling hot.

岁太阳在泉，寒淫所胜，则凝肃惨慄。民病少腹控睾，引腰脊，上冲心痛，血见，嗌痛颔肿。

"In the year when Taiyang is affecting the earth energy, the cold energy is partial overabundant, The weather will be desolate, solemn and very cold. People will often contract pain in the lower abdomen radiating to the testis, loins and kidney, heartache caused by the rushing up of the cold evil, bleeding, pain in the pharynx and swelling of the chin."

帝曰：善。治之奈何？岐伯曰：诸气在泉，风淫于内，治以辛凉，佐以苦〔明抄本"苦"下有"甘"字〕，以甘缓之，以辛散之。热淫于内，治以咸寒，佐以甘苦，以酸收之，以苦发之。湿淫于内，治以苦热，佐以酸淡，以苦燥之，以淡泄之。火淫于内，治以咸冷，佐

以苦辛，以酸收之，以苦发之。燥淫于内，治以苦温，佐以甘〔林校云："'甘'字疑当作'酸'"〕辛，以苦下之。寒淫于内，治以甘热，佐以苦辛，以咸写之，以辛润之，以苦坚之。

Yellow Emperor said: "Good. Then, how to treat it? Qibo said: "When the energy is affecting the earth energy, if the internal body is injured by the excessive wind energy, it should apply the medicine of acrid taste and cool nature mainly for treating, assist with the medicine of bitter and sweet taste, moderate the liver wood with the medicine of sweet taste, and disperse the wind evil with the medicine of acrid taste; if the internal body is injured by the excessive heat energy, apply the medicine of salty taste and cold nature mainly for treating, assist with the medicine of sweet and bitter taste, collect the Yin energy with the sour taste and disperse the heat-evil with the medicine of bitter taste; if the internal body is injured by the excessive wetness energy, apply the medicine of bitter taste and hot nature mainly for treating, assist with the medicine of sour and flat taste, dry the wetness with the medicine of bittter taste and discharge the wetness-evil with medicine of flat taste. If the internal body is injured by the excessive fire energy, apply the medicine of salty taste and cold nature mainly for treating, assist with the medicine of bitter and acrid taste, collect the Yin energy with the medicine of sour taste, and diffuse the fire-evil with the medicine of bitter taste; if the internal body is injured by the excessive dryness energy, apply the medicine of bitter taste and warm nature mainly for treating, assist with the medicine of sour and acrid tastes, discharge the heat-evil with the medicine of bitter taste and cold nature and purge the fire-evil with the medicine of salty taste; if the internal body is injured by the excessive cold energy, apply the medicine of sweet taste and hot nature mainly for treating, assist with the medicine of bitter and acrid tastes, warm and moisten the energy with the medicine of acrid taste, and substantialize the energy with the medicine of bitter taste."

帝曰：善。天气之变何如？岐伯曰：厥阴司天，风淫所胜，则太虚埃昏，云物以扰，寒生春气，流水不冰。民病胃脘当心而痛，上支两胁，鬲咽不通，饮食不下，舌本强，食则呕，冷泄腹胀，溏泄，瘕水闭，蛰虫不去〔吴本，明抄本"去"并作"出"《类经》移此句于上文"流水不冰"句下似是〕，病本于脾。冲阳绝，死不治。

Yellow Emperor said: "Good. What is the condition when the heaven energy is changing?" Qibo said: "When Jueyin is controlling the heaven energy, the wind energy is partial overabundant. The sky will be dusty and hazy, the clouds and all things are stirred and swayed by the wind energy, as the spring decree is implemented in the cold season, the flowing water can not freeze, and the hibernants are still hiding. People will contract stomachache by the position of heart, the proping feeling in the hypochondria, dysphagia, fail to take food and drink, stiffness of the root of tongue, vomiting after taking food, cold-type diarrhea, abdominal swelling, diarrhea with loose stools, stagnation of energy to become abdominal mass and dysuria, and these diseases are stemmed from the spleen. If the Chongyang pulse is severed, it shows the stomach energy has been injured, the patient can by no means to be cured and die.

少阴司天，热淫所胜，怫热至，火行其政。民病胸中烦热，嗌乾，右胠满，皮肤痛，寒热

咳喘，大雨且至，唾血血泄，鼽衄嚏呕，溺色变，甚则疮疡胕肿，肩背臂臑及缺盆中痛，心痛肺䐜，腹大满，膨膨而喘咳，病本于肺，尺泽绝，死不治。

" In the year when Shaoyin is controlling the heaven energy, the heat energy is partial overabundant. The monarch fire is playing its role, the weather is depressed and hot, and the heavy rain will arrive. People will often contract the disease of irritability and heat in the chest, dry pharynx, fullness of the right hypochondrium, pain of skin, cold and fever, cough, rapid breathing, spitting blood, hematochezia, epistaxis, sneezing, vomiting, deep-coloured urine, pyogenic infection and ulceration of skin, edema, pain in the shoulder, back, lower and upper arms, heartache, distention of the lung, fullness and enlargement of the abdomen, rapid breathing and cough, and these diseases are stemmed from the lung. If the Chize pulse is severed, it shows the lung energy has been injured, the patient can by no means to be cured and die.

太阴司天，湿淫所胜，则沉阴且布，雨变枯槁。胕肿骨痛阴痹，阴痹者按之不得，腰脊头项痛，时眩，大便难，阴气不用，饥不欲食，咳唾则有血，心如悬，病本于肾。太谿绝，死不治。

" In the year when Taiyin is controlling the heaven energy, the wetness energy is partial overabundant. The dismal energy will be spreading, the excessive rain, on the contrary, causes the grasses and woods to become withered. People will often contract edema, pain in the bone, and the yin-type bi-syndrome of which the location can hardly be distinguished when pressing. The patient will have pain in the loin, neck and head, frequent dizziness, dyschesia, disfunction of the Yin energy, reluctant to eat when hungry, spitting blood and uneasiness of heart as if it is hanging in the air, and these diseases are from the kidney. If the Taixi pulse is severed, it shows the kidney energy has been injured, the patient can by no means to be cured and die.

少阳司天，火淫所胜，则温气流行，金政不平。民病头痛，发热恶寒而疟，热上皮肤痛，色变黄赤，传而为水，身面胕肿，腹满仰息，泄注赤白，疮疡咳唾血，烦心胸中热，甚则鼽衄，病本于肺。天府绝，死不治。

"In the year when shaoyang is controlling the heaven energy, the fire-energy is partial overabundant. The energies of warmness and heat will be prevailing, the metal has lost its cool and restraining energy, it fails to play its role. People will contract the diseases of headache, fever and chillness and malaria; when the heat is in the upper part of the body, the skin will be painful and turn into yellowish-red, when the heat is transmitted inside and uncontrolled, edema in the face and the body, abdominal fullness, sighing, watery diarrhea with purulent and bloody stools, pyogenic infection and ulceration of skin, spitting blood, oppressive feeling over the chest, heat in the chest and epistaxis will occur; and these diseases are stemmed from the lung. If the Tianfu pulse is severed, it shows the lung energy has been injured, the patient can by no means to be cured and die.

阳明司天，燥淫所胜，则木乃晚荣，草乃晚生，筋骨内变。民病左胠胁痛，寒清于中，感而疟，大凉革候，咳，腹中鸣，注泄鹜溏，名木敛，生菀于下，草焦上首，心胁暴痛，不可

反侧，嗌乾面尘腰痛，丈夫㿗疝，妇人少腹痛，目昧眦，疡疮痤痈，蛰虫来见，病本于肝。太冲绝，死不治。

" In the year when Yangming is controlling the heaven energy, the dryness energy is partial overabundant. The grasses and woods will be recovered behind schedule. People will contract the diseases of the muscle and bone. The weather will become abnormal due to the great coolness, the tips of one branches of the big trees will become withered, the tips of the grasses will become shrivelled due to the lying below the generative energy, and the hibernants which should be hiding, on the contrary, will be appearing outside. People will contract the diseases of pain in the left hypochronium if the viscera are is invaded by the external cold again, malaria will occur. Besides, people will contract the diseases of cough, borborygmus watery diarrhea, loose stools, sudden acute pain in the heart and the hypochondria causing the patient unable to turn around; dry throat, dusty complexion, lumbago, disorder of head and hernia in man and pain in the lower abdomen in woman, dark in the canthi, pyogenic infection and ulceration of skin and carbuncle will occur, and these diseases are stemmed from the liver. If the Taichong pulse is severed, it shows the liver energy has been injured, the patient will by no means to be cured and die.

太阳司天，寒淫所胜，则寒气反至，水且冰，血变于中，发为痈疡。民病厥心痛，呕血血泄鼽衄，善悲，时眩仆，运火炎烈，雨暴乃雹，胸腹满，手热肘挛掖冲，心澹澹大动，胸胁胃脘不安，面赤目黄，善噫，嗌乾，甚则色炲，渴而欲饮，病本于心。神门绝，死不治。所谓动气知其藏也。

"In the year when Taiyang is controlling the heaven energy, the cold energy which is overabundant comes all of a sudden, and the water will be frozen. If the motion's energy of Wu Gui year in which the assimilated fire is flaming strongly, the cold and fire will be combating, and the torential rain and the hail will occur. In man, the variation of blood will take place and the diseases of carbuncle, ulceration, heartache due to the attack of the cold-evil, hematochezia, epistaxis, melancholy, falling down often due to dizziness, fullness of chest and abdomen, hot hand, convulsion of the elbow, swelling of the armpit, palpitation, restlessness, uneasiness of the chest, hypochondria and the gastric cavity, red face, yellow eyes, eructation, dry throat, burn-black complexion and desire for drinking due to thirsty will occur. These diseases are stemmed from the heart. If the Shenmen pulse is severed, it shows the heart energy has been injured, the patient can by no means to be cured and die.

"Thus, from the the pulsation of the channel-energy, one can know the existence of the visceral energies. "

帝曰：善。治之奈何？岐伯曰：司天之气，风淫 所胜，平以辛凉，佐以苦甘，以甘缓之，以酸写之。热淫所胜，平以咸寒，佐以苦甘，以酸收之。湿淫所胜，平以苦热，佐以酸辛，以苦燥之，以淡泄之。湿上甚而热，治以苦温，佐以甘辛，以汗为故而止。火淫所胜，平以酸冷，佐以苦甘，以酸收之，以苦发之，以酸复之，热淫同。燥淫所胜，平以苦湿，佐以酸辛，以苦下之。寒淫所胜，平以辛热，佐以甘苦，以咸写之。

Yellow Emperor said: " Good. But how to treat it ?" Qibo said: " In the diseases caused

by the energy that controls the heaven energy, if it is overcome by the wind-evil, apply medicine of acrid taste and cool nature as the main medicine to calm the overcoming energy and apply the medicine of bitter and sweet taste as the assistant medicine, buffer the urgency of the disease with the medicine of sweet taste, and discharge the evil energy with the medicine of sour taste; if it is overcome by the heat evil, apply the medicine of salty taste and cold nature mainly to moderate the overcoming energy, assist with the medicine of bitter and sweet taste, collect the Yin energy with the medicine of sour taste; if it is overcome by the wetness-evil, apply the medicine of bitter taste and hot nature mainly to moderate the overcoming energy, assist with the medicine of sour and acrid tastes, dry the wetness with the medicine of bitter taste and purge the wetness-evil with the medicine of flat taste; if the wetness-evil is overabundant in the upper part of the body with fever, it should be treated mainly with bitter warm medicine and assist with the medicine of sweet and acrid taste and treat with the diaphoresis therapy until the normal condition is resumed; if it is overcome by the fire-evil, apply the medicine of sour taste and coold nature mainly to moderate the overcoming energy, assist with the medicine of bitter and sweet tastes, collect the Yin energy with the medicine of sour taste, disperse the fire-evil with the medicine of bitter taste, and resume the Yin fluid with the medicine of sour taste; if it is overcome by the heat-evil, the treating should be likewise; if it is overcome by the dryness-evil, apply the medicine of bitter taste and wet nature to mainly moderate the overcoming energy and assist with the medicine of sour and acrid taste, purge the dryness retention with the medicine of bitter taste; if it is overcome by the cold-evil, apply the medicine of acrid taste and hot nature mainly to moderate the overcoming energy, assist with the medicine of sweet and bitter taste and purge the cold-evil with the medicine of salty taste."

帝曰：善。邪气反胜，治之奈何？岐伯曰：风司于地，清反胜之，治以酸温，佐以苦甘，以辛平之。热司于地，寒反胜之，治以甘热，佐以苦辛，以咸平之。湿司于地，热反胜之，治以苦冷，佐以咸甘，以苦平之。火司于地，寒反胜之，治以甘热，佐以苦辛，以咸平之。燥司于地，热反胜之，治以平〔《素问校讹》引古抄本“平”作“辛”〕寒，佐以苦甘，以酸平之，以和为利，寒司于地，热反胜之，治以咸冷，佐以甘辛，以苦平之。

Yellow Emperor said: " Good. How to treat the disease caused by the excessive overcoming evil energy?" Qibo said: " When the insufficient wind energy is affecting the earth energy, and the wood wind is overcome by the overcoming cool metal excessively, it should be treated with the medicine of sour taste and warm nature mainly, assist with the medicine of bitter and sweet taste and recuperate the weakened health energy with the medicine of acrid taste; when the insufficient heat is affecting the earth energy and heat is overcome by the overcoming cold energy excessively, treat mainly with the medicine of sweet taste and hot nature and assist with the medicine of bitter and acrid tastes and recuperate the weakened healthy energy with the medicine of salty taste; when the insufficient wetness energy is affecting the earth energy and heat is overcome by the overcoming cold water excessively, it should treat mainly with the medicine of bitter taste and cool nature, assist with the medicine

of salty and sweet tastes, and recuperate the weakened healthy energy with the medicine of bitter taste; when the insufficient fire energy is affecting the earth energy and fire is overcome by the overcoming cold water excessively, treat mainly with the medicine of sweet taste of hot nature, assist with the medicine of of bitter and acrid taste and recuperate the weakened healthy energy with the medicine of salty taste; when the insufficient energy of dryness is affecting the earth energy and dryness is overcome by the overcoming heat energy excessively, treat mainly with the medicine of acrid taste and cold nature, assist with the medicine of bitter and sweet taste, recuperate the weakened healthy energy with the medicine of sour taste, and the medicines applied should be of mild nature; when the insufficient cold energy is affecting the earth energy and the heat energy is overcoming, treat mainly with the medicine of salty taste and cool nature, assist with the medicine of sweet and acrid taste, and recuperate the weakened healthy energy with the medicine of bitter taste."

帝曰：其司天邪胜何如？岐伯曰：风化于天，清反胜之，治以酸温，佐以甘苦；热化于天，寒反胜之，治以甘温，佐以苦酸辛；湿化于天，热反胜之，治以苦寒，佐以苦酸；火化于天，寒反胜之，治以甘热，佐以苦辛；燥化于天，热反胜之，治以辛寒，佐以苦甘；寒化于天，热反胜之，治以咸冷，佐以苦辛。

Yellow Emperor asked: "How to treat the disease caused by the insufficient energy that controls the heaven energy and the evil energy is overcoming?" Qibo said: "When the insufficient wind energy of Jueyin is controlling the heaven energy and the cool energy is overcoming it excessively, it should treat mainly with the medicine of sour taste and warm nature and assist with the medicine of bitter and sweet taste; when the insufficient energy of heat is controlling the heaven energy and the cold energy is overcoming it excessively, it should be treated mainly with the medicine of sweet taste and warm nature and assist with the medicine of bitter, sour and acrid taste ; when the insufficient energy of wetness is controlling the heaven energy and the heat energy is overcoming it excessively. it should treat mainly with the medicine of bitter taste and cold nature and assist with the medicine of bitter and sour taste; when the insufficient energy of fire is controlling the heaven energy and the cold energy is overcoming it excessively, treat mainly with the medicine of sweet taste and hot nature and assist with the medicine of bitter and acrid tastes; when the insufficient energy of dryness is controlling the heaven energy and the heat energy is overcoming it excessively, treat mainly with the medicine of acrid taste and cold nature and assist with the medicine of bitter and sweet taste; when the insufficient energy of cold is controlling the heaven energy and the heat energy is overcoming it reversely, treat mainly with the medicine of salty taste and cold nature, and assist with the medicine of bitter and acrid taste."

帝曰：六气相胜奈何？岐伯曰：厥阴之胜，耳鸣头眩，愦愦欲吐，胃鬲如寒，大风数举，倮虫不滋，胠胁气并，化而为热，小便黄赤，胃脘当心而痛，上支两胁，肠鸣飧泄，少腹痛，注下赤白，甚则呕吐，鬲咽不通。

Yellow Emperor asked: "What is the condition when six-energy takes chance to invade and causes disease?" Qibo said: "When the wind energy of Jueyin is invading due to partial

overabundance and invades, people will have tinnitus, dizziness, feeling of oppression over the chest, desire for vomiting, cold feeling above the gastric cavity and under the diaphram. When the strong wind is blowing, the naked worms can not multiply. By this time, people will often contract the syndromes of fever due to merging of the hypochondria's energy to the liver energy, and the deep-coloured urine, stomachache by the location of heart, distention of hypochondria and upper limbs, tinnitus, lienteric diarrhea, pain in the lower abdomen and dysentery will occur. If the disease is severe, the patient will vomit and has dysphasia.

少阴之胜，心下热善饥，齐下反动，〔读本，吴本“动”作“痛”〕气游三焦，炎暑至，木乃津，草乃萎，呕逆躁烦，腹满痛，溏泄，传为赤沃。

" When the heat energy of Shaoyin is partial overabundant and invades, the patient will have heat over the epigastric region, feeling hungry often, pain under the navel and the spreading of heat all over the triple warmer. As the hot summer arrives, the fluid of the woods flows and the grasses become withered. People will contract the diseases of vomiting, irritability, pain and distention of the abdomen, loose stools and even to have hematuria.

太阴之胜，火气内郁，疮疡于中，流散于外，病在胠胁，甚则心痛热格，头痛 喉痹项强，独胜则湿气内郁，寒迫下焦，痛留顶，互引眉间，胃满，雨数至，燥〔张介宾说：“‘燥’当作‘温’”〕，化乃见，少腹满，腰脽重强，内不便，善注泄，足下温，头重足胫胕肿，饮发于中，胕肿于上。

" When the wetness energy of Taiyin is partial overabundant and invades, if the fire energy is stagnated inside of the body it will ferment into pyogenic infection and ulcer, if it is spreading outside, it will cause disease in the hypochondria or even to cause heartache. When the heat is hindered in the upperpart of the body, people will contract the diseases of headache, sore throat and the stiffness of the neck. When the wetness energy is overabundant solely and stagnates inside, and the lower warmer is pressed by the cold-wetness energy, then, the radiated pain in the top of head and brows and distention of stomach will occur. The frequent appearance of the scaled worms on the ground shows the phenomenon of warmness is emerging. People will have distention of the lower abdomen, heaviness and stiffness of the lumbar vertebra, difficulty of stretching and bending the extremities due to the retention of wetness inside, watery diarrhea, warm in the feet, heaviness of the head, swelling of the tibia of foot, and edema in the upper part of the body due to the fluid retention inside.

少阳之胜，热客于胃，烦心心痛，目赤欲呕，呕酸善饥，耳痛溺赤，善惊谵妄，暴热消烁，草萎水涸，介虫乃屈，少腹痛，下沃赤白。

" When the fire energy of Shaoyang is partial overabundant and invades, if the heat-evill retains in the stomach, the syndromes of irritability, heartache, red eyes, desire for vomiting, sour vomiting, frequent hungry, pain in the ears, deep-coloured urine, apt to be frightened and delirium will occur. The sudden heat drys up all things and cause the grasses to become withered, the waters dry up and exhausted, and the cyprid lies still. People will contract pain in the lower abdomen and dysentery with purulent and bloody stools.

阳明之胜，清发于中，左胠胁痛溏泄，内为嗌塞，外发𩓣疝，大凉肃杀，华英改容，毛虫乃殃，胸中不便，嗌塞而咳。

" When the dryness energy of Yangming is partial overabundant and invades, the cool energy will be sent out from inside causing pain in the left hypochondrium and diarrhea. The cool energy causes the obstruction of pharynx inside, and causes swelling of the scrotum outside. As the great cool energy causes desolution, the grasses and woods will be withered, some of the caterpillars will die. People will contract the diseases of uneasiness in the chest, obstruction of the larynx and cough.

太阳之胜，凝溧且至，非时水冰，羽乃后化，痔疟发，寒厥入胃，则内生心痛，阴中乃疡，隐曲不利，互引阴股，筋肉拘苛，血脉凝泣，络满色变，或为血泄，皮肤否肿，腹满食减，热反上行，头项囟顶脑户中痛，目如脱，寒入下焦，传为濡写。

" When the cold energy of Taiyang is partial overabundant and invades, the condensed and very cold weather will be arriving. The water will freeze in advance, and the growing of the insects with wings will be postponed. People will contract the diseases of hemorrhoid and malaria. When the cold energy invades the stomach, the energy will reverse up to cause heartache. People will also contract the sores in the genital organs, dysuria, radiated pain in the inner side of the thigh, convulsion and contraction of the muscle, discolouration of the complexion due to stagnation and fullness of the channels, hematochezia, edema of skin due to the retention of body fluid, abdominal fullness, reduction of food and drink, pain on the top of head due to the up-rising of heat, pain in the eyeball like falling off and watery diarrhea caused by the cold energy which invades the lower warmer. "

帝曰：治之奈何？岐伯曰：厥阴之胜，治以甘清，佐以苦辛，以酸写之。少阴之胜，治以辛寒，佐以苦咸，以甘写之。太阴之胜，治以咸热，佐以甘辛，以苦写之，少阳之胜，治以辛寒，佐以甘咸，以甘泻之。阳明之胜，治以酸温，佐以辛甘，以苦泄之。太阳之胜，治以甘〔林校云："详此为治，皆先泻其不能，而后泻其来胜，疑'甘'字苦之误也"〕热，佐以辛酸，以咸写之。

Yellow Emperor asked: " How to treat it ?" Qibo said: " when treating the disease caused by the overcoming energy of Jueyin, apply the medicine of sweet taste and cool nature mainly for treating, assist with the medicine of bitter and acrid taste, and purge the overcoming energy with the medicine of sour taste; When treating the disease caused by the overcoming heat energy of Shaoyin, apply the medicine of acrid taste and cold nature mainly for treating, assist with the medicine of bitter and salty taste, and purge the overcoming energy with the medicine of sweet taste ; when treating the disease caused by the overabundant wetness energy of Taiyin, apply the medicine of salty taste and hot nature mainly for treating, assist with the medicine of acrid and sweet taste, and purge the overcoming energy with the medicine of bitter taste; when treating the disease caused by the fire energy of Shaoyang, apply the medicine of acrid taste and cold nature mainly for treating, assist with the medicine of sweet and salty tastes and purge the overcoming energy with the medicine of sweet taste; when treating the disease caused by the dryness energy of Yangming, apply the medicine of

sour taste and warm nature mainly for treating, assist with the medicine of acrid and sweet tastes, and purge the overcoming energy with the medicne of bitter taste; when treating the disease by the cold energy of Taiyang, apply the medicne of bitter taste and hot nature mainly for treating, assist with the medicine of acrid and sour tastes, and purge the overcoming energy with the medicine of salty taste."

帝曰：六气之复何如？岐伯曰：悉乎哉问也？厥阴之复，少腹坚满，裹急暴痛，偃木飞沙，倮虫不荣，厥心痛，汗发呕吐，饮食不入，入而复出，筋骨掉眩，清厥，甚则入脾，食痹而吐。冲阳绝，死不治。

" Yellow Emperor asked:" what is the condition when the disease is caused by the retaliating energy of the six-energy?" Qibo said:" What an exhaustive question you have asked. When the energy of Jueyin is retaliating, it will cause mass and flatulence of the lower abdomen, muscular stiffness in the abdomen and hypochondria will have sudden pain. In the natural world, the trees will lie flat, the dust will be flying and the worms with naked body will not multiply. People will contract the diseases of syncope due to the disorder of vital energy, heartache, sweating, vomiting, can hardly eat, vomit after taking food, trembling of muscle and bone, dizziness and cold extremities. When the disease is severe, the wind-evil will invade the spleen to cause stomachache and vomiting after food intake. When the Chongyang pulse is severed, the patient can by no means to be cured and die .

少阴之复，燠热内作，烦躁鼽嚏，少腹绞痛，火见燔焫，嗌燥，分注时止，气动于左，上行于右，咳，皮肤痛 ，暴瘖心痛，郁冒不知人，乃洒淅恶寒，振栗谵妄，寒已而热，渴而欲饮，少气骨痿，隔肠不便，外为浮肿，哕噫，赤气后化，流水不冰，热气大行，介虫不复，病痱胗疮疡，痈疽痤痔，甚则入肺，咳而鼻渊。天府绝，死不治。

"When the energy of Shaoyin is retaliating, the feverish sensation accompanied with restlessness will produce inside, and the diseases of irritability, epistaxis, sneezing, angina of the lower abdomen, firing heat outside and burning heat of the body, dry pharynx, ceasing now and then of the urination and stool, moving about of the energy on the left side and reversing up to the right side, cough, pain of the skin, sudden dysphonia, heartache, unconciousness, has aversion to cold feeling like the sprinkling of cold water over the body, rigor, speaking nonsence, fever after chillness, thirsty and desire for drink, short of breath, flaccidity of bone, intestinal obstruction, retention of feces, edema outside, hiccup and eructation will occur. If the heat energy of Shaoyin monarch-fire is lagging behind in retaliating, the flowing water will not freeze, the heat energy will be prevailing and the cyprid will not hibernate. People will often contract the superficial lesions of miliaria, papule, pyogenic infection and ulceration of skin, carbuncle, acne and hemorrhoid, when the heat-evil is excessive, it will invade into the lung and cause cough and sinusitis. If the Tianfu pulse is severed, the patient can by no means to be cured and die.

太阴之复，湿变乃举，体重中满，食饮不化，阴气上厥，胸中不便，饮发于中，咳喘有声。大雨时行，鳞见于陆，头顶痛重，而掉瘛尤甚，呕而密默，唾吐清液，甚则入肾，窍写无度。太豀绝，死不治。

"When the energy of Taiyin is retaliating, the disease of wetness energy will occur, the patient will contract heaviness of the body, fullness of the chest, indigestion of food, adveresness of Yin energy, uneasiness of chest, unceasing cough and the fluid retention inside. If the heavy rains fall often and the fish appears on the ground, people will feel pain and heaviness of the head and neck, and the disease will become even more severe when being frightened. As the wetness is abundant inside, the patient will be reluctant to move and like to spit water. If the wetness invades the kidney, the diarrhea of the patient will be out of control. If the Taixi pulse is severed, the patient can by no means to be cured and die.

少阳之复，大热将至，枯燥燔爇，介虫乃耗，惊瘛咳衄，心热烦燥，便数憎风，厥气上行，面如浮埃，目乃瞤瘛，火气内发，上为口糜，呕逆，血溢血泄，发而为疟，恶寒鼓慄，寒极反热，嗌络焦槁，渴引水浆，色变黄赤，少气脉萎，化而为水，传为胕肿，甚则入肺，咳而血泄。尺泽绝，死不治。

"When the energy of Shaoyang is retaliating, the extreme heat will be coming soon. It causes all things to become dry and scorching hot, and the cyprid will be injured. People will contract the diseases of terror, pain on the top, cough, hemorrhage, heat in the heart, irritability, frequent micturition and have aversion to wind. When the heat-evil is reversing up, the patient will have dusty complexion and the heating of eyes. When the fire energy enters inside, it will cause thirsty, vomiting or hemorrhage of the patient; when the fire energy is falling down, it causes hematochezia, malaria, chillness and shivering with cold; when the extreme cold energy turns into heat energy, the patient will have dry throat, thirst, desire for drinking, yellowish-red complexion, short of breath with vascular flaccidity-syndrome. When the assimilated heat energy turns into watery disease, edema will occur; when the evil energy invades further the lung, hemoptysis will occur. If the Chize pluse is severed, the patient will by no means to be cured and die.

阳明之复，清气大举，森木苍乾，毛虫乃厉。病生胠胁，气归于左，善太息，甚则心痛否满，腹胀而泄，呕苦咳哕，烦心，病在鬲中头痛，甚则入肝，惊骇筋挛。太冲绝，死不治。

"When the energy of Yangming is retaliating, the cool and restrained energy will be prevailing, many trees will become grey and withered and many animals will contract the epidemic disease. People will contract the disease on the hypochondria, the syndrome of slanting on the left side of the energy to cause frequent sigh. When the condition is severe, it will cause heartache, feeling of fullness and oppression of the chest, abdominal distention, diarrhea, vomiting, cough, hiccup and irritability. When the evil energy is in the diaphram, headache will occur, if the evil energy enters into the liver, people will have the disease of terrifying and muscular stiffness. If the Taichong pulse is severed, the patient can by no means to be cured and die.

太阳之复，厥气上行，水凝雨冰，羽虫乃死，心胃生寒，胸膈不利，心痛否满，头痛善悲〔《史载之方》引"悲"作"恐"〕，时眩仆，食减，腰脽反痛，屈伸不便，地裂冰坚，阳光不治，少腹控睾，引腰脊，上冲心，唾出清水，及为哕噫，甚则入心，善忘善悲。神门绝，死不治。

"When the energy of Taiyang is retaliating, the cold energy ascends, the water freezes and the snow falls. Most of the insects with wings will die. People will contract the diseases of production of cold energy from the heart and stomach, uneasiness of the chest, heartache, feeling of fullness and oppression of the chest, headache, frequent frightening, frequent dizziness and falling down, reduction of food intake, pain in the lumbar vertebra and difficulty in stretching and bending the extremities. If the ground is craked, the ice is thick and firm, and the sun is not hot at all, people will contract the diseases of pain in the lower abdomen and radiated pain to the testes, loins and spine. When the reverse energy rises up to attack the heart, the syndromes of spitting clear saliva, hiccup and eructation will occur, If the Shenmen pulse is severed, the patient can by no means to be cured and die."

帝曰：善。治之奈何？岐伯曰：厥阴之复，治以酸〔林校引别本"酸"作"辛"〕寒，佐以甘辛，以酸写之，以甘缓之。少阴之复，治以咸寒，佐以苦辛，以甘写之，以酸收之，辛苦发之，以咸软之。太阴之复，治以苦热，佐以酸辛，以苦写之，燥之，泄之。少阳之复，治以咸冷，佐以苦辛，以咸软之，以酸收之，辛苦发之，发不远热，无犯温凉，少阴同法。阳明之复，治以辛温，佐以苦甘，以苦泄之，以苦下之〔四库本作"以甘发之"〕，以酸补之。太阳之复，治以咸热，佐以甘辛，以苦坚之。治诸胜复，寒者热之，热者寒之，温者清之，清者温之，散者收之，抑者散之，燥者润之，急者缓之，坚者耎之，脆者坚之，衰者补之，强者写之，各安其气，必清必静，则病气衰去，归其所宗，此治之大体也。

Yellow Emperor said: "Good. But how to treat it?" Qibo said: "When treating the disease caused by retaliating energy of Jueyin, it should apply the medicine of acrid taste and cold nature mainly for treating, and assist with the medicine of sweet and acrid tastes, purge the evil energy with the medicine of sour taste and buffer its urgeney with the medicine of sweet taste.

"When treating the disease caused by the retaliating anergy of Shaoyin, apply the medicine of salty taste and cold nature mainly for treating and assist with the medicine of bitter and acrid tastes, purge the evil energy with the medicine of sweet taste, collect the evil energy with the medicine of sour taste, disperse the evil-energy with the medicine of bitter taste and dissipate the mass with the medicine of salty taste.

"When treating the disease caused by the retaliating energy Taiyin, apply the medicine of bitter taste and hot nature, assist with the medicine of sour and acrid tartes, apply bitter medicine to purge the evil, dry the wetness and purgate the wet-evil.

"When treating the disease caused by the retaliating energy of Shaoyang, apply the medicine of salty taste and cold nature mainly for treating and assist with the medicine of bitter and acrid tastes, dissipate the mass with the medicine of salty taste, collect the evil energy with the medicine of sour taste and apply the diaphoresis therapy with the medicine of bitter taste. When applying diaphoresis therapy, it is not necessary to avoid the contraindication of using the medicine of hot nature in hot weather or of cold nature in cold weather, but the medicine of warm or cool nature must not be used.

"When applying the diaphoresis therapy in treating the disease caused by the retaliating

energy of Shaoyin, it should be applied in the same way.

"When treating the disease caused by the retaliating energy of Yangming, apply the medicine of acrid taste and warm nature mainly for treating and assist with the medicine of bitter and sweet tastes, apply the medicine of bitter taste for slow purgation, disperse with the medicine of sweet taste and recuperate the deficiency with the medicine of sour taste.

"When treating the disease caused by the retaliating energy of Taiyang, apply the medicine of salty taste and hot nature mainly for treating, assist with the medicine of sweet and acrid tastes and stabilize the energy with the medicine of bitter taste.

"When treating the diseases caused by the various overcoming and retaliating energies, apply the medicine of hot nature to the cold disease, apply the medicine of cold nature to the hot disease, apply the medicine of cool nature to the wet disease and apply the medicine of warm nature to the cool disease, when the primordial energy or the patient is exhausting, apply the medicine for collecting, when the energy of the patient is oppressed and stagnated, apply the medicine for dispersing, when the patient is invaded by the dryness evil, apply the medicine for moistening, when the patient's energy is pressing, apply the medicine to ease up, when the evil energy of the patient is substantial, apply the medicine for softening and dissipating, when the energy of the patient is weak, apply the medicine for stabilizing, when the energy of the patient is hyperactive, apply the medicine for purging. In this way, the five viscera will each get to its due position without disturbing each other, the evil energy will be diminishing in due course, and the other energies will be each to its category without partial overabundance and resume its own normal state. These are the treating methods on the whole."

帝曰：善。气之上下，何谓也？岐伯曰：身半以上，其气三矣，天之分也，天气主之。身半以下，其气三矣，地之分也，地气主之。以名命气，以气命处，而言其病。半，所谓天枢也。故上胜而下俱病者，以地名之，下胜而上俱病者，以天名之。所谓胜至，报气屈服而未发也。复至则不以天地异名，皆如复气为法也。帝曰：胜复之动，时有常乎？气有必乎？岐伯曰：时有常位，而气无必也。帝曰：愿闻其道也。岐伯曰：初气终三气，天气主之，胜之常也。四气尽终气，地气主之，复之常也。有胜则复，无胜则否。帝曰：善。复已而胜何如？岐伯曰：胜至则复，无常数也，衰乃止耳。复已而胜，不复则害，此伤生也。帝曰：复而反病何也？岐伯曰：居非其位，不相得也。大复其胜则主胜之，故反病也。所谓火燥热也。

Yellow Emperor said: "Good. In the energies, some are in the upper part and some are in the lower part of the body, and why is it so?" Qibo said: "There are three energies in the upper part of the body (ie., the energy that controls the heaven energy and the left and right intermediate energies) which are the parts of human body that correspond to heaven and are controlled by the heaven energy, and there are three energies in the lower part of the body (ie., the energy that affects the earth energy and the left and right intermediate energies) which are the parts of human body that correspond to the earth and are controlled by the energy that affects the earth energy. The overcoming energy and the retaliating energy are indicated by the upper part and the lower part, and the sections of body showing the diseases are

indicated by the six energies. The demarcation of the upper body and the lower body is the Tianshu point (around the navel).

"When the three energies in the upper body are overabundant and the three energies in the lower body are deficient, the disease is in the lower part, and the contracted diseases are named according to the earth energy; when the three energies in the lower body are overabundant and the three energies in the upper body are deficient, the disease is in the upper part, and the contracted diseases are named according to the heaven energy. The above statement refers to the condition when the overcoming energy has arrived and the retaliating energy is still hiding. When the retaliating energy has arrived, the disease will not be named according to the energies that control the heaven energy or affects the earth energy, but are named according to the variation of the retaliating energy."

Yellow Emperor asked: "Is there a regular time in the changes of the overcoming and retaliating energies and is there any regular pattern in the coming or not coming of the energy?" Qibo said: "Although there are regular postitions in the four seasons, yet the coming or not coming of the overcoming energy and the retaliating energy are uncertain." Yellow Emperor said: "I hope to know the reason." Qibo said: "The stages which are from the initial energy to the third energy are controlled by the heaven energy, and they appear to be the common seasonal positions of the overcoming energy; the stages which are from the fourth energy to the terminal energy are affected by the earth energy, and they appear to be the common seasonal positions of the retaliating energy. The retaliating energy can only occur when the overcoming energy is existing, if there is no overcoming energy, there will be no retaliating energy."

Yellow Emperor said: "Good. But sometimes, the overcoming energy occurs again after the retaliating energy has already retreated, and what is the reason?" Qibo said: "The retaliating energy comes after the overcoming, and after the retaliating, the overcoming energy can occur again, the times of the overcoming and the retaliating are not definite, and they will stop when both of them become debilitating. The overcoming energy occurs again after the retaliating energy, and if the retaliating does not occur after the overcoming energy in correspond, it will injure the life of a man."

Yellow Emperor asked: "There is the case of after the retaliating energy arrives, the retaliating energy itself causes the disease, and why is it?" Qibo said: "This is because of the arrival of the retaliating energy is not in the proper seasonal time and the retaliating energy does not agree with the proper position of the season, when the overcoming energy is retaliated by the retaliating energy excessively, the retaliating energy will become deficient, and if it is overcome again by the energy that dominated the season, the retaliating energy itself will cause the disease. These are the cases in the fire, dryness and heat."

帝曰：治之何如？岐伯曰：夫气之胜也，微者随之，甚者制之。气之复也，和者平之，暴者夺之。皆随胜气，安其屈伏，无问其数，以平为期，此其道也。

Yellow Emperor asked: "How to treat it?" Qibo said: "In treating the disease caused by

the overcoming energy, if the disease is light, one must suit its property, when it is severe, one must stop it by applying the medicine of overcoming. when treating the disease caused by the retaliating energy, if the disease is moderate, one must adjust it to become calm, if the disease is violent, one must weaken it. In a word, suit the overcoming energy and stabilize the suppressed energy. The times of applying medicine are not limited, but must stop applying when the energy is being eased up. This is the general rule for treating."

帝曰：善。客主之胜复奈何？岐伯曰：客主之气，胜而无复也。帝曰：其逆从何如？岐伯曰：主胜逆，客胜从，天之道也。

Yellow Emperor said: "Good. What are the overcoming and retaliating conditions of the dominating energy of the host energy (dominating energy of the year) and the guest energy?" Qibo said: "There is only the condition of overcoming without retaliating between the host energy and the guest energy." Yellow Emperor asked: "How to distinguish the adverse and agreeable conditions?" Qibo said: When the host energy is overcoming, it is the adverse condition, when the guest energy is overcoming, it is the agreeable condition, and this is the common rule of heaven and earth."

帝曰：其生病何如？岐伯曰：厥阴司天，客胜则耳鸣掉眩，甚则咳；主胜则胸胁痛，舌难以言。少阴司天，客胜则鼽嚏，颈项强，肩背瞀热，头痛少气，发热耳聋目瞑，甚则胕肿血溢，疮疡咳喘；主胜则心热烦躁，甚则胁痛支满。太阴司天，客胜则首面胕肿，呼吸气喘；主胜则胸腹满，食已而瞀。少阳司天，客胜则丹胗外发，及为丹熛疮疡，呕逆喉痹，头痛嗌肿，耳聋血溢，内为瘛疭；主胜则胸满咳仰息，甚而有血，手热。阳明司天，清复内余，则咳衄嗌塞，心鬲中热，咳不止而白血出者死。太阳司天，客胜则胸中不利，出清涕，感寒则咳；主胜则喉嗌中鸣。

Yellow Emperor said: "What are the diseases caused by them?" Qibo said: "When Jueyin is controlling the heaven energy, if the guest energy is overcoming, people will contract tinnitus and dizziness, or even cough; if the host energy is overcoming, people will contract pain in the chest and hypochondrium, and also difficulty in speaking due to stiff tongue.

"When Shaoyin is controlling the heaven energy, if the guest energy is overcoming, people will contract sneezing, stiffness of the neck, fever in the shoulder and back, headache, short of breath, fever, deafness, blur eyes, even to have edema, hemorrhage, pyogenic infection and ulceration of skin, cough and rapid breathing; if the host energy is overcoming, people will contract heart-heat, restlessness, even to have pain and fullness of hypochondria.

"When Taiyin is controlling the heaven energy, if the guest energy is overcoming, people will contract edema in the head and face, and rapid breathing; if the host energy of the year is overcoming, people will contract fullness of the chest and abdomen, and mental confusion after food intake.

"When Shaoyang is controlling the heaven energy, if the guest energy is overcoming, people will contract papule with redness of skin, pyogenic infection and ulceration of skin, vomiting, sore throat, headache, swelling of pharynx, deafness, hemorrhage and convulsion

of extremities; if the host energy is overcoming, people will contract fullness of the chest, cough, sigh, even to have hemoptysis and hot hand.

"When Yangming is controlling the heaven energy, if the guest energy of coolness is having a surplus inside and controls the heaven energy, people will contract cough, hemorrhage, obstruction of the pharynx, heat in the diaphram, unceasing cough with white complexion. If the patient is bleeding continuonsly, he will die.

"When Taiyang is controlling the heaven energy, if the guest energy is overcoming, the patient will feel uneasy in the chest, having a running nose, and cough when feeling cold; if the host energy of the year is overcoming, the wheezing sound of the throat will be heard.

厥阴在泉，客胜则大关节不利，内为痉强拘瘛，外为不便；主胜则筋骨繇并，腰腹时痛。少阴在泉，客胜则腰痛，尻股膝髀腨骺足病，瞀热以酸，胕肿不能久立，溲便变；主胜则厥气上行，心痛发热，鬲中众痹皆作，发于胠胁，魄汗不藏，四逆而起。太阴在泉，客胜则足痿下重，便溲不时，湿客下焦，发而濡写，及为肿隐曲之疾；主胜则寒气逆满，食饮不下，甚则为疝。少阳在泉，客胜则腰腹痛而反恶寒，甚则下白溺白；主胜则热反上行而客于心，心痛发热，格中而呕。少阴同候。阳明在泉，客胜则清气动下，少腹坚满而数便写；主胜则腰重腹痛，少腹生寒，下为鹜溏，则寒厥于肠，上冲胸中，甚则喘不能久立。太阳在泉，寒复内余，则腰尻痛，屈伸不利，股胫足膝中痛。

"When Jueyin is affecting the earth energy, if the guest energy is overcoming, the patient will find difficulty in moving his joints, when the energy is inside, it causes spasm, rigidity and convulsion of the musele, when it is outside, it causes the inconvenience of actions; if the host energy is overcoming, the patient will contract swaying and stiffness of the muscle and bone, frequent pain in the loins and abdomen.

"When Shaoyin is affecting the earth energy, if the guest energy is overcoming, the patient will contract lumbago, uneasiness of the sacrococcygeal region, thigh, knee, upper half of the thigh, tibia, fibula and foot, feeling of hotness and aching pain now and then, edema causing the patient can hardly stand long, discolouring of the urine and feces; if the host energy is overcoming, the adverse energy will be rising up to cause heartache, fever and the bi-syndrome in the diaphram. As the disease breaks out from the hypochondrium, the sweat can hardly be retained, the patient will have cold extremities.

"When Taiyin is affecting the earth energy, if the guest energy is overcoming, the diseases of flaccidity of foot, heaviness of the lower limbs, and abnormal in urination and defecation will occur. As the wetness is retained in the lower warmer, the syndromes of diarrhea due to wetness-evil, edema and the disease of the external genitals and anus will occur; if the host energy is overcoming, the cold energy will reverse upward, the feeling of fullness and oppression, reduction of food and drink and even the hernia pain will occur.

"When Shaoyang is affecting the earth energy, if the guest energy is overcoming, the patient will have pain in the loins and abdomen, chilliness and even to have white urine and feces; if the host energy is overcoming, the heat will, on the contrary, rise up to attack the heart, the diseases of heartache, internal contention of fever and vomiting will occur. The

other syndromes occurred are the same with those when Shaoyin is affecting the earth energy.

"When Yangming is affecting the earth energy, if the guest energy is overcoming, the cool energy will be stirring below, the lower abdomen will be hard and full and diarrhea will occur often; if the host energy is overcoming, the patient will have heaviness of the loins, abdominel pain and diarrhea with loose stools due to the descent of cold energy from the lower abdomen; when the cold energy in the intestine and stomach rises up to attack the chest, it will cause rapid breathing of the patient and he can hardly stand long.

"When Taiyang is affecting the earth energy, the cold energy of water will cause pain in the loins and the sacrococcygeal region, difficulty in stretching and bending the extremities and pain in the thigh, tibia, foot and knee."

帝曰：善。治之奈何？岐伯曰：高者抑之，下者举之，有余折之，不足补之，佐以所利，和以所宜，必安其主客，适其寒温，同者逆之，异者从之。

Yellow Emperor said: "Good. But how to treat it?" Qibo said: "Suppress the up-rising energy to cause it falling down, lift the bogging down energy to cause it rising up, purge the sthenie energy which is having a surplus, and invigorate the asthenic energy which is insufticient, besides, apply the favourable medicine and proper food to stabilize the guest energy and the host energy and suit the coldness and hotness of the energies. When the host energy is similar with the guest energy, if the overcoming energy is excessive, it should be stopped by treating reversely, when the host energy is different from the guest energy, one of them should be followed and adjusted according to the conditions of the partial strong or the partial weak of them."

帝曰：治寒以热，治热以寒，气相得者逆之，不相得者从之，余以知之矣。其于正味何如？岐伯曰：木位之主，其写以酸，其补以辛。火位之主，其写以甘，其补以咸。土位之主，其写以苦，其补以甘。金位之主，其写以辛，其补以酸。水位之主，其写以咸，其补以苦。厥阴之客，以辛补之，以酸写之，以甘缓之。少阴之客，以咸补之，以甘写之，以咸收之〔明抄本"咸"作"酸"〕。太阴之客，以甘补之，以苦写之，以甘缓之。少阳之客，以咸补之，以甘写之，以咸软之。阳明之客，以酸补之，以辛写之，以苦泄之。太阳之客，以苦补之，以咸写之，以苦坚之，以辛润之。开发腠理，致津液，通气也。

Yellow Emperor said: "When treating the cold disease, apply the hot medicine, when treating the hot disease, apply the cold medicine, when the host energy is similar with the guest energy, treat the disease reversely, when the host energy is different from the guest energy, treat agreeably to follow one of them, These are all known to me. But what is the specific taste for invigorating and purging when treating the disease caused by the energy activities of the five elements?" Qibo said: "When treating the disease caused by the years dominating wind wood host energy of Jueyin (the wood position is in the initial energy which is in the sixty one days period before Spring Equinox), purge with the medicine of sour taste and invigorate with the medicine of acrid taste. When treating the disease caused by the year's dominating monarch-fire host energy of Shaoyin (the monarch-fire position is in the second

energy which is in the sixty one days period after Spring Equinox) and the prime minister-fire energy of Shaoyang (the prime minister-fire position is in the third energy which is in the thirty days period before and thirty days after the Summer Solstice), purge with the medicine of sweet taste and invigorate with the medicine of salty taste. When treating the disease caused by the year's dominating wetness earth host energy of Taiyin (the earth position is in the fourth energy which is in the sixty one days period before Autumnal Equinox), purge with the medicine of bitter taste and invigorate with the medicine of sweet taste. When treating the disease caused by the year's dominating dryness metal host energy of Yangming (the metal's position is in the fifth energy which is in the sixty one days period after Autumnal Equinox), purge with the medicine of acrid taste and invigorate with the medicine of sour taste. When treating the disease caused by the year's dominating cold water host energy of Taiyang (the water's position is in the terminal energy which is in the period of thirty days before and thirty days after the Winter Solstice), purge with the medicine of salty taste and invigorate with the medicine of bitter taste.

"When treating the disease caused by the guest energy of Jueyin, invigorate with the medicine of acrid taste, purge with the medicine of sour taste, and disperse with the medicine of sweet taste. When treating the disease caused by the guest energy of Shaoyin, invigorate with the medicine of salty taste, purge with the medicine of sweet taste, and weaken the evil energy with the medicine of sour taste. When treating the disease caused by the guest energy of Taiyin, invigorate with the medicine of sweet taste, purge with the medicine of bitter taste, and moderate the energy with the medicine of sweet taste. When treating the disease caused by the guest energy of Shaoyang, invigorate with the medicine of salty taste, purge with the medicine of sweet taste, and soften the firmness with the medicine of salty taste. When treating the disease caused by the guest energy of Yangming, invigorate with the medicine of sour taste, purge with the medicine of acrid taste, and purgate with the medicine of bitter taste. When treating the disease caused by the guest energy of Taiyang, invigorate with the medicine of bitter taste, purge with the medicine of salty taste, stabilize with the medicine of bitter taste, and moisten with the medicine of acrid taste. These treatments are all for dredging the striae, inducing the body fluid and driving through the Yang energy."

帝曰：善。愿闻阴阳之三也何谓？岐伯曰：气有多少，异用也。帝曰：阳明何谓也？岐伯曰两阳合明也。帝曰：厥阴何也？岐伯曰：两阴交尽也。

Yellow Emperor said: "Good. I am told there are three Yins and three Yangs, and what is the reason?" Qibo said: "This is because the energies of Yin and Yang may be more or may be less in quantity, and they are different in functions." Yellow Emperor asked: "What is the meaning of Yangming?" Qibo said: "When the two Yangs of Taiyang and Shaoyang are both bright, it is called Yangming (bright Yang)."

Yellow Emperor asked: "What is the meaning of Jueyin?" Qibo said: "When the two Yins of Taiyin and Shaoyin are both diminishing, it is called Jueyin (the last stage of Yin)."

帝曰：气有多少，病有盛衰，治有缓急，方有大小，愿闻其约奈何？岐伯曰：气有高下，

病有远近，证有中外，治有轻重，适其至所为故也。《大要》曰：君一臣二，奇之制也；君二臣四，偶之制也；君二臣三，奇之制也；君二臣六：偶之制也。故曰：近者奇之，远者偶之，汗者不以奇，下者不以偶，补上治上制以缓，补下治下制以急，急则气味厚，缓则气味薄，适其至所，此之谓也。病所远而中道气味之者，食而过之，无越其制度也。是故平气之道，近而奇偶，制小其服也。远而奇偶，制大其服也。大则数少，小则数多。多则九之，少则二之。奇之不去则偶之，是谓重方。偶之不去，则反佐以取之，所谓寒热温凉，反从其病也。

Yellow Emperor said: "Since the energies are different in quantities, the diseases are different in prosperity and decline, some of the treatings should be urgent and some can be treated slowly, and the prescriptions are different in large and small, I hope you can tell me the standard in distinguishing them." Qibo said: "As the evil energies are different in upper and lower locations, the focuses are different in distances, and the appearances of syndrome are different in the interior and the exterior, thus, the treating can be heavy or light according to the specific condition which takes the medicine's effect reaching the focuses as the criterion. It was stated in the《Essentials》: 'When applying one monarch medical herb and two courtier medical herbs, it is the method of making an odd prescription; when applying two monarch medical herbs and four courtier medical herbs, it is the method of making an even prescription; when applying two monarch medical herbs and three courtier medical herbs, it is the method of making an odd prescription; when applying two monarch medical herbs and six courtier medical herbs, it is the method of making an even prescription.'

"When the focus is high, use the odd prescription, when the focus is far, use the even prescription; in diaphoresis, the even prescription must not be used, in purgation, the odd prescription must not be used; when invigorating, the prescription for treating the upper part of the body should be slow, and the prescription for invigorating the lower part should be urgent; most medicine in urgent property are having a heavy taste and most of the medicines with moderate property are having a flat taste. But in any case, the prescription should reach precisely to the focus of the disease. If the focus is remote, the taste of the medicine may become lacking by halfway, so, taking the medicine after or before the meal should be taken into consideration. In any case, the medical effect must reach the focus and this rule must not be violated.

"When adjusting the energy to become moderate, if the focus is high, no matter using the odd or even prescription, it should be small, if the focus is remote, no matter using the odd or even prescription, it should be large. A large prescription means a few medical herbs in a large quantity, a small prescription means many medical herbs in a small quantity. When the kinds of medical herbs are many, it may be nine of them, when the kinds of medical herbs are few, it may be only two of them.

"When after applying the odd prescription and the disease is still remaining, apply the even prescription, and it is called the complex prescription; when applying the even prescription and the disease is still remaiming, apply the method of adverse assisting (the agreeable treating), such as when treating the cold disease with hot medicine, add cold medicine which

is agreeable with the cold disease as the assisting medicine; when treating the hot disease with cold medicine, add hot medicine which is agreeable to the hot disease as the assisting medicine, when treat the cool and warm diseases, add warm and cold medicines as the assisting medicines."

帝曰：善。病生于本，余知之矣。生于标者，治之奈何？岐伯曰：病反其本，得标之病，治反其本，得标之方。

Yellow Emperor said: "Good. I have known the disease stemming from the root energies (the six energies of wind, heat, wetness, fire, dryness and cold), but how to treat the diseases stemming from the branch energies (the energies of three Yins and three Yangs)?" Qibo said: "When the syndromes are contrary to the root, it can be ascertained to be the disease from the branch. When treating, distinguish what is urgent and what is not, if the branch disease is urgent, then the branch should be followed and the branch disease should be treated first."

帝曰：善。六气之胜，何以候之？岐伯曰：乘其至也。清气大来，燥之胜也，风木受邪，肝病生焉。热气大来，火之胜也，金燥受邪、肺病生焉。寒气大来，水之胜也，火热受邪，心病生焉。湿气大来，土之胜也，寒水受邪，肾病生焉。风气大来，木之胜也，土湿受邪，脾病生焉。所谓感邪而生病也。乘年之虚，则邪甚也。失时之和，亦邪甚也。遇月之空，亦邪甚也。重感于邪，则病危矣。有胜之气，其必来复也。

Yellow Emperor said: "Good. What is the symptom when the six-energy is overabundant?" Qibo said: "It can be known when the six-energy arrives. When the cool energy comes in large scale, the dryness energy will be partial overabundant to injure the wind wood energy, and the liver disease will occur. When the heat energy comes in large scale, the fire energy will be partial overabundant to injure the metal energy, and the lung disease will occur. when the cold energy comes in large amount, the water energy will be partial overabundant to injure the fire, and the heart disease will occure, when the wetness energy comes in large scale, the earth energy will be partial overabundant to injure the cold water, and the kidney disease will occur, when the wind energy comes in a large scale, the wood energy will be partial overabundant to injure the earth wetness energy, and the spleen disease will occur. These diseases are affected by the evil energies. In the case of when the dominating energy of the year (host energy) is insufficient, when it is disharmonious with the guest energy, and when the moon is vacant (before the first quarter, and after the last quarter of the month when the energy and blood of human body is deficient), the evil energy will be even more severe. If the evil energy is contracted during the above three cases, the disease will be a dangerous one. Whenever the overcoming energy appears, the retaliating energy will certainly come in the wake of it."

帝曰：其脉何如？岐伯曰：厥阴之至其脉弦，少阴之至其脉钩，太阴之至其脉沉，少阳之至大而浮，阳明之至短而濇，太阳之至大而长。至而和则平，至而甚则病，至而反者病，至而不至者病，未至而至者病，阴阳易者危。

Yellow Emperor asked: "What are the pulse conditions when the six-energy arrives?"

Qibo said: "On the arrival of Jueyin energy, the pulse condition is wiry, on the arrival of Shaoyin energy, the pulse condition is hooked. On the arrival of Taiyin energy, the pulse condition is sunken, on the arrival of Shaoyang energy, the pulse condition is gigantic and floating, on the arrival of Yangming energy, the pulse condition is short and choppy, on the arrival of Taiyang energy, the pulse condition is gigantic and long. When the pulse condition is calm on the arrival, the man is normal. When the pulse is exceedingly prosperous on the arrival, it shows there is disease, when the pulse condition is on the contrary to the energy of the four-season it shows there is disease. When the pulse fails to arrive when the energy arrives, it shows there is disease, when the energy fails to arrive when the pulse has arrived already, it shows there is disease. When Yin pulse is seen in the Yang disease or Yang pulse is seen in the Yin disease, the patient will be in danger."

帝曰：六气标本，所从不同奈何？岐伯曰：气有从本者，有从标本者，有不从标本者也。帝曰：愿卒闻之。岐伯曰：少阳太阴从本，少阴太阳从本从标，阳明厥阴，不从标本从乎中也。故从本者，化生于本，从标本者有标本之化，从中者以中气为化也。帝曰：脉从而病反者，其诊何如？岐伯曰：脉至而从，按之不鼓，诸阳皆然。帝曰：诸阴之反，其脉何如？岐伯曰：脉至而从，按之鼓甚而盛也。

Yellow Emperor asked: "The changes of the six energies are different in folowing the root or following the branch, and what is the reason?" Qibo said: "In the changes of the six energies, some are following the root and some are following the branch, some do not change with the root nor with the branch. Yellow Emperor said: "I hope to know it thoroughly". Qibo said: "The changes of Shaoyang and Taiyin follow the root (in Shaoyang, fire is the root and Yang is the branch; in Taiyin, wetness is the root and Yin is the branch. Both Shaoyang and Taiyin are having the similar property in roots and branches, so, the diseases caused by both the two channels are changing with the root); the changes of Shaoyin and Taiyang follow the root and the branch (in Shaoyin, heat is the root and Yin is the branch, and the intermediate energy is the cold energy of Taiyang, in Taiyang, cold is the root, Yang is the branch, the intermediate energy is the heat energy or Shaoyin. Both Shaoyin and Taiyang are different in root and branch, and the root of one being the intermediate energy of the other, besides, they are different in water and fire, and different in Yin and Yang, the root and branch can not be assimilated, thus, in changing, they follow either the root or the branch); the changes of Yangming and Jueyin do not folow the root or the branch, but follow the intermediate energy (in Yangming, dryness is the root and Yang is the branch and the intermediate energy is the wetness earth of Taiyin, in Jueyin, wood is the root and Yin is the branch, the intermediate energy is prime minister-fire of Shaoyang. The dryness energy assimilates with the wetness energy, and the wood energy assimilates with the fire energy, thus, both Yangming and Jueyin do not follow the root nor the branch, but follow the intermediate energy). When the change follows the root, it is because the evil energy is stemmed from the root; when the change follows the root or the branch, it is because some of the diseases are stemmed from the root and some are stemmed from the branch. When the change

follows the intermediate energy, it is because the disease is stemmed from the intermediate energy."

Yellow Emperor asked: "How to diagnose the disease when the pulse condition following the root or branch but is contrary to the disease?" Qibo said: "When the pulse condition is similar with the disease, such as when the gigantic, floating and slippery pulse conditions are seen in Yang disease they are the agreeable pulses, but if the pulsation is so weak that it can hardly be felt when pressing, then, it is not a genuine Yang disease and the condition of all the Yang pulses in Yang syndromes are the same." Yellow Emperor asked: "What about the pulse condition when it is contrary to the Yin disease?" Qibo said: "When the pulse condition is similar with the syndrome, but the pulsation under the finger is very strong when pressing, then, it is not a genuine Yin disease.

是故百病之起，有生于本者，有生于标者，有生于中气者，有取本而得者，有取标而得者，有取中气而得者，有取标本而得者，有逆取而得者，有从取而得者。逆，正顺也；若顺，逆也。故曰：知标与本，用之不殆，明知逆顺，正行无问。此之谓也。不知是者，不足以言诊，足以乱经。故《大要》曰：粗工嘻嘻，以为可知，言热未已，寒病复始，同气异形，迷诊乱经。此之谓也。夫标本之道，要而博，小而大，可以言一而知百病之害，言标与本，易而勿损，察本与标，气可令调，明知胜复，为万民式，天之道毕矣。

"Therefore, in the starting of the various diseases, some of them stem from the root energy, some stem from the branch energy, and some of them from the intermediate energy. Some of the diseases are cured by treating the root energy, some are cured by treating the branch energy, some are cured by treating the intermediate energy, some are cured by treating both the root energy and the branch energy, some are cured by treating reversely and some are cured by treating agreeably. The so called adverse treating means to treat against the condition of the disease, and in fact, it is the positive treating; in the so called agreeable treating, it seems to be agreeable superficially, but in fact, it is a negative treating. When one knows the reasons of the root and branch, there will be no danger in treating, when one understands the principles of agreeable and adverse treating, he can treat properly without flaws; when one knows not the principles, he can by no means diagnose, and can only disturb the channel energies. It was stated in the《Essentials》'A physician of lower level thinks he has known all things complacently, but when he comes in contact with the treating, before his argument about the fever ends, the phenomena of cold begin to manifest. He does not understand the diseases from the same energy may be different, he can hardly make a clear diagnosis due to the perplexity in mind, and thus, he can only disturb the channel energy.'

"The principle of root and branch is concise but can be applied extensively, and all the changes of the diseases can be understood through a single example. When one understands the principles of root and branch, his treating can hardly cause injury, when determining whether the disease belongs to the root or branch by observing, he can adjust the evil energy to become calm. When one understands clearly the principle of the overcoming and the retaliating energies of the six energies, he can set an example to common physicians and he can al-

so understand thoroughly the change of heaven and earth."

帝曰：胜复之变，早晏何如？岐伯曰：夫所胜者，胜至已病，病已愠愠，而复已萌也。夫所复者，胜尽而起，得位而甚，胜有微甚，复有少多，胜和而和，胜虚而虚，天之常也。帝曰：胜复之作，动不当位，或后时而至，其故何也？岐伯曰：夫气之生，与其化衰盛异也。寒暑温凉盛衰之用，其在四维。故阳之动，始于温，盛于暑；阴之动，始于清，盛于寒。春夏秋冬，各差其分。故《大要》曰：彼春之暖，为夏之暑，彼秋之忿，为冬之怒，谨按四维，斥候皆归，其终可见，其始可知，此之谓也。帝曰：差有数乎？岐伯曰：又凡三十度也。帝曰：其脉应皆何如？岐伯曰：差同正法，待时而去也。《脉要》曰：春不沉，夏不弦，冬不濇，秋不数，是谓四塞。沉甚曰病，弦甚曰病，濇甚曰病，数甚曰病，参见曰病，复见曰病，未去而去曰病，去而不去曰病，反者死。故曰：气之相守司也，如权衡之不得相失也。夫阴阳之气，清静则生化治，动则苛疾起，此之谓也。

Yellow Emperor asked: "Sometimes, the change of the overcoming energy or the retaliating energy is early, sometimes, it is late, and what is the reason?" Qibo said: "When the overcoming energy arrives, the patient would have contracted disease already. When the evll energy is accumulating, the retaliating energy would have germinated already. The retaliating energy takes the opportunity to rise when the overcoming energy is coming to the end. When the retaliating energy gets into its position, it will become intensified. In the overcoming energies, there are differences in heavy and light extents, in the retaliating energies, there are the differences in the large and small quantities. When the overcoming energy is moderate, the retaliating energy will be moderate also, when the overcoming energy is deficient, the retaliating energy will be deficient also, and this is the common rule of the change in the heaven energy."

Yellow Emperor asked: "In the breaking out of the overcoming energy or the retaliating energy, sometimes it is not on its seasonal position exactly, and is sometimes lagging behind, and what is the reason?" Qibo said: "This is because of the changes of the six-energy have the different conditions of being deficient and overabundant. The effects of the coldness, hotness, coolness and warmness, prosperily and deficiency are displayed in the last month of each season. So, when the Yang energy starts up, it begins with warmness and becomes extremely prosperous in summer heat; when the Yin energy starts up, it begins with coolness and becomes extremely prosperous in winter cold, and the weathers of spring, summer, autumn and winter are all different. It was stated in the《Essentials》: 'The warmness of spring developes into the heat of summer, the coolness of autumn developes into the cold of winter'. When one observes the change of the last month in every season and scouts the returning back of the weather, he can see the terminal of the energy and know the beginning of the energy."

Yellow Emperor asked: "In the weather changes of the four seasons, is there any difference in days?" Qibo said: "The difference is about thirty and odds days."

Yellow Emperor asked: "What is the correspondding condition in the pulse?" Qibo said: "The pulse with time difference is similar with that of the normal condition, only, when

judging, the time difference must be deducted. It was stated in the《Pulse Essentials》: 'When the pulse condition in spring is not sunken in the least, when the pulse condition in autumn is not rapid in the least, when the pulse condition in summer is not wiry in the least, when the pulse condition in winter is not choppy in the least, they are called the obstruction of the seasonal energy. When it is excessively sunken, it is the sick pulse, when it is excessively wiry, it is the sick pulse, when it is excessively rapid, it is the sick pulse, when it is excessively choppy, it is the sick pulse, when the pulse is disorderly and uneven, it is the sick pulse, when the energy has gone and the pulse reappears, it is the sick pulse. When the energy is still remaining and the pulse has gone already, it is the sick pulse, when the energy has gone but the pulse is still remaining, it is the sick pulse, when the pulse condition is contrary to the energy, it is the fatal pulse'. Therefore, the energies of the four seasons are mutually related, each keeps to its own position and each has its own duty, like the sliding weight and the steelyard, not one of them can be excluded. When the energies of Yin and Yang are quiet, they produce calmness to cause the generation and transformation, when they are changing, they will cause disease."

帝曰：幽明何如？岐伯曰：两阴交尽故曰幽，两阳相合故曰明，幽明之配，寒暑之异也。帝曰：分至何如？岐伯曰：气至之谓至，气分之谓分，至则气同，分则气异，所谓天地之正纪也。

Yellow Emperor asked: "What is the meaning of 'Gloomy and Bright?' Qibo said: "When the energies of the two Yins are diminished, it is called 'Gloomy', when the energies of the two Yangs combine together, it is called 'Bright', and the coordination of gloomy and bright causes the difference of the cold and hot weather." Yellow Emperor asked: "What is the equinox and the solstice?" Qibo said: "When the energy arrives, it is solstice, when the energy divides, it is equinox. In solstice, the energies are the same, in equinox, the energies are different, and this is the common law of heaven and earth."

帝曰：夫子言春秋气始于前，冬夏气始于后，余已知之矣。然六气往复，主岁不常也，其补写奈何？岐伯曰：上下所主，随其攸利，正其味，则其要也，左右同法。《大要》曰：少阳之主，先甘后咸；阳明之主，先辛后酸；太阳之主，先咸后苦；厥阴之主；先酸后辛；少阴之主，先甘后咸；太阴之主，先苦后甘。佐以所利，资以所生，是谓得气。

Yellow Emperor said: "I have known what you said that the energies of spring and autumn start formerly, and the energies of summer and winter start later, but since the six-energy is moving reciprocally and the dominating energy of the year is changing constantly, how to apply the therapies of invigorating and purging?" Qibo said: "In treating the disease caused by the energy that controls the heaven energy and the energy that affects the earth energy, since the energies are controlled from above and below respectively, the applying of invigorating or purging therapy should be based on the benefitial for curing the disease, and the main point is the applying the medicine of proper taste. To the disease caused by the left and right intermediate energies, the treatment should be the same. It was stated in the《Essentials》: 'When Shaoyang is dominating the year, apply the medicine of sweet taste first,

and then, apply the medicine of salty taste; when Yangming is dominating the year, apply the medicine of acrid taste first, and then apply the medicine of sour taste; when Taiyang is dominating the year, apply the salty taste first and then the medicine of bitter taste; when Jueyin is dominating the year, apply the medicine of sour taste first and then apply the medicine of acrid taste; when Shaoyin is dominating the year, apply the medicine of sweet taste first and then apply the medicine of salty taste; when Taiyin is dominating the year, apply the medicine of bitter taste first and then apply the medicine of sweet taste. Besides, one should assist with the favourable medicine to help the mechanism of generation and transformation. In this way, the tastes can be in conformity with the six-energy.'"

帝曰：善。夫百病之生也，皆生于风寒暑湿燥火，以之化之变也。经言盛者写之，虚者补之，余锡以方士，而方士用之，尚未能十全，余欲令要道必行，桴鼓相应，犹拔刺雪汙，工巧神圣，可得闻乎？岐伯曰：审察病机，无失气宜，此之谓也。帝曰：愿闻病机何如？岐伯曰：诸风掉眩，皆属于肝。诸寒收引，皆属于肾。诸气膹郁，皆属于肺。诸湿肿满，皆属于脾。诸热瞀瘛，皆属于火。诸痛痒疮，皆属于心。诸厥固泄，皆属于下。诸痿喘呕，皆属于上。诸禁鼓慄，如丧神守，皆属于火。诸痉项强，皆属于湿。诸逆冲上，皆属于火。诸胀腹大，皆属于热。诸躁狂越，皆属于火。诸暴强直，皆属于风。诸病有声鼓之如鼓，皆属于热。诸病胕肿疼酸惊骇，皆属于火。诸转反戾，水液浑浊，皆属于热。诸病水液，澄澈清冷，皆属于寒。诸呕吐酸，暴注下迫，皆属于热。故《大要》曰：谨守病机，各司其属，有者求之，无者求之，盛者责之，虚者责之，必先五胜，疏其血气，令其调达，而致和平，此之谓也。

Yellow Emperor said: "Good. Most of the diseases are stemmed from the healthy and evil changes of the six-energy of wind, cold, heat, wetness, dryness and fire. It was stated in the medical books that it should be purged when the energy is overabundant, and should be invigorated when the energy is deficient. I have instructed the physicians with these methods but they can not obtain a satisfactory result. I would like to have the important theory be put into use and obtain a relating effect like the drumstick relating to the hitting of the drum, produce an immediate effect like pulling off the thorn and clear away the foul, and cause the common physicians to attain a higher level of treating. Can you tell me how to do it?" Qibo said: "When one observes carefully the mechanism of the disease and treat without violating the principle of the harmonization of the six-energy, the aim can be achieved."

Yellow Emperor said: "I hope to hear about the mechanism of disease you said." Qibo said: "All the syndromes of trembling and dizziness caused by the wind evil are pertaining to the liver; all syndromes of muscular stiffness caused by the cold evil are pertaining to the kidney; all the feelings of irritability and oppression caused by the disease of vital energy are pertaining to the lung; all the syndromes of edema and fullness caused by the wetness evil are pertaining to the spleen, all the blur sighted of eyes and convulsion of extremities caused by the heat evil are pertaining to the fire; all the syndromes of pain, itching, pyogenic infection and ulceration of skin are pertaining to the heart; all the syndromes of cold extremeties, retention or incontinence of feces and urine are pertaining to the lower warmer; all the syndromes of rapid breathing, hiccup and vomiting are pertaining to the upper warmer; all the

syndromes of trismus, shivering with cold, percussion of the teeth are pertaining to the fire; all the syndromes of convulsive disease and stiffness of neck are pertaining to wetness, all the syndromes of adverseness of vital energy are pertaining to the fire; all the syndromes of abdominal distention and fullness are pertaining to the heat; all the syndromes of irritability, uneasiness, mania and acting rashly are pertaining to the fire; all syndromes of sudden muscular stiffness are pertaining to the wind evil; all the diseases with sound , such as borborgmus and the sound like drum beating in percussion are pertaining to heat; all the diseases of edema, aching pain, frightening, uneasiness are pertaining to the fire; all the syndromes of cramp, muscular stiffness, turbidness of the excreted fluid are pertaining to the heat; in all the cases of excreting clear and cold fluid are pertaining to the cold; all the syndromes of acid eructation, sudden diarrhea with urgent sensation are pertaining to the heat. Thus, it was stated in the《Essentials》: 'Pay good attention to the mechanism of the diseases and know well the belongings of various syndromes, investigate the reason of the disease and the related syndromes, and the reason or the disease which is without the expected syndromes, find out the reason when the evil energy is overabundant and the reason when the energy is deficient. Find out the overcoming energy of the five-element motion. Dredge the energy and blood to become calm and circulate fluently according to the mechanism of the disease'".

帝曰：善。五味阴阳之用何如？岐伯曰：辛甘发散为阳，酸苦涌泄为阴，咸味涌泄为阴，淡味渗泄为阳，六者或收或散，或缓或急，或燥或润，或软或坚，以所利而行之，调其气使其平也。帝曰：非调气而得者，治之奈何？有毒无毒，何先何后？愿闻其道。岐伯曰：有毒无毒，所治为主，适大小为制也。

Yellow Emperor said: "Good. What are the functions of the five tastes of the medicine and their belongings to Yin and Yang?" Qibo siad: "The medicine of acrid and sweet tastes are for dispersing, they belong to Yang; the sour and bitter tastes are used in emetic and purgating therapies, they belong to Yin; the medicine of salty taste is also used in emetic and purgating therapy, they belong to Yin; the medicine of flat taste is for sweating and purgating, it also belongs to Yang. Among the six kinds of medicine, their functions are different in colleting, dispersing, moderating, urging, drying, moistening, softening and enforcing. When in treating, apply the medicine according to its specific funciton, so as the energy can be adjusted and become calm."

Yellow Emperor asked: "Some of the diseases can not be cured by adjusting the energy, and how to treat it? Which of the medicines are toxicant and which are not? Which should be used first and what is the reason?" Qibo said: "In applying the medicine with toxicity or without toxicity, it should be applied according to the case of which one is effective to the disease. The dosage should be determined according to the condition of the disease."

帝曰：请言其制。岐伯曰：君一臣二，制之小也；君一臣三佐五，制之中也；君一臣三佐九，制之大也。寒者热之，热者寒之，微者逆之，甚者从之，坚者削之，客者除之，劳者温之〔胡本，读本，吴本“温”并作“益”〕，结者散之，留者攻之，燥者濡之，急者缓之，散

者收之，损者温之，逸者行之，惊者平之。上之下之，摩之浴之，薄之劫之，开之发之，适事为故。帝曰：何谓逆从？岐伯曰：逆者正治，从者反治，从少从多，观其事也。帝曰：反治何谓？岐伯曰：热因寒用，寒因热用，塞因塞用，通因通用，必伏其所主，而先其所因，其始则同，其终则异，可使破积，可使溃坚，可使气和，可使必已。帝曰：善。气调而得者何如？岐伯曰：逆之从之，逆而从之，从而逆之，疏气令调，则其道也。

Yellow Emperor said: "Please tell me the institution of the prescription." Qibo said: "When using one monarch medical herb and two courtier medical herbs, it is the formation of a small prescription; when using one monarch medical herb, three courtier medical herbs and five assistant medical herbs, it is the formation of a medium prescription; when using one monarch medical herb, three courtier medical herbs and nine assistant medical herbs, it is a formation of a large prescription.

"In treating the cold disease, apply the medicine of hot nature, in treating the hot disease, apply the medicine of cold nature. When the disease is light, apply the medicine which is against the condition of the disease, when the disease is severe, apply the medicine which is agreeable to the condition of the disease. To the evil energy which is firm and substantial, weaken it; to the evil energy that retains in the body, dispel it; to the disease caused by fatigue, nourish the healthy energy by the medicine of warm nature, to the disease caused by the stagnation of energy and blood, disperse it; to the disease caused by the retention of evil energy, attack and dispel it; to the disease of dryness, moisten it; to the disease which is acute, remit it, to the disease caused by the exhaustion of energy and blood, collect it; to the consumptive disease, invigorate it; to the disease caused by the stagnation due to easy life, dredge it; to the disease of terror, calm it; when the primordial energy is bogging down, lift it up; when the evil energy is reversing up, depress it down. Apply massage, bathe, driving away the evil energy, stopping the out-burst of the evil energy, purgating or dispersing therapies to fit the condition of the disease."

Yellow Emperor asked: "What is the meaning of adverse treating and agreeable treating? Qibo said: "To treat reversely is actually the positive treating, such as treat the cold disease with hot medicine or treat the hot disease with cold medicine, it is the case of treating against the diseases condition and it is the positive treating. To follow agreeably in treating is actually the adverse treating, such as treat the cold disease with hot medicine and assist with cold medicine or treat the hot disease with cold medicine and assist with hot medicine, it is the case of assisting with the medicine which follows the condition of the disease, and it is the adverse treating. As to the quantity of the medicine for positive treating, it should be determined by the condition of the disease."

Yellow Emperor asked: "What is the condition of the adverse treating?" Qibo said: "When treating the real cold inside and the pseudo heat outside, when treating the real heat inside and the pseudo cold outside, when using the invigorating medicine to hinder the pseudo syndrome, and when using the medicine of promoting circulation to treat the disease of circulation, the adverse treating can be used, so as to subdue the main disease. One must find

out the reason of the disease first, then, the disease may be subdued. In the adverse treating, the cold and hot nature of the medicine seems to be similar with that of the disease, but the curative effect is entirely different, such as, treat with hot medicine and assist differently, such as, treat with hot medicine and assist with cold medicine in cold disease, the curative effect is mainly from the hot medicine. It is only in this way, the protracted disease can be broken through, the substantiality of the disease can be dissipated, the energy and blood can be adjusted and the patient can be recovered."

Yellow Emperor said: "Good. Some diseases are contracted when the six energies are harmonious, and how to treat them?" Qibo said:" One can apply the adverse treating or the agreeable treating, one can apply the main medicine for adverse treating and assistant medicine for the agreeable treating, or apply the main medicine for the agreeable treating and the assistant medicine for adverse treating to dredge the functional activities of vital energy to become harmonious, and this is the proper way of treating."

帝曰：善。病之中外何如？岐伯者：从内之外者，调其内；从外之内者，治其外；从内之外而盛于外者，先调其内而后治其外；从外之内而盛于内者，先治其外而后调其内，中外不相及，则治主病。

Yellow Emperor asked: "Some internal diseases and external diseases are affecting each other, how to treat them?" Qibo said: "When the disease is produced inside and then developed outside, treat the interior first; when the disease is produced from outside and then developes into inside, treat the exterior first; when the disease is produced inside, then affects the outside and the disease is emphasizing on the exterior, treat the internal part first and then the external part; when the disease is produced outside and then affects inside and the disease is emphasizing on the interior, treat the external part first and then the internal part; when the internal disease and the external disease have no relation with each other, it should be treated according to the main syndrome."

帝曰：善。火热复，恶寒发热，有如疟状，或一日发，或间数日发，其故何也？岐伯曰：胜复之气，会遇之时，有多少也。阴气多而阳气少，则其发日远；阳气多而阴气少，则其发日近。此胜复相薄，盛衰之节，疟亦同法。

Yellow Emperor said: "Good. When the fire heat energy is retaliating, it causes people to have chilliness and fever like in malaria, sometimes it bursts out every day, sometimes it bursts out after an interval of several days, and why is it?" Qibo said: "This is because the overcoming energy and the retaliating energy are sometimes plenty and sometimes few. When the Yin energy is plenty and the Yang energy is few, the interval of the bursting will be long; when the Yang energy is plenty and the Yin energy is few, the interval of the bursting will be short. This is the condition of the mutual combat of the overcoming and retaliating energies, and the mutual regulation of abundance and deficency. In malaria, the condition is the same."

帝曰：论言治寒以热，治热以寒，而方士不能废绳墨而更其道也。有病热者寒之而热，有病寒者热之而寒，二者皆在，新病复起，奈何治？岐伯曰：诸寒之而热者取之阴，热之而寒

者取之阳，所谓求其属也。帝曰：善。服寒而反热，服热而反寒，其故何也？岐伯曰：治其王气，是以反也。帝曰：不治王而然者何也？岐伯曰：悉乎哉问也！不治五味〔胡本，吴本"五味"并作"王味"《素问校讹》引古抄本作"王气"〕属也。夫五味入胃，各归所喜，故酸先入肝，苦先入心，甘先入脾，辛先入肺，咸先入肾，久而增气，物化之常也。气增而久，夭之由也。

Yellow Emperor said: "It was stated in the treatise that one should treat the cold disease with the hot medicine, treat the hot disease with the cold medicine and a physician must not annul this rule to treat in some other ways. But sometimes, the hot disease becomes even more hot after adminitstering the cold medicine, and the cold disease becomes even more cold after administering the hot medicine, not only the cold disease or hot disease is still remaining, but some new diseases are induced, how to treat it?" Qibo said: "When the disease becomes even hotter after administering the cold medicine, the Yin should be nourished; when the disease becomes even colder after administering the hot medicine, the Yang should be invigorated, and this is the way of seeking the energy of the same kind."

Yellow Emperor said: "Good. What is the reason of the disease becoming hot after administering the cold medicine and becoming cold after administering the hot medicine?" Qibo said: "When the hyperactive energy is treated solely, the result will be on the contrary."

Yellow Emperor asked: "Sometimes the condition occurs when the hyperactive energy is not treated, and what is the reason?" Qibo said: "What an exhausted question you have asked. It is the kind of neglecting to treat the addiction to a certain taste. When the five-taste enters into the stomach, it goes first to the viscus which it delights: the sour taste enters into the liver first, the bitter taste enters into the heart first, the sweet taste enters into the spleen first, the acrid taste enters into the lung first, and the salty taste enters into the kidney first. When the accumulation is protracted, the energy of the due viscus will be promoted. It is the common rule of the activity of the energies of the five tastes after the taste entering into the stomach, and it is the reason when the protracted disease of the visceral energy to become overabundant and finally comes to the contrary."

帝曰：善。方制君臣何谓也？岐伯曰：主病之谓君，佐君之谓臣，应臣之谓使，非上下三品之谓也。帝曰：三品何谓？岐伯曰：所以明善恶之殊贯也。

Yellow Emperor said: "Good. In the medical prescriptions, there are the differences of the monarch medical herb and the courtier medical herb, what is the reason?" Qibo said: "The main medical herb for treating the disease is the monarch herb, the assistant medicine for helping the monarch medicine is the courtier herb, and the medicine for supporting the courtier medicine is the envoy herb. They do not mean the three grades of upper, medium and lower ones."

Yellow Emperor asked: "What is the meaning of the three grades?" Qibo said: "The term of three grades is for showing whether the medicine is toxic or not."

帝曰：善。病之中外何如？岐伯曰：调气之方，必别阴阳，定其中外，各守其乡，内者内治，外者外治，微者调之，其次平之，盛者夺之，汗者下之，寒热温凉，衰之以属，随其

攸利，谨道如法，万举万全，气血正平，长有天命。帝曰："善。"

Yellow Emperor said: "Good. How to treat the interior disease and the exterior disease?" Qibo said: "When treat by adjusting the energies, it must distinguish the Yin and Yang and ascertain whether it belongs to the interior or the exterior first. Treat according to the location of the focus of the disease. When it is inside, treat internally, when it is ontside, treat externally. When the disease is light, adjust it, when the disease is severe, moderate it, and when it is abundant, attack and consume it. Apply the diaphoresis or purgative therapies according to the cold, hot, warm or cool property of the evil energy asnd dissipate it according to the categorical property of the evil energy. When one observes the rules above carefully, the treating will be absolutely satisfactory, the energy and blood can be calmed down and the patient may live long." Yellow Emperor said: "Good."

著至教论篇第七十五

Chapter 75
Zhu Zhi Jiao Lun
(The Supreme Principle Which Relates to Heaven, Earth and Man)

黄帝坐明堂，召雷公而问之曰：子知医之道乎？雷公对曰：诵而颇〔《太平御览》卷七百二十一《方术部》引“颇”作“未”〕能解，解而未能别，别而未能明，明而未能彰，足以治群僚，不足至〔吴本“至”作“治”〕侯王，愿得受树天之度，四时阴阳合之，别星辰与日月光，以彰经术，后世益明，上通神农，著至教，疑于二皇。帝曰：善！无失之，此皆阴阳表里上下雌雄相输应也，而道上知天文，下知地理、中知人事，可以长久，以教众庶，亦不疑殆，医道论篇，可传后世，可以为宝。

When Yellow Emperor sat in the Bright Hall, he summoned Lei Gong and asked: "Do you understand the principle of medicine?" Lei Gong said: "I have read the medical books, but I can hardly explain it; even though I can explain it, I can hardly analyse it clearly; even though I can analyse it, I do not understand the reasons of it; even though I can understand the reasons of it, I can hardly practise it in clinic. Therefore, with my knowledge of medicine, I can only treat the diseases of my colleagues, and I am not capable to treat the diseases of the kings and the nobles. I hope you can tell me the way of surveying the heavens degree, enable me to comprehend fully the mysteries of the four seasons, Yin and Yang, stars, sun and moon, and integrating them with the medical theory and practice which may be promoted and become ever so obvious in the later generations. In this way, the most brilliant skill of medicine which is inherited from the remote medical master Shen Nọng, and can reach the medical level of the two kings (Baoxi and Nuiwo)."

Yellow Emperor aid: "Good." These principles must not be lost. They are the inter-relations and mutual responses between the Yin and Yang, superficies and interior, ups and downs, male and female. The medical theory and skill can only last long when the astronomy above, the geography below and the human affairs in the middle are known, and it is only under this condition can the medical instructions be taught to people without perplexion. It will be really valuable to write down the theories of medicine in books and pass them to the later generations."

雷公曰：请受道，讽诵用解。帝曰：子不闻《阴阳传》乎！曰：不知。曰：夫三阳天为业，上下无常，合而病至，偏害阴阳。雷公曰：三阳莫当，请闻其解。帝曰：三阳独至者，是三阳并至，并至如风雨，上为巅疾，下为漏病，外无期，内无正，不中经纪，诊无上下，以书别。雷公曰：臣治疏愈，说意而已。帝曰：三阳者，至阳也，积并则为惊，病起疾风，至

如礔砺，九窍皆塞，阳气滂溢，干嗌喉塞，并于阴，则上下无常，薄为肠澼，此谓三阳直心，坐不得起，卧者便身全〔林校引《甲乙经》“便身全”作“身重”〕。三阳之病，且以知天下，何以别阴阳，应四时，合之五行。

Lei Gong said: "Please impart the medical theory to me, and I will read it aloud until I can comprehend, it." Yellow Emperor asked: "Have you ever heard of the book《Yin Yang Zhuan》?" Lei Gong said: "No." Yellow Emperor said: "When the three Yang energies do not follow the common law and move up and down, they will combine to cause the partial over-abundance of Yin or Yang to form disease."

Lei Gong asked: "When the energies of the three Yangs arrive simultaneously, they can hardly be stopped, and why is it?" Yellow Emperor said: "In the simultaneous arrival of the three Yang energies, it is swift like the storm, when it invades the upper part of the body, it will cause disorder of the head, when it invades the lower part of the body, it will cause the incontinence of feces and urine. The disease contracted has no evident symptom outside, and has no definite criterion for distinguishing inside. As the infection does not follow the common law, it can hardly be determined whether the disease is pertaining to the upper part or to the lower part."

Lei Gong said: "When I treat this kind of disease, only a few of them can be cured, please tell me the reason and remove my perplexion." Yellow Emperor said: "When the energies of the three Yangs arrive simultaneously, it is the condition of the utmost abundance of Yang, and the accumulation of Yang causes frightening. The onset of the disease is swift like wind, and it is vigorous like the thunderbolt which can even shut the nine orifices. As the Yang energy is overflowing outside, it causes dry larynx and the obstruction of the throat. If the energies of the three Yangs combine with Yin, the Yin energy will be stirred and the upper and the lower part of the body will become disorderly, if the evil retains in the lower warmer, the intestinal bi-syndrome (syndrome due to the dysfunction of the large or small intestine) will occur. As the evil energy of the three Yangs accumulates to effect the channels, the patient will not be able to stand up after sitting, and the body will feel heavy when lying down. Although the diseases stated above are pertaining to the three Yangs, yet, through them, one can understand further the relation between heaven and man, the ways of distinguishing Yin and Yang to suit the four seasons and to coordinate with the five elements."

雷公曰：阳言不别，阴言不理，请起受解，以为至道。帝曰：子若受传，不知合至道以惑师教，语子至道之要，病伤五藏，筋骨以消，子言不明不别，是世主学尽矣。肾且绝，惋惋日暮，从容不出，人事不殷。

Lei Gong said: "I can not distinguish it even when you speak it plainly, not to say comprehending it when you speak it indistinctly. Let me stand up to hear your explanation, so that I may understand the most profound principle."

Yellow Emperor said: "Although you have received the impartation from your teacher, but you do not know how to integrate it with the supreme principle, so, there are still some-

thing perplexing with your teacher's teaching. Now, let me tell you the essentials about the supreme principle. If the five viscera of man are injured by the evil energy, the muscle and bone will be wasting away day after day. If the principles of medicine are not distinguished nor comprehended as you have said, the supreme principle would have had lost long ago. For instance, if the kidney pulse is severing, the patient will feel oppressive in heart, and become even worse in the evening, the patient will feel slothful in the body, unwilling to go out and reluctant to contact people."

示从容论篇第七十六

Chapter 76
Shi Cong Rong Lun
(Diagnose According to the Established Norm in a Leisured Way)

黄帝燕坐，召雷公而问之曰：汝受术诵书者，若能览观杂学，及于比类，通合道理，为余言子所长，五藏六府，胆胃大小肠脾胞膀胱，脑髓涕唾，哭泣悲哀，水所从行，此皆人之所生，治之过失，子务明之，可以十全，即不能知，为世所怨。雷公曰：臣请诵《脉经·上下篇》甚众多矣，别异比类，犹未能以十全，又安足以明之。

When Yellow Emperor was sitting and resting leisurely, he summoned Lei Gong and said: "You have read many medical books and learned many medical skills, you must have understood the medical principle thoroughly and be able to reason the diseases by analogy. Now tell me your understanding from study. As the five solid organs, the six hollow organs, gallbladder, stomach, the large and small intestine, spleen, uterus, urinary bladder, brain and spinal cord, nasal mucus and saliva, crying, sorrow and the operation of the body fluid are all dispensable to the existence of man, and it is easy to make mistake in treating, you must understand the medical principles in advance, so that the treating may not have a chance of error, and not be blamed by."

Lei Gong said: "I have read a lot of contents in the first and last volumes of the book 《On Channels》, but I still can not reason the disease by analogy, so, in treating, I can not achieve complete curative effect. How can you say that I have understood it thoroughly?"

帝曰：子别试通五藏之过，六府之所不和，针石之败，毒药所宜，汤液滋味，具言其状，悉言以对，请问不知。雷公曰：肝虚肾虚脾虚，皆令人体重烦冤，当投毒药刺灸砭石汤液，或已，或不已，愿闻其解。帝曰：公何年之长而问〔于鬯说"问"当作"闻"〕之少，余真问以自谬也。吾问子窈冥，子言《上下篇》以对，何也？夫脾虚浮似肺，肾小浮似脾，肝急沉散似肾，此皆工之所时乱也。然从容得之。若夫三藏土木水参居，此童子之所知，问之何也？

Yellow Emperor said: "Then you can tell me what you have understood besides the first and last volumes of 《On Channels》, such as the disease pertaining to the affections of the five viscera, the disharmony of the six bowels, the deteriorated case of acupuncture, the proper application of the toxicant, and the tastes of the decoctions. You may relate them in details so that I can explain to you in details. Now, bring up the questions what you do not understand."

Lei Gong said: "All the liver asthenia, kidney asthenia and spleen asthenia cause the heaviness of the body, restlessness, and mental depression. I have treated them with toxi-

cant, acupuncture, stone needle and decoctions, some of the treatments are effective, but some are not, please explain the reason to me."

Yellow Emperor said: "You are advanced in years, but why the medical theory you have heard is so superficial?

"May be I have made an improper question. The question I asked is pertaining to the more profound medical theory, and why do you answer me with the words of asthenia of liver, kidney and spleen in the first and last volumns of 《On Channels》?

"When the condition of the spleen pulse is empty and floating like the lung pulse, when the kidney pulse is weak and floating like the spleen pulse and when the liver pulse is rapid and sunken like the kidney pulse, they are often confused by the common physicians. But if one sets his mind at ease and diagnoses leisurely, he can distinguish them one by one.

"The viscera of spleen, liver and kidney are all under the diaphram, and their positions to each other are quite near, they can be distinguished even by a child, why do you ask me?"

雷公曰：于此有人，头痛，筋挛骨重，怯然少气，哕噫腹满，时惊，不嗜卧，此何藏之发也？脉浮而弦〔《针灸资生经》第六《头痛》引作"其脉举之则弦"〕，切之石坚，不知其解，复问所以三藏者，以知其比类也。帝曰：夫从容之谓之也。夫年长则求之于府，年少则求之于经，年壮则求之于藏，今子所言皆失。八风菀熟，五藏消烁，传邪相受。夫浮而弦者，是肾不足也，沉而石者，是肾气内著也，怯然少气者，是水道不行，形气消索也，咳嗽烦冤者，是肾气之逆也，一人之气，病在一藏也，若言三藏俱行，不在法也。

Lei Gong said: "Here is a patient who has headache, convulsion of muscle and tendon, heaviness of the bone joints, being timid, short of breath, has abdominal distention, being terrified often, reluctant to sleep, to which viscus does this disease belong? His pulse condition is wiry when holding up, and is hard like stone when being pressed, and I do not know the reason. Now I ask again the conditions of the above three viscera, because I want to know the way of analogy."

Yellow Emperor said: "In analogizing, one should diagnose in a leisure way. Generally speaking, to the elder people, as they often are addicted in delicious food, their disease should be seeked from the six bowels; to the young people, as they are often overstrained in physical labor, their diseases should be seeked from the channels; to the people in the prime of life, as they often indulge in sexual life, their diseases should be seeked from the five viscera. Now, you only state the pulses of the three viscera, and neglect to seek its source, so, you are wrong. The accumulated evil from the eight winds can form heat and consume the five viscera. Besides, the variation of the evil energy can be passed to one another in regular order. The floating and wiry pulse condition you have said shows the insuffciency of the kidney energy; the pulse is as hard as stone instead of sunken when being pressed heavily shows the kidney energy is stagnated inside without moving; in this case, the turbid Yin will not descend, the body fluid will not be spread to cause dissipation to the physique and vital energy, and the up-reversing of the kidney energy causes cough and disquietude. Therefore, the disease should be in the kidney. If you hold that the disease is in all the three viscera of liver,

spleen and kidney, it is not tally with the medical classics."

雷公曰：于此有人，四支解堕，喘咳血泄，而愚诊之，以为伤肺，切脉浮大而紧，愚不敢治，粗工下砭石，病愈多出血，血止身轻，此何物也？帝曰：子所能治，知亦众多，与此病失矣。譬以鸿飞，亦冲于天，夫圣人之治病，循法守度，援物比类，化之冥冥，循上及下，何必守经。今夫脉浮大虚者，是脾气之外绝，去胃外归阳明也，夫二火不胜三水，是以脉乱而无常也。四支解堕，此脾精之不行也。喘咳者，是水气并阳明也。血泄者，脉急血无所行也，若夫以为伤肺者，由失以狂也，不引比类，是知不明也。夫伤肺者，脾气不守，胃气不清，经气不为使，真藏坏决，经脉傍绝，五藏漏泄，不衄则呕，此二者不相类也。譬如天之无形，地之无理，白与黑相去远矣。是失，吾过矣。以子知之，故不告子，明引比类、从容，是以名曰诊轻，是谓至道也。

Lei Gong said: "Here is a patient who has slothful and weak extremities, rapid breathing, cough and hematochezia. I diagnosed and thought the disease was caused by the lung injury, but his pulse condition was floating, gigantic and empty, so I dare not treat him. A physician of lower level treated him with stone needle and the bleeding was plenty. But after the bleeding, the patient felt relaxed in the whole body. What is the disease?" Yellow Emperor said: "Although you have known and cured many diseases, yet you are wrong regarding this one. The phycician of a lower level can cure the disease occasionally like the aquatic bird can fly into the sky occasionally.

"The superior physician adheres to the standing orders, reasons the disease by analogy, analyses it through pondering and treating according to the changing situation. When he inspects the upper part of the body, the lower part can also be known, and he may not adhere to the condition of channel rigidly.

"When the pulse condition of the patient is floating, gigantic and empty, it shows the spleen energy is pouring into the stomach, and the body fluid joins the Yang solely.

"When the second fire (stomach) is incapable to control the third water (the third Yin or the spleen), the pulse condition will become disorderly.

"The slothful and weak extremities show the inability of spreading the essence of the spleen, the rapid breathing and cough shows the combination of the water energy to the Yangming channel, the hematochezia shows the shrinking of the channel which obstructs the blood circulation to cause the blood overflowing outside. If you think it is due to the lung injury, it is an error of wantonness. The reason of which you can not reason by analogy is because you do not have a clear comprehension about it.

"If the disease is caused by the lung injury, the spleen energy will not be maintained, the stomach energy will not be clear, the lung energy will be damaged and deteriorated and the refined energy will not be able to be spread by the channels. As the refined energies of the five viscera are leaking, the diseases of hemorrhage or hematemesis will occur.

"There is a large difference between the disease of lung injury, and that of the spleen injury. They are different like the heaven and earth, and like black and white.

"Your failure in diagnosis is also my fault, I thought you have understood it well al-

ready, and I did not remind you the standing orders of the analogy and the diagnosis in a leisure way which are surely the brilliant theory and the quintessence in diagnosis."

疏五过论篇第七十七

Chapter 77
Shu Wu Guo Lun
(The Five Faults in Diagnosis and Treating)

黄帝曰：呜呼远哉！闵闵乎若视深渊，若迎浮云，视深渊尚可测，迎浮云莫知其际，〔于鬯说："际字当依《六微旨大论》作'极'"〕圣人之术，为万民式，论裁志意，必有法则，循经守数，按循医事，为万民副，故事有五过四德〔"四德"二字疑衍，全篇只论"五过"〕，汝知之乎？雷公避席再拜曰：臣年幼小，蒙愚以惑，不闻五过与四德，比类形名，虚引其经，心无所对。

Yellow Emperor said: "Alas. How profound and far-reaching is the medicine. It is like probing an abyss or facing the floating cloud when studying it. One may survey the abyss but can hardly know the ultimate of the floating cloud. The medical technique of the sage is the model of the masses, and when he studied and determined the knowledge of medicine, it was based on a certain standing order. It is only to follow the routine and the standing order, and treat the disease according to the medical principle, can one benefit the patient. Do you know the stipulated five faults in diagnosis and treating?"

Lei Gong stood up, bowed and said: "I am young, dull-witted and muddled, and I have not heard the five faults in diagnosis and treating. I can only analogize according to the appearance and the name of the disease, quote the text from the medical classics vaguely. I can not answer it with my inner heart."

帝曰：凡未诊病者，必问尝贵后贱，虽不中邪，病从内生，名曰脱营；尝富后贫，名曰失精；五气留连，病有所并。医工诊之，不在藏府，不变躯形，诊之而疑，不知病名；身体日减，气虚无精，病深无气，洒洒然时惊，病深者，以其外耗于卫，内夺于荣。良工〔"良"字疑误，似应作"粗"〕所失，不知病情，此亦治之一过也。

Yellow Empperor said: "When treating, one must inquire the conditions of the patient's daily life. If the patient was noble in the past and is now humble, although he had not attacked by the evil energy, yet he has disease produced from the interior, and it is called the 'exhaustion of nutrition'. If the patient was rich in the past and is now poor that causes the disease, it is called the 'depletion of essence'. Both the diseases are due to the depression of spirit and the gradual accumlation of the stagnated energy and blood. The physician is often perplexed and can not be ascertaind what the disease is in diagnosing as the disease is not in the viscera, and the body appears to have nothing different. But the patient is getting thinner and thinner, his energy is debilitating and his essence is consuming day after day. When the

condition of the disease becomes severe, the patient will be exhausted, afraid of cold, be terrified and restless. As the disease is caused by the depression of the spirit, the Wei energy will be wasted outside, and the Rong energy which nourished the blood will be depleted inside, and the condition will become worse day after day. The physician of lower level neglects the condition of the disease and treats it carelessly. This is the first fault in diagnosis and treating.

凡欲诊病者，必问饮食居处，暴乐暴苦，始乐后苦，皆伤精气。精气竭绝，形体毁沮。暴怒伤阴，暴喜伤阳，厥气上行，满脉去形。愚医治之，不知补写，不知病情，精华日脱，邪气乃并，此治之二过也。

"In diagnosis, the physician must ask the patient about his food, drink and daily life, and find out whether there is any sudden joyfulness or sudden sorrow happened to him, whether he enjoyed a happy life or suffered a hardship in the past, as all these conditions can injure the refined energy, debilitate the refined energy and do harm to the body. The sudden onset of fury can injure the Yin energy, and the sudden onset of joy can injure the Yang energy. When the Yin or Yang energy is injured, the Jueyin energy will ascend to cause the distention and fullness of the channels, and the body of the patient will become emaciated. When a physician of lower level diagnoses, he does not know whether the patient should be invigorated or be purged, neither he knows the condition of the disease causing the consumption of the patient and the prosperity of the evil energy. This is the second fault in diagnosis and treating.

善为脉者，必以比类奇恒从容知之，为工而不知道，此诊之不足贵，此治之三过也。

"The physician who is good in diagnosis, can certainly distinguish the disease by analogy, analyse the extraordinary and ordinary disease, handle leisurely and carefully the rule of the changing condition of the disease. If a physician is ignorant about these principles, his diagnosis and treating will be of nothing commendable. This is the third fault in diagnosis and treating.

诊有三常，必问贵贱，封君败伤，及欲侯王。故贵脱势，虽不中邪，精神内伤，身必败亡。始富后贫，虽不伤邪，皮焦筋屈，痿躄为挛。医不能严，不能动神，外为柔弱，乱至失常，病不能移，则医事不行，此治之四过也。

"In diagnosis, one must inquire in advance the three states of the noble or humble, rich or poor, happy or miserable of the patient. Such as, when a former prince or duke who has been dismissed from office and demoted, although he is not attacked by the outer evil, yet his spirit is injured already. His body will be harmed and he can even die.

"When a formerly rich man has become poor, although he has no injury of outer evil, yet his hair wil become withered, his muscle will be contractive and he will contract the disease of flaccidity of his feet. When treating this kind of disease, if the physician can not deal with it carefully to transform the patient's mental idea, but submits to the will of the patient and treats it in a perfunctory way, the disease can by no means be recovered, not to say to have any curative effect. This is the fourth fault in diagnosis and treating.

凡诊者，必知终始，有知余绪。切脉问名，当合男女，离绝菀结，忧恐喜怒，五藏空虚，血气离守，工不能知，何术之语，尝富〔富”似应作“负”〕大伤，斩筋绝脉，身体复行，令泽不息，故伤败结，留薄归阳，脓积寒炅，粗工治之，亟刺阴阳，身体解散，四支转筋，死日有期，医不能明，不问所发，唯言死日，亦为粗工，此治之五过也。

“In diagnosis, one must know the whole proccess of the development of the disease, and be able to know the end by inspecting the beginning. In the palpation and the inquiry, one must notice the difference of male and female.

“All the factors of separation between the loved ones in life or death, depression in sentiment, sorrow, terror, joy and anger can empty the five viscera causing them the inability of maintaining the energy and blood. If a physician does not know these things, how can he know what to do in treating?

“Such as a seriously wounded man, the nutrition to his muscle is almost severed, although his body can still move, yet his body fluid can no more be generated. So, his physique is ruined and his energy and blood which are stagnated inside can no more nourish the whole body through circulation as before. Since the old injury has not yet been recovered, the energy and blood retain inside, and finally join the Yang channel, they change into pus and the stagnated blood causing the alternate onset of cold and heat of man. The physician of lower level treats it with common method as he knows not the syndrome of cold and heat is caused by the pus and stagnated blood, he pricks the Yin and Yang channels again and again causing the consumption of the channel-energy. When the channel energy of the patient being dissipated, the convulsion of the extremities will occur, and the patient will soon die. When a physician can not distinguish the disease, not caring the reason of the disease, but can only determine the date of the patient's death, he is also a physician of lower level. This is the fifth fault in diagnosis and treating.

凡此五者，皆受术不通，人事不明也。故曰：圣人之治病也，必知天地阴阳，四时经纪〔“经纪”疑应作“经络”〕；五藏六府，雌雄表里；刺灸砭石，毒药所主：从容人事，以明经道，贵贱贫富，各异品理，问年少长，勇怯之理；审于分部，知病本始，八正九候，诊必副矣。

“The five faults stated above are due to the physician's inability of comprehending the medical skill what he learned, neither knows the noble or humble, rich or poor, and happy or miserable conditions of the patient.

“Therefore, for a cultivated physician, before he diagnoses and treating, he must know the relation between the Ying and Yang, heaven and earth , the four seasons, the channels and collaterals, the five solid organs and the six hollow organs, the female (the six Yins) and the male (the six Yangs), the pulse conditions of the superficies and interior, the main diseases that can be cured by acupuncture, moxibustion, stone needle and toxicant. He must be able to analogize the changes of human affairs so that he can handle the routine of diagnosis and treating. The patients are different in noble and humble, rich and poor, strong and weak in physiques, and loose and dense of striae of skin. One must analyse the bold and timid char-

acter of the patient and inspect the belongingness of the disease, so as to know the reason of the disease. Refer further to the eight solar terms of the year (the four equinoxes and the four solstices) and the conditions of the nine sub-parts of the pulse. In this way, the diagnosis and treating can certainly be precise.

治病之道，气内为宝，循求其理，求之不得，过在表里；守数据治，无失俞理，能行此术，终身不殆。不知俞理，五藏菀熟，痈发六府，诊病不审，是谓失常。谨守此治，与经相明。《上经》、《下经》，揆度阴阳，奇恒五中，决以明堂，审于终始，可以横行。

"In the way of treating, one must seek the reason of the evil and healthy energy-change through the operations of the Rong and Wei energies inside. If the reason can not be found, seek it from the relation between the superficies and interior.

In treating, the pricking depth must be in accordance with the more or less energy and blood of the patient and must not prick against the rule. If a physician can abide to the rule, he may make no medical mishap in his whole life.

"If the physician does not know the rule of acupuncture but prick the acupoint rashly, it will cause the five viscera to retain heat and the six bowels to have carbuncle and pyogenic infection. When one fails to treat the disease carefully, it is called the "deviation from routine"; when one abides to the routine and treats carefully, it is in conformity to the medical classics.

"The books of the《Upper Classics》and the《Lower Classics》are discussing the principles of Yin, Yang, extraordinary and ordinary diseases. The diseases of the five viscera are manifested on the complexion. When inspecting, one must be shrewd and keen. When one can understand the beginning and the end of the disease by inspecting, his treating will be invincible."

徵四失论篇第七十八

Chapter 78
Zheng Si Shi Lun
(The Four Reasons in the Failure of Treating)

黄帝在明堂，雷公侍坐。黄帝曰：夫子所通书受事众多矣，试言得失之意，所以得之，所以失之。雷公对曰：循经受业，皆言十全，其时有过失者，请〔吴本“请”作“愿”〕闻其事解〔按“事”字衍〕也。

Yellow Emperor was sitting in the Bright Hall and Lei Gong was keeping accompany. Yellow Emperor asked: “You have been reading medical books and learning medicine for a long time, can you tell me your opinion about the reasons of the success and failure in treating, and what disease can be cured and what disease can not be cured?” Lei Gong answered: “In the proccess of receiving the medical education, I heard only the treating could achieve a complete curative effect, but in practice, I had failure often, I hope to know the reason.”

帝曰：子年少智未及邪，将言以杂合耶？夫经脉十二，络脉三百六十五，此皆人之所明知，工之所循用也。所以不十全者，精神不专，志意不理，外内相失，故时疑殆。诊不知阴阳逆从之理，此治之一失也。

Yellow Emperor said: “It is because you are still young, and your intelligence is not enough, or you have some miscellaneous theories in your mind and you can not concentrate your thought in learning. There are twelve channels and three hundred and sixty five collaterals in human body, they are known to all and they are followed and applied by physicians in treating. The failure of achieving a perfect curative effect is due to the inability of concentrating one's mind, fail to do any mental analysis and unable to know the channels' conditions by inspecting the complexion. Thus, perplexity and trouble often occur.

“When one does not understand the principle of Yin and Yang and the agreeable and adverse property of the disease, it is the first reason of the failure in treating.

受师不卒，妄作杂术，谬言为道，更名自功，妄用砭石，后遗身咎，此治之二失也。

“When one abandons his medical learning by half way and treats the disease in some other way, exaggerates his treating as the truth, or to plagiarizes the achievement of the predecessors as his own skill by changing its name, applies the needle indiscriminately, and as a result, it will bring troubles to himeslf. This is the second reason of the failure in treating.

不适贫富贵贱之居，坐〔高注本“坐”作“土”〕之薄厚，形之寒温，不适饮食之宜，不别人之勇怯，不知此类，足以自乱，不足以自明，此治之三失也。

“When one knows not the poor or rich, noble or humble situation of the patient, not knowing the thickness of earth in his living location, not knowing the cold and heat of the

patient's body, not knowing what food and drink the patient should take, unable to distinguish the bold and timid character of the patient, nor can analyse the disease by analogy, it can only muddle one's head without having a clear mind concerning the disease. This is the third reason of the failure in treating.

诊病不问其始，忧患饮食之失节、起居之过度，或伤于毒，不先言此，卒持寸口，何病能中，妄言作名，为粗所穷，此治之四失也。

"When one fails to ask the time of the onset of the disease, not knowing whether the disease is due to the stimulation of the spirit, out of order of the daily life or due to poisoning, and palpate the pulse of the patient rashly without knowing the reason of the disease, how can he diagnose the disease accurately? He can only talk at random, fabricate the name of the disease, and finally bogs himself down in trouble due to carelessness. This is the fourth reason of the failure in treating.

是以世人之语者，驰千里之外，不明尺寸之论〔"论"字与下"诊"字误倒，应作"不明尺寸之诊，论无人事"〕，诊无人事。治数之道，从容之葆，坐持寸口，诊不中五脉，百病所起，始以自怨，遗师其咎。是故治不能循理，弃术于市，妄治时愈，愚心自得。呜呼！窈窈冥冥，孰知其道？道之大者，拟于天地，配于四海，汝不知道之谕，受以明为晦。

"Thus, some physicians of lower level exaggerate his talking like a horse galloping in a remote distance of thousand miles away, but in fact, he does not even understand the way of the palpation of the Cun and Chi pulses, how can he know the astronomy above, the geography below and the human affairs in the middle which are related to the treating? The principle of Yin and Yang, the agreeable and adverse conditions of the disease, viscera and channels can only be mastered through leisureliness, stableness and tardiness.

"If one knows only the way of inspecting the Cun Kou pulse but does not know how to integrate it with the five viscera, he will not be able to know the reason of the disease. When a medical accident occurs, he will first complain himself as he has not learned profoundly, then he blames the poor teaching of his teacher. So. if one practises medicine, but he can not treat patients according to the medical principle, he can only flaunt in the market and treat diseases rashly. When a patient is cured occasionally, he brags about his ability.

"Alas! How subtle and profound is the principle of the medicine, and who can understand its reasons. The theory of medicine can compare favourably with heaven and earth, and match the deep sea. If one does not understand the importance of the medical principle, he will remain muddled even he has been imparted by the one who understands the medical principle."

阴阳类论篇第七十九

Chapter 79
Yin Yang Lei Lun
(On the Three Yin Channels and the Three Yang Channels)

孟春始至，黄帝燕坐，临观八极，正八风之气，而问雷公曰：阴阳之类，经脉之道，五中所主，何藏最贵？雷公对曰：春、甲乙青、中主肝，治七十二日，是脉之主时，臣以其藏最贵。帝曰：却念上下经，阴阳从容，子所言贵，最其下也。

On the day of the Beginning of Spring, Yellow Emperor sat leisurely by the window and watched the scenery of the eight directions and inspected the orientations where the eight winds come from. He asked Lei Gong: "According to the analysis of Yin and Yang channels theory and the Law of the five viscera dominating the seasons, which viscus do you think is the most important one?" Lei Gong answered: "The spring season belongs to Jia and Yi in the decimal cycle, it is of wood and green colour, and it is liver among the five viscera. The liver is prosperous in the seventy two days period of spring and it is the period when the liveris implementing its decree. So, I think liver is most important among the five viscera."

Yellow Emperor said: "You should recall the contents you learned in the chapter of analogy and analysis to Yin and Yang by leisureliness in the 《Upper and Lower Classics》. What you think the most important one is actually the most unimportant one."

雷公致斋七日，旦复待坐。帝曰：三阳为经，二阳为维，一阳为游部，此知五藏终始。三阳〔张介宾说："三阳误也当作'三阴'，三阴，太阴也，太阴为诸阴之表，故曰三阴为表"〕为表，二阴为里，一阴至绝作朔晦，却具合以正其理。雷公曰：受业未能明。

Lei Gong fasted for seven days consecutively and sat by the side of Yellow Emperor in an early morning. Yellow Emperor said to him: "In the Yin and Yang channels of man, the third Yang (the Foot Taiyang Channel) is running along with the longtitude, it lies along the back and reach the top of head above verticaily and it controls the Yang energy of human body. The second Yang (the Yangming Channel) is running along with the latitude, which spreads over the face and head above, covering the chest and abdomen horizontally. The first Yang (the Shaoyang Channel) is the traveling channel, it starts from the outer canthus, lying along the superclavicular fossa and the lateral side of the body, travelling between the Taiyang and Yangming channels. One can determine the beginning and the terminal of the visceral energy by inspecting the coming in and going out of the circulation of the various Yang channels. The third Yin (the Taiyin Channel) which controls the lung, hair and skin is the superficies of Yin channels. The second Yin (the Shaoyin Channel) sinking inside which controls the kidney and bone is the interior. The first Yin (the Jueyin Channel) is the last

stage of Yin which is prior to the beginning of Yang, like the demarcation of the dark moon in the last day of the lunar month and the new moon of the first day of the lunar month. The growth and decline of one another is conform to the condition of the channel's circulation and the Yin and Yang operations in human body." Lei Gong said: "I don't think I have understood what you meant."

帝曰：所谓三阳者，太阳为经，三阳脉，至手太阴，弦浮而不沉，决以度，察以心，合之阴阳之论。所谓二阳者，阳明也，至手太阴，弦而沉急不鼓炅至以病皆死。一阳者，少阳也，至手太阴，上连人迎，弦急悬不绝，此少阳之病也，专阴则死。

Yellow Emperor said: "The so called the third Yang is indicating the Taiyang Channel of the body its pulse appears on the Cunkou (located along the radial artery proximal to the wrist of hand) of the Hand Taiyin Channel. The pulse condition should be full and gigantic. If it is wiry, floating and not sunken on the Cunkou of Hand Taiyin, it is the sick pulse. By this time, One should observe the prosperous or the debilitating condition of the patient's energy and blood, and deliberate the disease by heart by inferring the theory of Yin and Yang. The so called second Yang is indicating the Yangming Channel which appears on the Cunkou of the Hand Taiyin Channel of lung. The pulse condition should by floating, gigantic and short. If it is wiry, sunken and urgent without agitating on the Cunkou Hand Taiyin, it shows the primordial energy of the patient is declining. If this pulse condition appears when the patient has a fever, the primordial energy of the patient will be consumed by the heat and causes death of the patient. The pulse of the first Yang (the Shaoyang channel) appears on the Cunkou of the Hand Taiyin connects the above Renying pulse (located in the cervical arteries lateral to the thyroid cartilage). It should be of a little wiry and harmonious, If it is wiry, but suspending and continuous, it is the sick pulse of the Shaoyang energy of wood. If the wood energy is extremely prosperous and the pulse condition is extremely wiry without any symptom of relaxation, it is called the 'Yin pulse without Yang' which shows the fatal disease of the patient.

三阴者，六经之所主也，交于太阴；伏鼓不浮，上空志心〔《甲乙》"志"作"至"，按"空"误应作"控"〕。二阴至肺，其气归膀胱，外连脾胃。一阴独至，经绝，气浮不鼓，钩而滑。此六脉者，乍阴乍阳，交属相并，缪通五藏，合于阴阳，先至为主，后至为客。

"The pulse of third Yin (Spleen) appears on the Cunkou of the Hand Taiyin Channel of lung and it dominates the six channels. It connects the pulse of heart above and its pulse condition is sunken agitating without floating. The second Yin is the Shaoyin Channel which connects the lung. Its energy goes to the bladder and it connects the stomach and spleen out side. When the energy of the first Yin appears on the Cunkou of the Taiyin Channel solely, it shows the channel energy has been severed causing it to become floating and fails to become agitating, and its pulse condition is like hook and is slippery. The six pulse conditions stated above may appear to be changing into Yin or Yang abruptly, but they are all related and they all appear in the Cunkou. They connect with the five viscera inside and they conform with the changes of Yin and Yang. In the arrival of the six channel energy on the Cunk-

ou; some are early and some are late, the energy that appears early is the host energy and the energy that appears late is the guest energy."

雷公曰：臣悉尽意，受传经脉，颂得从容之道、以合《从容》，不知阴阳，不知雌雄。帝曰：三阳为父，二阳为卫，一阳为纪；三阴为母，二阴为雌，一阴为独使。

Lei Gong said: "Now I understand what you mean. The knowledge of channel you imparted to me before, and the principle of leisureliness I read in books are similar to the way of treating leisurely you have just said, but I do not understand the meaning of Yin and Yang, and male and female." Yellolw Emperor said: "The third Yang is equivalent to the honorable father, the second Yang is equivalent to the guard outside, and the first Yang is equivalent to the pivot; the third Yin is equivalent to the mother who is good at breeding, the second Yin is equivalent to the female who watches inside, and the first Yin is equivalent to the messenger who communicates the Yin and Yang."

二阳一阴，阳明主病，不胜一阴，软〔《甲乙》"软上有"脉"字〕而动，九窍皆沉。三阳一阴，太阳脉胜，一阴不能止，内乱五藏，外为惊骇。二阴二阳，病在肺，少阴脉沉，胜肺伤脾，外伤四支。二阴二阳皆交至，病在肾，骂詈妄行，巅疾为狂。二阴一阳，病出于肾，阴气客游于心脘，下空窍堤，闭塞不通，四支别离。一阴一阳代绝，此阴气至心，上下无常，出入不知，喉咽干燥，病在土脾。二阳三阴，至阴皆在，阴不过阳，阳气不能止阴，阴阳并绝，浮为血瘕，沈为脓胕。阴阳皆壮，下至阴阳。上合昭昭，下合冥冥，诊决死生之期，遂合岁首。

"The second Yang is the Yangming Channel of stomach earth, the first Yin is the Jueyin Channel of liver wood, when the liver-evil bully the stomach, it causes the disease of Yangming. As the second Yang of Yangming can not overcome the first Yin of wood, the Yangming pulse is soft and stirring and the stomach will fail to nourish the nine orifices which will be obstructed.

"When the energy of the third Yang of Foot Taiyang bladder and the first Yin of Jueyin liver cause the disease alternately, the liver can not overcome the bladder. It is because the liver wood produces the fire and the bladder cold water can precisely overcome the fire. So, the Taiyang channel is overcoming. The inability of the Jueyin energy of liver to control the Taiyang energy of cold water causes the partial overabundant of the cold energy which will confuse the five viscera inside and causes restlessness and terror outside of the patient.

"When the second Yin of Shaoyin heart energy and the second Yang of Yangming stomach energy cause the disease, the heart fire flames up to injure the lung and the disease is in the lung. The overabundant fire counter-subjugates the kidney causes the sunken condition of the Shaoyin pulse. The evil energy of heart above and the evil energy of stomach below overcome the lung outside and injure the spleen inside. As the spleen controls the four extremities, the failure of spreading the spleen energy causes the injury of the four extremities.

"When the second Yin of Shaoyang heart fire and the second Yang of Yangming stomach earth cause the disease, the kidney will be attacked and cause the deficiency of the kidney water. When the dryness is excessive, it causes the diseases of head, the swearing at people

wantonly and mania of the patient.

"When the second Yin of Foot Shaoyin kidney and the first Yang of Hand Shaoyang tripple warmer cause the disease, the kidney will be sick. The kidney of Yin ascends to reach the pericardium and descends to control the lower abdomen and bladder below to cause heart-channel collic, and the four extremities of the patient feel like being scattered.

"When the first yin of Jueyin liver and the first Yang of Shaoyang gallbladder are extremely weak and sever now and then, it is due to the up-rising of the Jueying energy to attack the heart. As the wood wind is mobile, it goes up and down without definite direction. The patient will have the symptoms of reluctant to eat and drink, incontinence of faeces and urine and dry throat. The disease is in the spleen.

"When the second Yang of Yangming stomach, the third Yin of Hand Taiyin Lung and the utmost Yin spleen cause the disease, including the disease of the utmost Yin of spleen, the Yin energy will not be able to exceed the Yang, and the Yang energy will not be able to control the Yin. If both the Yin and Yang energies are severed, the out floating Yang will cause the abdominal mass due to blood stasis outside, and the sunken Yin will cause pus and erosion inside. If both the Yin and Yang energies are overabundant, they will turn down to cause the disease of penis in a man and the disease of vagina in a woman. In diagnosis, one must inspect the pulse carefully to tally with the obvious principle of heaven above and coordinate with the profound principle of earth below. In this way, can the date of the patient's survival or death be anticipated, but one must count it from the beginning of the year."

雷公曰：请问短期。黄帝不应。雷公复问。黄帝曰：在经论中。雷公曰：请闻短期。黄帝曰：冬三月之病，病合于阳者，至春正月脉有死征，皆归出春。冬三月之病，在理已尽，草与柳叶皆杀，春阴阳皆绝，期在孟春。春三月之病，曰阳杀，阴阳皆绝，期在草干。夏三月之病，至阴不过十日；阴阳交，期在溓水。秋三月之病，三阳俱起，不治自已。阴阳交合者，立不能坐，坐不能起，三阳独至，期在石水；二阴独至，期在盛水。

Lei Gong said: "Some diseases can cause the death of the patient in a very short time, and why is it?" Yellow Emperor did not answer. When Lei Gong asked again, Yellow Emperor said: "It was stated in the ancient medical books." Lei Gong asked: "What are the contents concerning the disease of death in a short time in the ancient medical books?" Yellow Emperor said: "The Yin energy is prosperous in the three months of winter season. If the disease contracted is of Yang property, it shows the Yin energy of the patient is quite insufficient. The disease will become worse in the first month of spring when the Yang energy becomes prosperous. If the death symptom is seen in the pulse condition, the patient will die by the end of spring and before the beginning of summer when the Yang energy is even more prosperous and the Yin energy is even more on the wane.

"For the disease in the three months of winter, if the death symptom is seen in the pulse condition, the patient will die in spring.

"In winter, when the grasses and willow leaves are dead, if both the Yin and Yang pulses are severed, the patient will die in the first lunar month.

"The disease in the three months of spring is called the Yang being killed disease. If both the Yin and Yang pulses are severed, the patient will die at the time when the grasses dry.

"The Yang enegy is prosperous in the three months of summer. If, by this period, the disease of utmost Yin (spleen) is contracted, it shows the Yin energy of the patient is extremely weak, he will die within ten days. If the Yin pulse appears on the Yang position or the Yang pulse appears in the Yin position, it shows the spleen energy has not yet entirely exhausted then, the patient will die when the water begins to ice up in early winter.

"For the disease in the three months of autumn, if there are improvements in all the three Yin channels, the patient can be recovered even not being treated. If the Yin and Yang energies cause diseases alternately, there must be the condition of partial abundant or partial decline in Yin and Yang, if the Yang energy is overabundant, the patient will not be able to sit down after standing; if the Yin energy is overabundant, the patient will not be able to stand up after sitting. If all the three Yangs arrive without Yin, it shows the Yang energy is hyperactive and the Yin energy is exhausting. The exhaustion of Yin energy is a fatal disease, the patient will die at the time when the water freezes and hard as stone. When all the three Yins arrive without Yang, it is also a fatal disease, the patient will die in the raining season in summer."

方盛衰论篇第八十

Chapter 80
Fang Sheng Shuai Lun
(On the Prosperity and Debility of the Yin and Yang Energies)

雷公请问气之多少，何者为逆，何者为从。黄帝答曰：阳从左，阴从右，老从上，少从下。是以春夏归阳为生，归秋冬为死，反之，则归秋冬为生，是以气多少，逆皆为厥。

Lei Gong asked: "In the prosperity and debility of the energies, what is adverse and what is agreeable?" Yellow Emperor said: "The Yang energy moves from the left to the right, the Yin energy moves from the right to the left; the energy of the elders moves from below to above, and the energy of juveniles moves from below to above. So, when the Yang energy returns to spring and summer, it is agreeable and causes survival, when the Yang energy returns to autumn and winter, it is adverse and causes death. In the vice versa, when the Yin energy returns to autumn and winter, it is agreeable and causes survival, when the Yin energy returns to spring and summer, it is adverse and causes death. Therefore, no matter the energy is prosperous or debilitating, the jueni-syndrome (coldness of extremities) will occur whenever the energy is adverse."

问曰：有余者厥耶？答曰：一上不下，寒厥到膝，少者秋冬死，老者秋冬生；气上不下，头痛巅疾，求阳不得，求阴不审，五部隔无征，若居旷野，若伏空室，绵绵乎属不满日。

Lei Gong asked: "Can a man contract jue-syndrome when his energy is having a surplus?" Yellow Emperor said: "If the Yang energy ascends continuously without descending, it will cause the cold feet under the knees. If this disease happens to a youth in autumn or winter, he will die; if it happens to an elder people in autumn or winter, he will survive. When the Yang energy ascends without descending, it will cause headache and the diseases of head. When you take the jue-syndrome as a Yang disease, you can not find the Yang heat, when you take it as a Yin disease, you can not distinguish the cold energy of Yin. It is a syndrome like Yang and also like that of Yin. Besides, the viscera seem quite remote and there are no prominent syndromes manifested for verifying. It seems that the patient is in the wilderness or hiding himself in an empty room where he can hardly see things clearly even with a concentrated mind.

是以少气之厥，令人妄梦，其极至迷，三阳绝，三阴微，是为少气。

"Thus, when one's energy is deficient in the jue-syndrome, he will have nonsensical dreams, when the energy is extremely deficient, the dreams will be fantastic and perplexing. When the energies of the three Yang channels are severed, and the energies of the three Yin channels are fine when diagnosing, it is the symptom of the deficiency of energy.

是以肺气虚，则使人梦见白物，见人斩血藉藉，得其时则梦见兵战。肾气虚，则使人梦见舟船溺人，得其时则梦伏水中，若有畏恐。肝气虚则梦见菌香生草，得其时则梦伏树下不敢起。心气虚则梦救火阳物，得其时则梦燔灼。脾气虚则梦饮食不足，得其时则梦筑垣盖屋。此皆五藏气虚，阳气有余，阴气不足，合之五诊，调之阴阳，以在经脉。

"When the lung energy is deficient, the patient will see white things in the dream, or dream of the slaughtering and bleeding of men, when the lung metal energy is prosperous, he will dream of war.

"When the energy of kidney water is deficient, he will dream of boat and the drowning of men, when the energy of kidney water is prosperous, he will dream of the hiding of himself in the water like encountering something dreadful.

"When the energy of liver wood is deficient, he will dream of fragrant grasses and trees, when the energy of liver wood is prosperous, he will dream of his hidding under a tree, daring not to get up.

"When the energy of the heart fire is deficient, he will dream of putting out a fire and dream of lightening, when the energy of the heart fire is prosperous, he will dream of a big fire is burning.

"When the energy of the spleen earth is deficient, he will dream of the insufficiency of his food and drink, when the energy of the spleen earth is prosperous, he will dream of building the wall and house.

"All these cases are caused by the deficienty of the five solid organ's energy and the having a surplus of the six hollow organ's energy. When the Yin energy of the five-viscera is insufficient, the deficiency of Yin leads to hyperactivity of Yang, It causes the dreams to become disorderly. When treating, one should infer the outer appearance of the visceral disease and adjust the Yin and Yang and the twelve channels.

诊有十〔"十"疑当作"五"〕度度人：脉度、藏度、肉度、筋度、俞度，阴阳气尽〔按主注："诊备尽阴阳虚盛之理"，细译其意，似本句应作"诊备阴阳"〕，人病自具。脉动无常，散阴颇阳，脉脱不具。诊无常行，诊必上下，度民君卿。受师不卒，使术不明，不察逆从，是为妄行，持雌失雄，弃阴附阳，不知并合，诊故不明，传之后世，反论自章。

"There are standards of five aspects in measuring the disease of the patient: they are the pulse standard, the viscera standard, the muscle standard, the tendon standard and the shu point standard. If one can understand thoroughly the principle of Yin and Yang through diagnosis, he can know the disease comprehensively. There is no regular pattern in the pulsation, the Yin pulse may be scattered, the Yang pulse may be partial-abundant and the condition of the pulsation may not be obvious, so, in diagnosis, no regular routine can be followed. When treating, both the Renying pulse and the Fuyang (Chongyang) pulse must be inspected both, and the social status and the happy or miserable situation of the patient must be taken into consideration. If the physician has not been graduated in his medical study, he has only a lower level in medical treating, and unable to distinguish the adverse or agreeable condition of the energy, he can only injure the Yang by invigorating the Yin, or consumes the Yin by

invigorating the Yang. As he does not understand the reasons of the balance of Yin and Yang, he can by no means to have an accurate diagnosis. When he imparts his ways of diagnosis and treating to the later generations, he will expose his defects of violating the ancient teaching.

至阴虚，天气绝，至阳盛，地气不足；阴阳并交，至人之所行；阴阳并交者，阳气先至，阴气后至。是以圣人持诊之道，先后阴阳而持之，《奇恒之势》乃六十首，诊合微之事，追阴阳之变，章五中之情，其中之论，取虚实之要，定五度之事，知此乃足以诊。是以切阴不得阳，诊消亡。得阳不得阴，守学不湛，知左不知右，知右不知左，知上不知下，知先不知后，故治不久，知醜知善，知病知不病，知高知下，知坐知起，知行知止，用之有纪，诊道乃具，万世不殆。

"When the utmost Yin energy (the earth energy) is deficient, the Yang energy will not descend due to severing; when the utmost Yang energy (the heaven energy) is prosperous, the Yin energy will become weak and not ascending; but a cultivated physician can mingle and communicate the energies of Yin and Yang. In the mingling and communicating of the Yin and Yang energies, the Yang energy comes first, and the Yin energy comes next.

"Thus, when a physician of higher level diagnoses and palpates, he always notices the order of priority of Yin and Yang, infers to the sixty conditions of the ordinary and extraordinary diseases, synthesizes the small and fragmentary cases obtained from diagnosis, and weighs the changes in Yin and Yang to know clearly the location of the disease in the five viscera, then, infers the medical principle and the outline of sthenia and asthenia to judge according to the five standards. When a physician knows all these things, he is capable in diagnosis and treating.

"When a physician knows only the Yin but not knowing the Yang, he is not capable in diagnosing, when he knows only Yang but not knowing the Yin, the medical knowledge he learned is not profound, when he knows only the left side but not knowing the right, knowing the right side only but not knowing the left, knowing what is above but not knowing what is below or knowing what comes early but not knowing what comes late, the curative effect will not be enduring. When treating, one must know the good through the evil, know the healthy condition through the disease, know what is below through what is above, know the standing condition through the sitting condition, know the ceasing condition through the moving condition. Only in this way, can the treating be in perfect order, the diagnosis be all-exclusive, and the treating may always not get into trouble.

起所有余，知所不足，度事上下，脉事因格。是以形弱气虚，死；形气有余，脉气不足，死。脉气有余，形气不足。生。是以诊有大方，坐起有常，出入有行，以转神明，必清必净，上观下观，司八正邪，别五中部，按脉动静，循尺滑濇，寒温之意，视其大小，合之病能逆从以得，复知病名，诊可十全，不失人情。故诊之，或视息视意，故不失条理，道甚明察，故能长久；不知此道，失经绝理，亡言妄期，此谓失道。

"When inspecting the aspect which is having a surplus, one can know the aspect which is insufficient, when considering the upper and lower parts of the patient, one can probe the

reason through diagnosis. Such as, when the patient's physique is weak and his energy is debilitating, it shows death of the patient; when the energy of the physique is overabundant and the energy of the channel is deficient, it also shows death of the patient; when the channel energy is overabundant and the physique energy is insufficient, it shows the patient will survive.

"Therefore, in diagnosis and treating, the physician should abide with the medical principle, in his sitting, standing and acting, he should do it according to a definite rule. He should inspect the upper and lower parts with a sensitive mind, to distinguish the four seasons and the eight solar terms and the part of the five viscera which is atacked by the evil energy soberly. Press and observe the condition of the pulse, inspect the slippery, choppy, cold and warm pulse condition on the skin of anterolateral side of the forearm, examine the change of the stool and urine of the patient to know whether the energy is adverse or agreeable and ascertain the name of the disease. When one diagnoses and treats in this way, it will be flawless and agree with the human feelings. So, in treating, one can always keep the orderliness by inspecting the breath and the mental attitude of the patient. When one's medical theory is extremily superior, he can naturally avoid the malpractices. If one does not understand these things, but violates the principle and fundamental tenet, talks about the disease and draws conclusion rashly, he is running counter to the law."

解精微论篇第八十一

Chapter 81
Jie Jing Wei Lun
(Interpretation of the Subtle Reason of the Falling of Tears)

黄帝在明堂。雷公请曰：臣受业，传之行教以经论，从容形法，阴阳刺灸，汤药所滋，行治有贤不肖，未必能十全。若先言悲哀喜怒，燥湿寒暑，阴阳妇女，请问其所以然者，卑贱富贵，人之形体所从，群下通使，临事以适道术，谨闻命矣。请问有毚愚仆漏之问，不在经者，欲闻其状。帝曰：大矣。

When Yellow Emperor was sitting in the Bright Hall, Lei Gong said to him: "The medical principles you imparted me which I imparted to others were all based on the medical treatises, such as the principle of leisureliness, the theories of Yin and Yang, acupuncture and moxibusion, the way of applying decoctions and tonics, etc., but some of the treatings are effective and some are not, and the curative effects are not entirely perfect. You have told me to treat differently when the patients are in different situations of sorrow, melancholy, joy and anger, when the weathers are different in dryness, wetness, coldness and hotness, and when the patients of different sexes in different states of prosperity and debility in Yin and Yang. When I inquire the reasons of them, you told me the treatings should be discriminative according to the noble or humble, rich or poor and strong or weak conditions of the patient to suit the medical principle in the clinic practice. You have told me these contents already. Now I have some foolish and simple questions which are not found in the medical classics, and I hope you can tell me about them." Yellow Emperor said: "The question you put forward is quite important."

公请问：哭泣而泪不出者，若出而少涕，其故何也？帝曰：在经有也。复问：不知水所从生，涕所从出也。帝曰：若问此者，无益于治也，工之所知，道之所生也。夫心者，五脏之专精也，目者其窍也，华色者其荣也，是以人有德也，则气和于目，有亡，忧知于色。是以悲哀则泣下，泣下水所由生。水宗者积水也，积水者至阴也，至阴者肾之精也，宗精之水所以不出者，是精持之也，辅了裹之，故水不行也。

Lei Gong asked: "When one crys, both the tear and the nasal mucus come out, and what is the reason?! Yellow Emperor said: "It is written in the medical classics." Lei Gong said: "I do not understand how the tear produces and where does the nasal mucus come from." Yellow Emperor said: "This question you put forward will not benefit the treating, but it should be known by physicians as it is a part of the medical theory. The heart is the chief of the viscera and the body, the eyes are the apertures and the face complexion is the manifestation outside. So, when a man has something complacent, the energy is concentrated in the

two eyes with a radiant look; if he has something disappointing, the melancholy will be manisfested in the eyes. The tears of crying are produced from water. The source of water is the body fluid. It is the utmost Yin that accumultes the body fluid, and the utmost Yin is the essence of the kidney. The water which stems from the essence of kidney does not flow out usually as it is protected, encircled and controlled by the essence of kidney. Therefore, normally, the tears can not go so far as to come out automatically.

夫水之精为志，火之精为神，水火相感，神志俱悲〔《太素》无“水火”八字〕》，是以目之水生也。故谚言曰：心悲名曰志悲，志与心精，共凑于目也。是以俱悲则神气传于心精，上不传于志而志独悲，故泣出也。泣涕者脑也，脑者阴〔《太素〕、《甲乙》“阴”并作“阳”〕也。髓者骨之充也，故脑渗为涕。志者骨之主也，是以水流而涕从之者，其行类也。夫涕之与泣者，譬如人之兄弟，急则俱死，生则俱生，其志以早悲，是以涕泣俱出而横行也，夫人涕泣俱出而相从者，所属之类也。

“The retained energy of water is the will, and the refined energy of fire is the spirit, as the saying goes: ‘The melancholy of heart is actually the melancholy of will’! When one is in melancholy, the will of kidney and the essence of heart will assemble in the eyes at the same time.

“Thus, when the heart and the kidney are both in melancholy, the spirit and the energy will be transferred to the essence of heart but not to the will of kidney below, causing the sole melancholy of the will of kidney. When the will of kidney fails to be supported by the essence of life which can control the water, the tears will flow out.

“The nasal mucus belongs to the brain, the brain belongs to the Yin, and the marrow is that which fills the cavity of the bone. When the marrow seeps out, it becomes the mucus. The will of kidney dominates the bone, so when the tears come out, the mucus comes out in the wake of it. The mucus and the tear are like brothers, they die together when in danger and live together when in joy. If there is melancholy in the will of kidney, the mucus and tear will spring up together. The reason of the coming out of the tear and mucus in accompany is because they all belong to water.”

雷公曰：“大矣。请问：人哭泣而泣不出者，若出而少，涕不从之何也？帝曰：夫泣不出者，哭〔“哭”是似乎作“志”不悲也〕。不泣者，神不慈者。神不慈则志不悲，阴阳相持，泣安能独来。夫志悲者，惋惋则冲阴，冲阴则志去目，志去则神不守精，精神去目，涕泣出也。

Lei Gong said:“Your explanation is splendid. Some one wants to cry but fails to cry out, or he has only a few tears without mucus, and what is the reason?” Yellow Emperor said: “When one cries without tears, it is because his will is not sad, when he fails to cry out, it is because his spirit is not being moved, when one's spirit is not moved, his will will not be sad. Since the Yin (the will) and the Yang (the spirit) stalemate without any mutual responses, how can the tears come out by itself?

且子独不诵不念夫经言乎，厥则目无所见。夫人厥则阳气并于上，阴气并于下，阳并于上，则火独光也；阴并于下则足寒，足寒则胀也。夫一水不胜五〔《太素》“五”作“两”〕火，

素　问

PLAIN QUESTIONS
（SU WEN）

故目眦〔明抄本“目”下无“眦”字〕盲。

“When one's will is sad, he will have a sentiment of sorrow which will stir the Yin energy causing the will of kidney to give up the keeping guard of the eyes. When the will of kidney leaves the eyes, the spirit will not guard the refined energy. If both the spirit and the refined energy leave the eyes, the tears and mucus will come out at the same time.

“What is more, haven't you read the texts in the medical classics? It was stated in t medical classics: 'When one contracts the jue-syndrome, the Yang energy will be accumu ed in the upper part of the body and the Yin energy in the lower part. When the Yang en accoumulated above, the Yang energy will be hyperactive in the upper part; when the energy accumulates in the lower part, it will cause the disease of cold feet and thereupon tention. Since one water can not overcome two fires, it will cause the eyes to see nothing

是以冲风，泣下而不止。夫风之中目也，阳气内守于精，是火气燔目，故见风则泣下也。有以比之，夫火疾风生乃能雨，此之类也。

“The fact of the flowing out unceasingly of tears when one is facing the wind is because when the eyes are attacked by the wind evil, the Yang energy descends to guard the essence of life. When the Yang energy is absent, the fire energy will burn the eyes which causes the flowing of tears. For instance, a strong wind can cause the rain, and this condition in human body is about the same.”

附录

原文校注据本书名：

素问王冰注　　四部丛刊影印明顾氏本
黄帝内经太素　　东洋医学丛书影印本　　简称太素
难经集注　　四部丛刊影印佚存丛书本
伤寒论　　重庆人民出版社排印本
脉经　　四部丛刊影印元广勤书堂刊本
甲乙经　　人民卫生出版社刘衡如校本　　简称甲乙
鬼遗方　　人民卫生出版社影印本
中藏经　　丛书集成本
诸病源候论　　人民卫生出版社影印本　　简称病源
备急千金要方　　人民卫生出版社影印本　　简称千金
千金翼方　　人民卫生出版社影印本
外台秘要　　人民卫生出版社影印本　　简称外台
太平圣惠方　　人民卫生出版社排印本
铜人针灸腧穴图经　　人民卫生出版社影印本　　简称图经
医心方　　人民卫生出版社影印本
校证活人书　　丛书集成本
伤寒补亡论　　梁园豫医双璧本

灵　　　枢

SPIRITUAL PIVOT
(LING SHU)

叙

昔黄帝作《内经》十八卷，《灵枢》九卷，《素问》九卷，乃其数焉，世所奉行唯《素问》耳。越人得其一二而述《难经》，皇甫谧次而为《甲乙》，诸家之说悉自此始。其间或有得失，未可为后世法。则谓如《南阳活人书》称：咳逆者，哕也。谨按《灵枢经》曰：新谷气入于胃，与故寒气相争，故曰哕。举而并之，则理可断矣。又如《难经》第六十五篇，是越人标指《灵枢·本输》之大略，世或以为流注。谨按《灵枢经》曰：所言节者，神气之所游行出入也，非皮肉筋骨也。又曰：神气者，正气也。神气之所游行出入者流注也，井荥输经合者本输也，举而并之，则知相去不啻天壤之异。但恨《灵枢》不传久矣，世莫能究。夫为医者，在读医书耳，读而不能为医者有矣，未有不读而能为医者也。不读医书，又非世业，杀人尤毒于梃刃。是故古人有言曰：为人子而不读医书，犹为不孝也。仆本庸昧，自髫迄壮，潜心斯道，颇涉其理。辄不自揣，参对诸书，再行校正家藏旧本《灵枢》九卷，其八十一篇，增修音释，附于卷末，勒为二十四卷。庶使好生之人，开卷易明，了无差别。除已具状经所属申明外，准使府指挥依条申转运司选官详定，具书送秘书省国子监。今崧专访请名医，更乞参详，免误将来。利益无穷，功实有自。

Preface

In the past, Yellow Emperor wrote the《Canon of Internal Medicine》in 18 rolls of which comprising 9 rolls of "Plain Questions" and 9 rolls of "Spiritual Pivot", but only the "Plain Questions" was in vogue. According to a small part of the "Plain Questions", Qin Yueren wrote the《Classic on Difficulty》, and Huangpu Mi wrote the《Jia Yi》and from then on, the scholars in various views occurred. Among the different opinions, some were defective which were not suitable to be followed by the later generations, such as, in the《Nan Yang Huo Ren Shu》(The Nanyang Book of Saving Lives) stated: "cough is vomiting". But in "Spiritual Pivot", it was stated precisely: "When the cereal energy newly enters into the stomach, the cold energies combat with each other causing the vomit." Through the statement, the reason is made clear. Again, in the sixty-fifth chapter of the《Classic on Difficulty》, Qin Yueren summarized the general outline of the "Ben Shu" On acupoints of "Spiritual Pivot" of which people thought it was an annotation to the text. But in "Spiritual Pivot" it was stated precisely: "The acupoints are the places where the spirit and the energy flowing in and flowing out, they are not skin, muscle, tendon and bone." Again, it stated: "The spirit energy is the healthy energy, its flowing in and out is the pouring, and the Jing, Xing, Shu, Jing and He points are the acupoints." One can see the statement is much more exquisite than that in the《Classic of Difficulty》, and the difference is like the high sky and the low land. It is a pity that the "Spiritual Pivot" has been missed for long and people could do nothing about it.

It is necessary for a physician to read medical books. Sometimes, although one reads the medical books, yet he is not capable to be a physician, but no one can be a physician without reading medical books. When one does not read medical books and has not received any medical education from his family, he might kill the patient so cruelly like putting him to death with a stick or sword. Thus, the old saying goes: "When a son of man does not read the medical books, he is unfilial".

I am a mediocre man, but I have been interested in medicine since my youth and robust age and I have understood some principles about it. So, I venture to infer various books and rectify the "Spiritual Pivot" which is of eighty-one chapters in nine rolls stored in my home with some additions, deletions and interpretations, and appended them at the end of the book, arranging the whole book as twenty-four rolls, so that when one who is interested in preserving health reads it, he can understand it easily without perplexion.

This edition, according to the stipulation, has been sent to the related authorites for examination and will be sent to the National Education Department. Now I visit and consult some prominent physicians to ask their helps for correcting the errors in details, so that it may not do any harm to the future and can render inexhaustible benefit.

时宋绍兴乙亥仲夏望日。锦官史崧题

This preface is written by the government officer Shi Song of Jinguan city on the fifteenth of the seven lunar month in Yi Hai year of the Shaoxing (1155 A. D.) of Song Dynasty.

九针十二原第一

Chapter 1
Jiu Zhen Shi Er Yuan
(The Nine Kinds of Needle and the Twelve Source Points)

黄帝问于岐伯曰：余子万民，养百姓，而收其租税。余哀其不给，而属有疾病。余欲勿使被毒药，无用砭石，欲以微针通其经脉，调其血气，营其逆顺出入之会，令可传于后世。必明为之法令，终而不灭，久而不绝，易用难忘；为之经纪，异其章，别其表里；为之终始，令各有形，先立针经，愿闻其情。

Yellow Emperor said to Qibo："I love all the people, and I want to maintain all the officials, so, I levy duties from them. I have compassion for the people when they can not die a natural death. What is more, they fall ill constantly. I want to treat them with a fine needle inserting into the skin instead of giving them any medicine or applying any stone needle for to dredge the channel, adjust the energy and blood, promote the circulation of the blood, causing the agreeable and adverse conditions of the channels and the coming and going of the energy and blood be complementary with each other. I hope to have a standing order of acupuncture so that it may be handed down to the later generations. Therefore it is necessary to draw up a statue for acupuncture, to facilitate its application and made it unlikely to be forgotten, so that the acupuncture method may not be obliterated and lost. In the statue, it should regulate the depth criterion of the forwardness and the backwardness of the fine needle, distinguish the acupoints of the solid organs and the hollow organs with analystic paragraphs and chapters and stipulate the length of the different kinds of needle. In a word, to comply a classic of acupuncture, and I hope to hear from you the substantial contents of it."

岐伯答曰：臣请推而次之，令有纲纪，始于一，终于九焉。请言其道。小针之要，易陈而难入，粗守形，上守神，神乎神，客在门，未睹其疾，恶知其原。刺之微在速迟，粗守关，上守机，机之动，不离其空，空中之机，清静而微，其来不可逢，其往不可追，知机之道者，不可挂以发，不知机道，叩之不发，知其往来，要与之期，粗之暗乎，妙哉工独有之。往者为逆，来者为顺，明知逆顺，正行无问，逆〔逆而夺之：胡本，藏本，日抄本"逆"作"迎"〕而夺之，恶得无虚，追而济之，恶得无实，迎之随之，以意和之，针道毕矣。

Qibo said："I like to tell you the essentials commencing from the first kind of needle to the ninth kind of needle according to the order systematically. Concerning the essentials of acupuncture, it is easy to be talked about, but it is difficult to attain the standard of being exquisite. A physician adheres to the bodily position rigidly and prick the focus, but a superior physician treats according to the various expressions of the patient which shows the patient's state of mind. A physician of lower level is like the one who is standing outside of the door, he can not even perceive what the disease is, how could he know the source of the disease? The skill in pricking is in the application of the swift and slow pricking and pulling of the needle. A physician of lower level can only adhere to the acupoints on the joints of the limbs rigidly, but a superior physician can observe the flexible change of the channel's energy, and the flexible change can by no means divorce from the acupoint. The reasons contained in acupuncture are rather subtle. When the evil energy is overabundant, one must not make a head-on invigoration, when the evil energy is debilitative, one must not purge pursuantly. When one knows the principle of the functional activities of vital energy change, he will not make even a tiny mistake, when he knows not the principle, it is like the arrow fastened on the bow string which can not be shot out. Thus, one must handle the mechanism of the agreeable and adverse, coming and going, abundant and debilitative of the channels and the energies, then, can a curative effect be expected. A physician of lower level is ignorant about these things, and it is only a superior physician knows the subtle device. As to the agreeable and adverse condition: when the healthy energy is moving away, it is the adverse condition, when the healthy energy is retaliating, it is the agreeable condition, when one understands the principle of the agreeable and adverse conditions, he will be able to prick daringly and straightforwardly without consulting others. When the patient's healthy energy is already in debility, but, on the contrary, the purge therapy is applied, how can the patient separate himself from becoming even more asthenic? When the evil energy is already abundant, but, on the contrary, the invigorating therapy is applied, how can the patient be separated from becoming even more sthenic? One must purge when facing the evil energy, and invigorate when the healthy energy has moved away. If one can think over and analyse the patient's condition before applying invigorating or purging, the pricking will fit the principle of acupuncture.

凡用针者，虚则实之，满则泄之，宛陈则除之，邪胜则虚之。大要曰：徐而疾则实，疾而徐则虚。言实与虚，若有若无，察后与先，若存若亡，为虚与实，若得若失。虚实之要，九针最妙，补泻之时，以针为之。泻曰：必持内之，放而出之，排阳〔排阳得针：《甲乙》郑五第四“阳”作“扬”，“得”作“出”〕得针，邪气得泄。按而引针，是谓内温，血不得散，气不得出也。补曰随之，随之，意若妄之，若行若按，如蚊虻止，如留如还，去如弦绝，令左属右，其气故止，外门已闭，中气乃实，必无留血，急取诛之。持针之道，坚者为宝，正指直刺，无针〔无针：覆刻《太素》卷二十一“无针”作“针无”〕左右，神在秋毫，属意病者，审视血脉，刺之无殆。方刺之时，必在悬阳，及与两衡，神属勿去，知病存亡，血脉者〔血脉者：《甲乙》卷五第四“血”上有“取”字〕，在腧横居，视之独澄〔“澄”《太素》卷二十一作“满”〕，切之独坚。

“In pricking, when the healthy energy is a sthenic, apply the invigorating therapy, when the evil energy is sthenic, apply the purging therapy, when there is stagnated blood, apply the blood-letting therapy, when the evil energy is overwhelming, apply the purgative therapy. Generally speaking, when applying the needle in invigoration, it should be slow in inserting and quick in drawing, and press the needle hole hastly after drawing; in purging, it should be quick in inserting and slow in drawing without pressing the needle hole. In invigorating and purging, the patient seems to feel it yet seems to feel nothing; one should inspect the advanced and the lagging behind of the energy arrival to ascertain whether the needle should be retained or be pulled out immediately. In short, whatever the invigorating or purging therapy is used, it must cause the patient to feel something obtainned when in invigorating and to feel something being lost when in purging. The nine kinds of needles are different in functions, one can realize the invigorating or purging with different techniques. In purging, one should hold the needle tight and then insert, when the patient has got the acupuncture feeling, wave the needle and enlarge the needle hole, and then pull out the needle with twist so that the evil energy can be excreted along with the pulling out of the needle. if the needle hole is pressed right after the pulling of the needie, it will cause the evil energy to retain inside, the stagnated blood will not be dispersed, and the evil energy will not be excreted. In invigorating, the pricking can be carried out at any time, the pricking should be like wittingly yet unwittingly, the insertion is like advancing yet stopping, and the feeling of the patient is like a mosquito bite on the skin. When the needle has been inserted into the skin, stop and linger inside to wait for the desired acupuncture feeling, when it arrives, pull out the needle swiftly like an arrow getting off from the bow string; pull out the needle with the right hand and press to close the needle hole with the left hand quickly, in this way, the channel energy can be retained inside, and when the needle hole is closed, the middle warmer energy can be substantialized. If there is bleeding under the skin, it must not be left alone, but should eliminate it promptly. In holding the needle, it is valuable to keep a resolute mind, aiming at the acupoint accurately and prick promptly, the needle should not be slanting to the right or to the left, the acupuncturist should concentrate his mind at the needle point, take good notice of the patient, inspect his channel and take care of keeping away from it, in this way, the inserting will be of no danger. Just before pricking, watch the location between the patient's nose, eyes and brows with a concentrated mind without any negligence, so that the prognosis of the disease can be estimated. The so called 'inspect the channel' is to watch the channel by the side of the acupoint which is quite full when watching. and quite substantial when pressing.

九针之名，各不同形：一曰镵针，长一寸六分；二曰员针，长一寸六分；三曰鍉针，长三寸半；四曰锋针，长一寸六分；五曰铍针，长四寸，广二分半；六曰员利针，长一寸六分，七曰毫针，长三寸六分；八曰长针，长七寸；九曰大针，长四寸。镵针者，头大末税，去泻阳气。员针者，针如卵形〔针如卵形：《太素》杨注作“锋如卵”〕，揩摩分间，不得伤肌肉，以泻分气。鍉针者，锋如黍粟之锐，主按脉勿陷，以致其气。锋针者，刃三隅，以发痼疾。铍针者，末如剑锋，以取大脓。员利针者，大如氂，且员且锐，中身微大，以取暴气〔以取暴气《太素·九针所主》杨注“气”作“痹”〕。毫针者，尖如蚊虻喙，静以徐往，微以久留之而养，以取痛痹。长针者，锋利身薄，可以取远痹。大针者，尖如梃，其锋微员，以泻机关之水也。九针毕矣。

“In the nine kinds of needle, each of them has the different shape. The first kind is called the sagital needle of which the length is 1.6 inches; the second kind is called the ovoid-tip needle of which the length is 1.6 inches; the third kind is called the blunt-tip needle of which the length is 3.5 inches, the fourth kind is called the ensiform needle of which the length is 1.6 inches; the fifth kind is called the sword-shaped needle of which is 4 inches in length and 0.25 inches in width; the sixth kind is called the round-sharp needle of which the length is 1.6 inches; the seventh kind is called the filiform needle of which the length is 3.6 inches; the eighth kind is called the long needle of which the length is 7 inches; the ninth kind is called the large needle of which the length is 4 inches. The sagital needle is large and sharp which is used in shallow pricking for to excrete the heat of the skin; the point of the ovoid-tip needle is like an egg, it is used to rub between the muscles which not only do no harm to the muscles, but also can disperse the evil energy of the muscles; the point of the blunt-tip needle is somewhat round like glutinous millet, it is used to press the channel for inducing the healthy energy and excreting the evil energy; the ensiform needle has blades on its three sides for treating the protracted and refractory diseases; the point of the sword-shaped needle is sharp like the point of a sword which is used to prick the carbuncle and discharge the pus; the point of the round-sharp needle is long and sharp like hair, the body of the needle is somewhat thick which can be used to treat the bi-syndrome ;the point of the filiform needle is like the probocis of a mosquito, when the needle is inserted slowly into the skin and retains inside, it can repose one's mind, it can be used to treat the cold-type arthralgia also; the point of the long needle is sharp and the body of the needle is rather long which can be used to treat the protracted bi-syndrome; the point of the large needle is like the bamboo stubble and is somewhat round which can be used to excrete the accumulated water wich accumulated in the joint. These are the conditions of the nine kinds of needle.

夫气之在脉也，邪气在上，浊气在中，清气在下。故针陷脉则邪气出，针中脉则浊气出，针太深则邪气反沉，病益。故曰：皮肉筋脉各有所处，病各有所宜〔病各有所宜：《甲乙》卷五第四“宜”作“舍”〕，各不同形，各以任其所宜。无实无虚，损不足而益有余，是谓甚病，病益甚。取五脉者死，取三脉者恇；夺阴者死，夺阳者狂，针害毕矣。刺之而气不至，无问其数；刺之而气至，乃去之，勿复针。针各有所宜，各不同形，各任其所为。刺之要，气至而有效，效之信，若风之吹云，明乎若见苍天，刺之道毕矣。

"As to the channel-energy of human body, the evil energy of Yang is usually on the upper part of the body, the drossy energy usually stays in the middle and the cold-wetness remains in the lower part, thus, the pricking position must not be the same. Such as, when pricking the bone cavity in the cave in of the head, it will cause the evil energy of Yang to come out; when pricking the Yangming channel, it will cause the drossy energy to come out, when the disease is in the superficies and the pricking is too deep, it will cause the evil energy to go inside and aggravate the disease. Since the skin, muscle, tendon and channel are all having their own positions, the diseases are all having their points for residing, and the conditions of diseases are different, the pricking must be cautious. One must not invigorate the sthenic disease and must not purge the asthenic disease, as any measure of injuring the deficiency or profit the surplus will aggravate the pain of the patient, and causes the disease becoming even more severe. When pricking the acupoints of the five solid orgns of the patient whose refined energy is debilitative, it may cause the death of the patient, when pricking the acupoints of the three Yang's channel, it may cause the patient to become cowardly; when the Yin channel is injured, the patient may contract the jue-syndrome, when the Yang channel is injured, the patient may contract mania. In pricking, one must wait for the patient to get the acupuncture feeling, if the feeling is not felt after pricking, it must be kept waiting until it comes, disregard of the times of the patient's respiration; when the acupuncture feeling is felt, the needle can be pulled out and no more pricking is necessary. The nine kinds of needle have different functions and they are different in shapes, in acupuncture, the kind of needle should be selected according to the different conditions of the disease respectively. The most important thing in acupuncture is to get the acupuncture feeling, when it appears, the curative effect will appear in the wake of it, and the curative effect is so reliable as the blue sky appearing when the clouds are blown away by the wind. These are the principles of acupuncture."

黄帝曰：愿闻五脏六腑所出之处。岐伯曰：五脏五腧，五五二十五腧；六腑六腧，六六三十六腧。经脉十二，络脉十五，凡二十七气以上下，所出为井，所溜为荥，所注为腧，所行为经，所入为合，二十七气所行，皆在五腧也。节之交，三百六十五会，知其要者，一言而终，不知其要，流散无穷。所言节者，神气之所游行出入也，非皮肉筋骨也〔《素问·调经论》王注《针经》作"非骨节也"〕。

Yellow Emperor said: " I hope to hear the exits of the channel-energy of the viscera." Qibo said: In each channel of the five solid organs, there are the five acupoints of Jing, Xing, Shu, Jing and He, they are altogether twenty five acupoints; in each channel of the six hollow organs, there are the six acupoints of Jing, Xing, Shu, Yuan, Jing and He, they are altogether thirty six acupoints. In each of the twelve channels of the viscera, there is a collateral branch, together with each collateral branch on the Ren, Du and spleen channels, they are fifteen collateral branches. The energies of the twenty seven channels (of twelve channels and fifteen collateral branches) circulate around the whole body, going out and coming in between the upper and the lower extremities. The channel-energy turns from weak to strong gradually and finally enters into the He point, which is the so called 'the energy initiats from the Jing point, flows to the Xing point, pours into the Shu point, passes through the Jing point, and enters into the He point'. The twenty seven energies flow and pour into the five acupoints unceasingly day and night. There are three hundred and sixty five acupoints where the joints of the human body connect, they are all the locations where the energy and blood going out and coming in and the places where the channel-energy permeat the joints, they are not the bone joints. When one knows the essentials, it can be concluded by a single sentence, if knows not, it will be slack and irrelevant.

睹其色，察其目，知其散复；一其形，听其动静，知其邪正。右主推之，左持而御之，气至而去之。凡将用针，必先诊脉，视气之剧易，乃可以治也。五脏之气已绝于内，而用针者反实其外，是谓重竭，重竭必死，其死也静，治之者辄反其气，取腋与膺；五脏之气已绝于外，而用针者反实其内，是谓逆厥，逆厥则必死，其死也躁，治之者，反取四末。刺之害，中而不去，则精泄；害〔复刻《太素》卷二十一《九针要道》"害"并作"不"〕中而去，则致气。精泄则病益甚而恇，致气则生为痈疡。

In the course of pricking, one must inspect the patient's complexion and the eyes' expression to survey the dispersion and the restoration of the patient's blood and energy, differentiate the strong or weak physique of the patient, listen to the volumn of the voice to infer the healthy energy, evil energy, asthenia and sthenia of the patient, insert the needle with the right hand and guard the needle with the left hand, when getting the acupuncture feeling after the pricking, the needle should be pulled out. Before pricking, one must observe and know whether the channel-energy is harmonious or not. If one invigorates the Yang energy outside of the patient whose visceral energy is already severed inside and who is of Yin-deficiency, his Yang energy will be even more abundant and his Yin energy will become even more debilitative, in this condition, it is called the double exhaustion, and the patient with double exhaustion will die, when he dies, he appears to be calm, This is because the physician runs against the channel-energy, pricks the acupoints on the armpit and chest erroneously to cause the visceral energy to become debilitative and exhausting. If one invigorates the internal Yin energy of the patient whose visceral energy is debilitative outside and who is of Yang-deficiency, the Yin energy will become even more abundant and the Yang energy becomes even more debilitative to cause cold extremities, it is called the adverse jue-syndrome, the patient with adverse jue-syndrome will die, and when he dies, he appears to be irritable. This is because the physician pricks the tips of the patient's four limbs causing the exhaustion of the Yang energy.

The fundamentals of the pricking are: when the needle has already reached the focus, but not being pulled out, it will injure the energy; when the needle fails to reach the focus, the evil energy will be detained inside. When the energy is injured, the disease will be aggravated and the patient will become debilitative, when the evil energy is detained, the patient will apt to contract carbuncle and ulceration.

五脏有六腑有十二原，十二原出于四关，四关主治五脏。五脏有疾，当取之十二原，十二原者，五脏之所以禀三百六十五节气味〔气味：孙鼎宜曰："味"当作"会"〕也。五脏有疾也，应出十二原，而原各有所出，明知其原，睹其应，而知五脏之害矣。阳中之少阴，肺也，其原出于太渊，太渊二。阳中之太阳，心也，其原出于大陵，大陵二。阴中之少阳，肝也，其原出于太冲，太冲二。阴中之至阴，脾也，其原出于太白，太白二。阴中之太阴，肾也，其原出于太溪，太溪二。膏之原，出于鸠尾，鸠尾一。肓原，出于脖胦，脖胦一。凡此十二原者，主治五脏六腑之有疾者也。

Outside of the five solid organs, there are the six hollow organs, outside of the six hollow organs, there are the twelve source points, The twelve source points issued from the four large joints of the limbs and the source points of the four large joints are mainly the locations for to treat the infections of the five viscera, Thus, when the five-viscera is ill, the twelve source points should be pricked. The twelve source points are the points where the channle-energy of the three hundred and sixty five acupoints assemble, when the five viscera have disease, it will reflect on the twelve source points, and each of the source points belongs to a certain viscus. When one understands the attribute of the source point and perceive its response, be can comprehend the disease condition of the viscus.

The lung and heart situate above the diaphragm in the position of Yang. The lung is a Yin viscus situates in Yang position, and it is Shaoyin in Yang, its source points are the left and right Taiyuan points (LU. 9). The heart is a Yang viscus situates in the Yang position, it is Yang in Yang, its source points are the left and right Daling points (PC. 7). The liver, spleen and kidney situate below the diaphragm, they situate in the position of Yin. The liver is a Yang viscus situates in the position of Yin, it is Shaoyang in Yin, its source points are the left and right Taichong points (LR. 3); the spleen is a Yin viscus situates in the position of Yin, its source points are the left and right Taibai points (SP. 3); the kidney is a Yin viscus situates in the position of Yin, it is Taiyin in Yin, its source points are the left and right Taixi points (KI. 3). The source point of the diaphragm is the single Jiuwei point (RN. 15) which belongs to the Ren channel. The source point of the area below the heart and above the diaphragm is the single Qihai point (RN. 6) which belongs to the Ren channel. The twelve source points above are the crucial locations for the energies of viscera, channels and collaterals to pour in and communicate with, so, through treating the points, the diseases of the five solid organs and the six hollow organs can be cured.

胀取三阳，飧泄取三阴。

When the patient has abdominal distention, prick the three Yang Channels of foot; when the patient has diarrhea, prick the three Yin Channels of foot.

今夫五脏之有疾也，譬犹刺也，犹污也，犹结也，犹闭也。刺虽久，犹可拔也；污虽久，犹可雪也；结虽久，犹可解也；闭虽久，犹可决也。或言久疾之不可取者，非其说也。夫善用针者，取其疾也，犹拔刺也，犹雪污也，犹解结也，犹决闭也。疾虽久，犹可毕也。言不可治者，未得其术也。

When the five-viscera contracts the disease, it is like a sting on the muscle, a stain on a thing, a tie on a piece of string or a stretch of silt on the river. Although the sting has remained for many days, it can still be removed, although the stain has existed for a long time, it can still be washed away, although the knot has been tied for a long time, it can still be untied, although the river has been silted up for a long time, the silt can still be cleared away. Some people think that a protracted disease can not be cured by acupuncture, the opinion is not right. A physician who is good at acupuncture can cure the disease, even it is a protracted disease, just like pulling a sting, removing a stain. untie a knot or clear away the silt in the river flow. Those who think a protracted disease can not be cured by acupuncture is that they do not have the acupuncture technique。

刺诸热者，如以手探汤；刺寒清者，如人不欲行。阴有阳疾者，取之下陵三里，正往无殆，气下乃止，不下复始也。疾高而内者，取之阴之陵泉；疾高而外者，取之阳之陵泉也。

When pricking the fever, the hand should be like dipping in the boiling soup, the needle should be lifted up instantly after pricking; when pricking the cold, the pricking should be like one relunctants to leave home before traveling. When there is heat phenomenon of Yang evil in Yin, the Zusanli point (ST. 36) should be pricked, when pricking, one must concentrate his mind to prick the acupoint accurately, when the evil energy has retreated, the pricking should be stopped, if the evil energy does not retreat, it should be pricked again. When the disease is on the upper part of the body pertaining to the internal solid organ, prick the Yinlingquan point (SP. 9), when the disease is on the upper part of the body pertaining to the external hollow organ, prick the Yangligquan (G B. 34).

本输第二

Chapter 2
Ben Shu
(On Acupoints)

黄帝问于岐伯曰：凡刺之道，必通十二经络〔十二经络：《太素》卷十一《本输》“经络”作“经脉”。〕之所终始，络脉之所别处〔《太素》卷十一《本输》“处”作“起”〕，五输之所留〔《太素》卷十一《本输》“留”下有“止”字〕，六腑之所与合，四时之所出入，五脏〔《太素》卷十一《本输》“六腑”上有“五脏”二字〕之所溜处，阔数之度，浅深之状，高下所至。愿闻其解。

Yellow Emperor asked Qibo and said: “In pricking, one must understand the beginnings and the terminals of the twelve channels, the extra branches of the collaterals, the places where the five kinds of Jing, Xing, Shu, Jing and He acupoints stop, the corresponding relations of the five solid organs and the six hollow organs, the going out and the coming in of the Yin and Yang energies in different seasons, the energy-circulations of the five viscera, the width and the depth of the channels, collaterrals, and minute collaterals from head to foot. I hope you can explain them to me.”

岐伯曰：请言其次也。肺出于少商，少商者，手大指端〔《太素》卷十一《本输》“指”下无“端”字〕内侧也，为井木；溜于鱼际，鱼际者，手鱼也，为荥；注于太渊，太渊，鱼后一寸陷者中也，为腧；行于经渠，经渠，寸口中也，动而不居，为经；入于尺泽，尺泽，肘中之动脉也，为合，手太阴经也。

Qibo said: “Let me tell you in order. The channel-energy of lung channel issues from Shaoshang point (LU. 11), the Shaoshang point is on the inner flank of the thumb, and it is called Jing Wood; from here, the channel-energy flows into the Yuji point (LU. 10), the Yuji point is behind the hand thenar eminence, and it is called Xing; from here, the channel-energy pours into Taiyuan point (LU. 9), the Taiyuan point is in the cave-in one inch behind the thenar eminence, and it is called Shu; from here, the channel-energy passes through the Jingqu point (LU. 8), the Jingqu point is in the cave-in of Cunkou where the Taiyin Channel pulsates unceasingly, and it is called Jing; from here, the channel-energy gets into the Chize point (LU. 5), Chize is on the artery of the elbow, and it is called He. These are the five acupoints belonging to the Hand Taiyin Channel of Lung.

心出于中冲，中冲，手中指之端也，为井木；溜于劳宫，劳宫，掌中中指本节之内间也，为荥；注于大陵，大陵，掌后两骨之间方下者也，为腧；行于间使，间使之道，两筋之间，三寸之中也，有过则至，无过则止，为经；入于曲泽，曲泽，肘内廉下陷者之中也，屈而得之，为合，手少阴也。

"The channel-energy of the Heart Channel issues from the Zhongchong point (PC. 9), the Zhongchong point is on the tip of the middle finger, and it is called Jing Wood; from here, the channel-energy flows into Laogong point (PC. 8), the Laogong point is on the inner side of the basic joint of middle finger in the centre of the palm, and it is called Xing; from here, the channel-energy pours into the Daling point (PC. 7), the Daling point is in the cave-in between the two bones behind the palm, and it is called Shu; from here, the channel-energy passes through the Jianshi point (PC. 5), the Jianshi point is in the cave-in between the two tendons three inches behind the palm, when the associated viscus is ill, reactions will appear, and when there is no disease in the related viscus, the channel is calm, and it is called Jing; from here, the channel-energy gets into the Quze point (PC. 3), the Quze point is in the cave-in of the elbow, it can be found when the patient is bending his elbow, and it is called He. These are the five acupoints belonging to the Hand Shaoyin Channel of Heart (Pericardium).

肝出于大敦，大敦者，足大指之端及三毛之中也，为井木；溜于行间，行间，足大指间也，为荥；注于太冲，太冲，行间上二寸陷者之中也，为腧；行于中封，中封，内踝之前一寸半，陷者之中，使逆则宛，使和则通，摇足而得之，为经；入于曲泉，曲泉，辅骨之下，大筋之上也，屈膝而得之，为合，足厥阴也。

"The channel-energy of the Liver Channel issues from the Dadun point (LR. 1), the Dadun point is between the outer flank of the toe and the clump hair (hair growing in the thick cluster on the skin of the dorsal aspect of the proximal phalanges of the toe), and it is called Jing Wood; from here, the channel-enengy flows into the Xingjian point (LR. 2); the Xingjian point is in the cave-in of the artery between the toe and the second toe, and it is called Xing; from here, the channel-energy pours into the Taichong point (LR. 3), the Taichong point is in the cave-in two inches above the Xingjian point, and it is call Shu; from here, the channel-enengy passes through the Zhongfeng point (LR. 4), the Zhongfeng point is in the cave-in one inch in front of the inner ankle, when pricking it reversely, the channel-energy will be blocked, when the pricking is in harmony with it, the channel-energy will be flowing fluently, the point can be found when the patient is stretching his foot, and it is called Jing; from here, the channel-energy gets into the Ququan point (LR. 8), the Ququan point is below the fibula in the knee, above the large tendon and below the small tendon, it can be found when the patient is bendig his knee, and it is called He. These are the five acupoints belonging to the Foot Jueyin Channel of Liver.

脾出于隐白，隐白者，足大指之端内侧也，为井木；溜于大都，大都，本节之后，下陷者之中也，为荥；注于太白，太白，腕骨之下也，为腧；行于商丘，商丘，内踝之下，陷者之中也，为经；入于阴之陵泉，阴之陵泉，辅骨之下，陷者之中也，伸而得之，为合，足太阴也。

"The channel-energy of the Spleen Channel issues from the Yinbai point (SP、1), the Yinbai point is on the inner flank of the big toe, and it is called Jing Wood; from here, the channel-enengy flows into the Dadu point (SP. 2), the Dadu point is in the cave-in behind the basic joint of the big toe, and it is called Xing; from here, the channel-energy pours into the Taibai point (SP. 3), the Taibai point is below the bony nodule of the inner flank of the foot, and it is called Shu; from here, the channel-energy passes through the Shangqiu point (SP. 5), the Shangqiu point is in the cave-in below and in front of the inner ankle, and it is called Jing; from here, the channel-energy enters into the Yinlingquan point (SP. 9), the Yinlingquan point is in the cave-in below the fibula on the inner flank of the knee, it can be found when the patient is stretching his foot, and it is called He. These are the five acupoints belonging to the Foot Taiyin Channel of Spleen.

肾出于涌泉，涌泉者，足心也，为井木；溜于然谷，然谷，然骨之下者也，为荥；注于太溪，太溪，内踝之后，跟骨之上，陷中者也，为腧；行于复留，复留，上内踝二寸，动而不休，为经；入于阴谷，阴谷，辅骨之后，大筋之下，小筋之上也，按之应手，屈膝而得之，为合，足少阴经也。

"The channel-energy of the kidney issues from the Yongquan point (KI. 1), the Yongquan point is at the centre of the sole, and it is called Jing Wood; from here, the channel-energy flows into the Rangu point (KI. 2), the Rangu point is in the cave-in of the large bone in front of the inner ankle, and it is called Xing; from here, the channel-energy flows into the Taixi point (KI. 3), the Taixi point is in the cave-in of the small bone of the heel behind the inner ankle, and it is called Shu; from here, the channel-energy passes through the Fuliu point (KI. 7), the Fuliu point is two inches above the inner ankle where the artery is pulsating unceasingly, and it is called Jing; from here, the channel-energy gets into the Yingu point (KI. 10), the Yingu point is behind the fibula on the inner flank of the knee, below the large tendon and above the small tendon, which can be felt when being pressed, it can be found when the patient is bending his knee and the point is at the terminal of the horizontal line of poplitea between the two tendons, the point is called He. These are the five acupoints belonging to the Foot Shaoyin Channel of Kidney.

膀胱出于至阴，至阴者，足小指之端也，为井金；溜于通谷，通谷，本节之前外侧也，为荥；注于束骨，束骨，本节之后，陷者中也，为腧；过于京骨，京骨，足外侧大骨之下，为原；行于昆仑，昆仑，在外踝之后，跟骨之上，为经；入于委中，委中，腘中央，为合，委而取之，足太阳也。

"The channel-energy of Bladder Channel issues from the Zhiyin point (BL. 67), the Zhiyin point is on the outer flank of the little toe, and it is called Jing Metal; from here, the channel-energy flows into the Tonggu point (BL. 66), the Tonggu point is in the cave-in in front of the basic joint of the outer flank of the small toe, and it is called Xing; from here, the channel-energy pours into the Shugu point (BL. 65), the Shugu point is in the cave-in behind the basic joint in the outer flank of he small toe, and it is called Shu; from here, the channel-energy goes through the Jinggu point (BL. 64), the Jinggu point is in the cave-in on the dorso-ventral boundary of the foot below the large bone on the outer flank of the foot, and it is called Yuan; from here, the channel-energy passes through the Kunlun point (BL. 60), the Kunlun point is in the cave-in of the small bone of the heel on the outer ankle, and it is called Jing; from here, the channel-energy gets into the horizontal line of poplitea behind the knee, it can be found when the patient is bending his knee, and it is called He. These are the five acupoints belonging to the Foot Taiyang Channel of Bladder.

胆出于窍阴，窍阴者，足小指次指之端也，为井金；溜于侠溪，侠溪，足小指次指之间也，为荥；注于临泣，临泣，上行一寸半陷者中也，为腧；过于丘墟，丘墟，外踝之前下，陷者中也，为原；行于阳辅，阳辅，外踝之上，辅骨之前，及绝骨之端也，为经；入于阳之陵泉，阳之陵泉，在膝外陷者中也，为合，伸而得之，足少阳也。

"The channel-energy of the Gallbladder Channel issues from the Qiaoyin point (GB. 11), the Qiaoyin point is on the outer flank of the next toe to the small toe, and it is called Jing Metal; from here, the channel-energy flows into the Xiaxi point (GB. 43), the Xiaxi point is in the cave-in in front of the basic joint between the small toe and its next toe, and it is called Xing; from here, the channel-energy pours into the Linqi point (GB. 15), the Linqi point is in the cave-in between and behind the basic joint of the small toe and its next toe, 1.5 inches above the Xiaxi point, and it is called Shu; from here, the channel-energy goes through the Qiuxu point (GB. 40), the Qiuxu point is in the cave-in of the outer ankle, and it is called Yuan; from here, the channel-energy passes through the Yangfu point (GB. 38), the Yangfu point is on the lower end of the fibula four inches above the outer ankle, and it is called Jing; from here, the channel-energy gets into the Yanglingquan point (GB. 34), the Yangligquan point is in the cave-in of the outer fibula, one inch under the knee, it can be found when the patient is stretching his foot, and it is called He. These are the five acupoints and the source points which belong to the Foot Shaoyang Channel of Gallbladder.

胃出于厉兑，厉兑者，足大指内次指之端也，为井金；溜于内庭，内庭，次指外间也，为荥；注于陷谷，陷谷者，上中指内间上行二寸陷者中也，为腧；过于冲阳，冲阳，足跗上五寸陷者中也，为原，摇足而得之；行于解溪，解溪，上冲阳一寸半陷者中也，为经；入于下陵，下陵，膝下三寸，胻骨外三里也，为合；复下三里三寸为巨虚上廉，复下上廉三寸为巨虚下廉也，大肠属上，小肠属下，足阳明胃脉也，大肠小肠，皆属于胃，是足阳明也。

"The channel-energy of the Stomach Channel issues from the Lidui point (ST. 45), the Lidui point is on the tip of the second toe, and it is called Jing Metal; from here, the channel flows into the Neiting point (ST. 44), the Neiting point is in the cave-in of the outer flank of the second toe and it is called Xing; from here, the channel-energy pours into the Xiangu point (ST. 43), the Xiangu point is in the cave-in two inches above the Neiting point on the inner side of the middle toe, and it is called Shu; from here, the channel-energy goes through the Chongyang point (ST. 42), the Chongyang point is on the artery between the bones five inches above the dorsum, it can be found when the patient waves his foot, and it is called Yuan; from here, the channel-energy passes through the Jiexi point (ST. 41), the Jiexi point is behind the cave-in of the joint of dorsum, 1.5 inches above the Chongyang point, and it is called Jing; from here, the channel-energy gets into the Xialing point, the Xialing point is the Zusanli point (ST. 36), which is on the outer flank of the tibia three inches below the knee, and it is called He; three inches from here below, it is the Shangjuxu point (ST. 37), another three inches below is the Xiajuxu point (ST. 39), the large intestine belongs to the Shangjuxu point, the small intestine belongs to the Xiajuxu point, and they are both related with the Yangming Channel of Stomach. These are the five acupoints and the source points which belong to the Foot Yangming Channel of Stomach.

三焦者，上合手少阳，出于关冲，关冲者，手小指次指之端也，为井金；溜于液门，液门，小指次指之间也，为荥；注于中渚，中渚，本节之后陷者中也，为腧；过于阳池，阳池，在腕上陷者之中也，为原；行于支沟 支沟，上腕三寸，两骨之间陷者中也，为经；入于天井，天井，在肘外大骨之上陷者中也，为合，屈肘乃得之；三焦下腧，在于足大指之前，少阳之后，出于腘中外廉，名曰委阳，是太阳络也，手少阳经也。三焦者，足少阳太阴〔足少阳太阴之所将：《太素》卷十一无"足少阳"三字，"太阴"作"太阳"〕（一本作阳）之所将，太阳之别也，上踝五寸，别入贯腨肠，出于委阳，并太阳之正，入络膀胱，约下焦，实则闭癃，虚则遗溺，遗溺则补之，闭癃则泻之。

"The circulation of the channel-energy of the triple warmer conforms with the Hand Shaoyin Channel above, its channel issued from the Guanchong point (SJ. 1), the Guanchong point is on the tip of the ring finger beside the small finger, and it is called Jing Metal; from here, the channel-energy flows into the Yemen point (SJ. 2), the Yemen point is between the small finger and the ring finger, and it is called Xing; from here, the channel-energy flows into the Zhongzhu point (SJ. 3), the Zhongzhu point is in the cave-in between the two bones behind the small finger and the ring finger, and it is called Shu; from here, the channel-energy goes through the Yangchi point (SJ. 4), the Yangchi point is in the cave-in on the horizontal line of the wrist, and it is called Yuan; from here, the channel-energy passes through the Zhigou point (SJ. 6), the Zhigou point is in the cave-in between the two bones three inches behind the wrist, and it is called Jing; from here, the channel-energy gets into the Tianjing point (SJ. 10), the Tianjing point is above the large bone on the outer side of the elbow, it can be found when the patient is bending his elbow, and it is called He. The channel-energy of the triple warmer has another branch to connect the lower acupoint on the foot, it branches out from the outer flank of the poplitea in front of the Foot Taiyang Channel and behind the Foot Shaoyang Channel of Gallbladder, it is the Weiyang point and it is also the place where the Foot Taiyang Channel and Collaterals branch out. These are the general conditions of the five acupoints, the source points and the lower acupoint belonging to the Hand Shaoyang Channel of the Triple-warmer. The channel-energy of the Triple-warmer is connecting the Foot Taiyang channel, it is the another branch of the Foot Taiyang Channel, its channel-energy pours into the calf from the location five inches above the ankle, and comes out from the Weiyang point, and from here, it merges into the main channel of Foot Taiyang and goes inside to net the bladder and the Triple-warmer. When the Triple- warmer is sthenic, dysuria will occur, when the Triple-warmer is asthenic, the enuresis of the incontinence of urine will occur; when treating the enuresis which is of asthenic, invigorating therapy should be applied, when treating dysuria which is of sthenic, purging therapy should be applied.

手太阳〔手太阳：按“手太阳”三字，与各脏腑之文不类，应据《太素》卷十一删〕小肠者，上合手太阳，出于少泽，少泽，小指之端也，为井金；溜于前谷，前谷，在手外廉本节前陷者中也，为荥；注于后溪，后溪者，在手外侧本节之后也，为腧；过于腕骨，腕骨，在手外侧腕骨之前，为原；行于阳谷，阳谷，在锐骨之下陷者中也，为经；入于小海，小海，在肘内〔在肘内；顾《校记》云：“内”乃“外”之误字〕大骨之外，去端半寸陷者中也，伸臂〔伸臂《甲乙》卷三第二十九“伸臂”并作“屈肘”〕而得之，为合，手太阳经也。

“The circulation of the channel-energy of the Small Intestine conforms with the Hand Taiyang Channel above. Its channel-energy comes out from the Shaoze point (SI. 1), the Shaoze point is on the outer flank of the tip of the small finger, and it is called Jing Metal; from here, the channel-energy flows into the Qiangu point (SI. 2), the Qiangu point is in the cave-in in front of the basic joint on the outer flank of the small finger, and it is called Xing; from here, the channel-energy pours into the Houxi point (SI. 3), the Houxi point is in the cave-in behind the basic joint on the outer flank of the small finger, and it is called Shu; from here, the channel-energy goes through the Wangu point (SI. 4), the Wangu point is in the cave-in in front of the wrist bone on the outer flank of the hand, and it is called Yuan; from here, the channel-energy passes through the Yanggu point (SI. 5), the Yanggu point is in the cave-in below the wrist on the outer flank of the hand, and it is called Jing; from here, the channel-energy gets into the Xiaohai point (SI. 8), the Xiaohai point is in the cave-in five inches from the outer terminal of the large bone outside of the elbow, it can be found when the patient bends his elbow, and it is called He. These are the five acu-points and the source points belonging to the Hand Taiyang Channel of the Small Intestine.

大肠上合手阳明，出于商阳，商阳，大指次指之端也〔之端：《甲乙》卷三第二十七作“内侧”〕，为井金；溜于本节之前二间〔溜于本节之前二间：《太素》卷十一作“溜于二间”，二间在本节之前〕，为荥；注于本节之后三间〔注于本节之后三间：《太素》卷十一作“注于三间”，三间在本节之后〕，为腧；过于合谷，合谷，在大指岐骨〔在大指歧骨之间：《太素》卷十一“大指”下无“歧骨”二字，“指下”并有“二指”二字〕之间，为原，行于阳溪，阳溪，在两筋间陷者中也，为经；入曲池，在肘外辅骨陷者中，屈臂〔屈臂而得之：《太素》卷十一“臂”作“肘”〕而得之，为合，手阳明也。

“The circulation of the channel-energy of the large intestine conforms with the Hand Yangming Channel above. Its channel-energy issues from the Shangyang point (LI. 1), the Shangyang point is on the forefinger's inner flank beside the thumb, and it is called Jing Metal; from here, the channel-energy flows into the Erjian point (LI. 2), the Erjian point is in the cave-in in front of the basic joint on the inner flank of the forefinger, and it is called Xing; from here, the channel-energy pours into the Sanjian point (LI. 3), the Sanjian point is in the cave-in behind the basic joint on the inner flank of the forefinger, and it is called Shu; from here, the channel-energy goes through the Hegu point (LI. 4), the Hegu point is on the bone junctute between the thumb and the forefinger, and it is called Yuan; from here, the channel-energy passes through the Yangxi point, (LI. 5), the Yangxi point is in the cave-in between the two tendons on the horizontal line of the wrist, and it is called Jing;

from here, the channel-energy gets into the Quchi point (LI. 11), the Quchi point is in the cave-in in the end of the horizontal line appearing when bending the elbow on the fibula outside of the elbow, it can be found when the patient is touching his breast, and it is called He. These are the five acupoints and the source points belonging to the Hand Yangming Channel of large intestine.

是谓五脏六腑之腧，五五二十五腧，六六三十六腧也。六腑皆出足之三阳，上合于手者也。

"The acupionts stated above are: the five acopoints of Jing, Xing, Shu, Jing and He of each of the five solid organs which are altogether twnety five points, the six acupoints of Jing, Xing Shu, Yuan, Jing and He of each of the six hollow organs which are altogether thirty six points; the channel-energy of the six hollow organs issues from the Foot Taiyang, Foot Yangming and Foot Shaoyang channels, and at the same time, they conform with the three Hand Channels.

缺盆之中，任脉也，名曰天突，一。次任脉侧之动脉，足阳明也，名曰人迎，二。次脉手阳明也，名曰扶突，三。次脉手太阳也，名曰天窗，四。次脉足少阳也，名曰天容，五。次脉手少阳也，名曰天牖，六。次脉足太阳也，名曰天柱，七。次脉颈中央之脉，督脉也，名曰风府。腋内〔内："内"当作"下"，应据本经《寒热篇》改〕动脉，手太阴也，名曰天府。腋下三寸，手心主也，名曰天池。

"Right in the middle between the left and right Quepen points is the Tiantu point (RN 22) which belongs to the Ren Channel; beside it, where the artery is responding to the fingers near the Ren Channel, it is the Reying point (ST. 9) which belongs to the Foot Yangming Channel of stomach. On the further side of it, it is the Futu point (ST. 32) which belongs to th Hand Yangming Channel. On the further side of it, it is the Tianchuang point (SI. 16) which belongs to the Hand Taiyang Channel. On the further side of it, it is the Tianrong point (SI. 17) which belongs to the Foot Shaoyang Channel. On the further side of it, it is the Tianyou point (SJ. 16) which belongs to the Hand Shaoyang Channel. On the further side of it, it is the Tianzhu point (BL. 10) which belongs to the Foot Taiyang Channel. On the further side of it, in the middle of the neck, it is the Fengfu point (DU. 16) which belongs to the Du Channel. On the artery under the armpit is the Tianfu point (LU. 3). Three inches under the armpit is the Tianchi pont (PC. 1) which is controlled by the Hand shaoyin heart.

刺上关者，呿不能欠；刺下关者，欠不能呿。刺犊鼻者，屈不能伸；刺两关者，伸不能屈。

"When pricking the Shangguan point, the patient's mouth should be opened and must not be closed, when pricking the Xiaguan, the patient's mouth should be closed and must not be opened. When pricking the Dubi point, the patient's foot should be bent and must not be stretched, when pricking the Neiguan point, the patient should open his palm and must not be held.

足阳明挟喉之动脉也〔足阳明挟喉之动脉也，其腧在膺中：《太素卷》十一无此十四字〕，其腧在膺中。手阳明次在其腧外，不至曲颊一寸。手太阳当曲颊。足少阳在耳下曲颊之后。手少阳出耳后，上加完骨之上。足太阳挟项大筋之中发际。阴尺动脉在五里，五腧之禁也。

"The Renying point of the Yangming Channel is beside the Adam's apple where the artery responds the fingers. Its channel-energy descends to the front part of the chest and the Qihu point (ST. 13). The Futu point of the Hand Yangming is one inch short of reaching the curved cheek, the Tianchuang point of the Hand Taiyang Channel is right below the curved cheek, one inch behind the Futu point. The Tianchuang point of the Foot Shaoyang Channel is behind the curved cheek below the ear. The Tianyou point of the Hand shaoyang channel is behind the ear and right above it is the Wangu point (GB. 12). The Tianzhu point of the Taiyang Channel is in the cave-in outside of the large tendon by the rear hair line of the neck. The Wuli point is three inches above the elbow, it is where the chi pulse of Yin locates, it must not be pricked, if it is pricked erroneously, it will cause the visceral energy by which the acupoints transporting inside to become exhausting, so, it is a point of contraindication.

肺合大肠，大肠者，传道之腑。心合小肠，小肠者，受盛之腑。肝合胆，胆者，中精之腑。脾合胃，胃者，五谷之腑。肾合膀胱，膀胱者，津液之腑也。少阳〔少阳：《太素》卷十一，《甲乙》卷一第三，"阳"并作"阴"〕属肾，肾〔肾：《灵枢略·六气论》"肾"下有"气"字〕上连肺，故将两藏。三焦者，中〔口：孙鼎宜曰："'中'当作'四'"，形误〕渎之腑也，水道出焉，属膀胱，是孤之腑也。是六腑之所与合者。

"The lung coordinates with the large intestine, the intestine is a hollow organ for to transport the dross. The heart coordinates with the small intestine, the small intestine is a hollow organ for receiving the digested water and cereals. The liver coordinates with the gallbladder, and the gallbladder ia a clean hollow organ which rejects all the turbids. The spleen coordinates with the stomach, the stomach is a hollow organ to accommodate the water and cereals. The kidney coordinates with the bladder, the bladder is a hollow organ where the water and fluid assemble. The Shaoyin Channel belongs to the kidney, its channel energy connects the lung above, so, the energy of the kidney channel passes through the viscera of bladder and lung. The hollow organ of the triple warmer is like a water gutter which leads to all sides, it dredges the water and connects the bladder below, as it has no coordinating viscus, it is called the solitary hollow organ. These are the coordinate relations between the six hollow organs and the five solid organs.

春取络脉诸荥大经分肉之间，甚者深取之，间者浅取之。夏取诸腧孙络肌肉皮肤之上。秋取诸合，余如春法。冬取诸井诸腧之分，欲深而留之。此四时之序，气之所处，病之所舍，藏之所宜。转筋者，立而取之，可令遂已。痿厥者，张而刺之，可令立快也。

"In spring, it should prick the the collaterals on the superficies and the spaces between various Xing points, large tendons and muscles, prick deeply when the disease is severe, and prick shallowly when the disease is slight. In summer, it should prick the Shu points of the twelve channels and the shallow parts of muscles and skin. In autumn, it should prick the He points of the twelve channels, other things in pricking should like that in spring. In winter, it should prick the Jing points of the twelve channels and the Shu points of the hollow and solid organs, the pricking should be deep and the needle should be retained. These are the most proper places for adapting the sequence of the weather change of the four seasons, the locations where the channel energy concentrates and the sites of diseases in various seasons. As to treating the patient with constriction of the muscles, the patient must be standing upright when pricking, and the disease can be recovered very soon. To the patient of muscular flaccidity and coldness of extremities, the patient should lie down, and he will feel easy after pricking."

小针解第三

Chapter 3
Xiao Zheng Jie
(Explanation on Small Needle)

所谓易陈者，易言也。难入者，难著于人也。粗守形者，守刺法也。上守神者，守人之血气有余不足，可补泻也。神客者，正邪共会也。神者，正气也。客者，邪气也。在门者，邪循正气之所出入也。未睹其疾者，先知邪正何经之疾也。恶知其原者，先知何经之病，所取之处也。

The so called "easy to relate" means it is easy to talk about the disease. The so called "hard to enter" means a common man can hardly understand clearly the subtleness of the disease. The so called "the physician of lower level adheres to the outer appearance" means a physician of lower level can only treat according to the routine of pricking. The so called "the physician of advanced level treats according to the essentials of the disease" means a superior physician can perceive the sthenic or asthenic conditions of the patient to determine the treating of invigorating or purging. The so called "spirit and guest" means the co-existence of the healthy energy and the evil energy in the channel. The so called "spirit" means the healthy energy, and "guest" means the evil energy. The so called "by the door" means the evil energy comes in and goes out along with the healthy energy through the striae. The so called "missing the disease" means the physician has no idea where the disease is. The so called " how can the source of the disease be known?" means how can one know to which channel the disease belongs and with which acupoint should the disease be treated.

刺之微在数迟者，徐疾之意也。粗守关者，守四肢而不知血气正邪之往来也。上守机者，知守气也。机之动，不离其空中者，知气之虚实，用针之徐疾也。空中之机，清净以微者，针以得气，密意守气勿失也。其来不可逢者，气盛不可补也。其往不可追者，气虚不可泻也。不可挂以发者，言气易失也。扣之不发者，言不知补泻之意也，血气已尽而气〔而气不下：“气”似应作“病”〕不下也。

The so called "the clue of pricking is in the speed" means it is important to master the fast and slow speed of inserting and drawing the needle. The so called " the physician of lower level sticks to the joint" means a physician of lower level adheres only to the pricking acupoints on the extremities without knowing the abundant or deficient energy condition, the coming and going of the blood and the healthy energy. The so called " a superior physician accords with the mechanism of the disease" means a physician of advanced level knows the general rule of the change of the functional activities of vital energy so that he can invigorate or purge properly by pricking. The so called "in treating the different conditions of the vital energy, it can not divorce from invigoration and purging" means one must know first the abundance or deficiency of the energy in the acupoint, then can he apply the therapy of invigoration or purging. The so called "be sure to examine the energy carefully and calmly" means examine the coming and going of the energy carefully after getting the acupuncture feeling so as not to miss the opportunity of invigorating or purging. The so called "do not oppose diametrically the energy that is coming" means one must not invigorate when the evil energy is overabundant. The so called "do not pursue the energy that is going" means do not purge when the healthy energy is debilitative. The so called "one must not make light of the acupuncture feeling" means the feeling of acupuncture after pricking can easily fade away. The so called "fails to shoot out as if the arrow is fastened on the bow string" means when one knows not the meaning of invigorating and purging and prick erroneously, it will cause the energy and blood to become exhausting and the discease will not be cured.

知其往来者，知气之逆顺盛虚也。要与之期者，知气之可取之时也。粗之暗者，冥冥不知气之微密也。妙哉！工独有之者，尽知针意也。往者为逆者，言气之虚而小，小者逆也。来者为顺者，言形气之平，平者顺也。明知逆顺，正行无问者，言知所取之处也。迎而夺之者，泻也。追而济之者，补也。

The so called "knowing the coming and the going of the energy" means knowing the adverse and agreeable, deficient and abundant condititons of the energy which is in circulation. The so called "the time of pricking is important" means when one knows the importance of the waiting of energy, he will be able to know the proper time of pricking. The so called " the ignorance of the physician of lower level" means the physician of lower level is ignorant who knows not the subtle function of the energy's circulation. The so called "only a superior physician can treat wonderfully" means a superior physician understands thoroughly the way of pricking and the importance of waiting the energy. The so called " when the energy has gone, it is adverse" means the energy will become debilitative and tiny when the evil energy has faded away, and tiny means adverse. The so called " when the energy comes it is agreeable" means when the healthy energy comes gradually, it is harmonious and calm, and harmonious and calm means agreeable. The so called" when knowing the conditions of agreeable and adverse clearly, one can prick without asking others" means when one understands the agreeable and adverse relation of the energy's circulation, he can select the proper acupoint without hesitating. The so called " snatch against it" means prick against the direction of the channel's circulation and it is the purging therapy. The so called "assist along with it" means to prick in the direction similar with the channel's circulation, and it is the invigorating therapy.

所谓虚则实之者，气口虚而当补之也。满则泄之者，气口盛而当泻之也。宛陈则除之者，去血脉也。邪胜则虚之者，言诸经有盛者，皆泻其邪也。徐而疾则实者，言徐内而疾出也。疾而徐则虚者，言疾内而徐出也。言实与虚，若有若无者，言实者有气，虚者无气也。察后与先，若亡若存者，言气之虚实，补泻之先后也，察其气之已下与常存也。为虚与实，若得若失者，言补者佖然若有得也，泻则怳然若有失也。

The so called "substantialize when it is deficient" means apply the invigorating therapy by pricking when the energy of Cunkou (the common position for pulse palpation) is deficient. The so called " purge when it is full" means apply purging therapy by pricking when the energy on Cunkou is overabundant. The so called "eliminate the protracted stagnation" means it should remove the stagnated blood in the collaterals. The so called "when the evil energy is excessive, empty it" means when the evil energy is abundant in the channel, purging therapy should be applied to let out the evil energy along with the needle. The so called "to invigorate with the slow and swift pricking" means when applying the invigorting therapy, insert the needle slowy and draw swiftly. The so called " to purge with the swift and slow pricking" means when applying the purging therapy, insert the needle swiftly and draw slowly. The so called "the sthenia and the asthenia are like being and not being" means the invigorating can cause the retaliating of the healthy energy, and the purging can cause the disappearing of the evil energy. The so called"take note of the pricking order and observe the existing and not existing of the evil energy" means diagnose to know the sthenia and asthenia of the energy to ascertain the order of the invigorating and purging, and examine whether the evil energy has retreated or still retaining. The so called "the sthenia and asthenia can cause gain and loss" means the patient feels fullness as if acquiring something when being invigorated, and feels like losing something when being purged.

夫气之在脉也，邪气在上者，言邪气之中人也高，故邪气在上也。浊气在中者，言水谷皆入于胃，其精气上注于肺，浊溜于肠胃，言寒温不适，饮食不节，而病生于肠胃，故命曰浊气在中也。清气在下者，言清湿地气之中人也，必从足始，故曰清气在下也。针陷脉则邪气出者，取之上。针中脉则浊气出者，取之阳明合也。针太深则邪气反沉者，言浅浮之病，不欲深刺也，深则邪气从之入，故曰反沉也。皮肉筋脉各有所处者，言经络各有所主也。取五脉者死，言病在中，气不足，但用针尽大泻其诸阴之脉也。取三阳之脉者，唯言尽泻三阳之气，令病人恇然不复也。夺阴者死，言取尺之五里五往者也。夺阳者狂，正言也。

The so called "when the energy is in the channel, the evil energy is above" means after the invasion of evil energy to the channel, the wind-heat injures the head most probably, so it is the evil energy above. The so called "the turbid energy is in the middle" means after the water and cereals enter into the stomach, their refined energy pours into the lung above, and the thick and turbid part remains in the stomach and abdomen, if cold and heat is encountered, and the patient can not practise temperance in eating and drinking, the disease of the stomach and the intestine will occur, so, it is the turbid energy in the middle. The so called "the lucid enegy is on below. " means when cold, cool or wet energy causes the disease, it initiates from the foot, so, it is called the lucid energy is on below. The so called " when prick the channels on the head, the evil energy will come out" means when the evil energy of wind-heat injures the upper part of a man, it should prick the acupoints on the head, and the evil energy will be let out. The so called"when the needle hits the channel, the turbid energy will come out" means prick Zusanli which is the He point of the stomach channel to treat the disease caused by the turbid energy of stomach and intestine. The so called "when the pricking is too deep, the evil energy will, on the contrary, become sunken" means to the disease of which its evil energy is on a shallow position, do not prick deeply, otherwise, it will, cause the evil energy to penetrate inside, so, it is on the contrary to become sunken. The so called "the skin, muscle, tendon and channel are having their regular position" means the skin, muscle, tendon are on their regular positions respectively, and there are the definite positions in the channels and collaterals for treating the various diseases. The so called "the patient will die when the five-channel is pricked" means when the disease is in the five viscera and the patient's primordial energy is deficient, if excessive purging is applied by pricking the acupoints of the five viscera, the patient will die. The so called "prick the three channels" means when one spares no effort to purge the energy of the acupoints of the six hollow organs, it will cause the patient to turn cowardly and can hardly be recovered. The so called "when Yin is seized, the patient will die" means when pricking the Wuli point which is behind the Chize point to purge for five times, the Yin energy in the five viscera will be exhausted, and the patient will die. The so called "when Yang is seized, the patient will die" means when the energies of the three Yang channel of the six hollow organs are purged greatly, it will cause the mental change of the patient and mania will occur.

睹其色，察其目、知其散复，一其形、听其动静者，言上工知相五色于目，有知调尺寸小大缓急滑涩，以言所病也。知其邪正者，知论虚邪与正邪之风也。右主推之、左持而御之者，言持针而出入也。气至而去之者，言补泻气调而去之也。调气在于终始一者，持心也。节之交三百六十五会者，络脉之渗灌诸节者也。

The so called "watch the complexion and examine the eyes of the patient to know the dispersion and assembling of the disease and apprehend the changes of the channels by palpation" means a superior physician not only knows how to inspect the complexion and the change of eye-lustre of the patient, but can also observe the large or small, slow or rapid, slippery or choppy pulse conditions on the position of the skin of anterolateral side of the forearm and Cunkou, so that to understand the pathogenesis. The so called "to know the debilitating evil and the wind evil" means to know whether the patient has contracted the debilitating evil or the wind-evil. The so called " insert with the right hand and guard with the left hand" indicates the different actions in inserting and drawing the needle. The so called "relinquish when the energy has arrived" means when the functional activities of vital energy has become harmonious after invigorating or purging, the pricking should be stopped. The so called "when adjusting the energy, be concentrated from the beginning to the end" means when the physician is adjusting the energy with the needle, he must keep his mind concentrative and not to excrete his spirit. The so called "the three hundred and sixty five points on the junctures" means the three hundred and sixty five acupoints are the places for the energy and blood of the channels and collaterals to permeate the various joints.

所谓五脏之气已绝于内者，脉口气内绝不至，反取其外之病处与阳经之合，有留针以致阳气，阳气至则内重竭，重竭则死矣，其死也无气以动，故静。所谓五脏之气已绝于外者，脉口气外绝不至，反取其四末之输，有留针以致其阴气，阴气至则阳气反入，入则逆，逆则死矣，其死也阴气有余，故躁。所以察其目者，五脏使五色循明，循明则声章，声章者，则言声与平生异也。

The so called "the energy of the five-viscera is exhausted inside" means when the pulse condition is week, floating and asthenic, as if the pulse is not existing when palpating, if the asthenic Yin syndrome is treated, on the contrary, by pricking the superficies of the focus and the He points of the Yang channel, and also retains the needle to induce the Yang energy, The Yin energy will become even exhausting inside when the Yang energy comes, as the Yin energy is exhausting again and again, the patient will certainly die.

The so called "the energy of the five-viscera is exhausted outside" means when the pulse condition is sunken and tiny as if the pulse is not existing when palpating lightly, if treat, on the contrary, by pricking the acupoints on the tips of the extremities, and also retains the needle to induce the Yin energy, the Yang energy will be bogged down when the Yin energy arrives, and when the Yang energy bogs down, the diesase of Jueni will occur and cause death of the patient. This is due to the Ying energy is having a surplus.

The reason of examining the eyes is that the refined energy of the five-viscera can cause the five colours of the complexion and the eyes to become clear and bright, it also causes one to have a loud and prominent voice. The loud and prominent voice means the voice which is different from ordinary.

邪气脏腑病形第四

Chapter 4
Xie Qi Zang Fu Bing xing
(The Visceral Diseases Caused by Evil Energy)

黄帝问于岐伯曰：邪气之中人也奈何？岐伯答曰：邪气之中人高〔高也：《医学纲目》卷一《五脏类》“高”下有“下”字〕也。黄帝曰：高下有度乎？岐伯曰：身半已上者，邪中之也；身半已下者，湿中之也。故曰：邪之中人也，无有常，中于阴则溜于腑，中于阳则溜于经。

Yellow Emperor asked Qibo and said: “What is the condition when the exogenous evil invades a man?” Qibo answered: “It depends on whether the invasion is in the upper part or in the lower part.” Yellow Emperor asked: “Is there any difference when invading the upper part and the lower part?” Qibo said: “When the upper part of the body contracts the disease, it is caused by the wind-cold and the exogenous evil, when the lower part of the body contracts disease, it is caused by the wetness-evil, thus, when the exogenous evil invades the body, it is not necessary in a fixed way. When the exogenous evil invades the Yin channel, it can be transmitted to the six hollow organs, when the exogenous evil invades the Yang channel, it can cause diseases on the location along the route where the Yang channel passes.”

黄帝曰：阴之与阳也，异名同类，上下相会，经络之相贯，如环无端。邪之中人，或中于阴，或中于阳，上下左右，无有恒常，其故何也？

Yellow Emperor said: “Although the Yang channel and the Yin channel are different in names, yet they all belong to the system of the channel and collateral, they connect each other in the upper part and the lower part, and the channel and the collaterals are linking to become an entirety like a ring without end. But when the evil injures a man, some are on the Yin channel and some are on the Yang channel; sometimes the disease is in the upper part, sometimes it is in the lower part, sometimes it is on the left side, and sometims it is on the right side, and what is the reason?”

岐伯曰：诸阳之会，皆在于面。中人也〔中人也：孙鼎宜曰：“‘中人’上当脱‘邪之’二字〕，方乘虚时，及新用力，若饮食汗出〔若饮食汗出：《太素》卷二十七《邪中》“若”后并有“热”字〕腠理开，而中于邪。中于面则下阳明，中于项则下太阳，中于颊则下少阳，其中于膺背两胁亦中〔亦中其经：史崧《音释》云：“一本作下其经”〕其经。

Qibo answered: “The three Yang channels of hand and foot are converging on the face and head. The evil energy often takes the advantage to invade when the body is in debility, fatigue right after hard labour and perspiration after taking hot food and drink when the striae of skin are open. When the face is hit by the evil energy, it will shift down to the Foot

Yangming Channel of stomach. When its neck is hit by the evil energy, it will shift down to the Foot Taiyang Channel of bladder. When the cheek is hit by the evil energy, it will shift down to the Foot Shaoyang Channel of gallbladder. If the chest, back and the hypochondria are hit by the evil energies, they will shift down to the subordinative Yangming Channel, Taiyin Channel and Shaoyang Channel respectively."

黄帝曰：其中于阴奈何？岐伯答曰：中于阴者，常从臂胻始。夫臂与胻，其阴，皮薄，其肉淖泽，故俱受于风，独伤其阴。

Yellow Emperor asked: "What is the condition when the Yin channel is invaded by the evil energy?" Qibo answered: "When the evil energy hits the Yin channel, the disease often starts from the arm and the leg. As the arm humerus and the leg tibia are on the inner side where the skin is thinner and the muscle is softer, so, when the body contracts the evil energy, it is the Yin channel that is apt to be injured."

黄帝曰：此故伤其脏乎？岐伯答曰：身之中于风也，不必动脏。故邪入于阴经，则其脏气实，邪气入而不能客，故还之于腑。故中阳则溜于经，中阴则溜于腑。

Yellow Emperor asked: "Can the evil energy injure the five-viscera?" Qibo answered: "When one contracts the evil energy, the five-viscera is not necessary to be injured, if the Yin channel is invaded by the exogenous evil, and the visceral energy of the patient has been substantial all the time, the evil energy can by no means to retain in the viscera, and it can not but return to the six-hollow-organ. Therefore, when the Yang channel is invaded by the evil energy, it will retain in the related channel and cause disease, when the Yin channel is invaded by the evil energy, it will retain in the six-hollow-organ and cause disease."

黄帝曰：邪之中人脏，奈何？岐伯曰：愁忧恐惧〔愁忧恐惧：《难经·四十九难》作"忧愁思虑"〕则伤心。形寒寒饮则伤肺，以其两寒相感，中外皆伤，故气逆而上行。有所堕坠，恶血留内；若有所大怒，气上而不下，积于胁下，则伤肝。有所击仆，若醉入房，汗出当风，则伤脾。有所用力举重，若入房过度，汗出浴水，则伤肾。黄帝曰：五脏之中风奈何？岐伯曰：阴阳俱感，邪乃得往，黄帝曰：善哉。

Yellow Emperor asked: "some evil energies can injure the five-viscera, and what is the reason?" Qibo said: " Melancholy and anxiety can injure the heart. When the body catches cold and the cold water is drunken, the lung will be injured, as the two kinds of cold-evil can injure both the interior and the exterior, the disease of up-reversing of the lung energy will occur. If one falls from a high place causing the stagnated blood to retain inside or the patient flies into a fury, causing the vital energy rushes up without descending, the energy will be stagnating under the hypochondria and injures the liver. When one falls down or being hit, and he also fails to practise temperance in eating an drinkng, or being overstrained in labour, his spleen will be injured. When one lifts the weight with difficulty, conducts sexual activities excessively or takes a bath or soaks in the water after sweating, his kidney will be injured." Yellow Emperor asked: "Why is it that the five-solid organs can be injured by the wind-evil? Qibo said: "Both the solid organs and the hollow orgons can be invaded, but it is only the external evil and the internal evil can cause the retention of the disease." Yellow

Emperor said: "Good."

黄帝问于岐伯曰：首面与身形也，属骨连筋，同血合于气耳。天寒则裂地凌冰，其卒寒或手足懈惰，然而其面不衣何也？岐伯答曰：十二经脉，三百六十五络，其血气皆上于面而走空窍，其精阳气上走于目而为睛，其别气走于耳而为听，其宗气上出于鼻而为臭，其浊气出于胃，走唇舌而为味。其气之津液皆上熏于面，而皮〔而皮：《太素》卷二十七《邪中》"而"作"面"〕又厚，其肉坚，故天气〔故天气"胡本、熊本、周本、藏本，"气"并作"热"〕甚，寒不能胜之也。

Yellow Emperor asked Qibo and said: "The head, face and the whole body are connecting the bone, tendon, blood and energy. In the cold season when the earth is frozen to become cracking, and the ice is accumulating, if the weather becomes even more cold suddenly, the hands and feet of a man will be shivering with cold and reluctant to move about, but the face is not necessary to be covered with clothes to keep away from the cold, and what is the reason?" Qibo answered: "The circulation of energy and blood in the twelve channels and the three hundred and sixty five collaterals are reaching the head and face first, and then enter into the various apertures. The refined energy pours up in to the eyes to enable the sight seeing. The channel energy moves aside reaching the ears below to enable the hearing. The air being sent to the nose to enable the smelling. The essential substance from cereals produces from stomach reaches up to contact the lips and tongue to enable the tasting. All the fluids of the energies can rise up to fumigate the face which is thick with firm muscle. As the Yang on the face is very hot, it can not be surpassed by the cold weather."

黄帝曰：邪之中人，其病形何如？岐伯曰：虚邪之中身也，洒淅动形。正邪之中人也微，先见于色，不知于身，若有若无，若亡若存，有形无形，莫知其情。黄帝曰：善哉。

Yellow Emperor asked: "what is the pathosis when the evil energy invades a man?" Qibo said: "When the asthenic evil injures a man, the patient will have shivers and chilliness. When the wind of the four seasons injures a man, the disease is light, the patient appears to have slight change in the complexion, but his body is normal, it seems the disease has already disappeared yet seems the disease is still remaining inside; it seems that the patient is having a disease and seems to have no disease, and the condition of the disease can hardly be known." Yellow Emperor said: "Good."

黄帝问于岐伯曰：余闻之，见其色，知其病，命曰明；按其脉，知其病，命曰神；问其病，知其处，命曰工。余愿闻见而知之，按而得之，问而极之，为之奈何？岐伯答曰：夫色脉与尺之〔夫色脉与尺之：《甲乙》卷四第二上"之"下有"皮肤"二字〕相应也，如桴鼓影响之相应也，为之奈何？岐伯答曰：夫色脉与尺之相应也，如桴鼓影响之相应也，不得相失也，此亦本末根叶之出候也，故根死则叶枯矣。色脉形肉不得相失也，故知一则为工，知二则为神，知三则神且明矣。

Yellow Emperor asked Qibo: "I am told when a physician can know the pathosis of the patient by examining his complexion, it is called explicitness; when he can know the pathosis of the patient by palpating, it is called marvelousness; when one can know the pathosis of the patient by inquiring and hearing the patient's anamnesis, it is called skillfulness. I like to know why is it that the disease's condition can be known by examining the complexion, the pathosis can be known by palpation, and the location of the disease can be known by inquiring?" Qibo answered: " There are corresponding relations between the patient's complexion, pulse condition and the skin of anterolateral side of the forearm and the disease, they are like the responding sound when the drum is hit by the drumstick which can by no means fail to sound. They are correlated like the root and stem of a tree with its branches and leaves, but the diagnosis must not be identical with the common method, when the root dies, the leaves will be withered. Thus, none of the three aspects of the complexion examining, the pulse palpating and the skin of anterolateral side of the forearm diagnosing should be excluded. When one knows one aspect, he is skillful, when one knows two aspects he is marvelous, when one knows three aspects, he is an ingenious and ingenious physician. "

黄帝曰：愿卒闻之。岐伯答曰：色青者，其脉弦也；赤者，其脉钩也；黄者，其脉代也；白者，其脉毛；黑者，其脉石。见其色而不得其脉，反得其相胜之脉，则死矣；得其相生之脉，则病已矣。

Yellow Emperor said; "I hope to hear your explanation about the complexion and the pulse. " Qibo said: "When the complexion is green, the pulse condition should be wiry; when the complexion is red, the pulse condition should be hooked; when the complexion is yellow, the pulse condition should be intermittent; when the complexion is white, the pulse condition should be floating and slippery; when the complexion is black, the pulse condition should be stony. These are the regular patterns of the corespondances of the complexions and pulses. When the complexion is not in conformity with the pulse condition, and when, on the contrary, a subjugating pulse condition is seen, the patint will die; but when a producing pulse condition is seen, the disease of the patient will be cured. "

黄帝问于岐伯曰：五脏之所生，变化之病形何如？岐伯答曰：先定其五色五脉之应，其病乃可别也。黄帝曰：色脉已定，别之奈何？岐伯曰：调其脉之缓、急、小、大、滑、涩，而病变定矣。

Yellow Emperor asked Qibo: "What are the changes and the appearance of the disease caused by the five-viscera?" Qibo answered: "It must ascertain first the correspondant relation between the five-colour of complexion and the five-condition of pules, then can the disease be distinguished. " Yellow Emperor asked: "How can one distinguish the disease's condition after the complexion and the pulse condition are ascertained?" Qibo answered: "When the slow or urgent, gigantic or small, slippery or choppy pulse condition is found after examining, the pathosis can be ascertained. "

黄帝曰：调之奈何？岐伯答曰：脉急者，尺之皮肤亦急；脉缓者，尺之皮肤亦缓；脉小者，尺之皮肤亦减而少气；脉大者，尺之皮肤亦贲而起；脉滑者，尺之皮肤亦滑；脉涩者，尺之皮肤亦涩，凡此变者，有微有甚。故善调尺者，不待于寸，善调脉者，不待于色。能参合而行之者，可以为上工，上工十全九；行二者，为中工，中工十全七；行一者，为下工，下工十全六。

Yellow Emperor asked: "How to examine the changes of the pulse conditions and the skin of anterolateral side of the forearm?" Qibo said: "When the pulse is urgent, and the skin of anterolateral side of the forearm is also pressing, when the pulse is slow and the skin of anterolateral side of the forearm is also thin and deficient, when the pulse is gigantic and the skin of anterolateral side of the forearm is also large and protruding, when the pulse is slippery and the skin of anterolateral side of the forearm is also slippery, when the pulse is choppy and the skin of anterolateral side of the forearm is also choppy. In all the six kinds of changes, some are obscure and some are quite obvious. Thus, he who is good at examining the skin of anterolateral side of the forearm needs not wait until the palpation of the Cunkou pulse and he who is good at examining the pulse condition needs not wait until examining the patient's complexion. When a physician can diagnose according to the three aspects of examining the complexion, palpating the pulse and inspecting the skin of anterolateral of the forearm, he is supposed to be a superior physician, and he can cure nine patients out of ten; when one can diagnose according to two aspects, he is supposed to be a physician of medium level, and he can cure seven patients out of ten; when one can diagnose according to one aspect only, he is supposed to be a physician of lower level, and he can cure six patients out of ten."

黄帝曰：请问脉之缓、急、小、大、滑、涩之病形何如？岐伯曰：臣请言五脏之病变也。心脉急甚者为瘛疭；微急为心痛引背，食不下。缓甚为狂笑；微缓为伏梁，在心下，上下行，时唾血。大甚为喉吤；微大为心痹引背，善泪出。小甚为善哕，微小为消瘅。滑甚为善渴；微滑为心疝引脐，小腹鸣。涩甚为瘖；微涩为血溢，维厥，耳鸣，颠疾。

Yellow Emperor asked: "What is the pathosis when the pulse condition is slow, urgent, small, gigantic, slippery and choppy respectively?" Qibo said: "I will comment from the pathosis of the five viscera: when the heart pulse is very urgent, muscular spasm will occur; when it is slighly urgent, heartache drawing the back and the syndrome of the patient can hardly take in the food will occur. When the heart pulse is very slow, uneasiness and boisterous laughing will occur; when it is slightly slow, the disease of fuliang (disease with epigastric fullness and mass due to stagnation of vital energy and blood) will occur, its energy can move upwards or downwards, and sometimes, it causes the patient to spit blood. When the heart pulse is gigantic, the patient feels like a sting obstructing in the throat, when it is slightly gigantic, the cardiac bi-syndrome with pain drawing the back will occur, and the tears of the patient fall often. When the heart pulse is very small, hiccup of the patient will occur, when it is small, diabetes will occur. When the heart pulse is very slippery, the patient will be very thirsty, when it is slightly slippery, heart-channel colic with pain drawing the naval and causing sound in the lower abdomen will occur, When the heart pulse is very choppy, the patient will become dumb, when it is slightly choppy, the spitting blood, hemorrhage and reverseness of the Yang pulse causing tinnitus and headache will occur.

肺脉急甚为癫疾；微急为肺寒热，怠惰咳唾血，引腰背胸，若鼻息肉不通。缓甚为多汗；微缓为痿瘘、偏风，头以下汗出不可止。大甚为胫肿；微大为肺痹，引胸背起，恶日光。小甚为泄，微小为消瘅。滑甚为息贲上气，微滑为上下出血。涩甚为呕血；微涩为鼠瘘，在颈支腋之间，下不胜其上，其应善痠矣。

“When the lung pulse is very urgent，‘dian disease’ on head will occur，when it is slightly urgent，cold and heat syndrome will occur，the patient will be tired and weak，spitting blood，becoming uncomfortable with pain drawing the loins，back and chest，and is troubled by the wart obstructing the nose. When the lung pulse is very slow，the patient will have hidrosis，when it is slightly slow，the syndroms of flaccidity，omalgia and unceasing sweating below the head will occur. When the lung pulse is very gigantic，swelling of the foot tibia will occur，when it is slightly gigantic，the lung-bi-syndrome drawing the chest and back to become uneasy will occur，and the patient detests the sunlight. When the lung pulse is very small，diarrhea will occur，when it is slightly small，diabetes will occur. When the lung pulse is very slippery，rapid respiration and the reversing of the lung energy will occur，when it is slight slippery，hemorrhage of mouth，nose，the front private part and the anus will occur. When the lung pulse is very choppy，hematemesis will occur，when it is slightly choppy，scrofula on the neck or under the armpit，and the pulse condition of asthenia in the lower part which can not withstand the sthenia in the upper part will occur；as metal can subjugate wood，the patient likes to take the sour taste extremely.

肝脉急甚者为恶言〔恶言：《甲乙》卷四第二下校注“恶言”一作“忘言”，按“忘”误，应据《千金》改作“妄”〕；微急为肥气，在〔在《难经·五十六难》“在”下并有“左”字〕胁下如覆杯。缓甚为善呕，微缓为水瘕痹也。大甚为内痈，善呕衄；微大为肝痹，阴缩，咳引小腹。小甚为多饮，微小为消瘅。滑甚为㿗疝，微滑为遗溺。涩甚为溢饮，微涩为瘛挛筋痹。

When the liver pulse is very urgent，the mood of the patient will become abnormal and he talks rashly and talks nonsense，when it is slightly urgent，swelling mass due to the stagnation of lung like a bottom-up cup under the left hypochondrium will occur. When the lung pulse is very slow，vomiting will occur，when it is slightly slow，bi-syndrome due to accumulation of fluid will occur. When the liver pulse is very gigantic，internal carbuncle，often vomiting and epistaxis will occur，when it is slightly gigantic，hepatic bi-syndrome will occur，and the patient will have shrinkage of the external genitals and will feel pain in the lower abdomen when being drawn by coughing. When the liver pulse is very small，the patient will be thirsty and will drink a lot，when it is slightty small，the patient will eat a lot but often hungry and has the syndrome of muscular emaciation. When the liver pulse is very slippery，the scrotum will be swelling，when it is slightly slippery，enuresis will occur. When the liver pulse is very choppy，phlegm-retention syndrome will occur，when it is slightly choppy，convulsion and contracture of the muscle will occur.

脾脉急甚为瘛疭；微急为膈中，食饮入而还出，后沃沫。缓甚为痿厥；微缓为风痿，四肢不用，心慧然若无病。大甚为击仆；微大为疝〔疝：《脉经》卷三第三作“痞”〕气，腹裹大脓血，在肠胃之外。小甚为寒热，微小为消瘅。滑甚为㿗癃，微滑为虫毒蛕蝎腹热。涩甚为肠㿗；微涩为内溃，多下脓血。

“When the spleen pulse is very urgent，convulsion of the extremities will occur，when it is slightly urgent, vomiting after food intake and thick foam in stool will occur. When the spleen pulse is very slow, the four limbs will be weak and cold, when it is slightly slow, flaccidity caused by wind evil and inconvenient of moving the extremities will occur, but the patient is quite clear and seems to have no disease. When the spleen pulse is very gigantic, the patient will fall all of a sudden due to coma, when it is slightly gigantic, the syndrome of piqi (mass formation due to asthenia of the spleen and stagnation of vital energy) wrapping with a lot of pus and blood outside of the intestine and stomach will occur. When the spleen pulse is very small, the syndrome of cold and heat will occur, when it is slightly small, emaciation of muscle will occur. When the spleen pulse is very slippery, the scrotum will be swelling and dysuria will occur, when it is slightly slippery, various parasitic infestation will occur, and the patient feels hot in the abdomen. When the spleen pulse is very choppy, gynecopathy of a woman will occur, when it is slightly choppy, internal ulcer and bloody stool will occur.

肾脉急甚为骨癫疾；微急为沉厥奔豚〔沉厥奔豚：《太素》卷十五《五脏脉诊》无“奔豚”二字〕，足不收，不得前后。缓甚为折脊；微缓为洞，洞者，食不化，下嗌还出。大甚为阴痿；微大为石水，起脐以下至小腹腄腄然，上至胃脘，死不治。小甚为洞泄，微小为消瘅。滑甚为癃㿉；微滑为骨痿，坐不能起，起则目无所见。涩甚为大痈，微涩为不月沉痔。

"When the kidney pulse is very urgent, flaccidity-syndrome involving the bone and "dian disease" (disease on head) will occur, when it is slightly urgent, the patient will feel heavy and cold of feet which can hardly be stretched and bent, and he will have retention of feces and urine. When the kidney pulse is very slow, the spine of the patient will be painful like being broken, when it is slightly slow, dong-disease of which the food can not be digested and vomit after intake will occur. When the kidney pulse is very gigantic, impotence will occur, when it is slightly gigantic, indurated edema which causes swelling from under the navel to the lower abdomed will occur, if the swelling reaches the gastric cavity, the patient will by no means to be cured and die, When the kidney pulse is very small, diarrhea out of control will occur when it is slightly small, diabetes will occur. When the kidney pulse is very slippery, dysuria and swelling of the scrotum will occur, when it is slightly slipery, flaccidity-syndrome involving the bone will occur, the patient can not get up after sitting down, and sees nothing when he gets up. When the kidney pulse is very choppy, large carbuncle will occur, when it is slightly choppy, internal hemorrhoid and menoxenia of a woman will occur."

黄帝曰：病之六变者，刺之奈何？岐伯答曰：诸急者多寒；缓者多热；大者多气少血；小者血气皆少；滑者阳气盛，微有热；涩者多血〔多血：“多”误，应作“少”〕少气，微有寒。是故刺急者，深内而久留之。刺缓者，浅内而疾发针，以去其热。刺大者，微泻其气，无出其血。刺滑者，疾发针而浅内之，以泻其阳气而去其热。刺涩者，必中其脉，随其逆顺而久留之，必先按而循之，已发针，疾按其痏，无令其血出，以和其脉。诸小者，阴阳形气俱不足，勿取以针，而调以甘药之。

Yellow Emperor asked: "How to treat the six kinds of pulse conditions caused by various diseases by pricking?" Qibo answered: "When the pulse condition is urgent, it is mostly pertaining to the cold; when the pulse condition is slow, it is mostly pertaining to the heat, when the pulse condition is gigantic, it is mostly pertaining to the energy which is having a surplus and the blood which is deficient; when the pules condition is small, it is mostly pertaining to the deficiency of both the energy and the blood; when the pulse condition is slippery, it is due to the abundant Yang energy with slight hotness; when the pulse condition is choppy, it is due to the deficiency of energy and blood with slight cold. Thus, when pricking the disease with urgent pulse, the pricking should be deeper and the needle retention should be longer. When pricking the disease with slow pulse, the pricking should be shallow, and the pulling out of the needle should be swift. When pricking the disease with gigantic pulse, the energy can be let out slightly, but the bleeding is not permissible. When pricking the disease with slippery pulse, the insertion should be swift and the pricking should be shallow so as the Yang can be purged and the heat-evil can be removed. When pricking the disease with choppy pulse, the channel must be hit, manipulate the needle according to the agreeable or adverse direction movement of the energy and the retention of the needle should be longer, press in advance the route of the energy circulation to make the energy to become smooth, press and knead the needle hole immediately after the pulling of the needle to stop the bleeding and adjust the channel. To the disease of small pulse condition, and the patient is weak in Yin, Yang, physique and energy, pricking is not advisable, it may be treated with medicine of mild nature."

黄帝曰：余闻五脏六腑〔五脏六腑：孙鼎宜曰："五脏"二字衍。〕之气，荥输所入为合，令〔令：《太素》卷十一《腑病合输》作"今"〕何道从入，入安连过〔连过：《甲乙》卷四第二下作"从道"〕，愿闻其故。岐伯答曰：此阳脉之别入于内，属于腑者也。黄帝曰：荥输与合，各有名乎。岐伯答曰：荥输治外经，合治内腑。

Yellow Emperor said: "I am told that the channel-energy of the six hollow organs enters into the He point from the Xing point, through which channel does it enter into the He point? After the energy enters into the channel, how can it communicate with other channel? I hope to know the reason." Qibo said: "This is the condition of the various Hand and Foot Yang Channels of the six hollow organs enter into inside through the large collaterals." Yellow Emperor asked: "Can the Xing points and the He points be distinguished?" Qibo answered: "The Xing points are for treating the external channels and the He points are for treating the internal hollow organs."

黄帝曰：治内腑奈何？岐伯曰：取之于合。黄帝曰：合各有名乎？岐伯答曰：胃合于三里，大肠合入于巨虚上廉，小肠合入于巨虚下廉，三焦合入于委阳，膀胱合入于委中央〔委中央："央"是衍文〕，胆合入于阳陵泉。

Yellow Emperor asked: "How to treat the diseases of the hollow organs inside of the body?" Qibo said: "The He points should be pricked," Yellow Emperor asked: "Do all the He points have their names?" Qibo answered: "The He point of the stomach is Sanli (ST. 36), the He point of large intestine is Shangjuxu (ST. 37), the He point of small intestine is

Xiajuxu (ST. 39), the He point of the triple warmer is Weiyang (BL. 39), the He point of the bladder is Weizhong (BL. 40) and the He point of the gallbladder is Yanglingquan (GB. 34)."

黄帝曰：取之奈何？岐伯答曰：取之三里者，低跗；取之巨虚者，举足；取之委阳者，屈伸而索之；委中者，屈〔屈：《甲乙》卷四第二下"屈"下有"膝"字〕而取之；阳陵泉者，正〔正：《甲乙》卷四第二下"正"下并有"立"字〕竖膝予之齐，下至委阳〔下至委阳：张介宾曰："委阳当作委中"〕之阳取之；取诸外经者，揄申而从之。

Yellow Emperor asked: "How to prick the He points?" Qibo answered: "When pricking the Sanli point, the dorsum of the foot should be kept low and flat; when pricking the Shangjuxu and Xiajuxu point, the foot should be lifted; when pricking the Weiyang point, the knee should be bent and the foot should be stretched; when pricking the Weizhong point, the knee should be bent; when pricking the Yanglingquan point, the patient should stand upright to keep the two knees at the same level, and the point is on the outer flank of the Weizhong point. To all the Xing points and Shu points of the external channels, it should apply the method of waving and stretching in pricking."

黄帝曰：愿闻六腑之病。岐伯答曰：面热者足阳明病，鱼络血者手阳明病，两跗之上脉竖〔竖：张注本"竖"作"坚"〕陷者足阳明病，此胃脉也。

Yellow Emperor said: "I hope to know the disease conditons caused by the six hollow organs." Qibo said: "When the face is hot, it shows the Foot Yangming Channel is affected; when the stagnated blood spots appear on the thenar eminence of hand, it shows the Hand Yangming Channel is affected; when the Chongyang pulse appears to be firm and quite hidden on the dorsum of foot, it also shows the Foot Yangming Channel is affected. These are the methods for examining the channel of stomach energy.

大肠病者，肠中切痛而鸣濯濯，冬日重感于寒即泄，当脐而痛，不能久立，与胃同候，取巨虚上廉。

"When the large intestine is affected, there will be acute pain in the abdomen with borborygmus now and then, if the cold-evil is contracted again in winter, diarrhea will occur, the patient will have pain by the navel and will not be able to stand long during the pain. As the intestine is close related with the stomach, it can be treated by pricking the Shangjuxu point of the stomach channel.

胃病者，腹䐜胀，胃脘当心而痛，上支两胁，膈咽不通，食饮不下，取之三里也。

"In the stomach disease, the patient will feel distention of the stomach and has pain of the gastric cavity by the position of heart which is propping the hypochondria. As the passage from the pharynx to the chest is obstructed, the patient can hardly take food and drink. It can be treated by pricking the Zusanli point (ST. 36).

小肠病者，小腹痛，腰脊控睾而痛，时窘之後，当耳前热，若寒甚，若独肩上热甚，及手小指次指之间热，若脉陷者，此其候也，手太阳病也〔手太阳病也：《脉经》卷六第四无此五字〕，取之巨虚下廉。

In the disease of small intestine, there will be fullness and distention in the stomach and the scrotum is painful due to the drawing of the loins and back. The patient is often distressed, feeling hot and cold in front of the ears, feeling hot above the brows and the location between the small finger and the ring finger. When the pulse condition is asthenic and bogging down, it is the syndrome of the affection of the small intestine which can be treated by pricking the Xiajuxu point.

三焦病者，腹〔腹：《千金》卷二十第四“腹”下并有“胀”字〕气满，小腹尤坚，不得小便，窘急，溢则水，留即为胀，候在足太阳之外大络，大络在太阳少阳之间，亦〔亦：《脉经》卷九第九“亦”作“赤”〕见于脉，取委阳。

“In the disease of the triple warmer, there will be distention and fullness in the abdomen, and the lower abdomen is rather firm due to distention. The patient will have dysuria and will feel very uncomfortable. When the fluid retains in the skin, it becomes edema, when it accumulates in the abdomen, it causes distention. The disease of the triple warmer can also appear on the large collateral on the outer flank of the Foot Taiyang Channel, this large collateral is situated between the Taiyang Channel and the Shaoyang Channel. When the triple warmer is affected, the large collateral will be red. It can be treated by pricking the Weizhong point.

膀胱病者，小腹偏肿而痛，以手按之，即欲小便而不得，肩上热，若脉陷，及足小指外廉及胫踝后皆热，若脉陷，取委中央。

“In the disease of bladder, the lower abdomen is swelling and painful. When the site of pain is pressed by hand, the patient will like to pass urine but can hardly begin the urination, and he is also hot on the shoulder. If the patient has a bogging pulse with hotness in foot, hotness in the outer flank of the small finger, tibia and behind the ankle, it can be treated by pricking the Weizhong point.

胆病者，善太息，口苦，呕宿汁，心下澹澹，恐人将捕之，嗌中吩吩然，数唾，在足少阳之本末，亦视其脉之陷下者灸之；其寒热者，取阳陵泉。

“In the disease of gallbladder, the patient often sighs, has bitter taste in the mouth, vomits clear water, has palpitation as if someone is going to arrest him, and it seems something is obstructing the throat which causes frequent cough and spitting saliva. In this case, the circulating route of the Foot Shaoyang Channel should be inspected, besides, it should also find out which collateral is bogging to which can be treated with moxibustion; if the syndrome of alternating episodes of chills and fever appears, the Yanglingquan point should be pricked.”

黄帝曰：刺之有道乎？岐伯答曰：刺此者，必中气穴，无中肉节，中气穴则针染〔染：《甲乙》卷五第一下作“游”〕于巷，中肉节即皮肤痛。补泻反则病益笃。中筋则筋缓，邪气不出，与其真相搏，乱而不去，反还内著〔著：“著”字疑误，据杨注，应作“病”〕，用针不审，以顺为逆也。

Yellow Emperor asked: “Is there any rule in pricking the points stated above?” Qibo answered: “When pricking these points, the acupoint connecting the energy must be hit, and the muscle or the joint must not be hit. When the acupoint connecting the energy is hit, the needle will promote the circulation of energy under the needle hole and can cause the channel unimpeded. If the muscle or joint is hit erroneously, it can only injure the healthy muscle and cause pain of it. If purge is applied when it should be invigorted or invigoration is applied when it should be purged, it will aggravate the disease. If the tendon is hit erroneously, the tendon will become flaccid, and the evil energy will not be excreted, and, as a result, the evil energy will be contending with the healthy energy. As the healthy enetgy has not been removed, it will return inside to causc disease. This is due to the careless applying of the needle and taking the agreeable energy as the adverse one."

根结第五

Chapter 5
Gen Jie
(The Beginning and End of the Channel)

岐伯曰：天地相感，寒暖相移，阴阳之道，孰少孰多？阴道偶，阳道奇。发于春夏，阴气少，阳气多，阴阳不调，何补何泻？发于秋冬，阳气少，阴气多，阴气盛而阳气衰，故茎叶枯槁，湿雨下归，阴阳相移，何泻何补？奇邪离经，不可胜数，不知根结，五脏六腑，折关败枢，开阖而走，阴阳大失，不可复取。九针之玄，要在终始，故能知终始，一言而毕，不知终始，针道咸绝。

Qibo said: "The energies of heaven and earth are correspondent with each other and the cold and hot weathers are shifting from one to another. It is hard to understand the rule of the Yin and Yang changes and know which is the deficient side with less energy and which is the abundant side with more energy. The number of Yin is even, and the number of Yang is odd. When one falls sick in spring and summer, the Yin energy is less and the Yang energy is more and the Yin and Yang energies are not in harmony, to this kind of disease, how to treat with purging and invigorating? When one falls sick in autumn and winter, the Yang energy is less and the Yin energy is more, and the Yin and Yang are interchanging, to this kind of disease, how to purge with purging and invigorating? When the unhealthy energy invades the channels and collaterals, the diseases occurred will be numerous, if one does not know the beginnig and end of the channels and acupoints, once the energy's mechanism is damaged, the pivot becomes deteriorated, the function of opening and closing is out of order, and the energy is excreted, the Yin and Yang will be greatly injured and the refined energy will not be able to be collected again. As to the main point of applying the needles, it is in the comprehension of the beginning and end of the channel. When one knows the facts of the beginning and end of the channedl, the principle of acupuncture can be known by a few words. When one knows not the importance of them, the principle of acupuncture will become extinct to him.

太阳根〔于至阴：《素问·阴阳离合论》“根”下有“起”字〕于至阴，结于命门，命门者目也〔命门者目也《太素》卷十《经脉根结》并无此五字〕。阳明根于厉兑，结于颡大，颡大者钳耳也。少阳根于窍阴，结于窗笼，窗笼者耳中也。太阳为开〔开：《太素》卷五《阴阳合》卷十《经脉根结》作“关”〕，阳明为阖，少阳为枢。故开〔故开折：“开”误，应作“关”〕折则肉节渎而暴病起矣，故暴病者取之大阳，视有余不足，渎者皮肉宛膲而弱也。阖折则气无所止息而痿疾起矣，故痿疾者，取之阳明，视有余不足，无所止息者，真气稽留，邪气居之也。枢折即骨繇而不安于地，故骨繇者取之少阳，视有余不足，骨繇者，节缓而不收也，所谓骨繇者摇故也，当穷其本也。

"The Foot Taiyang Channel begins from the Zhiyin point (BL. 67) on the outer flank of the small toe, and ends at the Jingming point (BL. 11) on the inner canthus of face. The Foot Yangming Channel begins from the Lidui point (ST. 45) at the tip of the second toe beside the big toe, and ends at Touwei point (ST. 8) on the frontal eminence. The Foot Shaoyang Channel begins from the Qiaoyin point (GB. 44) at the tip of the toe next to the small toe, and ends at the Tinggong point (SI. 19) on the ear. The Taiyang Channel in the body is like a bolt of the outer door, the Yangming Channel in the body is like the plank of the outer door, and the Shaoyang Channel in the body is like the pivot of the outer door. If the bolt of Taiyang fails to achieve its function of bolting the door, the sudden onset of disease due to the ulceration in the spaces of muscles will occur; thus, when treating the sudden onset of disease, the Foot Taiyang Channel of Bladder should be pricked, purge when it is having a surplus and invigorate when it is deficient according to the condition of the disease; the so called alternation means the emaciation of muscle and the withering of skin. If Yangming fails to achieve its function of closing the door, the Yang energy will rest nowhere and the flaccidity syndrome will occur; thus, when treating flaccidity, the Yangming Channel of Stomach should be pricked, purge when it is having a surplus and invigorate when it is deficient according to the condition of the disease; the so called rest in nowhere means when the healthy energy is impeded, the evil energy will be retained inside. If Shaoyang fails to achieve its function of pivoting, the syndrome of wavering of the bone will occur and the patient can not walk on the ground safely, thus, when treating the syndrome of wavering of the bone, the Shaoyang Channel of Bladder should be pricked, purge when it is having a surplus and invigorate when it is deficient according to the condition of the disease; the so called wavering of the bone means the joints of bone can not be controlled due to flaccidity. One should probe the source of the conditions stated above.

太阴根于隐白〔根：《素问·阴阳离合论》"根"下有"起"字〕，结于太仓。少阴根于涌泉，结于廉泉。厥阴根于大敦，结于玉英，络于膻中。太阴为开〔开：应作"关"〕，厥阴为阖，少阴为枢。故开〔"开"应作"关"〕折则仓廪无所输膈洞，膈洞者取之太阴，视有余不足，故开折者气不足而生病也。阖折即气绝而喜悲，悲〔悲者："悲"上脱"善"字，应据《甲乙》卷二第五补〕者取之厥阴，视有余不足。枢折则脉有所结而不通，不通者取之少阴，视有余不足，有结者皆取之不足〔皆取之不足：按"不足"衍，应据《甲乙》卷二第五删〕。

"The Foot Taiyin Channel begins from the Yinbai point (SP. 1) at the inner tip of the big toe, and ends at Taicang point (Zhongwan RN 12) of the upper abdomen. The Foot Jueyin Channel begins from Dadun point (LR. 1) at the outer tip of the big toe, and ends on the Yuying point (Yutang RN 18) and nets the Tanzhong point (RN 17) below. The Foot Shaoyin Channel begins from the Yongquan point (KI. 1) of the sole, and ends at the Lianquan point (RN 23) on the neck and throat. The Taiyin Channel in the body is like the bolt of the inner door, the Jueyin Channel in the body is like the flank of the inner door, and the Shaoyin Channel in the body is like the pivot of the inner door. If the Taiyin Channel fails to achieve its function of bolting the door, the spleen will be unable to convey and transform, the water and cereals will not be transported, and the syndromes of obstruction in chest and diarrhea will occur. The syndromes can be treated by pricking the acupoints on the Foot Taiyin Channel of Spleen, purge when it is having a surplus and invigorate when it is deficient according to the condition of the disease. The main reason of failing to bolt of the Taiyin Channel is due to the deficiency of energy. When the Jueyin Channel fails to achieve its function of closing, the retardation of the functional activities of vital energy will occur, the patient will often be sorrow stricken. The syndrome can be treated by pricking the acupoints on the Foot Jueyin Channel of Liver, purge when there is a surplus and invigorate when it is deficient according to the condition of the disease. When the Shaoyin Channel fails to achieve its function of pivoting, the kidney channel will be stagnated and obstructed. The syndrome can be treated by pricking the acupoints on the Foot Shaoyin Channel of Kidney, purge when there is a surplus and invigorte when it is deficient. Whenever there is stagnation in the channel, the pricking methods stated above should be applied.

足太阳根于至阴，溜于京骨，注于昆仑，入于天柱、飞扬也。

足少阳根于窍阴，溜于丘墟，注于阳辅，入于天容、光明也。

足阳明根于厉兑，溜于冲阳，注于下陵（马莳曰："下陵当作解谿"），入于人迎、丰隆也。

手太阳根于少泽，溜于阳谷，注于少海，入于天窗、支正也。

手少阳根于关冲，溜于阳池，注于支沟，入于天牖、外关也。

手阳明根于商阳，溜于合谷，注于阳溪，入于扶突、偏历也。此所谓十二经者，盛络皆当取之。

"The Foot Taiyang Channel of Bladder begins from the channel's Jing (Well) point of Zhiyin (BL. 67), flows to the Yuan (Source) point of Jinggu (BL. 64), pours into Jing (River) point of Kunlun (BL. 60), reaches Tianzhu point (BL. 10) on the neck above and reaches Feiyang (BL. 58) on the foot below.

"The Foot Shaoyang Channel of Gallbladder begins from the channel's Jing (Well) point of Qiaoyin (GB. 44), flows to the Yuan (Source) point of Qiuxu (GB. 40), pours into the Jing (River) point of Yangfu (GB. 39), reaches the Tianronog point (SI. 17) on the neck above, and reaches the collateral point of Guangming (GB. 37).

"The Foot Yangming Channel of Stomach begins from the channel's Jing (Well) point of Lidui (ST. 45), flows to the Yuan (Source) point of Chongyang (ST. 42), pours into the Jing (River) point of Jiexi (ST. 41), reaches to the Renying point (ST. 9) on the neck above and reaches the collateral point of Fenglong (ST. 40) on foot below.

"The Hand Taiyang Channel of Small Intestine begins from the channel's Jing (Well) point of Shaoze (SI. 1), flows to the Jing (River) point of Yanggu (SI. 5), pours into the He (Sea) point of Xiaohai (SI. 8), reaches the Tianchuang point (SI. 7) of the arm above, and reash the Zhizheng point of the arm below.

"The Hand Shaoyang Channel of Triple Warmer begins from the channel's Jing (Well) point of Guanchong (SJ. 1), flows to the Yuan (Source) point of Yangchi (SJ. 4), pours into the Jing (River) point of Zhigou (SJ. 6), reaches to Tianyou point (SJ. 18) on the head above, and reaches the collateral point of Waiguan (SJ. 5)

"The Hand Yangming Channel of Large Intestine begins from the channel's Jing (Well) point of Shangyang (LI. 1), flows to the Yuan (Source) point of Hegu (LI. 4), pours into the Jing (River) point of Yangxi (LI. 5), reaches the Futu point (LI. 18) on the neck, and reaches the Collateral point of Pianli (LI. 6). These are the locations where the twelve channels and collaterals flow and pour into, when the collateral is overabundant and full, it should be purged by pricking.

一日一夜五十营，以营五脏之精，不应数者，名曰狂生。所谓五十营者，五脏皆受气。持其脉口，数其至也，五十动而不一代者，五脏皆受气；四十动一代者，一脏无气；三十动一代者，二脏无气，二十动一代者，三脏无气；十动一代者，四脏无气；不满十动一代者，五脏无气。予之短期，要在终始。所谓五十动而不一代者，以为常也，以知五脏之期〔期：疑当作“气”〕。予之短期者，乍数乍疏也。

"The channel-energy circulates in the body fifty cycles in a day and night. If the circulation of the refined energy of the five viscera is not in conformity with the fifty cycles to be faster or slower, one will be sick, and it is called 'getting ill'. The criterion of the fifty cycles can be used to observe the substantiality of deficiency of the five viscera, to count the times of the pulse beats when palpating, and to determine the robustness and the feebleness of the patient's body. When the pulse does not stop once within fifty beats, it shows the refined energy of the five viscera is prosperous; when the pulse stops once within fourty beats, it shows the energy fails to reach one of the viscera; when the pulse stops once within thirty beats, it shows the energy fails to reach two of the viscera; when the pulse stops once within twenty beats, it shows the energy fails to reach three of the viscera; when the pulse stops once within ten beats, it shows the enegy fails to reach four of the viscera; when the pulse stops within less than ten beats, it shows the energy fails to reach all the viscera, and the patient will die in a short period. So, it is important to observe the condition of the pulse. When the pulse beats fifty times without stopping, it is the normal pules condition of the five viscera from which one can know the refined energy in the five viscera is normal. As to whether the patient will die in a short period, it is determined by the fast and slow conditions by turns of the pules beats."

黄帝曰：逆顺五体者，言人骨节之小大，肉之坚脆，皮之厚薄，血之清浊，气之滑涩，脉之长短，血之多少，经络之数，余已知之矣，此皆布衣匹夫之士也。夫王公大人，血食〔血食之君：“血”字应作“肉”〕之君，身体柔脆，肌肉软弱，血气慓悍滑利，其刺之徐疾浅深多少，可得同之乎？岐伯答曰：膏粱菽藿之味，何可同也。气滑即出疾，其气涩则出迟，气悍则针小而入浅，气涩则针大而入深，深则欲留，浅则欲疾〔疾：张注本作“迟”〕。以此观之，刺布衣者深以留之，刺大人者微以徐之，此皆因气慓悍滑利也。

Yellow Emperor said: " There are five kinds of normal and abnormal physiques in men, in the various physiques, there are large or small sizes in the joints, firm or crisp of the muscle, thick or thin of the skin, clear or turbid of the blood, slippery or choppy of the circulation of energy, long or short of the channel, different in the density of blood and different number in the channel and collateral, and I have understood all the conditions already. But they are denoting the conditions of the labouring people. As to the princes and nobles who take meat every day, their bodies are feeble, and their blood circulation is rapid and slippery, can the treating to them such as swift or slow inserting, deep or shallow pricking and the number in pricking the acupoints be the same with that of treating the labouring people?" Qibo answered: "When treating the people who usually take meat, fine flour and rice, must not be the same with the people who take coarse grain . To the patient who has a slippery energy, the pulling of needle should be swift; to the patient who has a choppy energy, the pulling of needle should be slow; to the patient who has a slippery energy, it should prick shallowly with a small needle, to the people who has a choppy energy, it should prick deeply with a large needle; when pricking deeply, the needle should be retained, when pricking shallowly, the pricking of needle should be slow. According to the principle stated above, the pricking to the labouring people should be deep and the needle should be retained, to the princes and nobles, the pricking should be shallow, and the inserting should be slow, as their energies are rapid and slippery which are apt to induce the abnormal conditions."

黄帝曰：形气之逆顺奈何？岐伯曰：形气不足，病气有余，是邪胜也，急泻之。形气有余，病气不足，急补之。形气不足，病气不足，此阴阳气俱不足也〔"气"字衍〕不可刺之，刺之则重不足，重不足则阴阳俱竭，血气皆尽，五脏空虚，筋骨髓枯，老者绝灭，壮者不复矣。形气有余，病气有余，此谓阴阳俱有余也，急泻其邪，调其虚实。故曰有余者泻之，不足者补之，此之谓也。

Yellow Emperor asked: "How to treat when the physique and function are deficient or having a surplus?" Qibo said: "When the physique and function are deficient and the evil energy is having a surplus, it is the condition of sthenia of the evil energy, and the evil energy should be purged hastily; when the physique and function are having a surplus and the evil energy is deficient, it should be invigorated hastily; when the physique and function are deficient and the evil energy is also deficient, it shows both the Yin and Yang are deficient, when treating, it must not treat by pricking, if it is pricked erroneously, the healthy energy of the patient will be deficient all the more to cause exhaustion of both the Yin and Yang, the blood and energy will all be used up, the energy of the five viscera will be emptied and the tendon and marrow will be withered, In this case, an old man will die, and the disease of a man in his prime of life can hardly be recovered. If the physique and function are having a surplus, and the evil energy is also having a surplus, it should purge the sthenic evil and adjust the asthenia and sthenia to keep them in balance. So, purge when there is having a surplus and invigorate when there is a deficiency.

故曰刺不知逆顺，真邪相搏。满〔满：《甲乙》卷五第六作"实"〕而补之，则阴阳四溢，肠胃充郭，肝肺内膜，阴阳相错。虚而泻之，则经脉空虚，血气竭枯，肠胃僈辟，皮肤薄著，毛腠夭膲〔膲：《太素》卷二十二《刺法》作"焦"〕，予之死期。故曰用针之要，在于知调阴与阳，调阴与阳，精气乃光，合形与气，使神内藏。故曰上工平气，中工乱脉，下工绝气危生。故曰下工不可不慎也。必审五脏变化之病，五脉之应，经络之实虚，皮之柔粗，而后取之也。

"Therefore, when one knows not the treating principle of purging and invigorating, adverse and agreeable, it will cause the contention of the healthy energy and the evil energy. If the disease of sthenic evil is treated erroneously with invigorating therapy, both the Yin and Yang will be overabundant which will cause the fullness of the intestine and the stomach, distention of the liver and lung inside and the disorder of Yin and Yang. If the disease of asthenia of healthy energy is treated erroneously with purging therapy, the channel will be emptied, the blood and energy will be exhausted, the intestine and stomach will be emaciated with the skin attaching the bone, the fine hair becomes short and the striae become dried, and the patient will die in a short period. Thus, the main clue of acupuncture is in the knowing of the principle of adjusting. When Yin and Yang are adjusted, the refined energy of the patient will be abundant, the physique and function will be unified, and the spirit will be able to store inside. The physician of higher level can keep the energies in balance, the physique of medium level can treat the patient according to the pulse condition, and the physician of lower level can only exhaust the energy and cause danger to the patient's life. So, in pricking, it must be very cautious. One must observe the changes of the five viscera, the corresponding relation between the pulse condition of the five-viscera and the disease, the asthenia and sthenia of the channels and the soft and coarse of the skin first, then, treat by pricking the proper acupoint.

寿夭刚柔第六

Chapter 6
Shou Yao Gang Rou
(On the Relation Between Firmness and Softness of Body and One's Life-span)

黄帝问于少师曰：余闻人之生也，有刚有柔，有弱有强，有短有长，有阴有阳，愿闻其方。少师答曰：阴中有阴〔有阴：《甲乙》卷六第六作“有阳”〕，阳中有阳〔有阳《甲乙》卷六第六作“有阴”〕，审知阴阳，刺之有方，得病所始，刺之有理，谨度病端，与时相应，内合于五脏六腑，外合于筋骨皮肤。是故内有阴阳，外亦有阴阳。在内者，五脏为阴，六腑为阳；在外者，筋骨为阴，皮肤为阳。故曰病在阴之阴者，刺阴之荥输；病在阳之阳者，刺阳之合；病在阳之阴者，刺阴之经；病在阴之阳者，刺络脉。故曰病在阳者命〔命：与注本，张注本并作“名”〕曰风，病在阴者命曰痹，阴阳俱病命曰风痹。病有形而不痛者，阳之类也；无形而痛者，阴之类也。无形而痛者，其阳完而阴伤之也，急治其阴，无攻其阳；有形而不痛者，其阴完而阳伤之也，急治其阳，无攻其阴。阴阳俱动，乍有形〔乍有形，乍无形：《甲乙》卷六第六无两“形”字〕，乍无形，加以烦心，命曰阴胜其阳，此谓不表不里，其形不久。

Yellow Emperor asked Shaoshi: "I am told the human bodies are different in character: some are firm and some are soft; in constitution, some are strong and some are weak; in the type of build, some are tall and some are short; and some are of Yin and some are of Yang; I hope to know the reason." Shaoshi answered: "There is Yin in Yang and there is Yang in Yin, when one knows the law of Yin and Yang and the mutual relation between them, he can treat the disease by pricking properly, know the initial condition of the disease and apply the pricking technique properly. In treating, one should also estimate the corresponding relation between the course of disease and the weather changes of the four seasons conscientiously. In human body, the Yin and Yang conform with the five solid and six hollow organs inside, and conform with the tendon, bone and skin outside, so, in human body, there are Yin and Yang inside and there are also Yin and Yang outside. The five solid organs are Yin and the six hollow organs are Yang inside, the tendon and bone are Yin and the skin is Yang outside. So, when treating the disease of Yin in Yin, it should prick the Xing points on the Yin channel; when treating the disease of Yang in Yang, it should prick the He point of the Yang channel; when treating the disease of Yin in Yang, it should prick the Jing (River) point of the Yin channel; when treating the disease of Yang in Yin, it should prick the collateral points of the Yang channel. This is the fundamental rule of selecting the acupoints for pricking according to the relation between the disease and the internal and external Yin and Yang. The diseases can also be classified into Yin and Yang categories, when the disease is of the Yang channel, it is called wind, when it is of the Yin channel, it is called bi (disease due to blocking of extremities, meridians and viscera by evils), when the disease is in both the Yin and Yang channels, it is called arthralgia due to wind-evil. When the disease has formal change but the patient has no pain, it belongs to the category of Yang channel, when the disease has no formal change but the patient is painful, it belongs to the category of Yin channel. When there is no formal change but the patient is painful, it shows only the Yin channel is injured, but the Yang is unharmed, so it should treat the acupoints on the Yin channel hastily by pricking, and the Yang channel must not be attacked. When there is formal change but the patient has no pain, it shows only the Yang channel in injured, but the Yin channel is unharmed, it should treat the acupoints on the acupoints on the Yang channel hastily, but the Yin channel must not be attacked. When the superficies and the interiors of both the Yin and Yang are diseased, the formal change appears all of a sudden and missing all of a sudden, and the patient is irritable, it is the so called Yin surpassing Yang and it is a disease of neither superficies nor interior which is hard to be cured. In this case, the physique of the patient can hardly exist long."

黄帝问于伯高曰：余闻形气病之先后，外内之应奈何？伯高答曰：风寒伤形，忧恐忿怒伤气。气伤脏，乃病脏；寒伤形，乃应形〔应形："应"误，当作"病"〕，风伤筋脉，筋脉乃应〔乃应，"应"误，当作"病"〕。此形气外内之相应也。

Yellow Emperor asked Bogao: "I am told there are the early or late and interior or exterior corresponding relations between the physique and function and the disease, and what is the reason?" Bogao answered: "When the wind-evil invades from outside, it injures the physique first, the respond is outside; when the melancholy, terror and anger cause the excitation of the spirit, it injures the internal energy first, the respondence is inside, When the energies are not coordinate to violate the harmony of the five viscera, it causes the disease of the five viscera. when the wind-evil injures the physique, the muscular surface and skin will be diseased. When the wind-evil injures the muscle which is between the exterior and the interior, the muscle will be diseased. These are the internal and external relations between the physique and function and the disease."

黄帝曰：刺之奈何？伯高答曰：病九日者，三刺而已。病一月者，十刺而已。多少远近，以此衰之。久痹不去身者，视其血络，尽出其血。黄帝曰：外内之病，难易之治奈何？伯高答曰：形先病而未入脏者，刺之半其日；脏先病而形乃应者，刺之倍其日。此月〔月：胡本、统本、藏本，日抄本并作"外"〕内难易之应也。

Yellow Emperor asked: "How to determine the course of treating?" Bogao said: "When the disease has lasted for nine days, it can be recovered by pricking three times; when the disease has lasted for a month, it can be recovered by pricking ten times. The number of the lasting days of disease and the remote and recent of the course of disease can all be determined by the progressive standard of pricking once for three lasting days in the course of the disease. In the protracted bi-syndrome of which the evil energy is retaining, it should inspect the superficial venules and remove the extravasated blood as far as possible." Yellow Emperor said: "Since in human body, some diseases are of internal and some are of external, when treat by pricking, some diseases can be cured easily and some can not, how to distinguish them?" Bogao answered: "When the physique is diseased first, and the disease has not yet transmitted into the internal organ, it is a disease of superficies, the times of pricking can be reduced by half; when the internal organ is diseased first and then the physique is also diseased, it shows the disease is in both inside and outside, the times of pricking should be doubled. These are the rules of the corresponding relation in the internal and external disease and the easiness and difficulty in treating the disease by pricking."

黄帝问于伯高曰：余闻形有缓急，气有盛衰，骨有大小，肉有坚脆，皮有厚薄，其以立寿夭奈何？伯高答曰：形与气相任则寿，不相任则夭。皮与肉相果〔果：《甲乙卷六第十一》作“裹”〕则寿，不相果〔果：《甲乙卷六第十一》作“裹”〕则夭。血气经络胜形则寿，不胜形则夭。

Yellow Emperor asked Bogao: "I am told in human body, there are the conditions of slow and fast in form, prosperous and deficient in disposition, large and small in skeleton, firm and crisp in muscle and thick and thin in skin, can they be used to determine the life span of a man?" Bogao answered: " When one's physique is equivalent to his energy, he will live long, otherwise, he will die young. When one's skin attaches the muscle tightly, he will live long, otherwise, he will die young. When one's energy, blood, channel and collaterals are abundant to surpass his physique, he will live long, otherwise, he will die young, when they are deficient and can hardly surpass the physique, he will die young."

黄帝曰：何谓形之缓急？伯高答曰：形充而皮肤缓者则寿，形充而皮肤急者则夭。形充而脉坚大者顺也，形充而脉小以弱者气衰，衰则危矣。若形充而颧不起者骨小，骨小则夭矣。形充而大肉䐃坚而有分者肉坚，肉坚则寿矣；形充而大肉无分理不坚者肉脆，肉脆则夭矣。此天之生命，所以立形定气而视寿夭者。必明乎此立形定气，而后以临病人，决死生。

Yellow Emperor asked: " What is the meaning of the moderate and acute conditions of the physique?" Bogao answered "When one's physique is substantial and his skin is soft, he will live long, when his physique is substantial and his skin is firm, he will die young. When one's physique is substantial and his channel-energy is firm and gigantic, the superficies and interior are in conformity which is called agreeable; when one's physique is substantial and his channel-energy is weak and small, it is the debility of energy which is a dangerous phenomenon. When one's physique is substantial and his cheekbone is not protruding, his skeleton must be small, and a man with small skeleton will die young. When one's physique is substantial and the muscles of his legs and buttocks are protruding with lines on the skin, it is called the firm muscle, and a man with firm muscle will live long. When one's physigue is substantial and the muscles of his arms, legs and buttocks have no lines on the skin, it is called the crisp muscle, and the man with crisp muscle will die early. This is the law of nature to maintain the life. According to the firm and soft, strong and weak of the physique, one can determine to Yin or Yang the energy belongs, and perceive the life span of a man. For a physician, he must understand the points stated above, so that he can treat the disease, perceive the prognosis and judge the survival and death of the patient."

黄帝曰：余闻寿夭，无以度之。伯高答曰：墙基卑，高不及其地者，不满三十而死；其有因加疾者，不及二十而死也。黄帝曰：形气之相胜，以立寿夭奈何？伯高答曰：平人而气胜形者寿；病而形肉脱，气胜形者死，形胜气者危矣。

Yellow Emperor said: "I am told some people live a long life and some people die early, but their condition can hardly be inferred." Bogao said: "When inferring the life span of a man, it can be observed from the face, when one's bones around the ear are flat and bogging down and fail to reach the muscle level in front of the ear, he will die before thirty, if he contracts exogenous evil or internal disease again and becomes sick, he may die before twenty." Yellow Emperor asked: "How to determine the long or short life of a man when the energy surpasses the physique or vice versa?" Bogao answered: "For a healthy man, when his energy is surpassing the physique, he will live long; for the one whose physique and muscle are very thin, even though his energy surpasess the physique, yet his physique and muscle are exhausted, he will die very soon as well. If one's physique is not very emaciated, but his primordial energy is already fallen into a decline, although his physique is surpassing the primordial energy, the disease is still a dangerous one."

黄帝曰：余闻刺有三变，何谓三变？伯高答曰：有刺营者，有刺卫者，有刺寒痹之留经者。黄帝曰：刺三变〔刺三变：《太素》卷二十二《三变赖篇》"三"下无"变"字〕者奈何？伯高答曰：刺营者出血，刺卫者出气，刺寒痹者内热〔内热："内热"应作"内熨"〕。黄帝曰：营卫寒痹之为病奈何？伯高答曰：营之生病也，寒热少气，血上下行。卫之生病也，气痛时来时去，怫忾贲响，风寒客于肠胃之中。寒痹之为病也，留而不去，时痛而皮不仁。黄帝曰：刺寒痹内热〔内热：应作"内熨"〕奈何？伯高答曰：刺布衣者，以火焠之。刺大人者，以药熨之。

Yellow Emperor asked: "I am told there are three kinds of pricking, and what are they?" Bogao said: "They are the Ying-energy pricking, the Wei-energy pricking and the cold-type arthralgia pricking." Yellow Emperor asked: "What are the three kinds of pricking like?" Bogao answered: "The Ying-energy pricking is to prick the vein to cause bleeding, the Wei-energy pricking is to disperse the Wei-energy, and the cold-type arthralgia pricking is to carry on hot application of medicine after pricking." Yellow Emperor asked: "What are the syndromes caused by the Ying-energy, the Wei-energy and the cold-type arthralgia respectively?" Bogao answered: "The main syndroms of the Ying disease are: the alternating episodes of chills and fever, short of breath and the running up and down rashly of blood; the main syndromes of Wei diseases are: the pain due to the disorder of vital energy coming and going now and then, being painful and painless by turns, the fullness and distention of the abdomen caused by external invasion of the wind-cold, and the retention of evil energy in the intestine and stomach; the syndromes of cold-type arthralgia are: often painful of the muscle and the numbness of the skin due to the protracted retention of the cold evil in between the channel and the collaterals." Yellow Emperor asked: "In the cold-type arthralgia pricking, how to carry on the hot application of medicine after pricking?" Bogao answered:

"The treating should be different according to the different constitutions of the patients: to common people, acupuncture with heated needle should be applied; to the nobles, hot application of medicine after pricking should be applied."

黄帝曰：药熨奈何？伯高答曰：用淳酒〔淳：《甲乙》卷十第一上作"醇"〕二十升，蜀椒一升〔一升：张注本"升"作"斤"〕，干姜一斤，桂心一斤，凡四种，皆㕮咀，渍酒中。用绵絮一斤，细白布四丈，并内酒中。置酒马矢煴中，盖封涂，勿使泄。五日五夜，出布绵絮，曝干之，干复渍，以尽其汁，每渍必晬其日，乃出干〔干：《甲乙》卷十第一上并无"干"字〕。干〔干：《太素》卷二十二《三变刺》无此"干"字〕，并用滓与绵絮，复布为复巾，长六七尺，为六七巾。则用之生桑炭炙巾，以熨寒痹所刺之处，令热入至于病所，寒复炙巾以熨之，三十遍而止。汗出，以巾拭身，亦三十遍而止。起步内中，无见风。每刺必熨，如此病已矣，此所谓内热也。

Yellow Emperor asked: "How to conduct the hot application of medicine?" Bogao answered: "Take twenty litres of wine without any impurities, one catty (1/2 kilogramme) of pepper, one catty of dried ginger and one catty of laurel, chew the four ingredients into coarse granules and soak them in wine; take one catty of cotton fiber, fourty feet of fine white cloth and soak them also into the wine with the ingredients; put the utensil of the wine on the warm horse dung, seal the mouth of the utensil with mud to avoid the letting out of air; take out the white cloth and fiber from the wine after five days and nights, dry them in the sun and soak them again in the wine until all the wine are absorbed. Each time of the soaking should be a day and a night before drying in the sun; put the ingredients' dregs and the cotton fiber into a bag of six or seven feet made of double layers of cloth, and the bags should be six of them ready for use. When using, scorch the bag with fillings on the burning mulberry charcoal and warm the location where the cold-type arthralgia is more serious with the heated bag to cause the heat transmitting directly into the focus. When the bag becomes cold, scorch it again on fire and warm the focus again until thirty times and wipe away the sweat of the patient's body after each warming for thirty times also. After the treating, the patient should take a stroll in the room and keep away from the wind. Each pricking should cooperate together with the hot application of medicine, and in this way, the disease can be cured. This is the method of the hot application of medicine."

官针第七

Chapter 7
Guan Zhen
(On the Application of Needles)

凡刺之要，官针最妙。九针之宜，各有所为〔之宜、所为："宜""为"二字，上下误倒〕，长短大小，各有所施也，不得其用，病弗能移。疾浅针深，内伤良肉，皮肤为痈；病深针浅，病气不泻，支〔支：《甲乙》卷五第二作"反"〕为大脓。病小针大，气泻太甚，疾必为害；病大针小，气不泄泻，亦复为败〔亦复为败：《甲乙》卷五第二作"亦为后败"〕。失针之宜，大者泻，小者不移，已言其过，请言其所施。

The most important clue of acupuncture is in the application of the nine needles. The application of the nine kinds of needle has a proper scope respectively, and the applications of the long, short, large and small needles are different. If the application is not correct, the disease will not be removed. Such as, when one pricks deeply to the focus which is in a shallow location, it will injure the good muscle inside to cause the suppuration of the skin; when pricks shallowly to the focus which is in a deeper location, the evil-energy will not be removed and finally causing a big ulcer; when applyng a large needle to a slight disease and the energy is purged excessively, the condition of the disease will become worse; when one applies a small needle to a serious disease, the evil-energy will not be purged, and it will cause trouble later. Thus, the application of the needle must be appropriate. When the size of the needle is bigger than enough, it will injure the healthy energy; when it is smaller than it ought to be, the disease will not be removed. These are the conditions when applying the needle erroneously, Here we discuss the proper applications of the needle.

病在皮肤无常处者，取以镵针于病所，肤白勿取。病在分肉间，取以员针于病所。病在经络痼痹者，取以锋针，病在脉，气少当补之者，取以鍉针于井荥分输。病为大脓者，取以铍针。病痹气暴发者，取以员利针。病痹气痛而不去者，取以毫针。病在中者，取以长针，病水肿不能通关节者，取以大针。病在五脏固居者，取以锋针，泻于井荥分输，取以四时。

When the disease is in the surface of the skin without a definite location, it can be treated with the sagital needle. If the diseased location of the skin is pale, the sagital needle must not be used. When the disease is in the muscle or between the muscles, it can be treated with the ovoid-tip needle. When the disease is in the channel and the patient's energy is deficient which needs invigoration, treat with the blunt-tip needle by pressing the Jing (Well), Xing and Shu points respectively. To the patient with the disease of serious suppurative ulcer, it can be treated with the sword-shaped needle to eliminate the pus. When treating the bi-syndrome, it can be treated with the horse-tail-shaped needle. When treating the bi-syndrome with unceasing pain, it can be treated with the filiform needle. When the disease has penetrated inside, it can be treated with the long needle. When treating edema and the joints of the patient are choppy, it can be treated with the large needle. When treating the protracted disease retaining in the five-viscera, it can be treated with the ensiform needle. When pricking the Jing (Well) and Xing points for purging, it must treat them respectively according to the different weathers of the four seasons.

凡刺有九，以应九变。一曰输刺；输刺者，刺诸经荥输脏输也。二曰远道刺；远道刺者，病在上，取之下，刺府输也。三曰经刺；经刺者，刺大经之结络经分也。四曰络刺；络刺者，刺小络之血脉也。五曰分刺；分刺者，刺分肉之间也。六曰大泻刺；大泻刺者，刺大脓以铍针也。七曰毛刺；毛刺者，刺浮痹皮肤也。八曰巨刺；巨刺者，左取右，右取左。九曰焠刺；焠刺者，刺燔针则取痹也。

There are nine kinds of needling to suit the nine kinds of pathological change. The first kind is called the shu-needling which is to prick the shu points on the various Jing (Well), Xing, Shu, Jing (River) and He points of the twelve channels on the extremities and the visceral acupoints on the back and the two latteral sides. The second kind is called the distant-needling which is to prick the acupoint on lower part when the disease is in the upper part, and prick the acupoints of the three Yang channels. The third kind is called the channel-needling which is to prick the knots or hardness that connect the deep lying channel. The fourth kind is called the blood-letting-needling which is to prick the superficial and small vien beneath the skin. The fifth kind is called the intermuscular-needling which is to prick the pace of the low-lying muscular layers, The sixth kind is called the drainage-needling which is to prick the suppurative ulcer. The seventh kind is called the skin-needling which is to prick the superficial bi-syndrome of skin without injuring the muscle. The eighth kind is called the opposing-needling which is to prick the points contralateral to the affected side. The ninth kind is called the red-hot-needling which is to treat the bi-syndrome with the needle heated by the burning fire.

凡刺有十二节，以应十二经。一曰偶刺；偶刺者，以手直心若背，直痛所，一刺前，一刺后，以治心痹，刺此者傍针也。二曰报刺；报刺者，刺痛无常处也，上下行者，直内无拔针，以左手随病所按之，乃出针复刺之也。三曰恢刺；恢刺者，直刺傍之，举之前后，恢筋急，以治筋痹也。四曰齐刺〔齐：孙鼎宜曰：“‘齐’当作‘参’”〕；齐刺者，直入一，傍入二，以治寒〔寒气：《甲乙》卷五第二“寒”下有“热”字〕气小深者。或曰三刺；三刺者，治痹气小深者也〔或曰三刺，三刺者治痹气小深者也；《针灸大成》卷一引无“或曰”以下十四字〕。五曰扬刺；扬刺者，正内一，傍内四，而浮之，以治寒气之博大者也。六曰直针刺；直针刺者，引皮乃刺之，以治寒气之浅者也。七曰输刺；输刺者，直之直出，稀发针而深之〔稀发针而深之：按“稀”“深”二字疑误，似应分作“疾”“浅”二字〕，以治气盛而热者也。八曰短〔短：“短”字疑误，似应作“竖”〕刺；短刺者，刺骨痹稍摇而深之，致针骨所，以上下摩骨也。九曰浮刺；浮刺者，傍入而浮之，以治肌急而寒者也。十曰阴刺；阴刺者，左右率刺之，以治寒厥，中寒厥〔中寒厥：《圣济总录》卷一百九十二引无“中寒厥”三字〕，足〔足：《圣济总录》卷一百九十二“足”上有“取”字〕踝后少阴也。十一曰傍针刺；傍针刺者，直刺傍刺各一以治留痹久居者也。十二曰赞刺；赞刺者，直入直出，数发针而浅之出血，是谓治痈肿也。

There are twelve methods in pricking to treat the various diseases of the twelve channels. The first kind is calld the paired-needling, and in the needling, prick the painful location on the chest first, and then, prick the painful location on the back, so as to treat the diseases of the obstruction of the heart-energy kind, and the pricking should be shallow to avoid hurting the internal organ, The second kind is called the trigger-puncture which is to treat the unlocalized pain which is now up and now down, prick straightly but do not pull out the needle immediately, press the location of the pain with the left hand and then pull out the needle, and prick likewise again when another painful point is found. The third kind is called the relaxing-needling which is to prick straightly beside the painful muscle and manipulate the needle up and down, anteriorly and posteriorly to relax the muscle so as to relieve the muscular aching and spasm. The fourth kind is called the uneven-puncture which is to prick the centre of the affected part with one needle and both sides with two needles respectively ,it is also called triple-puncture which is for treating the protracted but slight cold and heat. The fifth kind is called the Yang-puncture which is to prick the centre of the affected part with one needle and prick the four sides with four needles in shallow pricking to treat the disease of which the cold and heat are extensive. The sixth kind is called the perpendicular-needling which is to hold the skin up with fingers first, and then prick with needle along with the skin to treat the bi-syndrome attacked by slight cold-evil. The seventh kind is called the Shu-point-needling of which the thrusting and lifting of the needle are perpendicular with swift insersting and shallow pricking to treat the disease with abundant energy and high fever. The eighth kind is called the vertical-needling which is to treat the bone bi-syndrome, after the insertion, wave the needle slightly to advance the needle and cause the needle tip to approach the bone, apply the lifting and thrusting method of the needle so as it can treat the bone bi-sydrome. The ninth kind is called the superficial-puncture which is to prick shallowly lateral to the surface of the muscle to treat the bi-syndrome due to muscular spasm. The tenth kind is called the Yin-puncture which is to prick the inner sides of the left and right thighs to treat the cold-type jue-syndrome, the Taixi point of Foot Shaoyin behind the inner ankle should be pricked. The eleventh kind is called the nearby-needle puncture which is to prick straightly the affected part with one needle and prick the nearby location with another needle to treat the protracted bi-syndrome. The twelfth kind is called the repeated-shallow-puncture of which the thrusting and lifting of needle are perpendicular, and the pricking is swift and shallow to treat the carbuncle and swelling.

脉之所居深不见者，刺之微内针而久留之，以致其空脉气也。脉浅者勿刺，按绝其脉乃刺之，无令精出〔无令精出：《圣济总录》卷一百九十二引“精”下有“气”字〕，独出其邪气耳。所谓三刺则谷气出者，先浅刺绝皮，以出阳邪；再刺则阴邪出者，少益深，绝皮致肌肉，未入分肉间也；已入分肉之间，则谷气出。故《刺法》曰：始刺浅之，以逐邪气而来血气；后刺深之，以致阴气之邪；最后刺极深之，以下谷气。此之谓也。故用针者，不知年之所加，气之盛衰，虚实之所起，不可以为工也。

When the channel is lying low and can not be seen, when pricking, it should thrust the needle gently and retain it longer to guide the channel energy into the acupoint. When pricking the channel which is in a shallow location, do not prick hastily, it must be pressed to sever the flow of the channel and keep away from the blood vessel first, then can the needle be thrusted. The pricking is for eliminating the evil energy only, and the refined energy must not be excreted. The so called the three-stage of pricking is ultimately to get the needling response. The way of doing it is: firstly, prick shallowly through the skin to purge the evil-energy of Wei; secondly, prick and purge the evil-energy of Ying, and the pricking should be more deeply, penetrating through the skin and approaching the muscle but not reaching the flesh adherent to the bone; lastly, when the needle finally reaches the flesh adhering to the bone, the needling response will occur. So it was stated in the《Pricking Therapy》: "In the beginning, prick the skin shallowly, it can dispel the evil energy of Yang and promote the circulation of the healthy energy; next, prick more deeply to dispel the evil-energy of Yin; finally, prick very deeply to produce the needling response so as to invigorate the asthenia or purge the sthenia." Therefore, when one knows not the rule of the age-adding of man, being ignorant about the diseases caused by the abundance or deficiency, asthenia or sthenia of the blood and energy, he will not be considered to be a good physician.

凡刺有五，以应五脏。一曰半刺；半刺者，浅内而疾发针，无针伤肉，如拔毛状，以取皮气，此肺之应也。二曰豹文刺；豹文刺者，左〔左：《太素》卷二十二《五刺》"左"上有"刺"字〕右前后，针之中脉为故，以取经络之血者，此心之应也。三曰关刺；关刺者，直刺左右，尽筋上，以取筋痹，慎无出血，此肝之应也。或曰渊刺，一曰岂刺。四曰合谷刺；合谷刺者，左右鸡足，针于分肉之间，以取肌痹，此脾之应也。五曰输刺；输刺者，直入直出，深内之至骨，以取骨痹，此肾之应也。

There are five kinds of pricking therapy for suiting the related affections of the five viscera. The first kind is called the shallow-needling of which the insertion should be swift without injuring the muscle like plucking a piece of fine hair; it can purge the energy of the skin, and it is the pricking therapy corresponding to the lung. The second kind is called the leopard-spot-needling which is to prick the left, right, front and rear, and the collaterals must be hit. It can be used to disperse the stagnated blood in the channel and collaterals, and it is the pricking therapy corresponding to the heart. The third kind is called the joint-needling which is to prick around the joints of the extremities straightly to treat the tendinous bi-syndrome. In pricking, it must cause bleeding and it is the pricking therapy corresponding to the liver. The pricking is also called the Yuan-pricking or Qi-pricking. The fourth kind is called the multi-direction-needling which is to prick right forward with one needle and prick slantingly on the left and right sides with two needles like the pattern of a chicken's claw. When the texture and interspace of muscles is pricked, it can cure myalgia, and it is the pricking therapy corresponding to the spleen. The fifth kind is called the Shu-point-needling of which the thrusting and lifting of the needle are perpendicular to reach the location near the bone. It can cure rheumatism involving the bone, and it is the pricking therapy corresponding to the kidney.

本神第八

Chapter 8
Ben Shen
(The Diseases Caused by Spiritual Activities)

黄帝问于岐伯曰：凡刺之法，先必本于神。血、脉、营、气、精神，此五脏之所藏也，至其淫泆，离藏则精失、魂魄飞扬、志意恍乱、智虑去身者，何因而然乎？天之罪与？人之过乎？何谓德气，生精、神、魂、魄、心、意、志、思、智、虑？请问其故。

Yellow Emperor asked Qibo："Acccording to the principle of acupuncture, one must examine the patient carefully first and then treat according to the conditions of his spiritual activities. As the blood, channel, Ying-energy, vital energy and the essence of life are all stored by the five viscera, when they become abnormal and be divorced from the storing viscus, the refined energy of the fiver viscera will be lost, the soul and the inferior spirit will be rising in the air, the will will be vexed and the patient himself will lose his intelligence and fail to ponder, and why is it so? Is it due to the natural morbidity or due to the artificial fault of man? Besides, what is the original substance? How can it produce the essence of life, spirit, soul, inferior spirit, mind in heart, idea, will, pondering, wisdom and consideration? I hope to hear the reason about it."

岐伯答曰：天之在我者德也，地之在我者气也，德流气薄而生者也。故生之来谓之精，两精相搏谓之神，随神往来者谓之魂，并精而出入者谓之魄，所以任物者谓之心，心有所忆谓之意，意之所存谓之志，因志而存变谓之思，因思而远慕谓之虑，因虑而处物谓之智。

Qibo answered："The human being comes of existence when receiving the original substance and energy of heaven and earth, and the interflow and the combat of the original substance and energy cause the shaping of man. The original substance which enables the evolution of human body is called the essence of life; when the Yin essence and the Yang essence combine, it produces the activities of life which is called the spirit; the function of consciousness appears along with the spiritual activities is called the soul; the faculty of motion produced along with the coming and going of the refined energy is called the inferior spirit; when one makes a settlement to a matter from outside, it is by the heart (mind); when the heart recalls something and leaves an impression, it is called the idea; when one studies the changing conditions repeatedly according to the understanding, it is calld the pondering; when one has a remote inferring acquired from pondering, it is call the consideration; when one makes a corresponding decision to settle the matter after pondering, it is called wisdom.

故智者之养生也，必须四时而适寒暑，和喜怒而安居处，节阴阳而调刚柔，如是则僻邪不至，长生久视。

"Thus, when a wise man preserves his health, he always adapt himself to the cold and hot weather agreeably with the four seasons, keep the moods of overjoy and anger in harmony to maintain his motion and rest in daily life at ease, so that he can control the over-abundance of Yin and Yang and regulates the firmness and softness. In this way, the debilitating and thief evil will not invade, and one will not likely to become decrepit and he will live a long life.

是故怵惕思虑者则伤神，神伤则恐惧流淫而不止。因悲哀动中者，竭绝而失生。喜乐者，神惮散而不藏。愁忧者，气闭塞而不行。盛怒者，迷惑而不治。恐惧者，神荡惮而不收。

"Excessive terror and pondering cause the wastage of Yin energy to become unstable of the patient. Excessive sorrow injures the internal viscera, causing the functional activities of vital energy to become exhausted and the death of the patient. Excessive overjoy causes the dispersion of the energy which can no more be stored. Excessive melancholy causes the impediment and stagnation of the functional activities of vital energy. Fury causes mania and the abnormality of the patient. Excessive terror causes the unrestraint of the refined energy due to the unrest of the spirit.

心〔心怵惕：《素问·宣明五气篇》王注引无"心"字〕怵惕思虑则伤神，神伤则恐惧自失，破䐃脱肉，毛悴色夭，死于冬。

"Excessive terror and pondering will injure the spirit, when the spirit is hurt, one will not be able to control himself, when the condition is protracted, the muscular prominence will become deteriorative and the muscle will be consuming and falling; when the disease developes further to cause the patient's hair to become withered and the complexion to become abnormal, he will die in winter.

脾〔脾：《素问·宣明五气篇》王注引《五运行大论》新校正引均无"脾"字〕愁忧而不解则伤意，意伤则乱，四肢不举，毛悴色夭，死于春。

"When the excessive melancholy can not be removed, the idea will be injured, when it is injured, the patient will become depressed, disquieted and reluctant to lift the limbs due to the weakness of them; when the disease developes further to cause the patient's hair to become withered and the complexion to become abnormal, he will die in spring.

肝〔肝《素问·宣明五气篇》王注引无"肝"字〕悲哀动中则伤魂，魂伤则狂忘〔忘《甲乙》卷一第一，《千金》卷十一第一并作"妄"〕不精〔不精：《甲乙》卷一第一作"其精不守"〕，不精则不正当人〔不精则不正当人：《甲乙》卷一第一并无"不精则不正当"六字，"人"上并有"令"字，连下读〕，阴缩而挛筋，两胁骨不举，毛悴色夭，死于秋。

"When the excessive melancholy affects the internal organs, it will injure the soul, when the soul is hurt, the syndrome of abalienation will occur, it will cause failure of storing the blood of the liver, atrophy of the external genitals, spasm of muscles and pain of bones in both hypochondria; when the disease developes further to cause the patient's hair to become withered and the complexion to become abnormal, he will die in autumn.

肺〔肺：《素问·宣明五气篇》王注引无"肺"字〕喜乐无极则伤魄，魄伤则狂，狂者意不存人〔人：《甲乙》卷一第一作"其人"属下读〕，皮革焦，毛悴色夭，死于夏。

Excessive overjoy will injure the inferior spirit, when it is hurt, the syndrome of mania will occur, it will cause the patient's consciousnesss to become disorderly, he will not be able to observe anything and his skin will become withered; when the disease developes further to cause the patient's hair to become withered and the complexion to become abnormal, he will die in summer.

肾〔肾:《素问·举痛论》王注引无"肾"字〕盛怒而不止则伤志，志伤则喜忘其前言，腰脊〔腰脊:《千金》卷十九第一"腰脊"下并有"痛"字〕不可能俯仰屈伸，毛悴色夭，死于季夏。

When the fury is not restrained, it will injure the will which may cause the oblivion of what he has said time and again, pain in the loins and spine and is unable to face up and down willingly; when the disease developes further to cause the patient's hair to become withered and the complexion to become abnormal, he will die in late summer.

恐惧而不解则伤精，精伤则骨酸痿厥，精时自下。是故五脏，主藏精者也，不可伤，伤则失守而阴虚，阴虚则无气，无气则死矣。是故用针者，察观病人之态，以知精神魂魄之存亡得失之意，五者以伤，针不可以治之也。

"When the excessive terror is not relieved, it will injure the essence of life, arthralgia and syncope with flaccidity will occur, and the patient will often have nocturnal emission. Therefore, the five-viscera is to store the refined energy which must not be injured, otherwise, the refined energy will lose its proper place of storing to cause Yin-deficiency, in this case, the activity of vital energy will be lacking, and the patient will die very soon. Thus, when apply the needling, one must observe the appearance of the patient so as to know the overabundant and deficient condition of the essence of life, spirit, inferior spirit, etc. of the patient, if the patient's refined energy in the five-viscera has already been injured, he can by no means be cured by acupuncture.

肝藏血，血舍魂，肝气虚则恐，实则怒。脾藏营，营舍意，脾气虚则四肢不用，五脏不安，实则腹胀经溲不利。心藏脉〔脉:《医经正本书》第一作"神"〕，脉舍神，心气虚则悲，实则笑不休。肺藏气，气舍魄，肺气虚则鼻塞，不利少气，实则喘喝，胸盈仰息。肾藏精，精舍志，肾气虚则厥，实则胀，五脏不安。必审五脏之病形，以知其气之虚实，谨而调之也。

"The liver stores the blood, and soul adheres to the blood. When the liver energy is deficient, the mood of terror will occur; when the liver energy is overabundant, one will apt to get angry. The spleen stores the Ying-energy, and idea adheres to the Ying-energy. When the spleen energy is deficient, it will cause dullness of the motions of the four limbs and the inharmony of the five viscera, when the spleen energy is obstructed, it will cause abdominal distention, menoxenia, dyschesia and dysuria. The heart stores the spirit, and the spirit adheres to the blood, when the heart energy is deficient, the mood of sorrow will occur; when the heart energy is overabundant, the syndrome of unceasing laughing will occur. The lung stores the energy, and the inferior spirit adheres to the primordial energy of a man. When the lung energy is deficient, one will have stuffy nose, dyspnea, short of breath; when the lung energy is substantial and full, rapid breathing, fullness feeling in the chest even go so far as to breath rapidly while facing up will occur. The kidney stores the essence of life, and the will of a man adheres to the refined energy. When the kidney energy is deficient, one will have cold hands and feet, when there is sthenic-evil in the kidney, abdominal distention will occur, and the five viscera can hardly be harmonious. Therefore, when treating, it must observe the syndromes caused by the five viscera to know the asthenia and sthenia of the primordial energy and then treat the disease cautiously."

终始第九

Chapter 9
Zhong Shi
(The Beginning and Terminal of the Channels)

凡刺之道，毕于终始，明知终始，五脏为纪，阴阳定矣，阴者主脏，阳者主腑〔阴者主脏，阳者主腑：注有浩曰："二句据韵互易，当作'阳者主腑，阴者主脏"〕，阳受气于四末，阴受气于五脏。故泻者迎之，补者随之，知迎知随，气可令和。和气之方，必通阴阳，五脏为阴，六腑为阳，传之后世〔传之后世，《甲乙》卷第五无"传之"以下二十四字〕，以血为盟，敬之者昌，慢之者亡，无道行私，必得夭殃。

The regulations of acupuncture are all written on the chapter of《Beginning and Terminal of the Channel》, when one understands the meaning of the beginning and terminal of the channel, he will be able to determine the relation between the Yin channel and the Yang channel. The Yin channel is interlinked with the five solid organs and the Yang channel is interlinked with the six hollow organs. The Yang channel inherits the channel-energy of the four extremities, and the Yin energy inherits the channel-energy from the five viscera. So, when one twists the needle against the running direction of the channel, it is the purging therapy; when one twists the needle along with the running direction of the channel, it is the invigorating therapy. When one knows the way of twisting the needle to purge the coming sthenic energy and to invigorate the going asthenic energy , the channel energies can be harmonized, thus, the clue of harmonizing the channel energy is in the understanding of the law of Yin and Yang. The five solid organs are Yin inside, and the six hollow organs are Yang outside.

谨奉天道，请言终始，终始者，经脉为纪，持其脉口人迎，以知阴阳有余不足，平与不平，天道毕矣。所谓平人者不病，不病者，脉口人迎应四时也，上下相应而俱往来也，六经之脉不结动也，本末之寒温之相守司也，形肉血气必相称也，是谓平人。少气者，脉口人迎俱少而不称尺寸也。如是者，则阴阳俱不足，补阳则阴竭，泻阴则阳脱。如是者，可将以甘药，不〔不："不"下脱"愈"字〕可饮以至剂。如是者，弗灸〔弗灸："灸"当作"久"〕，不已者，因而泻之，则五脏气坏矣。

Now, let us discuss the meaning of the beginning and terminal of channels prudently according to the principle of overabundance and deficiency of Yin and Yang in heaven and earth. The so called the beginning and terminal is to examine whether the Yin and Yang, asthenia and sthenia are keeping balance by palpating the Cunkou (radial artery proximal to the wrist) and Renying (cervical arteries lateral to the thyroid cartilage), taking the twelve channels as the guiding principle, in this way, the reasons of the overabundance and deficiency of Yin and Yang can be understood. The so called a healthy person is the one who has no disease and the Cunkou and Renying pulse-condition of a healthy man is corresponding with the seasons; the Cunkou and Renying pulse conditions are in consonance with each other, they come and go continuously and the pulsations of the six channels are unceasing; although there are changes of cold and heat in the four seasons, yet the Cunkou and Renying are each having the specific pulse condition without interfering each other, the physique, muscle, blood and energy are harmonious and are keeping in line with each other. These are the conditions of a healthy man. When a man is short of breath, his Cunkou and Renying pulse conditions will appear to be fine, and his skin of the anterolateral side of the forearm is not matching the pulse condition, which shows both his Yin and Yang are deficient. When treating the disease of deficiency in both Yin and Yang, if Yang is invigorated, it will cause the exhaustion of Yin energy; if Yin is purged, it will cause the exhaustion of Yang energy. So, to the patient of this kind, it can only be invigorated with a slow-acting prescription. If the disease is not cured, the quick-acting prescription may be used. The disease of this kind can by no means be cured in a short time. When one does not treat in this way, but treat with acupuncture, it will injure the healthy energy of the five viscera.

人迎一盛，病在足少阳，一盛而躁，病在手少阳。人迎二盛，病在足太阳，二盛而躁，病在手太阳。人迎三盛，病在足阳明，三盛而躁，病在手阳明。人迎四盛，且大且数，名曰溢阳，溢阳为外格。脉口一盛，病在足厥阴，厥阴一盛而躁，在手心主。脉口二盛，病在足少阴，二盛而躁，在手少阴，脉口三盛，病在足太阴，三盛而躁，在手太阴。脉口四盛，且大且数者，名曰溢阴，溢阴为内关，内关不通死不治。人迎与太阴脉口俱盛四倍以上，命名关格，关格者，与之短期。

When the Renying pulse is twice as large as the Cunkou pulse, the disease is in the Foot Shaoyang Channel of Gallbladder. When it is twice as large and impetuous, the disease is in the Hand Shaoyang Channel of Triple Warmer. When the Renying pulse is three times as large as the Cunkou pulse, the disease is in the Foot Taiyang Channel of Bladder. When it is three times as large and impetuous, the disease is in the Hand Taiyang Channel of Small Intestine. When the Renying pulse is four times as large as the Cunkou pulse, the disease is in the Foot Yangming Channel of Stomach. When it is four times as large and impetuous, the disease is in the Hand Yangming Channel of Large Intestine. When the Renying pulse is five times as large as the Cunkou pulse, being gigantic and rapid, it is called the overflowing of Yang which shows the six Yang channels are all partial-overabundant and the Yang fails to communicate with the Yin energy, it is also called "rejecting from outside".

When the Cunkou pulse is twice as large as the Renying pulse, the disease is in the Foot Jueyin Channel of Liver. When it is twice as large and impetuous, the disease is in the Hand Jueyin Channel of Pericardium. When the Cunkou pules is three times as large as the Renying pulse, the disease is in the Foot Shaoyin Channel of Kidney. when it is three times as large and impetuous, the disease is in the Hand Shaoyin Channel of Heart. When the Cunkou pulse is four times as large as the Renying pulse, the disease is in the Foot Taiyin Channel of

Spleen. When it is four times as large and impetuous, the disease is in the Hand Taiyin Channel of lung. When the Cunkou pulse is five times as large as the Renying pulse, being gigantic and rapid, it is called the overflowing of Yin which shows the six Yin channels are all partial overabundant and fail to communicate with the Yang energy, it is also called "closing from inside." When the superficies and the interior are being obstructed due to the closing from inside, it is a fatal disease. When the Renying pulse and the Cunkou pulse are both more then five times as large as usual, it is called "Guan Ge" (close and reject). When one has Guan Ge, he will soon die.

人迎一盛，泻足少阳而补足厥阴，二泻一补，日一取之，必切而验之，疏取之上，气和乃止。人迎二盛，泻足太阳，补足少阴，二泻一补，二日一取之，必切而验之，疏取之上，气和乃止。人迎三盛，泻足阳明而补足太阴，二泻一补，日二取之，必切而验之，疏取之上，气和乃止。脉口一盛，泻足厥阴而补足少阳，二补一泻，日一取之，必切而验之，疏而取之上，气和乃止。脉口二盛，泻足少阴而补足太阳，二补一泻，二日一取之，必切而验之，疏取之上，气和乃止。脉口三盛，泻足太阴而补足阳明，二补一泻，日二取之，必切而验之，疏而取之上，气和乃止。所以日二取之者，太阳主胃，大富于谷气，故可日二取之也。人迎与脉口俱盛三倍以上，命曰阴阳俱溢，如是者不开，则血脉闭塞，气无所行，流淫于中，五脏内伤。如此者，因而灸之，则变易而为他病矣。

When the Renying pulse is twice as large as the cunkou pulse, the Foot Shaoyang Channel of Gallbladder should be purged and the Foot Jueyin Channel of Liver should be invigorated; when purging, one acupoint should be pricked, when invigorating, two acupoints should be pricked, and the pricking should be once a day; besides, one must feel the Renying and cunkou pulses to test whether the disease is relieving or aggravating, if the patient has irritation or unquietness, the channel on the upper part of the body should be pricked, and cease the pricking when the channel energies become harmonious. When the Renying pules is three times as large as the Cunkou pules, it should purge the Foot Taiyang Channel of Bladder and invigorate the Foot Shaoyin Channel of Kidney; when purging, two acupoints should be pricked, when invigorating, one acupoint should be pricked, and the pricking should be once in two days; besides, one must feel the Renying and Cunkou pulses to test whether the disease is relieving or aggravating, if the patient has irritation or unquietness, the channel of the upper part of the body should be pricked, and cease the pricking when the channel energies become harmonious. When the Renying pulse is four times as large as the Cunkou pulse, it should purge the Foot Yangming Channel of Stomach and should invigorate the Foot Taiyin Channel of Spleen; when purging, two acupoints should be pricked, when invigorating, one acupoint should be pricked, and the pricking should be twice a day; besides, one should feel the Renying and Cunkou pulses to test whether the disease is relieving or aggravating, if the patient has irritation and unquietness, the channel in the upper part of the body should be pricked, and cease the pricking when the channel energies become harmonious. When the Cunkou is twice as large as th Renying pulse, it should purge the Foot Ju yin Channel of Liver and invigorate the Foot Shaoyang Channel of Gallbladder; when invigorating, two acupoints should be pricked, when purging, one acupoint should be pricked, and the pricking should be once a day; besides, one should feel the Cunkou and Renying pulses to test whether the disease is relieving or aggravating, if the patient has irritation and unquietness, the channel of the upper part of the body should be pricked, and cease the pricking when the channel energies become harmonious. When the Cunkou pulse is three times as large as the Renying pulse, it should purge the Foot Shaoyin Channel of Kidney and invigorate the Taiyang Channel of Bladder; when in vigorating, two acupoints should be pricked, when purging, one acupoint should be pricked; and the pricking should be once in two days; besides, one should feel the Cunkou and Renying pulses to test whether the disease is relieving or aggravating, if the patient has irritation and unquietness, the channel of the upper part of the body should be pricked, and cease the pricking when the channel energies become harmonious. When the Cunkou pulse is four times as large as the Renying pulse, it should purge the Foot Taiyin Channel of Spleen and invigorate the Foot Yangming Channel of stomach; when invigorating, two acupoints should be pricked, when purging, one acupoint should be pricked, and the pricking should be twice in a day; besides, one should feel the Cunkou and Renying pulses to test whether the disease is relieving or aggravating, if the patient has irritation and unquietness, the channel of the upper part of the body should be pricked, and cease the pricking when the channel energies become harmonious. The reason of the pricking twice a day is that the Yangming Channel controls the condition of the stomach, and in the stomach, the essential substance from cereals is abundant, and the energy and blood are plenty, so, the pricking may be twice a day. When the Renying and Cunkou pulses are both more than four times larger than usual, it is called the "overflowing of Yin and Yang"; if the channel is not dredged, it will cause the functional activities of vital energy to become blocked, the circulation of the vital energy hindered, the energy and blood unimpeded, and the five viscera will be harmed. In this case, if moxibustion is aplied erroneously, change will occur to cause disease.

凡刺之道，气调而止，补阴泻阳，音气〔气：《甲乙》卷五第五作“声”〕益彰，耳目聪明，反此者血气不行。

Generally, in pricking, when the Yin and Yang energies have kept in harmony, the pricking should be ceased. Besides, one should pay attention to the invigoration of Yin and the purging of Yang, in this way, can the patient have a loud voice, keen ears and bright eyes. If one runs to the contrary, purge the Yin and invigorate the Yang, the blood and energy of the patient will not operate normally.

所谓气至而有效者，泻则益虚，虚者脉大如其故而不坚也，坚如其故者，适虽言故，病未去也。补则益实。实者脉大如其故而益坚也，夫如其故而不坚者，适虽言快，病未去也。故补则实，泻则虚，痛虽不随针〔针：“针”下脱“减”字，应据《甲乙》卷五第五补〕，病必衰去。必先通十二经脉之所生病，而后可得传于终始矣。故阴阳不相移，虚实不相倾，取之其经。

The so called there will be curative effect when the energy arrives under the needle means when the sthenic syndrome is treated with the purging therapy, sthenia will turn into asthenia, and the asthenic pulse condition will remain gigantic but not firm. If the pulse condition remains to be firm, the disease is not alleviated although the patient feels comfortable for the time being, When the asthenic syndrome is treated with the invigorating therapy, the asthenia will turn into sthenia, and the sthenic pulse condition will remain gigantic and even more firm. If the pulse condition remains gigantic but not firm, the disease is not alleviated although the patient feels comfortable for the time being. So, when one applies the invigorating therapy accurately, the healthy energy can be substantialized, when one applies the purging therapy accurately, the evil energy will become debilitative. Even though the pain can not be removed immediately along with the prickings of the needle, yet the disease can certainly be somewhat relieved. One must understand the relations between the twelve channels and the disease first, then can he achieve the condition of well begun and well ended. The Yin channel and Yang channel can by no means be interchanged, and the sthenic syndrome can by no means be reversed, thus, when treating, prick the acupoints of the related channel.

凡刺之属，三刺至谷气，邪僻妄合，阴阳易居，逆顺相反，沉浮异处，四时不得，稽留淫泆，须针而去。故一刺则阳邪出，再刺则阴邪出，三刺则谷气至，谷气至而止。所谓谷气至者，已补而实，已泻而虚，故以知谷气至也。邪气独去者，阴与阳未能调，而病知愈也。故曰补则实，泻则虚，痛虽不随针，病必衰去矣。

In pricking. one should take note of applying the three-pricking method to cause the healthy energy coming slowly. All the affections such as: the mixing of the evil energy with the blood and energy disorderly, the slipping of the internal Yin to outside, the bogging of the external Yang to inside, the reverse circulation of energy and blood, the abnormal sinking and floating of the pulse condition, the inconsistency of the channel with the four seasons, the stagnation of the energy and blood of the patient and the running rashly of the blood and energy should be removed by pricking. so, it must pay attention to the three pricking method. In the method, the initial pricking will expel the evil energy in Yang; the second pricking will expel the evil energy of Yin; the third pricking will cause the healthy energy to come slowly, and by this time, the needle can be pulled out. The so called the arrival of the healthy energy means one can know the arrival of the healthy energy when the patient feels the energy is more substantial after invigoroting and feels the evil-energy is somewhat retreated after purging, When the evil energy is removed, although the blood and energy of Yin and Yang have not yet been harmonized, yet, one can know the disease will be rcovered soon. Thus, the saying goes: "Invigorating causes the substantialness and purging causes the deficiency, although the pain is not reduced along with the time of pricking, yet the disease will be declined."

阴盛而阳虚，先补其阳，后泻其阴而和之。阴虚而阳盛，先补其阴，后泻其阳而和之。

When the evil energy in the Yin channel is overabundant and the healthy energy in the Yang channel is deficient, it should invigorate the healthy energy of the Yang channel first and then purge the evil energy of the Yin channel, so as to adjust the surplus and deficiency of them. When the healthy energy of the Yin channel is deficient and the evil energy of the Yang channel is overabundant, it should invigorate the healthy energy of the Yin channel first, and then purge the evil energy of the Yang channel, so as to adjust the surplus and deficiency of them.

三脉动于足大指之间，必审其实虚。虚而泻之，是谓重虚，重虚病益甚。凡刺此者，以指按之，脉动而实且疾者疾泻之，虚而徐者则补之，反此者病益甚。其动也，阳明在上，厥阴在中，少阴在下。

The three channels of Foot Yangming, Foot Jueyin and Foot Shaoyin are all having their arteries spreading in between the big toe and the second toe; when pricking, one must examine whether the syndrome is of asthenic or sthenic, if the purging is applied erroneously to asthenic syndrome, it is called double asthenia, the asthenia will become all the more, and the disease will be aggravated. Generally, when pricking this kind of disease, press the artery with fingers first, if the pulsation is sthenic and fast, the purging therapy should be applied; when the pulsation is asthenic and slow. the invigorating therapy should be applied. If one applies the invigorating or purging erroneously, the disease will be aggravated. As to the locations of the arteries, the artery of Foot Yangming is on the dorsum of foot, the artery of Foot Jueyin is in the dorsum of foot and the artery of Foot Taiyin is under the dorsum of foot.

膺腧中膺，背腧中背，肩髆虚者，取之上。

When pricking the acupoints of the chest, the chest must be hit; when pricking the acupoints of the back, the back must be hit. When the arm has aching pain, distention and numbness, the acupoints on the channel of upper limb should be pricked.

重舌，刺舌柱以铍针也。

To the patient of sublingual swelling, prick the large vein under the tongue to cause bleeding.

手屈而不伸者，其病在筋，伸而不屈者，其病在骨，在骨守骨，在筋守筋。

When one fails to stretch his fingers after bending, the disease is in the tendon; when one fails to bend his fingers after stretching, the disease is in the bone. When the disease is in the bone, treat the acupoints which control the bone; when the disease is in the tendon, treat the acupoints which control the tendon.

补须〔补须:"须"是误字，应作"泻"〕一方实，深取之，稀按其痏，以极出其邪气；一方虚，浅刺之，以养其脉，疾按其痏，无使邪气得入。邪气来也紧而疾，谷气来也徐而和。脉实者，深刺之，以泄其气；脉虚者，浅刺之，使精气无得出，以养其脉，独出其邪气。刺诸痛者〔刺诸痛者:《太素》卷二十二《三刺》"痛者"下并有"深刺之，诸痛者"六字〕，其脉皆实。

The important rule of invigorating and purging is: when purging, pay attention to find out the sthenic side of the channel energy and prick deeply with purging therapy. after pulling the needle, press the needle hole softly with hand to excrete the evil energy to the full; when invigorating, pay attention to find out the asthenic side of the channel energy and prick shallowly to maintain the channel pricked with invigorating therapy, after pulling out the needle, press the needle hole with hand hastily to avoid the incursion of the evil energy. When the evil energy arrives, there will be the urgent feeling under the needle and when the healthy energy arrives, there will be the slow and harmonious feeling under the needle. When the channel energy is overabundant and sthenic, deep pricking should be applied; when the channel energy is deficient and asthenic, shallow pricking should be applied to prevent the excretion of the refined energy and thus maintain the channel. It is only the evil energy should be let out. To all kinds of disease with pain, prick deeply as all the pulse condition indicating the disease with pain are of sthenic.

故曰：从腰以上者，手太阴阳明皆主之；从腰以下者，足太阴阳明皆主之。病在上者下取之，病在下者高〔高："高"是"上"的误字，应据《针灸问对》卷上改〕取之，病在头者取之足，病在足者取之腘。病生于头者头重，生于手者臂重，生于足〔足：胡本，熊本，周本，统本并作"腰"〕者足重，治病者先刺其病所从生者也。

All the diseases above the loins can be treated with the acupoints of the Hand Taiyin Channel of Lung and the Hand Yangming Channel of Large Intestine; all the diseases under the loins can be treated with the acupoints of Foot Taiyin channel of Spleen and the Foot Yangming Channel of Stomach. When the disease is on the upper part, the acupoints down below can be pricked, when the disease is on the lower part, the acupoints on the upper can be pricked, when the disease is on the loins, the acupoints on the popliteal fossa can be pricked when the disease is in the head, the patient will feel heavy on the head; when the disease is in the hand, the patient's arm must be feeling heavy; when the disease is in the foot, his foot must be feeling heavy. When treating, one must analyze carefully the resons of the disease first, and then carry on the pricking.

春气在〔在：《太素》卷二十二《三刺》"在"下有"豪"字〕毛，夏气在皮肤，秋气在分肉，冬气在筋骨，刺此病者各以其时为齐。故刺肥人者，以秋冬之齐；刺瘦人者，以春夏之齐。病痛者〔病痛者：《甲乙》卷五第五作"刺之痛者"〕阴也，痛而以手按之不得者阴也，深刺之。病在上者阳也，病在下者阴也。痒者阳也，浅刺之。

In spring, the evil energy is in the fine hair, in summer, the evil energy is in the skin, in autumn, the evil energy is in the muscle, and in winter, the evil energy is in the tendon and bone. When treating the diseases which are related with seasons, the pricking should be different in deep or shalow according to the changes of the season. To a fleshy person, the deep pricking which is suitable in autumn and winter should be applied; to a thin and feeble person, the shallow pricking which is suitable in spring and summer should be applied. When the patient has pain in pricking, it is mostly the syndrome of Yin, when the pain can not be relieved after pressing by hand, it is also a syndrome of Yin which should be treated with deep pricking. When the patient is itching, it shows the evil is outside and it should be treated with shallow pricking. When the disease is on the upper part of the body, it belongs to Yang, when it is on the lower part, it belongs to Yin.

病先起阴者，先 治其阴而后治其阳；病先起阳者，先治其阳而后治其阴。刺热厥者，留针反为寒；刺寒厥者，留针反为热。刺热厥者，二阴一阳；刺寒厥者，二阳一阴。所谓二阴者，二刺阴也；一阳〔一阳：《甲乙》卷七第三并作“二阳”，“二阳”上有“所谓”二字〕者，〔一：《甲乙》卷七第三并作“二”〕一刺阳也。久病者邪气入深，刺此病者，深内而久留之，间日而复刺之，必先调其左右，去其血脉刺道毕矣。

When the disease starts from the Yin channel first, it should treat the Yin channel first, and then, treat the Yang channel; when the disease starts from the Yang channel first, it should treat the Yang channel first and then treat the Yin channel. When pricking the cold extremities due to heat-evil, the retention of the needle can cause the heat to turn into cold; when pricking the cold type jue-syndrome, the retention of the needle can cause the cold to become heat. When pricking the cold extremities due to heat-evil, the Yin channel should be pricked twice and the Yang channel once. The so called Yin twice means to prick the Yin channel twice, and the Yang twice means to prick the Yang channel twice. When the disease is protracted and the evil has penetrated into the viscera, it should prick deeply and retain the needle longer, and the pricking should be proceeded every other day. One must prick the channel perpendicularly when the evil is in the channel, and prick the collateral in contralateral when the disease is in the collateral, and the stagnated blood in the vessel should be removed. These are the principles of acupuncture.

凡刺之法，必察其形气，形肉〔肉：《甲乙》卷五第五“肉”作“气”〕未脱，少气而脉又躁，躁厥〔厥：《甲乙》卷五第五校注云：“‘厥’一作‘疾’字”〕者，必为缪刺之，散气可收，聚气可布，深居静处，占〔占：《灵枢略·六气论》并作“与”〕神往来，闭户塞牖，魂魄不散，专意一神，精气之〔之：《灵枢略·六气论》并作“不”〕分，毋闻人声，以收其精，必一其神，令志在针，浅而留之，微而浮之，以移其神，气至乃休。男内女外，坚拒勿出，谨守勿内，是谓得气。

Generally, when pricking, one must examine the physique and vital energy of the patient. If the physique of the patient is not emaciated, but he is short of breath and his pulse condition is impetuous and rapid, it should apply the contralateral pricking to collect the dispersing energy and disperse the accumulating evil energy. When pricking, the physician should like staying in a secluded place and deal with the spirit only, he should also like shutting himself in a room with the doors and windows closed, he must be clear in consciousness, pure in thought with consistent mind and concentrating energy; he can hear no voice of the people beside, keeping a sound mind and concentrates his attention on the pricking only. He should apply the twisting and lift the needle softly to shift away the fearful feeling of the patient until getting the acupuncture feeling under the needle. When the patient is a man, wait for the Wei-energy to have the acupuncture feeling; when the patient is a woman, wait for the Ying-energy to have the acupuncture feeling. One must resist resolutely the coming out of the healthy energy, and guard against strictly the going in of the evil energy, and this is the so called getting the acupuncture feeling.

凡刺之禁：新内勿刺，新刺勿内。已醉勿刺，已刺勿醉。新怒勿刺，已刺勿怒。新劳勿刺，已刺勿劳。已饱勿刺，已刺勿饱。已饿勿刺，已刺勿饿。已渴勿刺，已刺勿渴。大惊大怒，必定其气，乃刺之。乘车来者，卧而休之。如食顷乃刺之。出〔出：《甲乙》卷五第一上，《千金》卷二十九第三并作“步”〕行来者，坐而休之，如行十里顷乃刺之。凡此十二禁者，其脉乱气散，逆其营卫，经气不次，因而刺之，则阳病入于阴，阴病出为阳，则邪气复生，粗工勿察，是谓伐身，形体淫泆，乃消脑髓，津液不化，脱其五味，是谓失气也。

The contraindications in pricking are: one must not be pricked right after sexual intercourse, and one must not conduct sexual intercourse right after the pricking; one must not be pricked after drunken, and one must not be drunken after the pricking; one must not be pricked right after getting angry, and one must not get angry after the pricking; one must not be pricked right after fatigue due to hard labour, and one must not do hard labour after the pricking; one must not be pricked right after eating his fill, and one must not eat his fill after the pricking; one must not be pricked when being hungry, and one must not be hungry after the pricking; one must not be pricked when being thirsty, and one must not be thirsty after the pricking; one must not be pricked when one is terrified greatly or flying into a fury, the pricking must wait until his energy has become calm. To the patient who comes by car, he should lie on the bed for the period of taking a meal before pricking. To the patient who comes by walk, he should sit and rest for the period of a ten li walk (an hour) before pricking. Generally, all the patients who have the conditions of contraindication above are having a confusing pulse condition, dispersed healthy energy, abnormal operations of the Ying-energy and Wei-energy and the deficiency of the energy and blood of the channel, if one pricks perfunctorily, the disease of Yang channel will penetrate into the internal organs, the disease of Yin channel will encroach the Yang channel, and the evils will create disturbances. A physician of lower level pays no attention to these contraindications, and actually, he is injuring the body of the patient, it causes the patient to become aching and painful of the physique, consumption of the marrow, failing to spread the body fluid, and the patient will not be able to obtain the refined substances from the five tastes of food. In this way, the healthy energy of the patient will be diminished very soon, and this is the so called the forfeiture of energy.

太阳之脉〔太阳之脉：《甲乙》卷二第一上作“太阳脉绝”〕，其终也，戴眼，反折，瘈疭，其色白，绝皮乃绝汗，绝汗则终矣。少阳终者，耳聋，百节尽纵，目系绝，目系绝一日半则死矣，其死也，色青白乃死。阳明终者，口目动作，喜惊，妄言，色黄，其上下之经盛而不行则终矣。少阴终者，面黑，齿长而垢，腹胀闭塞，上下不通而终矣。厥阴终者，中热嗌干，喜溺心烦，甚则舌卷，卵上缩而终矣。太阴终者，腹胀闭不得息，气噫，善呕，呕则逆，逆则面赤，不逆则上下不通，上下不通则面黑皮毛燋而终矣。

When the Hand and Foot Taiyang Channels are severing, the eyes of the patient will be staring up, and he will have opisthotonos, convulsion of hands and feet, pale complexion and perspiration with sudden onset. When the Hand and Foot Shaoyang Channels are severing, the patient will become deaf, his joints of the whole body become loose and weak and his eyes are staring; when the channel energy connecting the brain is severed, he will die in one and half days, and before dying, his complexion turns to white from green. When the Hand and Foot Yangming Channels are severing, the patient will have distortion of the face, he is frightened often, talking nonsense with a yellow complexion. When the arteries of the hand channels above and the foot channels below are having the hyperactive beats, the patient will die. When the Hand and Foot Shaoyin Channels are severing, the patient will have a black complexion, and his teeth become longer with tartars. When the patient has abdominal fullness and distention, impediment of the upper functional activities of vital energy with that of the lower, he will die. When the Hand and Foot Jueyin Channels are severing, the patient will have heat in the chest, dry throat, frequent micturition, irritation and even go so far as to have the syndrome of curled tongue, testicle was contracted from above and then he dies. When the Hand and Foot Taiyin Channels are severing, the patient will have abdominal distention, dyspnea, frequent eructation, frequent vomiting, up-reversing of vital energy when vomiting, red complexion due to the up-reversing of vital energy, and if the vital energy fails to reverse up, the energy above and the energy below will be blocked to cause the black complexion; finally, the patient's skin and fine hair will become withered and die.

经脉第十

Chapter 10
Jing Mai
(On Channels)

雷公问于黄帝曰：禁脉〔禁脉：张注本“脉”作“服”〕之言，凡刺之理，经脉为始，营其所行，制其度量，内次五脏，外别六腑，愿尽闻其道。黄帝曰：人始生，先成精，精成而脑髓生，骨为干，脉为营，筋为纲，肉为墙，皮肤坚而毛发长，谷入于胃，脉道以通，血气乃行。雷公曰：愿卒闻经脉之始生。黄帝曰：经脉者，所以能决死生，处百病，调虚实，不可不通。

Leigong asked Yellow Emperor and said: "It was stated in the《Jing Fu Chapters》: 'In acupuncture, channel is most important, one must estimate the condition of the beginning and the end of its operation, know its length, its relations with the five solid organs inside and different relations with the six hollow organs outside.' I hope to hear the reasons about it." Yellow Emperor said: "In the beginning of human life the essence of life is formed first, then it developes into the brain and the spinal cord, and finally, the human body is shaped. The skeletons are like the wooden pillars on the two sides of the wall, the channels are like the barracks connecting each other, the tendons are like the strings the muscles are like the walls, and the skins and hairs are protecting the bones, channels, tendons and muscles. When the five-cereal enters into the stomach, it produces the refined substances which causes the unimpediment of the vessels and the unceasing operations of the blood and energy." Leigong said: "I hope to hear about the condition of the initial occurrence of the channel." Yellow Emperor said: "One can determine the survival or death of the patient, can treat various diseases and find out whether the disease is of sthenic or asthenic according to the condition of the channel, and one must understand it."

肺手太阴之脉，起于中焦，下络大肠，还循胃口，上膈属肺，从肺系横出腋下，下循臑内，行少阴心主之前，下肘中，循臂内上骨下廉，入寸口，上鱼〔《圣济总录》卷一百九十一引“上”下无“鱼”字，“上”字连下读〕，循鱼际，出大指之端；其支者，从腕后直出次指内廉，出其端。是动则病肺胀满，膨膨而喘咳，缺盆中痛，甚则交两手而瞀，此为臂厥。是主肺所生病者，咳，上气喘渴，烦心胸满，臑臂内前廉痛厥，掌中热。气盛有余，则肩背〔背：守校本作“臂”。〕痛，风寒，汗出中风，小便数而欠。气虚则肩背痛寒，少气不足以息，溺色变。为此诸病，盛则泻之，虚则补之，热则疾之，寒则留之，陷下则灸之，不盛不虚，以经取之。盛者寸口大三倍于人迎，虚者则寸口反小于人迎也。

"The Hand Taiyin Channel of Lung starts from the abdomen of the middle warmer, winds the large intestine below, returns to pass the upper entrance of the stomach, ascends through the diaphragm and links the lung; then it runs horizontally from the trachea to the location under the armpit, passes along the inner flank of the upper arm, in front of the Hand Shaoyin and the Hand Jueyin Channels to reach the inside of the elbow, then it runs along the inner side of the forearm and the lower end of the radius to reach the Cunkou pulse, and then, runs along the thenar eminence to reach the tip of the thumb; its branch starts from the rear of the wrist and runs to the tip of the inner side of the forefinger (Lieque point) and connects with the Hand Yangming Channel of Large Intestine. The diseases stem from Hand Taiyang Channel energy are: distention of the lung, stagnation of the vital energy, rapid breathing, cough and pain in the supraclavicular fossa: when the case is severe, the patient will press his chest with his two hands intersecting. These syndromes are caused by the up-reversing of the channel energy of the arm. The diseases of Hand Taiyin Channel are related to the lung, they are: cough, short of breath, rapid breathing with sound, feeling oppression over the chest, sensation of fullness in the chest, pain in the front of the inner side of the upper arm and hotness in the centre of the palm. When the evil energy is having a surplus, pain in the shoulder and arms, frequent micturition but has reduction of urine will occur, when the healthy energy is deficient, pain and cold in the shoulder and back, short of breath and changing colour of the urine will occur. When treating, apply purging therapy when the syndrome is sthenic, apply invigorating therapy when the syndrome is asthenic, apply swift pricking when it is a heat syndrome, apply retention of the needle when it is a cold syndrome and apply moxibustion when the pulse is deficient and bogging. As to the syndrome which is not sthenic nor asthenic, prick the acupoints of the Hand Taiyin Channel. When the Cunkou pulse is four times as large as the Renying pulse, it is the sthenic syndrome of the Hand Taiyin Channel, when the Cunkou pulse is smaller than the Renying pulse, it is the asthenic syndrome of the Hand Taiyin Channel.

大肠手阳明之脉，起于大指次指之端，循指上廉，出合谷两骨之间，上入两筋之中，循臂上廉，入肘外廉，上臑外前廉，上肩，出髃骨之前廉，上出于柱骨之会上，下入缺盆，络肺，下膈，属大肠；其支者，从缺盆上颈，贯颊，入下齿中，还出挟口，交人中，左之右，右之左，上挟鼻孔。是动则病齿痛颈肿。是主津液所生病者，目黄口干，鼽衄，喉痹，肩前臑痛，大指次指痛不用。气有余则当脉所过者热肿，虚则寒栗不复。为此诸病，盛则泻之，虚则补之，热则疾之，寒则留之，陷下则灸之，不盛不虚，以经取之。盛者人迎大三倍于寸口，虚者人迎反小于寸口也。

"The Hand Yangming Channel of Large Intestine starts from the tip of the forefinger, runs along the upper side of the forefinger (Erjian and Sanjian points), passes the Hegu point in the forked bone between the thumb and the forefinger to reach the cave-in betwen the two tendons on the wrist (Yangxi point), then runs along the upper part of the forearm (Pianli, Wenliu, Xialian and Shanglian points) to reach the outer flank of the upper arm (Zhouliao, Wuli, and Binao points) to reach the shoulder (Jianyu) and the scapula, and then converges with the various Yin channels at the Dazhui point, then, it descends to the supraclavicular fossa, communicates with the lung, crosses through the diaphragm and links the large intestine; its branch ascends to the neck from the supraclavicular fossa, passes the cheek to reach the seam of the lower teeth, then turns back to make a detour to the upper lip and converges with the symmetrical Hand Yangming Channel of the other side at the nasolabial groove, then the left channel goes to the right and the right channel goes to the left to clip the two sides of the nostrils and connect the Foot Yangming Channel of stomach. The diseases stem from the Hand Yangming Channel are toothache and the swelling of the neck. The diseases of Hand Yangming Channel are related with the body fluid, they are: yellow eyes, dry mouth, running clear nasal mucus or having epitaxis, sore throat, pain in the shoulder and the upper arm, pain of the forefinger which can hardly be used. When the channel energy of Hand Yangming is having a surplus and has sthenic syndrome, heat and swelling on the locations where the channel passes will occur, when the channel energy of Hand Yangming is deficient and has asthenic syndrome, the patient will be shivering with cold, and can hardly to become warm again. When treating, apply purging therapy when the syndrome is sthenic, apply invigorating therapy when the syndrome is asthenic, apply swift pricking when it is a heat-syndrome, apply retention of the needle when it is a cold-syndrome and apply moxibustion when the pulse is deficient and bogging down, As to the syndrome which is not sthenic nor asthenic , prick the Hand Yangming Channel. When the Renying pulse is four times as large as the Cunkou pulse, it is the sthenic syndrome of Hand Yangming Channel, when the Renying pulse is smaller than the Cunkou pulse, it is the asthenic syndrome of the Hand Yangiming Chaanel.

胃足阳明之脉，起于鼻之交頞中，旁纳太阳之脉，下循鼻外，入上齿中，还出挟口还唇，下交承浆，却循颐后下廉，出大迎，循颊车，上耳前，过客主人，循发际，至额颅；其支者，从大迎前下人迎，循喉咙入缺盆，下膈，属胃，络脾；其直者，从缺盆下乳内廉，下挟脐，入气街中；其支者，起于胃口，下循腹里，下至气街中而合，以下髀关，抵伏兔，下膝膑中，下循胫外廉，下足跗，入中指内间；其支者，下廉〔下廉：《太素》卷八，《脉经》卷六第六“廉”并作“膝”〕三寸而别，下入中指外间；其支者，别跗上，入大指间，出其端。是动则病洒洒振寒，善呻〔呻：《太素》卷八作“伸”〕数欠，颜黑，病至则恶人与火，闻木声则惕然而惊，心欲动，独闭户塞牖而处，甚则欲上高而歌，弃衣而走，贲响腹胀，是为骭厥。是主血〔血：《脉经》卷六第六校注云：“‘血’”一作‘胃’〕所生病者，狂疟温淫汗出，鼽衄，口喎〔口喎：莫文泉曰：“按口喎属筋病，与脉病不干，口喎当为‘病’，谓口生病疮，与‘唇胗’”同为疡证〕唇胗，颈肿喉痹，大腹水肿，膝膑肿痛，循膺、乳、气街、股、伏兔、骭外廉、足跗上皆痛，中指不用。气盛则身以前皆热，其有余于胃，则消谷善饥，溺色黄。气不足则身以前皆寒栗胃中寒则胀满。为此诸病，盛则泻之，虚则补之，热则疾之，寒则留之，陷下则灸之，不盛不虚，以经取之。盛者人迎大三倍于寸口，虚者人迎反小于寸口也。

“The Foot Yangming Channel of Stomach starts from the Yingxiang point beside the nostril and runs into the Foot Taiyang Channel beside, then, descend along the outer flank of the nose to enter into the seam of the upper teeth and comes out to encircle the lips and meets the symmetrical Foot Yangming Channel of the other side at the Chengjiang point, then, it runs along the rear of the cheek, passes the Daying and Jiache points to reach the front of the ear, and then, passes the Kezhuren point and runs along the hair line to reach the forehead; its branch starts from the front of the Daying point, descends to the Renying point, passing the throat (Shuitu and Qishe points) to enter into the supraclavicular fossa, then, descends again to cross the diaphragm, links the stomach and communicates with the spleen. Another Foot Yangming Channel which runs straightly forward , starts from the supraclavicular fossa to reach the inner side of the breast and near the naval (passing Tianshu, Wailing, Daju, Shuidao and Guilai points) to reach the Qijie point (Qichong) beside the pubic hair margin; another branch starts from the lower outlet of the stomach, runs along the inside of the abdomen and joins the channel which runs straightly forward stated above in front of the Qijie point (Qichong), then it runs along the thigh, passes the Futu point then along the knee cap and the outside of the tibia, passing the dorsum of the foot and reaches the inner side of the middle toe; another branch starts from the location three inches beneath the knee, and descends to the outer side of the second toe; another branch starts from the dorsum of the foot, runs into the big toe to connect the Foot Taiyang Channel of Spleen. The diseases stem from Foot Yangming Channel are: shivering with cold, yawns and stretches oneself often, black colour of the forehead, detestation of man and fire when becoming ill, afraid of hearing the sound made by wood, palpitation and prefering to stay alone with the doors and windows closed. When the disease is severe, the patient may sing loudly in a high place and runs about with his clothes taken off, and he has abdominal distention and borborygmus. These syndromes are due to the up-reversing of the channel energy of the foot tibia. The diseases of Foot Yangming are related to the stomach are: mania, malaria, excessiveness of warm-heat, perspiration, running clear nasal mucus, epistaxis, aphtha, swelling of the neck, sore throat, abdominal distention, swelling above the navel, pain in the kneecap, pain along the breast、the Qijie point、the frontal leg、the Futu point、the outer flank of tibia and the dorsum of foot, and the middle toe can not move. When the Hand Yangming Channel energy is overabundant, the patient will have hotness in the chest and abdomen, he will often get hungry due to rapid digestion and will have deep coloured urine: when his energy is deficient, the chest and abdomen will be cold and the cold in the stomach may cause distention and fullness. When treating, apply purging therapy when the syndrome is sthenic, apply invigorating therapy when the syndrome is asthenic, apply swift pricking when it is a heat-syndrome, apply retention of the needle when it is a cold-syndrome and apply moxibustion when the pulse is deficient and bogging down. As to the syndrome which is neither asthenic nor sthenic, prick the Foot Yangming Channel. When the Renying pulse is four times as large as the Cunkou pulse, it is the sthenic syndrome of the Foot Yangming Channel; when the Renying pulse is smaller than the Cunkou pulse, it is the asthenic syndrome of the Foot Yangming Channel.

脾足太阴之脉，起于大指之端〔起于大指之端：《病沅》卷十六《心腹相引痛候》卷三十《舌肿强候》“起于”下并有“足”字〕，循指内侧白肉际，过核骨后，上内踝前廉，入腨内，循胫骨后，交出厥阴之前。上膝股内前廉，入腹属脾络胃，上膈，挟咽，连舌本，散舌下；其支者，复从胃，别上膈，注心中〔中：《病沅》卷十六《心腹相引痛候》作“经”〕。是动则病舌本〔舌本：《太素》卷八“舌”下无“本”字〕强，食则呕，胃脘痛，腹胀善噫，得后与气〔得后与气：《太素》卷八，《伤寒论》卷一成注引并作“得后出余气”〕，则快然如衰，身体皆重。是主脾所生病者，舌本痛，体不能动摇，食不下，烦心，心下急痛〔急痛：《脉经》卷六第五，《图经》卷二“急痛”下并有“寒疟”二字〕，溏、瘕、泄、水闭，黄疸，不能卧，强立，股膝内肿厥，足大指不用。为此诸病，盛则泻之，虚则补之，热则疾之，寒则留之，陷下则灸之，不盛不虚，以经取之。盛者寸口大三倍于人迎，虚者寸口反小于人迎也。

“The Foot Taiyin Channel of Spleen starts from the tip of the big toe, runs along the white flesh on the inner side of the big toe, passes the bony nodule and ascends to the front of the inner ankle, then, ascends again to the calf, runs along the rear of the tibia to intersect the Foot Jueyin Channel and runs in front of it, then ascends along the front of the inner side of the knee, enters into the thigh, links the spleen and communicates with the stomach, then crosses the diaphragm above, and ascends to press close to the throat, links the tongue and spreads under the tongue; another branch reached up from the stomach to connect the Hand Shaoyin Channel of Heart. The diseases stem from the Spleen Channel are: stiff tongue, vomiting after food intake, pain in the gastric cavity, abdominal distention, frequent eructation and relief of the abdominal distention after loosening the bowel and discharge the remainder energy of the dreg, but the body is still heavy. The diseases of Foot Taiyin Channel are related with the spleen, they are: pain in the root of the tongue, failing to wave the body, failing to take food, feeling of oppression over the chest, acute pain below the heart, cold-type malaria, diarrhea with loose stool dysentery, dysuria, jaundice, and the desire of lying down of the patient; when the patient stands with difficulty, there will be swelling along the inner side of the thigh and knee, causing the inability of moving the big toe. When treating, apply purging therapy when the syndrome is asthenic, apply invigorating therapy when the syndrome is asthenic, apply swift pricking when it is a heat-syndrome, apply retention of the needle when it is a cold-syndrome and apply moxibustion when the pulse is deficient and bogging down. As to the syndrome which is neither asthenic nor sthenic, prick the Foot Taiyin Channel of Spleen. When the Cunkou pulse is four times as large as the Renying pulse, it is the sthenic syndrome of the Foot Taiyin Channel; when the Cunkou pulse is smaller than the Renying pulse, it is the asthenic syndrome of the Foot Taiyin Channel.

心手少阴之脉，起于心中，出属心系，下膈络小肠〔肠：《素问·诊要经终论》王注作“腹”〕；其支者，从心系上挟咽，系目系，其直者，复从心系却上肺，下出腋下，下循臑内后廉，行〔行：与注本，张注本，营校本“行”下并有“手”字〕太阴心主之后，下肘内，循臂内后廉，抵掌后锐骨之端，入掌内后廉〔入掌内后廉：《太素》卷八“内”下无“后”字〕，循小指之内出其端。是动则病嗌干心痛，渴而欲饮，是为臂厥。是主心所生病者，目黄胁痛，臑臂内后廉痛厥，掌中热痛〔热痛：《图经》卷二“热”下无“痛”字〕。为此诸病，盛则泻之，虚则补之，热则疾之，寒则留之，陷下则灸之，不盛不虚，以经取之。盛者寸口大再倍于人迎，虚者寸口反小于人迎也。

"The Hand Shaoyin Channel of Heart starts from the heart, it connects the heart system, descends to cross the diaphragm to communicate with the lower abdomen; its branch ascends from the heart system to press close to the throat and links the ocular connections (the structure connecting the eyeballs with the brain, including blood vessels and optic nerves); another heart channel which is running straightly forward ascends from the heart system to the lung and reaches the armpit horizontally, then descends along the rear of the inner side of the upper arm (Qingling point) and passes the rear of the Hand Taiyin Channel of Lung and the Hand Jueyin Channel of Pericardium to reach the inner side of the elbow, then, passes along the inner flank of the forearm to reach the point of the eminent head of the radius behind the palm to reach the tip of the small finger. The diseases stem from the Hand Shaoyin Channel are: dry pharynx, heartache and desire to drink due to thirst. These syndromes are due to the chaotic channel energy of the arm . The diseases of Hand Shaoyin are related with the heart, they are: yellow eyes, fullness and pain in the hypochondria, pain in the rear of the inner sides of the upper arm and the forearm, and hotness in the palm. When treating, apply purging therapy when the syndrome is sthenic, apply invigorating therapy when the syndrome is asthenic, apply swift pricking when it is a heat-syndrome, apply retention of the needle when it is a cold-syndrome and apply moxibustion when the pulse is deficient and bogging down. As to the syndrome which is neither asthenic nor sthenic, prick the Hand Shaoyin Channel of Heart. When the Cunkou pulse is three times as large as the Renying pulse, it is the sthenic syndrome of Hand Shaoyin Channel; when the Cunkou pulse is smaller than the Renying pulse, it is the asthenic syndrome of the Hand Shaoyin Channel.

小肠手太阳之脉，起于小指之端，循手外侧上腕，出踝中，直上循臂骨下廉，出肘内侧两筋之间，上循臑外后廉，出肩解，绕肩胛，交肩上，人缺盆，络心，循咽下膈，抵胃属小肠；其支者，从缺盆循颈上颊，至目锐眦，却入耳中；其支者，别颊上出页抵鼻，至目内眦，斜络于颧〔斜络于颧：《太素》卷八无此四字〕。是动则病嗌痛颔肿，不可以顾，肩似拔，臑似折。是主液所生病者，耳聋目黄颊〔颊：《脉经》卷六第四，《图经》卷二"颊"下并有"颔"字〕肿，颈颔肩臑肘臂外后廉痛。为此诸病，盛则泻之，虚则补之，热则疾之，寒则留之，陷下则灸之，不盛不虚，以经取之。盛者人迎大再倍于寸口，虚者人迎反小于寸口也。

"The Hand Taiyang Channel of Small Intestine starts from the tip of the small finger, it runs along the outer flank of the hand to enter into the wrist above and comes out from the styloid process of ulna, runs along the ulna side of the arm to reach the middle of the bones beside the elbow (Xiaohai point), then, ascends along the rear and the outer flank of the upper arm, comes from the seam posterior to the bone (Jianzheng point), bypasses the shoulder and meets the symmetrical Taiyang Channel of the other side above the shoulder (Dazhui point), passes the supraclaviclar fossa and the armpit to communicate with the heart; the Hand Taiyang Channel that runs straightly forward descends along the pharynx to cross the diaphragm below and links the stomach and the small intestine; its branch separates from the supraclavicular fossa, ascends along the neck (Tianchuang, Tianrong and Quanliao points) to reach the outer canthus and turns into the ear; another branch starts from the upper orbit, the cheek to reach the nose and then, reaches the inner canthus. The diseases stem from the Hand Taiyang Channel are: pain in the pharynx, swelling of the chin, inability of turning back the head, pain in the shoulder as if being hauled and pain in the arm as if being broken. The diseases of Hand Taiyang are related to the body fluid are: deaf, yellow eyes, swelling of the cheek and chin and pain along the outer flank of the neck, shoulder, elbow and arm. When treating, apply purging therapy when the syndrome is sthenic, apply invigorating therapy when the syndrome is asthenic, apply swift pricking when it is a heat-syndrome, apply retention of the needle when it is a cold-syndrome and apply moxibustion when the pulse is deficient and bogging down. As to the syndrome which is neither asthenic nor sthenic, prick the Hand Taiyang Channel. When the Renying pulse is three times as large as the Cunkou pulse, it is the sthenic syndrome of the Hand Taiyang Channel; when the Renying pulse is smaller than the Cunkou pulse, it is the asthenic syndrome of the Hand Taiyang Channel.

膀胱足太阳之脉，起于目内眦，上额，交巅；其支者，从巅至耳上角；其直者，从巅入络脑，还出别下项，循肩髆内，挟脊，抵腰中，入循膂，络肾，属膀胱；其支者，从腰中下挟脊，贯臀，入腘中；其支者，从髆内左右，别下，贯胛，挟脊内，过髀枢，循髀外，从后廉，下合腘中，以下贯踹内，出外踝之后，循京骨，至小指外侧。是动则病冲头痛，目似脱，项如拔，脊痛，腰似折，髀不可以曲，腘如结，踹如裂，是为踝厥。是主筋所生病者，痔疟狂癫疾，头颅项痛，目黄，泪出，鼽衄，项背腰尻腘踹脚皆痛，小指不用。为此诸病，盛则泻之，虚则补之，热则疾之，寒则留之，陷下则灸之，不盛不虚，以经取之。盛者人迎大再倍于寸口，虚者人迎小于寸口也。

"The Foot Taiyang Channel of Bladder starts from the inner canthus, it passes the forehead above and joins the symmetrical Foot Taiyang Channel of the other side on the top of head; its branch starts from the top of head to reach the upper part of the ear; the Foot Taiyang Channel runs straightly forward and communicates with the brain from the top of head; it branches to reach the neck below, runs along the lower part of the shoulder to press close to the vertebrae and enters into the body, then, penetrates into the muscle of the spine to communicate with the kidney and links the bladder; another branch runs along the loin, descends to the anus, passes through the buttock and reaches the popliteal fossa; another branch starts from the inner side of the shoulder, descends to pass the greater trochanter, runs along the rear of the outer flank of the thigh to reach the popliteal, then, passes the calf to the rear of the outer ankle, then, runs along the fifth metatarsal bone on the lateral aspect of the foot to reach the tip of the outer flank of the small toe, and then, connects the Foot Shaoyin Channel. The diseases stem from the Foot Taiyang Channel are: pain between the two eyebrows, pain in the eyeball which seems falling off, pain in the neck seems being dragged, pain in the loins and spine seems to be broken and the leg fails to bend, the popliteal fossa of the patient seems to be fastened and the calf seems to be split, These syndromes are due to the up-rising of the channel energy from the outer ankle. The diseases of Foot Taiyang Channel are related to the tendon, they are: hemorrhoid, malaria, mania, epilepsy, pain on the top of head and neck, falling tears, running clear nasal mucus, epistaxis, pain in the neck, loins, buttocks, poplitea, calf and foot, and failure of moving the small toe. When treating, apply the purging therapy when the syndrome is sthenic, apply invigorating therapy when the syndrome is asthenic, apply swift pricking when it is a heat-syndrome, apply retention of the needle when it is a cold-syndrome and apply moxibustion when the pulse is deficient and bogging down, As to the syndrome which is neither asthenic nor sthenic, prick the Foot Taiyang Channel. When the Renying pulse is three times as large as the Cunkou pulse, it is the sthenic syndrome of the Foot Taiyang Channel, when the Renying pulse is smaller than the Cunkou pulse, it is the asthenic syndrome of the Foot Taiyang Channel.

肾足少阴之脉，起于小指〔小指：《素问·厥论》王注“小指”下有“之端”二字〕之下，邪走足心，出于然谷之下，循内踝之后，别入跟中，以上踹内，出腘内廉，上股内后廉，贯脊，属肾，络膀胱；其直者，从肾上贯肝膈，入肺中，循喉咙，挟舌本；其支者，从肺出络心〔从肺出络心：《外台》卷七《胸胁痛及妨闷方门》“从”作“起”，汪琥曰“心”字当作“心包”〕，注胸中。是动则病饥不欲食，面如漆柴，咳唾则有血，喝喝〔喝喝：《脉经》卷六第《千金》卷十九第一作“喉鸣”〕而喘，坐而欲起，目䀮䀮如无所见，心如悬若饥状，气不足则善恐，心惕惕如人将捕之，是为骨厥。是主肾所生病者，口热舌干，咽肿上气，嗌干及痛，烦心心痛，黄疸，肠澼，脊股内后廉痛，痿厥嗜卧，足下热而痛。为此诸病，盛则泻之，虚则补之，热则疾之，寒则留之，陷下则灸之，不盛不虚，以经取之。灸则强食生肉，缓带，披发，大杖，重履而步。盛者寸口大再倍于人迎，虚者寸口反小于人迎也。

“The Foot Shaoyin Channel of Kidney starts from the tip of the small toe, slants into the sole and comes out beneath the navicular bone anterior to the medial malleolus, then, runs along the rear of the inner ankle, passes the heel and ascends to the inner side of the calf, then comes from the inner side of the poplitea, ascends along the rear of the inner side of the thigh, reaches the spine and communicates with the bladder; the Foot Shaoyin Channel which runs straightly forward starts from the kidney, ascends to reach the lung, runs along the throat to link the root of the tongue; its branch starts from the lung to communicate with the pericardium, reaches the chest and connects the Hand Jueyin Channel of pericardium. The diseases stem from the Foot Shaoyin Channel of Kidney are: the patient is reluctant to eat when hungry, black complexion like charcoal, spitting blood when coughing, rapid breathing with sound, irritation, wanting to stand up when sitting due to restlessness, the eyes are in a dazed and seem to see nothing. suspension of heart and deficiency of energy. These syndromes are due to the disorder of the channel energy of the kidney. The diseases of Foot Shaoyin Channel are related to the kidney, they are: bitter taste in the mouth, dry tongue, swelling of the pharynx, up-reversing of the vital energy, dry larynx with pain, feeling oppression of the chest, heartache, jaundice, intestinal bi-syndrome, pain in the rear of the spine and the inner side of the thigh, weak of the feet, cold extremities, somnolence and having pain and heat in the sole. When treating, apply purging therapy when the syndrome is sthenic, apply invigorating therapy when the syndrome is asthenic, apply swift pricking when it is a heat-syndrome, apply retention of the needle when it is a cold-syndrome and apply moxibustion when the pulse is deficient and bogging down. As to the syndrome which is neither asthenic nor sthenic, prick the Foot Shaoyin Channel. If the moxibustion therapy is applied, the patient should take the uncooked meat even with difficulty, loosen his clothes and ribbons, spread his hair, lean on a large stick, wear the heavy shoes and walk slowly, and these were the five measures for curing the disease of kidney in ancient times. When the Cunkou pulse is three times as large as the Renying pulse, it is the sthenic syndrome of the Foot Shaoyin Channel; when the Renying pulse is smaller than the Cunkou pulse, it is the asthenic syndrome of the Foot Shaoyin Channel.

心主手厥阴心包络〔心包络:《太素》卷八“心包”下无“络”字〕之脉，起于胸中，出属心包络，下膈，历络三焦，其支者，循胸出胁，下腋三寸，上抵腋，下循臑内，行太阴少阴之间，入肘中，下臂，行两筋之间，入掌中，〔入掌中:《甲乙》卷二第一上无“入掌中”三字〕，循中指出其端；其支者，别掌中，循小指次指出其端。是动则病手心热，臂肘挛急，腋肿，甚则胸胁支满，心中憺 憺大动，面赤目黄，喜笑不休〔喜笑不休:《太素》卷八无此四字〕。是主脉所生病者，烦心心痛，掌中热。为此诸病，盛则泻之，虚则补之，热则疾之，寒则留之，陷下则灸之，不盛不虚，以经取之。盛者寸口大一倍于人迎，虚者寸口反小于人迎也。

"The Hand Jueyin Channel of Pericardium starts from the chest. It links the pericardium, descends to cross the diaphragm and connects the upper warmer, middle warmer and the lower warmer one by one; its branch starts from the chest, runs to the hypochodrium, passes the location three inches below the armpit and ascends to the armpit, then, runs along the inner side of the upper arm, passes between the Hand Taiyin Channel of Lung and the Hand Shaoyin Channel of Heart to enter into the elbow, then descends along the forearm, passes between the two tendons (Jianshi point) and reaches the tip of the middle finger; another branch starts from the palm, runs along the ring finger to reach its tip and connects with the Hand Shaoyin Channel of Triple Warmer. The diseases stem from Hand Jueyin Channel are: hotness in the palm, muscular stiffness of the elbow, swelling under the armpit, fullness and distention of the chest, uneasiness and wavering of the heart, red complexion and yellow eyes. The diseases of Hand Jueyin Channel are related to the pericardium, they are: restlessness, heartache and hotness in the centre of the palm. When treating, apply the purging therapy when the syndrome is sthenic, apply invigorating therapy when the syndrome is asthenic, apply swift pricking when it is a heat-syndrome, apply retention of the needle when it is a cold-syndrome and apply moxibustion when the pulse is deficient and bogging down, As to the syndrome which is neither asthenic nor sthenic, prick the Hand Jueyin Channel. When the Cunkou pulse is twice as large as the Renying pulse, it is the sthenic syndrome of the Hand Jueyin Channel; When the Cunkou pulse is smaller than the Renying pulse, it is the asthenic syndrome of the Hand Jueyin Channel.

三焦手少阳之脉，起于小指次指端，上出两指之间，循手表腕，出臂外两骨之间，上贯肘，循 臑外，上肩，而交出足少阳之后，入缺盆，布膻中，散落〔落:日刻本，《太素》卷八，

《脉经》卷六十一并作“络”〕心包，下膈，循属三焦；其支者，从膻中上出缺盆，上项，系耳后直上，出耳上角，以屈下颊至䪼；其支者，从耳后入耳中，出走耳前，过客主人前，交颊，至目锐眦。是动则病耳聋浑浑焞焞，嗌肿喉痹。是主气所生病者，汗出，目锐眦痛，颊痛〔痛：当注本作“肿”〕，耳后肩臑肘臂外皆痛，小指次指不用。为此诸病，盛则泻之，虚是补之，热则疾之，寒则留之，陷下则灸之，不盛不虚，以经取之。盛者人迎大一倍于寸口，虚者人迎反小于寸口也。

“The Hand Shaoyang Channel of Triple Warmer starts from the tip of the ring finger, runs between the small finger and the ring finger (Yemen and Zhongzhu points) and the dorsum of the hand to reach the middle of the two bones of the outer flank of the forearm (Zhigou point), then ascends to cross the elbow, and runs along the outer flank of the upper arm and the shoulder (passing the Naohui, Jianliao and Tianliao points) crosses and runs behind the Foot Shaoyang Channel of Gallbladder, then runs into the supraclavicular fossa, crosses the Tanzhong point and communicates with the pericardium, then descends to the diaphragm and links the upper, middle and the lower warmers comprehensively; another branch separates from the location of the Tanzhong point, passes the supraclavicular fossa and the neck, ascends behind the ear to reach the upper part of the ear (passing Yifeng, Chimai and Luxi points), then turns down to reach the forehead and under the orbit; another bracnh starts from the rear of the ear, runs into the ear and comes out from the front of the ear, passes the front of the Kezhuren point and joins the branch stated above on the cheek, then it reaches the outer canthus and connects the Foot Shaoyang Channel of Gallbladder. The diseases stem from the Hand Shaoying Channel are: deafness causing the patient can not hear clearly, swelling of the pharynx and sore throat. The diseases of Hand Shaoyang Channel are related to the triple warmer, they are: pain in the outer canthus, swelling of the cheek, pain in the rear of ear、shoulder、upper arm、elbow and arm, and the ring finger can hardly move. When treating, apply purging therapy when the syndrome is sthenic, apply invigorating therapy when the syndrome is asthenic, apply swift pricking when it is a heat-syndrome, apply retention of the needle when it is a cold-syndrome and apply moxibustion when the pulse is deficient and bogging down. As to the syndrome which is neither asthenic nor sthenic, prick the Hand Shaoyang Channel. When the Renying pulse is twice as large as the Cunkou pulse, it is the sthenic syndrome of the Hand Shaoyang Channel; When the Renying pulse is smaller than the Cunkou pulse, it is the asthenic syndrome of the Hand Shaoyang Channel.

胆足少阳之脉，起于目锐眦，上抵头角，下耳后循颈行手少阳之前，至肩上，却交出手少阳之后，入缺盆；其支者，从耳后入耳中，出走耳前，至目眦后；其支者；别〔别锐眦：《太素》卷八，《十四经发挥》“别”下并有“目”字〕锐眦，下大迎，合于手少阳，抵于䪼，下加颊车，下颈合缺盆以下胸中，贯膈络肝属胆，循胁里，出气街，绕毛际，横入髀厌中；其直者，从缺盆下腋，循胸过季胁，下合髀厌中，以下循髀阳，出膝外廉，下外辅骨之前，直下抵绝骨之端，下出外踝之前，循足跗上，入小指次指之间，其支者，别跗上，入大指之间，循大指岐骨内出其端，还贯爪甲，出三毛。是动则病口苦，善太息，心胁痛不能转侧，甚则面微有尘，体无膏泽，足外反热，是为阳厥。是主骨所生病者，头痛，颔痛，目锐眦痛，缺盆中肿痛，腋下肿，马刀侠瘿，汗出振寒，疟，胸胁肋髀膝外至胫绝骨外踝前及诸节皆痛，小指次指不用。为此诸病，盛则泻之，虚则补之，热则疾之，寒则留之，陷下则灸之，不盛不虚，以经取之。盛者人迎大一倍于寸口，虚者人迎反小于寸口也。

"The Foot Shaoyang Channel of Gallbladder starts from the outer canthus. It ascends to the corner of the forehead, then turns down to the rear of the ear and runs along the neck, crosses the Hand Shaoyang Channel of Triple Warmer and runs behind it to reach the shoulder, and then, enters into the supraclavicular fossa; its branch starts from the outer canthus, descends to the location near the Daying point and connects the Hand Shaoyang Channel of Triple Warmer, then runs to the lower orbit, passes the Jiache point, descends to the neck and joins the channel which enters the supraclavicular fossa stated above, then it descends to the chest, crosses the diaphragm, communicates with the liver, links the gallbladder, runs along the hypochondrium, passes the Qijie point, bypasses the pubic hair margin to reach the greater trochanter horizontally; the Foot Shaoyang Channel which runs straightly forward starts from the Quepen point to the armpit, passes along the chest and ribs to join the branch stated above at the greater trochanter, then runs along the outer side of the upper thigh to reach the Yanglingquan point, and descends in front of the fibula to reach the Yangfu point below, then comes out from the front of the outer ankle to run along the dorsum of the foot and reach the middle between the small toe and the fourth toe; its branch starts from the dorsum of foot to pass along the forked bone of the big toe to reach the tip of the big toe, then, turns back to penetrate into the nail and comes out from the rear of the toe's nail to connect the Foot Jueyin Channel of Liver. The diseases stem from the Foot Shaoyang Channel are: bitter taste in the mouth, frequent sighing, pain in the heart and the hypochondrium, failing to toss and turn the body, dusty complexion, lost of lustre of the muscles and skins of the whole body and hotness in the outer flank of the foot. These syndromes are due to the evil energy in the Shaoyang Channel. The diseases of Foot Shaoyang Channl are related to the tendon, they are: pain on the face, pain in the forehead, pain in the outer canthus, pain and swelling of the supraclavicular fossa, swelling and pain under the armpit, scrofula, sweating, shivering with cold, malaria, pain in the chest, hypochondrium、rib、thigh and knee, and pain in the joints of the tibia, lower end of fibula and the outer ankle, and the fourth toe can hardly move. When treating, apply purging therapy when the syndrome is sthenic, apply invigorating therapy when the syndrome is asthenic, apply swift pricking when it is a heat-syndrome, apply retention of the needle when it is a cold-syndrome and apply moxibustion when the pulse is deficient and bogging down. As to the syndrome which is neither asthenic nor sthenic, prick the Foot Shaoyang Channel. When the Renying pulse is twice as large as the Cunkou pulse, it is the sthenic syndrome of the Foot Shaoyang Channel; when the Renying pulse is smaller than the Cunkou pulse, it is the asthenic syndrome of the foot Shaoyang Channel.

肝足厥阴之脉，起于大指丛毛之际，上循足跗上廉，去内踝一寸，上踝八寸，交出太阴之后，上腘内廉，循股阴，入〔入：《脉经》卷六第一“入”下有“阴”字〕毛中，过阴器，抵小腹，挟胃属肝络胆，上贯膈，布胁肋，循喉咙之后，上入颃颡，连目系，上出额，与督脉会于巅；其支者，从目系下颊里，环唇内；其支者，复从肝别贯膈，上注肺。是动则病腰痛不可俯仰，丈夫㿗疝，妇人少腹肿，甚则嗌干，面尘脱色。是肝所生病者，胸满呕逆飧泄，狐疝遗溺闭癃。为此诸病，盛则泻之，虚则补之，热则疾之，寒则留之，陷下则灸之，不盛不虚，以经取之。盛者寸口大一倍于人迎，虚者寸口反小于人迎也。

“The Foot Jueyin Channel of Liver starts from the Dadun point on the clustered hair of the toe. It ascends along the upper side of the dorsum of foot (Xingjian and Taichong points) to reach the location one inch in front of the inner ankle, and ascends to the location eight inches above the ankle, intersects with the Foot Taiyin Channel of Spleen and runs behind it, then ascends to the inner side of the poplitea and thigh to reach the pubic hair margin, after encircling the external genitals, it ascends to the lower abdomen, then presses close to the stomach, links the liver and comunicates with the gallbladder (Zhangmen and Qimen points); its branch crosses through the diaphragm and spreads around the hypochondrium and the armpit, then, runs along the rear of the throat and passes the upper opening of the throat to link the ocular connectors, and then, ascends to the forehead to converge with the Du Channel on the Baihui point on the top of head; another branch starts from the ocular connectors to reach the inner side of the cheek and surround the lips; another branch starts from the liver, crosses through the diaphragm, ascends to reach the lung and connects the Hand Taiyin Channel of Lung. The diseases stem from Foot Jueyin Channel are: lumbago, failing to face up and down, swelling of the scrotum in a man and swelling of the lower abdomen and loin in a woman. The patient can go so far as to have dry throat and the losing lustre of the complexion. The diseases of Foot Jueyin Channel are related to liver, they are: fullness of the chest, vomiting, diarrhea, inguinal hernia, enuresis and dysuria. When treating, apply purging therapy when the syndrome is sthenic, apply invigorating therapy when the syndrome is asthenic, apply swift pricking when it is a heat-syndrome, apply retention of the needle when it is a cold-syndrome and apply moxibustion when the pulse is deficient and bogging down. As to the syndrome which is neither asthenic nor sthenic, prick the Foot Jueyin Channel. When the Cunkou pulse is twice as large as the Renying pulse, it is the sthenic syndrome of the Foot Jueyin Channel; When the Cunkou pulse is smaller than the Renying pulse, it is the asthenic syndrome of Foot Jueyin Channel.

手太阴气绝则皮毛焦，太阴者行气温于皮毛者也，故气不荣则皮毛焦，皮毛焦则津液去皮节〔皮节：此二字是衍文〕，津液去皮节者，则爪〔则爪：《难经·二十四难》“则”字上有“皮节伤”三字，“爪”作“皮”〕枯毛折，毛折者则毛〔毛：《脉经》卷三第四并作“气”〕先死，丙笃丁死，火胜金也。

“When the channel energy of Hand Taiyin of lung is exhausted, the skin and the hair will be withered, as the Hand Taiyin channel of lung can soften the skin and hair with its energy. If its energy is not flowing and not being kept harmonious, it will cause the skin and hair to become dry and withered, and it is the appearance of the wastage of the body fluid. If the body fluid is wasted, it will injure the surface of the skin, and when the surface of the skin is hurt, the skin will be dried and the hair lost, and it is the symptom of the death of the Lung channel energy in advance. The disease will become aggravated on the day of Bing, and the patient will die on the day of Ding. This is because the lung belongs to metal in the five elements, Bing and Ding belong to fire, and fire overcomes the metal.

手少阴气绝则脉不通，脉不通则血不流；血不流，则髦色不泽，故其面黑如漆柴者，血先死，壬笃癸死，水胜火也。

"When the channel energy of Hand Shaoyin of heart is obstructed, the heart channel will become unimpeded and the blood will not flow fluently causing the lost of lustre of the complexion, and it is the appearance of the death of blood in advance. The disease will become aggravated on the day of Ren, and the patient will die on the day of Gui. This is because the heart belongs to fire in the five elements, Ren and Gui belong to water, and water overcomes the fire.

足太阴气绝者，则脉不荣肌肉〔则脉不荣肌肉，《难经》二十四难，《甲乙》卷二第一上并作"则脉不营其口唇"〕，唇舌者〔唇舌者：《脉经》卷三第三，《甲乙》卷二第一上并作"口唇者"〕肌肉之本也，脉不荣则肌肉软；肌肉软则舌萎人中满；人中满则唇反，唇反者肉先死，甲笃乙死，木胜土也。

"When the channel energy of Foot Taiyin of spleen is exhausted, the channel energy will not be able to nourish the lips. The lip is the root of the muscle. when the muscle is not nourished, it will become unsmoothed causing the swelling of the nasolabial groove; when the nasolabial groove is swelling and the lips are turning outside, it is the appearance of the death of the muscle in advance. The disease will become aggravated on the day of Jia, and the patient will die on the day of Yi. This is because the spleen belongs to earth in the five elements, Jia and Yi belong to wood, and wood overcomes the earth.

足少阴气绝则骨枯，少阴者冬〔冬：《太平圣惠方》卷二十六作"肾"〕脉也，伏行而濡骨髓者也，故骨不濡则肉不能著〔著："著"下脱"骨"字，应据《脉经》卷三第五补〕也，骨肉不相亲则肉软却，肉软却故齿长而垢，发无泽，发无泽者骨先死，戊笃己死，土胜水也。

"When the channel energy of Foot Shaoyin of kidney is exhausted, the bone will be withered. This is because the Foot Shaoyin is the kidney channel which is deep lying to harmonize the marrow and moisten the bone, if the bone fails to obtain the nourishment from the kidney energy, the muscle will not be able to attach closely to the bone, and when the bone and the muscle are not attaching closely together, the muscle will become shrinked and soft, the patient's teeth will become longer and withered and the hair will have no lustre at all. When the hair loses it lustre, it is the appearance of the death of bone in advance. The disease will become aggravated on the day of Wu, and the patient will die on the day of Ji. This is because the kidney belongs to water in the five elements, Wu and Ji belong to earth, and the earth overcoms water.

足厥阴气绝则筋绝，厥阴者肝脉也，肝者筋之合也，筋者聚于阴气〔阴气：《素问·诊要经络论》王注作"阴器"〕，而脉〔脉《难经·二十四难》无"脉"字〕络于舌本也，故脉弗荣则筋急，筋急则引舌与卵，故唇青〔唇青：《难经·二十四难》无“唇青”二字〕舌卷卵缩则筋先死，庚笃辛死，金胜木也。

“When the channel energy of Foot Jueyin of liver is exhausted, it will cause the severing of the vital energy of the tendon. It is because the Foot Jueyin is the channel of liver, and the tendon's condition agrees with that of the liver; all tendons assemble in the external genitals and communicate with the root of tongue above, when the liver can no more nourish the tendons, the contracture of tendons will ocur causing the curled tongue and the shrinking of testes, and they are the appearances of the death of the tendon in advance. The disease will become aggravated on the day of Geng and the patient will die on the day of Xin. This is because the liver belongs to wood in the five elements, Geng and Xin belong to metal, and the metal overcomes the wood.

五阴气俱绝，则目系转，转则目运，目运者为志先死，志先死则远一日半死矣。

“When all the Yin channel energies of the five solid organs are exhausted, the ocular system will be revolving and the patient will have dizziness, and it is the appearance of the death of the five moods in advance. Since the five moods have died in advance, the patient will die within one and half days.

六阳气绝，则阴与阳相离，离则腠理发泄，绝汗乃出，故旦占夕死，夕占旦死。

“When all the Yang channel energies of the six hollow organs are exhausted, the Yin and Yang will be divorced to cause the instability of the striae, excretion of the refined energy and the sweating of the critical stage. When the conditions occur in the morning, the patient will die in the evening; when the conditions occur in the evening, the patient will die in the morning.

经脉十二者，伏行分肉之间，深而不见；其常见者，足太阴过于外〔外：《太素》卷九《经络别异》作“内”〕踝之上，无所隐故也。诸脉之浮而常见者，皆络脉也。六经络手阳明少阳之大络，起于五指间，上合肘中。饮酒者，卫气先行皮肤，先充络脉，络脉先盛，故卫气已平，营气乃满，而经脉大盛。脉之卒然动者，皆邪气居之，留于本末；不动则热，不坚则陷且空，不与众同，是以知其何脉之动〔动：《太素》卷九《经络别异》作“病”〕也。

“The twelve channels lying concealed run deeply between the muscular layers which can hardly be seen; the Foot Taiyin Channel of Spleen can be seen often when it passes the upper part of the inner ankle without any covering. When the collaterals branched off from the channel they can be seen on the surface of the body. In the hand and foot six channels, the large collaterals of the Hand Yangming Channel of Large Intestine and the Hand Shaoyang Channel of Triple Warmer start from the middle of the five fingers respectively and reach the elbow above. For a man who drinks wine, the energy of wine runs to the skin along with the Wei-energy to fill the collaterals, causing the collaterals to become full and abundant first, then, the Wei-energy becomes even and the Ying-energy becomes abundant as well. When the channel of a man is fully filled all of a sudden, it is due to the invasion of the evil energy and its retention in the root and branch of the channel without moving, and the retention of evil energy will be transformed into heat. If the superficial collaterals of a man are not substantial, it shows the evil energy has penetrated inside and the channel is emptied. Since the condition is quite different from the ordinary ones, one can know which channel has been affected."

雷公曰：何以知经脉之与络脉异也？黄帝曰：经脉者常不可见也，其虚实也以气口知之，脉之见者皆络脉也。雷公曰：细子无以明其然也。黄帝曰：诸络脉皆不能经大节之间，必行绝道而出，入复合于皮中，其会皆见于外。故诸刺络脉者，必刺其结上，甚血者虽无结，急取之，以泻其邪而出其血，留之发为痹也，凡诊络脉，脉色青则寒且痛，赤则有热。胃中寒，手鱼之络多青矣；胃中有热，鱼际络赤；其暴黑者，留久痹也；其有赤有黑有青者，寒热气也；其青短者，少气也。凡刺寒热者皆多血络，必间日而一取之，血尽而止，乃调其虚实；其小而短者少气，甚者泻之则闷，闷甚则仆，不得言，闷则急坐之也。

Leigong asked: "How can one know the difference of the channel with its collaterals?" Yellow Emperor said: "Commonly, one can not see the channel, its condition of asthenia or sthenia can only be determined by palpating the Cunkou pulse, and the channel appearing outside are all collaterals." Leigong said: "I don't see their difference." Yellow Emperor said: "All the collaterals do not pass through the large joints but run to the skins and striae where the channels are absent, they pour in and out, join the superficial collaterals of the skin and appear on the superficies with them together. So, when treating the disease which affects the collaterals, one must prick and hit the juncture of the collaterals. When the disease is severe, even if there is no stagnated blood, it should also prick hastily to purge the evil energy and let out the blood, if the blood is retained inside, it will cause bi-syndrome; When inspecting the collateral, if it is green, it shows there are cold evil and pain; if it is red, it shows there is fever. When there is cold in the stomach, the collaterals on the thenar eminence will be green; when there is heat in the stomach, the collaterals on the thenar eminence will be red; when the collaterals on the thenar eminence is black, it is the protracted bi-syndrome, if the red, black and green colours appear at the same time, it is the disease of cold and heat; if it is green and short, it is the symptom of the deficiency of the Yang energy. When treating the disease with cold and heat in the stomach, the superficial venules must be pricked for many times, it should prick every other day and cease the pricking when the stagnated blood is emptied. One should also inspect whether the disease is asthenic or sthenic, if the channel is green and short, it shows the deficiency of the patien's energy, if excessive purging is applied, it will cause the patient to become uneasy and disquiet, when the condition is severe, the patient will fall down and unable to talk, it should help him to sit dowvn to avoid stumbling.

手太阴之别，名曰列缺，起于腕上分间，并太阴之经直入掌中，散人于鱼际。其病实则手锐掌热，虚则欠故，小便遗数，取之去腕半寸〔半寸：二字误倒，应乙作“寸半”〕，别走阳明也。

"The large collateral branches off from the Hand Taiyin Channel of Lung to connect other channel is called Lieque. It starts from the muscular layers of the wrist, runs in parellel with the Hand Taiyin Channel and enters into the thenar eminence and then spreads on the skin. When the large collateral is affected, and if it is a sthenic syndrome, the location of the processus styloideus radius on the wrist and the palm will become hot; if it is an asthenic syndrome, yawning with open mouth, incontinence of urine or frequent micturition of the patient will occur. When treating, prick the Lieque point which is one and half inches behind the wrist. The Large collateral of Hand Taiyin Channel connects the Hand Yangming Channel of Large Intestine here.

手少阴之别，名曰通里，去腕一寸半，别而上行，循经入于心中，系舌本，属目系。其实则支膈，虚则不能言，取之掌后一寸，别走太阳也。

"The Large collateral branches off from the Hand Shaoyin of Heart to connect other channel is called Tongli. It starts from one inch behind the wrist, descends along the Hand Shaoyin Channel to enter into the pharynx, connects the tongue and links the ocular connectors. When the large collateral is affected, and if it is an a sthenic syndrome, the patient will feel uneasy with proping feeling between the chest and the diaphragm, if it is asthenic syndrome, the patient will not be able to talk. When treating, prick the Tongli point which is one inch behind the wrist. The Large collateral of Hand Shaoyin Channel connects the Hand Taiyang Channel of Small Intestine here.

手心主之别，名曰内关，去腕二寸，出于两筋之间，循经以上，系于心包络，心系实则心痛，虚则为头强，取之两筋间也。

"The large collateral branches off from the Hand Jueyin Channel of Pericardium to connect other channel is called Neiguan. It starts from two inches above the wrist, passes the middle of the two tendons and descends along the Hand Jueyin Channel to link the pericardium. When the large collateral is affected, and if it is a sthenic syndrome of the heart system, heartache will occur, if it is asthenic, feeling of oppression over the chest will occur. When treating, prick the Neiguan point which is between the two tendons two inches above the wrist.

手太阳之别，名曰支正，上腕五寸，内注少阴；其别者，上走肘，络肩髃。实则节弛肘废，虚则生肬，小者如指痂疥，取之所别也。

"The large collateral branches off from the Hand Taiyang Channel of Small Intesine to connect other channel is called Zhizheng. It starts from five inches above the wrist to connect the Hand Shaoyin Channel of Heart; another branch ascends to pass the elbow and reach the Jianyu Point. When the large collateral is affected, and if it is a sthenic syndrome, the tendons of the patient will be loose and flaccid and the elbow will become stiff, if it is an asthenic syndrome, the superfluous verruca will occur, and the small ones are like the scabs between the fingers. When treating, prick the collateral point of the Hand Taiyang Channel.

手阳明之别，名曰偏历，去腕三寸，别入太阴；其别者，上循臂，乘肩髃，上曲颊偏齿；其别者，入耳，合于宗脉。实则龋聋〔龋：《甲乙》卷二第一下有"齿耳"二字〕，虚则齿寒痹隔，取之所别也。

The large collateral branches off from the Hand Yangming Channel of Large Intestine to connect other channel is called Pianli. It separates from three inches above the wrist to connect the Hand Taiyin Channel; its branch ascends to the arm, passes the Jianyu point and the curved jaw and nets all over the teeth; another channel enters into the ear and converges with the general assemblage of the Hand Taiyang, Hand Shaoyang, Foot Shaoyang and Foot Yangming collateral. When the large collateral is affected, and if it is a sthenic syndrome, caries and deafness will occur; if it is an asthenic syndrome, cold of teeth and block of diaphragm will occur. When treating, prick the collateral point of Pianli of the Hand Yangming Channel.

手少阳之别，名曰外关，去腕二寸，外绕臂，注胸中，合心主。病实则肘挛，虚则不收，取之所别也。

"The large collateral branches from the Hand Shaoyang Channel of Triple Warmer to connect other channel is called Waiguan. It starts from two inches above the wrist, ascends to bypass the inner side of the arm, runs into the chest and connects the channel of Pericardium. When the large channel is affected, and if the syndrome is sthenic, the joint of the elbow of the patient will become stiff; if the syndrome is asthenic, the joint of the elbow will become loose and flaccid. When treating, prick the collateral point of Waiguan of the Hand Shaoyang Channel.

足太阳之别，名曰飞阳，去踝七寸，别走少阴。实则鼽窒头背痛，虚则鼽衄，取之所别也。

"The large collateral branches off from the Foot Taiyang Channel of Bladder to connect other channel is called Feiyang. It separates from seven inches above the outer ankle and connects the Foot Shaoyin Channel. When the large collateral is affected, and if the syndrome is sthenic, stuffy nose and pain on the head and back will occur; if the syndrome is asthenic, running of the clear nasal mucus and epitaxis will occur. When treatig, prick the collateral point of Feiyang point of the Foot Taiyang Channel.

足少阳之别，名曰光明，去踝五寸，别走厥阴，下络足跗。实则厥，虚则痿躄，坐不能起，取之所别也。

"The large collateral branches off from the Foot Shaoyang Channel of Gallbladder to connect other channel is called Guangming. It separates from five inches above the outer ankle and connects the Foot Jueyin Channel of Liver and spreads on the dorsum of foot. If the large collateral is affected. and if the syndrome is sthenic, the jueni syndrome will occur; if the syndrome is asthenic, the patinet can hardly walk and can not stand up after sitting. When treating, prick the collateral point of Guangming of the Foot Shaoyang Channel.

足阳明之别，名曰丰隆，去踝八寸，别走太阴；其别者，循胫骨外兼，上络头顶，合诸经之气，下络喉嗌。其病气逆则喉痹瘁瘖，实则狂巅，虚则足不收，胫枯，取之所别也。

"The large collateral branches off from the Foot Yangming Channel of stomach to connect other channel is called Fenglong. It separates from eight inches above the outer ankle and connects the Foot Taiyin Channel of Spleen; its branch ascends along the outer flank of tibia to communicate with the head , and converges the energies of various channels there, and then, descends to reach the throat. If the large collateral is affected and the vital energy is up-reversing, the patient will have obstruction of the throat and dysphonia all of a sudden. when the syndrome is sthenic, the patient will have mania; when the syndrome is asthenic, the tendons and feet of the patient will become loose and flaccid, and the muscle of the tibia will become withered. When treating, prick the collateral point of Fengling of the Foot Yangming Channel.

足太阴之别，名曰公孙，去本节之后一寸，别走阳明；其别者，入络肠胃。厥气上逆则霍乱，实则肠〔肠:《脉经》卷六第五,《千金》卷十五上第一并作“腹”〕中切痛，虚则鼓胀，取之所别也。

"The large collateral branches off from the Foot Taiyin Channel of Spleen to connect other channel is called Gongsun. It separates from one inch behind the basic joint of the big toe and connects the Foot Yangming Channel of Stomach; another branch penetrates into the abdomen and communicates with the intestine and stomach. When the large collateral is affected and the chaotic energy reverses up to cause the disorder of the spleen energy, of cholera will occur. If the syndrome is sthenic, abdominal pain like being cut will occur, if the syndrome is asthenic, abdominal distention will occur. When treating, prick the collateral point of Gongsun of the Foot Taiyin Channel.

足少阴之别，名曰大鍾〔大鍾:《千金》卷十九第一“大”并作“太”〕，当踝后绕根，别走太阳；其别者，并经上走于心包，下外贯腰脊。其病气逆则烦闷，实则闭癃，虚则腰痛，取之所别者也。

"The large collateral branches from the Foot Shaoyin Channel of Kidney to connect other channel is called Taizhong. It separates from the rear of the inner ankle, winds the heel and connects the Foot Taiyang Channel of Bladder; its branch runs in parallel with the Foot Shaoyin Channel of Kidney to reach below the pericardium and descends to link the loin and back . If the large collateral is affected, the patient will have adverseness of vital energy and restlessness. When the syndrome is sthenic, retention of urine will occur; when the syndrome is asthenic, the patient will have lumbago. When treating, prick the collateral point of Taizhong of the Foot Shaoyin Channel.

足厥阴之别，名曰蠡沟，去内踝五寸，别走少阳；其别者，径胫，上睾，结于茎。其病气逆则睾肿卒疝，实则挺长，虚则暴痒，取之所别也。

"The large collateral branches off from the Foot Jueyin Channel of Liver to connect other channel is called Ligou. It separates from five inches above the inner ankle to connect the Foot Shaoyang Channel of Gallbaldder; its branch ascends along the Foot Jueyin Channel to reach the testis and the penis. If the large collateral is affected, pain with sudden onset of hernia due to the adverseness of the vital energy will occur. when the syndrome is sthenic, the penis will erect; When the syndrome is asthenic, itching with sudden onset of the external genitals will occur. When treating, prick the collateral point of Ligou of the Foot Jueyin Channel.

任脉之别，名曰尾翳，下鸠尾，散于腹。实则腹皮痛，虚则痒搔，取之所别也。

"The large collateral branches off from the Ren Channel and Chong Channel is called

Weiyi. It separates from the xiphoid process and descends to spread on the abdomen. When the large collateral is affected, and if the syndrome is sthenic, the skin of the abdomen will be painful, if the syndrome is asthenic, the anus will be itching. When treating, prick the collateral point of Weiyi of the Ren Channel.

督脉之别，名曰长强，挟膂〔膂：张注本用“脊”〕上项，散头上，下当肩胛左右，别走太阳，入贯膂。实则脊强，虚则头重，高摇之〔高摇之，挟脊之有过者：《甲乙》卷二第一下校语云：“《九墟》无‘高摇之’以下九字〕，挟脊之有过者，取之所别也。

“The large channel branches off from the Du Channel to connect other channel is called Changqiang. It ascends to press close to the spine and reaches the neck, spreads on the head, descends to the scapula and connects the Foot Shaoyin Channel and Taiyang, and then penetrates along the side of the spinal column. When the large collateral is affected, and if the syndrome is sthenic, rigidity of spine will occur; when the syndrome is asthenic, the heaviness of the head will occur. When treating, prick the collateral point of Changqiang of the Du Channel.

脾之大络，名曰大包，出渊腋下三寸，布胸胁。实则身尽痛，虚则百节尽皆纵，此脉若罗络之血者，皆取之脾之大络脉也。

“The large collateral of the spleen is called Dabao. It starts from three inches under the Yuanye point and spreads over the chest and hypochondrium. When the large collateral is affected, and if the syndrome is sthenic, the patient will feel painful all over the body; if the syndrome is asthenic, the joints of the whole body will become loose and flaccid. This large collateral is containing the bloods of the various collaterals. When treating, prick the collateral point of Dabao of the spleen channel.

凡此十五络者，实则必见，虚则必下，视之不见，求之上下，入经不同。络脉异所别也。

“All the fifteen large collaterals branching off from the large channels above can be seen when the evil energy is sthenic and the blood is fully filled in the vessel. They can not be seen when the healthy energy is asthenic and the pulse is bogging down. So, in treating, it should be seeked from the various acupoints from the collaterals. As the conditions of the channels in different persons are different, the conditions of the collateral are different also.”

经别第十一

Chapter 11
Jing Bie
(Branches of the Twelve Channels)

黄帝问于岐伯曰：余闻人之合于天道〔天道：《甲乙》卷二第一下"道"作"地"〕也，内有五脏，以应五音五色五时五味五位也；外有六腑，以应六律，六律建阴阳诸经而合之十二月、十二辰、十二节、十二经水、十二时、十二经脉者，此五脏六腑之所以应天道。夫十二经脉者，人之所以生，病之所以成，人之所以治，病之所以起，学之所始，工之所止也，粗之所易，上之所难也。请问其离合出入奈何？岐伯稽首再拜曰：明乎哉问也！此粗之所过，上之所息也，请卒言之。

Yellow Emperor asked Qibo："I am told the human body agrees with the natural world; the five solid organs of Yin correspond to the five tones，five colours，five seasons，five tastes and the five orientations respectively inside，and the rule of the six hollow organs of Yang correspond to the six-rule of music of Yang outside，and the established of the six music-rule is pertaining to Yang. The channels coordinate with the twelve months，twelve branches of the duodecimal cycle，twelve solar terms，twelve rivers，twelve two-hour periods and the twelve channels. These are the general conditions of the five solid organs and the six hollow organs to adapt the phenomena of the natural world，the twelve-channel is the passage of the flowing of the blood and energy in human body，it has close relation with the existence of man，the forming of disease，the human health and the recovery of disease. For a beginner of treating the disease，he must learn the theory of the channel，and for a good physician，he must also take good attention to it. A physician of lower level thinks the theory of channel is easy to learn，but a physician of higher level deems that the study of it can hardly be proficient. Now，I want to know what is the condition of the divorce and combine of the channel branch，in human body，can you tell me all about it?" Qibo bowed respectively and said："What a brilliant question you have asked! The condition of channel is what the imprudent physician neglects and what an astute physician studies carefully. Now，let me tell you in details.

足太阳之正，别入于腘中，其一道下尻五寸，别入于肛，属于膀胱，散之肾，循膂当心入散；直者，从膂上出于项，复属于太阳，此为一经也。足少阴之正，至腘中，别走太阳而合，上至肾，当十四椢，出属带脉；直者，系舌本，复出于项，合于太阳，此为一合。成以〔成以诸阴之别，皆为正也：《甲乙》卷二第一下无"成以"十字〕诸阴以之别，皆为正也。

"The main channel-branch of the Foot Taiyang Channel of Bladder separates from the popliteal fossa of a man，the channel branch descends to reach five inches below the sacrococcygeal region, enters into the anus and the inside of the abdomen to connect the hollow organ of bladder of its same channel and spreads on the kidney, then ascends along the inside of the spine and scatters by the position of the heart; another channel branch of the Foot Taiyang Channel runs straightly forward, ascends from the spine to reach the top of head, then connects its same channel of Foot Taiyang.

The main channel-branch of from the Foot Shaoyin Channel of Kidney starts from the popliteal fossa and connects the Foot Taiyang Channel, then ascends to the kidney and connects the Belt Channel at the location of the fourteenth vertabra; the other channel-branch off from Foot Shaoyin, runs straightly forward to link the root of tongue, comes out from the neck and connects the Foot Taiyang Channel of Bladder. This is the first coordination of the colocation of the superficies and interior of the Foot Taiyang Channel and the Foot Shaoyin Channel.

足少阳之正，绕髀入毛际，合于厥阴；别者，入季胁之间，循胸里属胆，散之上〔散之上：丹波元简曰："上"字衍〕肝，贯心，以〔以：《太素》卷九《经脉正别》杨注无"以"字〕上挟咽，出颐颔中，散于面，系目系，合少阳于〔于：张注本"于"下有"目"字〕外眦也。足厥阴之正，别跗上，上至毛际，合于少阳，与别俱行，此为二合也。

"The main channel-branch of the Foot Shaoyang Channel of Gallbladder separates and winds the thigh, enters into the pubic hair margin and connects the Foot Jueyin Channel of Liver. Another channel-branch enters into the soft ribs on the lateral side of the chest, runs along the chest and connects the hollow organ of gallbladder of its same channel, then scatters on the liver, passes the heart, presses close to the throat, comes out from the location between the cheek and the chin, spreads on the face, links the ocular connectors and connects the Foot Shaoyang Channel of Gallbladder at the outer canthus. The main channel-branch of the Foot Jueyin Channel of Liver, separates from the dorsum of the foot, ascends to reach the pubic hair margin and connects the Foot Shaoyang Channel of Gallbladder and runs along with the other main channel-branch of the Gallbladder Channel. This is the second coordination of the colocation of the superficies and interior of Foot Shaoyang Channel and the Foot Jueyin Channel.

足阳明之正，上至髀，入腹里，属胃，散之脾，上通于心，上循咽出于口，上頞顑〔頞：周本"頞"作"额"〕，还系目系，合于阳明也。足太阴之正，上至髀，合于阳明，与别俱行，上结于咽，贯舌中〔舌中：《太素》卷九《经脉正别》"中"作"本"〕，此为三合也。

"The main channel-branch of Foot Yangming Channel of Stomach ascends to reach the thigh, enters into the abdomen, links the hollow organ of stomach and scatters on the spleen, then, ascends to reach the heart, runs along the throat, comes out from the mouth to reach the forehead and the skull, then, encircles the ocular connectors and connects the Foot Yangming Channel of Stomach. The main channel-branch of the Foot Taiyin Channel ascends above to connect the Yangming Channel and runs along with the other channel-branch of the Stomach Channel, then ascends to communicate the pharlynx and links the root of tongue. This is the third coordination of the collocation of the superficies and interior of the Foot Yangming Channel and the Foot Taiyin Channel.

手太阳之正，指地，别于肩解，人腋走心，系小肠也。手少阴之正，别入于渊腋两筋之间，属于心，上走喉咙，出于面，合目内眦，此为四合也。

"The main channel-branch of the Hand Taiyang Channel of Small Intestine descends from above to below. It separates from the joint behind the shoulder, enters into the armpit, reaches the heart and connects the hollow organ of the small intestine of its same channel. The main channel branch of the Hand Shaoyin Channel of Heart enters into the Yuanye point which is between the two tendons under the armpit, links the heart, then ascends to the throat, reaches the face and connects with one of the branches of the Hand Taiyang Channel at the inner canthus. This is the fourth coordination of the collocation of the superficies and interior of the Hand Taiyang Channel and the Hand Shaoyin Channel.

手少阳之正，指天，别于巅，入缺盆，下走三焦，散于胸中也。手心主之正，别下渊腋三寸，入胸中，别属三焦，出循喉咙，出耳后，合少阳完骨之下，此为五合也。

"The main channel-branch of the Hand Shaoyang Channel of Triple Warmer descends from above to below. It starts from the top of the head and enters into the supraclavicular fossa, then, descends again to reach the triple warmer and scatters on the chest. The main channel-branch of the Hand Jueyin Channel of Pericardium separates from three inches below the armpit, enters into the chest, links the triple warmer, runs along the throat to reach the location behind the ear, and connects the Hand Shaoyang Channel of Triple warmer below the Wangu point. This is the fifth coordination of the collocation of the superficies and interior of the Hand Shaoyang Channel and the Hand Jueyin Channel.

手阳明之正，从手循膺乳，别于肩髃，人柱骨下，走大肠，属于肺，上循喉咙，出〔出：张注本作"入"〕缺盆，合于阳明也。手太阴之正，别人渊腋少阴之前，入走肺，散之太阳〔太阳：曰刻本作"大肠"〕，上出缺盆，循喉咙，复合阳明，此六合也。

"The main channel-branch of the Hand Yangming Channel of Large Intestine starts from the hand and ascends along the location between the lateral side of the chest and the breast to reach the Jianyu point, passes the clavicle, reaches the large intestine of its same channel, then it links the lung, runs along the throat to enter the supraclavicular fossa and connects the Hand Yangming Channel. The main channel-branch of Hand Taiyin Channel of Lung separates to reach the front of the Yuanye point of the Hand Shaoyin Channel, runs to the lung, scatters on the large intestine, ascends to pass the supraclavicular fossa, runs along the throat and connects the Hand Yangming Channel of Large Intestine. This is the sixth coordination of the collocation of the superficies and interior of the Hand Yangming Channel and the Hand Taiyin Channel."

经水第十二

Chapter 12
Jing Shui
(The Water of Channels)

黄帝问于岐伯曰：经脉十二者，外合于十二经水，而内属于五脏六腑。夫十二经水者，其有大小、深浅、广狭、远近各不同，五脏六腑之高下、大小、受谷之多少亦不等，相应奈何？夫经水者，受水而行之；五脏者，合神气魂魄而藏之；六腑者，受谷而行之，受气而扬之；经脉者，受血而营之〔营：《灵枢略·六气论篇》作"荣"〕合而以治奈何？刺之深浅，灸之壮数，可得闻乎？

Yellow Emperor asked Qibo ："When viewing the twelve channels of a man from outside，they are like the twelve waters，when viewing them from inside ，they link the five solid organs and the six hollow organs. The twelve channels receive water from the source and flow to various places，the five solid organs combine and store the spirit，energy，soul，and inferior spirit respectively；the six hollow organs receive the five cereals，transfer and transform them，and spread the energy of the refined substances all over the body；the channels receive the blood and pass the blood to nourish the whole body. When treating，how to coordinate with these conditions such as controlling the depth of pricking，managing the times of moxibustion，etc.，can you tell me about them?"

岐伯答曰：善哉问也！天至高，不可度，地至广，不可量，此之谓也。且夫人生于天地之间，六合之内，此天之高、地之广也，非人力之所能度量而至也。若夫八尺之士，皮肉在此〔在此：据《太素》卷五《十二水》杨注"在此"二字似应作"色脉"〕，外可度量切循而得之，其死可解剖而视之，其脏之坚脆，腑之大小，谷之多少，脉之长短，血之清浊，气之多少，十二经之多血少气，与其少血多气，与其皆多血气，与其皆少血气，皆有大数。其治以针艾，各调其经气，固其常有合乎？

Qibo answered；"What a good question you have asked！The sky is so high that one can hardly infer，the earth is so vast that one can hardly measure，and this is the saying that has always been so. When a man exists between the heaven and earth and situates within the three dimensions ，he can hardly measure the acurate height of heaven and the extent of earth artificially. The body of a grown-up man has the skin，muscle and channel；to a living man，one can inspect him by touching，to a dead body，one can examine it carefully by autopsy；there is a definite standard of the firm and fragile in each of the five solid organs，the sizes of the six hollow organs，the quantity of the cereals received，the length of the channels，the clearness or turbidity of blood，the abundance or deficiency of the channel energy and the different conditions of the blood and energy in the channel. In the channels，some have plenty of blood and less energy, some have less blood and plenty of energy, some have plenty of blood and plenty of energy and some have less blood and less energy. When one adjusts the asthenic or sthenic channel energy of a patient with acupuncture or moxibustion, the handling of the depth of pricking and the times of moxibustion should correspond with the deep or shallow, and the plenty or less of the water of the twelve channels."

黄帝曰：余闻之，快于耳，不解于心，愿卒闻之。岐伯答曰：此人之所以参天地而应阴阳也，不可不察。足太阳外合清水，内属膀胱，而通水道焉。足少阳外合于渭水，内属于胆。足阳明外合于海水，内属于胃。足太阴外合于湖水，内属于脾。足少阴外合于汝水，内属于肾。足厥阴外合于渑水，内属于肝。手太阳外合淮水，内属小肠，而水道出焉。手少阳外合于漯水，内属三焦。手阳明外合于江水，内属于大肠。手太阴外合于河水，内属于肺。手少阴外合于济水，内属于心。手心主外合于漳水，内属于心包。凡此五脏六腑十二经水者，外有源泉而内有所禀，此皆内外相贯，如环无端，人经亦然。故天为阳，地为阴，腰以上为天，腰以下为地。故海以北者为阴，湖以北者为阴中之阴，漳以南者为阳，河以北至漳者为阳中之阴，漯以南至江者为阳中之太阳〔阳中之太阳：《甲乙》卷一第七“阳中之”下并无“太”字〕，此一隅之阴阳也，所以人与天地相参也。

Yellow Emperor said: "Your speech is pleasing to the ears, but it is still perplexing me. I hope you can tell me in details." Qibo said: "This is the fact of human being coordinates with the heaven and earth and adapting the Yin and Yang, and one must understand it. The Foot Taiyang Channel coordinates with the water of Jing River outside and links the hollow organ of bladder inside, and it communicates with the watercources which run all over the body. The Foot Shaoyang Channel coordinates with the water of Wei River outside, and links the hollow organ of gallbladder inside. The Foot Yangming coordinates with the water of the sea outside, and links the hollow organ of stomach inside. The Foot Taiyin Channel coordinates with the water of the lake outside, and links the solid organ of spleen inside. The Foot Shaoyin Channel coordinates with the water of Ru River outside, and links the solid organ of kidney inside. The Foot Jueyin Channel coordinates with the water of the Mian River outside, and links the solid organ of liver inside. The Hand Taiyang Channel coordinates with the water of the Huai River outside and links the hollow organ of small intestine inside, and the small intestine separates the lucid and turbid substances and leads out the turbids through the watercource. The Hand Shaoyang Channel coordinates with the water of the Luo River outside and links the triple warmer inside. The Hand Yangming Channel coordinates to the water of the river outside and links the hollow organ of large intestine inside. The Hand Taiyin Channel coordinates with the water of the stream outside and links the solid organ of lung inside. The Hand Shaoyin Channel coordinates to the water of Ji River outside and links the solid organ of heart. The Hand Jueyin coordinates to the water of Zhang River outside and links the pericardium. In a word, the water of the twelve channels of the five solid organs and the six hollow organs all have sources outside and they receive water respectively inside. They connect and communicate with each other outside and inside, like a ring goes round without end, and the condition of the human channel is the same. The heaven is above and it is Yang, the earth is down below and it is Yin; the upper part of the body above the loins is heaven and it belongs to Yang, the lower part of the body below the loins is earth and it belongs to Yin. Therefore, the location north of the water of the sea (stomach) is called Yin, the location north of the water of the lake (spleen) is called Yin in the Yin, the location south of the water of Zhang River (pericardium) is called Yang, the region from north of the water of the stream (lung) to the water of Zhang River is called Yin in the Yang, the region from south of the water of Luo River (triple warmer) to the water of the streem is called Yang in the Yang. These are the examples illustrated with part of the waters in certain location, and it is the principle of the correspondence of a man to the heaven and earth."

黄帝曰：夫经水之应经脉也，其远近浅深，水血之多少各不同，合而刺之奈何？岐伯答曰：足阳明，五脏六腑之海也，其脉大血多，气盛热壮，刺此者不深弗散，不留不泻也。足阳明刺深六分，留十呼。足太阳深五分，留七呼。足少阳深四分，留五呼。足太阴深三分，留四呼。足少阴深二分，留三呼。足厥阴深一分，留二呼。手之阴阳，其受气之道近，其气之来疾，其刺深者皆无过二分，其留皆无过一呼。其少长大小肥瘦，以心撩之，命曰法天之常。灸之亦然。灸而过此者得恶火，则骨枯脉涩；刺而过此者，则脱气。

Yellow Emperor asked: "The energy of channels corresponds with the channels of a man, but the conditions of the remote and near, shallow or deep and plenty or less in the energy and blood between them are different, how to do it when combining their conditions with the applying of the acupuncture therapy?" Qibo answered: "In the five solid organs and the six hollow organs, the Foot Yangming Channel of Stomach is like the sea among the twelve channels, it is the channel which has a large pulse, plenty of blood, abundant energy and intense heat. So, when pricking the channel, it must be pricked deeply, or else, the evil can not be dispelled; the needle must be retained, or else, the evil can not be purged. When pricking the Foot Yangming Channel, which has plenty of blood and energy , the depth of pricking should be six fen (0. 6 inch) , and the period of the needle retention should be of ten exhalations. When pricking the Foot Taiyang Channel, which has plenty of blood and little energy, the depth of the pricking should be five fen (half inch), and the period of the needle retention should be of seven exhalations. When pricking the Foot Shaoyang Channel which has plenty of blood and plenty of energy, the depth of the pricking should be four fen and the period of the needle retention should be of five exhalations. When pricking the Foot Taiyin Channel which has plenty of blood and little energy, the depth of the pricking should be three fen, and the period of the needle retention should be of four exhalations. When pricking the Foot Shaoyin Channel which has little blood and little energy, the depth of the pricking should be two fen, and the period of the needle retention should be of three exhalations. When pricking the Foot Jueyin Channel which has plenty of blood and little energy, the depth of the pricking should be one fen, and the period of the needle retention should be of two exhalations. As to the Hand channels of Yin and Yang, they are closer to the heart and the lung from which to receive the energy, and the energies flowing in them are faster, so, generally, the depth of the pricking should not exceed two fen, and the period of the needle retention should not exceed one exhalation; nevertheles, the patients are different in old and young, tall and short, and fat and thin, one must deliberate carefully to treat reasonably. When treating with moxibustion, it should be in the same way. When the moxibustion is excessive to injure the human body, it is called the evil fire which will cause the withering of the marrow and the stagnation of the blood. When the pricking is excessive, it will injure the healthy energy of the patient."

黄帝曰：夫经脉之小大，血之多少，肤之厚薄，肉之坚脆，及䐃之大小，可为度量乎？岐伯答曰：其可为度量者，取其中度也，不甚脱肉而血气不衰也。若失度之人，痟瘦而形肉脱者，恶可以度量刺乎。审切循扪按，视其寒温盛衰而调之，是谓因适而为之真也。

Yellow Emperor asked: "Is there any standard for measuring the plenty or less quantity of the blood, the thickness or the thinness of the skin the firmness or fragility of the muscle and the size of the protruding part of the muscle?" Qibo answered: "They can be measured when the patient is of a medium stature, not very emaciated in the muscle and his blood and his energy are not declined. As to the patient who is abnormal in size, very emaciated and his muscle is bogging down, one can only determine the depth of the pricking through inspection, palpating the Cunkou pulse, pressing the skin of anterolateral side of the forearm and massage the skin and the muscle, then treat accordingly after examining the cold and heat, asthenic and sthenic conditions of the patient. This is the so called treat prudently according to different cases by pricking."

经筋第十三

Chapter 13
Jing Jin
(The Tendons Distributed Along the Channels)

足太阳〔足太阳：按《脉经》、《经别》、《经水》等篇例之，"足太阳"上疑脱"黄帝曰"三字〕之筋，起于足小指，上结于踝，邪上结于膝，其下循足外踝〔其下者循足外踝：周本"踝"作"侧"〕，结于踵，上循跟，结于腘；其别者，结于踹外，上腘中内廉与腘中并上结于臀，上挟脊上项；其支者，别入结于舌本；其直者，结于枕骨，上头下颜〔颜：《甲乙》卷二第六作"额"〕，结于鼻；其支者，为目上网〔网：《甲乙》卷二第六并作"纲"〕，下结于九页〔頄：《太素》卷十三《经筋》并作"鼽"。王注："鼽，面顴也〕；其支者，从腋后外廉，结于肩髃；其支者，入腋下，上出缺盆，上结于完骨；其支者，出缺盆，邪上出于頄。其病小指支〔支：圣济总录〕卷一百九十一作"及"〕，跟肿〔肿：《太素》卷十三《经筋》，《甲乙》卷二第六并作"踵"〕痛，腘挛，脊反折，项筋急，肩不举，腋支〔腋支：按"支"疑亦"及"之误字〕，缺盆中纽痛，不可左右摇。治在燔针劫刺，以知为数，以痛为输，名曰仲春痹也。

Yellow Emperor said: "The tendon distributed along the channel (the channel tendon) of the Foot Taiyang Channel of Bladder starts from the small toe, assembles on the outer ankle and ascends slantingly to the knee; another branch below runs along the outer flank of the foot and assembles on the heel, then, runs along the heel to reach the popliteal fossa; another branch assembles on the outer flank of the calf to reach the inner side of the popliteal fossa and runs in parallel with the other branch on the popliteal stated above, then it ascends to assemble on the buttock above and runs along the spinal column to reach the top of head; from here, another branch separates out to link the root of the tongue; the branch which runs straightly forward assembles in the occipital bone to reach the top of head above and reach the forehead below, then, assembles by the two sides of the nose; from here, it separates to become the fine tendons around the eyelash and the eye socket above and assembles on the cheekbone below; another branch separates from the outer side behind the armpit and ascends to assemble at the Jianyu point; another branch enters into the lower part of the armpit, ascends to the supraclavicular fossa and ascends again to assemble on the Wangu point behind the ear; another branch separates from the supraclavicular fossa, slanting up to reach the cheekbone above. The diseases stem from this channel tendon are: pain in the small finger and the heel, contracture of the popliteal, reverse bending of the spinal column, tightness of the tendon in the neck, pain in the armpit and the supraclavicular fossa causing the patient to become restless and the inability of waving the shoulder. When treating, prick with the heated needle and pull out the needle instantly after pricking, the times of the pricking are not limited but must stop the pricking as soon as the disease is remitted, and prick the painful location only . This is the so called bi-syndrome of mid-spring.

足少阳之筋，起于小指次指，上结外踝，上循胫外廉，结于膝外廉；其支者，别起外辅骨，上走髀，前者结于伏兔之上，后者结于尻；其直者，上乘眇季胁，上走腋前廉，系于膺乳，结于缺盆；直者，上出腋，贯缺盆，出太阳之前，循耳后，上额角，交巅上，下走颔，上结于頄；支者，结于目眦为外维。其病小指次指以转筋，引膝外转筋，膝不可屈伸，腘筋急，前引髀，后引尻，即上乘眇季胁痛，上引缺盆膺乳颈，维筋急，从左之右，右目不开，上过右角，并跻脉而行，左络于右，故伤左角，右足不用，命曰维筋相交。治在燔针劫刺，以知为数，以痛为输，名曰孟春痹也。

"The tendon of the Foot Shaoyang Channel of Gallbladder starts from the tip of the fourth toe, it assembles on the outer ankle above and runs along the outer flank of the tibia, assembles at the Yanglingquan point on thc outer flank of the knee; its branch joins the outer fibula, ascends to reach the upper thigh, its frontal branch assembles on the femoral rectus muscle and its rear branch assembles on the sacrococcygeal region; the channel tendon that runs straightly forward ascends to reach the soft and empty location under the hypochondrium, and then, ascends to reach to the front of the armpit, runs along the breast beside the chest and assembles on the supraclavicular fossa above; another branch which runs straightly foward separates from the armpit, passes the supraclavicular fossa and runs in front of the channel tendon of the Foot Taiyang Channel, then, runs along the rear of the ear, ascends to the forehead corner, converges at the top of head, descends to reach the chin and ascends to assemble at the cheekbone; another branch assembles on the outer canthus to become the outer fine tendons of the eye. The diseases stem from this channel tendon are: spasm in the fourth toe, spasm of the outer flank of the knee drawn by the fourth toe, inability of bending and stretching the knee joint, stiffness of the popliteal fossa, drawing pain of the thigh in the front and drawing pain of the sacrococcygeal region in the rear, pain in the soft and empty location under the armpit and the soft ribs, contracture of the supraclavicular fossa, breast, neck and all the locations where the channel tendon link, When there is contracture in the channel tendon which runs from the left side to the right side, the right eye will not be able to open, and this channel tendon ascends to pass the right forehead corner and runs in parallel with the Jiao Channel; the channel tendon of the left side is connecting the right side, so, when the channel tendon of the left side is injured, the right foot will not be able to move, and it is called the phenomenon of the intersection of the joint and the tendon. When treating, prick with the heated needle and pull out the needle instantly after the pricking, the times of the pricking are not limited but must stop the pricking as soon as the disease is remitted, and prick the painful location only. This is the so called the bi-syndrome of early-spring.

足阳明之筋，起于中三指〔中三指：廖平曰："'三'字衍，'中'亦误字，当作'次'"〕，结于跗上，邪外上加于辅骨，上结于膝外廉，直上结于髀枢，上循胁，属脊，其直者，上循骭，结于膝；其支者，结于外辅骨，合少阳，其直者，上循伏免，上结于髀，聚于阴器，上腹而布，至缺盆而结，上颈，上挟口，合于烦，下结于鼻，上合于太阳，太阳〔太阳为目上网：《太素》卷十三《经筋》无"太阳"二字，"为"字属上读。"网"作"纲"〕为目上网；其支者，从颊结于耳前。其病足中指支，胫转筋，脚跳坚，伏免转筋，髀前肿，㿉疝腹筋急，引缺盆及颊，卒口僻，急者目不合。热则筋纵，目不开。颊筋有寒，则急引颊移口〔移口：按"移"似误字，应作"哆"，《说文·口部》"哆，此口也"〕；有热则筋弛纵缓，不胜收〔不胜收《太素》卷十三《经筋》"胜"下无"收"字〕故僻，治之以马膏，膏〔膏：按此"膏"字蒙上误衍〕其急者，以白酒和桂，以涂其缓者，以桑钩钩之，即以生桑灰置之坎中，高下以坐等，以膏熨急颊，且饮美酒，噉美炙肉，不饮酒者，自强也，为之三拊而已。治在燔针劫刺，以知为数，以痛为输，名曰季春痹也。

"The tendon of the Foot Yangming Channel of Stomach starts from the outer flank of the second toe, assembles on the dorsum of the foot, slanting up to the fibula and assembles on the outer flank of the knee, then assembles on the hip joint and links the spinal column; the branch that runs straightly forward runs along the tibia and assembles on the knee; another branch separates to assemble in the outer fibula and connects the channel tendon of the Foot Shaoyang Channel; another branch that runs straightly forward along the femoral rectus muscle, and assembles on the thigh, then, converges in the external genitals and scatters when reaches the abdomen, then ascends to assemble in the supraclavicular fossa, passes the neck, presses close to the mouth, links the cheekbone and assembles on the nose to connect the channel tendon of the Foot Taiyang Channel, the fine tendons of the upper eyelid belong to the Foot Taiyang Channel and the fine tendons of the lower eyelids belong to the Foot Yangming Channel; another branch starts from the cheek and assembles in front of the ear. The diseases stem from this channel tendon are: pain in the middle toe and the tibia, contracture of the dorsum of foot, spasm of the femoral rectus muscle, swelling in the frontal part of the thigh, swelling of the scrotum, contracture of the tendon of the abdomen which draws the supraclavicular fossa to become painful and sudden onset of the distortion of the face; when the contracture is due to cold, the eyes will not be able to close, when it is due to heat, the eyes will not be able to open. When there is cold in the cheek tendon, it will draw the cheek to become painful and the mouth will not be able to shut when being opened; when there is heat in the cheek tendon, the tendon will be loose and flaccid causing the distortion of the face. When treating, the horse fat should be applied. If the disease is an acute one, smear the flaccid side of the tendon with the cinnamon powder mixed with spirit; if the disease is a chronic one, hook the patient' s mouth corner with a hook of mulbery wood, then put some burning charcoal of mulberry wood in a pit on the ground , and the depth of the pit should be the same with the length fit for the patient to sit on the ground. Press the part of the cheek contracture with the horse fat, and the patient should drink some wine of good quality and eat some roast mutton. If the patient does not drink, he should drink the wine even with difficulty. Then massage time after time to accomplish the treating. When treating the patient with the disease of the tendon, prick with the heated needle and pull out the needle instantly after the pricking, the times of the pricking are not limited but must stop the pricking as soon as the disease is remitted, and prick the painful location only. This is the so called the bi-syndrome of late spring.

足太阴之筋，起于大指之端内侧，上结于内踝；其直者，络于膝内辅骨，上循阴股，结于髀，聚于阴器，上腹，结于脐，循腹里，结于肋〔肋：《太素》卷十三《经筋》《甲乙》卷二第六并作“胁”〕，散于胸中；其内者，著于脊，共病足大指支，内踝痛，转筋痛，膝内辅骨痛，阴股引髀而痛，阴器纽痛，下引脐两胁痛，引膺中脊内痛。治在燔针劫刺，以知为数，以痛为输，命曰孟秋〔孟秋：《太素》卷十三《经筋》“孟”作“仲”〕痹也。

"The tendon of the Foot Taiyin Channel of Spleen starts from the inner side of the tip of the big toe and assembles on the inner ankle; its branch which runs straightly forward ascends to assemble on the knee beside the fibula, then, ascends along the inner flank of the thigh and assembles in the upper part of the thigh and converges in the external genitals, then ascends to the abdomen, assembles in the navel, runs along the abdomen, assembles in the hypochondrium and spreads on the chest; the branch inside attaches to the spinal column. The diseases stem from the channel tendon are: pain in the big toe and the inner ankle, spasm of muscle , pain in the upper part of the thigh drawn by the inner side of the thigh, pain in the external genitals to cause restless, pain of the navel, hypochondria, the lateral sides of the chest and the spine drawn from above. When treating, prick with the heated needle and pull out the needle instantly after the pricking, the times of the pricking are not limited but must stop the pricking as soon as the disease is remitted, and prick the painful location only. This is the so called the bi-syndrome of mid-autumn.

足少阴之筋，起于小指之下〔起于小指之下：《甲乙》卷二第六“小指之下”并有“入足心”三字〕，并足太阳之筋，邪走内踝之下，结于踵，与太阳之筋合，而上结于内辅之下，并太阴之筋而上循阴股，结于阴器，循脊内挟膂，上至项，结于枕骨，与足太阳之筋合。其病足下转筋，及所过而结者皆痛及转筋。病在此者，主痫瘛及痉，在外者不能俯，在内者不能仰。故阳病者腰反折不能俯，阴病者不能仰。治在燔针劫刺，以知为数，以痛为输，在内者熨引饮药。此筋折纽，纽〔此筋折纽，纽发：《圣济总录》卷一百九十一无“此筋折纽纽”五字〕数甚者，死不治，名曰仲秋〔仲秋：《太素》卷十三《经筋》作“孟秋”〕痹也。

"The tendon of the Foot Shaoyin Channel of Kidney starts from under the small toe and enters into the sole, it connects the channel tendon of the Taiyin Channel, slanting to reach the lower side of the inner ankle, assembles on the ankle and joins the Foot Taiyin Channel of Bladder, then ascends to assemble in the lower part of the fibula, runs along the channel tendon of the Foot Taiyin Channel of Spleen to reach the inner side of the thigh, assembles in the external genitals, runs along the inner side of the spine to the neck, assembles on the occipital bone and connects the channel tendon of the Taiyang Channel. The diseases stem from this channel tendon are: spasm of the muscle of foot and pain and spasm in the locations where the channel tendon passes and assembles. The diseases occurred are mainly of the epilepsy, spasm of the muscle and the convulsion kind, when the tendon of the back is affected, the body can hardly stoop down, when the tendon of the abdomen is affected, the body can hardly face upward, when the back has contracture, the lumbus will not be able to stoop down due to the reverse-bending of the spine , and when the abdomen has contracture, one will not be able to face upward. When treating, prick with the heated needle and pull out the needle instantly after the pricking, the times of the pricking are not limited but must stop the pricking as soon as the disease is remitted, and prick the painful location only. When the disease is inside, apply the topical application of heated drugs, physical and breathing exercises and the administration of the medical decoction; when the attack of the disease is too frequent and is very serious, the patient can by no means to be cured. This is the so called the bi-syndrome of early autumn.

足厥阴之筋，起于大指之上，结于内踝之前，上循胫，上结内辅之下，上循阴股，结于阴器，络诸筋。其病足大指支，内踝之前痛，内辅痛，阴股痛转筋，阴器不用，伤于内则不起，伤于寒则阴缩入，伤于热则纵挺不收。治在行水清阴气。其病转筋者，治在燔针劫刺，以知为数，以痛为输，命曰季秋痹也。

"The tendon of the Foot Jueyin Channel of Liver starts from the upper part of the toe, ascends to assemble at the Zhongfeng point in front of the inner ankle, then runs along the tibia and assembles in front of the fibula on the knee, then runs along the inner side of the thigh, assembles on external genitals and joins the various Channel tendons of other channels. The diseases stem from this channel tendon are: pain of the inner ankle drawn by the toe, pain in the inner fibula, pain and spasm of the inner flank of the thigh and inability of using the external genitals. If the disease is caused by excessive sexual intercourse, impotence will occur, if the disease is caused by heat, the penis will be erect without contracting. When treating, wash the penis with water to reduce the energy of Jueyin. If the disease is of the spasm kind, prick with the heated needle and pull out the needle instantly after the pricking, the times of the pricking are not limited but must stop the pricking as soon as the disease is remitted, and prick the painful location only. This is the so called the bi-syndrome of late autumn.

手太阳之筋，起于小指之上，结于腕，上循臂内廉，结于时内锐骨之后，弹之应小指之上，入结于腋下；其支者，后走腋后廉，上绕肩胛，循 颈出走太阳之前〔出走太阳之前：《太素》卷十三《经筋》并作“足”，“之”下并有“筋”字〕，结于耳后完骨；其支者，入耳中；直者，出耳上，下结于颔，上属目外眦。其病小指支，肘内锐骨后廉痛，循臂阴入腋下，腋下痛，腋后廉痛，绕肩胛引颈而痛，应耳中鸣痛，引颔目瞑，良久乃得视，颈〔颈：《圣济总录》卷一百九十一作“头”〕筋急则为筋瘘颈肿。寒热在颈者，治在燔针劫刺之，以知为数，以痛为输，其为肿者，复而锐之。本支者，上曲牙，循耳前，属目外眦，上颔〔颔：《太素》卷十三《经筋》作“额”〕，结于角。其痛〔痛：为注本作“病”〕当所过者支转筋。治在燔针劫刺，以知为数，以痛为输，名曰仲夏痹也。

"The tendon of the Hand Taiyang Channel of Small Intestine starts from the tip of the small finger, it assembles on the wrist, runs along the inner side of the arm and assembles behind the eminent head of the elbow, and there will be some feeling in the small finger when the location is flicked with the finger, then it ascends and assembles in the armpit; its branch separates from the rear of the armpit, ascends to wind the scapula, runs along the neck and passes the front of the channel tendon of the Foot Taiyang Channel and assembles on the Wangu point behind the ear; another branch separates from here to enter into the ear; the channel tendon that runs straightly forward starts from above the ear, descends to assemble on the chin and then ascends to link the outer canthus. The diseases stem from this channel tendon are: pain of the small finger and the rear of the eminent head of the radius at the inner side of the elbow, pain along the inner side of the arm and the armpit, pain in the rear of the armpit, pain in the neck drawn by the scapula, tinnitus, pulling pain is the chin to cause the shutting of the eyes and the patient can not see anything for quite a long time. When there is cold in the neck, there will be constracture of tendon in the head, scrofula and swelling of the neck. When treating, prick with the heated needle and pull out the needle instantly after the pricking, the times of the pricking are not limited but must stop the pricking as soon as the disease is remitted, and prick the painful location only. If the swelling is not reduced after pricking, prick again with the sagittal needle. This is the so called bi-syndrome of mid-summer.

手少阳之筋，起于小指次指之端，结于腕，中循臂结于肘，上绕臑外廉，上肩走颈，合手太阳；其支者，当曲颊入系舌本；其支者，上曲牙，循耳前，属目外眦，上乘颔〔颔：张介宾曰："'颔'当作'额'〕，结于角，其病当所过者即支转筋，舌卷。治在燔针劫刺，以知为数，以痛为数，名曰季夏痹也。

"The tendon of the Hand Shaoyang Channel of Triple Warmer starts from the tip of the ring finger, assembles in the wrist, runs along the arm and assembles in the elbow, then, winds the outer flank of the upper arm, ascends to the shoulder and reaches the neck, then connects the channel tendon of the Hand Taiyang Channel of Small Intestine; its branch enters into the cheek bone deeply and links the root of the tongue; another branch ascends to reach the top of ear, runs along the upper forehead and links the outer canthus, then, passes the forehead to assemble in the forehead angle. The diseases stem from this channel tendon are: curled tongue and pain and spasm of the muscles along the locations where the channel tendon passes. When treating, prick with the heated needle and pull out the needle instantly after the pricking, the times of the pricking are not limited but must stop the pricking as soon as the disease is remitted, and prick the painful location only. This is the so called the bi-syndrome of late sumer.

手阳明之筋，起于大指次指之端，结于腕，上循臂，上结于肘外〔肘外：《甲乙》卷二第六"肘"下无"外"字〕，上臑，结于髃；其支者，绕肩胛，挟脊；直者，从肩髃上颈；其支者，上颊，结于頄；直者，上出手太阳之前，上左角，络头，下右颔。其病当所过者支痛及转筋〔支痛及转筋：《甲乙》卷二第六"支"下无"痛及"二字，"筋"下有"痛"字〕，肩不举，颈不可左右视。治在燔针劫刺，以知为数，以痛为输，名曰孟夏痹也。

"The tendon of the Hand Yangming Channel of Large Intestine starts from the tip of the forefinger, it assembles on the wrist , then, ascends along the forearm and assembles at the elbow, then ascends along the upper arm and assembles at the Jianyu point; another branch bypasses the scapula and runs along the spine; the channel tendon that runs straight-forward, ascends from the Jianyu point to reach the neck; another branch ascends to the cheek and assembles on the cheekbone; another channel tendon that runs straightly forward ascends along the channel tendon of the Hand Taiyang Channel and then it is divided into two branches , one of it reaches the left forehead corner, communicates with the head and descends to the right of chin, the other one reaches the right forehead corner, communicates the top of head and descends to the left of chin. The diseases stem from this channel tendon are: pain and spasm along the locations where the channel tendon passes, inability of lifting the shoulder and inability of turning the neck. When treating, prick with the heated needle and pull out the needle instantly after the pricking, the times of pricking are not limited but must stop the pricking as soon as the disease is remitted, and prick the painful location only. This is the so called the bi-syndrome of early summer.

手太阴之筋，起于大指之上，循指上行，结于鱼后〔鱼后：《甲乙》卷二第六“鱼”下有“际”字〕，行寸口外侧，上循臂〔上循臂：按“臂”下似应有“内”字〕，结肘中，上臑内廉，入腋下，出缺盆，结肩前髃〔前髃：《千金》卷十七第一作“髃前”〕上结缺盆，下结胸里，散贯贲，合贲下，抵季胁。其病当所过者支转筋痛，甚成息贲，胁急吐血。治在燔针劫刺，以知为数，以痛为输，名曰仲冬痹也。

“The tendon of the Hand Taiyin Channel of Lung starts from the tip of the thumb, ascends along finger and assembles behind the thenar eminence, runs along the outer flank of the Cuukou pulse, then, ascends along the forearm and assembles in the elbow, then, ascends along the inner side of the upper arm, passes the armpit and the supraclavicular to reach the front of the Jianyu point, then, ascends again to the supraclavicular fossa and assembles there, then, descends to communicate with the chest, scatters and penetrates under the cardia to reach the location of the soft ribs. The diseases stem from this channel tendon are the pain and spasm of the muscles in the lower extremities where the channel tendon passes , if the disease developes into the lumps located on the right hypochondrium, the patient will have acute pain in the hypochondrium and the syndrome of spitting blood. When treating, prick with the heated needle and pull out the needle instantly after the pricking, the times of the pricking is not limted but must stop the pricking as soon as the disease is remitted, and prick the painful location only. This is the so called the bi-syndrome of mid-winter.

手心主之筋，起于中指，与太阴筋并行，结于肘内廉，上臂阴，结腋下，下散前后挟胁；其支者，入腋，散胸中，结于臂。其病当所过者，支转筋，前及胸痛息贲。治在燔针劫刺，以知为数，以痛为输，名曰孟冬痹也。

“The channel tendon of the Hand Jueyin Channel of Pericardium starts from the middle finger and runs in parallel with the Hand Taiyin Channel of Lung, it assembles in the inner side of the elbow, ascends along the inner side of the arm and assembles under the armpit, then descends to spread in the front and the rear to clip the channel tendon of the hypochondrium; its branch enters into the armpit, spreads into the chest and assembles in the cardia. The diseases stem from this channel tendon are: pain and spasm of muscles along the locations where the channel tendon passes and the pain of chest which causes the lumps. When treating, prick with the heated needle and pull out the needle instantly after the pricking, the times of the pricking are not limited but must stop the pricking as soon as the disease is remitted, and prick the painful location only, This is the so called bi-syndrome of early winter.

手少阴之筋，起于小指之内侧，结于锐骨，上结肘内廉，上入腋，交太阴，挟乳里，结于胸中，循臂，下系于脐。其病内急，心承伏梁，下为肘网。其病当所过者支转筋，筋痛。治在燔针劫刺，以知为数，以痛为输。其成伏梁唾血脓者，死不治。经筋之病，寒则反折筋急，热则筋弛纵不收，阴痿不用。阳急则反折，阴急则俯不伸。焠刺者，刺寒急也，热则筋弛纵不收，无用燔针。名曰季冬痹也。

"The tendon of the Hand Shaoyin Channel of Heart starts from the inner flank of the small finger, assembles in the sharp bone along the small finger's side behind the palm, then ascends to the inner side of the elbow, reaches the armpit and intersects with the Hand Taiyin Channel of Lung, then, slips into the breast, and assembles in the chest and descends along the cardia and connects the navel below. The diseases stem from this channel tendon are the contracture of the chest and the mass under the position of heart which is called fuliang. As this tendon is the main tendon for bending and stretching the elbow so there will be pain and spasm of the muscle along all the locations where the channel tendon passes. When treating, prick with the heated needle and pull out the needle instantly after the pricking, the times of the pricking are not limited but must stop the pricking as soon as the disease is remitted, and prick the painful location only . When the patient has the syndrome of spitting blood and pus and has the disease of fuliang, he can by no means to be cured and dies. This is the so called the bi-syndrome of late winter. All the diseases are caused by the channel tendon, if the disease belongs to cold, contracture of the channel tendon will occur, if it belongs to heat, the channel tendon will be loose and the patient will be impotent. When the channel tendon contracture is in the back, it will cause the back to bend reversely; when the channel tendon contracture is in the abdomen, the patient will be stooping and fails to stretch up the body. The heated needle is for treating the contracture caused by cold, to the syndrome of loose and flaccid channel tendon, the heated needle must not be used.

足之阳明，手之太阳，筋急则口目为噼，眦，急不能卒视，治皆如右方也。

"When there is spasm in the Foot Yangming Channel of stomach and the Hand Yangming Channel of Small Intestine, distortion of the face and inability to see things completely will occur. When treating, prick with the heated needle as the method stated above."

骨度第十四

Chapter 14
Gu Du
(Measurement of the Bone)

黄帝问于伯高曰：脉度言经脉之长短，何以立之？伯高曰：先度其骨节之大小广狭长短，而脉度定矣。

Yellow Emperor saked Bogao and said: "How to determine the length of the channels of the three Yins and the three Yangs?" Bogao answered: "One must measure the size, width and the length of the bones first, then can the lengths of the channel be determined."

黄帝曰：愿闻众人之度，人长七尺五寸者，其骨节之大小长短各几何？伯高曰：头之大骨围二尺六寸，胸围四尺五寸，腰围四尺二寸。发所复者颅至项尺二寸；发以下至颐长一尺，君子终折。

Yellow Emperor said: "I hope to know the bone size of a man in ordinary stature. Since a man in normal stature is seven and half feet tall, what about the size and length of his bone?" Bogao said: "The circumference of the skull when measuring on the level of the peaks of the ears is two feet and six inches, the circumference of the chest measuring on the level of the nipples is four feet and five inches, the circumference of the loin measuring on the level of the navel is four feet and two inches, the length from the frontal hairline to the location of neck covered by the hair is one foot and two inches, the length from the frontal hairline to the bottom of the cheek is one foot, and a wise and reasonable person still has to infer and check the data with other factors.

结喉以下至缺盆中长四寸，缺盆以下至髑骬长九寸，过则肺大，不满则肺小。髑骬以下至天枢长八寸，过则胃大，不及则胃小。天枢以下至横骨长六寸半，过则回肠广长，不满则狭短。横骨长六寸半，横骨上廉以下至内辅之上廉长一尺八寸，内辅之上廉以下至下廉长三寸半，内辅下廉下至内踝长一尺三寸，内踝以下至地长三寸，膝腘以下至跗属长一尺六寸，跗属以下至地长三寸，故骨围大则太过，小则不及。

"The length from the Adam's apple to the middle point between the two Quepen points is four inches. The length from the Quepen point to the sternal xiphoid process is nine inches, when it is more than nine inches, the lung is comparatively larger than the ordinary ones, when it is less than nine inches; the lung is comparatively smaller than the ordinary ones. The length from the sternal xiphoid process to the Tianshu point (on the level of the navel) is eight inches, when it is more than eight inches, the stomach is comparatively larger than the ordinary ones, when it is less than eight inches, the stomach is comparatively smaller than the ordinary ones. The length from the Tianshu point to the pubic bone is six and half inches, when it is more than six and half inches, the large intestine is large and long, when it is less than six and half inches, the large intestine is shorter. The length of the pubic bone is six and half inches, the length from the pubic bone to the bone process beside the knee is one foot and eight inches, the length from below the upper edge of the bone process beside the knee to its lower edge is three and half inches. The length from the lower edge of the bone process beside the knee to the inner ankle is one foot and three inches, the length from the inner ankle to the ground is three inches, the length from the popliteal to the level of the ankle is one foot and six inches, and the length from the ankle to the ground is three inches. So, when the circumference of the bone is long, the size of the bone is large, when the circumference of the bone is short, the size of the bone is small.

角以下至柱骨长一尺〔《甲乙》卷二第七校语："尺一作寸"〕，行腋中不见者长四寸，腋以下至季胁长一尺二寸，季胁以下至髀枢长六寸，髀枢以下至膝中长一尺九寸，膝以下至外踝长一尺六寸，外踝以下至京骨长三寸，京骨以下至地长一寸。

"The length from the forehead corner to the spinous process of the seventh cervical vertebra is one foot, and from the spinous process of the seventh vertebra to the horizontal line of the armpit which can not be seen due to its hiding in the armpit is four inches. The length from under the armpit to the hypochondrium is one foot and two inches, from the hypochondrium to the hip joint is six inches, from the hip joint to the level of the middle point of the knee cap is one foot and nine inches, from the level of the middle of the knee cap to the outer ankle is one foot and six inches, from the outer ankle to the fifth metatarsal bone on the lateral aspect of the foot is three inches, and from the fifth metatarsal bone on the lateral aspect of the foot to the ground is one inch.

耳后当完骨者广九寸，耳前当耳门者广一尺三寸〔三寸：《甲乙》卷二第七"三"作"二"〕，两颧之间相去七寸，两乳之间广九寸半〔广九寸半：《图翼》，《医统》，《金十方六集》等俱当折八寸〕，两髀之间广六寸半。

"The width between the two Wangu points behind the ears is nine inches, the width between the two Tinggong points in front of the ears is one foot and two inches, the width between the two cheekbones is seven inches, the width between the two nipples is eight inches, and the width between the two thighs is six and half inches.

足长一尺二寸，广四寸半。肩至肘长一尺七寸，肘至腕一尺二寸半，腕至中指本节长四寸，本节至其末长四寸半。

"The length of the foot is one foot and two inches, its width is four and half inches. The length from the end of the shoulder to the elbow is one foot and seven inches, from the elbow to the wrist is 1.25 feet, from the wrist to the root of the basic joint of the middle finger (between the finger and the palm) is four inches, and from the basic joint to the tip of the middle finger is four and half inches.

项髮以下至背骨长二寸半，膂骨以下至尾骶二十一节长三尺，上节长一寸四分分之一，奇分在下，故上七节至于膂骨九寸八分分之七，此众人骨之度也，所以立经脉之短也。是故视其经脉之在于身也，其见浮而坚，其见明而大者，多血；细而沉者，多气也。

"From the hairline behind the neck to the Dazhui point is two and half inches; there are altogether twenty one vertebrae in the spine, including twelve thoracic vertebrae, five lumbar vertebrae and four coccygeal vertebrae and the length is three feet. Each of the seven cervical vertebrae above is 1. 41 inches and the remainder is allocated in the spine, so, the length of the seven cervical vertebrae is 9. 87 inches. These are the bone lengths of a man in common statue, and it is the base for one to establish the standard for examining the length of channels. When one examines the channel and the collaterals of the body, the superficial and shallow ones are the collaterals. When they are obvious and thick, it shows the blood is plenty, when they are thin and hidden, it shows the energy is lacking.

五十营第十五

Chapter 15
Wu Shi Ying
(The Fifty Cycles of the Channel-energy Circulation)

黄帝曰：余愿闻五十营奈何？岐伯答曰：天周〔天周：《甲乙》卷一第九作“周天”〕二十八宿，宿三十〔宿三十：《素问·八正神明论》王注“三十”上无“宿”字〕六分，人气行一周〔一周：《素问·八正神明论》王注“周”下有“天”字〕，千八分。日行二十八宿，人经脉上下、左右、前后二十八脉，周身十六丈二尺，以应二十八宿。

Yellow Emperor said: “I like to know the condition of the fifty cycle-circulation of the channel energy.” Qibo said: “There are twenty eight constellations in the sky and the distance between each of them is thirty six minutes. The channel energy in human body circulates fifty cycles in a day and night, and it takes one thousand and eight minutes. In a day and night, the globe rotates to pass the twenty eight constellations, and the channels of a man distributed on the upper and lower, left and right and front and rear are also twenty eight, and the total length of them is one hundred and sixty two feet when one cycle of circulation in the whole body is completed, and the twenty eight channels correspond to the twenty eight constellations.

漏水下百刻，以分昼夜。故人一呼，脉再动，气行三寸，一吸，脉亦再动，气行三寸，呼吸定息，气行六寸。十息气行六尺，日行二分。二百七十息，气行十六丈二尺，气行交通于中，一周于身，下水二刻，日行二十五分。五百四十息，气行再周于身，下水四刻，日行四十分。二千七百息，气行十周于身，下水二十刻，日行五宿二十分。一万三千五百息，气行五十营于身，水下百刻，日行二十八宿，漏水皆尽，脉终矣。所谓交通者，并行一数也，故五十营备，得尽天地之寿矣，凡行八百一十丈也。

“Take one hundred graduations of leaking water in the clepsydra as the standard to divide the day and night. In an exhalation of a man, the pulse pulsates twice, and the pulse energy moves on three inches in the channel; in an inhalation, the pulse also pulsates twice and the pulse energy moves on three inches; in an exhalation and an inhalation which is called one respiration, the pulse energy moves on six inches. In ten respirations, the pulse energy moves on six feet; in twenty seven respirations, the pulse energy moves on sixteen feet and two inches which is exactly the time for the globe to rotate the distance of two minutes; it takes two hundred and seventy respirations for the channel energy to travel a cycle in the body, and the length of the channels is one hundred and sixty two feet. In the period of the mutual communication of energies for the circulation of a cycle in the two hundred and seventy respirations, it takes two graduations under the water level of the clepsydra, and the rotation of the globe is twenty minutes; in five hundred and forty respirations, the circulation of the channel is two cycles, the mark under the water level of the clepsydra is four graduations, and the rotation of the globe is forty minutes odds; in two thousand and seven hundred respirations, the circulation of the channel energy is ten cycles, the mark under the water level of the clepsydra is twenty graduations, and the rotation of the globe is five constellations and twenty minutes odds; in thirteen thousand and five hundred respirations, the circulation of the channel is fifty cycles, the mark under the water level of the clepsydra is one hundred graduations exactly, and the rotation of the globe is twenty eight constellations; by then, the water in the clepsydra has exhausted, and the channel energy has completed the distance of fifty cycles. The so called 'mutual communication'means to illustrate the circulating condition of the channel energy of one side to represent the conditions of both sides as the hand and foot channels of both sides are the same and they are communicating. When the conditions of the fifty cycles circulation of the channel energy is illustrated, it is the comprehensive condition of heaven and earth."

营气第十六

Chapter 16
Ying Qi
(The Ying-energy)

黄帝曰：营气之道，内谷为宝。谷入于胃，乃传之肺，流溢于中，布散于外，精专者行于经隧，常营无已，终而复始，是谓天地之纪。故气从太阴出，注手阳明，上行注足阳明，下行至跗上，注大指间，与太阴〔与太阴合：按“与”下应补“足”字〕合，上行抵髀〔《甲乙》卷一第十“髀”并作“脾”〕。从脾注心中，循手少阴，出腋下臂，注小指，合手太阳，上乘腋出䪼内，注目内眦，上巅下项，合足太阳，循脊下尻，下行注小指之端，循足心注足少阴，上行注肾，从肾注心，外散于胸中。循心主脉，出腋下臂，出两筋之间，入掌中，出中指之端，还注小指次指之端，合手少阳，上行注膻中，散于三焦，从三焦注胆，出胁注足少阳，下行至跗上，复出跗注大指间，合足厥阴，上行至肝，从肝上注肺，上循喉咙，入颃颡之窍，究于畜门。其支别者，上额循巅下项中，循脊入骶，是督脉也，络阴器，上过毛中，入脐中，上循腹里，入缺盆，下注肺中，复出太阴。此营气之所行也，逆顺之常也。

Yellow Emperor said:“The most valuable thing in the Ying-energy is to receive the cereals. When the water and cereals enter the stomach, the refined substances transformed will be transferred to the lung, overflowed in the five solid organs and scattered in the six hollow organs; the essence circulates in the channel tunnel and operates unceasingly, reaches the terminal and begin again which is identical with the law of heaven and earth. The Ying-energy starts from the Hand Taiyin Channel of Lung, it runs along the inner side of the arm, pours into the Hand Yangming Channel of large Intestine, then pours into the Foot Yangming Channel of Stomach, descends to the dorsum of the foot, and pours into the big toe to join the Foot Taiyin Channel of Spleen and reaches the spleen, then, pours into the heart through the branch of the spleen channel; then, runs along the Hand Shaoyin Channel of Heart, passes the armpit, runs along the rear of the inner flank of the arm, flows to the tip of the small finger and joins the Hand Taiyang Channel of Small Intestine; then, it descends to pass the armpit to reach the inner side of the orbit, pours into the inner canthus, then ascends to reach the top of head, and descends to the neck to join the Foot Taiyang Channel of Bladder; then, descends along the spinal column, passes the sacrococcygeal region and pours into the tip of the small toe; then, runs along the sole, pours into the Foot Shaoyin Channel of Kidney, and runs along the channel to pour into the kidney, then ascends from the kidney to pour into the pericardium and spreads on the chest outside; then, runs along the channel of pericardium, enters into the armpit, descends along the forearm, enters into the palm and reaches the tip of the middle finger of the hand, then, turns back to pour into the tip of the ring finger and joins the Hand Shaoyang Channel of Triple Warmer; then, ascends to pour into the Tanzhong, spreads in the upper, middle and lower warmer, then, it pours into the hollow organ of gallbladder from the triple warmer, passes the armpit, pours into the Foot Shaoyang Channel of Gallbladder, descends to the dorsum of the foot, then pours into the toe from the dorsum of the foot and joins the Foot Jueyin Channel of Liver; then it ascends along the liver channel to reach the liver, pours into the lung from the liver, ascends along the rear of the throat to reach behind the inner orifices of the nose (the two orifices on the upper end of the epiglottis), the inner orifices belong to the Foot Jueyin Channel which are different with the outer nosetrils which belong to the Du Channel. Another branch ascends to reach the forehead, runs along the centre of the top of head, descends to the neck, runs along the spinal column and enters into the sacral bone where the Du Channel passes; then it passes the Ren Channel, communicates with the external genitals, passes the pubic hair margin and enters into the navel, then ascends to enter the supraclavicular fossa, then, descends to pour into the lung, then, it begins to circulate again from the Hand Taiyin Channel of Lung. This is the traveling route of the Ying-energy and the routine of the agreeable and adverse moving of the two kinds of hand and foot channels.

脉度第十七

Chapter 17
Mai Du
(The Length of Channels)

黄帝曰：愿闻脉度。岐伯答曰：手之六阳，从手至头，长〔长：《太素》卷五《十二水》杨注“长”下有“各”字〕五尺，五六〔五六：《难经·二十三难》“五六”下有“合”字〕三丈。手之六阴，从手至胸中，三尺五寸，三六一丈八尺，五六三尺，合二丈一尺。足之六阳，从足上至头，八尺，六八四丈八尺。足之六阴，从足至胸中，六尺五寸，六六三丈六尺，五六三尺，合三丈九尺。跻脉从足至目，七尺五寸，二七一丈四尺，二五一尺，合一丈五尺。督脉任脉各四尺五寸，二四八尺，二五一尺，合九尺。凡都合一十六丈二尺，此气之大经隧也。经脉为里，支而横者为络，络之别者为孙，盛而血者疾诛之，盛者泻之，虚者饮药以补之。

Yellow Emperor said: "I hope to hear about the length of the channels." Qibo said: "In the left and right six Yang channels of hand, the length from the hand to the head in each of them is five feet, and they are altogether thirty feet. In the left and right six Yin channels of hand, the length from the hand to the chest in each of them is three feet and five inches and they are altogether twenty one feet. In the left and right six Yang channels of foot from the hand to the top of head, the length in each of them is eight feet and they are altogether forty eight feet, In the left and right six Yin channels of foot from the foot to the chest, the length in each of them is six feet and five inches, and they are altogether thirty nine feet. In the left and right Jiao channel from the foot to the eye, the length in each of them is seven feet and five inches, and the length altogether is fifteen feet. The length in each of the Du channel and the Ren channel is four feet and five inches, and their length altogether is nine feet. The total length of the channels is one hundred and sixty two feet, These are the routes of channels for the channel energy to circulate. The channels lie deeply inside, and the branches separates from the channel which runs horizontally are the collaterals, and the branches from the collaterals are the minute collaterals. When the minute collaterals are full with stagnated blood, they should be treated immediately, when the evil energy is abundant, purge therapy should be applied, when the healthy energy is deficient, it should be invigorated with medical decoction.

五脏常内阅于上七窍也，故肺气通于鼻，肺〔肺：《太素》卷六《脏·腑气液》，《甲乙》卷一第四并作“鼻”〕和则鼻能和臭香矣；心气通于舌，心〔心：《太素》卷六《》脏腑气液作“舌”〕和则舌能知五味矣，肝气通于目，肝〔肝：《太素》卷六《脏腑气液》作目〕和则目能辨五色矣；脾气通于口，脾〔脾：《难经·三十七难》，《甲乙》卷一第四并作“口”〕和则口能知五谷矣；肾气通于耳，肾〔肾：《太素》卷六《脏腑气液》并作“耳”〕和则耳能闻五音矣。五脏不和则七窍不通，六腑不和则留为痈。故邪在腑则阳脉不和，阳脉不和的气留之，气留之则阳气〔气：《难经·三十七难》作“脉”〕盛矣。阳气太盛则阴不利，阴脉不利则血〔血：《太素》卷六《脏腑气液》作“气”〕留之，血留之则阴气〔气：《难经·三十七难》作“脉”〕盛矣。阴气太盛，则阳气不能荣也，故曰关。阳气太盛，则阴气弗能荣也，故曰格。阴阳俱盛，不得相荣，故曰关格。关格者，不得尽期而死也。

"The refined energy of the five-viscera often reaches the face through the body and appears on the seven orifices. The lung energy communicates with the nose orifices and when the energy of the nose is harmonious, the nose can distinguish the odour of fragrance and foul; the heart energy communicates with the tongue and when the energy of the tongue is harmonious the tongue can distinguish the five tastes; the liver energy communicates with the eye orifices and when the energy of the eyes is harmonious, the eyes can distinguish black and white; the spleen energy communicates with the mouth orifice, and when the energy of the mouth is harmonious, the mouth can distinguish the fragrances of the five cereals; the kidney comunicates with the ear orifices, and when the energy of the ear is harmonious, the ears can hear the five tones. When the five-viscera is inharmonious, the seven orifices will be obstructed, when the six-bowel is inharmonious, the carbuncle will occur due to the stagnation of the blood. Thus, when the evil is in the six-bowel, the Yang channel will be inharmonious to cause the stagnation of the Yang energy, and the stagnation of Yang energy causes the overabundance of the Yang channel; when the evil is in the five-viscera, the Yin channel will become disorderly to cause the stagnation of the Yin energy, and the stagnation of the the Yin energy causes the overabundance of the Yin channel. When the Yin energy is overabundant, it causes the inability of the operation of the Yang energy, and it is called 'Guan'; when the Yang energy is overabundant, it causes the inability of the operation of the Yin energy, and it is called 'Ge'; when both the Yin and Yang are overabundant to cause the inability of mutual operating, it is called 'Guange' (failure of the mutual independing of the superficies and interior). When the patient appears to have the syndrome of Guange, he will not be able to live his natural life and dies early."

黄帝曰：跻脉起安止？何气荣水〔荣水：《太素》卷十《阴阳乔脉》作“营此”〕？岐伯答曰：跻脉〔跻脉：《素问·刺腰痛篇》王注作：“阴跻〕者，少阴〔少阴：《素问·刺腰痛篇》王注“少阴”上有“足”字〕之别，起于然骨之后，上内踝之上，直上循阴股入阴，上循胸里入缺盆，上出人迎之前，人頄，属目内眦，合于太阳、阳跻而上行，气并相还，则为濡目，气不荣则目不合。

Yellow Emperor asked: "Where does the Qiao Channel start and stop? With the help of which channel does it operate?" Qibo answerd: "The Yin Qiao Channel is another channel of the Foot Shaoyin Channel of Kidney, it starts from the rear of the Zhaohai point, ascends to the upper side of the inner ankle, runs along the inner flank of the thigh and enters into the external genitals, then, ascends along the abdomen and the chest to enter into the supraclavicular fossa, then comes out from the Renying, enters to the cheekbone, communicates with the inner canthus, joins the Foot Taiyang Channel of Bladder, and then, ascends again. The two energies of Yin Qiao and Yang Qiao channels encircle the eyes, if the Yin energy is overabundant, the tears will be falling, if the Yang energy is overabundant, the eyes can hardly be closed."

黄帝曰：气独行五脏，不荣六腑，何也？岐伯答曰：气之不得无行也，如水之流，如日月〔如日月之行不休：《难经·三十七难》无“如日月”七字〕之行不休，故阴脉荣其脏，阳脉荣其腑，如环之无端，莫知其纪，终而复始。其流溢之气，内溉脏腑，外濡腠理。

Yellow Emperor asked: "when the energies of the Yin channels circulate in the five-viscera alone, it does not nourish the six-bowel, and why is it?" Qibo answered: "The flow of the channel energy is like the water-flow which never ceases. The Yin channel energies nourish the refined energy of the five-viscera and the Yang channel energies nourish the refined energy of the six-bowel, they pour into each other like a ring, terminates and starts again without end. As to the channel energy which is overflowing, it permeates the solid and hollow organs inside, and moistures the surface of the muscle and the skin outside."

黄帝曰：跻脉有阴阳，何脉当其数？岐伯答曰：男子数其阳，女子数其阴，当数者为经，其不当数者为络也。

Yellow Emperor asked: "In the Qiao Channels, the Yang Qiao and the Yin Qiao are different, which of them is fifteen feet in length stated above?" Qibo said: "In a man, his Yang Qiao channel should be counted, and in a woman, the Yin Qiao channel should be counted. When the counted length which is included in the total length of channel, it is called the channel, the length which is excluded is called the collaterals. So, in a man, the Yang Qiao is the channel and the Yin Qiao is the collateral; in a woman, the Yin Qiao is the channel and the Yang Qiao is the collateral.

营卫生会第十八

Chapter 18
Ying Wei Sheng Hui
(The Issue of Distribution and Operation of Ying-energy and Wei-energy)

黄帝问于岐伯曰：人焉受气？阴阳焉会？何气为营？何气为卫？营安从生？卫于焉会？老壮不同气，阴阳异位，愿闻其会。岐伯答曰：人受气于谷，谷入于胃，以传与肺〔肺：《难经·三十难》作"五脏六腑"〕，五脏六腑，皆以受气，其清者为营，浊者为卫，营在脉中，卫在脉外，营周不休，五十〔五十：《灵枢略·六气论篇》"五十"下有"周"字〕而复大会。阴阳相贯，如环无端。卫气行于阴二十五度，行于阳二十五度，分为昼夜，故气至阳而起，至阴而止。故曰：日中而阳陇〔陇：日刻本作"隆"〕为重阳，夜半而阴陇为重阴。故太阴主内，太阳主外，各行二十五度，分为昼夜。夜半为阴陇，夜半后而为阴衰，平旦阴尽而阳受气矣。日中为阳陇，日西而阳衰，日入阳尽而阴受气矣。夜半而大会，万民皆卧，命曰合阴，平旦阴尽而阳受气，如是无已，与天地同纪。

Yellow Emperor asked Qibo and said: "Where does a man receive the refined energy? Where do the Yin and Yang energies converge? What kind of energy is called Ying and what kind of energy is called Wei? From where does the Ying-energy issue? Where do the Ying-energy and the Wei-energy meet? The deficient or overabundant condition of energy in an old man and a man in his prime of life are different, and the locations where the energy travels are also different in day and night, I hope to hear about the condition when the energies meet." Qibo answered: "The refined energy of a man stems from the refined substance transformed by the cereals received, when the cereals enter into the stomach, the refined substance produced will be transferred to the five solid organs and the six hollow organs, and they can all obtain the nutrition, in the refined substance, the lucid part is called the Ying-energy, and the turbid part is called the Wei-energy, the Ying-energy flows within the channel, and the Wei-energy flows outside of the channel, and they operate in the whole body unceasingly, the Ying-energy and the Wei-energy circulates fifty cycles each and then they meet. The Yin and Yang are communicating with each other, they go round and begin again like a ring without end. The Wei-energy runs twenty five cycles in the Yin portion and runs twenty five cycles in the Yang portion, half of its circulation is in the day and half of it is in the night, its circulation starts from the head which belongs to Yang and terminates by the Yin channels of hand and foot. The Wei-energy travels by the Yin channels of hand and foot. The Wei-energy travels outside of the six Yang channels of hand and foot in day time, as the Yang energy is most prosperous at noon, it is called 'Yang in prosperity'. The Wei-energy travels outside of the six Yin channels of hand and foot in night time, and the Yin energy is most prosperous at midnight, after midnight, the Yin energy falls into a decline gradually, and at dawn, the Yin energy is exhausted and the Yang energy comes in the wake of it; in day time, the Yang energy is most prosperous at noon, the Yang energy falls into a decline when the sun sets, in the evening, the Yang energy becomes exhausted and the Ying-energy comes in the wake of it; at midnight, the Ying-energy and the Wei-energy converge, as both the Ying-energy and the Wei-energy are in the position of Yin at midnight, and people are sleeping then, it is called the 'combinatinon of Yin'; at dawn, the Yin-energy is exhausted and the Yang energy comes in the wake of it. In this way, it circulates unceasingly, and it agrees with the condition of the transferring of the sun and moon in the universe."

黄帝曰：老人之不夜瞑者，何气使然？少壮之人不昼瞑〔不昼瞑：《甲乙》卷一第十一作“不夜寤”〕者，何气使然？岐伯答曰：壮者之气血盛，其肌肉滑，气道通，荣卫之行，不失其常，故昼精而夜瞑。老者之气血衰，其肌肉枯，气道涩，五脏之气相搏，其营气衰少而卫气内伐，故昼不精，夜不瞑。

Yellow Emperor asked:"An old man can hardly fall into sleep in night time and what energy causes it? A healthy young man can hardly be awaken when he falls into sleep in night time and what energy causes it?" Qibo answered: "For a healthy young man, his energy and blood are abundant, his muscles are smooth and his energy passage is unobstructed, and the operations of his Ying-energy and Wei-energy are normal, so, his spirit is easy in day time and sleeps soundly in night time. For an old man, his energy and blood are falling into a decline, his muscles are emaciated, his energy passage is unsmooth, the energies of the five-viscera are combating and can hardly be kept harmonious, so his Ying-energy is deficient, and his Wei-energy is corrupted inside, and as a result, his spirit is not easy in daytime and can not sleep soundly in night-time."

黄帝曰：愿闻营卫之所行，皆何道从来？岐伯答曰：营出于中焦，卫出于下〔下：《太素》卷十二首篇，《灵枢略》“下”并作“上”〕焦。黄帝曰：愿闻三〔三：按“三”误，应作“上”〕焦之所出。岐伯答曰：上焦出于胃上口，并咽以上贯膈而布胸中，走腋，循太阴之分而行，还至阳明，上至舌，下足阳明，常与营俱行〔常与营俱行：《病沅》卷十五《三焦病候》“营”下有“部”字〕于阳二十五度，行于阴亦二十五度一周也，故五十度而复大会于手太阴矣〔于阳二十五度至手太阴矣：《病沅》卷十五《三焦病候》无“于阳”以下三十字〕。黄帝曰：人有热，饮食下胃，其气未定，汗则出，或出于面，或出于背，或出于身半，其不循卫气之道而出何也？岐伯曰：此外伤于风，内开腠理，毛蒸理泄，卫气走之，固不得循其道，此气慓悍滑疾，见开而出，故不得从其道，故命曰漏泄。

Yellow Emperor said:"I hope to hear the conditions of the issues of the Ying-energy and the Wei energy and their routes of operation." Qibo said: "The Ying-energy is issued from the middle warmer and the Wei-energy is issued from the upper warmer." Yellow Emperor said: "I hope to hear about the condition of the upper warmer-issue." Qibo answered: "The energy of upper issues from the upper opening of the stomach, it runs along the gullet, passes the diaphragm and spreads in the chest, then, it runs horizontally to reach the armpit, descends along the range of the Hand Taiyin Channel of Lung, returns to the Hand Yangming Channel of Large Intestine, ascends to reach the nose, and then descends to pour into the Foot Yangming Channel of Stomach, and it often runs side by side with the Ying-energy and the Wei-energy." Yellow Emperor asked: "When one has heat in the body, he perspires as soon as the food and drink have just entered into the stomach, and the refined energy has not yet been transformed then; the sweat comes out from the face, back and the lateral side of the body and does not come out along the locations of the operating route of the Wei-energy, and what is the reason?" Qibo said: "It is because the invasion of the wind-evil from outside causes the loosening of the striae, and when the fine hair and the skin are steamed by the wind-heat, the striae will be open, and the Wei-energy will not run along its regular route, but passes the locations where the muscular striae are loose; as the characteristic of the Wei-energy is valiant and slippery, it passes through the locations where the striae are loose, and it is called the 'leaking of energy'."

黄帝曰：愿闻中焦之所出。岐伯答曰：中焦亦并〔并：日刻本旁注："并"，一曰当作"出"〕胃中，出上焦之后，此所受气者，泌糟粕，蒸津液，化其精微，上注于肺脉，乃化而为血，以奉生身，莫贵于此，故独得行于经隧，命曰营气。黄帝曰：夫血之与气，异名同类，何谓也？岐伯答曰：营卫者精气也，血者神气也，故血之与气，异名同类焉。故夺血者无汗，夺气者无血，故人生有一死而无两生。

Yellow Emperor said: "I hope to hear about the conditions of the middle warmer-issue." Qibo said: "The energy of middle warmer also issues from the stomach and behind the upper warmer, it transforms and produces the tastes of the five cereals, it strains away the dross and retains the refined fluid and pours it into the lung, then, it is transformed into blood to nourish the whole body, so, it is most valuable, it can run within the tunnel of the channel and it is called 'Ying' (nourish)". Yellow Emperor asked: "The blood and energy are different in names, but in fact, they belong to the same category, and why is it?" Qibo answered: "The Wei-energy is transformed from the refined energy of water and cereals and the Ying-energy is the variation of the water and cereals, so, although they are different in names, yet they are of the same category. Therefore, when the patient collapes due to massive hemorrhage, he must not be treated with diaphoresis, when one has the consumption of the energy, he must not lose his blood; of course, death is inevitable in one's life, but one can not revive after death."

黄帝曰：愿闻下焦之所出。岐伯答曰：下焦者，别回肠，注于膀胱而渗入焉。故水谷者，常并居于胃中，成糟粕，而俱下于大肠，而成下焦，渗而俱下，济泌别汁，循下焦而渗入膀胱焉。黄帝曰：人饮酒，酒亦入胃，谷未熟而小便独先下何也？岐伯答曰：酒者熟谷之液也，其气悍以清，故后谷而人，先谷而液出焉。黄帝曰：善。余闻上焦如雾，中焦如沤，下焦如渎，此之谓也。

Yellow Emperor said: "I hope to hear about the conditions of the lower warmer-issue." Qibo said: "The lower warmer starts from the lower end of the small intestine, it sends the dross to the large intestine, and pours the water into the bladder, and they are completed by gradual permeance. So, the substance of the water and cereals kind are stored in the stomach regularly, and after digestion, the dross will be sent to the large intestine; in the course of digestion, the water is squeezed, the lucid fluid is retained, and the turbid fluid is drained to the bladder along the lower warmer." Yellow Emperor asked: "When wine is drunken it also enters into the stomach, but the wine can be excreted through urination before the rice is digested, and what is the reason?" Qibo answered: " The wine is a liquid formed after the fermentation of the cereals, its energy is valiant and slippery, so, even when it enters into the stomach later than the food, it can be excreted through urination prior to the food, "Yellow Emperor said: "Good. So the saying goes: 'in the functions of the triple warmer, the upper warmer is like mists, the middle warmer is like the pivot, and the lower warmer is like the gutter.'"

四时气第十九

Chapter 19
Si Shi Qi
(Application of Different Pricking Therapies in Different Seasons)

黄帝问于岐伯曰：夫四时之气，各不同形，百病之起，皆有所生，灸刺之道，何者为定？岐伯答曰："四时之气，各有所在，灸刺之道，得气穴为定。故春取经血脉分肉之间，甚者深刺之，间者浅刺之；夏取盛经孙络，取分间绝皮肤；秋取经腧，邪在府，取之合；冬取井荥，必深以留之。

Yellow Emperor asked Qibo："The weathers in the four seasons are different and the diseases affected by the weathers of the various seasons are different，how to set the principle of acupuncture and moxibustion in treating?"Qibo answered："When the various energies of the four seasons affect a man to have diseases，they are in the different locations of the body，the principle of acupuncture and moxibustion should be set at the standard of getting the acupuncture feeling. Therefore，in spring，it should prick the collateral and the space between the muscles，prick deeply when the disease is severe and prick shallowly when the disease is slight；in summer，prick the Yang channel，minute collateral，or prick the boundary between the muscles，and the pricking should be shallow to penetrate into the skin；in autumn，prick the Shu-points of the various channels，if the disease is in the six hollow organs，prick the He points；in winter，prick the Well points and the Xing points of the various channels，the pricking should be deeper and the retention of the needle should be longer.

温疟汗不出，为五十九痏。风𤸇肤胀，为五十七〔七：《太素》卷二十三《杂刺》并作"九"〕痏，取皮肤之血者，尽取之。

"To the warm-type malaria without sweat，there are fifty nine acupoints for treating，to edema caused by wind-evil and to the edema of the skin，there are fifty nine acupoints for pricking，if there are superficial venules on the skin of the abdomen，they should all be pricked.

飧泄，补三阴之〔补三阴之，按"补"字误，似应作"取"，"之"是"交"的误字〕，上补阴陵泉，皆久留之，热行乃止。

"To lienteric diarrhea，prick the Sanyinjiao point and invigorate the Yinlingquan point by pricking，the retention of the needle must be longer，and stop the pricking after the occurrence of heat under the needle.

转筋于阳治其阳，转筋于阴治其阴，皆卒刺之。

"To the spasm of the muscle on the outer flank，prick the Yang channels on the outer side of the hand and foot，to the spasm of the muscle in the inner flank，prick the inner side of the hand and foot, and both of them should be pricked with heated needle.

徒瘀，先取环谷下三寸，以铍针针之，已刺而筩之，而内之，入而复之〔之：《甲乙》卷八第四作“出”〕，以尽其瘀，必坚，〔必坚：应作“必急刺之”〕来缓则烦悗，来急则安静，间日一刺之，瘀尽乃止。饮闭药，方刺之时徒饮之，方饮无食，方食无饮，无食他食百三十五日。

“When the patient has edema, prick the Guanyuan point three inches below the navel with the sword-shaped needle, after pricking, put a bamboo tube on the needle hole to absorb the water, and it should be carried on again and again to remove the water inside, the pricking should be rapid, as slow pricking will cause the patient to become restless and depression, and the rapid pricking will cause calmness of the patient. The pricking should be carried on every other day, and stop the pricking when the water is exhausted. Besides, the patient should take some tonic after the beginning of the pricking. When the patient has taken the tonic, he must avoid food. When he has taken food, he must avoid tonic, he must not take the food which is not beneficial for treating the edema, and this contraindication should be observed for one hundred and thirty five days.

著痹不去，久寒不已，卒取其三里骨为干。肠中不便，取三里，盛泻之，虚补之。

“When the patient has the wet-type arthralgia and has protracted cold-wetness evil, it should prick the bone inside with the heated needle, if the patient has the tibia bi-syndrome and feels uncomfortable in the stomach, prick the Sanli point; apply purge therapy when the evil energy is overabundant, and apply invigorating therapy when the healthy energy is deficient.

疠风者，素刺其肿上，已刺，以锐针针其处，按出其恶气〔气：《甲乙》卷十一第九下作血.”〕，肿尽乃止，常食方食，无食他食。

“When treating the patient of leprosy, prick the swelling location frequently. After pricking, press around the pricking hole to squeeze out the malicious blood (or stagnated blood). The patient should take some proper food often and avoid to take the food disadvantageous to the recuperation of the disease.

腹中常鸣〔腹中常鸣：《脉经》卷六第八“腹”并作“肠”〕，气上冲胸，喘〔喘：《甲乙》卷九第七无“喘”字〕不能久立，邪在大肠，刺肓之原、巨虚上廉、三里。

“When the patient has borborygmus with a loud sound, the vital energy reverses up to attack the chest often, and he can not stand long, it is the syndrome of the evil energy in the large intestine; prick the Qihai, Shangjuxu and Foot Sanli points.

小腹控睾、引腰脊，上冲心，邪在小肠者，连睾系，属于脊，贯肝肺，络心系，气盛则厥逆，上冲肠胃，熏肝，散于肓〔肓：《甲乙》卷九第八作“胸”〕，结于脐〔脐：《脉经》卷六第六作“厌”〕。故取之肓原以散之，刺太阴以予之，取厥阴以下之，取巨虚下廉以去之，按其所过之经以调之。

“The lower abdomen controls the testes and links the spinal column, when the pain reverses up to attack the heart and chest, it is the syndrome of the evil energy in the small intestine. The small intestine connects the testicular system, links the spinal column, reaches the liver and lung and comunicates with the heart vessels, when the evil energy is overabundant, the chaotic energy will reverse up to attack the intestine and stomach, implicates the liver and lung , spreads on the chest and assembles on the pharynx. Thus, when treating the disease of the small intestine, it should prick the Source point of the chest to disperse the evil energy, prick the points on the Hand Taiyin Channel to raise the energy and prick the points of the Foot Jueyin Channel to lower the energy, prick the Xiajuxu point to remove the evil energy and prick the acupoints along the locations where the channel passes to adjust the energy.

善呕，呕有苦，长太息，心中憺憺，恐人将捕之，邪在胆，逆在胃，胆液泄则口苦，胃气逆则呕苦，故曰呕胆，取三里以下胃气逆，则刺〔则刺：《太素》卷二十三《杂否则》无“则”字。《千金》卷十二“刺”下并有“足”字〕少阳血络以闭胆逆，却调其虚实以去其邪。饮食不下，隔塞不通，邪在胃脘，在上脘则刺抑而下之，在下脘则散而去之。

"When the patient often vomits the bile, sighs frequently, becomes frightened and restless as if someone is going to arrest him, it is the syndrome of the evil energy in the gallbladder, and the disorder of the vital energy will affect the stomach; when the bile is overflowing, there will be bitter taste in the mouth, when the stomach energy reverses up, the bile will be vomited. When treating, prick the Sanli point to keep the adverse stomach energy downwards, prick the superficial venules of the Foot Shaoyang Channel to restrain the up-reversing of the bile, besides, one should inspect the sthenic or asthenic conditions of the disease and remove the evil energy accordingly. As to the patient who can not eat nor drink due to the obstruction around the diaphragm, it is the syndrome of evil energy on the gastric cavity. When the disease is in the upper part of the gastric cavity, prick the acupoints on the upper part of the gastric cavity to restrain the adverse energy of the stomach; when the disease is in the lower part of the gastric cavity, prick the acupoints on the lower part of the gastric cavity to dispel the stagnation.

小腹痛肿，不得小便，邪在三焦约，取之太阳〔取之：《太素》卷二十三《杂刺》“取之”下并有“足”字〕大络，视其络脉与厥阴小络结而血者，肿上及胃脘，取三里。

"When the lower abdomen of the patient is swelling and he has dysuria, it is the evil energy in the bladder, prick the acupoints on the large collateral of the Foot Taiyang Channel. When there is stagnated blood in the large collateral of the Foot Taiyang Channel and in the small collateral of the Foot Jueyin Channel, and the swelling is approaching the gastric cavity above, it should prick the Sanli point.

覩其色，察其以〔察其以：《太素》卷二十三《杂刺》“以”作“目”〕，知其散复者，视其目色，以知病之存亡也。一其形，听其动静者，持气口人迎以视其脉，坚且盛且滑者病日进，脉软者病将下，诸经实者病三日已。气口候阴，人迎候阳也。

"During the pricking, observe the complexion and the eyes of the patient to know whether the disease is aggravating or relieving, when watching the eyes and the complexion of the patient, one can know whether the disease is severe or slight; in diagnosing the condition of the disease, one must palpate the Cunkou and the Renying pulses with a concentrated mind, if the pulse condition is firm and slippery, it shows the disease will be aggravated day after day; if the pulse is soft in coming, the disease will be alleviated soon. When the disease is the various channel and the pulse condition is substantial and vigorous, the disease will be recovered in three days. The Cunkou pulse shows the conditions of the five solid organs which are Yin, and the Renying pulse shows the conditions of the six hollow organs which are Yang.

五邪第二十

Chapter 20
Wu Xie
(The Pricking Therapy for Treating the Evils in the Five Viscera)

邪在肺，则病皮肤痛，寒热，上气喘〔上气喘：《脉经》卷六第七“气”并重“气”字〕，汗出，咳动肩背。取之膺中外腧，背三节五脏〔背三节五脏：《甲乙》卷九第三作“椎”，无“五脏”二字〕之傍，以手疾按之，快然，乃刺之，取之缺盆中以越之。

When the evil energy is in the lung, the patient will feel painful of the skin, he will have cold and heat, adverseness of vital energy, rapid breathing, sweating and cough to cause the shoulder and the back to become uncomfortable. When treating, prick the Zhongfu and the Yunmen points which are on the upper part and the lateral side of the chest, and prick the Feishu point beside the third vertebra of the back; press with force by hand first until the patient feels comfortable, and then, prick the acupoint. The disease can also be treated by pricking the Quepen point.

邪在肝，则两胁中痛，寒中，恶血在内，行善掣，节时脚肿〔节时脚肿：《甲乙》卷九第四连上文“行善掣”作“胻节时肿善瘛”〕取之行间以引胁下，补三里以温胃中，取血脉以散恶血，取耳间青脉，以去其掣〔掣：《太素》卷二十二《五脏刺》作“痹”〕。

When the evil energy is in the liver, the patient will have asthenia-cold of the middle warmer, stagnation of blood inside and swelling of the tibia joint to cause spasm often. when treating, prick the Xingjian point to lower the energy of the hypochondria, invigorate the Sanli point to warm the middle warmer, prick the superficial venules of the same channel to scatter the malicious blood, prick the green collateral on the ear to remove the bi-syndrome.

邪在脾胃〔脾胃：《脉经》卷六第五“脾”下无“胃”字〕，则病肌肉痛。阳气有余，阴气不足，则热中善饥；阳气不足，阴气有余，则寒中肠鸣腹痛，阴阳俱有余，若俱不足，则有寒有热。皆调于三里。

When the evil energy is in the spleen, the muscle of the patient will be painful, if the Yang energy is overabundant and the Yin energy is deficient, there will be heat in the stomach and the patient will often get hungry; if the Yang energy is deficient and the Yin energy is overabundant, there will be cold in the stomach and the patient will have borborygmus and pain in the abdomen; if both the Yin and Yang are having a surplus or both of their energies are deficient, it shows some of the syndromes belong to cold and some of them belong to heat, when treating, all of them can be treated by pricking the Foot Sanli point.

邪在肾，则病骨痛阴痹。阴痹者，按之而不得，腹胀腰痛，大便难，肩背颈项痛。时眩。取之涌泉、昆仑，视有血者尽取之。

When the evil energy is in the kidney, pain in the bone, the yin-type bi-sydrome will occur. In the yin-type bi-syndrome, the painful location can hardly be detected by pressing with hand, the patient will have abdominal distention, lumbago, dyschesia, pain and stiffness in the shoulder, back and neck and he will have frequent dizziness. When treating, prick the Yongquan point and the Kunlun point, if the stagnated blood is seen, the superficial venules of the channel should also be pricked.

邪在心，则病心痛喜悲，时眩仆。视有余不足而调之其输也。

When the evil energy is in the heart, heartache will occur, the patient will be sorrowful and will often fall due to dizziness. When treating, observe the asthenic or sthenic condition of the disease first, then, prick the acupoint of the some channel.

寒热病第二十一

Chapter 21
Han Re Bing
(Cold and Heat)

皮寒热者，不可附席，毛发焦，鼻槁腊，不得汗。取三阳之络，以补手太阴。

When the exogenous evil invades the skin and the fine hair to cause cold and heat of the patient, his skin can not tolerate to attach the mattress, his skin and fine hairs are withered and his nostrils are dry without any sweat, it should be treated by pricking the collateral points of the Foot Taiyang Channel, and invigorate by pricking the Hand Taiyin Channel.

肌寒热者，肌痛，毛发焦而唇槁腊，不得汗，取三阳于下以去其血者，补足太阴以出其汗。

When the exogenous evil invades the muscle causing the patient to have cold and heat, he will have pain in the muscle, withering of the hair, dryness of the lips and he has no sweat. It should be treated by pricking the collateral points of the Foot Taiyang Channel on the lower extremities and let out the stagnated blood, then, invigorate by pricking the Foot Taiyin Channel to cause sweating.

骨寒热者，病无所安，汗注不休。齿未槁，取其少阴于阴股之络；齿已槁，死不治。骨厥亦然。

When the exogenous evil penetrates into the bone causing the patient to have cold and heat, the pain will have nowhere to rest, and the patient will perspire all over the body; if the teeth are not withered, it should prick the collateral points of Foot Shaoyin Channel on the inner side of the thigh; if the teeth are withered, it is a fatal disease. In diagnosing and treating the jue-syndrome of bone, it should treat after the same method.

骨痹，举节不用而痛，汗注烦心。取三阴之经补之。

In bone bi-syndrome, all the bone joints in the body of the patient are painful and the joints fail to move nimbly, the patient has pouring perspiration, and the depressinon of the chest. Prick the points of the Hand and Foot three Yin channels and apply the invigorating therapy.

身有所伤血出多，及中风寒，若有所堕坠，四以懈惰不收，名曰体惰。取其小腹脐下三结交。三结交者，阳明、太阴也，脐下三寸关元也。

When the body of the patient is hurt by a blade of metal, bleeds a lot and he has also contracted wind-evil, or the patient is emaciated in the four extremities, reluctant to move about due to falling from a high place which is called 'fatigue and flaccid of limbs', it should be treated by pricking the Sanjiejiao point of the Ren Channel (Guanyuan point) three inches below the navel. The San-jiejiao point means the triple conection, it is the place where Foot Yangming, Foot Taiyin and the Ren channels meet.

厥痹者，厥气上及腹。取阳明之络，视主病也，泻阳补阴经也。

When one has the Jueni and the bi-syndrome, the energy will reverse up from the foot to attack the lower abdomen. When treating, prick the collateral points of the Yin or Yang channel, but must find out first where the main disease is; when the main disease is in the Yang channel, apply purge therapy, when it is in the Yin energy, apply invigorating therapy.

颈侧之动脉人迎。人迎，足阳明也，在婴筋之前。婴筋之后，手阳明也，名曰扶突。次脉，足〔足少阳脉也：张注本“足少阳”下无“脉”字〕少阳脉也，名曰天牖。次脉，足太阳也，名曰天柱。腋下动脉，臂〔臂：《本输篇》作“手”〕太阴也，名曰天府。

The artery on the lateral side of the neck is the Renying point, it belongs to the Foot Yangning Channel of Stomach and locates in front of the neck's tendon. Behind the neck's tendon is the Futu point which belongs to the Hand Yangming Channel of Large Intestine. On the further side , it is the Tianyou point which belongs to the Foot Shaoyang Channel, and on the further side is the Tianzhu point which belongs to the Foot Taiyang Channel of Bladder. The point in the artery of the armpit is the Tianfu point which belongs to the Hand Taiyin Channel of Lung.

阳迎头痛，胸满不得息，取之人迎。暴瘖气鞕，取扶突与舌本出血。暴聋气蒙，耳目不明，取天牖。暴挛痫眩，足不任身，取天柱。暴瘅内逆，肝肺相搏，血溢鼻口，取天府。此为天牖五部。

When the Yang evil energy reverses in the Yang channel and causes headache to have fullness of the chest and dyspnea, prick the Renying point. When one has dysphonia all of a sudden and the blockage of energy, prick the Futu point and the root of tongue to cause bleeding. When one has sudden onset of deafness, over-abundant vital energy and can not see and hear things clearly, prick the Tianyou point. When one has contracture of the limbs suddenly, has epilepsy or spasm and the heel can hardly sustain the body, prick the Tianzhu point. When one is suddenly hot and thirsty, the abdominal energy reverses up, the fire evils of the lung and liver combat causing the blood to run rashly and overflows on the nose and mouth, prick the Tianfu point. These are the locations of the five window-acupoints related to the orifices of head and face.

臂阳明有人頄徧齿者，名曰大迎，下齿龋取之。臂恶寒补之，不恶寒泻之。足太阳有入頄徧齿者，名曰角孙，上齿龋取之，在鼻与頄前。方病之时其脉盛，盛则泻之，虚则补之。一曰取之出鼻外。

In the part of Hand Yangming Channel which ascends to enter into the cheekbone and spreads all over the roots of teeth, its acupoint is called Daying. When the dental caries is on the lower jaw, prick the Daying point. When ones arm has aversion to the cold, apply purging therapy. In the part of the Hand Taiyang Channel which enters into the cheek and spreads all over the roots of teeth, its acupoint is called Jiaosun. When treating the caries on the upper jaw, prick the Jiaosun point and other points in front of the nose and cheekbone. When the disease is at the beginning, if the pulse is overabundant, apply purging therapy, if the pulse is deficient, apply invigorating therapy. According to other version, the acupoints on the lateral side of the nose can also be pricked.

足阳明有挟鼻入于面者，名曰悬颅，属口，对入系目本，视有过者取之，损有余，益不足，反者益其〔张介宾曰："其"当作"甚"〕。足太阳有通项入于脑者，正属目本，名曰眼系，头目苦痛取之，在项中两筋间，入脑乃别阴跻、阳跻，阴阳相交，阳入阴，阴出阳，交于目锐眦，阳气盛则瞋目，阴气盛则瞑目。

The acupoint on the Foot Yangming Channel which runs closely to the nose and enters into the face is called Xuanlu. The channel that runs downwards belongs to the mouth and the channel that runs upwards connects the ocular connectors. Treat the abnormal location and purge when there is a surplus and invigorate when it is deficient. If the treating is on the contrary, the disease will be aggravated. The part of the Foot Taiyang Channel which reaches the neck and enters into the brain belongs directly to the ocular connectors which are the structures connecting the eyeballs with the brain, including the blood vessels and optic nerves. To headache caused by the ocular connectors, prick the acupoints between the two tendons on the neck. The Foot Taiyang Chanenl penetrates from the neck into the brain and then, divides into the Yinqiao Channel and the Yangqiao Channel respectively. These two channels intersect, and then, the Yang channel enters into the Yin one, and the Yin channel comes out from the Yang one, they intersect on the Jingming point on the inner canthus. When the Yang energy is overabundant, the eyes keep wide open frequently, when the Yin energy is overabundant, the eyes keep closed frequently.

热厥取足太阴、少阳，皆留之；寒厥取足阳明、少阴于足，皆留之。

To the syndrome of cold extremities due to heat-evil, prick the acupoint on the Foot Taiyin Channel of Spleen and that on the Foot Shaoyang Channel of Gallbladder; to the cold-type jue-syndrome, prick the acupoints on Foot Yangming Channel of Stomach and that on the Foot Shaoyin Channel of Kidney. It can also prick the points on the foot. In all the prickings, the needle should be retained.

舌纵涎下，烦悗，取足少阴。振寒洒洒，鼓颔，不得汗出，腹胀烦悗，取手太阴。刺虚者，刺其去也；刺实者，刺其来也。

When one's tongue is weak, unable to withdraw and curl, the saliva comes out spontaneously and he feels oppressive over the chest, prick the acupoints on the Foot Shaoyin Channel of Kidney. When one is cold, the two cheeks are trembling like beating a drum, and he has distention and oppression in the abdomen but has no sweat in the body, prick the acupoints on the Hand Taiyin Channel of Lung. When treating the asthenia-syndrome, prick the asthenic location where the Ying energy and the Wei energy have passed for invigorating, when treating the sthenia-syndrome, prick the sthenic location where the Ying energy and the Wei energy have come for purging.

春取络脉，夏取分腠，秋取气口，冬取经输，凡此四时，各以时为齐。络脉治皮肤，分腠治肌肉，气口治筋脉，经输治骨髓、五脏。

When treating in spring, prick the acupoints between the collateral branches of the large channel, when treating in summer, prick the acupoints between the muscle and the skin, when treating in autumn, prick the acupoints of the Cunkou area on the wrist over the radial artery, when treating in winter, prick the acupoints on the channel. In the four seasons, each has its definite sphere of pricking. When pricking the muscle and skin, it can cure the disease of the skin, when pricking the muscle, it can cure the disease of the muscle, when pricking the Cunkou, it can cure the disease of the tendon, when pricking the channel, it can cure the disease of the bone marrow and the five viscera.

身有五部：伏兔一；腓二，腓者腨也；背三；五脏之腧四；项五。此五部有痈疽者死。病始手臂者，先取手阳明、太阴而汗出；病始头首者，先取项太阳而汗出；病始足胫者，先取足阳明而汗出。臂太阴可汗出，足阳明可汗出。故取阴而汗出甚者，止之于阳；取阳而汗出甚者，止之于阴。

There are five crucial parts in the body to have carbuncle. They are: the musculus rectus fermoris (the most prominent portion of the muscle on the anterior aspect of the thigh resembling a prostrate hare when the knees are extended), the calf, the back, the shu-points of the five viscera and the neck. When the carbuncle is affected on the various parts stated above, the patient may die. When the disease is on the arm, prick the acupoints on the Hand Yangming Channel and that on the Hand Taiyin Channel to cause sweating; when the disease initiates from the head, prick the acupoints of Foot Taiyang Channel on the neck to cause sweating; when the disease is on the leg, prick the acupoints of Foot Taiyang Channel on the neck to cause sweating; when the disease is on the leg, prick the acupoints on the Foot Yangming channel first to cause sweating. Both pricking the acupoints of the Hand Taiyin Channel or that on the Foot Yangming Channel can cause sweating. As the Yin channel and the Yang channel are communicating, if the sweat is abundant when pricking the Yin channel, the sweat can be stopped by pricking the Yang channel; if the sweat is abundant when pricking the Yang channel, the sweat can be stopped by pricking the Yin channel.

凡刺之害，中而不去则精泄，不中而去则致气；精泄则病甚而恇，致气则生为痈疽也。

Generally, in pricking, when the focus is hit and the needle is retained, it will purge the refined energy of the patient; if the focus is not hit and the needle is pulled out instantly, it will cause the evil energy to stagnate without dispersing. When the refined energy is purged, the disease will be aggravated and causes falling into a decline of the body; when the evil energy is stagnated, it will cause carbuncle.

癫狂第二十二

Chapter 22
Dian Kuang
(Mania-depressive Syndrome)

目眦外决于面者，为锐眦；在内近鼻者为内眦；上为外眦，下为内眦。

The eye-corner which is on the outer side of the face is called the outer canthus, the eye-corner which is nearing the nose is called the inner canthus. The outer canthus belongs to Yang and the inner canthus belongs to Yin.

癫疾始生，先不乐，头重痛，视举目赤，甚作极〔甚作极：《甲乙》卷十一第二"甚"属上"赤"字之头，作"举目赤甚"〕，已而烦心，侯之于颜，取手太阳、阳明、太阴，血变而止。

In the beginnig of the dian disease (disorder of head), the patient appears to be unhappy, his head is heavy, his two eyes are red and stare straight forward. When the disease is severe, the patient will have the feeling of oppression over the chest and restless. When one examines the expression between the two eyes and the eyebows of the patient, he can predict the attack of the disease. When treating, prick the acupoints of the Hand Taiyang, Yangming and Taiyin channels, and cease the pricking after the colour of the patient's complexion has turned into normal.

癫疾始作，而引口啼呼喘悸者，侯之手阳明、太阳，左强者攻其右，右强者攻其左，血变而止。癫疾始作，先反僵，因而脊痛，侯之足太阳、阳明、太阴〔阳明，大阴：《太素》卷三十《癫疾》无阳明，大阴〕、手太阳，血变而止。

In the initiation of dian disease, the patient makes a crying sound in the mouth; one should examine and prick the acupoints along the Hand Yangming and Taiyang channels and apply contralateral insertion, when the left side is stiff, prick the right side; when the right side is stiff, prick the left side, and cease the pricking after the colour of the patient's complexion has turned into normal. In the initiation of dian disease, the patient's body is erect and stiff first like a bow bending in the adverse direction, then, he feels pain in the spine and the back. One should examnine and prick the acupoints along the Foot Taiyang Channel and that of the Hand Taiyang Channel, and cease the pricking after the colour of the patient's complexion has turned into normal.

治癫疾者，常与之居，察其所当取之处。病至，视之有过者泻之，置其血于瓠壶之中，至其发时，血独动矣。不动，灸穷骨二十壮。穷骨者，骶骨也。

When treating the patient with dian disease, the physician should often live with the patient together to find out which are the proper channels and acupoints for treating. When the disease attacks, let out the blood from the diseased channels and put the blood released into a gourd; when the disease attacks again, the blood in the gourd will be moving. If the blood in the gourd is not moving, apply moxibustion of twenty moxa-cones to the qiong bone which is also called the sacrum bone (the location of the Changqiang point).

骨癫疾者，顑、齿诸腧、分肉皆满而骨居，汗出烦悗。呕多沃沫，气下泄，不治。

In the depressive psychosis involving the bone, the patient will have the feeling of distention in the cheeks, teeth and the muscles between the shu-points, he will also have stiffness of the bones, perspiration and the feeling of oppression of the chest. If the patient vomits with plenty of saliva, it shows the kidney energy is purging, the disease can by no means to be cured.

筋癫疾者，身倦〔倦：《太素》卷十三《癫疾》作“卷”〕挛急大，刺项大经之大杼脉。呕多沃沫，气下泄，不治。

In the dian disease involving the tendon, the patient is tired with muscular stiffness and he has a gigantic pulse, The disease can be treated by pricking the Dazhu point behind the neck. If the patient vomits with plenty of saliva which shows the kidney energy is excreting, the disease can by no means to be cured.

脉癫疾者，暴仆，四肢之脉皆胀而纵。脉满，尽刺之出血；不满，灸之挟项太阳，灸带脉于腰相去三寸，诸分肉本输。呕多沃沫，气下泄，不治。

In the dian disease involving the channel, the patient may suddenly fall down during the onset of the disease; the vessels in the four extremities are swelling and loose; if the vessels are swelling and full, it should be pricked to let out the blood; if the vessels are not swelling and full, it can be treated by applying moxibustion to the Foot Taiyang Channel clipping the neck, and apply moxibustion to the acupoints three inches from the Belt Channel on the waist and the shu-points of the four extremities and between the muscles. If the patient vomits with plenty of white foams which shows the excreting of the energy, the disease can by no means to be cured.

癫疾者，疾发如狂者，死不治。

When one contracts the dian disease, if the onset of the disease is like mania, it can by no means to be cured.

狂始生，先自悲也，喜忘、苦〔苦：《太素》卷三十《惊狂》作“喜”〕怒、善恐者，得之忧饥，治之取〔取：《甲乙》卷十一第二“取”上有“先”字〕手太阴〔太阴：统本、金陵本“太阴并作“太阳”〕、阳明，血变而止，及取足太阴、阳明。狂始发，少卧不饥，自高贤也，自辩智也，自尊贵也，善骂詈，日夜不休，治之取手阳明、太阳、太阴、舌下少阴，视之盛者，皆取之，不盛，释之也。

In the initiation of mania, the patient has the mood of sadness first, he is prone to forget, easy to get angry, apt to be frightened, and the disease is caused by melancholy and hunger. When treating, prick the acupoints of the Hand Taiyang Channel and that of the Hand Yangming Channel first and cease the pricking when the colour of the patient's complexion has turned into normal, then prick the acupoints on the Foot Taiyin Channel and that on the Foot Yangming Channel. In the beginnig of mania, the patient can hardly sleep, and he is not hungry, he considers himself as a brilliant and wise person, a smart talker, a talented and noble man, and he is fond of scolding others regardless day or night. When treating, prick the acupoints on the Hand Yangming, Taiyang and Taiyin channels and the acupoints on the Shaoyin Channel under the tongue. To the channels that are overabundant, they can all be pricked, to those which are not overabundant, they can be left alone.

狂言〔言:《太素》卷三十《惊狂》作“喜”〕、惊、善〔善:《太平御览》卷七百三十九引作“妄”〕笑、好歌乐〔好歌乐:《太平御览》卷七百三十九“好”下无“歌”字〕、妄行不休者,得之大恐,治之取手阳明、太阳、太阴。狂,目妄见、耳妄闻、善呼者,少气之所生也,治之取手太阳,太阴、阳明、足太阴、头两顑。狂者多食,善见鬼神,善笑而不发于外者,得之有所大喜治之取足太阴、太阳、阳明,后取手太阴、太阳、阳明。狂而新发,未应如此者,先取曲泉左右动脉,及盛者见血,有顷已,不已,以法取之,灸骨骶二十壮。

When the patient is wild with joy, frightened, often laughs without a reason, apt to be joyous and acts rashly and unceasingly day and night, the syndromes are caused by being frightened greatly. When treating, prick the acupoints on the Hand Yangming, Taiyang and Taiyin channels. The patient with mania can often see things which can be rarely seen, hear sounds which can be rarely heard and he often scream with fear, they are the symptoms of amentia caused by the debility of the energy and the decline of the spirit. When treating, prick the acupoints on the Hand Taiyang, Taiyin and Yangming channels, acupoints on Foot Taiyang Channel and that on the two cheeks of the head. The patient with mania eats a lot, likely to have seen the gods and the ghosts, he often laughs but not in the presence of men and these phenomina are due to the injury of the spirit caused by overjoy. When treating, prick the acupoints on the Foot Taiyin, Taiyang and Yangming channels first, then, prick the acupoints on the Hand Taiyin, Taiyang and Yangming channels. When mania is in its initial stage, from which the symptoms stated above have not yet appeared, prick the arteries on the left and right sides of the Ququan point. If the channel is filled and full, the disease can be cured after the blood being let out; if the disease is not cured, apply the method of treating the dian disease psychosis above and treat with twenty moxa-cones on the sacrum bone.

风逆暴四肢肿〔肿:《甲乙》卷十第二下作“痛”〕,身漯漯,唏然时寒,饥则烦,饱则善变,取手太阴表里,足少阴、阳明之经,肉清取荥,骨清取井、经也〔取井、经也:《太素》卷三十《风逆》“井”下无“经”字,应据《太素》删〕。

When the wind-evil invades from outside of the body and the chaotic energy reverses inside, the four extremities of the patient will be painful all of a sudden, he has sweating of the body, and sometimes, the breath which comes out from the nose makes sound caused by cold. The patient feels irritative when he is hungry and becomes active and restless when he eats his fill. In treating, prick the superficies and interior of Hand Taiyin Channel of Lung and the Hang Yangming Channel of Large Intestine, besides, prick the Foot Shaoyin Channel of Kidney and the Foot Yangming Channel of Stomach. When the patient feels cold in the muscle, prick the Xing points on the four channels stated above; when the patient feels cold in the bone, prick the Jing point (well point) on the four channels stated above.

厥逆为病也，足暴清，胸若将裂，肠若将以刀切之，烦而不能食，脉大小皆涩，暖取足少阴，清取足阳明，清则补之，温则泻之。厥逆腹胀满，肠鸣，胸满不得息，取之下胸二胁咳而动手者，与背腧以手按之立快者是也。

In the Jueni disease, the patient's feet become cool all of a sudden, his chest seems to be split, his intestine seems to be scraped by a knife, the patient can hardly take food due to the distention and fullness of the abdomen, and the coming of both the large and small pulse conditions are appeared to be choppy. If the patient is warm in the body, prick the acupoints on the Foot Shaoyin Channel, if the patient is cool in the body, prick the acupoints of the Foot Yangming Channel of Stomach; to the patient with cool body, apply invigorating therapy, to the patient with warm body, apply purge therapy. To the patient with Jueni disease who has abdominal distention and fullness, borborygmus, fullness of the chest and expiratory dyspnea, prick the acupoints on the hypochondria under the chest, the acupoint for treating is on the responding location which can be felt by hand when the patient coughs. Besides, prick the back-shu point, of which the point is on the location of having a comfortable sensation when being pressed by the fingers.

内闭不得溲，刺足少阴、太阳与骶上以长针，气逆则取其太阴、阳明、厥阴〔厥阴：《甲乙》卷九第十并无“阴”字，“厥”字连下“甚”字断句〕，甚取少阴、阳明动者之经也。

When one has dysuria, prick the acupoints on the Foot Shaoyin Channel, the Foot Taiyang Channel and the Changqiang point on the sacrum bone with the long needle. When the patient has adverseness of vital energy, prick the acupoints of the Foot Taiyin Channel and that of the Foot Yangming Channel. When the onset of Jueni disease is severe, prick the acupoints of arteries of the Foot Shaoyin Channel and that of the Foot Yangming Channel.

少气，身漯漯也，音吸吸也，骨竣体重，懈惰不能动，补足少阴。短气，息短不属，动作气索，补足少阴，去血络也。

To the patient who is deficient in energy, sweating in the body, discontinuous in talking, sore in the bone joints, feeling heavy of the body and reluctant to move about, prick the acupoints of the Foot Shaoyin Channel of Kidney and apply invigorating therapy. To the patient who is short of breath with rapid, short and discontinuous respiration, and his breath seems to become exhausting even when he acts slightly, prick the acupoints of Foot Shaoyin Channel of Kidney, apply the invigorating therapy and let out the blood in the superficial venules.

热病第二十三

Chapter 23
Re Bing
(Febrile Disease)

偏枯，身偏不用而痛，言不变，志不乱，病在分腠之间，巨针刺之，益其不足，损其有余，乃可复也。痱为病也，身无痛者，四肢不收，智乱不甚，其言微知，可治；甚则不能言，不可治也。病先起于阳，后入于阴者，先取其阳，后取其阴，浮而取之。

In hemiplegia, when the patient is painful in the body but can talk as usual, and his consciousness is normal, the disease is caused by the evil which is on the site where the skin and the muscle joined. When treating, prick with the large needle. If the disease belongs to the deficient kind, apply the invigorating therapy, if the disease is of having a surplus, apply the the purging therapy, and the disease can be recovered. In paralysis, when the patient is not very painful but his extremities are loose and fail to withdraw, his consciousness is disorderly but the case is not severe, he talks in a low voice but his words can be understood by others, the disease has the possibility of being cured; when the case is severe and the patient can not talk, the disease can hardly be cured. When the disease initiates from Yang and then penetrates into Yin, the Yang channel (superficies) should be pricked first, and then, prick the Yin channel. The shallow needling should be applied.

热病三日，而气口静、人迎躁者，取之诸阳，五十九刺，以泻其热而出其汗，实其阴以补其不足者。身热甚，阴阳皆静者，勿刺也；其可刺者，急取之，不汗出则泄。所谓勿刺者，有死征也。

When the febrile disease has lasted for three days and the Cunkou pulse is calm but the Renying pulse is irritable, select and prick the acupoints from the fifty nine points for treating the febrile disease of the various Yang channels to purge the heat-evil of the superficies and induce the sweat, besides, the pricking for enriching the Yin channel to invigorate the deficiency of the three Yin channels should be applied. To the patient whose body is very hot, but on the contrary, the Yin and the Yang pulses are calm, the pricking must not be applied; when the disease can still be treated by pricking, it should prick immediately, through the pricking, even if the evil is not let out through sweating it can be purged by diarrhea. As to the diseases which can not be treated by pricking, they are the fatal diseases.

热病七日八日，脉口动喘而短〔短：日刻本作“眩”〕者，急刺之，汗且自出，浅刺手大〔手大：《太素》卷二十五《热病说》“手”下无“大”字〕指间。

When the febrile disease has lasted for seven or eight days, the patient's Cunkou pulse is stirring and he has rapid respiration and dizziness, it should prick immediately to cause spontaneous perspiration, prick mainly the acupoints between the fingers with shallow needling.

热病七日八日，脉微小，病者溲血，口中干，一日半而死，脉代者，一日死。热病已得汗出，而脉尚躁，喘且复热，勿刺肤〔勿刺肤：《甲乙》卷七第一中作“勿庸刺”〕，喘甚者死。

When the febrile disease has lasted for seven or eight days, if the pulse condition is tiny, the patient has hematuria and dryness in the mouth, he will die after one and half days; when the intermittent pulse condition occurs, the patient will die after one day. In febrile disease, when the sweat is induced but the pulse condition is still overabundant and the patient has dyspnea and fever, it must not be pricked. when the rapid respiration is severe, the patient will die.

热病七八日，脉不躁，躁不散数〔躁不散数：《脉经》卷七第二十“不”下无“散”字〕，后三日中有汗；三日不汗，四日死。未曾汗者，勿腠〔腠：《太素》卷二十五《热病说》《病沅》第九并作“庸”〕刺之。

When the febrile disease has lasted for seven or eight days, but the pulse condition is not irritable, or the pulse condition is irritable but not rapid, if the sweat is seen within three days the disease can be recovered; if there is no sweat within three days, the patient will die in the fourth day. To the patient with no sweat, pricking is no more necessary.

热病先肤痛，窒鼻充面，取之皮，以第一针，五十九，苛珍鼻，索皮于肺，不得索之火，火者心也。

In febrile disease, when the patient feels painful in the skin, the nostrils are obstructed like being stuffed by something, it should prick the skin by shallow needling with the sharp-tip needle, select and prick the acupoints among the fifty nine points for treating the febrile disease, if the nose of the patient is swelling, prick the Feishu (Lung-shu) point with shallow needling. The Xinshu (Heart-shu) point must not be pricked as the heart belongs to the fire and fire subjugates metal.

热病先身涩，倚而热，烦悗，干唇口嗌，取之皮，以第一针，五十九〔五十九：《甲乙》卷七第一中“九”下有“刺”字〕，肤胀口干，寒汗出，索脉于心，不得索之水，水者肾也。热病嗌干多饮，善惊，卧不能起，取之肤肉，以第六针，五十九，目眦青〔目眦青：《脉经》卷七第十三“青”作“赤”〕，索肉于脾，不得索之木，木者肝也。

When at the beginning of the febrile disease, the skin appears to be coarse and choppy, the patient has dysphoria and restlessness, has fullness and oppressinon in the chest, dryness in the lips and the throat, it should treat the channel by pricking the acupoints of the related channels among the fifty nine points for treating the febrile disease with the sharp-tip needle. In some of the febrile disease, the skin of the patient has the sensation of distention, the mouth is dry and the body has clammy sweat; in some of the febrile diseases, the throat of the patient is dry, he drinks plenty, apt to be frightened and reluctant to get up when lying; when treating, it should mainly prick the muscle by selecting the acupoints from the fifty nine points for treating the febrile disease with the horse -tail-shaped needle. When the canthus is red, prick the muscle in the Pishu (Spleen-shu) point. The Ganshu (Liver-shu) point must not be pricked as the liver belongs to wood and wood subjugates earth.

热病面青脑痛〔热病面赤脑痛:《素问·刺热篇》新校正引《灵枢》作"热病而胸胁痛"〕,手足躁,取之筋间,以第四针,于四逆,筋躄目浸,索筋于肝,不得索之金,金者肺也。

In febrile disease when the patient is not painful in the hypochondria and the limbs are stirring, it should prick the tendon with the three-edged needle; if the patient has constriction in the tendon and has nebula in the eye, it should also treat the tendon by pricking the Ganshu (Liver-shu) point. The Feishu (Lung-shu) must not be pricked as the lung belongs to the metal and metal subjugates wood.

热病数惊,瘛疭而狂,取之脉,以第四针,急泻有余者,癫疾毛发去,索血于心,不得索之水,水者肾也。

In febrile disease, when the patient has convulsion, spasm of the muscle and dysphoria, purge the overabundant heat-evil with the three-edged needle hastily, the disease of Dian disease and baldness can be cured also. As it is treating the disease of heart, the Xinshu (Heart-shu) point should be pricked. The Shenshu (Kidney-shu) point must not be pricked as kidney belongs to water and water subjugates fire.

热病身重骨痛,耳聋而好瞑,取之骨,以第四针,五十九刺,骨病不食,啮齿耳青,索骨于肾,不得索之土,土者脾也。

In febrile disease, when the patient is heavy in the body and painful in the bone, deaf in the ears and fond of sleep, the bone should be treated, select and prick the acupoints from the fifty nine points for treating the febrile disease with the three-edged needle. In the bone disease, the patient is reluctant to eat, grinding his teeth and feeling cool in the two ears, the bone should also be treated by pricking the Shenshu (Kidney-shu) point. The Pishu (Spleen-shu) point must not be pricked as the spleen belongs to earth and earth subjugates water.

热病不知所痛,耳聋不能自收,口干,阳热甚,阴颇有寒者,热在髓,死不可治。

In febrile disease, when the patient is not very painful but he is deaf, flaccid extrimities and thirsty, his external heat is extreme and his internal heat is also overabundant, since the heat is both inside and outside, it shows the heat has penetrated into the bone marrow and the patient can by no means to be cured.

热病头痛颞颥,目瘈脉痛,善衄,厥热病也,取之以第三针,视有余不足,寒热痔〔丹波元简曰:"寒热痔"三字,上下文不相续,似为衍文〕。

In febrile disease, when the patient has severe headache, the vessels in the eye-area are beating and he has epistaxis often, it is the Jueni syndrome of heat-evil which should be treated by pricking with the blunt-tip needle. Examine whether the disease is having a surplus or being deficient and treat accordingly.

热病体重,肠中热,取之以第四针,于其腧及下诸指间,索气于胃胳得气也。

In febrile disease, when the patient feels heavy in the body and hot in the intestine, it should be treated by pricking the Weishu (Stomach-shu) point and the acupoints between the fingers and the toes with the three-edged needle, it can also prick the collateral points of the

Stomach Channel until the needling sensation is felt.

热病、挟脐急痛，胸胁满，取之涌泉与阴陵泉，取以第四针，针嗌里。

In febrile disease, when the patient has sudden pain over the navel and has the propping fullness in the hypochondria, it should prick the Yongquan point and the Yinlingquan point, and also prick the Lianquan point with the three-edged needle.

热病而汗且出，及脉顺可汗者，取之鱼际、太渊、大都、太白、泻之则热去，补之则汗出，汗出太甚，取内踝上横脉以止之。

In febrile disease, when the patient is about to perspire, the Yin or Yang pulse agrees with the Yin or Yang of the syndrome, and the heat can be dispelled by sweating, prick the Yuji point and Taiyuan point of Taiyin Channel and the Dadu point and the Taibai point of the Foot Taiyin Channel. The heat can be dispelled when applying the invigoratig therapy, and the sweat can be induced when applying the purging therapy. If the sweat induced is too much, it can be stopped by pricking the Sanyinjiao point on the horizontal line of the ankle.

热病已得汗而脉尚躁盛，此阴脉之极也，死；其得汗而脉静者，生。热病者，脉尚盛躁而不得汗者，此阳脉之极也，死；脉盛躁得汗静者，生。

In febrile disease, if the patient has had perspiration and his pulse is still stirring and overabundant, it shows the Yin channel is extremely debilitating and the patient will die; if the patient has perspiration and the pulse condition is calm, the patient will survive. In febrile disease, when the pulse is irritating and the patient has no sweat, it shows his Yang channel is extremely debilitating and the patient will die; when the pulse is stirring and abundant but the Ying and Yang channel are calm after perspiration, he will survive.

热病不可刺者有九：一曰，汗不出，大颧发赤哕者死；二曰，泄而腹满甚者死；三曰，目不明，热不已者死；四曰，老人婴儿，热而腹满者死；五曰，汗不出，呕下血者死；六曰，舌本烂，热不已者死；七曰，咳而衄，汗不出，出不至足者死；八曰，髓热者死；九曰，热而痉〔痉：《太素》卷二十五《热病说》作“痓”。〕者死。腰折，瘛疭，齿噤齘也。凡此九者，不可刺也。

In febrile disease, there are nine kinds of fatal syndromes which must not be pricked. First: the patient has no sweat, red in the cheekbone and has hiccup, it is a fatal syndrome; second: the patient has diarrhea with severe abdominal distention and fullness, it is a fatal syndrome; third: the patient's eyes can not see things clearly and the fever does not coming down, it is a fatal syndrome; fourth: when an old man or a child has fever and abdominal distention, it is a fatal syndrome; fifth: the patient does not perspire but vomits and has bloody stool, it is a fatal syndrome; sixth: the root of the tongue festers and the fever does not come down, it is a fatal syndrome; seventh: the patient has cough, epistaxis without perspiration, or the perspiration can hardly reach the feet, it is a fatal syndrome; eighth: when the heat-evil penetrates into the bone marrow, it is a fatal syndrome; ninth: the patient has fever with zhi syndrome, it is a fatal syndrome, The so called fever with zhi syndrome is the syndrome of stiffness of the spine and back like a bow bending in the adverse direction, the patient has convulsion, trismus and gnashing of teeth. All the fatal syndromes stated above must not be treated by pricking.

所谓五十九刺者，两手外内侧各三，凡十二痏；五指间各一，凡八痏，足亦如是；头入髮一寸傍三分各三，凡六痏；更入髮三寸边五，凡十痏；耳前后口下者各一，项中一，凡六痏；巅上一，囟会一，髮际一，廉泉一，风池二，天柱二。

The so called fifty nine points for treating the febrile disease are: on the outer flanks of both hands are three points each, and on the inner flanks of both hands are three points each, they are altogether twelve points. In between the five fingers, there is one point each and they are altogether eight points. In between the five toes, there is one point each and they are altogether eight points. One inch inside of the hairline on the head, there are three locations on each lateral side, and each location has a point, so, in each lateral side, there are three points, and on both lateral sides, they are altogether six points. Three inches inside of the hairline, there are five points on each lateral side, and they are altogether ten points. In the front and rear of the ear, there is one point each, under the mouth, there is one point, in the middle of the neck, there is one point, they are altogether six points. On the top of head there is one point, the Xinhui is one point, inside of the front hairline there is one point, inside of the rear hairline there is one point, the Lianquan is one point, the Fengchi are two points and the Tianzhu are two points, they are altogether nine points.

气满胸中喘息，取足太阴大指之端，去爪甲如薤叶，寒则留之，热则疾之，气下乃止。

When one has adverseness of vital energy, stuffy in the chest and perspires rapidly, prick the tip of the toe one Chinese chives width from the nail. If it is a cold syndrome , retain the needle longer; if it is a heat syndrome, pull out the needle instantly after pricking; cease the pricking when the adverse energy has descended and the rapid respiration has relieved.

心疝暴痛，取足太阴、厥阴、尽刺去其血络。

In heart-channel colic with sudden onset of pain, prick the Foot Taiyin and the Jueyin Channels and let out the blood from the superficial venules.

喉痹舌卷，口中干，烦心心痛，臂内廉痛，不可及头，取〔取：《甲乙》卷九第二“取”下有“关冲在”三字〕手小指次指爪甲下，去端如韭叶。

In sorethroat when the patient curls his tongue and fails to stretch, has dryness in the mouth, oppressive feeling in the chest, heartache, pain in the inner flank of the arm and fails to raise his arm to the level of the head, prick the Guanchong point. The Guanchong point is in the outer flank of the ring finger (nearing the small finger) one fen (the width of Chinese chives) from the nail.

目中赤痛，从内眦始，取之阴跻。风痉身反折，先取足太阳及腘中及血络出血；中有寒，取三里。

When the patient's eyes are red and painful and the disease initiates from the inner canthus, prick the Zhaohai point of the Yinqiao Channel. In wind-type convulsive disease when the spine is stiff, bending like a bow in an adverse direction, prick the Weizhong point of Foot Taiyang Channel first, and then, prick the superficial venules until bleeding. If the patient has cold in the abdomen, prick the Sanli point in addition.

癃，取之阴跃及三毛上及血络出血。

When treating dysuria, prick the Yinjiao Channel and the acupoint on the clump hair of the outer flank of the toe, it should also prick the superficial venules on the liver and kidney channels until bleeding.

男子如蛊，女子如怚，身体腰脊如解，不欲饮食，先取涌泉见血，视跗上盛者，尽见血也。

When a man has contracted Shan Jia disease (abdominal pain due to stagnation of energy) or a woman has contracted morning sickness (nausea or vomiting during early pregnancy), the body and the spine are like being split and the patient is reluctant to eat, prick the Yongquan point until bleeding first, then, examine the dorsum of the foot and prick the superficial venules which are overabundant to let out the blood slightly.

厥病第二十四

Chapter 24
Jue Bing
(Jue-Syndrome)

厥头痛，而若肿起而烦心，取之足阳明、太阴。

In headache due to jue-syndrome, when the patient's head and face are like swelling and has oppressive feeling in the chest, prick the Foot Yangming Channel of Stomach and Foot Taiyin Channel of Spleen.

厥头痛，头脉痛，心悲善泣，视头动脉反盛者，刺尽去血，后调足厥阴。

In headache due to jue-syndrome, when the channels in the patient's head are painful, he feels sad, apt to cry, his head is trembling and the collaterals are overabundant, prick the collaterals and let out the blood, then, prick the Foot Jueyin Channel of Liver for adjusting.

厥头痛，贞贞头重而痛，泻头上五行，行五，先取手少阴，后取足少阴。

In headache due to jue-syndrome, when the patient's head is heavy and has acute pain, select and prick the acupoints on the five channels on the top of head (the Du Channel is in the middle, on the lateral sides are the two Foot Taiyang Channel of Bladder and on the further lateral sides are the two Foot Shaoyang Channel of Gallbladder) to purge the heat of the various Yang channels, but the acupoints of the Hand Shaoyin Channel of Heart should be pricked first, and then, prick the Foot Shaoyin Channel of Kidney.

厥头痛，意善忘，按之不得，取头面左右动脉，后取足太阴。

In headache due to jue-syndrome, when the patient often sighs and is forgetful, and the site of pain can hardly be traced by the pressing of hand, prick the left and right arteries on the head and face first, and then, prick the Foot Taiyin Channel of Spleen for adjusting.

厥头痛，项先痛，腰脊为应，先取天柱，后取足太阳〔足太阳：《甲乙》卷九第一作“足太阳少阴”〕。

In headache due to jue-syndrome, when the neck is painful first, then the waist and spine are painful accordingly, prick the Tianzhu point first, then, prick the acupoints of the Foot Taiyang Channel of Bladder.

厥头痛，头痛甚，耳前后脉涌有热（一本云有动脉），泻出其血，后取足少阳。

In headache due to jue-sydrome, when the patient has acute pain in the head, and the collaterals in the front and rear of the ear are hot, they should be pricked and let out the blood first, then, prick the acupoints of the Foot Taiyang Channel of Small Intestine and the Foot Shaoyan Channel of Kidney.

真头痛，头痛甚，脑尽痛，手足寒至节，死不治。

In headache which connecting the brain inside due to jue-syndrome, when the patient is painful all over the body, his limbs are cold and the cold reaches the elbows and knees, the patient can by no means to be cured and dies.

头痛不可取于腧者，有所击堕，恶血在于内，若肉伤，痛未已，可则刺，不可远取也。

In some of the cases of headache, it must not be treated by pricking the acupoints, such as wound by strikes or tumble with stagnated blood inside, if the patient has internal injury, and the pain has not yet eliminated, it can only prick the site of pain on the head by oblique insertion. The pricking of the remote acupoint is forbidden.

头痛不可刺者，大痹为恶，日〔日:《甲乙》卷九第一“日”上有“风”字〕作者，可令少愈，不可已。

When treating headache, it must not depend on the pricking only. Due to the mischief of the severe bi-syndrome, the patient will have headache in the windy days, the pricking can ameliorate the disease, but it can not be eliminated.

头半寒痛，先取手少阳、阳明，后取足少阳、阳明。

In headache, when the patient feels cold on one side, it can be treated by pricking the acupoints on the Hand Shaoyan Channel of Triple warmer and the Hand Yangming Channel of Large Intestine first, then, prick the acupoints on the Foot Shaoyang Channel of Gallbladder and the Foot Yangming Channel of Stomach.

厥心痛，与背相控，善瘛，如从后触其心，伛偻者，肾心痛也，先取京骨、昆仑，发狂不已，取然谷。

In precordial pain of yin-cold type with drawing pain on the back, the patient apts to be frightened like something is propping his heart from behind, and he dares not to extend his waist straightly to become somewhat hunchbacked, it is the disease of the pain in the heart and the kidney. When treating, prick the Jinggu point and the Kunlun point first, if the pain is still not relieved, prick the Rangu point.

厥心痛，腹胀胸满，心尤痛甚，胃心痛也，取之大都、太白。

In precordial pain of yin-type with abdominal distention and fullness of the chest, when the heart is painful particularly, it is the disease of pain in the stomach and the heart. When treating, prick the Dadu point and the Taibai point.

厥心痛，痛如以锥针刺其心，心痛甚者，脾心痛也，取之然谷、太溪。

In precordial pain of yin-type with acute pain in the heart like being pricked by a drill, it is the disease of pain in the spleen and the heart. When treating, prick the Rangu point and the Taixi point.

厥心痛，色苍苍如死状，终日不得太息，肝心痛也，取之行间、太冲。

In precordial pain of yin-type with green complexion like the dead ember and the patient has pain in the body all day long, it is the disease of pain in the liver and the heart. When treating, prick the Xingjian point and the Taichong point.

厥心痛，卧若徒居，心痛间，动作痛益甚，色不变，肺心痛也，取之鱼际、太渊。

In precordial pain of yin-type, when the patient's heartache is somewhat relieved when lying or staying leisurely, and the pain becomes acute when he moves about, and his complexion remains unchanged, it is the disease of pain in the lung and the heart. When treating, prick the Yuji point and the Taiyuan point.

真心痛，手足清至节，心痛甚，旦发夕死，夕发旦死。

In myocardial infarction, when the cold of the limbs reaches the joints and the heart has acute pain, the patient will die in the evening when the disease attacks in the morning, and will die in the next morning when the disease attacks in the evening.

心痛不可刺者，中有盛聚，不可取于腧。肠中有虫瘕及蛟蛕，皆不可取以小针。

In some of the heartaches which are caused by the abdominal mass inside, they must not be treated by needling. If there is parasite or roundworm inside, it must not be treated by pricking with the small needle.

心肠〔心肠：《病沅》卷十八《蚘虫候》作"腹中"〕痛，侬作痛，肿聚，往来上下行，痛有休止〔痛有休止：《中脏经》卷上第二十四"有"下有"时"字〕，腹热，喜渴涎出者，是蛟蛕也，以手聚按而坚持之，无令得移，以大针刺之，久持之，虫不动，乃出针也。恙腹侬痛，形中上者〔恙腹侬痛，形中上者：《甲乙》卷九第二无"恙腹"以下八字〕。

In abdominal pain, when the patient makes sound during the disease attacks, his abdomen is swelling with mass inside, the onset of the disease comes and goes upwards and downwards, sometimes the pain appears and sometimes it disappears in paroxysm, the patient has heat in the abdomen and slobbers, it shows there is roundworm inside. When treating, draw the fingers close together and press firmly the site of the worm which is painful to cause the worm remains unmoved and prick with the large needle. Keep the pressing for a longer time and be sure the worm is not moving, then draw the needle.

耳聋无闻，取耳中。

When the patient is deaf and can hear nothing, prick the acupoint in the ear (Tinggong and Jiaosun points).

耳鸣，取耳前动脉。

When the patient has tinnitus, prick the artery in front of the ear.

耳痛不可刺者，耳中有脓，若有干耵聍，耳无闻也。

Where there is pain in the ear with the pus-sore or the dry ear wax in the ear causing the patient to lose his sense of hearing, it must not be pricked.

耳聋，取手小指次指爪甲上与肉交者，先取手，后取足。

To deafness, prick the location where the nail and the flesh meet on the outer flank of the ring finger's tip. Prick the Guanchong point on hand first, then, prick the Qiaoyin point on foot.

耳鸣，取手中指爪甲上，左取右，右取左，先取手，后取足。

To tinnitus, prick the tips of the middle finger and the middle toe of hand and foot, when the tinitus is in the left ear, prick the acupoints on the right side; when the tinnitus is in the right ear, prick the acupoints on the left side. Prick the acupoints on the hand first, and then, prick the acupoint on the foot.

足髀〔足髀：《太素》卷三十《髀疾》"髀"上无"足"字〕不可举，侧而取之，在枢合中以员利针，大针不可刺。

When the thigh fails to lift, prick the Huantiao point on the greater trochanter when the patient is lying sideways with the horse-tail shaped needle, the large needle must not be used.

病注下血，取曲泉。

When the patient has bloody stool, prick the Ququan point.

风痹淫泺，病不可已者，足如履冰，时如入汤中，股胫淫泺，烦心头痛，时呕时悗，眩已汗出，久则目眩，悲以喜恐，短气不乐，不出三年死也。

In arthralgia due to wind-evil which fails to recover in a long time, sometimes, the patient's feet is cold like stepping on the ice, sometimes, the patient is hot in the abdomen like filling with hot soup, his thighs and legs are sore and weak, has the feeling of oppression in the chest and has headache, he vomits often, has perspiration after dizziness and his eyes become dazzled when the perspiration lasts long, he feels sad about the past and being frightened often and he is short of breath and dispirited. The patient with the appearances stated above will die within three years.

病本第二十五

Chapter 25
Bing Ben
(In Treating the Root and Branch of the Disease)

先病而后逆者，治其本。先逆而后病者，治其本。先寒而后生病者，治其本。先病而后生寒者，治其本。先热而后生病者，治其本。先泄而后生他病者，治其本，必且调之，乃治其他病。先病而后中满者，治其标。先病后泄者，治其本。先中满而后烦心者，治其本。有客气，有同气。大小便不利，治其标；大小便利，治其本。

When one contracts a disease first, then the syndrome of adverseness of the energy and blood occurs, it should mainly treat the root which is the disease itself; when one contracts the syndrome of adverseness of the energy and blood first, then, a certain disease occurs, it should mainly treat the root to adjust the energy and blood; when one contracts the syndrome of cold property first, and then, the other disease occurs, it should mainly treat the root which is the syndrome of cold property; when one contracts a disease first, and then, the syndrome of cold property occurs, it should mainly treat the root which is the disease; when one contracts the syndrome of hot property first, then another disease occurs, it should mainly treat the root which is the syndrome of hot property; when one contracts diarrhea first, and then, the other disease occurs, it should mainly treat the root which is diarrhea, and treat the other disease after the diarrhea has been cured; when one contracts other disease first, then, the abdominal flatulence occurs, it should adjust the abdominal flatulence which is the branch first; when one contracts other disease first, and then the diarrhea occurs, it should mainly treat the the root which is the disease; when one contracts abdominal flatulence first and then the feeling of oppression of the chest occurs, it should mainly treat the root which is the abdominal flatulence. In the diseases of man, some are caused by the guest energy which is the transmission of evil energies of different roots, and some are caused by the identical energy which is the transmission of evil energies of the same root. When the patient contracts a disease, if there is retention of feces and urine and the case is urgent, it should treat the branch which is the retention of feces and urine first; if there is no retention of feces and urine, it should treat the disease.

病发而有余，本而标之，先治其本，后治其标；病发而不足，标而本之，先治其标，后治其本。谨详察间甚，以意调之，间者并行，甚为〔为：《素问·标本病传论》《甲乙》卷六第二并作“者”〕独行。先小大便不利而后生他病者，治其本也。

When the disease is sthenic which is having a surplus during its attack, then, the surplus evil is the root and the syndrome is the branch, it should treat the evil energy first, then, treat the disease; when the disease is asthenic and the healthy energy appears to be deficient, then, the deficient energy is the branch and the syndrome is the root, it should support the healthy energy first and then treat the disease. Thus, when treating, one must examine carefully the severe and slight extent of the syndrome and adjust accordingly. To the slight disease, the root and branch can be treated simultaneously; to the severe disease, it should treat the root or the branch first merely.

杂病第二十六

Chapter 26
Za Bing
(Miscellaneous Diseases)

厥，挟脊而痛者，至顶，头沉沉然，目𥉂𥉂然，腰脊强，取足太阳腘中血络。

In the Jueni of channel, there are pains clipping along the two sides of the spine, the patient's head and neck are tightened with uncomfortable feeling, his eyes can hardly see things clearly, his waist and spine are stiff and he can not face up and down. When treating, prick the Weizhong point of the Foot Taiyang Channel and prick the superficial venules until bleeding.

厥，胸满面肿，唇漯漯然，暴言难，甚则不能言，取足阳明。

In the Jueni of channel, the patient has fullness in the chest and his face and lips are swelling, he finds difficulty in speaking suddenly or even unable to speak. When treating, prick the acupoints of the Foot Yangming Channel.

厥气走喉而不能言，手足清，大便不利，取足少阴。

In the Jueni of channel, when the chaotic energy reaches up to the throat, the patient will not be able to speak, his limbs will be cold and will have retention of feces. When treating, prick the acupoints of the Foot Shaoyin Channel.

厥而腹向向然，多寒气，腹中瞉瞉，便溲难，取足太阴。

In the Jueni of channel, when the patient's abdomen is expanding, the cold energy is overabundant with sound like that of the water in the abdomen, and he also has constipation and dysuria, prick the acupoints of the Foot Taiyin Channel.

嗌干，口中热如胶，取足少阴〔阴：《甲乙》卷七第一中作“阳”〕。

When one has dry throat, his mouth is hot and sticky like the glue, prick the acupoints of the Foot Shaoyang Channel.

膝中痛，取犊鼻，以员利针，发〔发：《太素》卷三十《膝痛》，《甲乙》卷十第一下“发”上并有“针”字〕而间之。针大如氂，刺膝无疑。

When one's knee-joint is painful, prick the Dubi point with the horsetail-shaped needle. It should wait for a little while before pricking again. As the body of the horsetail-shaped needle is large as a yak's tail, the application for treating the joint disease must not be hesitant.

喉痹不能言，取足阳明；能言，取手阳明。

When one has sorethroat, if he can not speak, it should be treated by pricking the acupoints of the Foot Yangming Channel; if he can speak, prick the acupoints of the Hand

Yangming Channel.

疟不渴，间日而作，取足阳明〔取足阳明：《素问・刺疟篇》并作"刺足太阳"〕；渴而日作，取手阳明。

When one contracts malaria, if he is not thirsty, and the disease attacks every other day, prick the acupoints of the Foot Taiyang Channel; if he is thirsty, and the disease attacks every other day, prick the acupoints of the Hand Shaoyang Channel.

齿痛，不恶清饮，取足阳明；恶清饮，取手阳明。

In toothache, if the patient has no aversion to the cold drink, it can be treated by pricking the acupoints of the Foot Yangming Channel; if he has aversion to the cold drink, prick the acupoints of the Hand Yangming Channel.

聋而不痛者，取足少阳；聋而痛者，取手阳明。

If one is deaf without pain, it can be treated by pricking the acupoints of the Foot Shaoyang Channel; if he is deaf with pain, it should be treated by pricking the acupoints of the Hand Yangming Channel.

衄而不止，衃血流，取足太阳，不已，刺宛骨下，不已，刺腘中出血。

In epistaxis, when the bleeding does not coagulate, it should be treated by pricking the acupoints of the Foot Taiyin Channel, if the syndrome is not recovered, prick the Wangu point; if it is not recovered again, prick the Weizhong point on the centre of the horizontal line on the popliteal until bleeding.

腰痛，痛上寒，取足太阳阳明；痛上热，取足厥阴；不可以俯仰，取足少阳；中热而喘，取足少阴，腘中血络。

In lumbago, if the patient's upper part of the body is cold, it should be treated by pricking the acupoints of the Foot Taiyang Channel and the Foot Yangming Channel; if the upper part of the body has fever, prick the acupoints of the Foot Jueyin Channel, when the patient has lumbago and he fails to face up and down, prick the acupoints of the Foot Shaoyang Channel. When one has lumbago with internal fever and his mouth moves like that in rapid respiration, it should be treated by pricking the acupoints of the Foot Shaoyin Channel and prick the superficial venules on the centre of the horizontal line on the popliteal.

喜怒而不欲食，言益小〔言益小：《甲乙》卷九第五"小"并作"少"〕，刺足太阴；怒而多言，刺足少阳〔少阳：《甲乙》卷九第五作"少阴"〕。

When one often gets angry, relucts at eating and rarely speaks, it should be treated by pricking the acupoints of the Foot Taiyin Channel; when one is angry and speaks a lot, it should be treated by pricking the acupoints of the Foot Shaoyin Channel.

颇〔颇：张注本作"颔"〕痛，刺手阳明与颇之盛脉出血。

When one's chin is painful, it should prick the acupoint of the Hand Yangming Channel (Shangyang point) and the channel which is overabundant near the chin (Jiache point) until bleeding.

项痛不可俯仰，刺足太阳；不可以顾，刺手太阳〔手太阳：《甲乙》卷九第一校语云："一云手阳明"〕也。

When one's head and neck are painful and he can not face up and down, prick the acupoints of the Foot Taiyang Channel; if the head and neck fail to turn back, prick the acupoints of the Hand Yangming Channel.

小腹满大，上走胃〔胃：《甲乙》卷九第九作“胸”〕，至心，淅淅身时寒热，小便不利，取足厥阴。

When the patient's lower abdomen is expanding, the energy reaches up to the chest and the position of heart, he will have chilliness, the alternation episodes of chill and fever and has dysuria, prick the acupoints of the Foot Jueyin Channel.

腹满，大便不利，腹大，亦上走胸嗌，喘息喝喝然，取足少阴。

When the patient has abdominal distention, constipation, swelling of the abdomen, adverseness of the vital energy up-reaching to the chest, laryngopharnx, and his breathing is heavy and rapid with sound, prick the acupoints of the Foot Shaoyang Channel.

腹满食不化，腹向向然，不能大便，取足太阴〔太阴：《甲乙》卷九第七作“太阳”〕。

When the patient has abdominal fullness, the food can not be digested, the abdomen has asthenia-type flatulence and the patient can hardly move the bowels, it should be treated by pricking the acupoints of the Foot Taiyang Channel.

心痛引腰脊，欲呕，取足少阴。

When the waist and the spine are drawn by the heartache to become painful and the patient wants to vomit, prick the acupoints of the Foot Shaoyin Channel.

心痛，腹胀。啬啬然，大便不利，取足太阴。

When one has heartache, abdominal distention and dry stool, prick the acupoints of the Foot Taiyin Channel.

心痛引背不得息，刺足少阴；不已，取手少阳〔少阳：《千金》卷十三第六作“少阴”〕。

When the back has unceasing pain drawn by heartache, prick the acoupoints of the Foot Shaoyin Channel, if it is not alleviated, prick the acupoints of the Hand Shaoyin Channel.

心痛引小腹满，上下无常处，便溲难，刺足厥阴。

When one has heartache, abdominal distention, pain in the upper and lower sides without a definite position with constipation and dysuria, prick the acupoints of the Foot Jueyin Channel.

心痛，但短气不足以息，刺手太阴。

When one has heartache, short of breath and dyspnea, prick the acupoints of the Hand Taiyin Channel.

心痛，当九节刺之，按，已〔按已：《太素》卷二十六《厥心痛》作“不已”〕刺按之，立已；不已，上下求之，得之立已。

When treating heartache, it should prick the position under the ninth vertebra (the Jinsuo point of Du Channel), before pricking, press and rub the acupoint, after pricking, press and rub it again, and the pain can be alleviated; if it is not alleviated, seek and prick the acupoint which is related to the disease from the shu-points of the back, when the proper point is pricked, the pain will be alleviated.

颇痛，刺足阳明曲周动脉见血，立已；不已，按人迎于经，立已。

When one's cheek is painful, prick the surrounding artery of the curved jaw which is the Foot Yangming Channel (Jiache point) until bleeding , and the pain will be relieved immediately; if it is not relieved, prick the Renying point and press the related channel, apply shallow puncture and avoid to prick the artery, the pain will be relieved.

气逆上，刺膺中陷者与下胸动脉。

When one has adverseness of vital energy, prick the acupoint in the cave-in which is beside the chest (Wuyi point of Foot Yangming Channel) and the artery under the chest.

腹痛，刺脐左右动脉，已刺按之，立已；不已，刺气街，已刺〔已刺：《甲乙》卷九第七无"已刺"二字〕按之，立已。

When one has abdominal pain, prick the arteries on the left and right sides of the navel and press after pricking, the pain can be relieved immediately; if it is not relieved, prick again the Qichong point and press it, the pain can be ceased.

痿厥为四末束悗，乃疾解之，日二，不仁者十日而知，无休，病已止。

When treating the muscular flaccidity and coldness of the extremities, bind the four extremities of the patient until he is disquieted, then untie him hastily, and it should be done twice a day. If the patient does not feel disquieted, he will feel so after ten days, the treating must not be discontinued before the disease is recovered.

哕，以草刺鼻，嚏，嚏而已；无息，而疾迎引之，立已；大惊之，亦可已。

When one hiccups, prick the nose with a piece of straw to cause him sneeze, and it will be ceased; it can also cause the patient to hold his breath and induce the up-reversing energy to descend rapidly, and the hiccup can be stopped; if the patient can be caused to have fright greatly, the hiccup can also be stopped.

周痹第二十七

Chapter 27
Zhou Bi
(The Bi-Syndrome all over the Body)

黄帝问于岐伯曰：周痹之在身也，上下移徙，随脉其〔随脉其：按："脉其"二字误倒〕上下〔上下：按"上下"二字误衍〕，左右相应，间不容空，愿闻此痛，在血脉之中邪？将在分肉之间乎？何以致是？其痛之移也，间不及下针，其慉痛之时，不及定治，而痛已止矣，何道使然？愿闻其故。岐伯答曰：此众痹也，非周痹也。

Yellow Emperor asked Qibo: "When one has the bi-syndrome all over the body, it runs here and there along the blood circulation on the left and right sides to reach everywhere, diffusing extensively which has almost left no pace for a hole. I hope to know whether the evil of this pain is in the channel or in the muscle and the reason of it. In the interval of the pain's transfering, the time is not enough for the pricking, in the period of the pain taking form, the time is not enough for one to determine the way of treating, and no sooner than the treatment starts, the pain has been ceased, I hope to know the reason about it." Qibo said: "In this case, it is the poly bi-syndrome, and it is not the bi-syndrome all over the body."

黄帝曰：愿闻众痹。岐伯对曰：此〔此：《古今医统》卷十一《痹证门》作"凡众痹"〕各在其处，更发更止，更居更起，以右应左，以左应右，非能周也，更发更休也。黄帝曰：善。刺之奈何？岐伯对曰：刺此者，痛虽已止，必刺其处，勿令复起。

Yellow Emperor said: "I want to know the condition of the poly bi-syndrome." Qibo said: "The poly bi-syndrome scatters on the various parts of the body respectively, it is easy to break out and easy to terminate, easy to become active and easy to become inactive, the disease on the left side can affect the right side and that of the right side can affect the left side, it can spread all over the body, its pain can easily burst out and can cease easily." Yellow Emperor said: "Good, but how to treat the disease by pricking?" Qibo answered: "When pricking the poly bi-syndrome, it should prick the site of the pain repeatedly even if the pain has stopped to avoid the coming back of the pain.

帝曰：善。愿闻周痹何如？岐伯对曰：周痹者，在于血脉之中，随脉以上，随脉以下，不能左右，各当其所。黄帝曰：刺之奈何？岐伯对曰：痛从上下者，先刺其下以过（一作遏下同）之，后刺其上以脱之；痛从下上者，先刺其上以过之，后刺其下以脱之。

Yellow Emperor said: "Good. I hope to hear the condition about the bi-syndrome all over the body." Qibo answered: "In bi-syndrome all over the body, the evil is in the channel, it runs up and down along the channel, unable to run to the left and right and it causes pain on the site where the evil energy locates." Yellow Emperor asked: "How to treat it by pricking?" Qibo answered: "If the pain is from above, prick below to stop the developement of the disease first, then, prick above to eliminate its root; if the pain is from below, prick above to stop the developement of the disease first, then, prick below to eliminate the root of the disease."

黄帝曰：善。此痛安生？何因而有名？岐伯对曰：风寒湿气，客于外分肉之间，迫切而为沫，沫得寒则聚，聚则排分肉而分裂也〔而分裂也：《千金》卷八第一《素问·痹论》王注无"而分裂也"四字〕，分〔分：《千金》卷八第一作"肉"〕裂则痛，痛则神归之，神归之则热，热则痛解，痛解则厥，厥则他痹发，发则如是。

Yellow Emperor said: "Good. How does the pain of the bi-syndrome all over the body come about? Why is it called the bi-syndrome all over the body?" Qibo answered: "When the wind-cold and the warm-pathogen invade the muscle and the skin, it forces the body fluid to become phlegm and saliva which will become condensed and stagnated due to cold, and the stagnated phlegm and saliva will be squeezed and split the muscles to cause pain, when one is painful, his attention will be concentrated on the painful location, the concentration of attention will produce heat which will cause the cold to disperse and the pain to become alleviated; after the alleviation of the pain, the chaotic energy will reverse up to cause pain in other locations where the bi-syndromes resides and forms the bi-syndrome all over the body.

帝曰：善。余已得其意矣〔帝曰善，余已得其意矣：此九字涉下误衍，应删〕。此内不在藏，而外未发于皮，独居分肉之间，真气不能周，故命曰周痹。故刺痹者，必先切循其下之六经，视其虚实，及大络之血结而不通，及虚而脉陷空者而调之，熨而通之，其瘛坚，转引而行之。黄帝曰：善。余已得其意矣。亦得其事也。九者，经巽之理，十二经脉阴阳之病也。

"It is the case when the evil has not yet penetrated into the viscera and it manifests nothing on the skin outside, the evil retains between the muscles can only cause the healthy energy fail to circulate all over the body, and in this way, it produces pain and becomes bi-syndrome. Thus, when treating the bi-syndrome, one must press and follow the allocated locations of the six channels, examine the conditions of sthenia and asthenia and whether there is any stagnation of blood in the large collaterals and any of the condition of the bogging-in of the channel due to asthenia first, then, treat by adjusting, and the topical application of heated drugs can be used to dredge the energy and blood; if there is the condition of muscular contracture, it can also induce the energy to become unimpeded." Yellow Emperor said: "Good. Now I know the condition of the bi-syndrome and the principle of its treating."

口问第二十八

Chapter 28
Kou Wen
(The Treating Therapy from Oral Inquiry)

黄帝闲居，辟左右而问于岐伯曰：余已闻九针之经，论阴阳逆顺六经已毕，愿得口问。岐伯避席再拜曰：善乎哉问也，此先师之所口传也。黄帝曰：愿闻口传。岐伯答曰：夫百病之始生也，皆生于风雨寒暑，阴阳喜怒，饮食居处，大惊卒恐。则血气分离，阴阳破败，经络厥绝，脉道不通，阴阳相逆，卫气稽留，经脉虚空，血气不次，乃失其常。论不在经者，请道其方。

When Yellow Emperor stayed leisurely, he sent away the people on both sides and said to Qibo: "I have heard about the conditions of the nine kinds of needle, the Yin and Yang, the adverse and agreeable conditions of the hand and foot six channels expounded in the 《Classics of Needle》 already, I hope to hear further the treating knowledge from the oral inquiry you obtained in the past." Qibo left his seat, bowed and said: "You have put forward an excellent question. It was passed to me through oral instructions by my teacher." Yellow Emperor said: "I hope to know the contents of the oral instruction." Qibo said: "In the initiation of various diseases, most of them happen in the periods of the wind, rain, cold and heat, in one's mood of overjoy and anger, in the times of eating, drinking and living of daily life, by the internal and external causes of great fright and sudden fear. The unexpected disturbances cause the energy and the blood divorce, the Yin and Yang separate, the connection between the channels and the collaterals become severing, the channels become obstructed, the Yin and Yang deviate from each other, the Wei-energy becomes stagnated, the channels become empty, the energy and blood fail to circulate in their regular patterns, and all of them become disorderly. All the cases stated above are not seen in the ancient medical classics, and I like to tell you about them."

黄帝曰：人之欠者，何气使然？岐伯答曰：卫气昼日行于阳，夜半则行于阴。阴者主夜，夜者卧。阳者主上，阴者主下。故阴气积于下，阳气未尽，阳引而上，阴引而下，阴阳相引，故数欠。阳气尽，阴气盛，则目瞑；阴气尽而阳气盛，则寤矣。泻足少阴，补足太阳。

Yellow Emperor asked: "What energy causes the yawn?" Qibo answered: "The Wei-energy moves about in the Yang portion in daytime and in the Yin portion in night time. Yin is pertaining to the night, and night is related to lying down and sleep. Yang is related to ascent and is pertaining to above. Yin is related to descent and pertaining to below, when one is about to sleep at night, the Yin energy accumulates on below, as one has not yet fallen into sleep and the Yang energy has not yet entered into the Yin portion entirely, the Yang energy is still ascending, but by this time, the Yin energy has begun to descend, the running up and down of the Yin and Yang energies causes one yawn. When the Yang energy is exhausted, and the Yin energy is abundant, one will close his eyes and falls into sleep; when in daytime, the Yin energy is exhausted and the Yang energy is abundant, one will awake. When treating, it should purge by pricking the acupoints of the Foot Shaoyin Channel of Kidney and invigorate by pricking the acupoints of the Foot Taiyang Channel of Bladder."

黄帝曰：人之哕者，何气使然？岐伯曰：谷入于胃，胃气上注于肺。今有故寒气与新谷气，俱还入于胃，新故相乱，真邪相攻，气并相逆，复出于胃，故为哕。补手太阴，泻足少阴。

Yellow Emperor asked: "What energy causes the hiccup?" Qibo answered: "When the cereals enter into the stomach, they transform into the stomach energy and then, transfer to the lung above. If the cold energy is already in the middle warmer, it can not harmonize with the newly entered cereal energy, they will mingle and combat each other, finally, they come out from the stomach and reach up to the diaphragm, and the hiccup occurs. When treating, invigorate by pricking the acupoints of the Hand Taiyin Channel of Lung, and purge by pricking the Foot Shaoyin Channel of Kidney."

黄帝曰：人之唏者，何气使然？岐伯曰：此阴气盛而阳气虚，阴气疾而阳气徐，阴气盛而阳气绝，故为唏。补足太阳，泻足少阴。

Yellow Emperor asked: "What energy causes one swallowing together with rapid respiration?" Qibo answered: "When one's Yin energy is overabundant and the Yang energy is deficient, the Yin energy moves swiftly and the Yang energy moves slowly, or even the Yin energy is overabundant and the Yang energy is severing, the syndrome of swallowing together with rapid respiration will occur. When treating, invigorate by pricking the Foot Taiyang Channel of Bladder, and purge by pricking the Foot Shaoyin Channel of Kidney.

黄帝曰：人之振寒者，何气使然？岐伯曰：寒气客于皮肤，阴气盛，阳气虚，故为振寒寒慄。补诸阳。

Yellow Emperor asked: "What energy causes the chilliness of a man?" Qibo answered: "When the cold energy invades the skin, the Yin energy becomes overabundant and the Yang energy becomes deficient, the patient will have chilliness and the shivering with cold. When treating, apply warming and recuperating therapy to various Yang channels."

黄帝曰：人之噫者，何气使然？岐伯曰：寒气容于胃，厥逆从下上散，复出于胃，故为噫。补足太阴、阳明。一曰补眉本也。

Yellow Emperor asked: "What energy causes the eructation?" Qibo answered: "When the cold energy enters into the stomach, the chaotic energy of the jue-syndrome diffuses, it runs from bottom to top and comes out from the stomach to cause eructation. When treating, apply invigorating therapy by pricking the acupoints of the Foot Taiyin Channel of Spleen and the Foot Yangming Channel of Stomach."

黄帝曰：人之嚏者，何气使然？岐伯曰：阳气和利，满于心〔心：孙鼎宜曰："心"当作"胸"〕，出于鼻，故为嚏。补足太阳荣〔荣：字误，应作"荥"断句〕。眉本，一曰眉上也

〔一曰补眉本也：《甲乙》卷十二第一无“一曰”六字〕。

Yellow Emperor asked："What energy causes one sneeze?" Qibo answered："When the harmonious Yang energy is filling the chest，it will come out from the nose above to cause sneeze. If the sneeze is due to deficiency of Yang，it should invigorate by pricking the Xing point of Tonggu of Foot Taiyang Channel."

黄帝曰：人之亸者，何气使然？岐伯曰：胃不实则诸脉虚，诸脉虚则筋脉懈惰，筋脉懈惰则行阴用力，气不能复，故为亸。因其所在，补分肉间。

Yellow Emperor asked："What energy causes the weakness of the whole body and the clumsiness of the limbs?" Qibo answered："When the stomach energy is asthenic with little cereal energy，it will cause the channels of the whole body to become empty，the emptiness of the various channels will cause the tendons to become loose，if the patients conduct sexual intercourse difficultly again，his healthy energy will not be recovered and the syndrome of muscular flaccidity and coolness of the extremities will occur. When treating，prick the site where the disease attacks，and apply invigorating therapy by pricking the spaces between the muscles."

黄帝曰：人之哀而泣涕出〔泣涕出：《甲乙》卷十二第一“涕”下无“出”字，按：“泣涕出”下脱“目无所见”四字〕者，何气使然？岐伯曰：心者，五脏六腑之主也；目者，宗脉之所聚也，上液之道也；口鼻者，气之门户也。故悲哀愁忧则心动，心动则五脏六腑皆摇，摇则宗脉感，宗脉感则液道开，液道开故泣涕出焉。液者，所以灌精濡空窍者也，故上液之道开则泣，泣不止则液竭，液竭则精不灌，精不灌则目无所见矣，故命曰夺精。补天柱经侠颈。

Yellow Emperor asked："What energy causes the tears and the nasal discharge to come out when one is in sorrow and he can see nothing?" Qibo answered："The heart dominates the five solid organs and the six hollow organs，the eyes are the places where various channels converge and they are the passages of the tears and the nasal discharge，the orifices of mouth and the nose are the gateways for the breath to go in and come out，thus，when one is sorrowful，his heart will palpitate with restlessness，and the five solid organs and the six hollow organs will be unseasy；as the converging channel is also stirring，it causes all the fluid passages of the eyes，mouth and nose to open and the fluids flow out. As the body fluid is for irrigating the refined energy and moisten the orifices，when the passageways of the tears and the nasal mucus are open，they will flow out unceasingly，as a result，the tears will soon be exhausted，the refined energy will not be able to pour upwards and the eyes will not be able to see things. It is called the exhaustion of essence of life. When treating，invigorate by pricking the Tianzhu point which is in the hairline behind the neck."

黄帝曰：人之太息者，何气使然？岐伯曰：忧思则心系急，心系急则气道约，约则不利，故太息以伸出之。补手少阴、心主、足少阳留之也。

Yellow Emperor asked："What energy causes one sigh?" Qibo answered："When one is melancholic and anxious，it will cause the channels and the collaterals maintaining the heart to become tight and urgent，the routes of the vital energy will be obstructed，thus，one must smooth it out by sighing. When treating, invigorate by pricking the acupoints of the Hand Shaoyin Channel of Heart, the Hand Jueyin Channel of Pericardium and the Foot Shaoyang Channel of Gallbladder and retain the needle."

黄帝曰：人之涎下者，何气使然？岐伯曰：饮食者皆入于胃，胃中有热则虫动，虫动则胃缓，胃缓则廉泉开，故涎下。补足少阴。

Yellow Emperor asked: "What energy causes one to slobber?" Qibo answered: "All foods and drinks enter into the stomach, when there is heat in the stomach, the cereal-worm in the stomach will wriggle causing the stomach energy to become loose, then, the Lianquan point under the tongue which is the passageway of saliva will be openned, and the saliva comes out. When treating, invigorate by pricking the Foot Shaoyin Channel of Kidney."

黄帝曰：人之耳中鸣者，何气使然？岐伯曰：耳者宗脉之所聚也，故胃中空则宗脉虚，虚则下，溜脉有所竭者，故耳鸣。补客主人，手大指爪甲上与肉交者也。

Yellow Emperor asked: "What energy causes one to have tinnitus?" Qibo answered: "The ear is the place where many channels converge (Hand and Foot Shaoyang and Taiyang Channels, Hand Yangming Channel). When the stomach is empty, it will cause the asthenia of the converging channel, when the converging channel is asthenic, the lucid Yang will descend and cause the liu channel (the channel leading to the ear) to become deficient, and tinnitus occurs. When treating, invigorate by pricking the kezhuren point of the Foot Shaoyang Channel and the Shaoshang point of the Hand Taiyin Channel on the tip of the thumb where the nail and the flesh meet."

黄帝曰：人之自啮舌者，何气使然？岐伯曰：此厥逆走上脉气辈至也。少阴气至则啮舌，少阳气至则啮颊，阳明气至则啮唇矣。视主病者则补之。

Yellow Emperor asked: "What energy causes one to bite his own tongue?" Qibo answered: "It is due to the ascent of the cold energy and the channels arrive to the location each according to its category, such as, when the adverse energy of Shaoyin reaches the root of tongue, the patient will bite his tongue; when the adverse energy of Shaoyang reaches the cheek, he will bite his cheek; when the adverse energy of Yangming reaches the lips, he will bite his lips. When treating, invigorate the channel related to the main disease."

凡此十二邪者，皆奇邪之走空窍者也。故邪之所在，皆为不足。故上气不足，脑为之不满，耳为之苦鸣，头为之苦倾，目为之眩；中气不足，溲便为之变，肠为之苦鸣；下气不足，则乃为痿厥心悗。补足外踝下留之。

In a word, the twelve diseases are due to the attack of the peculiar pathogen against the orifices on the head and face. All the places where the evil energies reside are the places where the healthy energies are insufficient. When the health energy is insufficient on the upper side, the cerebral marrow will not be full in the brain, and the frequent tinnitus in the ears, the slanting of the head and dizziness of the eyes will occur; when the healthy energy is insufficient in the middle, the retention of feces and urine and the frequent borborygmus will occur; when the healthy energy on the lower side is insufficient, the muscular flaccidity and coldness of the extremities and the oppressive feeling of the chest will occur. When treating these syndromes, they can all be treated by pricking the Kunlun point below the outer ankle of the foot; it should apply invigorating therapy and retain the needle."

黄帝曰：治之奈何？岐伯曰：肾主为欠，取足少阴。肺主为哕，取手太阴、足少阴。唏者，阴与〔与：《甲乙》卷十二第一作“盛”〕阳绝，故补足太阳，泻足少阴。振寒者，补诸阳。噫者，补太阴、阳明。嚏者，补足太阳、眉本。亸，因其所在，补分肉间。泣出，补天柱经侠颈，侠颈者，头中分也。太息，补手少阴、心主、足少阳留之。涎下，补足少阴。耳鸣，补客主人、手大指爪甲上与肉交者。自啮舌，视主病者则补之。目眩头倾，补足外踝下留之。痿厥心悗，刺足大指间上二寸留之，一曰足外踝下留之。

Yellow Emperor asked: "How to treat the syndromes?" Qibo answered: "The kidney dominates the yawn, when treating, it should prick the acupoints of the Foot Shaoyin Channel. The lung dominates the hiccup, when treating, it should prick the acupoints of the Hand Taiyin Channel and the Foot Shaoyin Channel. When one has the syndrome of swallowing together with rapid respiration, it is due to the Yin is overabundant and the Yang is severing. When treating, it should invigorate by pricking the acupoints of the Foot Taiyang Channel and purge by pricking the acupoints of the Foot Shaoyin Channel. When one has chilliness and the shivering with cold, invigorate the various Yang channels. When one has eructation, invigorate by pricking the acupoints of the Foot Taiyin Channel and the Foot Yangming Channel. When one sneezes, invigorate by pricking the acupoints of the Foot Taiyang Channel. When one has muscular flaccidity and coldness of the extremities, invigorate by pricking the space between the muscles on the site of the disease.

"When one's tears are falling during sorrow, invigorate by pricking the Tianzhu point in the centre within the headline behind the neck. When one sighs, invigorate by pricking the acupoints of the Hand Shaoyin Channel, the Hand Jueyin Channel, the Foot Shaoyang Channel and retain the needle.

"When one slobbers, invigorate by pricking the acupoints of the Foot Shaoyin Channel. When one has tinnitus, invigorate by pricking the Kezhuren point on the tip of the thumb where the nail and the flesh meet. When one bites his own tongue, invigorate by pricking the related channel to the main disease. When one has dizziness in the eyes and the slanting of the head, invigorate by pricking the Kunlun point below the outer ankle and retain the needle. When one has muscular flaccidity and the oppressive feeling in the chest, prick hastily two inches above the toe and retain the needle. There is another saying about the treating; invigorate by pricking the acupoints under the outer ankle of foot."

师传第二十九

Chapter 29
Shi Chuan
(Treating Instructions Imparted by Precedent Masters)

黄帝曰：余闻先师，有所心藏，弗著于方。余愿闻而藏之，则而行之，上以治民，下以治身，使百姓无病，上下和亲，德泽下流，子孙无忧，传于后世，无有终时，可得闻乎？岐伯曰：远乎哉问也。夫治民与自治，治彼与治此，治小与治大，治国与治家，未有逆而能治之也，夫惟顺而已矣。顺者，非独阴阳脉论气之逆顺也，百姓人民皆欲顺其志也。

Yellow Emperor said："I am told that the preceding masters had many personal understandings which were not recorded in the plate, and I hope to hear about these understandings. I will keep them with good care and will take it as the norm of my behavior to treat the people and myself, so that the people may be exempted from diseases, the people in the upper class and the lower class in the society may keep harmonious, to have kind relations and good will between them, as love and kindness are prevailing among the people, their descendants will live peacefully without mental and physical disturbances and the good tradition may pass to the future generations without end. Can I hear about them?" Qibo said："When one treats the people or himself, treats things which is nearby or far away, handles a trifle of a major task, manages a country or a family, the treating has always been a failure when the treating is in the reverse way, and one must only treat in the agreeable way. The so called agreeable way not only involves the conditions of the Yin and Yang channels and the Ying and Wei energies, but also involves the treatings which are agreeable to the wishes of the people."

黄帝曰：顺之奈何？岐伯曰：入国问俗，入家问讳，上堂问礼，临病人问所便。黄帝曰：便病人奈何？岐伯曰：夫中热消瘅则便寒，寒中之属则便热。胃中热，则消谷，令人悬心善饥，脐以上皮热；肠中热，则出黄如糜，脐以下皮寒。胃中寒，则腹胀；肠中寒，则肠鸣飧泄。胃中寒，肠中热，则胀而且泄，胃中热，肠中寒，则疾饥，小腹痛胀〔小腹痛胀：《太素》卷二《顺养》"小"作"少"，"痛"下无"胀"字〕。

Yellow Emperor asked："How to treat agreeably?"Qibo answered："When one enters into a country, he must ask the condition of the local custom first; when one enters into a family, he must ask what are the taboos in the family first; when one wants to enter into the hall, he must inquire about the etiquettes of the host first; when treating, the physician must ask and know the various conditions of the patient and then ascertain which way of treating will be suitable." Yellow Emperor asked："How to treat in a suitable way?" Qibo answered："When one has heat in the intestine and the stomach, he will consume a lot of food and has the Xiaodan syndrome, treating with drugs of cold nature will be suitable; when one has cold in the intestine and stomach, treating with drugs of hot nature will be suitable; when there is heat in the stomach, the cereals in it will be digested rapidly to cause one's heart like hanging and he is apt to get hungry; when there is hot feeling on the skin above the naval, it is because there is heat in the intestine, the patient will have thin stool like the gruel; when there is cold feeling on the skin under the naval, it is because there is cold in the intestine, the syndromes of borborygmus and diarrhea will occur; when there is cold in the stomach and heat in the intestine, the syndrome of getting hungry rapidly and distention of the lower abdomen will occur."

黄帝曰：胃欲寒饮，肠欲热饮，两者相逆，便之奈何？且夫王公大人血食之君，骄恣从欲，轻人，而无能禁之，禁之则逆其志，顺之则加其病，便之奈何？治之何先。

Yellow Emperor asked: "When the stomach has heat, one should take the cold drinks and when the intestine has heat, one should take the hot drinks, as cold and heat are on the contrary, how should this kind of disease be treated? Especially, to the patients who are princes and nobles who always have meat in their meals, they are proud, indulge in their desires, look down upon others and can hardly be persuaded, when one advises him to treat against his opinion, it will oppose his will, if one treats agreeing with his will, the disease will become aggravated. In treating, what should one do first?"

岐伯曰：人之情，莫不恶死而乐生，告之以其败，语之以其善，导之以其所便，开之以其所苦，虽有无道之人，恶有不听者乎？

Qibo answered: "Generally, everyone is afraid of death and prefers living, if the physician tells the patient what is beneficial and what is harmful to his body, shows him the proper way of treating which will benefit him and relieve his misgiving that causes him miserable, he will not neglect your advise even if he is a somewhat unreasonable man."

黄帝曰：治之奈何？岐伯曰：春夏先治其标，后治其本；秋冬先治其本，后治其标。

Yellow Emperor asked: "How to treat it?" Qibo answered: "In spring and summer, treat the branch which is outside first, and then, treat the root which is inside; in autumn and winter, treat the root which is inside first and then, treat the branch which is outside."

黄帝曰：便其相逆者奈何？岐伯曰：便此者，食饮衣服，亦欲适寒温，寒无凄怆，暑无出汗。食饮者，热无灼灼，寒无沧沧。寒温中适，故气将持。乃不致邪僻也。

Yellow Emperor asked: "How to treat the patient with the contrary condition stated above and causes him to become appropriate?" Qibo answered: "When one treats to suit the patient's condition of this kind, keep the cold and heat moderate in his food and clothing. In clothing, when the weather is cold, put on thick clothes to avoid catching cold; when the weather is hot, wear thin clothes to avoid perspiration. In taking food and drink, avoid taking that of excessive heat and cold, but keep them in moderate temperature, in this way, the healthy energy can be maintained in the body so that the invasion of the evil energy which causes disease may be avoided."

黄帝曰：《本藏》以身形支节䐃肉，候五脏六腑之大小焉。今夫王公大人、临朝即位之君而问焉，谁可扪循之而后答乎？岐伯曰：身形支节者，脏腑之盖也，非面部之阅也。

Yellow Emperor said："It was stated in the chapters of《On Viscera》：'The conditions of the five solid organs and the six hollow organs can be determined by the physique and by the sizes and shapes of the protruding muscles in the joints of the limbs.' If a prince or the king wants to know the conditions of his viscera，how can one stroke his body and muscles before answering?"Qibo said："The conditions of physique and the protruding muscles of the limbs are coincide with that of the viscera，but one can know them also by examining the face."

黄帝曰：五脏之气，阅于面者，余已知之矣，以肢节而阅之奈何？岐伯曰：五脏六腑者，肺为之盖，巨肩陷咽，候见其外。黄帝曰：善。

Yellow Emperor said："Now I have known the refined energy of the viscera can be examined from the physique and the face，but how to know the conditions of the internal organs by examining the joints?" Qibo answered："Among the five solid organs and the six hollow organs，the lung is in the highest position and it is like a canopy，the condition of the lung can be determined by examining the high or low position of the shoulder and the condition of cave-in of the pharynx and larynx outside." Yellow Emperor said："Good."

岐伯曰：五脏六腑，心为之主，缺盆为之道，骺骨有余，以候髑骬。黄帝曰：善。

Qibo said："In the five solid organs and the six hollow organs，the heart is dominating，and the supraclavicular fossa is the passageway，as the distance between the two ends of the shoulder bone is quite wide，it can be used to examine the location and the shape of the supraclavicular bone so that to know the high or low，firm or crisp condition of the heart." Yellow Emperor said："Good."

岐伯曰：肝者主为将，使之候外，欲知坚固，视目小大。黄帝曰：善。

Qibo said："In the five solid organs，the liver is like a general，it can be used to determine the symptoms outside of the body，when one wants to know the patient's health condition of liver，examine the brightness or dullness of his eyes."Yellow Emperor said："Good."

岐伯曰：脾者主为卫，使之迎粮，视唇舌好恶，以知吉凶。黄帝曰：善。

Qibo said："The spleen is to defend the whole body，it receives the refined substance of the cereals and transports it to the various parts of the body. When one examine the appearance of the lips showing likes or dislikes，the good or bad condition of the spleen can be known." Yellow Emperor said："Good."

岐伯曰：肾者主为外，使之远听，视耳好恶，以知其性。黄帝曰：善。愿闻之腑之候。

Qibo said："The kidney dominates the water and body fluid which enables one to hear afar. When examining whether one's hearing is acute or not，the strong or weak condition of his kidney can be known." Yellow Emperor said："Good." I hope to hear further about how to determine the conditions of the six hollow organs."

岐伯曰：六腑者，胃为之海，广骸、大颈、张胸，五谷乃容；鼻隧以长，以候大肠；唇厚、人中长，以候小肠；目下果大，其胆乃横；鼻孔在外，膀胱漏泄；鼻柱中央起，三焦乃约。此所以候六腑者也。上下三等，脏安且良矣。

Qibo said: "In the six hollow organs, the stomach is like the sea which accommodates foods, when one's muscle of the cheek is plump, his neck is sturdy and his breast is unfolding, his ability of accommodating the cereals must be good. When one's nasal tube is long, it can be used to determine the large intestine. When the lips are thick and the vertical groove on the middle of the upper lip is long, it can be used to determine the small intestine. When the lower part of the skin under the lower eyelid is large, it shows his liver is wilfully despotic. When one's nostrils are turning up which can be seen outside, it shows his bladder is apt to become leaking. When one's nose-bridge is not flat, it shows that his triple warmer is normal. There are the methods of determining the conditions of the six hollow organs. In a word, when the upper and the lower sides of one's physique and face are matching, it symbolizes his internal organs are in harmony and are having normal functions.

决气第三十

Chapter 30
Jue Qi
(The Energies)

黄帝曰：余闻人有精、气、津、液、血、脉，余意以为一气耳，今乃辨为六名，余不知其所以然。岐伯曰：两神相搏。合而成形，常先身生，是谓精。何谓气？岐伯曰：上焦开发，宣五谷味，熏肤，充身泽毛，若雾露之溉，是谓气。何谓津？岐伯曰：腠理发泄，汗出溱溱，是谓津。何谓液？岐伯曰：谷入气满，淖泽注于骨，骨属屈伸，泄泽，补益脑髓，皮肤润泽，是谓液。何谓血？岐伯曰：中焦受气取汁，变化而赤，是谓血。何谓脉？岐伯曰：壅遏营气，令无所避，是谓脉。

Yellow Emperor said: "I am told that there are essence of life, vital energy, thin fluid, fluid, blood and vessel in human body. Formerly, I thought they were all energy, now I know they are six and have different names and I do not know why they are divided into different kinds?" Qibo said: "When the Yin and Yang sexes approcaching each other, they combine and form a new body; the substance that produces the body exists prior to the body is called the essence of life." Yellow Emperor asked: "What is vital energy?" Qibo said: "When the upper warmer disperses the refined substances of the five cereals which warms the skin and the muscle, fills into the physique and moisten the fine hairs like the dew moistening the grasses and woods, it is called the vital energy." Yellow Emperor asked: "What is thin fluid?." Qibo said: "When the striae excrets plenty of sweat, it is called the thin fluid." Yellow Emperor asked: "What is fluid?" Qibo said: "When cereals enter into the stomach, the vital energy will fill the whole body, the moist juice permeates into the bone marrow causing the bone joints to become smooth and be able to bend and stretch freely, the refined energy of the cereal will invigorate the cerebral marrow inside and moisten the skin outside, it is called fluid." Yellow Emperor asked: "What is blood?" Qibo said: "When the stomach of the middle warmer receives the food, absorbs its refined substance and transforms it into red fluid, it is called blood." Yellow Emperor asked: "What is vessel?" Qibo said: "It is like setting a dyke to guard against the energy and blood to run rashly without scruple, it is called the vessel."

黄帝曰：六气者，有余不足，气之多少，脑髓之虚实，血脉之清浊，何以知之？岐伯曰：精脱者，耳聋；气脱者，目不明；津脱者，腠理开，汗大泄；液脱者，骨属屈伸不利，色夭，脑髓消，胫痠，耳数鸣；血脱者，色白，夭然不泽，其脉空虚，此其候也。

Yellow Emperor asked: "In the six kinds of energies stated above, some are having a surplus and some are insufficient, how can one know whether the vital energy is plenty or less, the fluid is asthenic or sthenic and the blood is lucid or turbid?" Qibo said: "When one's essence of life is asthenic, his ears will be deaf; when one's vital energy is asthenic, his eyes will be dull; when one's thin fluid is asthenic, his striae will be open to have a lot of sweat; when one's fluid is asthenic, it will cause his bone joints fail to bend and stretch nimbly, his complexion will have no lustre, his cerebral marrow will not full and his legs will be sore; when one's blood is asthenic, the colour of his skin will be pale and dark without lustre; when one's vessel is asthenic, his vessel will be empty. These are the methods of examining whether the six-energy is plenty or less, asthenic or sthenic and lucid or turbid.

黄帝曰：六气者，贵贱何如？岐伯曰：六气者，各有部主也，其贵贱善恶，可为常主，然五谷与胃为大海也。

Yellow Emperor asked: "In the six energies, which one is most important and which one is less important?" Qibo said: "In the six energies, each of them is dominated by a certain viscus respectively; generally, the status of the most important, less important, good or bad in each of them may not change constantly, but all the six energies take the five cereals as the source of existance."

肠胃第三十一

Chapter 31
Chang Wei
(The Intestine and Stomach)

黄帝问于伯高曰：余愿闻六腑传谷者，肠胃之小大长短，受谷之多少奈何？伯高曰：请尽言之，谷所从出入浅深远近长短之度：唇至齿长九分，口广二寸半。齿以后至会厌，深三寸半，大容五合。舌重十两，长七寸，广二寸半。咽门重十两，广一寸半；至胃长一尺六寸。胃纡曲屈，伸之，长二尺六寸，大一尺五寸，径五寸，大容三斗五升。小肠后附脊，左环回周迭积，其注于回肠者，外附于脐上，回运环十六曲，大二寸半，径八分分之少半，长三丈二尺。回肠当脐，左环，回周叶积而下回运环反十六曲，大四寸，径一寸寸之少半，长二丈一尺。广肠傅脊，以受回肠，左环叶脊，上下辟，大八寸，径二寸寸之大半，长二尺八寸。肠胃所入至所出，长六丈四寸四分，回曲环反，三十二曲也。

Yellow Emperor asked Bogao: "I like to hear about the transportation of the cereals in the six hollow organs, the size and length of stomach and intestine and the capacity of the accommodation of the cereals." Bogao said: "Let me tell you the length of the various parts from the mouth where the cereals enter to the anus where the feces is excreted: The length from the lips to the teeth is nine fen (0.9 inch); the width of the mouth is two and half inches; the depth from the rear of teeth to the epiglottis is three and half inches; it can hold five ge (0.05 litre) of food; the weight of the tongue is ten ounces, it is seven inches long and two and half inches wide; the weight of the laryngopharynx is ten ounces and its width is one and half inches; the length from the laryngopharynx to the stomach is one foot and six inches, the body of the stomach is tortuous, bending and stretching, its length is two feet and six inches, its circumference is one foot and five inches, its diameter is five inches and its capacity is three and half litres. The small intestine attaches to the spine behind, it goes around from left to the right and is overlapping, with sixteen turnings, the part of small intestine connecting the large intestine attaches on the location above the navel, its circumference is two and half inches, its diameter is eight and two third fen, and its length is thirty two feet. The large intestine turns left by the site of the navel, it descends overlapping in sixteen turnings, its circumference is four inches, its diameter is one and one third inches, and its length is twenty one feet. The wide intestine (rectum) is near the spinal cord, it receives the dregs from the large intestine, it descends to connect the anus somewhat slantingly, its circumference is eight inches, its diameter is two and two third inches and its length is two feet and eight inches. The total length of the digestive tract is sixty feet and four inches and four fen, the turnings in the small intestine and the large intestine are thirty two."

平人绝谷第三十二

Chapter 32
Ping Ren Jue Gu
(The Fast of an Ordinary Man)

黄帝曰：愿闻人之不食，七日而死何也？伯高曰：臣请言其故。胃大一尺五寸，径五寸，长二尺六寸，横屈受水谷三斗〔《太素》卷十三《肠度》无“五升”二字〕五升。其中之谷常留二斗，水一斗五升〔《太素》卷十三《肠度》无“五升”二字〕而满。上焦泄气，出其精微，慓悍滑疾，下焦下溉诸肠。小肠大二寸半，径八分分之少半，长三丈二尺，受谷二斗四升，水六升三合合之大半。回肠大四寸，径一寸寸之少半，长二丈一尺。受谷一斗，水七升半。广肠大八寸，径二寸寸之大半，长二尺八寸，受谷九升三合八分合之一。肠胃之长，凡五丈八尺四寸〔《太素》卷十三《肠度》作“六丈四寸四分”〕，受水谷九斗二升一合合之大半，此肠胃所受水谷之数也。

Yellow Emperor said: “I am told that when a man does not eat, he will die in seven days and what is the reason?” Bogao said: “Let me tell you the reason. The circumference of the stomach is one foot and five inches, its diameter is five inches and its length is two feet and six inches, its capacity of holding the cereals and water is thirty litres, constantly, there are twenty litres of food and ten litres of fluid filling in the stomach. Through the dispersing function of the upper warmer, the refined substance of food is transported outside, as its energy is valiant, slippery and swift, it spreads to nourish the whole body. The function of the lower warmer is washing and cleaning the food and then the food is transported into the small intestine. The small intestine is two and half inches in size, its diameter is eight and one eighth fen, and its length is thirty two feet, its capacity is twenty four litres for holding the food and six litres and three and two third ge for holding the fluid. The circumference of the large intestine is four inches, its diameter is one and one third inches, its length is twenty one feet, it capacity for holding the food is ten litres and that holding the fluid is seven and half litres. The circunference of the wide intestine (rectum) is eight inches, its diameter is two and two third inches, its length is two feet and eight inches and its capacity of holding the dregs is nine litres three ge eight and one eighth fen. The total length of the intestine and stomach is sixty feet four inches and four fen, the overall capacity of holding the cereals and water is ninety two litres one and two third ge.

平人则不然，胃满则肠虚，肠满则胃虚，更虚更满，故气得上下，五脏安定，血脉和利，精神乃居，故神者，水谷之精气也。故肠胃之中，当留谷二斗，水一斗五升。故平人日再后，后二升半，一日中五升，七日五七三斗五升，而留水谷尽矣。故平人不食饮七日而死者，水谷精气津液皆尽故也。

"For an ordinary man, when his stomach is filled with food, his intestine is still empty; when his intestine is filled with the food which is transported from the stomach, his stomach will be empty, as the stomach and the intestine are filled and become empty now and then, it enables the ascent and descent of the functional activities of vital energy, the stability of the five viscera, the harmony of the channels and the tranquility of the spirit. So, it is supposed that the spirit of man is converted from the essential substance of food. Therefore, for an ordinary man without disease, there are always twenty litres of food and fifteen litres of fluid retained in his intestine and stomach, he urinates twice a day, and in each urination, the urine is two and half litres, that is, in one day, the urination is five litres, and in seven days, it will be thirty five litres, thus, after seven days, the water and cereals in the intestine and stomach will be exhausted. Therefore, when one fails to take food and drink for seven days he will die, it is due to the exhaustion of the cereals and fluid in his intestine and stomach."

海论第三十三

Chapter 33
Hai Lun
(On the Four Seas)

黄帝问于岐伯曰：余闻刺法于夫子，夫子之所言，不离于营卫血气。夫十二经脉者，内属于腑脏，外络于肢节，夫子乃合之于四海乎？岐伯答曰：人亦有四海、十二经水。经水者，皆注于海，海有东西南北，命曰四海。黄帝曰：以人应之奈何？岐伯曰：人有髓海，有血海，有气海，有水谷之海，凡此四者，以应四海也。

Yellow Emperor asked Qibo："I have heard your lecture about the pricking therapy，and what you said was not divorced from the Ying，Wei and channel energies. Since the twelve channels connect the five solid and six hollow organs inside，and link the four extremities and joints outside，can you coordinate them with the four seas?" Qibo answered："In human body，there are also four seas and twelve channels. The twelve channels flow to all directions but finally converge into the four seas，there are the seas of east，west，south and north，so，they are called the four seas. "Yellow Emperor asked："In what way does the body correspond with the four seas?" Qibo answered："In human body，there are the sea of marrow，sea of blood，sea of energy and the sea of water and cereals，and they correspond to the four seas."

黄帝曰：远乎哉，夫子之合人天地四海也，愿闻应之奈何？岐伯答曰：必先明知阴阳表里荥输所在，四海定矣。

Yellow Emperor said："How profound your talking is！You have coordinated the human body with heaven，earth and the four seas. I hope to hear further how do they correspond?" Qibo said："When one knows explicitly the locations of the Yin or Yang，superficies or interior，Xing and Shu points，he will be able to determine the four seas of the marrow，blood，energy and that of the water and cereals."

黄帝曰：定之奈何？岐伯曰：胃者水谷之海，其输上在气街〔街：当注本，张注本并作"冲"〕，下至三里。冲脉者为十二经之海，其输上在于大杼，下出于巨虚之上下廉。膻中者为气之海，其输上在于柱骨之上下，前在于人迎。脑为髓之海，其输上在于其盖，下在风府。

Yellow Emperor asked："How to ascertain the important acupoints of the four seas in human body?"Qibo answered："The stomach is the sea of water and cereals，its upper important acupoint is the Qichong point，and the lower one is the Sanli point；the Chong Channel is the sea of the twelve channels and it is also the sea of blood，its upper important acupoint is the Dazhu point，and the lower ones are the Shangjuxu point and the Xiajuxu point，the Tanzhong (the middle part between two breasts) is the sea of energy，its important acupoints are the Yamen point above the cervical vertebrae，Dazhui point below the cervical vertebrae and the Renying point in the front; the brain is the sea of the marrow, its upper important acupoint is the Baihui point and the lower one is the Fengfu point."

黄帝曰：凡此四海者，何利何害？何生何败？岐伯曰：得顺者生，得逆者败；知调者利，不知调者害。

Yellow Emperor asked: "As for the four seas of human body, what treatment will cause it to become beneficial? What treatment will cause it to become harmful? How to make its viability to become prosperous and what will cause it to decline?" Qibo said: "When one treats with the way which is agreeable with the physiological law, the viability of the four seas in the human body will be prosperous, when one treats against it, it will cause decline; when one knows how to recuperate the four seas, it will benefit the body, otherwise, it will injure the body."

黄帝曰：四海逆顺奈何？岐伯曰：气海有余者，气满胸中，悗〔悗：《太素》卷五《四系合》作"急"〕息面赤；气海不足，则气少不足以言。血海有余，则常想其身大，怫然不知其所病；血海不足〔血海不足：《甲乙》卷一第八"不足"上无"血海"二字〕，亦常想其身小，狭然不知其所病。水谷之海有余，则腹满；水谷之海不足，则饥不受谷食。髓海有余，则轻劲多力，自过其度；髓海不足，则脑转耳鸣，胫痠眩冒，目无所见，懈怠安卧。

Yellow Emperor asked: "What is the adverse and agreeable conditions of the four seas?" Qibo answered: "When the sea of energy is having a surplus, it shows the evil energy is overabundant, one will have fullness of breath in the chest, rapid respiration and red complexion; when it is insufficient, one will be short of breath and incapable to talk. When the sea of blood is having a surplus due to the plentiness of blood and the overabundance of channel energy, the patient will imagine his body is becoming gigantic, he seems to have no disease although he is having a melancholic mood; when the sea of blood is insufficient, he will often feel his body is becoming small and light, he appears to have no disease although he has the mood of taking things too hard. When the sea of water and cereals is having a surplus, it will cause one to have abdominal distention, when the sea of water and cereals are insufficient, one will feel hungry but can hardly take in food. When the sea of marrow is having a surplus, it will cause one to feel light and vigorous in the body, and he can endure unusually hard work; when the sea of marrow is insufficient, one's brain will feel like turning and he will have the syndromes of tinnitus, sore legs, dizziness, seeing nothing, slothful and sleepiness."

黄帝曰：余已闻逆顺，调之奈何？岐伯曰：审守其输而调其虚实，无犯其害，顺者得复，逆者必败。黄帝曰：善。

Yellow Emperor said: "Now I have known the adverse and agreeable conditions of the four seas, but how to treat it?" Qibo said: "One must know the upper and lower acupoints communicating the four seas and adjusts by invigorating the asthenia, and purging the thenia to avoid the mistake of purging asthenia and invigorating sthenia. When one can abide by this law, the patient will be healthy, otherwise, the disease will become deteriorative." Yellow Emperor said: "Good."

五乱第三十四

Chapter 34
Wu Luan
(The Five Disturbances)

黄帝曰：经脉十二者，别有五行，分为四时，何失而乱？何得而治？岐伯曰：五行有序，四时有分，相顺则治，相逆则乱。

Yellow Emperor asked："The twelve channels of a man belong to the five elements respectively and they are also related to the four seasons, what are the conditions of missing to become disorderly and that of hits to become orderly?" Qibo said："The creation and the subjugation of the five elements are having a regular sequence, and there are changes in the four seasons, it will be normal and orderly when they are agreeable to each other, and will be abnormal and disorderly when they reverse against each other."

黄帝曰：何谓相顺？岐伯曰：经脉十二者，以应十二月。十二月者，分为四时。四时者，春秋冬夏，其气各异，营卫相随，阴阳已和，清浊不相干，如是则顺之而治。

Yellow Emperor asked："What is the meaning of agreeable to each other?" Qibo answered："The twelve channels of human body correspond to the twelve months of the year, the twelve months are divided into four seasons of spring, summer, autumn and winter of which the weathers are different. If the interior and the exterior of the Ying energy and the Wei energy are agreeable to each other, the superficies and interior of Yin and Yang tally with each other, and there is no disturbance in the ascent and descent of the lucid and turbid energies, the functions of the viscera, and the channels and the weathers of the four seasons will be harmonious and the human body will be eased and comfortable."

黄帝曰：何谓逆而乱？岐伯曰：清气在阴，浊气在阳，营气顺脉〔营气顺脉：《太素》卷十二《营卫气行》"顺"下有"行"字。按"脉"字是衍文〕，卫气逆行，清浊相干，乱于胸中，是谓大悗。故气乱于心，则烦心密嘿〔嘿：《甲乙》卷六第四作"默"〕，俯首静伏；乱于肺，则俯仰喘喝，接〔接：《甲乙》卷六第四作"按"〕手以呼；乱于肠胃，则为霍乱；乱于臂胫，则为四厥；乱于头，则为厥逆，头重〔重《甲乙》卷六第四作"痛"〕眩仆。

Yellow Emperor asked："What is the meaning of adverse and becoming disorderly?" Qibo said："The lucid energy belongs to Yang, but it situates, on the contrary, on the position of Yin, the turbid energy belongs to Yin, but it situates, on the contrary, in the position of Yang; the Ying energy runs agreeably in the Yang portion, but the Wei energy runs adversely in the Yin portion, and the lucid energy and the turbid energy are interfering each other to disturb the chest. In this case, it is the adverse condition, and it is called the great gloominess. When the evil energy is in the heart to cause disturbance, it will cause one to become gloomy, silient and speachless, and bending his head motionlessly; when the evil energy is in the lung to cause disturbance, the patient will face up and down restlessly, respires with sound and presses his chest while respiring; when the evil energy is in the intestine and stomach to cause disturbance, cholera morbus will occur; when the disturbing energy is in the arm and leg, it will cause the jue-syndrome of the extremities; when the disturbing energy is in the head, it will cause one to have Jueni, his head will be painful and will often fall down due to dizziness."

黄帝曰：五乱者，刺之有道乎？岐伯曰：有道以来，有道以去，审知其道，是谓身宝。黄帝曰：善。愿闻其道。岐伯曰：气在于心者，取之手少阴、心主之输。气在于肺者，取之手太阴荥、足少阴输。气在于肠胃者，取之足太阴，阳明（不）下者，取之三里。气在于头者，取之天柱、大杼；不知，取足太阳荥输。气在于臂足，取之先去血脉，后取其阳明、少阳之荥输。

Yellow Emperor asked: "Is there any principle for treating the five kinds of disturbances stated above by pricking?" Qibo said: "When the disease attacks, there is a way of coming, when the disease is removed, there is a way of going, when one knows precisely the ways of coming and going of the disease and treat properly, it is supposed to be the treasure of maintaining the bodily health." Yellow Emperor said: "Good. I hope to hear the principle of treating." Qibo said: "When the disturbing energy is in the heart, prick the Shenmen acupoint of the Hand Shaoyin Channel and the Daling acupoint of the Hand Jueyin Channel of Pericardium, when the disturbing energy is in the lung, prick the Yuji point which is the Xing point of the Hand Taiyin Channel and the Taixi acupoint of the Foot Shaoyin Channel; when the disturbing energy is in the intestine and stomach, prick the Taibai acupoint of the Foot Taiyin Channel and the Sanli point which is the lower acupoint of the Foot Yangming Channel; when the disturbing energy is in the head, prick the Tianzhu acupoint and the Dazhu acupoint, if the syndrome is not relieved, prick the Tonggu point which is the Xing-point of Foot Taiyang Channel and the Shugu acupoint of the Foot Taiyang Channel; when the evil energy is in the arm and the leg, when pricking, remove the partial stagnated blood first, then prick the Xing-point or the acupoint of the Foot Yangming and the Foot Shaoyang Channel respectively according to the specific conditions of the disease which is on the arm or the leg."

黄帝曰：补泻奈何？岐伯曰：徐入徐出，谓之导气，补泻无形，谓之同〔同：日抄本作“固”〕精，是非有余不足也，乱气之相逆也。黄帝曰：“允〔允：《太素》卷十二《营卫气行》作“光”〕乎哉道，明乎哉论，请著之玉版，命曰治乱也。

Yellow Emperor asked: "How to invigorate or purge?" Qibo said: "When one inserts and pulls out the needle slowly, it is called the inducement of the energy. When pricking without regular forms in invigorating and purging, it is called stablizing the essence of life, this is not for invigorating the insufficient energy nor purging the surplus energy, it is because the evil energies that cause disturbances are falling into loggerheads and they must be dredged." Yellow Emperor said: "How brilliant the principle of pricking is! I will write down what you said in the plate of jade and name it as the five disturbances."

胀论第三十五

Chapter 35
Zhang Lun
(On Distention)

黄帝曰：脉之应于寸口，如何而胀？岐伯曰：其脉大坚以涩者，胀也。黄帝曰：何以知脏腑之胀也？岐伯曰：阴为脏，阳为腑。

Yellow Emperor asked: "When the pulse condition appears on the Cunkou, what pulse condition indicates the syndrome of distention?" Qibo answered: "When the pulse condition is gigantic, firm and choppy in coming, it is the pulse condition of the syndrome of distention." Yellow Emperor asked: "How to determine the distention of the five solid organs from that of the six hollow organs?" Qibo answered: "When the pulse condition is of Yin, the distention is in the five solid organs, when the pulse condition is of Yang, the distention is in the six hollow organs."

黄帝曰：夫气之令人胀也，在于血脉之中耶，脏腑之内乎？岐伯曰：三（一云二字）者皆存焉，然非胀之舍也。黄帝曰：愿闻胀之舍。岐伯曰：夫胀者，皆在于脏腑之外，排脏腑而郭胸胁，胀皮肤，故命曰胀。

Yellow Emperor said: "When one has disorder of vital energy, it will cause one to have the syndrome of distention. I like to know whether the distention is in the channeles or in the viscera?" Qibo answered: "Both the channels and the viscera can retain the distention, but they are not the place where the distention resides." Yellow Emperor said: "I hope to hear about the residence of distention." Qibo said: "Generally, distention is beyond the viscera, it pushes aside the viscera and falls on the location around the chest and hypochondria or falls on the striae of skin to cause distention, and thus, it is called distention."

黄帝曰：脏腑之在胸胁腹裹之内也，若匣匮之藏禁器也，各有次舍，异名而同处，一域之中，其气各异，愿闻其故。黄帝曰：未解其意，再问〔黄帝曰，未解其意，再问：《太素》卷二十九《胀论》无此九字〕。岐伯曰：夫胸腹，脏腑之郭也。膻中者，心主之宫城也。胃者，太仓也。咽喉小肠者，传送也。胃之五窍者，闾里门户也。廉泉玉英者，津液之道也。故五脏六腑者，各有畔界，其病各有形状。营气循脉，卫气逆〔卫气逆：《太素》卷二十九《胀论》无此三字〕为脉胀，卫气并脉循分为肤胀。三里而泻〔三里而泻：《甲乙》卷八第三任务"取三里泻之"〕，近者一下，远者三下，无问虚实，工在疾泻。

Yellow Emperor said: "The viscera are in the inner layer of the chest, hypochondria and abdominal cavity like a confidential article hidden in a casket, each of the five solid organs and the six hollow organs has its own residence, they have different names but locate in the same region and their activities and functions in the same region are different. I hope to know the reason about it." Qibo said: "The chest and abdomen are the outer casings of the viscera; the Tanzhong is the middel palace of the pericardium; the stomach is the granary for storing the water and cereals; the pharynx, throat and the small intestine are the courses for transmission; the ears, eyes, nose, mouth and tongue are like the doors of the house; the Lianquan point and the Yuying point are the route of the body fluid. Thus, in the five solid and six organs, each has its boundary, and their appearances of affection are different. When the Ying-energy runs along the channel, the distention of channel will occur; when the Wei-energy merges into the channel and runs in the boundaries between muscles, the distention of skin will occur. When treating distention, prick the Sanli point with purging therapy, purge once to the disease newly contracted and purge three times to the protracted disease, the distention can be removed. No matter whether the disease belongs to asthenia or sthenia, apply purge therapy hastily will be effective."

黄帝曰：愿闻胀形。岐伯曰：夫心胀者，烦心短气，卧不安。肺胀者，虚满而喘咳。肝胀者，胁下满而痛引小腹。脾胀者，善哕，四肢烦悗，体重不能胜衣，卧不安〔卧不安：按此三字是衍文〕。肾胀者，腹满引背央央然，腰髀痛。六腑胀：胃胀者，腹满，胃脘痛，鼻闻焦臭，妨于食，大便难。大肠胀者，肠鸣而痛濯濯〔濯濯：《甲乙》卷六第八并无此二字〕，冬日重感于寒，则飧泄不化。小肠胀者，少腹䐜胀，引腰〔腰：《脉经》卷六第四作“腹”〕而痛，膀胱胀者，少腹满而气癃。三焦胀者，气满于皮肤中，轻轻然而不坚。胆胀者，胁下痛胀，口中苦，善太息。凡此诸胀者，其道在一，明知逆顺，针数不失。泻虚补实，神去其室，致邪失正，真不可定，粗之所败，谓之夭命。补虚泻实，神归其室，久塞其空，谓之良工。

Yellow Emperor said: "I hope to hear about the appearances of the syndrome of distention." Qibo said: "In the distention related to the heart, the patient will have oppression in the chest, short or breath, restless when sleeping; in the lung distention, the patient has oppression of deficiency type in the chest, rapid respiration and cough; in the distention due to liver disorder, the patient will have distention and fullness under the hypochondria and drawing pain in the lower abdomen; in the spleen-distention, the patient will hiccup often, his four extremities will be clumpsy and his body will be feeling heavy and will not likely to withstand wearing clothes; in the kidney-distention, the patient will have fullness in the abdomen which drawing the back to become uncomfortable, and the loins, joints of extremities to become painful. As to the distention of the six hollow organs: the stomach-distention will cause fullness of the abdomen and pain of the gastric cavity, the nose seems to have smelt the scorching odour which obstruct eating, and the patient will have dyschesia; in the flatulence of large intestine, the patient will have borborygmus and pain in the intestine, when catching cold in winter, he will have diarrhea with indigested food; in the flatulence of the small intestine, the patient will have distention and fullness in the lower abdomen and pain in the abdomen; in the distention of the urinary bladder, the patient will have distention and fullness in the lower abdomen and the retention of urine; in the triple warmer-distention, the patient will have plenty of air in the skin to cause swelling, and the skin is empty and soft when pressing; in the distending pain of the hypochondrium due to gallbladder disorder, the patient will have pain under the hypochondrium, bitter taste in the mouth and he sighs often.

The treating principle to the various diseases of distention stated above are the same. The treating will be proper when one knows clearly the agreeable and adverse relations with the disease and when the times of pricking (one or three times) are correct. If purging therapy is applied to asthenic syndrome or the invigorating therapy is applied to the sthenic syndrome, the spirit of the patient will be dispersed, the evil energy will penetrate to injure the healthy energy to cause unstableness. A physician of lower level often fails to treat in a proper way, and he is supposed to be the one to cause the patient die early; if one applies invigorating therapy to the asthenic syndrome and purging therapy to the sthenic syndrome, the spirit of the patient will be maintained inside, his orifices will be stable and filling with healthy energy, the physician is supposed to be a good one."

黄帝曰：胀者焉生？何因而有〔而有：《太素》卷二十九《胀论》“有”下并有“名”字〕？岐伯曰：卫气之在身也，常然〔然：《太素》卷二十九《胀论》并无此字〕并脉循分肉，行有逆顺，阴阳相随，乃得天和，五脏更始〔更始：《太素》卷二十九《胀论》“始”作“治”〕，四时循序，五谷乃化。然后厥气在下，营卫留止，寒气逆上，真邪相攻，两气相搏，乃合为胀也。黄帝曰：善。何以解惑？岐伯曰：合之于真，三合而得。帝曰：善。

Yellow Emperor asked: "Where does distention generate and why it has the name of distention?" Qibo answered: "The Wei-energy in the body usually runs between the boundaries of muscles along with the channel, if the Wei-energy runs agreeably along the three foot channels and runs adversely along the three hand channels to keep the Yin and Yang harmonious, one will receive the genial energy of nature, the five solid organs will be kept in order, the four seasons will elapse in regular sequence, and food in the stomach will be digested and be absorbed normally, and one will be healthy. If the cold energy is hidden below, retaining between the Ying-enery and the Wei-energy, then, the flowing of both the energies will be abnormal, the cold energy will reverse up, the healthy energy and the evil energy will be combating, and the disease of distention will be shaped." Yellow Emperor said: "Good. But how to remove my perplexion?" Qibo said: "It is correct to apply the purging therapy, and to the protracted disease, the purging of three times is suitable." Yellow Emperor said: "Good."

黄帝问于岐伯曰：胀论言无问虚实，工在疾泻，近者一下，远者三下。今有其三而不下者，其过焉在？岐伯对曰：此言陷于肉肓，而中气穴者也。不中气穴，则气内闭；针不陷肓，则气不行；上〔上：《太素》卷二十九《胀论》作“不”〕越中肉，则卫气相乱，阴阳相逐。其于胀也，当泻不泻，气故不下，三而不下，必更其道，气下乃止，不下复始，可以万全，乌有殆者乎。其于胀也，必审其胗〔胗：《甲乙》卷八第三并作“诊”〕，当泻则泻，当补则补，如鼓应桴，恶有不下者乎。

Yellow Emperor asked Qibo: "You have said that one can disregard whether the distention is of asthenic or sthenic, but only applies purging by pricking hastily will be effective, pricks once when the disease is newly contracted, and pricks three times when the disease is protracted. Now, I have purged for three times, but the distention has not relieved, where is the error?" Qibo answered: "The so called prick once or prick three times here means the pricking must reach the membrane which is under the skin and above the muscle and one must also hit the acupoint of distention. If the acupoint is not hit, the energy will be shut inside without excreting, when the needle fails to reach the membrane under the skin and above the muscle, the energy will not be running between the boundaries of muscles, when the pricking is not hitting the acupoint but hit the place between the muscles erroneously, the Wei-energy will run rashly and the Yin and Yang energies will be contending inside. When treating distention by pricking, if one fails to purge when it should be purged, the energy of distention will not be dissipated, under this condition, one must prick by changing the acupoint until the energy of distention is removed. If it is not removed, one should prick again, and no accident will occur. When treating distention, one must examine carefully whether the syndrome belongs to the solid organ or to the hollow organ, purge when it should be purged and invigorate when it should be invigorated, then, the curative effect will be as clear as the sound of drumsticks hitting the drum. When one treats like this, how could any distention be not cured?"

五癃津液别第三十六

Chapter 36
Wu Long Jin Ye Bie
(The Five Kinds of Body Fluids)

黄帝问于岐伯曰：水谷入于口，输于肠胃，其液别为五，天寒衣薄则为溺与气，天热衣厚则为汗，悲哀气并则为泣，中热胃缓则唾。邪气内逆，则气为之闭塞而不行，不行则为水胀，余知其然也，不知其何由生，愿闻其道。

Yellow Emperor asked Qibo: "When the water and cereals enter into the mouth and then, being transmitted into the intestine, they will divide into five kinds of fluid: when the weather is cold and one's clothes are thin, most of them will be changed into urine and vapour, when the weather is hot in summer and one's clothes are thick, most of them will be-wet; when one's mood is in sorrow and the energy merges into the heart, they will transform into tears; when there is heat in the middle warmer and the stomach energy is flaccid and slow, they will change into saliva. When the evil energy is blocking inside, the Yang energy is obstructed and fails to circulate, edema will occur. I know the conditions above, but I do not know whence does the body fluid generate, and I hope to hear about it."

岐伯曰：水谷皆入于口，其味有五，各注其海，津液各走其道。故三〔三：《甲乙》卷一第十三并作"上"〕焦出气，以温肌肉，充皮肤，为其津〔为其津：按"其"字衍，应据《甲乙》卷一第十三删〕；其流〔流：《太素》卷二十九《津液》作"留"〕而不行者，为液。

Qibo said: "When the food enters the mouth, it has different tastes of sour, bitter, sweat, acrid and salty, and they pour into the four seas respectively. The body fluids transformed from the water and cereals and spread along certain routes individually. The Wei-energy issued from the upper warmer which moistens the muscle and maintains the skin is called the thin fluid, and that which is retained unmoved is called the fluid.

天暑衣厚则腠理开，故汗出；寒留于分肉之间，聚沫则为痛。天寒则腠理闭，气湿〔湿：《甲乙》卷一第十三作"涩"〕不行，水下留〔留：《甲乙》作"流"〕膀胱，则为溺与气。

"When one's clothes in summer are rather thick, his sweat pores open and he will perspire. When the cold-evil retains between the boundaries of muscles, the body fluid will be condensed into foam and pain will occur. When one's sweat pores are closed in winter, his energy will be unsmooth due to obstruction, the fluid will flow into the bladder below to become urine and vapour.

五脏六腑，心为之主，耳为之听，目为之侯，肺为之相，肝为之将，脾为之卫，肾为之外。故五脏六腑之津液，尽上渗于目，心悲气并则心系急，心系急则肺举，肺举则液上溢。夫心系与肺，不能常举，乍上乍下，故咳〔咳：《太素》卷二十九《津液》作"呿"。杨注："呿者，泣出之时，引气此口也"〕而泣出矣。

"Among the five solid organs and the six hollow organs, the heart is the dominator and the activities of other viscera are under its control; the ears take charge of the hearing, the eyes take charge of the sight seeing, the lung takes charge of assisting like a prime minister, the liver takes charge of the scheming like a general, the spleen takes charge of defending, and the kidney which stores the essence of life takes charge of supporting the outer activities of the whole body. All the body fluids of the five solid organs and the six hollow organs ascend to pour into the eyes; when one has sorrow in heart, the energies of the five solid organs and the six hollow organs will ascend and merge into the heart causing the channels and collaterals of the heart to become tense, when they become tense, the lobes of lung will be lifted up and the body fluid will ascend to become overflowing. But the lobes of lung can not be lifted up constantly when the channels and collaterals of heart are tense, and the energy can only now rise, now fall, thus, when the fluid ascends along with the energy and become overflowing, the phenomenon of crying with breathing and open mouth will occur.

中热则胃中消谷，消谷则虫上下作，肠胃充郭故胃缓，胃缓则气逆，故唾出。

"When there is heat in the middle warmer, the food in the stomach will be digested more easily, after the digestion, the parasites in the intestine will be active to move upwards and downwards. When the intestine is full, the stomach energy will become flaccid and slow, when it is flaccid and slow, the energy will be reversing up and the saliva will be excreted along with it.

五谷之津液和合而为膏者，内渗入于骨空，补益脑髓，而下流于阴股〔而下流于阴股：六字误衍〕。阴阳不和，则使液溢而下流于阴，髓液皆减而下，下过度则虚，虚故腰背〔腰背：《甲乙》卷一第十三"背"作"脊"〕痛而胫痠。

"When the grease formed by the combination of the body fluids transformed from the five cereals permeates into the vacancy of the bone, it can invigorate the brain and profit the marrow. If the Yin and Yang energies are not harmonious, the body fluid will be overflowing and flows out from the anus causing the marrow and the body fluid to become decreasing; when one exercises sexual activities excessively, his body will be in debility to have pain in the spine and sore in the legs."

阴阳气道不通，四海闭塞，三焦不泻，津液不化，水谷并行肠胃之中，别于回肠，留于下焦，不得渗膀胱，则下焦胀，水溢则为水胀，此津液五别之逆顺也。

"When the energy routes of the viscera are impeded, the sea of energy, the sea of blood, the sea of marrow and the sea of water and cereals will all be obstructed; the triple warmer will fail to transport, the body fluid will fail to digest, the water and cereals will be accumulated in the stomach and intestine. When the water and cereals enter into the large intestine, they will remain in the lower warmer and will not be permeated into the bladder, in this way, it will cause the lower warmer to have distention and fullness, and the overflowing of the body fluid will cause edema. These are the adverse and agreeable conditions of the five kinds of the body fluid."

五阅五使第三十七

Chapter 37
Wu Yue Wu Shi
(Determining the Conditions of the Five Viscera by Examining the Five Sense Organs)

黄帝问于岐伯曰：余闻刺五官五阅，以观五气。五气者，五脏之使也，五时〔五时：按“时”字误，应作“使”〕之副也。愿闻其五使当安出？岐伯曰：五官者，五脏之阅也。黄帝曰：愿闻其所出，令可为常。岐伯曰：脉出其于气口，色见于明堂，五色更出，以应五时〔以应五时：本句应作“以应五使”〕，各如其常〔常：与注本，此张注本作“脏”〕，经气入脏，必当治里。

Yellow Emperor asked Qibo saying: “I am told in acupuncture, there is the method of examining the colours of complexion of the five sense organs outside for diagnosing the changes of the five viscera inside, the colours of complexion are dispatched by the five viscera, and they are also corresponding with the missions of the five viscera. I hope to hear from where do the five colours of complexion which correspond to the missions of the five viscera reflect?” Qibo said: “The five sense organs are the outer reflection of the five viscera.” Yellow Emperor said: “I want to hear the relation between the five sense organs and the changes of the five viscera so that one can use it as the routine for examining the disease.” Qibo said: “The pulse condition of the five viscera can be reflected on the Cunkou, the colours of complexion can be reflected on the nose. The changes of the five colours of complexion correspond with the missions of the five viscera and the complexion represents the condition of the related viscus. As to the disease which is penetrated into the inner organ through the channel, the interior should be treated.”

帝曰：善。五色独决于明堂乎？岐伯曰：五官已辨〔辨：张注本作“辩”〕，阙庭必张，乃立明堂。明堂广大，蕃蔽见外，方壁高基，引垂居外，五色乃治，平搏广大，寿中百岁。见此者，刺之必已，如是之人者，血气有余，肌肉坚致，故可苦以针。

Yellow Emperor said: “Good. Does the complexion which reflects the visceral condition appears only on the nose?” Qibo said: “If the colours of the five sense organs can be distinguished clearly and the part of the forehead is apparent, then can one make the determination from the observation of the nose. When one's nose is broad and large, his cheeks and the tragus are manifesting outside apparently, his face is square and plump, his gum is protecting the teeth from outside, his five colours of complexion are normal and his five sense organs are open and wide in proper positions, he can live a long life of one hundred years.

When treating this kind of people, pricking will certainly be effective. As the energy and blood of people of this kind are having a surplus, and their muscles are substantial and firm, thus, they can be treated by pricking hastily."

黄帝曰：愿闻五官。岐伯曰：鼻者，肺之官也；目者，肝之官也；口唇者，脾之官也；舌者，心之官也；耳者，肾之官也。

Yellow Emperor said: "I hope to hear about the functions of the five sense organs." Qibo said: "The nose belongs to the lung, it takes charge of the respiration; the eyes belong to the liver, they take charge of the sight seeing; the mouth belongs to the spleen, it takes charge of receiving the water and cereals; the tongue belongs to the heart, it takes charge of distinguishing the tastes; the ears belong to the kidney, they take charge of hearing."

黄帝曰：以官何候？岐伯曰：以候五脏。故肺病者，喘息鼻胀；肝病者，眦青；脾病者，唇黄；心病者，舌卷短〔舌卷短：《甲乙》卷一第四"舌"下无"卷"字〕，颧赤；肾病者，颧与颜黑。

Yellow Emperor asked: "How can one diagnose by examining the complexion?" Qibo siad: "One can diagnose the condition of the five viscera by examining the five sense organs. When the lung has disease, one will have rapid respiration and his nosetril will be stirring; when the liver has disease, one's canthus will be green; when the spleen has disease, one's mouth and lips will be dry and yellow; when the heart has disease, one's tongue will become short and his cheekbones are red; when the kidney has disease, one's cheeks and the forehead will be black."

黄帝曰：五脉安出，五色安见，其常色殆者如何？岐伯曰：五官不辨，阙庭不张，小其明堂，蕃蔽不见，又埤其墙，墙下无基，垂角去外，如是者，虽平常殆，况加疾哉。

Yellow Emperor asked: "It will be very dangerous when one's pulse condition and the complexion are normal but he has disease, what is the reason?" Qibo said: "When one's complexion is not distinct, his forehead is not broad, his nose is narrow, his cheeks and tragus are not apparent, his face is narrow without any flesh in the lower part, his frontal eminence is bogging down and the gum of teeth is revealing outside, he has the symptom of tending to live a short life even he has no disease, let alone he has disease."

黄帝曰：五色之见于明堂，以观五脏之气，左右高下，各有形乎？岐伯曰：府〔府：张注本作"五"〕脏之在中也，各以次舍，左右上下，各如其度也。

Yellow Emperor said: "The five complexions appear on the nose where one can observe the energies of the five viscera, is there any specific image in the middle, left, right, upper and lower positions?" Qibo said: "Each of the five viscera has a definite location in the chest and the abdominal cavity, when the complexions are reflected on the nose, there are also regular criterions in left, right, upper and lower positions."

逆顺肥瘦第三十八

Chapter 38
Ni Shun Fei Shou
(Different Acupuncture Therapies to People of Different Fat and Lean Physiques and the Adverse and Agreeable Conditions of the Twelve Channels)

黄帝问于岐伯曰：余闻针道于夫子，众多毕悉矣，夫子之道应若失〔失：按“失”应作“矢”〕，而据未有坚然者也，夫子之问学熟〔熟：“熟”当作“孰””，下脱“得”字〕乎，将审察于物而心〔心：《太素》卷二十二《刺法》无“心”字〕生之乎？岐伯曰：圣人之为道者，上合于天，下合于地，中合于人事，必有明法，以起度数、法式检押，乃后可传焉。故匠人不能释尺寸而意短长，废绳墨而起平木〔平木：《太素》卷二十二《刺法》“平木”作“水平”〕也，工人不能置规而为圆，去矩而为方。知用此者，固自然之物，易用之教，逆顺之常也。

Yellow Emperor asked Qibo saying: "I have heard the acupuncture therapy from you and I have known a lot about it. Although the curative effect by applying the method you said is so sure like an arrow hitting the target, yet I don't see your argument has a definite ground. Is your learning inherited from others or it is invented by yourself after observing things?" Qibo said: "The acupuncture theory is created by the saints, it agrees with heaven above, with earth below, and in accordance with human affairs in the middle, it has an explicit rule in establishing the criterion of length and size, so that, it can be passed to the later generations. Therefore, a craftsman can not cast away the stipulated length and set a length at will, nor can he give away the usual practice and set a causal standard, likewise, one can not draw a circle without a pair of compasses, or draw a square without a ruler. When one treats according to the rule, he is agreeable with the natural law of things and his teaching is applicable. This is also the routine of measuring the adverse or agreeable condition of a thing."

黄帝曰：愿闻自然奈何？岐伯曰：临深决水，不用功力，而水可竭也，循掘决冲，而经可通也。此言气之滑涩，血之清浊，行之逆顺也。

Yellow Emperor said: "I hope to hear about the natural law." Qibo said: "When one drains away the water into a deep valley, the water can be exhausted without much effort, when one digs a tunnel from a hole disregarding the firmness, he will finally open up a passage. This is to say that the energy of human body has the different conditions of slippery or choppy, the blood has the different conditions of lucid or turbid, and the circulation of the energy and blood has the different conditions of adverse and agreeable, and one must abide to its natural condition."

黄帝曰：愿闻人之白黑肥瘦小长，各有数乎？岐伯曰：年质壮大，血气充盈，肤革坚固，因加以邪，刺此者，深而留之，此肥人也〔此肥人也：《太素》卷二十二《刺法》无此四字〕。广肩腋项，肉薄厚皮而黑色，唇临临然，其血黑以浊，其气涩以迟，其为人也，贪于取与〔与：《甲乙》卷五第六作“予”〕，刺此者，深而留之，多益其数也。

Yellow Emperor asked: "I hope to know whether there should be any difference in pricking the people of different types, such as to black and white ones, to fat and thin ones and to young and old ones?" Qibo said: "When a tall and strong man in his prime of life contracts evil and asks for treating, since his blood is abundant, his energy is prosperous and his skin is firm and dense, it should prick deeply and retain the needle. When treating another type of man whose shoulder, armpit and neck are open and wide, has a thin muscle, thick and black skin, plump and thick lips, turbid and black blood, as this kind of people are keen on gaining but also like to present things to others, it should prick deeply, retain the needle and increase the times of pricking."

黄帝曰：刺瘦人奈何？岐伯曰：瘦人者，皮薄色少，肉廉廉然，薄唇轻言，其血清气滑，易脱于气，易损于血，刺此者，浅而疾之。

Yellow Emperor asked: "How to prick a thin man?" Qibo said: "For a thin man, his skin is thin and he is pale, his muscle is emaciated, he has thin lips, low voice, his blood is lucid and his energy is slippery. Thus, he is easy to collapse and his blood is easy to suffer loss. When pricking people of this kind, it should prick shallowly and pull out the needle rapidly."

黄帝曰：刺常人奈何？岐伯曰：视其白黑，各为调之，其端正敦厚者，其血气和调，刺此者，无失常数也。

Yellow Emperor asked: "How to prick a normal man?" Qibo said: "Examine the black or white of the patient and coordinate with the deep-puncture or shallow-puncture. If the patient is upright and kind, his energy must be harmonious. When pricking people of this kind, one can by no means exclude the normal acupuncture therapy."

黄帝曰：刺壮士真骨者〔真骨者：按此三字误衍〕奈何？岐伯曰：刺壮士真骨〔真骨：按“真”应作“者”，“骨”字属下读〕，坚肉缓节监监然，此人重则气涩血浊，刺此者，深而留之，多益其数；劲〔劲：按“劲”当作“轻”〕则气滑血清，刺此者，浅而疾之。

Yellow Emperor asked: "How to prick a strong man in his prime of life?" Qibo said: "The bone of a strong man in his prime of life is firm, his muscle is thick and he has strong and large joints. When treating this kind of people, if he is a prudent and steady man, his energy will be stagnant and his blood turbid, it should prick deeply, retain the needle and increase the times of the pricking; if he is light-headed and active, his energy will be slippery and his blood lucid, prick shallowly and pull out the needle rapidly."

黄帝曰：刺婴儿奈何？岐伯曰：婴儿者，其肉脆血少气弱，刺此者，以豪〔豪：周本，日刻本，张注本，并作“毫”〕针，浅刺而疾发针，日再可也。

Yellow Emperor asked: "How to prick an infant?" Qibo said: "The muscle of an infant is soft, his blood is few and his energy is deficient, when treating, apply shallow-puncture with a filiform needle, and the insertion must be rapid. The pricking should be twice a day."

黄帝曰：临深决水奈何？岐伯曰：血清气浊〔浊：《太素》卷二十二《刺法》作“滑”〕，疾泻之，则气竭焉。黄帝曰：循掘决冲奈何？岐伯曰：血浊气涩，疾泻之，则经〔经：《甲乙》卷五第六作“气”〕可通也。

Yellow Emperor asked："How to integrate the pricking with the draining away the water into a deep valley?"Qibo said："When applying the rapid-purging therapy to the patient of lucid blood and slippery energy, it will cause the healthy energy to become exhausted. "Yellow Emperor asked："How to integrate the pricking with the digging a tunnel from a hole?" Qibo said："When applying the rapid-purging therapy to the patient of turbid blood and choppy energy, it will cause the unimpediment of the healthy energy. "

黄帝曰：脉行之逆顺奈何？岐伯曰：手之三阴，从脏走手；手之三阳，从手走头。足之三阳，从头走足；足之三阴，从足走腹。

Yellow Emperor asked："What are the conditions of the adverse and agreeable circulations of the twelve channels?" Qibo said："The three Yin channels of hand start from the chest and end on the tips of the fingers; the three Yang channels of hand start from the arm and end in the head; the three Yang channels of foot start from the head and end on the tips of the toe, the three Yin channels of foot start from the foot and end at the abdomen. "

黄帝曰：少阴之脉独下行何也？岐伯曰：不然。夫冲脉者，五脏六腑之海也，五脏六腑皆禀焉。其上者，出于颃颡，渗诸阳，灌诸精〔精：《甲乙》卷二第二作“阴”〕；其下者，注少阴之大络，出于气街〔街：黄校本作“衔”〕，循阴股内廉，入〔入：《甲乙》卷二第二“入”上有“斜”字〕腘中，伏行骭骨内，下至内踝之后〔后：《太素》卷十《冲脉》无此字〕属而别；其下者，并于少阴之经，渗三阴；其前者，伏行出附属，下〔下：顾氏《校记》云：“‘下’乃‘上’之误”〕循跗入大指间，渗诸络而温肌肉。故别络结则跗上不动，不动则厥，厥则寒矣。黄帝曰：何以明之？岐伯曰：以言导之，切而验之，其非必动，然后乃可明逆顺之行也。黄帝曰：窘乎哉！圣人之为道也。明于日月，微于毫厘，其非夫子，孰能道之也。

Yellow Emperor asked："Why does the Foot Shaoyin Channel of Kidney descend solely?" Qibo said："It is not the Foot Shaoyin Channel of Kidney, but it is the side branch of the Chong Channel. The Chong Channel is the sea of the five solid organs and the six hollow organs, and they are all moistened and nourished by it. Its ascending channel stem from the upper orifice of the nasal meatus, permeates into the Yang channel and pour into the Yin channel; its descending channel pours into the large collateral of Hand Shaoyin Channel of Kidney (the Dazhong point), comes out to the Qichong point, runs along the inner side of the thigh, enters slantingly into the popliteal fossa and lies concealed in the inner side of the leg, it descends to the joint of the tibia and the tarsal bone of the inner ankle and then branches out. Its descending side branch runs along with the Foot Shaoyin Channel, permeates into the three Yin channels of liver, spleen and kidney; its side branch which runs forward, runs into hiding and then comes out near the outer ankle, descends to the dorsum of foot, enters into the side of the toe, permeates into the collaterals to warm and nourish the muscle. Thus, if there is impediment in the collateral branch of the Chong Channel in the lower extremities, the pulse on the foot dorsum will not pulsate, when it is not pulsating, the Wei-energy will stop running and jueni and the syndrome of cold limbs will occur." Yellow Emperor asked: "How can one understand the adverse and agreeable conditions of the Chong Channel and the Shaoyin Channel?" Qibo said: "It can be made understood by oral explanation, besides, it can be verified by pressing the pulse on the foot dorsum, if it is not the Shaoyin Channel, the pulse on the foot dorsum will be pulsating, and one can know the adverse and agreeable relations of the Shaoyin Channel and the Chong Channel." Yellow Emperor said: "How significant it is! The principle of acupuncture of the saints is as bright as the sun and moon, and is meticulous without a least deviation. If it were not you, who can explain it!"

血络论第三十九

Chapter 39
Xue Luo Lun
(On Superficial Venules)

黄帝曰：愿闻其奇邪而不在经者。岐伯曰：血络是也。

Yellow Emperor said: "I hope to know the condition when the evil is not in the channel." Qibo said: "It is the condition when the evil is in the superficial venules."

黄帝说：刺血络而仆者，何也？血出而射者，何也？血少〔少：《太素》卷二十三《量络刺》《甲乙》卷一第十四并作"出"〕黑而浊者，何也？血出清〔血出清：《太素》卷二十三《量络刺》作"血清"〕而半为汁者，何也？发针而肿者，何也？血出若多若少而面色苍苍者，何也？发针而面色不变而烦悗者，何也？多出血而不动摇者，何也？愿闻其故。

Yellow Emperor asked: "Some patients collapse after the letting out of blood from the superficial venules, and why is it? When letting out the blood, it is like spurting, and why is it? The blood lets out is black and thick, and why is it? When the blood let out is dilute, one half of it is liquid juice, and why is it? When the needle is pulled out, the skin is swelling, and why is it? The patient's complexion is green disregarding the bleeding is plenty or few, and why is it? After the pulling out of the needle, the complexion of the patient remains unchanged but has oppressive feeling in the chest, and why is it? When the bleeding is plenty but the patient is not painful, and why is it? I hope to know the various reasons about them."

岐伯曰：脉气盛而血虚者，刺之则脱气，脱气则仆。血气俱盛而阴气〔阴气：按"阴"应作"阳"〕多者，其血滑，刺之则射；阳气畜积，久留而不泻者，其血黑以浊，故不能射。新饮而液渗于络，而未合和于血也，故血出而汁别焉；其不新饮者，身中有水，久则为肿。阴气积于阳，其气因于络，故刺之，血未出而气先行，故肿。阴阳之气，其新相得而未和合，因而泻之，则阴阳俱脱，表里相离，故脱色而〔而：《太素》卷二十三《量络刺》作"面"〕苍苍然。刺之血出多，色不变而烦悗者，刺络而虚经。虚经之属于阴者，阴脱，故烦悗。阴阳相得而合为痹者，此为内溢于经，外注于络，如是者，阴阳俱有余，虽多出血而弗能虚也。

Qibo said: "When the patient's channel energy is excessive but his blood is deficient, if the superficial venule is pricked and the blood is let out, he will have exhaustion of vital energy and fall down with coma. When both the blood and energy are excessive, the Yang energy in the channel is abundant, and the circulation of blood is fluent and slippery, if the superficial venule is pricked, the blood will be spurting; when the Yang energy accumulated in the superficial venules and retained long without being purged, then the blood let out will be black and thick and will not be spurting. When the patient has just drunk water which has permeated into the superficial venules but has not yet mingled with the blood, by this time, if the superficial venule is pricked, part of the fluid will be of liquid juice; if the patient has not drunk water just then, it is the fluid retained in the body and will cause edema when it is protracted. When the Yin energy accumulates in the Yang collateral, then, the Yin energy will hide in the collateral. When the collateral is pricked and the energy moves away before the coming out of the blood, the Yin energy will be shut in the striae of the muscle and the location of pricking will be swelling. When the Yin and Yang energies have just met but have not yet combined, the purging therapy will cause the Yin and Yang energies to become dispersing and the superficies and the interior divorcing, as a result, the complexion of the patient will be fading to become green. When the superficial venule is pricked and the bleeding is plenty, the complexion of the patient is unchanged but he has an oppressive feeling in the chest, it is because the pricking of the collateral causes the debility of the channel; as the channel connects the five viscera which are Yin, and when the Yin is in debility, the oppressive feeling of the chest will occur. When the Yin evil and the Yang evil combine, bi-syndrome will occur, when the evil energy retains in the body, it will fill the channel inside and pour into the collateral outside, in this way, the evils in both the Yin and Yang will be excessive. Thus, when pricking the collateral, although the bleeding is plenty, the channel will not be deficient."

黄帝曰：相之奈何？岐伯曰：血脉者，盛〔血脉者，盛："者盛"二字误倒〕坚横以赤，上下无常处，小者如针，大者如筋，则而泻之万全也，故无失数矣〔矣：《太素》卷二十三《量络刺》并无此字〕；失数而反，各如其度。

Yellow Emperor asked: "How to examine the superficial venules?" Qibo said: "When the channel energy of the patient is excessive, one can perceive the superficial venule is firm, full and red, it can be up above or down below without a definite location, the small one is like a needle and the large one is like a chopstick, under this condition, it will be perfectly safe when applying the therapy of pricking the collateral and let out the blood, but the pricking must not divorce from the principle of the blood-letting puncture. If the pricking is divorced from the principle and violates the routine, the eight conditions anticipated above will occur."

黄帝曰：针入而肉著者，何也？岐伯曰：热气因于针则针热，热则肉著于针，故坚焉。

Yellow Emperor asked: "After insertion of the needle, the muscle attaches to the body of the needle, and why is it?" Qibo said: "It is because the muscle is hot and hotness causes the muscle to attach the needle tightly."

阴阳清浊第四十

Chapter 40
Yin Yang Qing Zhuo
(The Lucid and Turbid of the Yin and Yang Energies)

黄帝曰：余闻十二经脉，以应十二经水〔十二经水：《太素》卷十二《营卫气行》“十二经水”下重“十二经水”四字〕者，其五色各异，清浊不同，人之血气若一，应之奈何？岐伯曰：人之血气，苟能若一，则天下为一矣，恶有乱者乎。黄帝曰：余问一人，非问天下之众。岐伯曰：夫一人者，亦有乱气，天下之众，亦有乱人，其合为一耳。

Yellow Emperor said: "I am told that the twelve channels in human body correspond to the twelve water channels on earth. The colours of the twelve water channels are different, and the lucidity and the turbidity of them are diverse, but in human body, the conditions of the blood and energy in the twelve channels are the same, why people say they are corresponding?" Qibo said: "If the conditions of the blood and energy in human body were the same, then, all things in the world could be the same also, and how could any turmoils happen?" Yellow Emperor said: "What I said was indicating the conditions of the blood and energy in the channels of a man, I did not ask the conditions about the human affairs in the world." Qibo said: "There is the disorderly energy in a person and also in the masses of the world. Their conditions are the same."

黄帝曰：愿闻气之清浊。岐伯曰：受谷者浊，受气者清。清者注〔注：日抄本作“五”〕阴，浊者注阳。浊而清者，上出于咽；清而浊者，则下行〔则下行：《甲乙》卷一第十二作“下行于胃”〕。清浊相干〔清浊相干：4卷一第十二“清浊相干”句上有“清者上行，浊者下行”八字〕，命曰乱气。

Yellow Emperor said: "I like to hear about the lucid and turbid energies in human body." Qibo said: "The cereal one eats is of the turbid energy, and the air one inhales is of the lucid energy. The lucid energy pours into the lung, and the turbid energy pours into the stomach; the lucid energy dominates Yin and the turbid energy dominates Yang; the lucid energy transformed by the turbid energy ascends and comes out from the pharynx, the turbid energy which is contained in the lucid energy descends to the gastric cavity. If the ascent and the descent of the lucid energy and the turbid energy become disorderly and interfering each other, it is called the disorderly energy."

黄帝曰：夫阴清而阳浊，浊者〔者：《甲乙》卷一第十二作“中”〕有清，清者有浊，清浊〔清浊：应据《太素》《甲乙》删〕别之奈何？岐伯曰：气之大别，清者上注于肺，浊者下走〔走：《甲乙》卷一第十二并作“流”〕于胃。胃之清气，上出于口；肺之浊气，下注于经，内积于海。

Yellow Emperor asked: "As Yin is lucid and Yang is turbid, in the turbid energy, it contains the lucid energy, and in the lucid energy, it contains the turbid energy, how to distinguish it?" Qibo said: "The approximate difference of the energies are: the lucid energy ascends and pour into the lung and the turbid energy descends and flows into the stomach. The lucid energy transformed by the stomach ascends to exit from the mouth, and the turbid energy which is contained in the lung descends to pour into the channel and accumulates in the sea of energy inside."

黄帝曰：诸阳皆浊，何阳浊甚乎？岐伯曰：手太阳独受阳之浊，手太阴独受阴之清，其清者上走空窍，其浊者下行诸经。诸阳皆清，足太阴独受其浊。

Yellow Emperor saked: "Since all the hollow organs of Yang are the locations where the turbid energy situates, which one of the hollow organs is the most turbid one?" Qibo said: "It is solely the Hand Taiyang Channel of Small Intestine receives the turbid energy of Yang most, and it is solely the Hand Taiyin Channel of Lung receives the lucid energy of Yin most; the lucid energy ascends to reach the orificies, and the turbid energy descends to enter into the various channels. The five viscera which all belong to Yin receive the lucid energy, except the spleen of Foot Taiyin Channel receives the turbid energy of the stomach."

黄帝曰：治之奈何？岐伯曰：清者其气滑，浊者其气涩，此气之常也。故刺阴者，深而留之；刺阳者，浅而疾之；清浊相干者，以数调之也。

Yellow Emperor asked: "How to treat and adjust the lucid and turbid energies of Yin and Yang?" Qibo said: "The lucid energy is slippery and the turbid energy is choppy, and these are the normal conditions of energies. Thus, when treating the disease of solid organs which belong to Yin, prick deeply and retain the needle longer; when treating the disease of hollow organs which belong to Yang, prick shallowly and pull out the needle swiftly. If the lucid energy and the turbid energy are interfering each other, one should deliberate whether the treating should be emphasized on Yin or Yang according to the specific condition."

阴阳系日月第四十一

Chapter 41
Yin Yang Xi Ri Yue
(The Yin and Yang of Human Body Relate to Sun and Moon)

黄帝曰：余闻天为阳，地为阴，日为阳，月为阴，其合之于人奈何？岐伯曰：腰以上为天，腰以下为地，故天为阳，地为阴。故足之十二经脉，以应十二月，月生于水，故在下者为阴；手之十指，以应十日，日主火〔日主火：按“主”字系“生于”二字之误〕，故在上者为阳。

Yellow Emperor asked: "I am told that heaven is Yang and the earth is Yin; the sun is Yang and the moon is Yin. What is the condition when Yin and Yang coordinate with the human body?" Qibo said: "The part of human body which is above the loins is called heaven, the part which is below the loins is called earth, so, the heaven belongs to Yang and the earth belongs to Yin. The twelve channels of feet (the three Yin and three Yang channels in the left and right feet) correspond with the twelve months of the duodecimal cycle, as the moon which is the essence of Yin creates water, so, all things below are called Yin. The ten fingers of two hands correspond with the ten days of the decimal cycle, as the sun which is the essence of Yang creates fire, so, all things above are called Yang."

黄帝曰：合之于脉奈何?”岐伯曰：寅者，正月之生阳也，主左足之少阳；未者六月，主右足之少阳。卯者二月，主左足之太阳；午者五月，主右足之太阳。辰者三月，主左足之阳明；巳者四月，主右足之阳明；此两阳合于前，故曰阳明。申者，七月之生阴也，主右足之少阴；丑者十二月，主左足之少阴。酉者八月，主右足之太阴；子者十一月，主左足之太阴；戌者九月，主右足之厥阴；亥者十月，主左足之厥阴。此两阴交尽，故曰厥阴。

Yellow Emperor saked: "What are the conditions when the twelve months and the ten days coordinate with the channels?" Qibo said: "The first lunar month is the month of Yin, and it is the time for the Yang energy to generate, as Yang appears in the left first and then in the right, thus, the first lunar month dominates the Shaoyang Channal of the left foot; the sixth lunar month is the month of Wei, it dominates the Shaoyang Channel of the right foot. The second lunar month is the month of Mao, it dominates the Taiyang Channel of the left foot; the fifth lunar month is the month of Wu, it dominates the Taiyang Channel of the right foot. The third lunar month is the month of Chen, it dominates the Yangming Channel of the left foot; the fourth lunar month is the month of Si, it dominates the Yangming Channel of the right foot. The third and the fourth lunar months are between Shaoyang and Taiyang, they are bright in the both Yang, so, they are called Yangming. The seventh lunar month is the month of Shen, it is the time when the Yin energy generates, as the Yin energy appears in the right first and then in the left, so, the seventh lunar month dominates the Shaoyin Channel of the right foot; the twelfth lunar month is the month of Chou, it dominates the Shaoyin Channel of the left foot. The eigth lunar month is the month of You, it dominates the Taiying Channel of the right foot; the eleventh lunar month is the month of Zi, it dominates the Taiyin Channel of the left foot. The ninth lunar month is the month of Xu, it dominates the Jueyin Channel of the right foot; the tenth lunar month is the month of Hai, it dominates the Jueyin Channel of the left foot. The ninth and the tenth lunar months are the terminals of Yin, so, they are called Jueyin.

甲主左手之少阳，己主右手之少阳。乙主左手之太阳，戊主右手之太阳。丙主左手之阳明，丁主右手之阳明。此两火并合，故为阳阴。庚主右手之少阴，癸主左手之少阴。辛主右手之太阴，壬主左手之太阴。

"In the day of Jia, it dominates the Shaoyang Channel of the left hand, in the day of Ji, it dominates the Shaoyang Channel of the right hand. In the day of Yi, it dominates the Taiyang Channel of the left hand, in the day of Wu, it dominates the Taiyang Channel of the right hand. In the day of Bing, it dominates the Yangming Channel of the left hand, in the day of Ding, it dominates the Yangming Channel of the right hand. The Bing and Ding days are bright in the both fires, so, they are called Yangming. In the day of Geng, it dominates the Shaoyin Channel of the right hand, in the day of Gui, it dominates the Shaoyin Channel of the left hand. In the day of Xin, it dominates the Taiyin Channel of the right hand, in the day of Ren, it dominates the Taiyin Channel of the left hand.

故足之阳者，阴中之少阳也；足之阴者，阴中之太阴也。手之阳者，阳中之太阳也；手之阴者，阳中之少阴也。腰以上者为阳，腰以下者为阴。

"The Yang channels in the two feet are the Shaoyang in Yin; the Yin channels in the two feet are the Taiyin in Yin. The Yang channels in the two hands are the Taiyang in Yang; the Yin channels in the two hands are the Shaoyin in Yang. The parts above the loins are called Yang, and the parts below the loins are called Yin.

其于五藏也，心为阳中之太阳，肺为阴中〔阴中：《太素》作"阳中"〕之少阴，肝为阴中之少阳，脾为阴中之至阴，肾为阴中之太阴。

"In the five viscera, the heart is the Taiyang in Yang, the lung is the Shaoyin in Yang, the liver is the Shaoyang in Yin, the spleen is the extreme Yin in Yin, and the kidney is the Taiyin in Yin."

黄帝曰：以治之奈何？岐伯曰：正月、二月、三月，人气在左，无刺左足之阳；四月、五月、六月，人气在右，无刺右足之阳。七月、八月、九月，人气在右，无刺右足之阴；十月、十一月、十二月，人气在左，无刺左足之阴。

Yellow Emperor asked: "How to treat it?" Qibo said: "The Yang energy moves from left to the right, in the first, second and third lunar months, the energy of man is on the left, the three Yang channels of the left foot must not be pricked. In the fourth, fifth and sixth lunar months, the energy of man is on the right, the three Yang channels of the right foot must not be pricked. The Yin energy moves from the right to the left, in the seventh, eighth and the ninth lunar months, the energy of man is in the right, the three Yin channels of the right foot must not be pricked. In the tenth, eleventh and the twelfth lunar months, the energy of man is on the left, the three Yin channels of the left foot must not be pricked."

黄帝曰：五行以东方为甲乙木王〔王：周本作"主"〕春，春者苍色，主肝〔主肝：《太素》卷五《阴阳合》"主"作"有"，上重"苍色"二字〕。肝者，足厥阴〔足：《太素》卷五《阴阳合》"足"上有"主"字〕也。今乃以甲为左手之少阳，不合于数何也？"岐伯曰：此天地之阴阳也，非四时五行之以次行也。且夫阴阳者，有名而无形，故数之可十，离之可百，散之可千，推之可万，此谓也。

Yellow Emperor asked: "In the five elements, the Jia and Yi woods of east are dominating the spring season of which the colour is green, and it dominates the liver which is of the Foot Jueyin Channel. Now you take the day of Jia as the Shaoyang Channel of the left hand which is against the rule of the five elements coordinating the decimal cycle, and why is it?" Qibo said: "This is the law of the variation of heaven, earth, Yin and Yang which is not arranged according to the sequence of the four seasons and the five elements. The Yin and Yang are in names but not in shapes. Thus, when one deduces things with the principle of Yin and Yang, it can be counted into ten, but it can be divided into hundreds, can be scattered into thousands, and can be inferred into ten thousands, and one must not stick on it rigidly."

病传第四十二

Chapter 42
Bing Chuan
(The Transmission of Diseases)

黄帝曰：余受九针于夫子，而私览于诸方，或有导引行气，乔〔乔：《甲乙》卷六第十作“按”〕摩、灸、熨、刺、焫、饮药，之一者可独守耶，将尽行之乎？岐伯曰：诸方者，众人之方也，非一人之所尽行也。

Yellow Emperor said: "I have learned the knowledge of the nine kinds of needle from you, and I have read many medical books recording to the methods of treatment privately. In treating, there are also the extremities and breathing exercices, massage, moxibustion, topical application of heated drugs, acupuncture, burning therapy and the administration of prepared medical herb. When treating, should the pricking therapy be applied alone, or cooperate it with other therapies synthetically?" Qibo said: "The multiple treatments can be applied to the multitude, it may not fit in with a specific person."

黄帝曰：此乃所谓守一勿失万物毕者也。今余已闻阴阳之要，虚实之理，倾移之过，可治之属，愿闻病之变化，淫传绝败而不可治者，可得闻乎？岐伯曰：要乎哉问。道，昭乎其如日醒，窘乎其如夜瞑，能被而服之，神与俱成，毕将服之，神自得之，生神之理，可著于竹帛，不可传于子孙。

Yellow Emperor said: "This is the so called sticking to a single therapy without discarding it lightly, and the treating of various complicated disease can be comprehended by analogy. Now I have heard the essentials of Yin and Yang, the reasons of asthenia and sthenia, the affections due to unstable striae and insufficient healthy energy and the diseases which still have the chance to be cured. Besides all of them, I hope to hear about the interior change of the disease of which the evil is transmitted from one viscus to another viscus, the disease of which the healthy energy is deteriorating and severing, and the disease which can by no means to be cured. Can I hear about them?" Qibo said: "What you ask is very important. The medical principle is prominent as one sees things clearly when he is sober in daytime yet one can hardly perceive its profoundness like having a hazy view in night time. If one can abide to the medical principle, keep it close like wearing clothes and appreciate it thoroughly, one will be immerged into it, when applying it all along, one will see its marvellous effect. The medical principle should be carved on the bamboo slips so that it can be handed down to the later generations. It must not be imparted to the descendents privately."

黄帝曰：何谓旦醒？岐伯曰：明于阴阳，如惑之解，如醉之醒。黄帝曰：何谓夜瞑？岐伯曰：瘖乎其无声，漠乎其无形，折毛发理，正气横倾，淫邪泮衍，血脉传溜〔溜：《甲乙》

卷六第十作“留”〕，大〔大：《素问·标本病传论》新校正引《灵枢经》作“夫”〕气入藏，腹痛下淫，可以致死，不可以致生。

Yellow Emperor asked: “What is the meaning of ‘seeing things clearly when one being sober in daytime’?” Qibo said: “When one understands the law of Yin and Yang, the original perplexity seems to have been removed and one becomes sober from drunkenness.” Yellow Emperor asked: “What is the meaning of ‘having a hazy view in night time’?” Qibo said: “When the outside evil invades the body, it is silent without a sound, and it is quiet without a trace, but the fine hair of the patient is chilled, his striae are open and his health energy dissipated, the evil energy disperses and overflows all over his body and the four extremities, it retains in the channel, flows into the viscera and causing the abdominal pain and the infiltration to the lower warmer. In this case, the patient can by no means to be cured and die.”

黄帝曰：大气入藏奈何？岐伯曰：病先发于心〔于心：《千金》卷十三第一“心”下有“者”字〕，一日而之肺〔之肺：《千金》卷十三第一“之肺”下并有“喘咳”二字〕，三〔三：《素问·标本病传论》新校正引《甲乙》作“五”〕日而之肝〔之肝：《千金》卷十三第一“之肝”下并有“胁痛支满”〕，五日而之脾〔之脾：《千金》卷十三第一“之脾”下并有“闭塞不通，身痛体重”八字〕，三日不已，死，冬夜半，夏日中。

Yellow Emperor asked: “How does the evil energy transmit after entering into the viscera?” Qibo said: “When the disease begins from the heart, the disease will be transmitted to the lung after one day, and the patient will have cough and rapid breathing; after another five days, the disease will be transmitted to the liver, the patient will have proping pain in the hypochondria; after another five days, the disease will be transmitted to the spleen, the energy of the patient will be obstructed and he feels heavy in the body; after another three days, if the disease is not recovered, the patient will die; in winter, he will die at midnight, and in summer, he will die at noon.

病先发于肺〔于肺：《脉经》卷六第七“于肺”下并有“喘咳”二字〕，三日而之肝〔之肝：《脉经》卷六第七“之肝”下并有“胁痛支满”四字〕，一日而之脾〔之脾：《脉经》卷六第七“之脾”下并有“闭塞不通，身痛体重”八字〕，五日而之胃，十日不已，死，冬日入，夏日出。

“When the disease begins in the lung, the patient will cough and has rapid breathing; the disease will be transmitted to the liver in three days, and the patient will have proping pain in the hypochondria; after another one day, the disease will be transmitted to the spleen, and the energy of the patient will be obstructed and he feels heavy in the body; after another five days, the disease will be transmitted to the stomach, and the patient will have abdominal pain; after another ten days, if the disease is not removed, the patient will die; in winter, he will die when the sun sets, and in summer, he will die when the sun rises.

病先发于肝〔于肝：《脉经》卷六第一“于肝”下并有“头目眩，胁痛支满”七字〕，三日〔三日：《脉经》卷六第一作“一日”〕而之脾，五日〔五日：《脉经》卷六第一作“二日”〕而之胃〔之胃：《脉经》卷六第一“之胃”下并有“而腹胀”三字〕，三日而之肾〔之肾：《脉经》卷六第一下并有“少腹腰脊痛，胫痠”七字〕，三〔三：《脉经》卷六第一并作“十”〕日不已，死，冬日入，夏早食。

“When the disease begins in the liver, the patient will have dizziness and proping pain in the hypochondria; the disease will be transmitted to the spleen after one day; after another two days the disease will be transmitted to the stomach, and the patient will have abdominal obstruction; after another three days, the disease will be transmitted to the kidney and the patient will have pain in the lower abdomen, spine and tibia; if the disease is not recovered after another ten days, the patient will die; in winter, he will die when the sun sets, and in summer, he will die at the time of breakfast.

病先发于脾，一日而之胃〔之胃：《脉经》卷六第五“之胃”下并有“而腹胀”三字〕，二日而之肾〔之肾：《脉经》卷六第五“之肾”下并有“少腹腰脊痛，胫痠”七字〕，三日而之膂〔而之膂：《脉经》卷六第五并无“膂”字〕膀胱〔膀胱：《脉经》卷六第五“膀胱”下并有“脊膂筋痛，小便闭”七字〕，十日不已，死，冬人定，夏晏食。

“When the disease begins in the spleen, it will be transmitted to the stomach after one day, and the patient will have distention of the stomach; after another two days, the disease will be transmitted to the kidney, and the patient will have pain in the lower abdomen, spine and tibia; after another three days, the disease will be transmitted to the bladder, and the patient will have pain in the tendons of the spine and arms, and he will have dysuria; If the disease is not recovered after another ten days, the patient will die; in winter, he will die when people go to sleep (9: 00-11: 00Pm.), in summer, he will die at the time of supper.

病先发于胃〔于胃：《脉经》卷六第六“于胃”下并有“胀满”二字〕，五日而之肾，三日而之膂膀胱，五日而上之心，二日不已，死，冬夜半，夏日昳。

“When the disease begins in the stomach, the patient will have distention of stomach, the disease will be transmitted to the kidney after five days; after another three days, the disease will be transmitted to the bladder; after another five days, the disease will be transmitted to the heart; if the disease is not recovered after another two days, the patient will die; in winter, he will die after midnight, and in summer, he will die in the afternoon.

病先发于肾，三日而之膂〔而之膂：《脉经》卷六第九并无“而膂”二字〕膀胱，三日而上之心，三日而之小肠〔三日而上之心，三日而之小肠：《脉经》卷六第九并作“二日上之心，心痛，三日之小肠胀”〕，三日不已，冬大晨，夏早〔早：日刻本，马注本并作“晏”〕晡。

“When the disease begins in the kidney, it will be transmitted to the bladder after three days; after another two days, the disease will be transmitted to the heart above to cause heartache; after another three days, the disease will be transmitted to the small intestine, and the patient will have distention of the small intestine; if the disease is not recovered after another three days, the patient will die; in winter, he will die at dawn, and in summer, he will die after sun set.

病先发于膀胱，五日而之肾，一日而之小肠〔小肠：《甲乙》卷六第十“小肠”下有“腹胀”二字〕，一〔一：《甲乙》卷六第十作“二”〕日而之心，二日不已，死，冬鸡鸣，夏下晡。

“When the disease begins in the bladder, it will be transmitted to the kidney after five days; after another one day, the disease will be transmitted to the small intestine, and the patient will have abdomial distention; after another two days, the disease will be transmitted to the heart; if the disease is not recovered after another two days, the patient will die; in winter, he will die at cock crow (1: 00-3: 00Am.), and in summer, he will die in the afternoon.

诸病以次相传，如是者，皆有死期，不可刺也！间一藏〔一藏：《素问・标本病传论》“一藏”下有“止”字〕及二〔及二：《素问・标本病传论》“二”作“至”〕三四藏者，乃可刺也。

"The various diseases are transmitted according to the regular sequence. To the diseases with the transmission of this kind, the date of death of the patient can be anticipated, and they can not be cured by acupuncture. When the transmission is ceased after skipping over one viscus or skipping over three or four viscera, then, it can be treated by pricking.

淫邪发梦第四十三

Chapter 43
Yin Xie Fa Meng
(Dream induced by Evil Energy)

黄帝曰：愿闻淫邪泮衍奈何？岐伯曰：正〔正：《病沅》卷四虚劳喜劳萝候》无此字〕邪从外袭内，而未有定舍，反〔反：《灵枢略》并作“及”〕淫于藏，不得定处，与营卫俱行，而与魂魄飞扬，使人卧不得安而喜梦。气淫于府，则有余于外，不足于内；气淫于藏，则有余于内，不足于外。

Yellow Emperor asked: "What is the pathology of the dream induces by evil energy?" Qibo said: "When the evil energy which is harmful invades the body, it has no certain place to locate, when it reaches the internal organs, it circulates along with the Ying-energy and the Wei-energy, and loafs along with the spirit causing one can hardly sleep well and has dream often. Whenever the energy is in prosperity in the hollow organs, the Yang is overabundant, and the Yang energy which is outside is having a surplus, and the Yin energy which is inside is insufficient; when the energy is in prosperity in the solid organs, then Yin is overabundant, and the Yin energy which is inside is having a surplus and the Yang energy which is outside is insufficient."

黄帝曰：有余不足有形乎？岐伯曰：阴气盛则梦涉大水而恐惧，阳气盛则梦大火而燔焫，阴阳俱盛则梦相杀。上盛则梦飞，下盛则梦堕，甚〔甚：《医说》卷五《梦》条引无此字〕饥则梦取〔取：《病沅》卷四《虚劳喜梦候》作“卧”，“予”作“行”〕，甚饱则梦予。肝气盛则梦怒，肺气盛则梦恐惧、哭泣、飞扬〔哭泣、飞扬：《千金》卷一《序例诊候》“哭泣”下无“飞扬”二字〕，心气盛则梦善笑恐畏〔恐畏：《太平御览》卷三十九引无“恐畏”二字〕，脾气盛则梦歌乐、身体重不举，肾气盛则梦腰脊两解不属。凡此十二盛者，至而泻之，立已。

Yellow Emperor asked: "Is there any appearance manifesting the surplus or insufficiency of Yin and Yang of the internal organs?" Qibo said: "When the Yin energy is in prosperity, one will dream of wading across a broad river and be scared; when the Yang energy is in prosperity, one will dream of the blaze of a big fire; when both the Yin and Yang energies are in prosperity, one will dream of fighting and slaughtering; when the upper part is in prosperity, one will dream of flying up of oneself; when the lower part is in prosperity, one will dream of falling down; when one sleeps with hunger, he will dream of lying; when one sleeps after eating his fill, the will dream of walking; when the liver energy is in prosperity, one will dream of getting angry; when the lung energy is in prosperity, one will dream of being frightened and crying; when the heart energy is in prosperity, one will dream of laughing; when the spleen energy is in prosperity, one will dream of song and music, or becoming heavy of the body causing the inability of moving the extremities; when the kidney energy is in prosperity, one will dream of divorce and disconnection of the loins and the back. To the dream caused by the twelve energies which are in prosperity, if one knows on which organ the evil energy situates and prick with the purging therapy, it can be stopped.

厥〔厥:《中藏经》卷上第二十四作“邪”〕气客于心，则梦见丘山烟火。客于肺，则梦飞扬，见金铁之奇物。客于肝，则梦山林树木。客于脾，则梦见丘陵大泽，坏屋风雨。客于肾，则梦临渊，没居〔没居:《中藏经》卷中第三十作“投”〕水中。客于膀胱，则梦游行。客于胃，则梦饮食。客于大肠，则梦田野。客于小肠，则梦聚邑冲衢。客于胆，则梦斗讼自刳。客于阴器，则梦接内。客于项，而梦斩首。客于胫，则梦行走而不能前，及居深地窌苑〔《甲乙》宛:《病沅》卷四《虚劳喜梦候》无此二字〕中。客于股肱〔肱:《病沅》卷四《虚劳喜梦候》并无此字〕，则梦礼节拜起〔起:《甲乙》卷六第八并作“跪”〕。客于胞脜〔脜:《病沅》卷四《虚劳喜梦候》无此字〕，则梦溲便。凡此十五不足者，至而补之立已也。

“When the evil energy invades the heart, one will dream of smoke and fire in the hill; when it invades the lung, one will dream of the flying up of himself, and sees strange things made of metal; when it invades the liver, one will dream of trees, flowers and grasses in the woods; when it invades the spleen, one will dream of the hills and the waters in a large scale, and the houses destroyed by wind and rain; when it invades the kidney, one will dream of facing a deep abyss or pluging into the water; when it invades the bladder, one will dream of wandering; when it invades the stomach, one will dream of food and drinks; when it invades the large intestine, one will dream of the fields; when it invades the small intestine, one will dream of the crowded street; when it invades the gallbladder, one will dream of quarreling and litigation; when the evil invades the genitals, one will dream of sexual intercourse; when it invades the neck, one will dream of decapitation; when it invades the tibia, one will dream of failing to proceed when walking, or living under the ground; when it invades the thigh, one will dream of courteous kneeling; when it invades the bladder and rectum, one will dream of urination or loosening the bowels. To the dream caused by the fifteen kinds of insufficient energy, when one knows on which organ the evil energy situates and prick with the invigorating therapy, it can be stopped.”

顺气一日分为四时第四十四

Chapter 44
Shun Qi Yi Ri Fen Wei Si Shi
(The Human Healthy Energy in the Day and Night Corresponds with the Energies of the Four Seasons)

黄帝曰：夫百病之所始生者，必起于燥湿、寒暑、风雨、阴阳、喜怒、饮食、居处，气合而有形，得藏而有名，余知其然也。夫百病者，多以旦慧昼安，夕加夜甚，何也？岐伯曰：四时之气使然。

Yellow Emperor said："The initiation of the various diseases begins from the attack of exogenous evils, such as dryness, wetness, cold, summer-heat, wind and rain or from the internal damage such as disharmony of Yin and Yang, emotional upset, immorderate diet and abnormal daily life. When the evil energy invades into the body, it will be manifested in the pulse condition, when the evil energy enters into the internal organs, the disease with different names can be examined from the superficies and interior, and I have known them all. As to the various diseases, most of them are light in the morning, calm in the day, aggravates in the evening and become even worse in the night, and why is it?"Qibo said："They are caused by the different energies of the four seasons."

黄帝曰：愿闻四时之气。岐伯曰：春生夏长，秋收冬藏，是气之常也，人亦应之，以一日分为四时，朝则为春，日中为夏，日入为秋，夜半为冬。朝则人气始生，病气衰，故旦慧；日中人气长，长则胜邪，故安；夕则人气始衰，邪气始生，故加；夜半人气入藏，邪气独居于身，故甚也。

Yellow Emperor said："I hope to know how the energies of the four seasons influence the human body."Qibo said："The weather is normal when it generates in spring, grows in summer, collects in autumn and stores in winter, and the human energy corresponds with it. When one divides the day and night into four seasons, then, the morning is spring, the noon is summer, in the time of sunset, it is the autumn, and in the night, it is the winter. In the morning, the health energy of human body is like the generation of the spring energy and the evil energy is declining, thus, the patient is easy and the disease is light; at noon, the health energy of human body is prosperous like the growth energy of summer, as the prosperous growth energy can overcome the evil energy, thus, the disease is calm; in the evening, the health energy of human body is collecting like the autumn energy, the evil energy begins to generate, and the disease is aggravating; in the night, the health energy of human body is storing like the winter energy, and the evil energy resides alone in the body, thus, the disease becomes even worse in the night."

黄帝曰：其时有反者何也？岐伯曰：是不应四时之气，藏独主其〔主其：周本作“生甚”〕病者，是必以藏气之所不胜时者甚，以其所胜时者起也。黄帝曰：治之奈何？岐伯曰：顺天之时，而病可与期。顺者为工，逆者为粗。

Yellow Emperor said: "In some diseases, their conditions are not agreeable to what you said, and why is it?" Qibo said: "It is the case when the disease is not corresponding with the energies of the four seasons, and a single viscus has contracted a serious disease. When the energy of the viscus is subjugated by the energy of the day, such as: the spleen disease encounters the day of wood, the lung disease encounters the day of fire, the kidney disease encounters the day of earth, the liver disease encounters the day of metal and the heart disease encounters the day of water, the disease will be aggravated; when the energy of the viscus is supported or agreeable with that of the day, such as; the spleen disease encounters the days of fire and earth, the lung disease encounters the days of earth and metal, the kidney disease encounters the days of metal and water, the liver disease encounters the days of water and wood; and the heart disease encounters the days of wood and fire, the disease will be somewhat alleviated." Yellow Emperor asked: "How to treat it?" Qibo said: "When one can treat agreeably or treat with the weather change of nature, the aggravation and alleviation of the disease can be anticipated. When one treats agreeably, he is a good physician, when one treats reversely, he is a physician of lower level."

黄帝曰：善。余闻刺有五变，以主五输，愿闻其数。岐伯曰：人有五藏，五藏有五变，五变有五输，故五五二十五输，以应五时。

Yellow Emperor said: "Good. I am told in pricking, there are five variations which take the five kinds of acupoints as the main points, I hope to hear about the rules." Qibo said: "In human body, there are five solid organs, each of them has the different variations in colour, time, date, tone and taste, each of the variations can be occurred in the five kinds of acupoint of Well, Xing, Shu, Jing and He. In the five solid organs, there are altogether twenty five acupoints which correspond to the five seasons of spring, summer, long summer, autumn and winter."

黄帝曰：愿闻五变。岐伯曰：肝为牡藏，其色青，其时春，其音角，其味酸，其日甲乙〔其日甲乙：《甲乙》卷一第二“其日甲乙”在“其时春”下，应据移正〕。心为牡藏，其色赤，其时夏，其日丙丁，其音徵，其味苦。脾为牝藏，其色黄，其时长夏，其日戊己，其音宫，其味甘。肺为牝藏，其色白，其音商〔其音商，其时秋：按《甲乙》卷一第二“其音商”在“其日庚辛”下，应据移正〕，其时秋，其日庚辛，其味辛。肾为牝藏，其色黑，其时冬，其日壬癸，其音羽，其味咸。是为五变。

Yellow Emperor said: "I hope to hear about the five variations." Qibo said: "The liver is a viscus of Yang, among the five colours, it is green, among the seasons, it is spring, among the decimal cycles of a day, it is Jia and Yi, among the five tones, it is Jue, and among the five tastes, it is sourness. The heart is a viscus of Yang, among the five colours, it is red, among the seasons, it is summer, among the decimal cycles of a day, it is Bing and Ding, among the five tones, it is Zhi, and among the five tastes, it is bitterness. The spleen is a viscus of Yin, among the five colours, it is yellow, among the seasons, it is long summer, among the decimal cycles of a day, it is Wu and Ji, among the five tones, it is Gong, and among the five tastes, it is sweetness. The lung is a viscus of Yin, among the five colours, it is white, among the seasons, it is autumn, in the decimal cycles of a day, it is Geng and Xin, among the five tones, it is Shang, and among the five tastes, it is acridness. The kidney is a viscus of Yin, among the five colours, it is black, among the seasons, it is winter, in the decimal cycles of a day, it is Ren and Gui, among the five tones, it is Yu, and among the five tastes, it is saltiness. These are the five variations which are corresponding to the five solid organs."

黄帝曰：以主五俞奈何？岐伯曰：藏主冬，冬刺井；色主春，春刺荥；时主夏，夏刺俞；音主长夏，长夏刺经；味主秋，秋刺合。是谓五变，以主五俞。

Yellow Emperor asked: "What are the conditions of the five kinds of acupoint dominated by the five variations?" Qibo said: "The five solid organs dominate the winter, in winter, one should prick the Jing-points (well) of the various channels; the five colours dominate the spring, in spring, one should prick the Xing-points of the various channels; the five seasons dominate the summer, in summer, one should prick the Shu-points of the various channels; the five tones dominate the long summer, in long summer, one should prick the Jing-points (channel) of the various channels; the five tastes dominate the autumn, in autumn, one should prick the He-points of the various channels. These are the conditions of the five variations dominating the five kinds of acupoint respectively."

黄帝曰：诸原安合，以致六输？岐伯曰：原独不应五时，以经〔以经：孙鼎宜曰："以经当作"以脏"〕合之，以应〔以应：孙鼎宜曰："以应当作"不应"〕其数，故六六三十六输。

Yellow Emperor asked: "What about the Yuan-point, how should it be allocated to coincide with the number of six kinds of acupoint in the hollow organs?" Qibo said: "The Yuan-points in the hollow organs are not corresponding to the five seasons, they will not fit the number of the six hollow organs when one coordinates it with the five solid organs. In the six hollow organs, there are thirty six acupoints."

黄帝曰：何谓藏主冬，时主夏，音主长夏，味主秋，色主春？愿闻其故。岐伯曰：病在藏者，取之井；病变于色者，取之荥；病时间时甚者，取之俞；病变于音者，取之经，经满而血者〔经满而血者：《甲乙》卷一第二校注："经"一作"络"。按似应作"病变于音络血而满者，取之经"〕；病在胃，及以饮食不节得病者，取之于〔于：按"于"字衍，应据《甲乙》卷一第二删〕合。故命曰味主合。是谓五变〔变：周本，日刻本作"病"〕也。

Yellow Emperor asked: "What is the meaning of the five solid organs dominate the winter, the five seasons dominate the summer, the five tones dominate the long summer, the five tastes dominate the autumn and the five colours dominate the spring?" Qibo said: "When the disease is in the five solid organs, the Jing-points (well) of various channels should be pricked, when the disease manifested on the complexion, the Xing-points (channel) of various channels should be pricked, when the disease is alleviated and aggravated now and then, the Shu-points of various channels should be pricked, when the disease is manifested in the voice and when the collateral is full with stagnated blood, the Jing-points of various channels should be pricked, to the disease of stomach and the diseases caused by intemperance of food and drink, the He-points of various channels should be pricked, as the disease of stomach is due to foods taken from mouth, so, the He-point dominates the tastes. These are the principles of pricking in the five kinds of diseases stated above."

外揣第四十五

Chapter 45
Wai Chuai
(Determination from Outside)

黄帝曰：余闻九针九篇，余亲授其调〔余亲授其调：《太素》卷十九《要知道》“授”作“受”〕，颇得其意。夫九针者，始于一而终于九，然未得其要道也。夫九针者，小之〔之：《甲乙》卷五第七无此字〕则无内，大之则无外，深不可为下，高不可为盖〔深不可为下，高不可以盖：《甲乙》卷五第七无“深不”十字〕，恍惚无穷，流溢无极，余知其合于天道人事四时之变也，然余愿〔愿：《太素》卷十九《要知道》“愿”下有“闻”字〕杂之毫毛，浑束为一，可乎？岐伯曰：明乎哉问也，非独针道焉，夫治国亦然。

Yellow Emperor said: “I have heard the nine-chapter about the nine kinds of needle, I have grasped its meaning personlly and know the meaning from the first kind to the ninth kind of needles approximately, but I do not understand its meaning thoroughly. In the principle of the nine kinds of needle, its meticulousness contained inside can not be smaller, and its extensiveness involved outside can not be larger. Its profoundness seem dim and boundless, and its applications are overflowing without end. I know its conditions are changing along with the law of heaven, the affairs of man and the variations of the four seasons, but I want to know whether it is possible to sum up the details which are as fine as the fine hair into a general programme?”Qibo said: “You are asking a brilliant question, it is not only necessary to have a general programme in acupuncture, but also necessary to have one in ruling a country.”

黄帝曰：余愿闻针道，非国事也。岐伯曰：夫治国者，夫惟道焉，非道，何可小大深浅，杂合而为一乎？

Yellow Emperor said: “What I want to hear is about the principle of acupuncture, not ruling a country.” Qibo said: “When ruling a country, it must base on a principle, if there is no principle, how can one sum up the tremendous small and large, complex and simple things into a general programme?”

黄帝曰：愿卒闻之。岐伯曰：日与月焉，水与镜焉，鼓与响焉。夫日月之明，不失其影，水镜之察，不失其形，鼓响之应，不后其声，动摇则应和，尽得其情。

Yellow Emperor said: “I hope to hear the details about it.” Qibo said: “It can be analogized with the sun and moon, water and the mirror and the drum and the sound of the drumbeat; the sun and moon are bright, but they can by no means without shadow, the water and the mirror are limpid and clear, but they can by no means remove their physical form, the responding sound of the drum can by no means later than the drumstick hitting the drum, and one will know the existence whenever there is a response. When one understands all of them, he will be able to master the therapy of acupuncture."

黄帝曰：窘乎哉！昭昭之明不可蔽。其不可蔽，不失阴阳也。合而察之，切而验之，见而得之，若清水明镜之不失其形也。五音不彰，五色不明，五藏波荡，若是则内外相袭，若鼓之应桴，响之应声，影之似形。故远者司外揣内，近者司内揣外，是谓阴阳之极，天地之盖，请藏之灵兰之室，弗敢使泄也。

Yellow Emperor said: "How critical! The illuminating light can not be concealed as it can not be divorced from the principle of Yin and Yang opposing each other. In treating, one should examine the overall conditions of the patient, verify it through palpation and obtain the condition of the disease by inspection, in this way, the condition of the disease will be as clear as the water and mirror without distortion. The voice and the complexion of the patient are the reflections of the functions of the internal organs, when the five tones are not resounding, the five colours are not distinct, it shows the five solid organs are wavering; it is the case of the interior and the exterior affecting each other, the reflection outside will like the drum responding to the drumbeat, and like the shadow appearing simultaneously with the body. Therefore, when observing the voice and complexion of the patient from outside, one can determine the syndrome of the organ inside; when inspecting the conditions of internal organ from inside, one can determine the changes of the voice and complexion outside. It can be considered to be the extreme of Yin and Yang changes, and the principle involving heaven and earth. I will keep it in the library of orchid chamber and be careful not to lose it."

五变第四十六

Chapter 46
Wu Bian
(The Five Kinds of Affections)

黄帝问于少俞曰：余闻百疾之始期也，必生于风雨寒暑，循毫毛而入腠理，或复还，或留止，或为风肿汗出，或为消瘅，或为寒热，或为留痹，或为积聚，奇邪淫溢，不可胜数，愿闻其故。夫同时得病，或病此，或病彼，意者天之为人生风乎，何其异也？少俞曰：夫天之生风者，非以私百姓也，其行公平正直，犯者得之，避者得无殆，非〔非：孙鼎宜曰："'非'上脱'风'字"〕求人而人自犯之。

Yellow Emperor asked Shaoyu: "I am told at the beginnings of various diseases, they must be affected by exogenous evils of wind, rain, cold and summer-heat; when the evil-energy moves along the fine hair and enters into the striae, it can be transformed or retained at the same place; it may cause the swelling due to wind-evil with perspiration, or burst into diabetes, alternating episodes of chills and fever, protracted bi-syndrome and abdominal mass; when the abnormal evil energy disperses all over the body, the diseases will be in thousands of ways to be capricious, I hope to hear the reason about it. As the diseases are contracted by people simultanneously, why is it that the diseases are different since the diseases are all caused by the wind from nature?" Shaoyu said: "The wind from nature blows universally, it is fair and upright which will not be impartial to certain people, when one offends it, he will become ill, when one keeps away from it, he will have no danger; it is not the wind that seeks and injures the people, but the people who offend it on their own accord will become ill."

黄帝曰：一时遇风，同时得病，其病各异，愿闻其故。少俞曰：善乎哉问！请论以比匠人。匠人磨斧斤，砺刀削，斫材木。木之阴阳，尚有坚脆，坚者不入，脆者皮弛，至其交节，而缺斤斧焉。夫一木之中，坚脆不同，坚者则刚，脆者易伤，况其材木之不同，皮之厚薄，汁之多少，而各异耶。夫木之早花先生叶者，遇春霜烈风，则花落而叶萎；久曝大旱，则脆木薄皮者，枝条汁少而叶萎；久阴淫雨，则薄皮多汁者，皮溃而漉；卒风暴起，则刚脆之木，枝折杌伤；秋霜疾风，则刚脆之木，根摇而叶落。凡此五者，各有所伤，况于人乎。

Yellow Emperor said: "When different people encounter wind evil and contract diseases simultanneously, but the diseases contracted are different, I hope to hear the reason abut it." Shaoyu siad: "You have asked a very good question. Let me take the craftman to analogize it. When a craftman sharpens his axe and knife for chopping the wood, the firmness and the softnes of the Yang side (the side facing the sun of the tree) and the Yin side (the back side of the tree) are different, when chopping or cutting the wood, the firm part can hardly be split and the soft part can easily be cracked, as to the part which has knots, it can even damage the axe or knife. Among the pieces of wood, some are tough and some are crisp, the tough ones are strong and the crisp ones are easy to be broken, let alone the kinds of wood which are different, they have different thickness in the bark, and have different amount of juice inside. For a tree which blooms and grows the leaves early, when encounters the frost in spring or violent winds, the flowers will be falling and the leaves withered; when a tree is scorched by the violent sun or encounters the severe drought, if the wood is weak and the bark is thin, the moisture content in the branches will be reduced, causing the leaves to become withered; when the protracted cloudy days and the long spell of wet weather are encountered, if the bark is thin and has plenty moisture content in the trunk, the bark will become deteriorated with water seeping out; when the sudden gale is encountered, if the wood is hard and crisp, the branches will be broken and the trunk injured; when the autumn frost and swift wind are encountered, if the wood is hard and crisp, its root will be wavering and the leaves falling. In the five different conditions of wood stated above, all of them have different damages respectively, let alone man."

黄帝曰：以人应木奈何？少俞答曰：木之所伤也，皆伤其枝，枝之刚脆而坚〔刚脆而坚：按“脆”字疑误，似应作“刚而坚者”〕，未成伤也。人之有常病也，亦因其骨节皮肤腠理之不坚固者，邪之所舍也，故常为病也。

Yellow Emperor asked: "What is the condition when comparing the man with a tree?" Shaoyu said: "When a tree is injured, the injury is in the branches, if the branches are sturdy and firm, they may not be injured at all. When a man is ill often, it is usually due to the infirmity of the bone and the striae of skin, and the bone joint and the striae are the places where the evil-energy often retains to cause diseases."

黄帝曰：人之善病风厥漉汗者，何以候之？少俞答曰：肉不坚，腠理疏，则善病风。黄帝曰：何以候肉之不坚也？少俞答曰：䐃肉不坚，而无分理，理者粗理〔理者粗理：《甲乙》卷第二上作“肉不坚”〕，粗理而皮不致者，腠理疏。此言其浑然者。

Yellow Emperor asked: "How to examine the reasons when one contracts jue-syndrome due to wind-evil often?" Shaoyu answered: "When one's muscle is not firm and substantial and his striae of skin are loose, he will contract syndrome due to wind often." Yellow Emperor asked: "How to examine when the muscle is not firm and substantial?" Shaoyu answered: "When the muscles of the shoulder, elbow, thigh and knee are not firm and substantial without texture of skin, it shows the infirmity and insubstantiality of them. When one's muscle is not firm, and has coarse and thin skin, his striae of skin must be loose and he is apt to contract wind evil. This is the approximate condition about it."

黄帝曰：人之善病消瘅者，何以候之？少俞答曰：五藏皆柔弱者，善病消瘅。黄帝曰：何以知五藏之柔弱也？少俞答曰：夫柔弱者，必有刚强〔刚强：周本无此二字〕，刚强多怒，柔者易伤也。黄帝曰：何以候柔弱之与刚强？少俞答曰：此人薄皮肤而目坚固以深者，长冲〔冲：《甲乙》卷十一第六作“衡”〕直扬，其心刚，刚则多怒，怒则气上逆，胸中蓄积，血气逆留，𦡱皮充饥〔𦡱皮充饥：《甲乙》卷十一第六任务“腹皮充胀”〕，血脉不行，转而为热，热则消肌肤〔肤：《甲乙》卷十一第六无此字〕，故为消瘅，此言其人暴刚而肌肉弱者也。

Yellow Emperor asked: "How to examine the reasons when one is apt to contract diabetes?" Shaoyu answered: "When one's five solid organs are weak, he is apt to contract diabetes." Yellow Emperor asked: "How can one know the five solid organs of the patient are weak?" Shaoyu answered: "When one's five solid organs are weak, he must be resolute in temperament and often gets angry, and when one has weak solid organs, he is apt to contract diabetes." Yellow Emperor asked: "How to examine the characteristics of weakness and resoluteness?" Shaoyu answered: "The skin of this kind of people is thin, when seeing things, his sight is firm, his eyeballs are sunken deeply with erected eyebows and wide-openned eyes to stare straightly with beaming rays. This kind of people is having a firm character and often gets angry, causing the energy reversing up to acumulate in the chest, in this way, the blood will be retained and impeded, the abdomen will be swelling and the circulation of the blood will be abnormal to cause the syndrome of stagnated heat, when the stagnated heat scorches the muscle and skin, diabetes will occur. This is the case when one is resolute in temperament but weak in the muscle."

黄帝曰：人之善病热者，何以候之？少俞答曰：小骨弱肉者〔小骨弱肉：按："弱肉"下脱"色不一"三字〕，善病寒热。黄帝曰：何以候骨之小大，肉之坚脆，色之不一也。少俞答曰：颧骨者，骨之本也。颧大则骨大，颧小则骨小。皮肤薄而其肉无䐃，其臂懦懦然，其地色殆然，不与其天同色，污然独异，此其候也。然后臂薄者，其髓不满，故善病寒热也。

Yellow Emperor asked: "How to examine the reasons when one often contracts cold and heat?" Shaoyu answered: "When one's skeleton is small, his muscle is weak, and the colours in his complexion are different, he is apt to contract cold and heat often." Yellow Eperor asked: "How to examine the large or small size of the skeleton, the firm or weak build of the muscle and whether or not the colours in one's complexion is identical?" Shaoyu answered: "The cheekbone on the face is the foundation of the skeleton of the whole body. When one's cheekbone is large, his skeleton of the body will be large also, when his cheekbone is small, his skeleton of the body will be small also. When one's skin is thin without any protruding muscle, his arms will be weak. When one's colour of the chin is black which is different from the colour of the forehead like being covered with a sluggish and turbid coating causing its colour to be different with that of other parts on the face, the reason of the disease can be estimated. If one's arms and the muscles on the rear of thighs are not plump, his marrow and body fluid must be deficient, and he will contract cold and heat frequently."

黄帝曰：何以候人之善病痹者？少俞答曰：粗理而肉不坚者，善病痹。黄帝曰：痹之高下有处乎？少俞答曰：欲知其高下者，各视其部。

Yellow Emperor asked: "How to examine the reasons when one contracts bi-syndrome often?" Shaoyu answered: "When one's texture of the skin is coarse, and his muscle is not firm and substantial, he will contract bi-syndrome often." Yellow Emperor asked: "When the bi-syndrome occurs, is it certain to occur on the upper part or the lower part of the body?" Shaoyu answered: "When one wants to know whether the bi-syndrome will occur on the upper or the lower part, he should examine the conditions of the five solid organs."

黄帝曰：人之善病肠中积聚者，何以候之？少俞答曰：皮肤薄而不泽，肉不坚而淖泽〔而淖泽：按："而"下应有"不"字〕，如此则肠胃恶，恶则邪气留止，积聚乃伤〔伤：《甲乙》卷八第二并作"作"〕。脾胃之间，寒温不次，邪气稍至；稸积留止，大聚乃起。

Yellow Emperor saked: "How to examine the reasons when one is apt to contract the intestinal mass?" Shaoyu answered: "When one's skin is emaciated, thin and not smooth, and the muscle is not substantial nor moist, it is due to the injury of the stomach and the intestine causing the evil-energy retaining inside, and consequently, the syndrome of mass will occur. If the food is indigested in the stomach and intestine, or the temperature of the food is maladjusted, the evil energy will invade into the spleen and stomach, and its retention in the abdomen will form the serious disease of large mass."

黄帝曰：余闻病形，已知之矣，愿闻其时。少俞答曰：先立其年，以知其时，时高则起，时下则殆，虽不陷下，当年有冲通，其病必起，是谓因形而生病，五变之纪也。

(According to the note of Danboyuan, this paragraph is supposed to be positioned here wrongly, hence, the English translation here is omitted.)

本脏第四十七

Chapter 47
Ben Zang
(The Various Conditions of Internal Organs Relating Different Diseases)

黄帝问于岐伯曰：人之血气精神者，所以奉生而周于性命者也。经脉者，所以行血气而营阴阳，濡筋骨，利关节者也。卫气者，所以温分肉，充皮肤，肥腠理，司关合者也。志意者，所以御精神，收魂魄，适寒温，和喜怒者也。是故血和则经脉流行，营覆阴阳，筋骨劲强，关节清利矣。卫气和则分肉解利，皮肤调柔，腠理致密矣。志意和则精神专直，魂魄不散，悔怒不起，五藏不受邪矣。寒温和则六府化谷，风痹不作，经脉通利，肢节得安矣。此人之常平也。五藏者，所以藏精神血气魂魄者也。六府者，所以化水谷而行津液者也。此人之所以具受于天也，无愚智贤不肖，无以相倚也，然有其独尽天寿，而无邪僻之病，百年不衰，虽犯风雨卒寒大暑，犹有弗能害也；有其不离屏蔽室内，无怵惕之恐，然犹不免于病，何也？愿闻其故。

Yellow Emperor said to Qibo: "The blood, energy, essence of life and the spirit of man are the substances that maintain the body and abide with the life. The functions of the channels of man are to promote the circulations of blood and energy, to operate the Yin and Yang, to moisten the tendon and bone and to smooth the joints; the functions of the Wei-energy of man are to nourish the muscle, to substantialize the skin, to enrich the striae and to control the opening and closing of the striae of skin; the functions of the will of man are to rein the spirit, to assemble the soul and the inferior spirit, to accommodate the weather changes of cold and heat and to adjust the excitation of the mood. Thus, when the blood is harmonious, the channel will be unimpeded causing the nutrition to reach the interior and exterior of the body, and hence, the tendons and bones will be strong and the joints facile; when the Wei-energy is harmonious, one's muscle will be comfortable, his nails and tendons will be smooth, his skin will be soft and his striae will be dense; when one's will is harmonious, his mind will be concentrated, his soul and inferior spirit will not be dispersing, and the anger and hatred will not appear, as his five solid organs are all harmonious, he can hardly be invaded by the evil-energy; when one can adapt the changes of the cold and hot weathers, the functions of transporting and transforming of the six hollow organs will be normal, the arthralgia due to wind-evil will not occur, the channels will be unimpeded, and the activities of the four extremities will be normal. These are the common conditions when the body is harmonious. In a word, the functions of the five solid organs are to store the essence of life, spirit, blood, energy, soul and the inferior spirit; the functions of the six hollow organs are to transport and transform the cereals and food, and to spread the body fluid to the whole body. These functions are endowed to all people from heaven, disregarding they are wise or stupid, worthy or unworthy. Newertheless, some people can enjoy a long life, they do not contract serious diseases, their bodies are not feeble even when they are old, and the rain, wind, sudden cold and severe summer-heat will not injure his health; but some people are different, they can by no means to evade diseases even when they often-stay in the room sheltered from wind and has not encountered anything terrible. I hope to hear the reason of it."

岐伯对曰：窘乎哉问也！五藏者，所以参天地，副阴阳，而连四时，化五节者也。五藏者，固有小大高下坚脆端正偏倾者；六府亦有小大长短厚薄结直缓急。凡此二十五者，各不同，或善或恶，或吉或凶，请言其方。

Qibo said: "Your question is very important. The functions and the activities of the five solid organs are in accordance with the heaven and earth, coordinate with the Yin and Yang, suit with the four seasons and correspond to the changes of the five seasons of spring, summer, long summer, autumn and winter. In the five solid organs, they are different in large or small, above or below, firm or fragile, upright or not, slanting or not, and the six hollow organs are different in size, length, thickness, crooked or straight, and pressing or not. In a word, the twenty five changes (in hollow organs, the change of the triple warmer is not counted as it is similar with that of the bladder) are different, they may be good or bad, may be a disaster or a blessing. Now, let me tell you the differences.

心小则安，邪弗能伤，易伤以忧；心大则忧不能伤，易伤于邪。心高则满于肺中，悗而善忘，难开以言；心下则藏外，易伤于寒，易恐以言。心坚则藏安守固；心脆则善病消瘅热中。心端正则和利难伤；心偏倾则操持不一，无守司也。

"When one's heart is small, the heart energy will be stable, he can hardly be injured by external evil energy, but he is apt to be injured by internal disturbances; when one's heart is large, he can hardly be injured by internal disturbances, but he is apt to be injured by exogenous evils. When the position of the heart is high, it will be fully covered by the lung, one will often be oppressive and forgetful, and he can hardly be enlightened by words; when the position of the heart is low, the heart energy will be tight, one is apt to be injured by cold-evil, and he is apt to be frightened by words. When one's heart is firm and substantial, the spirit stored inside will be stable; when one's heart is fragile, he will often contract diabetes and will have the retention of heat-evil in the middle warmer. When the position of the heart is upright, the heart energy will be harmonious, and one can hardly be injured by the exogenous evils; when the position of the heart is slanting, one can hardly keep a sound mind and he will not be able to handle things in an unanimous way.

肺小则〔肺小则：丹波元简曰："以前后文例推之，'肺小则'下恐脱'安'字"〕少饮，不病喘喝〔喝：《甲乙》卷一第五无此字〕；肺大则多饮〔则多饮：《千金》卷十七第一"则"下有"寒喘鸣"三字〕，善病胸痹喉痹〔喉痹：《甲乙》卷一第五无此二字〕逆气。肺高则上气肩息咳；肺下则居〔居：《甲乙》卷一第五作"逼"〕贲迫肺〔孙鼎宜曰："按'贲'当作

'鬲'，'肺'当作'心'"〕，善胁下痛。肺坚则不病咳上气；肺脆则苦病消瘅易伤。肺端正则和利难伤；肺偏倾则胸〔胸：《甲乙》卷一第五"胸"下有"胁"字〕偏痛也。

"When one's lung is small, his lung energy will be stable, he drinks little water and can hardly contract the disease of rapid respiration; when one's lung is large, he will contract the disease of rapid respiration in cold weather and he is apt to contract chest bi-syndrome and the adverseness of vital energy. When the position of the lung is high, the syndrome of the reversing up of the vital energy, breathing with elevation of shoulders and cough will occur; when the position of the lung is low, it will oppress the diaphragm and the heart, the pain under the hypochondria will occur. When one's lung is firm, he will not contract the syndrome of cough and the adverseness of vital energy; when one's lung is fragile, he will contract diabetes and apt to contract rapid respiration and epistaxis in hot weather. When the position of one's lung is upright, his lung energy will be harmonious, and he can hardly be injured by exogenous evil; when the position of one's lung is slanting, it will cause one to have partial pain of the chest and hypochondria.

肝小则藏〔藏：《甲乙》卷一第五无"藏"字〕安，无胁下之病〔病：张注本作"痛"〕；肝大则逼胃迫咽，迫咽〔迫咽：统本，金陵本并不叠此"迫咽"二字〕则苦膈中，且胁下痛。肝高则上支贲，切胁悗，为息贲；肝下则逼〔逼：《太素》卷六《五脏命分》作"安"〕胃，胁下空，胁下空则易受邪。肝坚则藏安难伤；肝脆则善病消瘅易伤。肝端正则和利难伤；肝偏倾则胁下痛也。

"When one's liver is small, the liver energy will be stable, the pain under the hypochondria will not occur; when the liver is large, it will oppress the stomach and the pharynx, one will have obstruction in the chest and pain under the hypochondria. When the position of the liver is high, it will reach up to prop the cardiac part causing contracture under the hypochondrium to become lumps located at right hypochondrium; when the position of the liver is low, the stomach energy will be stable, but it will be empty under the hypochondria causing one apt to contract exogenous evil. When one's liver is firm, his liver energy will be stable, he can hardly be injured by the exogenous evil; when one's liver is fragile, he will often contract diabetes and apt to be injured by exogenous evil. When the position of the liver is upright, the liver energy will be harmonious, and one can hardly be injured by exogenous evil; when the position of the liver is slanting, pain will occur under the hypochondria.

脾小则藏〔藏：《太素》卷六《五脏命分》无此字，下"肾小"节，《太素》亦"藏"字〕安，难伤于邪也；脾大则苦凑䏚而痛，不能疾行。脾高则䏚引季胁而痛；脾下则下加于大肠，下加于大肠则藏苦受邪。脾坚则藏安难伤；脾脆则善病消瘅易伤。脾端正则和利难伤；脾偏倾则善满〔善满：《甲乙》卷一第五"善满"作"瘈疭"〕善胀也。

"When the spleen is small, the spleen energy will be stable, and one can hardly be injured by the exogenous evil; when the spleen is large, it will often cause pain in the empty and soft part under the hypochondria and one will not be able to walk fast. When the position of the spleen is high, it will have drawing pain under the hypochondria; when the position of the spleen is low to attach the large intestine, the spleen is apt to be injured by the exogenous evil. When the spleen is firm, the spleen energy will be harmonious and the spleen can hardly be injured by the exogenous evil; when the spleen is fragile, one will apt to contract diabetes and he is apt to be injured by exogenous evil. When the position of the spleen is upright, the spleen energy will be harmonious, and one can hardly be injured by exogenous evil; when the position of the spleen is slanting, one will apt to contract clonic convulsion and abdominal distention.

肾小则〔则：《千金》卷十建筑物第一"则"下有"耳聋或鸣，汗出"六字〕藏安难伤；肾大则善病腰痛，不可以俯仰，易伤以邪。肾高则苦背膂痛，不可以俯仰〔不可以俯仰：《千金》卷十九第一作"耳脓血出，或生肉塞耳"〕；肾下则腰尻痛，不可以俯仰，为狐疝。肾坚则不病腰背痛；肾脆则善病消瘅易伤〔易伤：《太素》卷六《五脏命分》并无此二字〕。肾端正则和利难伤；肾偏倾则苦腰尻痛也。凡此二十五变者，人之所苦常病。

"When the kidney is small, the kidney energy will be stable and one can hardly be injured by the exogenous evil; when the kidney is large, one will have deafness, tinnitus, perspiration and apt to contract lumbago often, he will not be able to face up and down and apt to be injured by the exogenous evil. When the position of the kidney is high, one will have pain in the back, pus and blood flowing out from the ear or to have a wart stopping the ear; when the position of the kidney is low, one will have pain in the loins and the buttocks, he can hardly face up and down and will have the syndrome of inguinal hernia. When one's kidney is firm, he will have no pain in the loins; when one's kidney is fragile, he will have diabetes often. When the position of the kidney is upright, the kidney energy will be harmonious, and one can hardly be injured by the exogenous evil; when the position of the kidney is slanting, one will have partial pain in the loin and buttock. In short, the twenty five variations in the size, height, firmness, uprightness and slant of the five solid organs are the reasons for the human body to contract various diseases."

黄帝曰：何以知其然也？岐伯曰：赤色小理者心小，粗理者心大。无髑骬者心高，髑骬小短举者心下。髑骬长者心下〔下：《甲乙》卷一第五并无此字〕坚，髑骬弱小〔小：《千金》卷十三第一并无此字〕以薄者心脆。髑骬直下不举者心端正，髑骬倚一方者心偏倾也。

Yellow Emperor asked: "How to know the conditions of the size, height, firmness, uprightness and slant of the five solid organs?" Qibo said: "When one's skin is red with fine texture, his heart will be small; when the texture is coarse, his heart will be large. When one's sternal xiphoid process is not seen, the position of his heart will be high; when one's sternal xiphoid process is small and he is of chicken breast, the position of his heart will be low. When one's sternal xiphoid process is long, his heart will be firm; when one's sternal xiphoid process is weak and thin, his heart will be fragile. When one's sternal xiphoid process is not protruding, the position of his heart will be upright; when one's sternal xiphoid process is slanting to one side, his heart will be slanting.

白色小理者肺小，粗理者肺大。巨肩反膺陷喉者肺高，合腋张胁者肺下。好肩背厚者肺坚，肩背薄者肺脆。背膺厚者肺端正，胁偏疏者肺偏倾也。

"When one's skin is white and the texture is fine, his lung will be small; when one's texture is coarse, his lung will be large. When one's shoulders are tall, the chest is protruding outside and the throat is drawing back, the position of his lung will be high; when one's armpits are restraining and his hypochondria are opening, the position of his lung will be low. When one's shoulders are broad and his back is thick, his lung will be firm; when one's shoulders and back are thin, his lung will be fragile. When one's back and shoulders are broad and thick, the position of his lung will be upright; when one's chest is slanting, his lung will be slanting.

青色小理者肝小，粗理者肝大。广胸反骹者肝高，合胁兔骹者肝下，胸胁好者肝坚，胁骨弱者肝脆。膺〔膺：《甲乙》卷一第五"膺"下有"胁"字〕腹好相得者肝端正，胁骨偏举者肝偏倾也。

"When one's skin is green with fine texture, his liver will be small; when one's texture is coarse, his liver will be large. When the breadth between the two hypochondria is wide and the ribs are protruding, the position of one's liver will be high; when the breadth between the two hypochondria is narrow and the flat bones between the chest and the hypochondrium are concealing low, the position of one's liver will be low. When one's ribs are firm, his liver will be firm; when one's ribs are soft, his liver will be fragile. When one's chest, hypochodria and abdomen are matching, his liver will be upright; when one's ribs are slanting and protruding, his liver will be slanting.

黄色小理者脾小，粗理者脾大。揭唇者脾高，唇下纵者脾下。唇坚者脾坚，唇大而不坚者脾脆。唇上下好者脾端正，唇偏举者脾偏倾也。

"When one's skin is yellow with fine texture, his spleen will be small; when one's texture is coarse, his spleen will be large. When one's lipe are pursing up, the position of his spleen will be high; when one's lips are dropping, large and infirm, the position of his spleen will be low. When one's lips are firm, his spleen will be firm; when one's lips are large and infirm, his spleen will be fragile. When one's upper lip and the lower one are even, the position of his spleen will be upright; when one's lips are pursing up slantingly, the position of his spleen will be slanting.

黑色小理者肾小，粗理者肾大。高耳者肾高，耳后陷者肾下。耳坚者肾坚，耳薄不坚者肾脆。耳好前居牙车者肾端正，耳偏高者肾偏倾也。凡此诸变者，持则安，减则病也。

"When one's skin is black with fine texture, his kidney will be small; when one's texture is coarse, his kidney will be large. When the positions of the two ears are high, the position of his kidney will be high; when one's ears are bogging behind, the position of his kidney will be low; when the skin and muscle of one's ear are substantial, his kidney will be firm, when the skin and muscle of one's ear are thin and infirm, his kidney will be fragile. When one's ears are plump and situate in front of the two forehead angles, his kidney will be upright; when one of the ear is higher than the other one, his kidney will be slanting. To the condition in the five variations above, if it is well-maintained according to its specific condition, it can be remained stable, if it is maladjusted to cause injury, disease will occur."

帝曰：善。然非余之所问也。愿闻人之有不可病者，至尽天寿，虽有深忧大恐，怵惕之志〔志：熊本作“至”〕，犹不能减〔减：《甲乙》卷一第五作“感”〕也，甚寒大热，不能伤也；其有不离屏蔽室内，又无怵惕之恐，然不免于病者，何也？愿闻其故〔愿闻其故：《甲乙》卷一第五无此四字〕。岐伯曰：五藏六府，邪之舍也，请言其故〔请言其故：《甲乙》卷一第五无此四字〕。五藏皆小者，少病，苦燋〔燋：《太素》卷六《五脏命分》并作“焦”〕心，大〔大：《太素》卷六《五脏命分》无此字〕愁忧；五藏皆大者，缓于事，难使以〔以：《太素》卷六《五脏命分》无此字〕忧。五藏皆高者，好高举措；五藏皆下者，好出人下。五藏皆坚者，无病，五藏皆脆者，不离于病。五藏皆端正者，和利得人心〔心：《太素》卷六《五脏命分》无此字〕；五藏皆偏倾者，邪心而善盗，不可以为人，平〔平：《甲乙》卷一第五作“卒”〕反复言语也。

Yellow Eperor said："Good. But these are not what I want to know. I want to know why can some people enjoy a long life even when they encounter great misery and great fright to have terrible moods, they remain healthy and not being injured even encountering the bitter cold or scorching heat, but some other people can by no means to evade diseases even when they stay in the room sheltered from wind without any stimulations of deep sorrow or great fright?" Qibo said："The five solid and the six hollow organs are the places where the exogenous evils retain, when one's five solid organs are all small, the disease contracted will be light, but this kind of people often pay attention to worrying things which will unevitably cause them to become grieve; when one's five solid organs are all large, he will be slow in doing things, and he can hardly become sorrowful. When the position of the five solid organs are all high, one will crave after somthing high and far-reaching which is out of touch with reality; when the position of the five solid organs are all low, one will be weak-willed to rest content with remaining under others. When the five solid organs are all firm, one will not contract disease; when the five solid organs are all weak, one will not divorce from the disease. When the positions of the five solid organs are upright, one's disposition will be gentle and amiable; when the five solid organs are slanting, one will be harbouring wicked intentions, hankering for stealing, and his words are fickle."

黄帝曰：愿闻六腑之应。岐伯答曰：肺合大肠，大肠者，皮其应。心合小肠，小肠者，脉其应。肝合胆，胆者，筋其应。脾合胃，胃者，肉其应。肾合三焦膀胱，三焦膀胱者，腠理毫毛其应。

Yellow Emperor said："I hope to hear the conditions of the six hollow organs when being examined." Qibo said："The lung coordinates with the large intestine, as they are superficies and interior, one will know the condition of the large intestine when examining the skin; the heart coordinates with the small intestine as they are the superficies and interior, the condition of the small intestine can be examined by the channel; the liver coordinates with the gallbladder, as they are superficies and interior, the condition of gallbladder can be examined by the tendon; the spleen coordinates with the stomach, as they are superficies and interior, the condition of the stomach can be examined by the muscle; the kidney coordinates with the bladder and triple warmer, as they are the superficies and interior, the condition of the bladder and the triple warmer can be examined by the fine hair and the striae."

黄帝曰：应之奈何？岐伯曰：肺应皮。皮厚者大肠厚，皮薄者大肠薄。皮缓腹裹大者大肠大〔大：《甲乙》卷一第五并作“缓”〕而长，皮急者大肠急而短。皮滑者大肠直，皮肉不相离者大肠结。

Yellow Emperor asked: "How to examine it?" Qibo said: "When examining the lung, one should examine the conditions of the skin as the lung and the large intestine are the superficies and interior, thus, when the skin is thick, the large intestine will be thick; when the skin is thin, the large intestine will be thin. When the skin is loose and the abdomen is large, the large intestine will be loose and long; when the skin is tight, the large intestine will be tight and short. When the skin is smooth and moist, the large intestine will be smooth; when the skin and the muscle are not pressed close to each other, the large intestine will not be smooth.

心应脉，皮厚者脉厚，脉厚者小肠厚；皮薄者脉薄，脉薄者小肠薄。皮缓者脉缓，脉缓者小肠大而长；皮薄而脉冲小者，小肠小而短。诸阳经脉皆多纡屈者，小肠结。

"When one wants to know the conditions of the heart, he should examine the channel first. The heart and the small intestine are the superficies and interior, and the channel is under the skin, thus, when the skin is thick, the channel will be thick, and when the channel is thick the small intestine will also be thick; when the skin is thin, the channel will be thin, and when the channel is thin, the small intestine will also be thin. When the skin is loose, the channel will be loose, and when the channel is loose, the small intestine will be large and long; when the skin is thin and the channel is deficient and small, the small intestine will be small and short. When the various Yang channels and collaterals appear to be tortuous, the energy of the intestine will be stagnated also.

脾应肉。肉䐃坚大者胃厚，肉䐃么者胃薄。肉䐃小而么者胃不坚；肉䐃不称身者胃下，胃〔胃：《太素》卷六《脏腑应候》无此字〕下者下管约不利〔下管约不利：《太素》作“下脘未约”〕。肉䐃不坚者胃缓，肉䐃无小裹累者胃急。肉䐃多少裹累者胃结，胃结者上管〔上管：《太素》卷六《脏腑应候》“上管”上有“胃”字〕约不利也。

"When one wants to know the conditions of the spleen, one should examine the protruding muscle. As the spleen and the stomach are the superficies and interior, and the spleen controls the condition of the muscle, so, when the protruding muscle is large and firm, the muscle of the stomach will be thick; when the protruding muscle is thin and small, the muscle of the stomach will will be infirm; when the protruding muscle is not matching the body, one's stomach will be drooping to have gastroptosis, when the stomach is drooping, the lower outlet of the stomach will be restricted to cause difficulties of urination and loosening bowels. When the protruding muscle is infirm, the stomach energy will be loose and slow; when no small particles appeare on the protruding muscle, the stomach energy will be pressing; when there are many small particles appear on the protruding muscle, the stomach energy will be stagnated, in this way, the upper entrance of the stomach will be restricted and will cause difficulty of taking food and drink.

肝应爪，爪厚色黄者胆厚，爪薄色红〔色红：《太素》卷六《脏腑应候》无此二字。下

“色青”、“色赤”、“色白”、“色黑”并无〕者胆薄。爪坚色青者胆急，爪濡色赤者胆缓。爪直色白无约者胆直，爪恶色黑多纹者胆结也。

“When one wants to know the conditions of the liver, one should examine the nails. As the liver and the gallbladder are the superficies and interior, the liver controls the conditions of the nail, and the nail is the extention of the tendon, so, when the nail is thick, the gallbladder will be thick; when the nail is thin, the gallbladder will be thin. When one's nail is hard, his energy of gallbladder will be pressing; when one's nail is soft, the energy of the gallbladder will be mild. When the nail is flat without any line, the energy of gallbladder will be straight forward; when the nail is deformed with plenty of lines, the energy of gallbladder will be stagnated.

肾应骨。密理厚皮者三焦膀胱厚，粗理薄皮者三焦膀胱薄。疏腠理者三焦膀胱缓，皮急而无毫毛者三焦膀胱急。毫毛美而粗者三焦膀胱直，稀毫毛直三焦膀胱结也。黄帝曰：厚薄美恶皆有形，愿闻其所病。岐伯答曰：视其外应，以知其内藏，则知所病矣。

“When one wants to know the conditions of the kidney, one should examine the bone. The kidney controls the condition of the bone, and it corresponds with the condition of the triple warmer and the bladder. When one's skin-texture is fine and his skin is thick, the triple warmer and the bladder will be thick; when one's skin-texture is coarse and his skin is thin, his triple warmer and bladder will be thin. When one's skin-striae are loose, the energies of triple warmer and bladder will be moderate; when the skin is tight without any fine hair, the energies of triple warmer and bladder will be pressing. When the fine hairs are good looking and coarse, the energies of triple warmer and the bladder will be unimpeded; when the fine hair are few, the energies of triple warmer and the bladder will be stagnated and uneasy.” Yellow Emperor said: “Since the solid and hollow organs have different shapes in thickness and thinness, different in good and bad looking, I hope to know what diseases they will cause?” Qibo said: “When one examines the corresponding conditions outside, one will be able to estimate the changes of the internal organs, and thereby, the disease contracted will be known.”

禁服第四十八

Chapter 48
Jin Fu
(Understand the Channels Thoroughly before Pricking)

雷公问于黄帝曰：细子得受业，通于九针六十篇，旦暮勤服之，近者编绝〔近者编绝：《太素》卷十四《人迎脉口诊》作“远”。按“近”与“久”，上下误倒，应作“久者编绝，近者简垢”〕，久者简垢，然尚讽诵弗置，未尽解于意矣。外揣〔外揣：周本“揣”下有“其”字〕言浑束为一，未知所谓也。夫大则无外，小则无内，大小无极，高下无度，束之奈何？士之才力，或有厚薄，智虑褊浅，不能博大深奥，自强于学〔于学：《太素》卷十四《人迎脉口诊》“于学”下有“未”字〕若细子，细子恐其散于后世，绝于子孙，敢问约之奈何？黄帝曰：善乎哉问也！此先师之所禁，坐私传之也，割臂歃血之盟也，子若欲得之，何不斋乎。

Leigong asked Yellow Emperor："I have learned from you and I have understood the nine kinds of needle expounded in the《Sixty Chapters》. I study the related books very hard every morning and evening, in the books of old ages, some of their strings binding the bamboo slips are broken due to the long-term flipping through, in the books of recent years, some of the bamboo slips are stained due to the constant turning over, and I have insisted to keep on the reading without giving it up. However, I still can not understand their meanings thoroughly, especially the 'summing up the details like the fine hairs into a general programme' in the chapter of Wai Chuai (Determining from Outside), I don't know what it indicates. Since the principle of the nine kinds of needle can not be larger as it embraces all things outside, and it can not be smaller as it is incapable to contain anything, it reaches the extreme extent of large and small, and the realm of unfathomable height and depth. When one wants to sum it up into a general programme, how to do it? Moreover, in the talents of people, it may be profound or shallow, but in intelligence, most people are radical and superficial, they can not attain to the state of extensiveness and profoundness, besides, they do not study hard as I do. I am afraid the learning of the nine kinds of needle will be lost in the later generations, and it will be by no means to be learned by the descendants. Now, what should one do when one wants to simplify the principle of the nine kinds of needle?" Yellow Emperor said: "You have asked a very good question. The late masters had exhorted that it would be a crime when one imparts the principle privately. Before the impartation, the disciple must cut his arm and smear his mouth with the blood and swear an oath. Now, if you want to have the genuine impartmant, why don't you fast to show your sincerity?"

雷公再拜而起曰：请闻命于是也〔请闻命于是也：《太素》卷十四《人迎脉口诊》作“也于是”。“于是”二字属下读〕。乃斋宿三日而请曰：敢问今日正阳，细子愿以受盟。黄帝乃与俱入斋室，割臂歃血。黄帝亲〔亲：《太素》卷十四《人迎脉口诊》无此字〕祝曰：今日正阳，歃血传方，有〔有：《太素》卷十四《人迎脉口诊》无此字〕敢背此言者，反〔反：《太素》卷十四《人迎脉口诊》作“必”〕受其殃。雷公再拜曰：细子受之。黄帝乃左握其手，右授之书，曰：慎之慎之，吾为子言之。

Leigong bowed and again stood up and said: "I hope to hear your instructions." So, Leigong fasted for three days, came again to Yellow Emperor and said: "I hope to take the oath and receive your impartation today at noon." So, Yellow Emperor took Leigong to the fast hall, cut his arm and smear the blood on his mouth, then, Yellow Emperor said: "Today, at noon, I impart the acupuncture principles to you under the ceremony of smearing blood, if the oath is violated, you will have great disaster." Leigong bowed and again and said: "I accept what you said respectively and attentively". Then, Yellow Emperor took Leigong's hand with his left hand and presented the book with his right hand and said: "You must be very prudent in dealing with it. Now, let me tell you something more"

凡刺之理，经脉为始，营其所行，知其度量，内刺五藏，外刺六府，审察卫气，为百病母，调其虚实，虚实乃止，泻其血络，血尽不殆矣。雷公曰：此皆细子之所以通，未知其所约也。

"In the principle of pricking, one should study carefully the channels, measure the routes of circulation and know well their lengths and the sizes, their relations with the five solid organs inside and differentiate the relations with the six hollow organs outside; examine the Wei-energy which can defend outside when the Yang energy is stable, and when the Yang is deficient, the Wei-energy will not be guarding outside and diseases will occur. Besides, adjust the asthenia and sthenia, if the disease is of sthenic, purge the superficial venulus to cause bleeding, and when the stagnated blood in the superficial venulus is exhausted, the disease will be of no danger." Leigong said: "I knew all these principles before, but I don't know how to sum them up."

黄帝曰：夫约方者，犹约囊也，囊满而弗约，则输泄，方成弗约，则神与弗〔与弗：《太素》卷十四《人迎脉口诊》作“弗与”〕俱。雷公曰：愿为下材者，勿满而约之。黄帝曰：未满而知约之以为工，不可以为〔以为：《太素》卷十四《人迎脉口诊》“以”下无“为”字〕天下师。

Yellow Emperor said: "The so called 'the fixed way of pricking' is like the tying of the mouth of a bag, when the bag is full and it is not tied , the things in the bag will be let out, as many things are excluded, the ingenious curative effect will not appear along with the pricking treatment." Leigong said: "For the physicians who rest content with remaining in a lower level, they tie the mouth of the bag to sum up a general programme when the bag is not full." Yellow Emperor said: "When one can tie the mouth of the bag which is not full to sum up a general programme, he can be a superior physician, but he is not supposed to be a person of great learning and exemplary virtue."

雷公曰：愿闻为工。黄帝曰：寸口主中，人迎主外，两者相应，俱往俱来，若引绳大小齐等。春夏人迎微大，秋冬寸口微大，如是者名曰平人。

Leigong said: "I hope to know how can one to be a superior physician?" Yellow Emperor said: “When a superior physician palpates, he emphasizes on examining the pulse conditions of the Cunkou and Renying pulses, the pulse condition of Cunkou reflects the conditions of Yin of the five solid organs, and that of Renying reflects the conditions of Yang of the six hollow organs, the two pulses are corresponding to each other, come and go unanimously and unceasingly, the come and go of the Cunkou and Renying pulses which are affected by the respiration manifest unanimously like in tug of war, the string and man are moving unanimously. The pulsation of the Renying pulse is comparatively larger in spring and summer, as spring and summer belong to Yang; the pulsation of the Cunkou pulse is comparatively larger in autumn and winter, as autumn and winter belong to Yin. People with this kind of pulse condition are the normal people without disease.

人迎大一倍于寸口，病在足〔足:《太素》卷十四《人迎脉口诊》并无“足”字，下同〕少阳，一倍而躁，在手少阳〔一倍而躁，在手少阳，二倍而躁，病在手太阳，三倍而躁病在手阳明:《太素》卷十四《人迎脉口诊》、《甲乙》卷四第一上并无疑后人依本书《终始篇》增衍〕。人迎二倍，病在足太阳，二倍而躁，病在手太阳。人迎三倍，病在足阳明，三倍而躁，病在手阳明。盛则为热，虚则为寒，紧则为痛痹，代则乍甚乍间。盛则泻之，虚则补之，紧痛〔紧痛:《甲乙》卷四第一上“紧”下无“痛”字〕则取之分肉，代则取血络且饮药，陷下则灸之，不盛不虚，以经取之，名曰经刺。人迎四倍者，且大且数，名曰溢阳，溢阳为外格，死不治。必审按其本末，察其寒热，以验其藏府之病。

“When the Renying pulse is twice as large as the Cunkou pulse, the disease is in the Shaoyang Channel. When the Renying pulse is three times as large as the Cunkou pulse, the disease is in the Taiying Channel. When the Renying pulse is four times as large as the Cunlou pulse, the disease is in the Yangming Channel. When the Renying pulse is overabundant, it is the phenomenon of heat, when it is deficient, it is the phenomenon of cold. When the pulse is pressing, the cold-type bi-syndrome will occur; when the pulse is intermittent, the syndrome of now serious, now slight will occur; when the pulse is overabundant, apply purge therapy; when the pulse is deficient, apply invigorating therapy; when the pulse is pressing, prick the acupoints between the muscles; when the pulse is intermittent, prick the superficial venulus and administer medicine to the patient; when the pulse is deficient and apbogging, apply moxibustion; as to the pulse condition which is not sthenic nor asthenic, apply the ordinary way of pricking the proper channel. When the Renying pulse is five times as large as the Cunkou pulse, as the pulse is gigantic and rapid, it is called ‘rejection of Yang outside’ which is a fatal disease. In treating, one must inspect and palpate carefully the pulse conditions of the Cunkou reflecting inside and that of Renying reflecting outside, and examine the cold and heat of the disease to verify the extent of seriousness of the internal organs.

寸口大于人迎一倍，病在足〔《甲乙》卷四第一上并无足字，下同〕厥阴，一倍而躁，在手心主。寸口二倍，病在足少阴，二倍而躁，在手少阴。寸口三倍，病在足太阴，三倍而躁，在手太阴。〔一倍而躁，在手心足，二倍而躁，在手少阴，三倍而躁在手太阴。《甲乙》卷四第一上并无，疑为后人增衍〕盛则胀满、寒中、食不化、虚则热中、出縻、少气、溺色变、紧则痛痹，代则乍痛乍止。盛则泻之，虚则补之，紧则先刺而后灸之，代则取血络而后调〔后调：《太素》卷十四《人迎脉口诊》作“泄”〕之，陷下则徒灸之，陷下者，脉血结于中，中有著血，血寒，故宜灸之，不盛不虚，以经取之。寸口四倍者，名曰内关，内关者，且大且数，死不治。必审察其本末之寒温，以验其藏府之病。

“When the Cunkou pulse is twice as large as the Renying pulse, the disease is in the Jueyin Channel. When the Cunkou pulse is three times as large as the renying pulse, the disease is in the Shaoyin Channel. When the Cunkou pulse is four times as large as the Renying pulse, the disease is in the Taiyin Channel. When the Cunkou pulse is overabundant, the syndromes of abdominal distention, retention of cold-evil in the middle warmer and indigestion of the food will occur; when the Cunkou pulse is deficient, the syndromes of retention of heat-evil in the middle warmer, having stool like thoroughly cooked gruel, short of breath and yellow urine will occur; when the Cunkou pulse is pressing, the cold-type bi-syndrome will occur, when it is intermittent, the syndrome of now painful, now ceased will occur. When the pulse is overabundant, apply purge therapy; when the pulse is deficient, apply invigorating therapy; when the pulse is pressing, apply acupuncture first and then, apply moxibustion; when the pulse is intermittent, purge after pricking the superficial venulus; when the pulse is deficient and bogging, apply moxibustion only, as the deficient and bogging pulse is due to the stagnated blood in the superficial venulus, and cold causes the stagnation of blood, the cold should be dispersed by moxibustion. As to the pulse condition which is not sthenic nor asthenic, treat with the ordinary way according to the specific condition respectively. When the Cunkou pulse is five times as large as the Renying pulse, it is called 'shutting from inside to resist Yang' of which its pulse condition is gigantic and rapid, and it is a fatal disease. In treating, one must inspect and palpate carefully the conditions of Cunkou pulse reflecting inside and that of Renying pulse reflecting outside, and examine the cold and heat of the disease to verify the extent of the seriousness of the internal organs.

通其营〔营：《太素》卷十四《人迎脉口诊》并作“荥”〕输，乃可转于大数〔数：《甲乙》卷四第一上无此字〕。大数曰：盛则徒泻之，虚〔虚：《甲乙》卷四第一上有“小日”二字〕则徒补之，紧则灸刺且饮药，陷下则徒灸之，不盛不虚，以经取之。所谓经治者，饮药，亦曰〔曰：《甲乙》卷四第一止作“用”〕灸刺。脉急则引，脉大〔大：《太素》卷十四《人迎脉口诊》并作“代”〕以弱，则欲安静，用力无劳也。

“One can only impart the great method of acupuncture and moxibustion to others when he understands thoroughly the Xing and Shu points. To the patient whose pulse condition is gigantic and overabundant, purge threapy should be applied only; to the patient with tiny and deficient pulse condition, invigorating therapy should be applied; when the pulse is pressing, both acupuncture and moxibustion should be applied and the patient should take medicine also; when the pulse condition is deficient and bogging, apply moxibustion only; as to the disease which is not asthenic nor sthenic, apply ordinary treatment, that is, to administer medicine to the patient or apply acupuncture; when the pulse is pressing, prick to lead away the evil; when the pulse is intermittent, the patient should remain calm and he must not overfatigue to exert his strength difficultly.”

五色第四十九

Chapter 49
Wu Se
(The Five Colours)

雷公问于黄帝曰：五色独决于明堂乎？小子未知其所谓也。黄帝曰：明堂者鼻也，阙者眉间也，庭者颜也，蕃者颊侧也，蔽者耳门也，其间欲方大，去之十步，皆见于外，如是者寿必中百岁。

Leigong asked Yellow Emperor and said: "When examining the five colours in one's complexion, are they only determined on the location of Mingtang? I do not understand the meaning." Yellow Emperor said: "Mingtang or Hall means the nose; Que or the buildings along side of the palace's gate means the location between the two eyebrows; Tianting or the imperial court means the forehead; Fan or the fence means the sides of the two cheeks; Bi or barrier means the tragus. When the locations between these parts of a man appear to be upright and plump and one can see them in a single sight beyond ten paces, people of this kind will enjoy a long life of one hundred years old."

雷公曰：五官之辨奈何？黄帝曰：明堂骨高以起，平以直，五藏次于中央，六府挟其两侧，首面上于阙庭，王宫在于下极，五藏安于胸中，真色以致，病色不见，明堂润泽以清，五官恶得无辨乎。雷公曰：其不辨者，可得闻乎？黄帝曰：五色〔五色：《甲乙》卷一第十五"五色"上有"五脏"二字〕之见也，各出其色〔色：《甲乙》卷一第十五无此字〕部。部骨〔部骨：《甲乙》卷一第十五"部骨"上有"其"字〕陷者，必不免于病矣。其色部〔色部：二字互倒〕乘袭者，虽病甚，不死矣。雷公曰：官五色奈何〔官五色奈何：《甲乙》卷一第十五作"五官具五色何也"〕？黄帝曰：青黑为痛，黄赤为热，白为寒，是谓五官。

Leigong asked: "How to distinguish the colours in various sense organs which indicate the diseases?" Yellow Emperor said: "The nasal bone should be high and bulgy, upright and straight, the parts indicating the five solid organs situate in the middle of the nose in order and the six hollow organs supplement on the two sides. The Que and the Tianting above indicate the head and the face, the Xiaji which is between the two eyes indicates the heart, as heart is the monarch, so, Xiaji is called the imperial palace. When the five solid organs in the chest are stable and harmonious, the colours of the corresponding parts will be normal without any diseased colour and the colour on the nose will be smooth, moist and lucid. Under such situation, how can the diseased colour in the five sense organs be neglected?" Leigong said: "When one distinguishes it, what are the details?" Yellow Emperor said: "The diseased colours of the five solid organs will be manifested on the corresponding positions respectively, if the locations beside the centre are bogging, one will not be exempted from the disease. If the colour indicating a certain viscus appears on the location indicating its promoting viscus, such as, when the yellow colour (spleen) appears on Xiaji (heart), the patient will not die even if the disease is quite critical." Leigong asked: "What do the five colours indicate?" Yellow Emperor said: "Green and black indicate pain, yellow and red indicate heat and white indicates cold."

雷公曰：病之益甚，与其方衰如何？黄帝曰：外内皆在焉。切其脉口滑小紧以沉者，病益甚，在中；人迎气大紧以浮者，其病益甚，在外。其脉口浮滑者，病日进；人迎沉而滑者，病日损。其脉口滑以沉者，病日进，在内；其人迎脉滑盛以浮者，其病日进在外。脉之浮沉及人迎与寸口气小大等者，病难已。病之在藏，沉而大者，易已，小为逆；病在府，浮而大者，其病易已。人迎盛坚〔坚：《太素》卷十四《人迎脉口诊》作“紧”〕者，伤于寒；气口盛坚者，伤于食。

Leigong asked: "How to know when the disease is becoming aggravated or the evil-energy is declining?" Yellow Emperor said: "Both the hollow organs outside and the solid organs inside may fall into decline. When palpating the Cunkou, if the pulse condition is slippery, tiny, pressing and sunken, the disease will become aggravated day after day, and the disease is in the five solid organs; when the Renying pulse condition is gigantic, pressing and floating, the disease will be aggravated day after day also, and the disease is in the six hollow organs. When the Cunkou pulse condition is floating and slippery, the disease will be aggravated day after day; when the Renying pulse condition is sunken and slippery, the disease will be relieved day after day. When the pulse condition of Cunkou is slippery and sunken, the disease will be aggravated day after day, and the disease is in the five solid organs; when the Renying pulse condition is gigantic, pressing and floating, the disease will be aggravated day after day also, and the disease is in the six hollow organs. When the pulse condition is sunken or floating, and the gigantic or tiny conditions of the Renying and Cunkou pulses are similar, the disease can hardly be recovered. When the disease is in the five solid organs and the pulse is sunken and gigantic, the disease can easily be recovered; when the pulse is sunken and tiny, it is the adverse condition. When the disease is in the six hollow organs and the pulse is floating and gigantic, the disease can easily be recovered; when the pulse is floating and tiny, it is the adverse condition. The Renying pulse determines the condition of the superficies, when the pulse is overabundant and pressing, it shows one's Yang channels are injured by the cold-evil (exogenous evil); the Cunkou determines the condition of the interior, when the pulse is overabundant and pressing, it shows one's Yin channels are injured by the food (internal damage)."

雷公曰：以色言病之间甚奈何？黄帝曰：其色粗以明〔其色粗以明：“明”下脱“者为坚”三字〕，沉夭者为甚，其色上行者病益〔益：《甲乙》卷一第十五作“亦”〕甚，其色下行如云彻散者病方已。五色各有藏部，有外部，有内部也。色从外部走内部者，其病从外走内；其色从内走外者，其病从内走外。病生于内者，先治其阴，后治其阳，反者益甚；其病生于阳者，先治其外，后治其内，反者益甚。其脉滑大以代而长者，病从外来，目有所见，志有所恶〔恶：《甲乙》卷四第一上作“存”〕，此阳气〔阳气：《甲乙》卷四第一上“阳”下无

“气”字〕之并〔并：日抄本“并”作“病”〕也，可变而已。

Leigong asked：“How to illustrate the extent of the seriousness of the disease by examining the diseased colour in the complexion?” Yellow Emperor said：“When the patient's complexion is somewhat lustrous，the disease is light，when it is sunken and dark，the disease is serious. If the diseased colour is moving upwards，the disease will be aggravated，if the diseased colour is moving downwards like the floating clouds which are dissipating，the disease will soon be recovered. In the five diseases colours reflecting the various parts of the internal organs，some belong to the six hollow organs which are outside，some belong to the five solid organs which are inside. When the diseased colour is running from outside to inside，it shows the disease is entering into the interior from the superficies；if the diseased colour is running from inside to outside，it shows the disease is coming out from the interior to the superficies. When the disease starts from inside，the solid organs should be treated first，and then treat the hollow organs，if the treating is in the reverse sequence，the disease will be aggravated；when the disease starts from outside，the superficies should be treated first，and then treat the interior；if the treating is in the reverse sequence，the disease will be aggravated. When the pulse condition is slippery and gigantic or intermittent and long，it shows the evil is from outside. When one has photism or apt to have impractical wishful thinking，it is the disease of the overabundance of Yang，and it can be recovered when the Yang is restricted.”

雷公曰：小子闻风者，百病之始也；厥逆〔逆：“逆”是误字，似应作“痹”〕者，寒湿之起〔起：日抄本作“气”〕也，别之奈何？黄帝曰：常〔常：《甲乙》卷一第十五作“当”〕候厥中〔厥中：《甲乙》卷一第十五任务“眉间”〕，薄泽为风，冲浊为痹，在地为厥，此其常也，各以其色言其病。

Leigong said：“I am told that the wind-evil is the source of all diseases，and the bi-syndrome is due to the attack of the cold-wetness evil，how to distinguish them from the complexion of one's face?”Yellow Emperor said：“One should inspect the complexion between the two eyebrows，when the complexion is floating and lustrous slightly，it is the disease of wind，when the complexion is sunken and turbid，it is the bi-syndrome；when the diseased colour is in the lower part of the face (chin)，it is the jue-syndrome. These are the common ways of distinguishing them. In a word，the disease should be distinguished according to the complexion respectively.”

雷公曰：人不病卒死，何以知之？黄帝曰：大气入于〔于：金陵本作“干”〕藏府者，不病而卒死矣。雷公曰：病小愈而卒死者，何以知之？黄帝曰：赤色出两颧，大如母〔母：《甲乙》卷一第十五作“拇”〕指者，病虽小愈，必卒死。黑色出于庭，大如母指，必不病而卒死。

Leigong asked：“Some people die suddendly without any symptom，how can one know it in advance?”Yellow Emperor said：“When the great evil invades the internal organs，one can die suddenly without any symptom.” Leigong said：“In the case when the disease has turned to the better already but the patient dies all of a sudden，how can one know it in advance?” Yellow Emperor said：“When red colour appears on the two cheeks in the size of the thumb， although the disease has turned to the better already, yet the patient may die suddenly; when black colour appears on the forehead in the size of the thumb, the patient may die all of a sudden without any prominent symptom."

雷公再拜曰：善哉！其死有期乎？黄帝曰：察色以言其时。雷公曰：善乎！愿卒闻之。黄帝曰：庭者，首面也。阙上者，咽喉也。阙中者，肺也。下极者，心也。直下者，肝也。肝左者，胆也。下者，脾也。方上者，胃也。中央者，大肠也。挟大肠〔挟大肠：《甲乙》卷一第十五作"侠傍"〕者，肾也。当肾者，脐也。面王以上者，小肠也。面王以下者，膀胱子处也。颧者，肩也。颧后者，臂也。臂下者，手也。且内眦上者，膺乳也。挟绳〔绳：孙鼎宜曰："'绳'当作'日关'"〕而上者，背也。循牙车以下者，股也。中央者，膝也。膝以下者，胫也。当胫以下者，足也。巨分者，股里也。巨屈者，膝膑也。此五藏六府肢节〔肢节：《甲乙》卷一第十五作"支局"〕之部也，各有部分〔有部分：按此三字衍〕。有部分，用阴和阳，用阳和阴，当明部分，万举万当，能别左右，是谓大道，男女异位，故曰阴阳，审察泽夭，谓之良工。

Leigong bowed and again and said: "Good. Is there any definite date when people die suddenly?" Yellow Emperor said: "When one examines the change of the patient's complexion, the date of his death can be anticipated." Leigong said: "Good. I hope to hear about it." Yellow Emperor said: "The forehead associates with the diseases on the head and the face; the location above the middle of the eyebrows associates with the diseases of the pharynx and the throat; the location between the eyebrows associates with the diseases of the lung; the location between the eyes associates with the diseases of the heart; the location from the middle of the eyes straight to the nasal bone associates with the diseases of the liver, on the left of the location associates with the diseases of the gallbladder; the location below the nasal bone to the apex of the nose associates with the diseases of the spleen; slightly above the two sides of the apex of the nose associates with the diseases of the stomach; the location of the centre of the face associates with the diseases of the large intestine; the locations along side of the two cheeks associate with the diseases of the kidney; the location below the cheek which reflects the condition of the kidney associates with the diseases of the navel; the locations above the two sides of the apex of the nose associate with the diseases of the small intestine; the location of the nasolabial groove below the apex of the nose associates with the diseases of the bladder and the uterus. As with the diseases related to the four extremities determined by the various parts are: the cheekbone determins the shoulder; the location behind the cheek determines the arm; the location below it determines the hand; the location above the inner canthus determines the chest and the breast; above the location press close to the pupil determines the back; below the Yache (under the ear) of the curved bone of jaw determines the thigh; the location in the center of the two jawbones determines the knee; the location below it determines the leg; the location below it determines the foot; the large line beside the corner of the mouth determines the inner flank of the thigh; the location of the curved bone under the cheek determines the knee cap. These are the allocated positions indicating various diseases of the five solid organs and the six hollow organs, and each of them has its own position. In treating, promote Yang to match the Yin or promote Yin to match the Yang. As long as one can examine and know clearly the colour shown on the certain part of the face, his diagnose and treating will always be suitable. When one can distinguish the running leftwards of Yang and the running rightwards of Yin, he will come to the thoroughfare of understanding the principle of Yin and Yang. Since the positions showing the agreeable and adverseness of diseases of a man or a woman are different, one must know the law of Yin and Yang, besides, one must examine the lustrous or gloomy complexion of the patient to diagnose the good or bad condition of the disease. When one can do it in this way, he is deserved to be called a good physician.

沉浊为内，浮泽〔泽：《甲乙》卷一第十五作“清”〕为外，黄赤为风〔风：按“风”当是“热”之误〕，青黑为痛，白为寒，黄而膏润为脓，赤甚者为血，痛甚为挛，寒甚为皮不仁。五色各见其部，察其浮沉，以知浅深，察其泽夭，以观成败，察其散抟，以知远近，视色上下，以知病处，积神于心，以知往今。故相气不微，不知是非，属意勿去，乃知新故。色明不粗，沉夭为甚〔沉夭为甚：按本句与下“其病不甚”句误倒，应乙作“色明不粗，其病不甚；不明不泽，沉夭为甚”〕；不明不泽，其病不甚。其色散，驹驹然，未有聚；其病散而气痛，聚未成也。

“When one's complexion is sunken and turbid, the disease is in the solid organs inside, when it is floating and lucid, the disease is in the hollow organs outside. When the colour is yellow and red, it shows heat, when the colour is green and black, it shows pain, when the colour is white, it shows cold. When the complexion is yellow and lustrous like oil, it shows the carbuncle will turn into suppuration; when the colour is dark, it shows there is the retention of blood; when the pain is severe, it will turn into contracture of muscle, and when the invasion of cold-evil is severe, the skin will be numb. The five colours manifest on various parts, when examining the floating or sunken condition of the colour, the extent of seriousness of the disease can be known; when examining the moistness and dryness of the colour, the condition of whether the disease will turn to better or worse can be estimated; when examining the scattering and the assembling condition of the colour, the condition of whether the contracted disease is recent or remote can be known; when examining the up and down position of the colour, the location of the disease can be known, when one is utterly concentrated in examining the colour, he will be able to know the present and the past condition of the disease. Therefore, if one does not examine the complexion carefully, he will not be able to know the sthenia and the asthenia of the disease, and one can only know the past and the present condition of the disease when examining whole-heartly. When the complexion of the patient is lustrous and not coarse, his disease will not be very serious; when his complexion is dark without any lustre and looks sunken and turbid, the disease will be serious. When the colour is dispersing, nice looking and not concentrated in a definite location, it shows the patient has no abdominal mass; when the disease of the patient is alleviating and he has pain due to the disorder of vital energy only, it shows the abdominal mass has not yet shapped.

肾乘心，心先病，肾为应，色皆如是。

"When the kidney subjugates the heart excessively, it is because the heart is diseased in advance, in this case, the black colour which corresponds to the kidney will appear on the location indicating the viscus which is subjugated excessively (heart) and the cases in other viscera are all the same.

男子色在于面王，为小腹痛，下为卵痛，其圜直为茎痛，高为本，下为首，狐疝㿉阴〔《甲乙》卷一第十五"阴"下有"病"字〕之属也。

"When the diseased colour of a man appears above the apex of the nose, it shows abdominal pain and the drawing pain of the testis; when the diseased colour appears on one's nasolabial groove (Shuigou point), his penis will be painful; when the pain is in the upper part of one's nasolabial groove, his root of penis will be painful; when the pain is in the lower part of one's nasolabial groove, his penis will be painful. These diseases are of the inguinal hernia and the pain on testes or penis kind.

女子〔女子："女子"下脱"色"字〕在于面王，为膀胱子处之病，散为痛，抟为聚，方员左右，各如其色形。其随而下至胝〔胝：《甲乙》卷一第十五作"骶"〕为淫，有润如膏状，为暴食不洁。

"When the diseased colour appears above the apex of the nose in a woman, it shows the diseases of the bladder and the uterus; when the diseased colour is scattered, it shows pain; when the diseased colour is assembling, it shows abdominal mass, and the shape of the mass will be square or round, on the left or on the right like the appearance manifested outside by the diseased colour. When the colour descends to the lip, the white secretion from one's vulva will occur. When one's complexion is bright and smooth like the lard, it is the symptom of glutton or the taking of the unclean food.

左为左，右为右，其色有邪，聚散而不端，面色所指者也。色者，青黑赤白黄，皆端满有别乡。别乡赤者，其色亦〔亦：与注本，张注本作"赤"〕大如榆荚，在面王为不日。其色上锐，首空上向，下锐下向，在左右如法。以五色命藏，青为肝，赤为心，白为肺，黄为脾，黑为肾。肝合筋，心合脉，肺合皮，脾合肉，肾合骨也。

"When the diseased colour is seen on the left side, it shows the disease is on the left, when the disease is seen on the right side, it shows the disease is on the right, when the diseased colour on the face is assembling or scattering in an abnormal way, if only the location of the diseased colour is distinguished, one will be able to know on which internal organ the disease locates. The so called the five colours are: green, black, red, white and yellow and they should be all lustrous, decent, substantial and moist, each of them appears on the location indicating a certain viscus; but sometimes, it appears on the location indicating other viscus, such as, the red colour of heart appears on the apex of the nose in the size of the elm's pod, however, when the condition of the disease changes in a few days, the shape of the colour changes along with it. If the diseased colour is sharp on the upper edge, it shows the energy in the head is deficient, and the evil energy will develope upwards; when the lower edge is sharp, the disease will develope downwards; when the sharp edge is on the left side or in the right side, one can determine the trend of development according to the examples above. As to the correspondance of the five viscera with the five colours, the green colour corresponds to the liver, the red colour corresponds to the heart, the white colour corresponds to the lung, the yellow colour corresponds to the spleen, and the black colour corresponds to the kidney. The liver coordinates with the tendon, the heart coordinates with the channel, the lung coordinates with the skin, the spleen coodinates with the muscle, and the kidney coordinates with the bone."

论勇第五十

Chapter 50
Lun Yong
(On Braveness)

黄帝问于少俞曰：有人于此，并行并立，其年之长少等也，衣之厚薄均也，卒然遇烈风暴雨，或病或不病，或皆病〔皆病：《甲乙》卷六第五作“皆死”〕，或皆不病〔或皆不病：《甲乙》卷六第五无此四字〕，其故何也？少俞曰：帝问何急？黄帝曰：愿尽闻之。少俞曰：春青〔青：《甲乙》卷六第五作“温”〕风，夏阳风，秋凉风，冬寒风。凡此四时之风者，其所病各不同形。

Yellow Emperor asked Shaoyu and said: "There are some people walking and standing here, they are all about the same age and the thickness of their clothes are about the same, but when they encounter the storm, they may sick or not sick, or they all die, and what is the reason?" Shaoyu said: "What do you want to know first?" Yellow Emperor said: "I hope to know all the cases." Shaoyu said: "The warm breeze dominates in spring, the summer breeze dominates in summer, the cool breeze dominates in autumn and the cold wind dominates in winter. The different winds in the various seasons will cause different diseases when affecting the body of a man."

黄帝曰：四时之风，病人如何？少俞曰：黄色薄皮弱肉者，不胜春之虚风；白色薄皮弱肉者，不胜夏之虚风；青色薄皮弱肉，不胜秋之虚风；赤色薄皮弱肉，不胜冬之虚风也。

Yellow Emperor asked: "What are the conditions when a man is affected by winds in the four seasons?" Shaoyu said: "When one's skin is yellow and thin, and his muscle is soft, he is the one whose spleen energy is deficient, and he will not be able to stand the abnormal wind (of wood) in spring; when one's skin is white and thin, and his muscle is soft, he is the one whose lung energy is deficient and he will not be able to stand the abnormal wind (of fire) in summer; when one's skin is green and thin and his muscle is soft, he is the one whose liver energy is deficient, and he will not be able to stand the abnormal wind (of metal) in autumn; when one's skin is red and thin and his muscle is soft, he is the one whose heart energy is deficient and he will not be able to stand the abnormal wind (of water) in winter."

黄帝曰：黑色不〔不：《甲乙》卷六第五“不”下有“能”字〕病乎？少俞曰：黑色而皮厚肉坚，固不伤于四时之风。其皮薄而肉不坚，色不一者，长夏至而有虚风者，病矣。其皮厚而肌肉坚者，长夏至而有虚风，不病矣。其皮厚而肌肉坚者，必重感于寒，外内皆然，乃病。黄帝曰：善。

Yellow Emperor asked: "Will people of black colour not contract disease?" Shaoyu said:

"People with black and thick skin and firm muscle will surely not easily be injured by the abnormal wind of the four seasons, if one's skin is thin without definite colour and his muscle is infirm, he will contract disease in long summer when encountering the abnormal wind, people of thick skin and firm muscle will not contract disease in long summer even when the abnormal wind is encountered. But, if the one who has thick skin and firm muscle is affected by wind-cold repeatedly and is injured from inside and outside, still, he can not be exempted from disease." Yellow Emperor said: "Good."

黄帝曰：夫人之忍痛与不忍痛者，非勇怯之分也。夫勇士之不忍痛者，见难则前，见痛则止；夫怯士之忍痛者，闻难则恐，遇痛不动。夫勇士之忍痛者，见难不恐，遇痛不动；夫怯士之不忍痛者，见难与痛，目转面〔面：刘校云："详文义应改为"而"〕盼，恐不能言，失气惊，颜色变化〔化：周本，日记本并作"更"〕，乍死乍生。余见其然也，不知其何由，愿闻其故。少俞曰：夫忍痛与不忍痛者，皮肤之薄厚，肌肉之坚脆缓急之分也，非勇怯之谓也。

Yellow Emperor said: "Some people can endure pain and some can not, and they are not distinguished by bravery and timidity. Some of the brave men can not endure pain, they stride bravely forward before difficulty, but stop when they encounter pain; some timid people can endure pain, they are afraid of difficulty, but they can remain unmoved perseivingly when encountering pain. As to the brave men who can endure pain, they are not afraid of difficulty and they can remain unmoved when encourtering pain as well; for the timid ones who can not endure pain, when they encounter the difficulty and pain, they only turn their eyes, stare angrily but dare not speak, they hold their breath, become startling, pale and harbouring all sorts of misgivings. I have seen all these conditions, but I don't know the reason, and I hope you can tell me." Shaoyu said: "Concerning the ability of enduring pain, it is due to whether the skin is thick or thin and whether the muscle is firm or crisp, loose or tight in different people, it can not be explained by bravery and timidity."

黄帝曰：愿闻勇怯之所由然。少俞曰：勇士者，目深以固，长衡〔衡：与注本，张注本并作"冲"〕直扬，三焦理横，其心端直，其肝大以坚，其胆满以傍，怒则气盛而胸张，肝举而胆横，眦裂而目扬，毛起而面苍，此勇士之由然者也。

Yellow Emperor said: "I hope to know what causes the difference of bravery and timidity." Shaoyu said: "For a brave man, his eyeballs are bogging deeply, his eyesight is firm when seeing things, his eyebrows are long and erecting, the textures of his muscle are coarse and striate, his heart is normal, his liver is large and firm, his gallbladder is full with bile and the bile is intense, when he gets angry, his breath is plenty and his chest is expanding, his gallbladder is horizontal when his liver is lifted, his eyesockets are busting and his eyes are flashing, his hairs are standing up and he has green complexion. These are the reasons of why he is a brave man."

黄帝曰：愿闻怯士之所由然。少俞曰：怯士者，目大而不减，阴阳相失，其焦理纵，䯏骭短而小，肝系缓，其胆不满而纵，肠胃挺，胁下空，虽方大怒，气不能满其胸，肝肺虽举，气衰复下，故不能久怒，此怯士之所由然者也。

Yellow Emperor said: "I hope to know the conditions of a timid man." Shaoyu said:

"For a timid man, his eyes are large but not bogging deeply, he often turns his eyes with fright, the textures of his muscle are loose and flaccid, his sternal xiphoid prccess is short and small, his liver is small and the bile in his gallbladder is not full and lacking, his intestine and stomach are rather straight with less curves, the locations under his ribs are empty, his liver energy is not substantial, when he is in a rage, his energy of anger can not fill his chest, even when the energies of the liver and the gallbladder rush up, they will fall into decline immediately, as his energy is deficient, he can hardly sustain the anger long. These are the reasons why he is a timid man."

黄帝曰：怯士之得酒，怒不避勇士者，何藏使然？少俞曰：酒者，水谷之精，熟谷之液也，其气慓悍，其入于胃中，则胃胀，气上逆，满于胸中，肝浮胆横。当是之时，固〔固：统本金陵本并作“同”〕比于勇士，气衰则悔。与勇士同类，不知避〔避：统本作“为”〕之，名曰酒悖也。

Yellow Emperor said:"When a timid man has drunk the spirit, his condition is about the same with a brave man when he gets angry, which one of the viscera causes it?"Shaoyu said: "The spirit is the essence of the water and cereals, and the property of the juice fluid of the matured cereals is light and swift, when it enters into the stomach, it will cause distention of the stomach, besides, it will cause the energy of the gallbladder to run amuck. By this time, the timid man seems similar with the brave man, but when he recovers from drunkenness, he will regret. A timid man is similar with a brave man after drunken, but the knows not what to do, it is called perplexion after drunken."

背腧第五十一

Chapter 51
Bei Shu
(The Back-shu Points of the Five Viscera)

黄帝问于岐伯曰：愿闻五脏之腧，出于背者。岐伯曰：胸〔胸：日刻本与注本，，终身注本并作“背”〕中大腧在杼骨之端，肺腧在三焦〔焦：《素问·血气形志篇》王注引作“椎”〕之间〔间：《素问·血气形志篇》王注引作“傍”〕，心腧在五焦之间，膈腧在七焦之间，肝腧在九焦之间，脾腧在十一焦之间，肾腧在十四焦之间，皆〔皆：周本，明本并作“背”〕挟脊相去三寸所，则欲得〔得：《太素》卷十一《气穴》无此字〕而验之，按其处，应在〔在：《太素》卷十一《气穴》无此字〕中而痛解，乃其腧也。灸之则可，刺之则不可。气〔气：《甲乙》卷三第八无此字〕盛则泻之，虚则补之。以火补者，毋吹其火，须自灭也；以火泻者，疾吹其火，传〔传：《太素》卷十一《气穴》“作傅”〕其艾，须其火灭也。

Yellow Emperor said to Qibo: "I hope to know the conditions of the shu-points of the five viscera on the back." Qibo said: "The main back-shu points (Dazhu BL. 11) are on the two sides of the first vertebra behind the neck; the Feishu points (back-shu points of the lung BL. 13) are on the two sides of the third vertebra; the Xinshu points (back-shu points of the heart BL. 15) are on the two sides of the fifth vertebra; the Ganshu points (back-shu points of the liver BL. 18) are on the two sides of the ninth vertebra; the Pishu points (the back-shu points of the spleen BL. 20) are on the two sides of the eleventh vertebra; the Shenshu points (back-shu points of the kidney BL. 23) are on the two sides of the fourteenth vertebra. These shu points are pressing close on the left and right sides to the spine, and each of them is one and half inches beside the spine. When one wants to find out the situation of the acupoint, press with the finger to seek the location of which the patient feels painful or the location where the pain is alleviated, and it is the situation of the shu-point. When treating the shu-point, apply moxibustion is permissible, and acupuncture must not be applied. In moxibustion, when the evil energy is overabundant, apply purge therapy; when the healthy energy is deficient, apply invigorating therapy. When invigorating with moxibustion, the fire of the moxa stick must not be blowed out, it should be extinguished all by itself after burning; when purging with moxibustion, the fire of the moxa stick should be blowed out swiftly, then pat the moxa floss with hand. The treating is accomplished only after the extinguishing of fire."

卫气第五十二

Chapter 52
Wei Qi
(On the Wei-energy)

黄帝曰：五脏者，所以藏精神魂魄者也。六腑者，所以受水谷而行化物者也。其气内干五脏，而外络肢节。其浮气之不循经者，为卫气；其精气之行于经者，为营气。阴阳相随，外内相贯，如环之无端，亭亭淳淳乎，孰能穷之。然其分别阴阳，皆有标本虚实所离之处。能别阴阳十二经者，知病之所生。候虚实之所在者，能得病之高下。知六腑〔府：《甲乙》卷二第四作"经"〕之气街者，能知解结契绍于门户。能知虚石之坚软者，知补泻之所在。能知六经标本者，可以无惑于天下。

Yellow Emperor said: "The five solid organs are to store the spirit, soul and the inferior spirit; the six hollow organs are to receive the water and cereals, and to transport the refined substances. The energy goes inside to the five solid organs and goes outside to the extremities. The energy that floats outside of the channel and does not run along the channel is called the Wei-energy; the refined energy that runs inside of the channel is called the Ying-energy. The Yin and Yang are following each other, and the interior and the exterior are communicating with each other like a ring which has no beginning and terminal. Who can exhaust the essence of its endless operation? Nevertheless, the Yin and Yang energies in the body have the different conditions of interior or superficies and asthenia or sthenia, when one can distinguish the twelve channels of Yin and Yang, he will be able to understand the reason of causing disease; when one can examine the situation of asthenia and sthenia, he will be able to know the upper or lower locations of the disease; when one knows the main routes of the coming and going of the six hollow organs, he will be able to know how to dissipate the mass and dredge the acupoints; when one knows the belongings of the sthenia and asthenia to the firmness and the softness, he will be able to know which channel should be invigorated and which channel should be purged; when one knows the root and branch of the six channels of hand and foot, he will be able to understand the diseases extensively without perplexion."

岐伯曰：博哉圣帝之论！臣请尽意〔尽意：《甲乙》卷二第四无此字〕悉言之。足太阳之本，在跟以上五寸中，标在两络命门。命门者，目也。足少阳之本，在窍阴之间，标在窗笼之前。窗笼者，耳也。足少阴之本，在内踝下上三寸〔上三寸：《千金》卷十九第一并作"二寸"〕中，标在背腧与舌下两脉也。足厥阴之本，在行间上五寸所，标在背腧也。足阳明之本，在厉兑，标在人迎颊挟颃颡也。足太阴之本，在中封前上四寸之中，标在背腧与舌本也。

Qibo said: "How extensive your comment is. I like to tell you all my views. The root of the Foot Taiyang Channel is the Fuyang point (BL. 59) which is five inches above the heel; its branch is the gate of life of the left and right collaterals which is the Jingming point (BL. 1). The root of Foot Shaoyang Channel is the Qiaoyin point (GB. 44); its branch is in front of the window shield, the so called window shield indicates the Tinggong point (SI. 19) in front of the ear. The root of the Foot Shaoyin Channel is the Jiaoxin point (KI. 8) which is two inches above the inner ankle of foot; its branches are the Shenshu point (BL. 23) on the back and the Lianquan point (RN. 23) in the two channels under the tongue. The root of the Foot Jueyin Channel is the Zhongfeng point (LR. 4) five inches above the Xingjian point; its branch is the Ganshu point (BL. 18) on the back; the root of Foot Yangming is the Lidiu point (ST. 45) its branch is the Renying point (ST. 9) which is the location where the cheek, pharynx, lower palate and the nose communicate. The root of the Foot Taiyin Channel is the Sanyinjiao point (SP. 6) in front and above the Zhongfeng point; its branch is the Pishu point (BL. 20) on the back and the root of the tongue.

手太阳之本，在外踝之后，标在命门之上一寸也。手少阳之本，在小指次指之间上二寸，标在耳后上角下外眦也。手阳明之本，在肘骨中，上至别阳，标在颜下合钳上也。手太阴之本，在寸口之中，标在腋内动也。手少阴之本，在锐骨之端，标在背腧也。手心主之本，在掌后两筋之间二寸中，标在腋下下三寸也。凡候此者，下虚则厥，下盛则热；上虚则眩，上盛则热痛。故石〔石：《太素》卷十《经脉标本》作“实”〕者绝而止之，虚者引而起之。

“The root of the Hand Taiyang Channel is the Yanglao point (SI. 6) behind the outer ankle of the hand; its branch is one inch above the Jingming point. The root of the Hand Shaoyang Channel is in the Yeman point (SJ. 2) which is two inches above the middle of the small finger and the ring finger; its branches are in the Jiaosun point (SJ. 20) on the upper corner behind the ear and the Sizhukong point (SJ. 23) beside the outer canthus. The root of the Hand Yangming Channel is in the Quchi point (LI. 11) from the elbow bone to the Binao point (LI. 14) above; its branch is in the Touwei point (ST. 18) below the forehead and beside the ear. The root of the Hand Taiyin Channel is in the Tainyuan point (LU. 9) in the Cunkou, its branch is Tianfu point (LU. 3) in the artery under the armpit. The root of the Hand Shaoyin Channel is in the Shenmen point (HT. 7) which is on the terminal of the acute bone; its branch is in the Xinshu point (BL. 15) on the back. The root of the Pericardium Channel is in the Neiguan point (PC. 6) which is in the middle of the two tendons two inches from the wrist behind the palm; its branch is in the Tainchi point (PC. 1) which is three inches under the armpit. In examining the root and the branch of the twelve channels, when the roots of the various Yang channels are deficient, the jueni syndrome will occur; when the roots of the various Yang channels are overabundant, the cold extremities due to heat-evil will occur. When the branches of the various Yin channels are deficient, dizziness will occur; when the branches of the various Yin channels are overabundant, pain due to the heat-evil will occur. Therefore, when treating the syndrome of sthenia, it will eliminate the evil-energy and check its development; when treating the syndrome of asthenia, it will induce the healthy energy and substantialize it.

请言气街：胸气有街，腹气有街，头气有街，胫气有街。故气在头者，止之于脑。气在胸者，此之膺与背腧。气在腹者，止之背腧，与冲脉于脐左右之动脉者。气在胫者，止之于气街，与承山踝上以下。取此者用毫针，必先按而在久〔在久：《甲乙》卷二第四作“久存之”〕应于手，乃刺而予之。所治者，头痛眩仆，腹痛中满暴胀，及有新积。痛可移者，易已也；积不痛，难已也。

"Now, let me tell you the routes of the energy: The energy of chest has its own route, the energy of abdomen has its own route, the energy of head has its own route, and the energy of leg has its own route. Thus, when the energy is in the head, prick the Baihui point (DU. 20) on the top of head to prevent the affection of the disease. When the energy is in the chest, prick the chest and the Feishu point (BL. 13) on the back to prevent the affection of the disease. When the energy is in the abdomen, pick the Pishu point (BL. 20) on the back, the route of the Chong Vessel, prick the the Huangshu point (KI. 16) around the arteries of the navel and the Tianshu point (ST. 25). When the energy is in the leg, prick the Qichong point (ST. 30), Chengshan point (BL. 57) and the locations above and below the ankle of foot to prevent the affection of the disease. When pricking, apply the filiform needle, and press the acupoint with a considerable long time in advance, and then, prick with invigorating therapy or purging therapy respectively until the energy has arrived and felt by the fingers. The diseases caused by the energies of various routes are: headache, fainting, abdominal pain, abdominal flatulence, sudden distention and mass of the initial stage. If the site of the pain is transferable, it can be cured easily; if the mass is not painful and the location is fixed, it can hardly be cured."

论痛第五十三

Chapter 53
Lun Tong
(On Pain)

黄帝问于少俞曰：筋骨之强弱，肌肉之坚脆，皮肤之厚薄，腠理之疏密，各不同，其于针石火焫之痛何如？肠胃之厚薄坚脆亦不等，其于毒药何如？愿尽闻之。少俞曰：人之骨强、筋弱〔《甲乙》卷六第十一“弱”作“劲”〕、肉缓、皮肤厚者耐痛，其于针石之痛、火焫亦然。

Yellow Emperor asked Shaoyu and said: “In human body, there are the differences in the toughness and fragility in the tendons and the bones, there are the differences of the firmness and crispness in the muscle, there are the differences of the thickness and thinness in the skin and there are the differences in the looseness and denseness in the striae. What are the conditions of the pain when they receive the treatments of acupuncture, stone needle and moxibustion? There are also the differences of the thickness and thinness, firmness and crispness in the intestine and stomach, what are the responses to the stimulations when they are treated with toxic drugs? I hope to hear the details.” Shaoyu said: “When a man has a strong bone, tough tendon, soft muscle and thick skin, he is capable to endure pain, and he can also endure the pain from the treatment of acupuncture, stone needle and moxibustion.”

黄帝曰：其耐火焫〔焫：《甲乙》卷六第十一作“执”〕者，何以知之？少俞答曰：加以黑色而美骨者，耐火焫。黄帝曰：其不耐针石之痛者，何以知之？少俞曰：坚肉薄皮者，不耐针石之痛，于火焫亦然。

Yellow Emperor asked: “Some people can endure the pain of the moxa cauterization and how can one know it?” Shaoyu said: “People of black skin and strong skeleton can withstand the moxa cauterization.” Yellow Emperor asked: “Some people can not withstand the pain of needling and how can one know it?” Shaoyu said: “People with firm muscle and thin skin can not withstand the pain of the acupuncture treatment, and he can not withstand the pain of moxibustion also.”

黄帝曰：人之病，或〔或：此字误衍〕同时而伤，或易已，或难已，其故何如？少俞曰：同时而伤，其身多热者易已，多寒者难已。

Yellow Emperor asked: “When people contract disease simultaneously, some of them can be recovered easily and some of them can hardly be recovered and what is the reason?” Shaoyu said: “For the disease contracted simultaneously, people with plenty heat can be recovered easily, and people with plenty of cold can hardly be recovered.”

黄帝曰：人之胜毒，何以知之？少俞曰：胃厚、色黑、大骨及〔及：《甲乙》卷六第十一作“肉”〕肥者，皆胜毒；故其瘦而薄胃〔薄胃：此应乙作“胃薄”〕者，皆不胜毒也。

Yellow Emperor asked: "Some people can sustain toxic drugs and how can one know it?" Shaoyu said: "When one has thick stomach, black skin, large bone and fleshy muscle, he can sustain the toxic drugs; when one is thin and has weak stomach, he can hardly sustain toxic drugs."

天年第五十四

Chapter 54
Tian Nian
(The Natural Span of Life)

黄帝问于岐伯曰：愿闻〔愿闻：《灵枢略》作“夫”〕人之始生，何气〔气：《灵枢略》无此字〕筑为基，何立而〔而：《灵枢略》无此字〕为楯，何失而死，何得而生？岐伯曰：以母为基，以父为楯，失神者死，得神者生也。黄帝曰：何者为神？岐伯曰：血气已和，荣卫已通，五藏已成，神气舍心，魂魄毕具，乃成为人。

Yellow Emperor asked Qibo and said: “What is the foundation in the initiation of one's life? How to set the periphery for guarding outside? What is the thing when being lost will cause death and what is the thing when being preserved will cause survival?” Qibo said: “The mother is the foundation and the father is the railing. which is guarding outside, when one's spirit is lost, he will die, when one's spirit exists, he will survive.” Yellow Emperor asked: “What is the spirit?” Qibo said: “When one's blood and energy are harmonious, his Rong-energy and Wei-energy are unimpeded, his five viscera being shaped and the spirit being stored in his heart causing him to have thought and will, then, he becomes a man.”

黄帝曰：人之寿夭各不同，或夭寿，或卒死，或病久，愿闻其道。岐伯曰：五脏坚固，血脉和调，肌肉解利，皮肤致密，营卫之行，不失其常，呼吸微徐，气以度行，六腑化谷，津液布扬，各如其常，故能长久。

Yellow Emperor said: “The life spans in different people are different, some die early and some can live a long life, some die suddendly and some have protracted disease, I hope to hear the reason about it.” Qibo said: “The structures of the five solid organs should be firm, the channels should be genial and harminious, the muscle should be smooth and moist, the skin should be fine and dense, the running of the Ying-energy and the Wei-energy should not divorce from their normal condition, the respiration should be light and slow, the energy should run in a moderate way with proper speed, the six hollow organs should convert the cereals and the body fluid should spread to the various orifices, when all the aspects above are normal, one's life span will be long.”

黄帝曰：人之寿百岁而死，何以致之？岐伯曰：使道隧以长，基墙高以方，通调营卫，三部三里，起骨高肉满，百岁乃得终。

Yellow Emperor asked: “Some people can live to the age of one hundred years old, how can they live such a long life?” Qibo said: “When one's nostrils are deep and long, his nose is high, large square and upright which can harmonize the channel-energies of the Ying, Wei, the triple warmer and that of the Sanli point, he will live long. Thus, when one's nasal bone is protruding and his nasal muscle is plump, he can live until one hundred years old."

黄帝曰：其气之盛衰，以至其死，可得闻乎？岐伯曰：人生十岁，五藏始定，血气已通，其气在下，故好走。二十岁，血气始盛，肌肉方长，故好趋。三十岁，五藏大定，肌肉坚固，血脉盛满，故好步。四十岁，五藏六腑十二经脉，皆大盛以平定，腠理始疏，荣华颓落，发颇斑〔斑：《太素》卷二《寿限》作"颁"〕白，平盛不摇，故好坐。五十岁，肝气始〔始：《太平圣惠方》卷一《论形气盛衰法》无此字〕衰，肝叶始薄，胆汁始灭〔灭：周本，日刻本并作"减"〕，目始不明。六十岁，心气始衰，苦忧悲，血气懈惰，故好卧。七十岁，脾气虚〔虚：太平圣惠方》卷一《论形气盛衰法》作"衰"〕，皮肤枯。八十岁，肺气衰，魄离〔魄离：《甲乙》卷六第十二作"魂魄离散"〕，故言善误。九十岁，肾气焦〔焦：《太平圣惠方》卷一《论形气盛衰法》"焦"下有"竭"字〕，四藏〔四藏：《太素》卷二《寿限》作"脏枯"〕经脉空虚。百岁，五藏皆虚，神气皆去，形骸独居而终矣。

Yellow Emperor asked: "Can you tell me the prosperous and declining conditions of one's energy from youth to the death?" Qibo said: "When one is ten years old, his five viscera begin to become perfect, his blood and energy are unimpeded and his energy is in the lower extremities, so, he prefers to run. When one is twenty years old, his blood and energy begin to become prosperous, his muscle is developing, so, he prefers to walk fast. When he is thirty years old, his five viscera are completely sound, his muscle is firm, his blood is prosperous and ample, so, he prefers to walk slowly. When one is fourty years old, his five solid organs, six hollow organs and the twelve channels are well-developed and stable, his stria begins to become loose and his lustre in the complexion begins to wane, his hair on head and the temples are becoming grey, he likes to deal with things simply, and he is reluctant to act, so, he prefers to sit. When one is fifty years old, his liver energy begins to decline, his liver leaf is thin and weak, his bile is reducing gradually and his eyesight begins to become dim. When one is sixty years old, his heart energy begins to decline, he often suffers from worriment and sorrow, as the operation of his blood and energy are slow, he prefers to lie down. When one is seventy years old, his spleen energy is weak and his skin is dry. When one is eighty years old, his lung energy is declinig, his soul and inferior spirit are dispersing, so, he often has erroneous speech. When one is ninety years old, his kidney energy is withered and exhausting, all the visceral energies of his liver, heart, spleen and lung and his channel energy are emptied. When one is one hundred years old, the energies of all his viscera are emptied, and he has no more spirit, by this time, he has only the body in substance and he may die at any time."

黄帝曰：其不能终寿而死者，何如？岐伯曰：其五藏皆不坚，使道不长，空外以张，喘息暴疾，又卑基墙，薄脉少血，其肉不石〔石：《太素》卷二《寿限》作"实"〕，数中风寒，血气虚，脉不通，真邪相攻，乱而相引，故中寿而尽也。

Yellow Emperor asked: "Some people die early, they can not live their full span of life and why is it?" Qibo said: "When one's five viscera are all infirm, his nasolabial is short, his nostrils turn facing outside, he has rapid respiration, his forehead is low, his channel is small with few blood in it, his muscle is infirm, he often has apoplexy, his blood and energy are deficient, his channels are unimpeded, his healthy energy and evil energy are attacking each other so as the blood and energy in the body are abnormal causing the evil energy to penetrate deeply inside, people of this kind will die in his middle age."

逆顺第五十五

Chapter 55
Ni Shun
(The Agreeableness and Adverseness)

黄帝问于伯高曰：余闻气有逆顺，脉有盛衰，刺有大约，可得闻乎？伯高曰：气之逆顺者，所以应天地、阴阳、四时、五行也；脉之盛衰者，所以候血气之虚实有余不足。刺之大约者，必明知病之可刺，与其未可刺，与其已不可刺也。

Yellow Emperor asked Bogao: "I am told that the energies have the difference of agreeableness and adverseness, the pulse conditions have the difference of overabundance and deficiency and the pricking has its general method, can you tell me about them?" Bogao said: "The agreeable and adverse running of energy in human body are corresponding to the heaven, earth, Yin, Yang, the four seasons and the five elements; when examining the overabundance and deficiency of the pulse condition, one can determine the sthenia or asthenia of the disease and the having a surplus or deficiency of the blood and energy; when one treats with needle according to the general mothod of acupuncture, he must know precisely which kind of disease can be treated by pricking, which kind of disease must not be pricked for the time being and what kind of disease must not be pricked."

黄帝曰：候之奈何？伯高曰：兵法曰：无迎逢逢之气，无击堂堂之阵。刺法曰：无刺熇熇之热，无刺漉漉之汗，无刺浑浑之脉，无刺病与脉相逆者。黄帝曰：候其可刺奈何？伯高曰：上工，刺其未生者也。其次，刺其未盛者也。其次，刺其已衰者也。下工，刺其方袭者也，与其形之盛者也，与其病之与脉相逆者也。故曰：方其盛也，勿敢毁伤，刺其已衰，事必大昌。故曰：上工治未病，不治已病。此之谓也。

Yellow Emperor asked: "How to treat the disease which must not be pricked after examining?" Bogao said: "According to the art of war, one must not make a head-on attack to the approaching army which is irresistible, and one must not launch an attack to a strong and grand battle array of the enemy. In the《Methods of Acupuncture》, it was stated: "Do not prick when the patient is suffering from fever excessively, do not prick when the patient is sweating all over, do not prick when the pulse condition of the patient is confusing and when the disease is contrary to the pulse condition. "Yellow Emperor asked: "How to treat the disease which can be pricked after examining?" Bogao said: "For a physician of higher level, he can treat the disease which has not been manifested outside; nextly, he can treat and prick the disease of which its evil energy has not yet become overabundant; and nextly, he can treat and prick the disease of which its evil energy is declining. For a physician of lower level, he dares not prick when the diseases are overlapping, when the evil energy is prevailing or when the disease is contrary to the pulse condition, he waits until the evil energy has become deficient and then, take the opportunity to prick to receive a good curative effect. Therefore, for a physician of higher level, he can not only treat the internal organ which is diseased, but can also treat the internal organ which has not contracted disease."

五味第五十六

Chapter 56
Wu Wei
(The Five Tastes)

黄帝曰：愿闻谷气有五味，其入五脏，分别奈何？伯高曰：胃者，五脏六腑之海也，水谷皆入于胃，五脏六腑皆禀气于胃。五味各走〔走：《类说》卷三十七引作“入”〕其所喜，谷味酸，先走肝，谷味苦，先走心，谷味甘，先走脾，谷味辛，先走肺，谷味咸，先走肾。谷气〔谷气：《甲乙》卷六第九“谷气”下有“营卫俱行”四字〕津液已行，营卫大通，乃化糟粕，以次传下。

Yellow Emperor said: "There are five tastes in the essence derived from food, when they enter into the five viscera of the body, what routes will they follow respectively?" I hope you can tell me." Bogao said: "The stomach is like the sea for converging the nutrition of the five solid organs and the six hollow organs, as all the water and cereals enter into the stomach, so, all the five solid organs and the six hollow organs will receive the refined energy formed by the digestion of the stomach, and each of the five tastes of food will enter into the viscus it prefers respectively. Therefore, the sour taste tends to enter into the liver first; the bitter taste tends to enter into the heart first; the sweet taste tends to enter into the spleen first; the acrid taste tends to enter into the lung first; the salty taste tends to enter into the kidney first. The body fluid converted by the refined substances of the essence derived from food is running in the body causing the unimpediment of the Ying-energy and the Wei-energy, the waste matters will turn into dross which will be eliminated to the outside of the body along with urination and defecation."

黄帝曰：营卫之行奈何？伯高曰：谷始入于胃，其精微者，先出于胃之两焦，以溉五脏，别出两〔两：《甲乙》卷六第九“两”下有“焦”字，断句〕行，营卫之道。其大气之抟而不行者，积于胸中，命曰气海，出于肺，循喉咽，故呼则出，吸则入。天地之精气，其大数常出三入一，故谷不入，半日则气衰，一日则气少矣。

Yellow Emperor asked: "What are the condition of the operation of the Ying-energy and Wei-energy?" Bogao said: "When the cereals have entered into the stomach, its refined substances produced spread to the upper warmer and the middle warmer from the stomach to irrigate and nourish the five viscera, and the other two branches are the two routes of the Ying-energy and the Wei-energy. Besides, there is also the natural air which is assembling without scattering, it accumulates in the chest, and it is called the sea of qi (air). The air of this kind comes out from the lung and runs along the throat, it goes out when one exhales and comes in when one inhales. The refined energy of the cereals is stored in the sea of qi, it is approximately three fourth exhaled and one fourth inhaled. So, if one does not take any food for half a day, he will be feeling deficiency of breath; when he does not take any food for one day, he will be feeling short of breath."

黄帝曰：谷之五味，可得闻乎？伯高曰：请尽言之。五谷：秔〔秔：《甲乙》卷六第九作"粳"〕米〔米：《太素》卷二《调食》"失"下有"饭"字〕甘，麻〔麻：《素问·藏气法时论》作"小豆"〕酸，大豆咸，麦〔麦：《甲乙》卷六第九"麦"上有"小"字〕苦，黄〔黄：《五行大义》卷三《论配气味》引《甲乙》无此字〕黍〔黍：《千金》卷二十九第四作"稻"〕辛。五果：枣甘，李酸，栗咸，杏苦，桃辛。五畜：牛甘，犬酸，猪咸，羊苦，鸡辛。五菜：葵甘，韭酸，藿咸，薤苦，葱辛。

Yellow Emperor asked: "Can you tell me about the five tastes of the cereals?" Bogao said: "I like to tell you in details: In the five cereals, the taste of the round-shaped rice is sweet, the taste of sesame is sour, the taste of soybean is salty, the taste of wheat is bitter and the taste of millet is acrid. In the five fruits, the taste of jujube is sweet, the taste of plum is sour, the taste of chestnut is salty, the taste of apricot is bitter and the taste of peach is acrid. In the five animals, the taste of beaf is sweet, the taste of dog's meat is sour, the taste of pork is salty, the taste of mutton is bitter and the taste of chicken is acrid. In the five vegetables, the taste of celery is sweet, the taste of the Chinese chives is sour, the taste of bean leaves is salty, the taste of leek is bitter and the taste of scallion is acrid.

五色：黄色宜甘，青色宜酸，黑色宜咸，赤色宜苦，白色宜辛。凡此五者，各有所宜。五宜〔五宜：周本与注本并无此二字〕：所言五色〔五色：《太素》卷二《调食》作"五宜"〕者，脾病者，宜食秔米饭牛肉枣葵；心病者，宜食麦羊肉杏薤；肾病者，宜食大豆黄卷猪肉栗藿；肝病者，宜食麻犬肉李韭。肺病者，宜食黄黍鸡肉桃葱。

"In the five colours, yellow is suitable to sweetness, green is suitable to sourness, black is suitable to saltiness, red is suitable to bitterness and white is suitable to acridness. In the five colours, each has its suitability respectively. The so called five suitabilities are: the patient of spleen disease is suitable to take round-shaped rice, beef, jujube and celery; the patient of heart disease is suitable to take wheat, mutton, apricot and leek; the patient of kidney disease is suitable to take soybean, millet, pork and bean leaves; the patient of liver disease is suitable to take sesame, dog's meat, plum and Chinese chives; the patient of lung disease is suitable to take millet, chicken, peach and scallion.

五禁：肝病禁辛，心病禁咸，脾病禁酸，肾病禁甘，肺病禁苦。

"The five contraindications are: When treating the disease of liver, applying acridness is forbidden; when treating the disease of heart, applying saltiness is forbidden; when treating the disease of spleen, applying sourness is forbidden; when treating the disease of kidney, applying sweetness is forbidden; when treating the disease of lung, applying bitterness is forbidden.

肝色青，宜食甘，秔米饭牛肉枣葵〔葵：《太素》卷二《调食》无此字〕皆甘。心色赤，宜食酸，大肉麻李韭皆酸〔大肉麻李韭皆酸：《太素》卷二《调食》"大"作"犬"，无"麻韭"二字〕。脾色黄，宜食咸，大豆豕肉栗藿〔藿：《太素》卷二《调食》无此字〕皆咸。肺色白，宜食苦，麦羊肉杏薤〔薤:《太素》卷二《调食》无此字〕皆苦。肾色黑，宜食辛，黄黍鸡肉桃葱〔葱:《太素》卷二《调食》无此字〕皆辛。

"The colour of liver is green, when the liver is sick, taking the sweet food is advisable, and the round-shaped rice, beaf and jujube are sweet. The colour of heart is red, when the heart is sick, taking the sour food is advisable, and the dog's meat, sesame, plum and Chinese chives are sour. The colour of spleen is yellow, when the spleen is sick, taking the salty food is advisable, and the soybean, pork and chestnuts are salty. The colour of lung is white, when the lung is sick, taking the bitter food is advisable, and the wheat, mutton and apricot are bitter. The colour of kidney is black, when the kidney is sick, taking the acrid food is advisable, and the millet, chicken and peach are acrid."

水胀第五十七

Chapter 57
Shui Zhang
(The Edema)

黄帝问于岐伯曰：水与肤胀、鼓胀、肠覃、石瘕、石水〔石水："石水"二字是衍文〕，何以别之。岐伯答曰：水始起也，目窠上微肿，如新卧起之状，其颈脉动，时咳，阴股间寒，足胫瘇〔瘇：藏本与注本并作"肿"〕，腹乃大，其水已成矣。以手按其腹，随手而起，如裹水之状，此其候也。

Yellow Emperor asked Qibo: "How to distinguish the edema, anasarca, distention of abdomen, intestinal mass and stony mass of uterus?" Qibo said: "In the initiation of edema, it appears on one's eyelid to be somewhat dropsy as if he has just awoke from sleep, his Renying pulse on the neck pulsates rapidly, he coughs frequently, he feels cold in the inner side of the thigh and has edema in the leg, if his abdomen is expanding, then, his edema has been formed. When one presses the swelling site with hand and then relieves the hand, the abdomen swells up in the wake of it, as if water is wrapped inside. These are the symptoms of edema."

黄帝曰：肤胀何以候之？岐伯曰：肤胀者，寒气客于皮肤之间，鼟鼟然不坚，腹大，身尽肿，皮厚，按其腹，窅〔窅：《甲乙》卷八第四作"腹陷"〕而不起，腹色不变，此其候也。

Yellow Emperor asked: "How to diagnose anasarca?" Qibo said: "The formation of anasarca is due to the retention of the cold-energy between the skins. If the abdomen is empty and infirm when being percussed and appears to be large, the body is swelling all over, the skin is thick, the bogging site of the abdomen when being pressed does not swell up along with the lifting up of the hand, and the colour of the skin remains unchanged, they are the symptoms of anasarca."

鼓胀何如？岐伯曰：腹胀身皆大〔腹胀身皆大：《甲乙》卷八第四作"腹身皆肿大"〕，大〔大："大"字衍〕与肤胀等也，色苍黄，腹筋起，此其候也。

Yellow Emperor asked: "What are the symptoms of the distention of abdomen?" Qibo said: "When the patient's abdomen is distending and full, the whole body is swelling and expanding like that in anasarca, the skin is green and yellow and the vessels on the abdomen are swelling up abruptly, they are the symptoms of abdominal distention."

肠覃何如？岐伯曰：寒气客于肠外，与卫气相搏，气〔气：《甲乙》卷八第四"气"上并有"正"字〕不得荣〔荣：《太素》卷二十九《胀论》作"营"〕，因有所系，癖而内著，恶气乃起，瘜肉乃生，其始生〔生："生"字衍〕也，大如鸡卵，稍以益大，至其成如怀子之状，久者离岁，按之则坚，推之则移，月事以时下，此其候也。

Yellow Emperor asked: "What are the symptoms of the intestinal mass?" Qibo said: "When the cold-energy retains outside of the intestine to combat with the Wei-energy, it causes the healthy energy fails to operate normally. As the cold-energy and the Wei-energy are connecting and can not be dispersed, the abdominal mass will be formed gradually inside, the filthy energy will begin to arise, the polypus will begin to grow, at the beginning, it is only in the size of an egg, but it becomes larger and larger gradually, when the disease has shaped, the patient is like a pregnant woman and the course of the disease will last for several years, when press it with hand, it is firm and hard, when push it with hand, it is somewhat movable, but the menstruation of the patient comes on schedual. These are the symptoms of the intestinal mass."

石瘕何如?岐伯曰:石瘕生胞中寒，寒气客于子门〔门:《千金》卷二十一第四作“宫”〕，子门闭塞，气不得通，恶血当泻不泻，衃以〔衃以:《甲乙》卷八第四作“血衃乃”〕留止，日以益大，状如怀子，月事不以时下。皆生于女子，可导而下。

Yellow Emperor asked: "What are the symptoms of the stony mass of uterus?" Qibo said: "The stony mass of uterus grows in the uterus. When the cold-energy invades the orifices of the uterus, it closes up to cause the obstruction of the energy, the malicious blood which should be excreted fails to excrete causing the corrupted blood retaining inside, and the stony mass will become larger and larger day after day, finally, the patient will like a pregnant woman, and her menstruation will not come on schedule. This disease is contracted by women, and it can be eleminated by applying the purging therapy.

黄帝曰:肤胀鼓胀可刺邪?岐伯曰:先泻〔泻:《太素》卷二十九《胀论》并作“刺”〕其胀〔胀:《太素》卷二十九《胀论》并作“腹”〕之血络，后调其经，刺去〔去:“去”字衍〕其血络〔络:《太素》卷二十九《胀论》并作“脉”〕也。

Yellow Emperor asked: "Can the anasarca and the distention of abdomen be treated with pricking?" Qibo said: "One must prick the superficial venules of the abdomen first, then, adjust the channel according to its condition of asthenia and sthenia, but the main treatment should be the pricking of the superficial venules."

贼风第五十八

Chapter 58
Zei Feng
(The Evil Wind)

黄帝曰：夫子言贼风邪气之伤人也，令人病焉，今有其不离屏蔽，不出空穴〔空穴：明本，，统本，日刻本，张注本“空”并作“室”〕之中，卒然病者，非不〔不：《太素》卷二十八《诸风杂论》作“必”〕离贼风邪气，其故何也？

Yellow Emperor said to Qibo: “You have said that when a man is injured by the evil wind, he will be sick. But someone contracts disease suddenly when he stays at home without leaving the screen, and he is not invaded by the evil wind. What is the reason?”

岐伯曰：此皆尝有所伤于湿气，藏于血脉之中，分肉之间，久留而不去；若有所堕坠，恶血在内而不去。卒然喜怒不节，饮食不适，寒温不时，腠理闭而不通。其开〔其开：《甲乙》卷六第五无此二字〕而遇风寒，则血气凝结，与故邪相袭，则为寒痹。其有热则汗出，汗出则受风，虽不遇贼风邪气，必有因加而发焉。

Qibo said: “It is due to the patient was injured by the wetness in the past, and the wetness evil retained in between the channels and the muscles which have not yet been removed; or the patient fell from a high place in the past to have stagnated blood in the body which has not yet been dissipated; or due to the patient has excessive overjoy or anger suddenly, has improper food or drink or encounters extreme cold or heat to cause the obstruction of the striae; or due to the patient encounters wind-cold when his striae are open causing the stagnation of the blood and energy. When the protracted wetness-evil combines with the new-contracted wind-cold, it will cause the hypochondriac protrusion due to cold. When the patient is hot, he will perspire, when wind invades during his perspiration, he will become sick. When the protracted evil joins the recent evil, it can cause disease even there is no thief-wind and evil-energy newly encountered.”

黄帝曰：今夫子之所言者，皆病人之所自知也。其毋所遇邪气，又毋怵惕之所〔所：此“所”字疑衍〕志，卒然而病者，其故何也？唯有因鬼神之事乎？

Yellow Emperor said: “What you have said is reasonable and can be comprehended by the patient. But there is the condition when no evil-energy of the four seasons is encountered, and no stimulation of fright occurs, but the patient falls sick all of a sudden, and what is the reason?” It is really the gods and the ghosts who are making the troubles?”

岐伯曰：此亦有故邪留而未发，因而志有所恶，及有所慕，血气内乱，两气相搏。其所从来者微，视之不见，听而不闻，故似鬼神。

Qibo said: “This is because the patient has protracted evil retained in the body which has not yet bursted out, or he might have something detestable or something admirable in his heart causing his blood and energy confusing. Since the protracted evil and the recent evil energies are combating, disease will occur suddenly. As the reason of the disease is quite subtle, one can hardly see and hear anything related, so, it is like the gods and the ghosts are making the troubles."

黄帝曰：其祝〔其祝：《甲乙》卷六第五作“其由祝由”〕而已者，其故何也？岐伯曰：先巫者，因〔因：《太素》卷二十八《诸风杂论》作“固”〕知百病之胜，先知其病知所从生者，可祝〔可祝：“祝”下脱“由”字〕而已也。

Yellow Emperor asked: "Some diseases can be cured by talisman and incantation, and what is the reason?" Qibo said: "The witch doctor in ancient times actually knew the various diseases were conditioning each other. So, one must know the reason of the disease in advance, then can he cure the disease with talisman and incantation."

卫气失常第五十九

Chapter 59
Wei Qi Shi Chang
(Treating the Abnormal Wei-energy)

黄帝曰：卫气之留于腹中，搐积不行，苑蕴不得常所，使人支胁胃中满，喘呼逆息者，何以去之？伯高曰：其气积于胸中者，上取之；积于腹中者，下取之；上下皆满者，傍取之。

Yellow Emperor asked："When the Wei-energy accumulates in the chest but the stagnation does not retain in a definite location，it causes the propping of the hypochondria，abdominal flatulence，dyspnea and the adverseness of vital energy. How to eliminate them?" Bogao said："When the energy is accumulated in the chest，treat by pricking the acupoints on the upper part of the body；when the energy is accumulated in the abdomen，treat by pricking the acupoints on the lower part of the body；when the energy is full and distending in both the chest and the abdomen，treat by pricking the near by acupoints.

黄帝曰：取之奈何？伯高对曰：积于上，泻人迎，天突、喉中；积于下者，泻三里与气街；上下皆满者，上下取之，与季胁之下一寸；重者〔重者：按"重者"与上"与季胁之下一寸"句似误倒，当作"重者，与季胁之下一寸，鸡足取之"〕，鸡足取之。诊视其脉大而弦急，及绝不至者，及腹皮急甚者，不可刺也。黄帝曰：善。

Yellow Emperor asked："How to treat them by pricking the acupoints?" Bogao said："When the wei-energy is accumulated in the chest，purge by pricking the Renying (ST. 60)，Tiantu (RN. 22) and Houzhong points；when the Wei-energy is accumulated in the abdomen，purge by pricking the Sanli (ST. 36) and Qijie (ST. 30) points；when the chest and the abdomen are both full and distending with the energy，prick the Renying，Tiantu and Houzhong points above，prick the Sanli and Qijie points below and prick the Zhangmen point (LR. 13) in the middle. If the distention is severe，prick slantingly in the pattern of the chicken's claw. If the patient's pulse condition is gigantic，wiry and urgent，or the pulse is severing and the skin of the stomach is very hard，it must not be treated by pricking." Yellow Emperor said："Good."

黄帝问于伯高曰：何以知皮肉、气血、筋骨之病也？伯高曰：色起两眉〔色起两眉：《千金翼方》卷二十五《诊气血法》作"白色起于两眉间"〕薄泽者，病在皮。唇色青黄赤白〔白：《千金翼方》卷二十五《诊气色法》无此字〕黑者，病在肌肉。营气濡然者，病在血气〔气：《千金翼方》卷二十五《诊气色法》作"脉"〕。目色青黄赤白黑者，病有筋。耳焦枯受尘垢，病在骨。

Yellow Emperor asked Bogao："How to know there is disease in the skin，muscle，energy，blood，tendon and bone by examining?" Bogao said："When the white colour appears between the two eyebrows without lustre, the disease is in the skin; when the colours of green, yellow, red and black appear in the lips, the disease is in the muscle; when the blood and energy of the patient is deficient, the disease is in the channel; when the colours of green, yellow, red, white and black appear in the eye, the disease is in the tendon; when the ear is dry with plenty of earwax, the disease is in the bone."

黄帝曰：病形何如，取之奈何？伯高曰：夫百病变化，不可胜数，然〔夫面病变化，不可胜数，然：《甲乙》卷六第六并无此十字〕皮有部，肉有柱，血气有输，肉有属。黄帝曰：愿闻其故。伯高曰：皮之部，输于四末。肉之柱，在臂胫诸阳分肉之间，与足少阴分间〔分间：《千金翼方》卷二十五第一作"分肉之间"〕。血气之输〔血气之输：《千金翼方》卷二十五第一作"气血之轮"〕，输于诸络，气血留居，则盛而起。筋部无阴无阳，无左无右，候病所在。骨之属者，骨空之所以受益〔《甲乙》卷六第六作"液"〕而益脑髓者也。

Yellow Emperor asked: "What are the appearances of the diseases and how to treat them by pricking?" Bogao said: "In skin, there is the sub-part, in muscle, there is the protruding part, in the energy and blood, there are the orbiculi, in bone, there is the connected tissue, and all these are their dominating parts." Yellow Emperor said: "I hope to hear the reasons about them." Bogao said: "The sub-part of the skin is in the four extremities. The protruding muscle is between the muscles of the various Yang channels in the lower arm and between the muscles of the Foot Shaoyin Channel. The orbiculi of energy and blood are in the collateral points of the various channels, if the energy and blood are stagnant, the channel energy will be obstructed. When the disease is in the tendon, prick the focus disregarding of the Yin, Yang, left and right of the disease. When the disease is in the bone, prick the connected tissue of the bone as the cavity of the bone joint is the place for receiving fluid for supplementing the cerebral marrow.

黄帝曰：取之奈何？伯高曰：夫病变化，浮沉深浅，不可胜穷，各在其处〔"黄帝曰"至"各在其处"：《千金翼方》卷二十五第一作"若取之者，必须候病间甚者也"〕。病间者浅之，甚者深之，间者小之，甚者众之〔甚者众之：《千金翼方》卷二十五第一无"甚者"二字，"众"作"多"，"多之"二字，移在上文"甚者深之"之下〕，随变而调气〔气：《千金翼方》卷二十五第一作"之"〕，故曰上工。

"When one treats by pricking, he must examine the severe and the slight extent of the disease. To the disease which is light, prick shallowly and make few prickings; to the disease which is severe, prick deeply and make more prickings. When one can treat according to the variation of the disease, he is supposed to be a good physician."

黄帝问于伯高曰：人之肥瘦大小寒温，有老壮少小，别之奈何？伯高对曰：人年五十已上为老，二十已上为壮，十八已上为少，六岁已上为小。

Yellow Emperor asked Bogao: "How to distinguish the fat or thin, large or small, cold or hot and the senile, robust, young and infantile conditions of a man?" Bogao said: "When one is more than fifty, he is old; when he is more than twenty, he is robust; when he is more than eighteen, he is young, when he is more than six, he is infantile."

黄帝曰：何以度知其肥瘦？伯高曰：人有肥有膏有肉。黄帝曰：别此奈何？伯高曰：䐃肉坚，皮满者，肥。䐃肉不坚，皮缓者，膏。皮肉不相离者，肉。

Yellow Emperor asked: "How to estimate them?" Bogao said: "There are three types of human body: the fat type, the puffy type and the muscular type." Yellow Emperor asked: "How to distinguish them?" Bogao said: "When one's protruding muscle is firm and his skin is full, he is of the fat type; when his protruding muscle is infirm and his skin is loose, he is of the puffy type; when his skin and muscle are connecting tightly, he is of the muscular type."

黄帝曰：身之寒温何如？伯高曰：膏者其肉淖，而粗理者身寒，细理者身热。脂者其肉坚，细理者热，粗理者寒。

Yellow Emperor asked: "How to distinguish the cold and heat types of the body?" Bogao said: "The muscle of the man of puffy type is moist, if his texture is coarse, he can stand the cold, if his texture is fine and dense, he can stand the heat. The muscle of the man of the fat type is firm and substantial, if his texture is fine and dense, he can stand the heat, if his texture is coarse, he can stand the cold."

黄帝曰：其肥瘦大小奈何？伯高曰：膏者，多气而皮纵缓，故能纵腹垂腴。肉者，身体容大。脂者，其身收小。

Yellow Emperor asked: "What are the conditions when one's body is fat or thin, large or small?" Bigao said: "For a man of the puffy type, his energy is overabundant, his skin is loose and flaccid, so, his abdominal muscles are loose and his belly is hanging down. For a man of muscular type, the capacity of his body is larger. For a man of the fat type, his muscle is tight and dense, and his type of build is smaller."

黄帝曰：三者之气血多少何如？伯高曰：膏者多气，多气者热，热者耐寒。肉者多血则充形，充形则平。脂者，其血清，气滑少，故不能大。此别于众人者也。黄帝曰：众人奈何？伯高曰：众人皮肉脂膏不能相加也，血与气不能相多，故其形不小不大，各自称其身，命曰众人。

Yellow Emperor asked: "What are the conditions of the plenty or few energy and blood in the fat, puffy and muscular types of people?" Bogao said: "A man of puffy type has plenty of energy, and his physique is hot, so he can stand the cold. A man of muscular type has plenty of blood which can substantialize the physique, so his temperament is moderate. For a man of the fat type, his blood is lucid, his energy is slippery and few, so his body can not be stout. These are the differences from that of a common man." Yellow Emperor asked: "What are the conditions of the energy and blood of a common man?" Bogao said: "Generally, the skin, muscle and fat can not be added to the body, the blood and energy are keeping balance, none of them can be partially overabundant, so, one's body can only be kept in the normal size to fit the skin, muscle, tendon and bone of the whole body, a man like this is supposed to be a common man."

黄帝曰：善。治之奈何？伯高曰：必先别其三形，血之多少，气之清浊，而后调之，治无失常经。是故膏人，纵腹垂腴；肉人者，上下容大；脂人者，虽脂不能大者。

Yellow Emperor asked: "How to treat them?" Bogao said: "One must distinguish the plenty or few of the blood and the lucid or turbid of the energy in the three types of body first before treating. When treating, one must not divorce from the principle of the normal circulation of the Wei-energy. It must be noted that the people of the puffy type, their abdominal muscles are loose and flaccid, their bellies are hanging down; in the people of the muscular type, their capacities in the upper and the lower body are larger; in the people of the fat type, although their fats are plenty, yet their bodies can not be as large as the people of the puffy type and the muscular type."

玉版第六十

Chapter 60
Yu Ban
(The Plate of Jade)

黄帝曰：余以小针为细物也，夫子乃言上合之于天，下合之于地，中合之于人，余以为过针之意矣，愿闻其故。岐伯曰：何物大于天〔天：《太素》卷二十三《疽痛逆顺刺篇》“天”作“针者”二字〕乎？夫大于针者，惟五兵者焉。五兵者，死之备也，非生之具〔具：《太素》卷二十三《疽痛逆顺刺篇》作“备也”二字〕。且夫人者，天地之镇也，其不〔不：是衍文〕可不参乎？夫治民者，亦惟针焉。夫针之与五兵，其孰小乎？

Yellow Emperor said to Qibo: “I thought the small needle is only a trifle before, but now you say the functions of the needle can match the heaven above, the earth below and the man in the middle. I think you have overestimated the original meaning of it, and I hope to know your reasons about it.” Qibo said: “What can be larger than the needle? There are only the five weapons are larger than the needle, but the weapons are used for slaughtering, they are not used to save the life of man. Since human being is the most precious thing between heaven and earth, why can not the needle match the heaven and earth? As to the affairs concerning the ruling of the people, they can also be induced by the principle of the needle. Under such consideration, when comparing the functions with that of the five weapons, which one do you think will be smaller?”

黄帝曰：病之生时，有喜怒不测，饮食不节，阴气不足，阳气有余，营气不行，乃发为痈疽。阴阳〔阴阳：《太素》卷二十三《疽痛逆顺刺》“阳”下并有“气”字〕不通，两〔两：黄校本作“而”〕热相搏，乃化为脓，小针能取之乎？岐伯曰：圣人不能使化者，为之邪不可〔不可：孙鼎宜曰：“‘不可’二字衍文”〕留也。故两军相当，旗帜相望，白刃陈于中野者，此非一日之谋也。能使其民，令行禁止，士卒无白刃之难者，非一日之教也，须臾之〔臾之：《太素》卷二十三《疽痛逆顺刺》作“久之方”〕得也。夫至使身被痈疽之病，脓血之聚者，不亦离道远乎。夫痈疽之生，脓血之成也，不从天下，不从地出〔不从天下，不从地出：《甲乙》卷十一第九下无“不从”八字〕，积微之所生也。故圣人自〔自：《太素》卷二十三《疽痛逆顺刺》作“之”〕治于未有形也，愚者遭其已成也。

Yellow Emperor asked: “In the course of the disease, if the patient is capricious, fails to practise temperance in eating and drinking, his Yin energy in the five solid organs will be insufficient and the Yang energy in the six hollow organs will be having a surplus to cause the impediment of the Ying and Wei energies and the carbuncle will occur. When the Yin and Yang erergies are obstructed, the accumulated heat evil will turn into pus. Can this kind of disease be treated by pricking with the small needle?” Qibo said: “Since the disease has retained inside for a long period, even a sage can not eliminate the evil-energy immediately. It is like two hostile armies facing each other, their banners are manifesting, their weapons are displaying by the soldiers in the field, the disposition can not be schemed in a single day; when the people in a country can observe the law to avoid being killed for doing the unlawful things, it is not a single day for the people to receive the education concerned. When one's body has the carbuncle with pus accumulating, isn't it not far away from following the principle of preserving health and keeping fit? In fact, the carbuncle and the accumulation of pus are formed by the graduate accumulation of the various trifle causes of disease. Therefore, a sage pays attention to the prevention of the disease and treats it when it is not yet visible, but a dull-witted man can only treat after the disease is shaped."

黄帝曰：其已〔已：周本人“以”〕形，不予遭，脓已成，不予见，为之奈何？岐伯曰：脓已成，十死一生，故圣人弗使已成，而明为良方，著之竹帛使能者踵而传之后世，无有终时者，为其不予遭也。

Yellow Emperor asked: "When the carbuncle has formed, it is not known by common people, and when the suppuration is completed, it is not understood by common people, what can one do about it?" Qibo said: "When the suppuration is completed, ten of the patient will die and only one can survive. So, the sage formulated a very good prescription in the past for treating the disease before the suppuration, it was written on the bamboo slip and the silk for imparting to the talented people and the later generations endlessly. The reason of the sage who did in this way was precisely due to the fact that the common people did not know it."

黄帝曰：其已〔其已：《甲乙》卷十一经九下“已”下有“成”字〕有脓血而后遭乎〔而后遭乎：《甲乙》卷十一第九下无此四字〕，不导之〔导之：守山阁《校本》注云：“导之”二字衍〕以小针治乎？岐伯曰：以小治小者其功小，以大治大者多害〔多害：《甲乙》卷十一第九下任务“其功大”。下有“以小治大者多害大”八字〕，故其已成脓血〔血：《太素》卷二十三《疽痛逆顺刺》无此字〕者，其唯砭石铍锋之所取也。

Yellow Emperor asked: "If the carbuncle has formed with pus, can it be treated by the small needle?" Qibo said: "When using a small needle to treat a small site, its effect will be small, when using a large needle to treat a large site, the effect will be large, thus, when the carbuncle is suppurated with pus, it is advisable to apply the stone needle, the sword-shaped needle or the ensiform needle to remove the pus."

黄帝曰：多害者其不可全乎？岐伯曰：其在逆顺焉。黄帝曰：愿闻逆顺。岐伯曰：以为伤者，其白眼〔眼：《甲乙》卷十一第九下任务“睛”〕青黑眼小，是一逆也；内药而呕者，是二逆也；腹痛渴甚，是三逆也；肩项中不便，是四逆也；音嘶色脱，是五逆也。除此五者为顺矣。

Yellow Emperor asked: "Is the carbuncle which causes many injuries to the patient can hardly be cured?" Qibo said: "It is according to the condition whether the syndrome is an agreeable or an adverse one." Yellow Emperor said: "I hope to hear about the conditions of the agreeable and adverse syndromes." Qibo said: "There are five kinds of adverse syndrome in the carbuncle: When the white of the eye is green and dark and the eye is small, they are the adverse syndromes of the first kind; when the patient vomits after administering the medicine, it is the adveres syndrome of the second kind; when the patient is painful and very thirsty, they are the adverse syndromes of the third kind; when the patient finds difficulty in turning his shoulder and neck, it is the adverse syndrome of the fourth kind; when the voice of the patient is hoarse and ghastly pale in the complexion, they are the adverse syndromes of the fifth kind. All other syndromes besides the adverse syndromes are the agreeable syndromes."

黄帝曰：诸病皆有逆顺，可得闻乎？岐伯曰：腹胀，身热，脉大，是一逆也；腹鸣而满，四肢清，泄，其脉大，是二逆也；衄而不止，脉大〔大：《甲乙》卷四第一下校注："一作小"〕，是三逆也；咳且溲血，脱形，其脉小劲，是四逆也；脱形身热，脉小以疾，是谓五逆也。如是者，不过十五日而死矣。

Yellow Emperor asked: "In the various diseases, there are all the agreeable and adverse syndromes, can I hear about them?" Qibo said: "When one has abdominal distention, hot feeling in the body and the small pulse condition, they are the adverse syndromes of the first kind; when one has borborygmus in the abdomen and has abdominal distention, cool in the extremities, diarrhea and gigantic pulse condition, they are the adverse syndromes of the second kind; when one has unceasing epistaxis and gigantic pulse condition, they are the adverse syndromes of the third kind; when one has cough, hematuria, emaciation of the muscle and tiny and urgent pulse condition, they are the adverse syndromes of the fourth kind; when one has cough, emaciation of the body, hotness in the body and tiny and rapid pulse condition, they are the adverse syndromes of the fifth kind. When one contracts these syndromes, he will die within fifteen days.

其腹大胀，四末清，脱形，泄甚，是一逆也；腹胀便血，其脉大，时绝，是二逆也；咳溲血，形肉脱，脉搏，是三逆也；呕血，胸满引背，脉小而疾，是四逆也；咳呕腹胀，且飧泄，其脉绝，是五逆也。如是者，不及〔及：与注本，张注本并作"过"〕一时而死矣。工不察此者而刺之，是谓逆治。

"When one's abdomen is large and distending, his four extremities are cool, his body is emaciated and has severe diarrhea, they are the adverse syndromes of the first kind; when one has abdominal distention and fullness, hematochezia, gigantic and intermittent pulse condition, they are the adverse syndromes of the second kind; when one has cough, hematuria, emaciation, strong respond to the fingers when palpating the pulse, they are the adverse syndromes of the third kind; when one has hematemesis, fullness and oppression of the chest to affect the back, and has tiny and rapid pulse condition, they are the adverse syndromes of the fourth kind; when one has cough and vomiting, abdominal distention, diarrhea and the hidden and severing pulse condition, they are the adverse syndromes of the fifth kind. When these syndromes occur, the patient will die within one day. When a physician pricks rashly disregarding these dangerous appearances, it is called the adverse treating."

黄帝曰：夫子之言针甚骏，以配天地，上数天文，下度地纪，内别五脏，外次六府，经脉二十八会，尽有周纪，能杀生人，不能起死者，子能反之乎？岐伯曰：能杀生人，不能起死者也。黄帝曰：余闻之则为不仁，然愿闻其道，弗行于人。岐伯曰：是明道也，其必然也，其如刀剑之可以杀人，如饮酒使人醉也，虽勿诊，犹可知矣。

Yellow Emperor said: "As you have said the functions of the needle are tremendous, it can approach the astronomical phenomena above, follow the geographical environment below. In human body, there are the differences of the five solid organs inside, and the orderly arrangement of the six hollow organs outside, the twenty eight channels are having their strict usual practice of circulation. Sometimes, one can only treat the patient by pricking with the needle, but he can not bring back the patient's life, can you alter the situation?" Qibo said: "When one treats in an improper way, it can cause death of the patient and can not bring back his life." Yellow Emperor said: "Your saying is not tally with humanity, I hope to hear the reasons of it so that one may not prick the patient rashly." Qibo said: "The reason is quite explicit and it will have an inevitable result. When one is not keen in applying the needle, it is like using a sword to kill a man, or make one to become drunken with spirit. Through the anology above, one can understand the reasons without diagnosing."

黄帝曰：愿卒闻之。岐伯曰：人之所受气者，谷也。谷之所注者，胃也。胃者，水谷气血之海也。海之所行云气者〔海之所行云气者，天下也：《甲乙》卷五第一下"气"作"雨"〕，天下也。胃之所出气血者，经隧也。经隧者，五脏六腑之大络也，迎而夺之而已矣〔迎而夺之而已矣：《灵枢略六气论篇》无"迎而夺之而已矣"七字〕。

Yellow Emperor said: "I hope to hear the details." Qibo said: "The refined energy of a man depends on the supply of the cereals, and the cereals are gathered in the stomach. The stomach is the sea of the water, cereals, energy and blood. When the sea water evaporates, it descends to become the clouds and rain which are spreading in the sky, and likewise, the energy and blood which are converted and generated from the stomach circulate along the channels. The channels are the large collaterals of the five solid organs and the six hollow organs."

黄帝曰：上下有数乎？岐伯曰：迎之五里，中道而止，五至而已，五往而藏之气尽矣，故五五二十五而竭其输矣，此所谓夺其天下者也，非能绝其命而倾其寿者也。黄帝曰：愿卒闻之。岐伯曰：阈门而刺之者，死于家中；入门而刺之者，死于堂上。黄帝曰：善乎方，明哉道，请著之玉版，以为重宝，传之后世，以为刺禁，令民勿敢犯也。

Yellow Emperor asked: "When pricking the hand and foot channels above and below, is there any contraindication?" Qibo said: "When one purges by pricking the Wuli point against the direction of the channel energy errorneously, the visceral energy will stop by the halfway of its operation. The visceral energy can only arrive for five times, if the pricking to a certain viscus is erroneous for five times, the energy of the said viscus will be exhausted, since the total arrivals of the five visceral energy before exhausting are twenty five, so, when the times of the erroneous pricking are twenty five, all the visceral energies in the five viscera will be exhausted and the patient will die. It is not the needle that causes the patient's death, but it is due to the ignorance of the one who pricks, and his not knowing the acupuncture contraindications." Yellow Emperor said: "I hope to hear the details." Qibo said: "When one pricks rashly, if the pricking is shallow, the patient will die when he arrives home; if the pricking is deep, he will die in the hall of the physician." Yellow Emperor said: "The principle you have said is excellent, and the reasons are quite explicit. I will carve them on a plate of jade and take it as a valuable treasure, I will hand it down to the later generations as the acupuncture contraindications so that people may not violate the rule."

五禁第六十一

Chapter 61
Wu Jin
(The Five Contraindications)

黄帝问于岐伯曰：余闻刺有五禁？岐伯曰：禁其不可刺也。黄帝曰：余闻刺有五夺。岐伯曰：无泻其不可夺者也。黄帝曰：余闻刺有五过。岐伯曰：补泻无过其度。黄帝曰：余闻刺有五逆。岐伯曰：病与脉相逆，命曰五逆。黄帝曰：余闻刺有九宜。岐伯曰：明知九针之论，是谓九宜。

Yellow Emperor said to Qibo: "I am told there is the so called five-contraindication in pricking, what is the meaning of it?" Qibo said: "It means some parts of the body must not be pricked in the five days of contraindication." Yellow Emperor said: "I am told in pricking, there is the so called five-depletion." Yellow Emperor said: "It means one should avoid to purge by pricking the five kinds of diseases of which the refined energy is deficient." Yellow Emperor said: "I am told in pricking, there is the so called five-excessiveness." Qibo said: "It means one must not purge or invigorate by pricking excessively." Yellow Emperor said: "I am told in pricking, there is the so called five adverse-syndrome." Qibo said: "It means the five kinds of syndrome which are contrary to the pulse conditions, and it is called the five-adverseness." Yellow Emperor said: "I am told in pricking, there is the so called nine-appropriatness." Qibo said: "When one understands thoroughly and follows the principle of the nine kinds of needle, it is called the nine-appropriateness."

黄帝曰：何谓五禁？愿闻其不可刺之时。岐伯曰：甲乙日自乘，无刺头，无发蒙于耳内。丙丁日自乘，无振埃于肩喉廉泉。戊己日自乘四季，无刺腹去爪泻水。庚辛日自乘，无刺关节于股膝。壬癸日自乘，无刺足胫。是谓五禁。

Yellow Emperor asked: "What are the five contraindications? I hope to know on what day one must not treat by pricking." Qibo said: "In the days of Jia and Yi, do not prick the head, nor to prick the inside part of the ear by applying the 'Fameng pricking method' (pricking the Tinggong point at noon). In the days of Bing and Ding, do not apply the 'Zhen-ai pricking method' (pricking the Tianrong and Lianquan points) on the shoulder and the throat. In the days of Wu and Ji and the days of Chen, Xu, Chou and Wei, do not prick the abdomen, nor to apply the 'Quzhao pricking method' (removing water with the sword-shaped needle) to purge the water. In the days of Ren and Gui, do not prick the leg. These are the so called five contraindications."

黄帝曰：何谓五夺？岐伯曰：形肉已夺，是一夺也；大夺血之后，是二夺也；大汗出之后，是三夺也；大泄之后，是四夺也；新产及大血〔大血：《甲乙》卷五第一"大"下有

“下”字〕之后，是五夺也。此皆不可泻。

Yellow Emperor asked：“What are the five depletions?” Qibo said：“When one has protracted disease and his muscle is very thin，it is the first kind of depletion；when the patient has suffered from massive hemorrhage，it is the second kind of depletion；when the patient has excessive sweating，it is the third kind of depletion；when the patient has severe diarrhea，it is the fourth kind of depletion；when the parturient woman has just delivered a child or after massive hemorrhage，it is the fifth kind of depletion. One must not treat by purging to the patients with these five depletions.”

黄帝曰：何谓五逆？岐伯曰：热病脉静，汗已出，脉盛躁，是一逆也；病泄，脉洪大，是二逆也；著痹不移，䐃肉破，身热，脉偏绝，是三逆也；淫而夺形，身热，色夭然白，及后下血衃，血衃笃重，是谓四逆也；寒热夺形，脉坚博，是谓五逆也。

Yellow Emperor asked：“What are the five adverseness?” Qibo said：“When the patient has fever but his pulse condition is calm，or when the patient has perspiration but his pulse condition is irritating，it is the first kind of adverseness；when the patient has diarrhea but his pulse condition is full and gigantic，it is the second kind of adverseness；when the patient has protracted localized arthralgia and his protruding muscles in the elbow and the knee are broken and have ulcerations，has fever in the body but his pulse condition tends to be severing，it is the third kind of adverseness；when the patient has intestinal bi-syndrome，nocturnal emission，emaciation of the body，pale and dark in the complexion，red and black blood clots occur in the stool and the disease condition is quite serious，it is the fourth kind of adverseness；when the patient has fever and thin body but his pulse condition is firm and vigorous，it is the fifth kind of adverseness.”

动输第六十二

Chapter 62
Dong Shu
(The Pulsation of Arteries)

黄帝曰：经脉十二，而手太阴、足少阴、阳明独动不休，何也？岐伯曰：是明胃脉也。胃为五脏六腑之海，其清气上注于肺，肺气从太阴而行之，其行也，以息往来，故人一呼脉再动，一吸脉亦再动，呼吸不已，故动而不止。

Yellow Emperor said: "In the twelve channels, there are only the Hand Taiyin Channel of Lung, the Foot Shaoyin Channel of Kidney and the Foot Yangming Channel of Stomach have the unceasing pulsations of the arteries, and what is the reason?" Qibo said: "This is due to the Foot Yangming Channel of Stomach associates with the pulsation of the pulse. The stomach is the convergent location of the energies of the five solid organs and the six hollow organs, the fresh air converted by the refined substances of the food ascends to pour into the lung, and the air which starts from the Hand Taiyin Channel spreads to the whole body. The air of the lung operates up and down by the inhalation and the exhalation, and when one exhales once, the pulse pulsates twice, and when one inhales once, the pulse pulsates twice also, when the respiration carries on unceasingly, the pulsation of the Cunkou pulse will not stop."

黄帝曰：气之过于寸口也，上十焉息？下八焉伏？何道从还？不知其极。岐伯曰：气之离藏也，卒然如弓弩之发，如水之下岸，上于鱼以反衰，其余气衰散以逆上，故其行微。

Yellow Emperor said: "When the channel energy of Hand Taiyin passes the Cunkou, it rests when it ascends to reach the lung, and hides when it descends to reach the finger's tips. From what place will it return to its own channel of Hand Taiyin? I don't know its reason." Qibo said: "When the channel energy divorces from the internal organs inside to reach the channels outside, it is irresistable like the arrow shot from the bow or the torrent wates rushing down the cliff. When the channel energy ascends to reach the hand thenear eminence, it turns weaker, when the remainder energy reverses up, it will become deficient and seattered, and its movement is also slow."

黄帝曰：足之阳明何因而动？岐伯曰：胃气上注于肺，其悍气上冲头者，循咽，上走空窍，循眼系，入络脑，出顑，下客主人，循牙车，合阳明，并下人迎，此胃气别走于阳明者也。故阴阳上下，其动也若一。故阳病而阳脉小者为逆，阴病而阴脉大者为逆。故阴阳俱静俱动，若引绳相倾者病。

Yellow Emperor asked: "Why is there the artery in the Foot Yangming Channel of Stomach?" Qibo said: "When the stomach energy ascends and pours into the lung, the main flow of the energy rushes up to the head, then, it runs along the throat to reach the seven orifices and runs along the inner collaterals of the eyeball to contact with the brain inside, then, come out from the temple, descends to join the Kezhuren point, runs along the Jiache point and joins its own channel of Foot Yangming and ascends to Renying. This is the reason the Renying pulse is pulsating unceasingly when the stomach energy branches out and then returns to the Foot Yangming Channel. Thus, the pulsations of the Cunkou of the Taiyin artery and Renying of the Yangming artery are identical. When the Yang pulse is small in the Yang disease, it is called adverseness; when the Yin pulse is gigantic in the Yin disease, it is also called adverseness. Under the normal condition, the extent of pulsations of the Cunkou and Renying pulses are keeping balance, if one of them is overabundant and the other is deficient, it will cause disease."

黄帝曰：足少阴何因而动？岐伯曰：冲脉者，十二经之海也，与〔与：《素问·离合真邪论》王注引《灵枢》"与"下有"足"字〕少阴之大络，起于肾下，出于气街，循阴股内廉，邪入腘中，循胫骨内廉，并少阴之经，下入内踝之后，入足下；其别者，邪〔邪：本经《逆顺肥瘦篇》无此字〕入踝，出属跗上，入大指之间，注诸络，以温足胫〔胫：《甲乙》卷二第一下作"附"〕，此脉之常动者也。

Yellow Emperor asked: "Why is there the artery pulsation in the Foot Shaoyin Channel of Kidney?" Qibo said: "The Chong Channel is the sea of the twelve channels. It starts from the Huiyin point together with the colaterals of the Foot Shaoyin Channel, it comes out from the Qichong point, runs along the inner side of the thigh, slanting into the poplitea of the knee, then, runs along the inner side of the tibia, joins its own Foot Shaoyin Channel of Kidney, enters into the rear of the inner ankle of the foot and comes out from the location near the outer ankle, enters into the toe and pours into the collateral of the Shaoyin Channel in the leg to warm and moisten the leg. This is the reason the pulsation is unceasing in the Foot Shaoyin Channel.

黄帝曰：营卫之行也，上下相贯，如环之无端，今有其卒然遇邪气，及逢大寒，手足懈惰，其脉阴阳之道，相输之会，行相失也，气何由还？岐伯曰：夫四末阴阳之会者，此气之大络也。四街者，气之径路也。故络绝则径通，四末解则气从合，相输如环。黄帝曰：善。此所谓如环无端，莫知其纪，终而复始，此之谓也。

Yellow Emperor said: "The Ying-energy and the Wei-energy pass through the whole body, they operate above and below like a ring without an end. When one encounters cold suddenly, his extremities will be strengthless, the Yin and Yang operations of his channels and the circulations of his energy and blood will become abnormal, under such situation, from which location will the energy turn back to keep the coming and going without stopping?" Qibo said: "The four extremities of the human body are the places for the Yin and Yang energies to converge, and they are the large collaterals of the channel energy; the head, chest, abdomen and the tibia and fibula are the passages of the channel energy, so, when the collaterals are blocked due to being invaded, the channels can still remain unimpeded. The channel energy will become harmony again after the evil-energies in the four extremities have been relieved and the transmission will go on like a ring without an end."

五味论第六十三

Chapter 63
Wu Wei Lun
(On the Five Tastes)

黄帝问于少俞曰：五味入于口也，各有所走，各有所病。酸走筋，多食之〔之：《千金》卷二十六《序论》作“酸”〕，令人癃；咸走血，多食之〔之：《千金》卷二十六《序论》作“咸”〕，令人渴；辛走气，多食之〔之：《千金》卷二十六《序论》作“辛”〕，令人洞心；苦走骨，多食之〔《千金》卷二十六《序论》作“苦”〕令人变呕；甘走肉，多食之〔《千金》卷二十六作“甘”〕令人悗心。余知其然也，不知其何由，愿闻其故。

Yellow Emperor asked Shaoyu and said："When the five tastes enter into the stomach，each of them prefers to go to the viscus of its similar property and each of them causes the specific disease；such as，the sour taste goes to the tendon，when one takes sour taste excessively，he will have dysuria；the salty taste goes to the blood，when one takes the salty taste excessively，he will be thirsty；the acrid taste goes to the energy，when one takes the acrid taste excessively，he will have the feeling of fumigation of the heart；the bitter taste goes to the bone，when one takes the bitter taste excessively，he will vomit；the sweet taste goes to the muscle，when one takes the sweet taste excessively，he will feel oppression of the heart. I have known the conditions already，but I don't understand what causes them，and I hope to hear the reasons about it."

少俞答曰：酸入于胃，其气涩以收，上之两焦〔上之两焦：《甲乙》卷六第九无此四字〕，弗能出入也，不出即留于胃中，胃中和温，则下注膀胱，膀胱之胞薄以懦〔懦：《太素》卷二《调食》作“濡”〕，得酸则缩绻，约而不通，水道不行，故癃。阴者，积筋之所终〔终：《甲乙》卷六第九“终下”并有“聚”字〕也，故酸入〔《甲乙》卷六第九“入”下有“胃”字〕而走筋矣。

Shaoyu answered："When the sour taste enters into the stomach，as it is puckery and harsh and has the function of restraint，it can not operate to go in and come out along with the activities of vital energy；since it can not come out，it retains in the stomach which is warm，and then permeats downwards and pours into the bladder. As the bladder is thin and soft，it will become shrinking when encountering the sour taste and the exit of the bladder will be controlled and obstructed，in this way，the urination will be unsmoothed and the syndrome of dysuria will occur. The external genital is the place where all the tendons of the body converge，and the sour taste enters into the stomach through the tendon."

黄帝曰：咸走血，多食之，令人渴，何也？少俞曰：咸入于胃，其气上走中焦，注于脉，则血气走之，血与咸相得则凝，凝则胃中汁注之〔注之：《千金》卷二十六第一《序论》作

"泣"〕，注之则胃中竭〔竭：《千金》卷二十六第一《序论》作"乾渴"〕，竭则咽路焦，故舌本干而善渴。血脉者，中焦之道也，故咸入而走血矣。

Yellow Emperor asked: "The excessive salty taste causes one thirsty and why is it?" Shaoyu said: "When the salty taste enters into the stomach, the energy transformed ascends to reach the middle warmer, and then, from the middle warmer, pours into the channel. The channel reflects the condition of the blood flow, when the channel encounters the salty taste, it will be obstructed and the fluid in the stomach will become stagnant and unsmoothed in the wake of it, when the fluid in the stomach is stagnant, the fluid in the stomach will be dry and exhausted, when the stomach fluid is dry and exhausted, the pharynx which is the passage of the saliva will be dry, and one will be thirsty and be swallowing dryly. The channel starts to communicate with the blood and energy from the middle warmer, when the salty taste enters into the stomach, it goes to the blood."

黄帝曰：辛走气，多食之，令人洞心，何也？少俞曰：辛入于胃，其气走于上焦，上焦者，受气而营诸阳者也，姜韭之气熏之〔熏之：《千金》卷二十六第一并作"熏至营卫"〕，营卫之气〔营卫之气：《甲乙》卷六第九并无"之气"二字，"营卫"二字连下读〕不时受之，久留心下，故洞心〔洞心：《千金》卷二十六第一作"愠愠痛也"〕。辛与气俱行，故辛入而与汗俱出。

Yellow Emperor asked: "The acrid taste goes to the energy, when one takes the acrid taste excessively, he will feel like the fumigation of smoke to the heart, and why is it?" Shaoyu said: "When the acrid taste enters into the stomach, its energy ascends to the upper warmer, as the upper warmer has the function of receiving the refined energy of the food and drink for circulating the Yang energy to the whole body, when the energies of ginger and Chinese chives fumigate the ying and wei energies, they are often stimulated by the acridness, when the acridness retains long in the stomach, one will have the feeling of the fumigation of the heart. The acridness goes to the Wei energy and it travels along with the Wei energy, thus, when the acrid taste enters into the stomach, it will be sent forth along with the sweat."

黄帝曰：苦走骨，多食之，令人变呕，何也？少俞曰：苦入于胃，五谷之气，皆不能胜苦，苦入下脘，三焦之道皆闭而不通，故变呕．齿者，骨之所终也，故苦入而走骨，故入而复出，知其走骨也。

Yellow Emperor asked: "The bitter taste goes to the bone, when one takes excessive bitter taste, the colour of his teeth will be changed, and what is the reason?" Shaoyu said: "When the bitter taste enters into the stomach, all energies of the five cereals in the stomach can not withstand the bitter taste. When the bitter taste enters into the lower part of the gastric cavity, the passageway of the triple warmer will be obstrucated and the colour of the teeth will be changed. The teeth is the terminal of the bone, so, when the bitter taste enters into the stomach, it goes to the bone first, then, it comes out from the teeth causing the teeth turn into black and yellow. It is from the appearance, people know that the bitter taste goes to the bone."

黄帝曰：甘走肉，多食之，令人悗心，何也？少俞曰：甘入于胃，其气弱小，不能上至于上焦，而与谷留于胃中者，令人柔润者也，胃柔则缓，缓则虫动，虫动则令人悗心。其气外通于肉，故甘走肉。

Yellow Emperor asked: "The sweet taste goes to the muscle, when one takes the sweet taste excessively, he will have the feeling of oppression of the heart, and why is it?" Shaoyu said: "When the sweet enters into the stomach, as its energy is rather weak, it can not ascend to the upper warmer but can only retain in the stomach with the cereals. The sweetness can soften and moisten the stomach, when the stomach energy is soft, the operation of its energy will be loose and slow which will cause the wriggle of parasites in the stomach and the intestine, and the wriggle of parasites causes one to feel oppression of the heart; besides, the sweet taste communicates with the muscle outside, so, there is the version of 'sweet taste goes to the muscle'."

阴阳二十五人第六十四

Chapter 64
Yin Yang Er Shi Wu Ren
(The Twenty Five Kinds of People in Different Characteristics of Yin and Yang)

黄帝曰：余闻阴阳之人何如？伯高曰：天地之间，六合之内，不离于五，人亦应之。故五五二十五人之政，而阴阳之人不与焉。其态又不合于众者五，余已知之矣。愿闻二十五人之形，血气之所生，别而以候，从外知内何如？岐伯曰：悉乎哉问也，此先师之秘也，虽伯高犹不能明之也。黄帝避席遵循而却曰：余闻之，得其人弗教，是谓重失，得而泄之，天将厌之。余愿得而明之，金柜藏之，不敢扬之。岐伯曰：先立五形金木水火土，别其五色，异其五形之人，而二十五人具矣。黄帝曰：愿卒闻之。岐伯曰：慎之慎之，臣请言之。

Yellow Emperor said: "I am told that some human body belongs to Yin or to Yang, what is the condition? Bogao said: "It was stated by Shaoshi that within the six directions (east, west, north, south, up and down) between heaven and earth, nothing can divorce from the five elements, and a man corresponds to it. So, the twenty five kinds of people which belong to the five elements are excluded from the people of Yin and Yang kinds. The shapes of the people of the Yin and Yang kinds which contain the Taiyang, Shaoyang, Taiyin, Shaoyin and Mild kinds of people respectively are different from that of the common people, and I have already understood them all. Now I want to hear about the various shapes of the twenty five kinds of people, their characteristis when born of blood and energy, and I want to understand the changes of the internal organs by examining from outside, what should I do?" Qibo said: "You have asked a very exhaustive question. It is the confidential impartation from the late master, even Bogao can not comprehend it thoroughly." Yellow Emperor left his seat, moved back modestly and said: "I am told when one does not impart to the one who is deserving, it is a great error; when one has acquired the genuine impartation and neglects it, heaven will detest him. I hope when I obtain the impartation, expound it, store it in a golden cabinet, and dare not to discard it." Qibo said: "One must set the five shapes of the metal, wood, water, fire and earth elements, distinguish the five colours and separate the five tones first, then the characteristic-shape of the twenty five kinds of people can all be known." Yellow Emperor said: "I hope to hear them all." Qibo said: "You must be very very careful about it. Now, let me tell you in details."

木形之人，比于上角，似于苍帝。其为人苍色，小头，长面，大肩背，直身，小手足，好有才，劳心，少力，多忧劳于事。能春夏不能秋冬，感而病生，足厥阴佗佗然。大角之人，比于左足少阳，少阳之上遗遗然。左角之人，比于右足少阳，少阳之下随随然。钛角之人，比于右足少阳、少阳之上推推然。判角之人，比于左足少阳，少阳之下栝栝然。

"The man in wood type when analogizing with the five tones, is like the Shangjue (Upper Jue), he is similar with the people of the east where the Green Emperor lives. He is green and small headed, has a long face, large shoulders, flat back, upright body and small limbs, he is talented, being a mental worker, has weaker physical strength, and he often worries about his work, he can withstand the weather of spring and summer but can not withstand the weather of autumn and winter, when he encounters the evil energy in autumn and winter, he will fall sick. People of the Shangjue kind belongs to the Foot Jueyin Channel of Liver and their outer appearances are always gracefully poised. In the tones of wood, people belong to the Taijue (Greater Jue) kind can be analogized as the Left Foot Shaoyang, and the upper part of Shaoyang appears to be self-satisfied; people belong to the Zuojue (Left Jue) kind can be analogized as the Right Foot Shaoyang, and the lower part of Shaoyang who appears to be amiable; people belong to the Taijue (Large Jue) can be analogized as the Right Foot Shaoyang, and the upper part of the Shaoyang who appears to be proceeding; people belong to the Panjue (Half Jue) kind can be analogized as the Left Foot Shaoyang, and the lower part of Shaoyang appears to be upright.

火形之人，比于上徵，似于赤帝，其为人赤色，广肕，锐面小头，好肩背髀腹，小手足，行安地，疾心〔疾心：《千金》卷十三第一大"心"字〕，行摇，肩背肉满，有气轻财，少信，多虑，见事明，好颜，急心，不寿暴死。能春夏不能秋冬，秋冬感而病生，手少阴核核然。质〔质：《甲乙》卷一第十六作"太"〕徵之人比于左手太阳，太阳之上肌肌然。少徵之人，比于右手太阳，太阳之下慆慆然。右徵之人，比于右手太阳，太阳之上鲛鲛然。质判（一日质徵）之人，比于左手太阳，太阳之下支支颐颐然。

"The man in fire type, when analogizing with the five tones is like the Shangzhi (Upper Zhi), he is similar with the people of the south where the Red Emperor lives. He has the characteristics of broad and revealing teeth, thin and sharp chin, small head, well developed shoulder, back, thigh and abdomen, small hands and feet, he is steady in his step, fast in walking with swaying of shoulder, his muscle is plump in the back, daring, neglecting money, break his word often, misgiving, clear in analysing, anxious in heart, fail to enjoy a long life and apt to die suddenly. He can withstand the weather of spring and summer but can not withstand the weather of autumn and winter, when the evil energy of autumn and winter is encountered, he will fall sick. People of the Shangzhi (Upper Zhi) kind belong to the Hand Shaoyin Channel of Heart, and they are modest. In the tones of fire, people belong to the Taizhi (Greater Zhi) kind can be analogized as the Left Hand Taiyang Channel of Small Intestine, and the upper part of Taiyang appears to be bright; people belong to the Shaozhi (lesser Zhi) kind can be analogized as the Right Hand Taiyang Channel of Small Intestine, and the lower part of Taiyang appears to be joyous; people belong to the Youzhi (Right Zhi) kind can be analogized as the Right Hand Taiyang Channel of Small Intestine, and the upper part of Taiyang appears to be progressive and bright; people belong to the Panzhi (Half Zhi) kind can be analogized as the Left Hand Taiyang, and the lower part of Taiyang appears to be optimistic and self-satisfied.

土形之人，比于上宫，似于上古黄帝。其为人黄色，圆面，大头，美肩背，大腹，美股胫，小〔小："小"疑应作"大"〕手足，多肉，上下相称，行安地，举足浮〔举足浮："浮"是"孚"的误字〕，安心，好利人，不喜权势。善附人也。能秋冬不能春夏，春夏感而病生，足太阴敦敦然。太宫之人，比于左足阳明，阳明之上婉婉然。加宫之人（一曰众之人），比于左足阳明，阳明之下坎坎然。少宫之人，比于右足阳明，阳明之上枢枢然。左宫之人（一曰众之人，一曰阳明之上），比于右足阳明，阳明之下兀兀然。

"The man is earth type when analogizing with the five tones, is like the Shanggong (Upper Gong), he is similar with people of the centraliry where the Yellow Emperor lives. He has the characteristics of yellow skin, round face, large head, well-developed shoulders and back, large abdomen, strong thighs and legs, large hands and feet, plump muscle, even and matching in the upper and the lower parts of the body, his steps are steady, he is honest, ease of heart, likes to do things benefiting others, detest of power and influence, but he tends to rely on others. He can withstand the weather of autumn and winter but he can not withstand the weather of spring and summer, when he encounters the evil energy of spring and summer, he will fall sick. People of the Shanggong kind belong to the Foot Taiyin Channel of Spleen, and they are earnest. In the tones of earth, people belong to the Taigong (Greater Gong) kind can be analogized as the Left Foot Yangming, and the upper part of Yangming who appear to be amiable; people belong to the Jiagong (Right Gong) kind can be analogized as the Left Foot Yangming, and the lower part of Yangming who appear to be joyous and pleasant; people belong to the Shaogong (Lesser Gong) kind can be analogized as the Right Foot Yangming, and the upper part of Yangming who appear to be slippery and slick; people belong to the Zuogong (Left Gong) kind can be analogized as the Right Foot Yangming, and the lower part of Yangming who appear to be kind.

金形之人，比于上商，似于白帝。其为人方面，白色，小头，小肩背，小腹，小手足，如骨发踵外，骨轻、身清廉，急心，静悍，善为吏〔善为吏：《千金》卷十七第一作"性喜为吏治"〕。能秋冬不能春夏，春夏感而病生，手太阴敦敦然。钛〔钛：《甲乙》卷一第十六作"大"〕商之人，比于左手阳明之上廉廉然。右〔右：日刻本作"左"〕商之人，比于左手阳明，阳明之下脱脱然。右商之人，比于右手阳明，阳明之上监监然。少商之人，比于右手阳明，阳明之下严严然。

"The man in metal type when analogizing with the five tones is like the Shangshang (Upper Shang), he is similar with people of the west where the White Emperor lives. He has the characterisics of square face, white colour, small head, small shoulder and back, small abdomen, small hands and feet, light in the body when acting, thin, capable and vigorous, impetuous, capable in either moving or motionless, and he is fond of being an officer. He can withstand the weather of autumn and winter, but can not withstand the weather of spring and summer, when he encounters the evil energy of spring and summer, he will fall sick. People of the Shangshang kind belong to the Hand Taiyin Channel of Lung and they are resolute. In the tones of metal, people belong to Taishang (Greater Shang) kind can be analogized as the Left Hand Yangming, and the upper part of Yangming who appears to be unamiable; people belong to the Youshang (Right Shang) kind can be analogized as the Left Hand Yangming, and the lower part of Yangming who appear to be easy and slow in motion; people belong to the zuoshang (Left Shang) kind can be analogized as the Right Hand Yangming, and the upper part of Yangming who appear to be keen in observing; people belong to the Shaoshang (Lesser Shang) kind can be analogized as the Right Hand Yangming, and the lower part of Yangming appears to be solemn and dignified.

水形之人，比于上羽，似于黑帝。其为人黑色，面不平，大头，廉〔廉：《甲乙》卷一第十六并作“广”〕颐，小肩，大腹，动〔动：《甲乙》卷一经十六作“小”，校语作“大”〕手足，发行摇身，下尻长，背延延然，不敬畏，善欺绐人，戮死。能秋冬不能春夏，春夏感而病生，足少阴汗汗然。大羽之人，比于右足太阳，太阳之上颊颊然。少羽之人，比于左足太阳，太阳之下纡纡然。众之为人比于右足太阳，太阳之下洁洁然。桎之为人，比于左足太阳，太阳之上安安然。是故五形之人二十五变者，众之所以相欺〔刘衡如曰：“疑当作“异”〕者是也。

“The man in water type when analogizing with the five tones is like the Shangyu (Upper Yu), he is similar with the people of the north where the Black Emperor lives. He has the characteristics of black skin, rough face, large head, wide cheek, small shoulder, large abdomen, large hands and feet, swaying of the body when acting, longer length from the loin to the buttock and longer back, he does not respect people nor afraid of people, he cheats others frequently, and ocassionally, he may be killed. He can withstand the weather of autumn and winter but can not withstand the weather in spring and summer, when he encounters the evil energy of spring and summer, he will fall sick. People of the Shangyu kind belong to the Foot Shaoyin Channel of Kidney and they are mean. In the tones of Yu, people belong to the Taiyu (Greater Yu) can be analogized as the Right Foot Taiyang, and the upper part of Taiyang appears to be complacent; people belong to the Shaoyu (Lesser Yu) kind can be analogized as the Left Foot Taiyang, and the lower part of Taiyang appears to be tortuous and not frank; people belong to the Zhongyu (Right Yu) kind can be analogized as the Right Foot Taiyang, and the lower part of Taiyang appears to be silent and calm; people belong to the Zhiyu (Left Yu) kind can be analogized as the Left Foot Taiyang, and the upper part of Taiyang appears to be slow and leisurely. Thus, the twenty five varieties in the five types of man are different from common people.”

黄帝曰：得其形，不得其色何如？岐伯曰：形胜色，色胜形者，至其胜时年加，感则病形，失则忧矣。形色相得者，富贵大乐。黄帝曰：其形色相胜之时，年加可知乎？岐伯曰：凡年忌下上之人〔凡年忌下上之人：“凡年”七字，应据《甲乙》卷一第十六改为“凡人之”三字连下“大忌”断句〕，大忌常加〔常加：《甲乙》卷一第十六“加”下有“九岁”二字。应据补〕七岁，十六岁，二十五岁，三十四岁，四十三岁，五十二岁，六十一岁，皆人之大〔大：《甲乙》卷一第十六无此字〕忌，不〔不：《永乐大典》卷三千七《阴阳二十五人》条引无此字〕可不自安也，感则病行〔行：《甲乙》卷一第十六无此字〕，失则忧矣。当此之时，无为奸事，是谓年忌。

Yellow Emperor asked: "When the human body suits the shape of the five-element but does not have the proper colour in the skin, what will be the condition?" Qibo said: "When the five-colour-belonging of the shape subjugates the five-colour-belonging of the skin colour or the five-colour-belonging of the skin colour subjugates the five-element-belonging of the shape, and again, the overcoming year is encountered, people will fall sick when being affected slightly, and if the patient is maltreated, something worrisome will happen. If the skin colour and the shape are suiting with each other, one will have great pleasure." Yellow Emperor said: "There is the condition of subjugation of shape or the skin colour which is the year of contraindication, can you tell me condition about it?" Qibo said: "Generally speaking, the contraindication year of a man is every other nine years, commencing from seven years old, then the sixteen years old, twenty five years old, thirty four years old, fourty three years old, fifty two years and sixty one year old are all the years of great contraindication of men, one must be careful in these years as any affection will cause disease, and if the disease is maltreated, trouble will occur. In these years, one must not do anything mischievous. This is the condition of the so-called year of contraindication."

黄帝曰：夫子之言，脉之上下，血气之候，以知形气奈何？岐伯曰：足阳明之上，血气盛则髯〔髯：《甲乙》卷一第十六任务"须"〕美长；血少气多〔血少气多：《甲乙》卷一第十六作"血多气少"〕则髯短；故气少血多〔气少血多：《甲乙》卷一第十六作"气多血少"〕则髯少；血气皆少则无髯，两吻多画。足阳明之下，血气盛则下毛美长至胸；血多气少则下毛美短至脐，行则善高举足，足指少肉，足善寒；血少气多则肉而善瘃；血气皆少无毛，有则稀〔稀：《甲乙》卷一第十六"稀"下有"而"字〕枯悴，善痿厥足痹。

Yellow Emperor said: "You said that when examining the energy and blood from the upper part and the lower part of the three Yang channels of hand and foot, one can know whether the shape and energy are strong or weak, and what is the condition?" Qibo said: "When the shape-characteristic of the Foot Yangming Channel is in the upper part, if his blood and energy are overabundant, his beard will be handsome and long; if the blood is plenty and the energy is little, his beard will be short; if the energy is plenty and the blood is little, his beard will be sparse; if both the energy and blood are little, he will have no beard on the cheeks and will have plenty wrinkles by the corners of the mouth; when the shape-characteristic of Foot Yangming Channel is on the lower part, if both the blood and energy are overabundant, his pubic hair will be good looking and long, and he has hair in the breast; if the blood is plenty and the energy is little, his pubic hair will be good looking and short, and its extention will stop by the navel, he often lifts his feet high when walking, the muscle in his thumb is thin and he feels cold of the feet often; if the blood is little and the energy is plenty, the muscle of his lower extremities will apt to contract chilblain; if both the blood and energy are little, he will have no pubic hair, if there is any, they will be little and dry, his feet are week and flaccid and has arthralgia pain in the feet often.

足少阳之上，气血盛则通髯美长；血多气少则通髯美短；血少气多则少髯；血气皆少则无鬚，感于寒湿则善痹，骨痛爪枯也。足少阳之下，血气盛则胫毛美长，外踝肥；血多气少则踝毛美短，外踝皮坚而厚；血少气多则胻毛少，外踝皮薄而软；血气皆少则无毛，外踝瘦无肉。

"When the shape-characteristic of the Foot Shaoyang Channel is on the upper part, if both the energy and the blood are overabundant, the beard on the ckeeks connecting the temples will be handsome and long; if the blood is plenty and the energy is little, the beard on the cheeks connecting the temples will be handsome and short; if the blood is little and the energy is plenty, his beard will be little; if both the blood and the energy are little, he will have no beard. When one contracts the cold-wetness, he will often have arthralgia, pain of bone and the withering of the nails. When the shape-characteristic of the Foot Shaoyang Channel is on the lower part, if both the blood and the energy are overabundant, his fine hair on the legs will be handsome and long and the outer ankles of the feet will be fat and large; if the blood is plenty and the energy is little, the fine hair on the legs will be handsome and short, and the skin of the outer ankles of the feet will be firm and thick; if the blood is little and the energy is plenty, the fine hair on the legs will be little, and the skin of the outer ankles of the feet will be thin and soft; if both the blood and energy are little, he will have no hair on the legs, and his outer ankles of the feet will be lean without muscle.

足太阳之上，血气盛则美眉，眉有毫毛；血多气少则恶眉，面多少〔少：《甲乙》卷一第十六作"小"〕理；血少气多〔气多：《甲乙》卷一第十六作"气盛"〕则面多肉；血气和则美色。足太阴〔阴：当注本，张注本作"阳"〕之下，血气盛则跟肉满，踵坚；气少血多则瘦，跟空；血气皆少则喜转筋，踵下痛。

"When the shape-characteristic of the Foot Taiyang Channel in on the upper side, if both the energy and blood are overabundant, his eyebrows will be handsome and mixed with long hair; if the blood is plenty and the energy is little, his eyebrows will be withered and not moisturized and there will be many small lines on the face; if the blood is little and the energy is plenty, he will have plenty muscle on the face; if the blood and energy are harmonious, his complexion will be good looking. When the shape-characteristic of the Foot Taiyang Channel is on the lower part, if both the blood and the energy are overabundant, the muscle on the heel will be plump and substantial; if the energy is little and the blood is plenty, his heel will be thin without any muscle; if both the blood and the energy are little, he will have spasm of muscle and pain in the heel.

手阳明之上，血气盛则髭美；血少气多则髭恶；血气皆少则无髭。手阳明之下，血气盛则腋下毛美，手鱼肉以温；气血皆少则手瘦以寒。

"When the shape-characteristic of the Hand Yangming Channel is on the upper part, if both the blood and energy are overabundant, one's beard beside the mouth will be good looking; if the blood is little and the energy is plenty, the beards beside the mouth will be poor looking; if both the blood and the energy are little, one will have no beard beside the mouth. When the shape-characteristic of the Hand Yangming Channel is on the lower part, if both the blood and the energy are overabundant, one's hair under the armpit will be handsome and flourishing, and the muscle of the thenar eminence will be warm; if both the blood and

the energy are little, the muscle of one's hand will be thin and emaciated, and he often feels cold.

手少阳之上，血气盛则眉美以长，耳色美；血气皆少则耳焦恶色。手少阳之下，血气盛则手卷多肉以温；血气皆少则寒以瘦；气少血多则瘦以多脉。

"When the shape-characteristic of the Shaoyang Channel is on the upper part, if both the blood and energy are overabundant, one's eyebrows will be elegant and long, and the colour of the ears will be fine; if both the blood and the energy are little, ones ears will be scorching with dark colour. When the shape-characteristic of the Hand Shaoyang Channel is in the lower part, if both the blood and energy are overabundant, the muscle in the hand and fist will be plenty and warm; if both the blood and energy are little, one's hands will be cold, emaciated with little muscle; if the energy is little and the blood is plenty, one's skin and muscle will be thin, and the collaterals will be revealing outside.

手太阳之上，血气盛则有多髯，面多肉以平；血气少则面瘦恶〔恶：《甲乙》卷一第十六作"黑"〕色。手太阳之下，血气盛则掌肉充满；血气皆少则掌瘦以寒。

"When the shape-characteristic of the Hand Taiyin Channel is in the upper part, if both the blood and energy are overabundant, one will have plenty beard above and below the mouth, and the muscle on the face will be plenty and smooth; if both the blood and energy are little, there will be no muscle on the face, and he will be black. When the shape-characteristic of the Hand Taiyang Channel is on the lower part, if both the blood and energy are overabundant, the muscle of ones palm will be full; if both the blood and energy are little, the muscle in the palm will be thin and cold."

黄帝曰：二十五人者，刺之有约乎？岐伯曰：美眉者，足太阳之脉，气血多；恶眉者，血气少；其肥而泽者，血气有余；肥而不泽者，气有余，血不足；瘦而无泽者，气血俱不足。审察其形气有余不足而调之，可以知逆顺矣。

Yellow Emperor asked: "Is there any criterion when treating the twenty five kinds of men with acupuncture?" Qibo said: "When ones eyebrows are elegant, it is due to both the energy and blood in the Foot Taiyang Channel are plenty; when one's eyebrows are not elegant, it is due to both the blood and energy of the Foot Taiyang Channel are little; if one's muscle is fleshy and the colour of his skin is not moist, he belongs to the category of having a surplus in the energy but deficient in the blood; when one's muscle is emaciated and his skin colour is not lustrous, he belongs to the category of deficient in both energy and blood. When examining the surplus or deficient appearance of the energy and blood from outside, and adjusts according to the principle of invigorating the asthenia and purging the sthenia, one will know the difference between the agreeableness and adverseness."

黄帝曰：刺其诸阴阳奈何？岐伯曰：按其寸口人迎，以调阴阳，切循其经络之凝涩，结而不通者，此〔此：《永乐大典》卷一三八七《痹类》引作"在"〕于身皆为痛痹，甚则不行，故凝涩。凝涩者，致气以温之，血和乃止。其结络者，脉结血不和，决之乃行。故曰：气有余于上者，导而下之；气不足于上者，推而休之；其稽留不至者，因而迎之；必明于经隧，乃能持之。寒与热争者，导而行之；其宛陈血不结者，侧而予之〔侧而予之：《甲乙》卷一第十六任务“即而取之”〕。必先明知二十五人，则血气之所在，左右上下，刺约毕也。

Yellow Emperor asked: "How to prick the Yin channels and the Yang channels?" Qibo said: "Press the Cunkou pulse and the Renying pulse to examine the overabundance or deficiency of Yin and Yang, and press along the channel route to see whether there is any stagnation, if there is stagnation and impediment, one will have arthralgia in the body, and he can not walk when the case is serious. Thus, to the patient of blood and energy stagnation, his Yang energy should be induced so that his blood and energy can be warmed and smoothed, and stop the treating when the blood becomes harmonious. To the disease of the channel congealement causing the unimpediment of blood, dredge it to become smooth. Therefore, when the evil energy is hyperactive in the upper part, induce it to become descending; when the healthy energy is insufficient in the upper part, prick the acupoints on the upper part, rub and press the muscle and skin to raise the energy; when the energy does not arrive after the long retaining of the needle, apple poly-manipulation to induce the energy. One must understand thoroughly the passages of the channels in advance, then he can treat with correct method. In the condition of the cold and heat contention, one should dredge the energy and blood; when there is the protracted accumulation and stagnation of blood, prick the acupoint on the focus. In a word, one must understand the types of the twenty five kinds of men and pricks according to the characteristics of whether the disease is in the energy, blood, left, right, upper part and the lower part.

五音五味第六十五

Chapter 65
Wu Yin Wu Wei
(The Five Tones and the Five Tastes)

右徵与少徵，调右手太阳上，左商与左徵，调左手阳明上。
少徵与大宫，调左手阳明上。右角与大角，调右足少阳下。
大徵与少徵，调左手太阳上。众羽与少羽，调右足太阳下。
少商与右商，调右手太阳下。桎羽与众羽，调右足太阳下。
少宫与大宫，调右足阳明下。判角与少角，调右足少阳下。
钛商与上商，调右足阳明下。钛商与上角，调左足太阳下。

To people who belong to the Youzhi (Right Zhi) and Shaozhi (Lesser Zhi) kinds in the five tones, it should treat the upper part of the right Hand Taiyang Channel. To people who belong to the Zuoshang (Left Shang) and Zuozhi (Left Zhi) kinds, it should treat the upper part of the left Hand Yangming Channel. To people who belong to the Shaozhi (Lesser Zhi) and Dagong (Greater Gong) kinds, it should treat the upper part of the left Hand Yangming Channel. To people who belong to the Youjue (Right Jue) and Dajue (Greater Jue) kinds, it should treat the lower part of the right Foot Shaoyang Channel. To people who belong to the Dazhi (Greater Zhi) and Shaozhi (Lesser Zhi) kinds, it should treat the upper part of the left Hand Taiyang Channel. To people who belong to the Zhongyu (Right Yu) and Shaoyu (Lesser Yu) kinds, it should treat the lower part of the right Foot Taiyang Channel. To people who belong to the Shaoshang (Lesser Shang) and Youshang (Right Shang) kinds, it should treat the lower part of the right Hand Taiyang Channel. To people who belong to the Zhiyu (Left Yu) and Zhongyu (Right Yu) kinds, it should treat the lower part of the right Foot Taiyang Channel. To people who belong to the Shaogong (Lesser Gong) and Dagong (Greater Gong) kinds, it should treat the lower part of the right Foot Yangming Channel. To people who belong to the Panjue (Half Jue) and Shaojue (Lesser Jue) kinds, it should treat the lower part of the right Foot Shaoyang Channel. To people who belong to the Daishang (Greater Shang) and Shangshang kinds, it should treat the lower part of the right Foot Yangming Channel. To people who belong to the Daishang (Greater Shang) and Shangjue (Upper Jue) kinds, it should treat the lower part of the left Foot Taiyang Channel.

上徵与右徵同，谷麦，畜羊，果杏，手少阴，藏心，色赤，味苦，时夏。上羽与大羽同，谷大豆，畜彘，果栗，足少阴，藏肾，色黑味咸，时冬。上宫与大宫同。谷稷，畜牛，果枣，足太阴，藏脾，色黄，味甘，时季夏。上商与右商同，谷黍，畜鸡，果桃，手太阴，藏肺，色白，味辛，时秋。上角与大角同，谷麻畜犬，果李，足厥阴，藏肝，色青，味酸，时春。

Both the people of the Shangzhi (Upper Zhi) and the Youzhi (Right Zhi) belong to the tone of fire, under this category, in the five cereals, it is wheat, in the five animals, it is sheep, in the five fruits, it is apricot, in the channels, it is the Hand Shaoyin Channel, in the five solid organs, it is the heart, in the five colours, it is red, in the five tastes, it is bitterness, in the four seasons, it is summer. Both the people of the Shangyu (Upper Yu) and the Dayu (Greater Yu) belong to the tone of water, under this category, in the five cereals, it is soybean, in the five animals, it is pig, in the five nuts; it is chestnuts, in the channels, it is the Foot Shaoyin Channel, in the five solid organs, it is kidney, in the five colours, it is black, in the five tastes, it is saltiness, in the four seasons, it is winter. Both the people of the Shanggong (Upper Gong) and the Dagong (Greater Gong) belong to the tone of earth, under this category, in the five cereals, it is grain, in the five animals, it is cow, in the five fruits, it is jujube, in the channels, it is the Foot Taiyin Channel, in the five solid organs, it is the spleen, in the five colours, it is yellow, in the five tastes, it is sweetness, in the four seasons, it is late summer. Both the people of the Shangshang (Upper Shang) and Youshang (Right Shang) belong to the tone of metal, under this category, in the five cereals, it is the glutinous millet, in the five animals, it is chicken, in the five fruits, it is peach, in the channels, it is the Hand Taiyin Channel, in the five solid organs, it is the lung, in the five colours, it is white, in the five tastes, it is acridness, in the four seasons, it is autumn. Both the people of the Shangjue (Upper Jue) and the Dajue (Greater Jue) belong to the tone of wood, under this category, in the five cereals, it is the sesame, in the five animals, it is dog, in the five fruits, it is plum, in the channel, it is the Foot Jueyin Channel, in the five solid organs, it is the liver, in the five colours, it is green, in the five tastes, it is sourness, in the four seasons, it is spring.

大宫与上角，同右足阳明上。左角与大角，同左足阳明上。

少羽与大羽，同右足太阳下。左商与右商，同左手阳明上。

加宫与大宫，同左足少阳上。质判与大宫，同左手太阳下。

判角与大角，同左足少阳下。大羽与大角，同右足太阳上。

大角与大宫，同右足少阳上。

To the people of the Dagong (Greater Gong) and the Shangjue (Upper Jue) belong to the five tones, it should treat the upper part of the right Foot Yangming Channel. To the people of the Zuojue (Left Jue) and the Dajue (Greater Yu), it should treat the upper part of the left Foot Yangming Channel of stomach. To the people of the Shaoyu (Lesser Yu) and the Dayu (Greater Yu), it should treat the lower part of the right Foot Taiyang Channel of Bladder. To the people of the Zuoshang (Left Shang) and the Youshang (Right Shang), it should treat the upper part of the left Hand Yangming Channel of Large Intestine. To the people of the Jiagong (Right Gong) and the Dagong (Greater Gong), it should treat the upper part of the left Shaoyang Channel of Gallbladder. To the people of the Panzhi (Half Zhi) and the Dagong (Greater Gong), it should treat the lower part of the left Hand Taiyang

Channel of Small Intestine. To the people of the Panjue (Half Jue) and the Dajue (Greater Jue), it should treat the lower part of the left Foot Shaoyang Channel of Gallbladder. To the people of the Dayu (Greater Yu) and the Dajue (Greater Jue), it should treat the upper part of the right Foot Taiyang Channel of Bladder. To the people of the Dajue (Greater Jue) and the Dagong (Greater Gong), it should treat the upper part of the right Foot Shaoyang Channel of Gallbladder.

右徵、少徵、质徵、上徵、判徵。右角、钛角、上角、大角、判角。

右商、少商、钛商、上商、左商。少宫、上宫、大宫、加宫、左角宫。

众羽、桎羽、上羽、大羽、少羽。

The Youzhi (Right Zhi), Shaozhi (Lesser Zhi), Zhizhi (Greater Zhi), Shangzhi (Upper Zhi) and Panzhi (Half Zhi) are the five different types belong to the tone of fire. The Youjue (Right Jue), Daijue (Large Jue), Shangjue (Upper Jue), Dajue (Greater Jue) and Panjue (Half Jue) are the five different types belong to the tone of wood. The Youshang (Right Shang), Shaoshang (Lesser Shang), Daishang (Large Shang), Shangshang (Upper Shang) and Zuoshang (Left Shang) are the five different types belong to the tone of metal. The Shaogong (Lesser Gong), Shanggong (Upper Gong), Dagong (Greater Gong), Jiagong (Right Gong) and Zuogong (Left Gong) are the five different types belong to the tone of earth. The Zhongyu (Right Yu), Zhiyu (Left Yu), Shangyu (Upper Yu), Dayu (Greater Yu) and Shaoyu (Lesser Yu) are the five different types belong to the tone of water.

黄帝曰：妇人无须者，无血气乎？岐伯曰：冲脉、任脉，皆起于胞中，上循背〔背：《素问·空骨论》王注引《针经》并作“脊”〕里，为经络之海。其浮而外者，循腹右上行，会于咽喉，别而络唇口。血气盛〔血气盛：谬平曰：“血字衍”〕则充肤热肉〔则充肤热肉：《素问·空骨论》王注引《针经》“充”作“皮”，热下无“肉”字〕，血独盛则澹渗皮肤，生毫毛。今妇人之生〔今妇人之生：《甲乙》卷二第二无“今之生”三字，“妇人”二字属下读〕，有余于气，不足于血，以其数〔以其《甲乙》卷二第二“以其”下有“月水下”三字〕脱血也，冲任之脉，不荣口唇，故须不生焉。

Yellow Emperor asked: “A woman has no beard, is it because she has no blood and energy?” Qibo said: “Both the Chong Channel and the Ren Channel are starting from the bladder, they ascend along the inner side of the spine and they are the sea of the channel. The superficial Chong and Ren Channels ascend along the abdomen respectively and meet in the pharynx, then they bypass around the mouth and the lips. When the energy is overabundant alone, one's skin will be hot, when the blood is overabundant alone, one's hair will grow. For a woman, when her energy is having a surplus, but her blood is insufficient due to the monthy menstruation, so, her Chong and Ren Channels can not nourish her mouth and lips, and she has no beard.”

黄帝曰：士人有伤于阴，阴气绝而不起，阴不用，然其须不去，其故何也？宦者独去何也？愿闻其故。岐伯曰：宦者去其宗筋，伤其冲脉，血泻不复，皮肤内结，唇口不荣，故须不生。

Yellow Emperor asked: “Someone whose genital organ has been injured to become impotent, his penis can hardly erect and becomes invalid, but he still has beard, whereas an eunuch when being castrated, he has no beard, and what is the reason?" Qibo said: One's Chong Channel will be injured after his testes being cut off, his blood is discharged and can hardly be recovered. As his energy stagnates in the skin, his lips and mouth can not receive the nutrition of the energy and blood, so, he has no beard".

黄帝曰：其有天宦者，未尝被伤，不脱于血，然其须不生，其故何也？岐伯曰：此天之所不足也，其任冲不盛，宗筋不成，有气无血，唇口不荣，故须不生。

Yellow Emperor asked : "Someone was born with genital defect, he has not been castrated by operation, neither has he menstruation, but he has no beard also, and what is the reason?" Qibo said: "This is due to the poor development of his congenital energy, his Ren Channel and Chong Channel are not ample, the function of his penis is not complete, he has some energy but his blood is lacking, so, his lips and mouth can hardly be nourished, and he has no beard".

黄帝曰，善乎哉！圣人这通万物也，若日月之光影，音声鼓响，闻其声而知其形，其非夫子，孰能明万物之精。是故圣人视其颜色〔颜色:《太素》卷十《任脉》"颜"作"真"〕,黄赤者多热〔热:按:"热"似为"血"之误字〕气，青白者少热气，黑色者多血少气。美眉者太阳多血，通髯极须者少阳多血，美须者阳明多血，此其时然也。夫人之常数，太阳常多血少气，少阳常多气少血，阳明常多血多气，厥阴常多气少血，少阴常多血少气，太阴常多血少气〔多血少气:周本，当注本并作"多气少血"〕,此天〔天:疑当作"人"字〕之常数也。

Yellow Emperor said: "Your speach is excellent. The saints know the principles of all things, bright and clear like the light and shadow of the sun and moon, it is explicit like the drum-beat, when one hears the sound, he will know its appearance, if it were not you, who can explain its quintessence. Thus, when a saint examines the complexion of a man, he can know whether the patient's blood and energy is plenty or little; when the complexion appears to be yellow and red, the energy and blood of the patient are plenty; when the complexion appears to be green and white, his energy and blood are little; when the complexion appears to be black, his blood is plenty but his energy is little; when the two eyebrows are elegant, he belongs to the Taiyang Channel with plenty of blood; when his whiskers are connecting the hair, he belongs to the Shaoyin Channel with plenty of blood; when the complexion is good looking, he belongs to the Yangming Channel with plenty of blood. The conditions are usually like this. In the channel of one's body, there is a definite proportion in the blood and energy: in the Hand and Foot Taiyang Channels, usually the blood is plenty and the energy is little; in the Hand and Foot Shaoyang channels, usually the energy is plenty and the blood is little; in the Hand and Foot Yangming Channels, usually the blood is plenty and the energy is also plenty; in the Hand and Foot Jueyin Channels, usually the energy is plenty and the blood is little; in the Hand and Foot Shaoyin Channels, usually the energy is plenty and the blood is little; in the Hand and Foot Taiyin Channels, usually the blood is plenty and the energy is little. These are the conditions of the definite proportion of blood and energy in the channels of the body."

百病始生第六十六

Chapter 66
Bai Bing Shi Sheng
(The Initiation of Various Diseases)

黄帝问于岐伯曰：夫百病之始生也，皆生于风雨寒暑，清湿喜怒。喜怒不节则伤脏，风雨则伤上，清湿则伤下。三部之气，所伤异类〔异类：《甲乙》卷八第二作“各异”〕，愿闻其会。岐伯曰：三部之气各不同，或起于阴，或起于阳，请言其方，喜怒不节，则伤脏，脏伤〔则伤脏，脏伤：按“则伤”五字误衍，此应作“喜怒不节则病起于阴”〕则病起于阴也；清湿袭虚，则病起于下；风雨袭虚，则病起于上，是谓三部。至于其淫泆，不可胜数。

Yellow Emperor asked Qibo and said: “The initiation of various diseases are all due to the wind, rain, cold, heat, coolness, wetness, overjoy and anger from inside and outside. When one's overjoy and anger are without temperance, his internal organs will be injured, when one is affected by exogenous wind and rain, the upper part of his body will be hurt, when one is affected by the wetness-cold, the lower part of his body will be hurt. Since the injuries from the upper, middle and the lower parts are different, I hope you can tell me their common reason.” Qibo said: The various energies from the three parts are different, some of them start from the arm, leg and buttock, some of them start from the face, neck, chest, back and hypochondrium, and I like to tell you their reasons. When one is joyous or angry without temperance, the disease will start from inside, when the wetness-evil invades the tendon and bone, the disease will start from the lower part, when the wind and rain invade the exterior muscle just when the patient is in debility, the disease will start from the upper part. These are the three main parts where the disease initiates. When the disease penetrates, the syndromes occurred will be uncountable.”

黄帝曰：余固不能数，故问先师〔先师：《太素》卷二十七《邪传》作“天师”〕，愿卒闻其道。岐伯曰：'风雨寒热，不得虚邪，不能独伤人。卒然逢疾风暴雨而不病者，盖无虚，故邪不能独伤人，此必因虚邪之风，与其身形，两虚相得〔得：《甲乙》卷八第二作“搏”〕，乃客其形。两实相逢，众人肉坚。其中于虚邪也，因于天时，与其身形，参以虚实，大病乃成，气有定舍，因此为名、上下中外，分为三员。

Yellow Emperor said: “It is precisely because I am not able to count the diseases, so, I ask Your Excellency about it, I hope to hear the reasons in detail.” Qibo said: “If one has no debilitating evil, the wind, rain, cold and heat can not injure him by themselves. Some people encounter the gale and torential rain suddenly but are not infected with any disease, it is because they have no debilitating evil, and the storm can not hurt them. In the formation of the disease, the debilitating evil and the body in debility must be existing at the same time, it is only under such situation can the evil invade the body. When the weather is normal and one's body is strong, of which the skin and muscle are usually substantial, the debilitating evil can by no means to invade the body. Whenever one is injured by the debilitating evil, the weather must be abnormal and the body must be debilitative, it is only when the evil is substantial and the body is debilitating, can the serious disease occur. The energy may dominate the superficies and the interior, and the disease is named according to the place where the evil retains. There are altogether three parts of the upper, lower, interior and exterior.

是故虚邪之中人也，始于皮肤，皮肤缓则腠理开，开则邪从毛髮入，入则抵深，深则毛髮立，毛髮立则淅然，故皮肤痛。留而不去，则传舍于络脉〔脉：《甲乙》卷八第二无此字〕，在络之时，痛于肌肉，其痛之时息〔其痛之时息：《太素》卷二十七《邪传》“时”下无“息”字〕，大经乃代。留而不去，传舍于经，在经之时，洒淅喜惊。留而不去，传舍于输，在输之时，六经不通，四肢则肢节痛〔四肢则肢节痛：《甲乙》卷八第二作“四节即痛”〕，腰脊乃强，留而不去，传舍于伏冲之脉、在伏冲之时，体重身痛。留而不去，传舍于肠胃，在肠胃之时，贲响腹胀，多寒则肠鸣飧泄，食不化，多热则溏出麋〔麋：张注本作“糜”〕。留耳不去，传舍于肠胃之外，募原之间，留著于脉稽留而不去，息而成积，或著孙脉〔《甲乙》卷八第二并作“络”〕或著络脉，或著输脉，或著于伏冲之脉，或著于膂筋，或著于肠胃之募原，上连〔上连：按：“上连”当作“或著”〕于缓筋，邪气淫泆，不可胜论。

"When the debilitating evil invades the human body, it commences from the skin, when the skin is loosened, the striae will open and the evil energy will penetrate from the hair, after the invasion, it reached deeply to the inner side causing the hair to stand up, when the hair stands up, the patient will be shivering with cold and has pain in the skin; when the evil energy retains and not being removed, it will transmit to the collaterals, when the evil is in the collaterals, one's muscle will be painful, when the pain ceases, the channels will be painful instead; when the evil is not removed, it will transmit to the channel, when the evil is in the channel, the patient will have chillness and startle; when the evil is not removed, it will transmit to the shu-channel (Foot Taiyang Channel), the six hand channels of the patient will be impeded, his four extremities become painful and he fails to stretch and bend the spine; when the evil is not removed, it will transmit to the hidden Chong Channel, when the evil is in the Chong Channel, the patient will feel heavy and painful in the body; when the evil is not removed, it will transmit to the intestine and stomach, when the evil is in the intestine and stomach, the patient will have the swelling of the abdomen, if he has more cold, he will have borborygmus, diarrhea and indigestion of food; when the evil is retained and not removed, it will transmit to the outside of the intestine and stomach, and between the membranes outside of the intestine and retains in the fine collaterals of the membrane; when the evil is not removed, it will retain to become abdominal mass. In a word, when the evil energy invades the body, it can retain in the minute collateral, or in the collateral, or in the channel, or in the shu-channel, or in the hidden Chong Channel, or in the tendons of the spine or arm, or in the membrane outside of the intestine and stomach, or in the penis; the evil energy can spread all over the body with many variations which can hardly be listed completely."

黄帝曰：愿尽闻其所由然。岐伯曰：其著孙络之脉而成积者，其积往来上下，臂手孙络之居也，浮〔浮："浮"上脱"落"字〕而缓，不能句积而止之，故往来移行肠胃之间，水、湊渗注灌，濯濯有音，有寒则䐜䐜满雷引，故时切痛。其著于阳明之经，则挟脐而居，饱食则益〔益："益"应作"脉"〕大，饥则益小。其著于缓筋也，似阳明之积，饱食则痛，饥则安。其著于肠胃之募原也，痛而外连于缓筋，饱食则安，饥则痛。其著伏冲之脉者，揣之应手而动，发手则热气下于两股，如汤沃之状。其著于膂筋在肠后者，饥则积见，饱则积不见，按之不得。其著于输之脉者，闭塞不通，津液不下，孔窍干壅。此邪气之从外入内，从上下也。

Yellow Emperof said: "I hope to hear about the reasons of forming the abdominal mass in detail." Qibo said: "When the abdominal mass is formed due to the retenton of the evil energy in the minute collaterals, the abdominal mass can move up and down, as the abdominal mass is in the collaterals and the collaterals are floating and loose, it can not detain and fix the mass, when the mass transfers here and there, it gradually enters in between the intestine and stomach, if there is water, it will permeate inside with the sound of water, if there is cold, one's abdomen will be distended with gurgling sound like thunder and the patient has acute pain often. When the evil energy is in the Yangming Channel, the abdominal mass will be clipping around the navel, if one is full up, his collaterals will be thick and large, if one is hungry, his collaterals will be thin and small. When the evil energy retains in the penis, its condition will be similar with that in the Yangming Channel, if one is full up, he will have distention and pain, if one is hungry, he will, on the contrary, feel comfortable. When the evil energy retains in the membranes between the intestine and the stomach, the pain may affect the penis, if one is full up, he will feel comfortable, if one is hungry, he will be painful. When the evil energy retains in the Chong Channel which is hidden, the pulsation will be rapid and urgent when press by hand, and when the hand is lifted, there will be hot currents descending along the thighs like pouring hot soup. When the evil energy retains in the tendon of the arm, if one is hungry, the mass will be quite obvious, if one is full up, it will not be apparrent, and it can hardly be detected even when press with hand. When the evil energy is in the shu-channel, it will cause obstruction of the channel passage, inability of spreading the body fluid and causes the dryness of the orifices. These are the common syndromes of the evil energy when transferring from outside to inside and from upward to downward."

黄帝曰：积之始生，至其已成奈何？岐伯曰：积之始生，得寒乃生，厥乃成积也。黄帝曰：其成积奈何？岐伯曰：厥气生足悗，悗生胫寒，胫寒则血脉凝涩，血脉凝涩则寒气上入于肠胃，入于肠胃则䐜胀，䐜胀则肠外之〔肠外之：《太素》杨注作"肠胃之外"〕汁沫迫聚不得散，日以成积。卒然多食饮则肠满，起居不节，用力过度，则络脉伤，阳络伤则血外溢，血外溢则衄血，阴络伤则血内溢，血内溢则后〔后：《甲乙》卷八第二并作"脉"〕血，肠胃〔《太素》卷二十七《邪传》作"外"〕之络伤，则血溢于肠外，肠外有寒汁沫与血相搏，则并合凝聚不得散而积成矣。卒然外中于寒，若内伤于忧怒，则气上逆，气上逆则六输不通，温〔温：按据《太素》杨注"温"应作"卫"〕气不行，凝血蕴里而不散，津液涩渗，著而不去，而积皆成矣。

Yellow Emperor asked: "What is the condition in the course from the beginning to the shaping up of the abdominal mass?" Qibo said: "In the initiation of the abdominal mass, the cold energy invades the foot first, then the evil energy of the cold-type jue-syndrome ascends to the intestine and the stomach, and this is the main reason of shaping up a mass." Yellow Emperor asked: "What is the condition in the course of the shaping?" Qibo said: The energy of the cold-type jue-syndrome causes pain and the inconvenience of walking, and consequently, the leg will be cold, the coldness of the leg will cause the stagnation of the blood, when the cold energy descends and enters into the intestine and stomach gradually, the abdomen will distend, when the abdomen has distention, the fluid and foam outside of the intestine and stomach will be accumulating without dispersing due to the pressing of the cold evil, when the condition is protracted, it will become abdominal mass. When one eats too much suddendly to fill his intestine with food, the intestine will be difficult to transform and transport the food, when one does not practise temperance in his daily life or being overstrained, his collaterals will be injured, the blood will be flowing outside, when the blood overflows outside, one will have epistaxis, when the Yin collaterale are injured, the blood will overflow inside, when the blood overflows inside, one will have bloody stool. When the intestine and stomach are injured, the blood will overflow to the outside of the intestine, if there is cold energy beyond the intestine, the fluid and foam will combate with the overflowing blood, and they will be combined and stagnated without dispersing, in this case, it can also cause abdominal mass. When one is injured by the exogenous cold-evil, and again, hurt by the internal moods of melancholy or anger, it will cause the energy to reverse up, when the energy is reversing up, the energies of the six channels will be impeded when the Wei energy is obstructed, the blood will be stagnated, being wrapped inside without dispersing, and the body fluid will be unsmoothed, when this condition is protracted, the abdominal mass will be shaped up."

黄帝曰：其生于阴者奈何？岐伯曰：忧思伤心；重寒伤肺；忿怒伤肝；醉以入房，汗出当风、伤脾；用力过度，若入房汗出浴，则伤肾。此内外三部之所生病者也。

Yellow Emperor asked: "What is the condition when the disease initiates from the internal organs?" Qibo said: "Melancholy will injure the heart; the double cold (external cold of food and drink, and internal cold of the body) will injure the lung; anger will injure the liver; when one catches cold after sweating due to the sex intercourse and drunken, it will injure the spleen; when one is overstrained, or bathes with sweat after sex intercourse, it will injure the kidney. These are the diseases from the upper middle and lower parts of the inside and outside of the body."

黄帝曰：善。治之奈何？岐伯答曰：察其所痛，以知其应，有余不足，当补则补，当泻则泻，毋逆天时，是谓至治。

Yellow Emperor said: "Good. But how to treat the diseases?" Qibo said: "Examine the reason that causes the disease to know the corresponding syndrome, to the evil energy which is having a surplus and the health energy which is insufficient, invigorate when it should be invigorated and purge when it should be purged, when one violates not the relations between the weathers of the four seasons and the human body, it is supposed to be the best principle of treating."

行针第六十七

Chapter 67
Xing Zheng
(Needle Transmission)

黄帝问于岐伯曰：余闻九针于夫子，而行之于百姓，百姓之血气各不同形，或神动而气先针〔针："针"字疑衍〕行，或气与针相逢，或针已出气独行，或数刺乃知，或发针而气逆，或数刺病益剧，凡此六者，各不同形，愿闻其方。

Yellow Emperor asked Qibo said: "I have applied the nine kinds of needle you said to treat the people, as the bloods and energies of them are differnet in abundance and deficiency, and their constitutions are different, so, their needling reponses to the prickings are different. Some of them are excited when being pricked, the needling response comes prior to the pricking; in some of them, the needling response arrives just in time with the pricking; in some of them, the needling response still remains after pulling out of the needle; in some of them, the needling response can only come after several prickings; in some of them, the needling response comes very slowly after the pricking; in some of them, the disease becomes even more serious after pricking for many times. In the six cases, the conditions after pricking are different, and I hope to hear the reason about it."

岐伯曰：重阳之人，其神易动，其气易往也。黄帝曰：何谓重阳之人？岐伯曰：重阳之人，熇熇高高，言语善疾，举足善高，心肺之藏气有余，阳气滑盛而扬，故神动而气先行。

Qibo said: "When one's Yang is having a surplus, he is irritable, and the needling response under the needle can be produced easily." Yellow Emperor asked: "What is the condition when one's Yang is having a surplus?" Qibo said: "When one's Yang is having a surplus, he will be gallant and overbearing, rapid in speaking, lifting his feet high while walking, and he appears to be complacent. His energies of the heart and lung are having a surplus, the operation of his Yang energy is smooth, substantial and exultant, thus, when he is touched slightly, there will be a response instantly."

黄帝曰：重阳之人而神不先行者，何也？岐伯曰：此人颇有阴者也。黄帝曰：何以知其颇有阴也？岐伯曰：多阳者多喜，多阴者多怒，数怒者易解，故曰颇有阴，其阴阳之离〔离：《太素》卷二十七《邪传》无此字〕合难，故其神不能先行也。

Yellow Emperor asked: "For the people whose Yang is having a surplus, they can not express the hypersensitiveness of their minds in advance, and what is the reason?" Qibo said: "People of this kind have somewhat Yin energy inside." Yellow Emperor asked: "How to know they have somewhat Yin energy inside? Qibo said: "When a man's Yang is having a surplus, he is often joyous, when a man's Yin is having a surplus, he often gets angry, when his anger is always readily to be eliminated, he belongs to the category of Yin in Yang, so, he has somewhat Yin energy inside. People of this kind have more Yang and little Yin, and the Yin and Yang can hardly conform to each other, so, they can not express the hypersensitiveness of mind in advance."

黄帝曰：其气与针相逢奈何？岐伯曰：阴阳和调〔和调：《甲乙》卷一第十六"调"下有"者"字〕而〔而：《甲乙》卷一第十六无此字〕血气淖泽滑利，故针入而气出，疾而相逢也。

Yellow Emperor asked: "What is the condition when the needling response arrives with the pricking in due time?" Qibo said: "When one's Yin and Yang are harmonious, the circulation of his blood and energy are moist and smooth, so, when the needle is inserted, the needling response will arrive along with the pricking in due time."

黄帝曰：针已出而气独行者，何气使然？岐伯曰：其阴气〔阴气，阳气：《甲乙》卷一第十六"阴阳"下并无"气"字〕多而阳气少，阴气沉而阳气浮者内藏〔浮者内藏：当注本，张注本"浮"字断句，下并有"沉"字〕，故针已出，气乃随其后，故独行也。

Yellow Emperor asked: "When the needling response still remains after the pulling off the needle, what energy causes it?" Qibo said: "This is due to the patient has more Yin and little Yang, his Yin energy is sinking and his Yang energy is floating, when the Yin energy is sinking, it harbours inside and can hardly respond, but after the needle is pulled out, the needling response will appear soon after it, so, it is called 'To arrive individually'."

黄帝曰：数刺乃知，何气使然？岐伯曰：此人之多阴而少阳，其气沉而气往难，故数刺乃知也。

Yellow Emperor asked: "When the disease can only be relieved after pricking for many times, what energy causes it?" Qibo said: "People of this kind have more Yin and little Yang, as Yang is harboured inside, the occurrence of the needling response is rather difficult, so, the disease can only be cured after frequent pricking."

黄帝曰：针入而气逆者〔而气逆者：丹波元简曰："按上下文例，'者'下似脱'其数刺病益甚者'七字〕，何气使然？岐伯曰：其气逆与其数刺病益甚者，非阴阳之气，浮沉之势也，此皆粗之所败，上〔上：日刻本，张注本，黄校本并作"工"〕之所失，其形气无过焉。

Yellow Emperor said: "When one has adverseness of vital energy after the insertion of the needle, or the disease becomes even worse after frequent pricking, what energy causes it?" Qibo said: "When the adverseness of vital energy occurs or the disease becomes worse after frequent pricking, it is not due to the various conditions of overabundant, deficient, floating or sunken of Yin and Yang, but it is the bad result due to the careless treating, it is the error of the physician and it has nothing to do with the body and energy."

上膈第六十八

Chapter 68
Shang Ge
(Vomiting Instantly after Food Intake)

黄帝曰：气为上膈者，食饮〔饮：《甲乙》卷十一第八无此字〕入而还出，余已知之矣。虫为下膈，下膈者，食晬时乃出，余未得其意，愿卒闻之。岐伯曰：喜怒不适，食饮不节，寒温不时，则寒汁流〔流：卷十一第八作“留”〕于肠中〔于肠中：《甲乙》卷十一第八无此三字〕，流于肠中则虫寒，虫寒则积聚，守于下管〔守于下管：《太素》卷二十六《虫痈》“下管”下重“守于下管”四字〕，则肠胃充郭，卫气不营，邪气居之。入食则虫上食，虫上食则下管虚，下管虚则邪气胜之，积聚以留，留则痈成，痈成则下管约。其痈在管内者，即〔即：《太素》卷二十六《虫痈》作“则沉”〕而痛深；其痈在〔在：《甲乙》卷十一第八“在”下有“脘”字〕外者，则痈外〔痈外：按：“痈”字疑衍〕而痛浮，痈上皮热。

Yellow Emperor said:"When one has detention of the functional activities of vital energy it causes one vomit as soon as he takes in the food, and I have known the condition. When one has worm inside to cause the deferable vomiting, he vomits in a day and night after taking in the food, I don't understand its reason, and I hope you can tell me in detail." Qibo said: "This kind of disease is formed by improper overjoy and anger, irregular eating and drinking and dressing at will not in accord with the weather, consequently, the stomach energy is injured, the cold fluid retains in the intestine causing the parasites to feel cold and accumulate in the lower part of the gastric cavity, in this way, the intestine and stomach will be expanded, the spleen energy will fail to operate, and the evil energy will be retaining. When one takes in the food, the parasites take food also, when they take food, the lower part of the gastric cavity will be empty, and the evil energy takes the opportunity to invade, due to the retention of the evil energy, the deep-sited abscess will be shaped up causing the lower gastric cavity to become hard to restrain. When the abscess is in the lower gastric cavity, it willl cause deep and acute pain; when the abscess is outside of the lower gastric cavity, the pain will be shallow and floating, and the skin on the site of the abscess will be hot."

黄帝曰：刺之奈何？岐伯曰：微按其痈，视气〔气：张注本作“其”〕所行，先浅刺其傍，稍内益深，还而刺之，毋过三行，察其沉浮，以为深浅。已刺必熨，令热入中，日使热内，邪气益衰，大痈乃溃。伍以参禁，以除其内，恬憺无为，乃能行气，后以咸苦〔以咸：《甲乙》卷十一第八作“服酸”〕，化谷乃下矣。

Yellow Emperor asked: "How to treat this kind of disease by pricking?" Qibo said: "Press slightly the site of the abscess with hand, examine the flowing direction of the energy, prick shallowly by the side of the focus first, then prick deeper gradually and finally insert the needle; the pricking must not exceed three times, prick shallowly or deeply according to the depth of the abscess. After the pricking, apply the topical application of heated drugs to cause the heat to penetrate inside, when the heat is penetrated inside every day, the evil energy received previously will decline gradually, and the large carbuncle with pus and blood will be relieved. Besides, one should aply the method of the Three and Five contraindications to remove the cause of disease in the body. The patient must completely free of wishes or ambition, indifferent to fame and gain and free from destracting thoughts, so as his health energy may be unimpeded; soon afterwards, the patient should be recuperated with medicine and food of sour and bitter tastes; when the food can be digested by the patient, the syndrome of deferable vomiting will be eliminated."

忧恚无言第六十九

Chapter 69
You Hui Wu Yan
(Dysphonia due to Melancholy and Resentment)

黄帝问于少师曰：人之卒然忧恚而言无音者，何道之塞，何气出〔出：《甲乙》卷十二第二作“不”〕行，使音不彰？愿闻其方。少师答曰：咽喉〔喉：按：“喉”字涉下衍〕者，水谷之道也。喉咙者，气之所以上下者也。会厌者，音声之户也。口唇〔口唇：《灵枢略无音论篇》“唇”上无“口”字〕者，音声之扇也。舌者，音声之机也。悬雍垂者，音声之关也。颃颡者，分气之所泄也。横骨者，神气所使，主发舌者也。故人之鼻洞涕出不收者，颃颡不开〔开：《甲乙》卷十二第二《灵枢略·无音论篇》并作“闭”〕，分气失也。是故厌小而疾薄〔是故厌小而疾薄：《甲乙》卷十二第二“是故”作“其”，“而”下无“疾”字〕，则发气疾，其开阖利，其出气易；其厌大而厚，则开阖难，其气出迟，故重言也〔故重言也：《甲乙》卷十二第二“言也”下有“所谓吃者，其言逆，故重之”十字〕。人卒然无音者，寒气客于厌，则厌不能发，发不能下至〔发不能下至：《灵枢略·无音论篇》无“下”字，“至”下有“其机扇”三字〕，其开阖不致〔其开阖不致：《甲乙》卷十二第三作“机扇开阖不利”〕，故无音。

Yellow Emperor asked Shaoshi and said: "When one has dysphonia suddendly due to melancholy and resentment, the routes of energy and blood are obstructed, and the voice fails to be loud and clear, what energy obstructs it? I hope to hear the reason." Shaoshi said: "The pharynx is the passage for water and cereals to enter into the stomach, the throat is for the breath to go up and down and in and out, the epiglottis is like the window for sending out the voice, the lips are like the door of giving off the voice, the tongue is like the organ that produces the voice, the uvula is like the pass of the voice, the upper orifice of the palate is to divide the breath to go to the mouth and nose respectively, the palate which is controlled by the nerve is for dominating the tongue to form language. Thus, when one has sinusities with unceasing nasal discharge, it is due to the upper orifice of the palate fails to close, and it can not divide the breath properly. When the epiglottis is small and thin, the coming out of the breath will be easy and swift, so, one will be brisk and neat in talking; if the epiglottis is large and thick, it will be difficult to open and close, the coming out of the breath will be low, and one will be stammer in talking. When one has dysphonia suddenly, it is due to the cold-evil attacks the epiglottis to work abnormally, when its opening and closing are ineffective, one will have dysphonia."

黄帝曰：刺之奈何？岐伯曰：足之少阴，上系于舌〔舌：《甲乙》卷十二第二“舌”下有“本”字〕，络于横骨，终于会厌。两泻其血脉，浊气乃辟。会厌之脉，上络任脉，取之天突，其厌乃发也。

Yellow Emperor asked: "How to treat dysphonia by pricking?" Qibo said: "The Foot Shaoyin Channel links the root of tongue above, it communicates the palate and terminates at the epiglottis. When one treats by purging the Foot Shaoyin Channel of Kidney and the Ren Channel respectively, the cold-evil and the turbid energy will be removed. As the channel of the epiglottis passes the Ren Channel above, when one pricks the Tiantu point further more, the voice will come out from the epiglottis."

寒热第七十

Chapter 70
Han Re
(Cold and Heat)

黄帝问于岐伯曰：寒热瘰疬在于颈腋者，皆〔皆：《甲乙》卷八第一并无此字〕何气使〔使：《甲乙》卷八第一作“所”〕生？岐伯曰：此皆鼠瘘寒热之毒气也，留于脉而不去者也。

Yellow Emperor asked Qibo and said："The scrofula of cold and heat grow on the neck and under the armpit，what energy causes it?" Qibo said："The scrofula is caused by the cold and heat retaining in the channel which is not removed."

黄帝曰：去之奈何？岐伯曰：鼠瘘之本，皆〔皆：《千金》卷二十三第一“皆”下有“根”字〕在于脏，其末上出于颈腋之间〔间：《千金》卷二十三第一作“下”〕，其浮于脉中，而未内著于肌肉，而外为脓血者，易去也。

Yellow Emperor asked："How to treat is?" Qibo said："The scrofula is stemmed from the internal organ，and its branches ascend along the channel to appear on the neck and under the armpit. If the toxic energy is floating in the channel，has not yet penetrated into the muscle，but turns into pus and blood outside only，it can be easily removed."

黄帝曰：去之奈何？岐伯曰：请从其本引其末，可使衰去而绝其寒热。审按其道以予之，徐往徐来〔徐往徐来：《千金》卷二十三第一“徐往”下无“徐”字〕以去之，其小如麦者，一刺知，三刺而已。

Yellow Emperor asked："How to remove it?" Qibo said："Substantialize the internal organs with the health energy，and then，induce the evil toxicity of the scrofula to outside，in this way，the attack of cold and heat will stop. Examine the location of the scrofula，prick properly according to the route of the channel and remove the toxicity of scrofula with the acupuncture manipulation of coming slowly and going slowly. When the scrofula is in the size of a seed of the wheat，it will be effective after one pricking，and the disease will be cured after three prickings."

黄帝曰：决其生死奈何？岐伯曰：反其目视之，其中有赤脉，上下贯瞳子，见一脉，一岁死；见一脉半，一岁半死；见二脉，二岁死；见二脉半，二岁半死；见三脉，三岁而死。见赤脉不下贯瞳子，可治也。

Yellow Emperor asked："How to diagnose the survival and death of the patient?" Qibo said："Stir open the eyelid and see，if there is a red line of vessel running through the pupil vertically，the patient will die after one year，when the vessel is one and a half，the patient will die after one and half year，when there are two red vessels，the patient will die after two years，when the red vessels are two and half of them，the patient will die after two and half years, when the red half vessels are three of them, the patient will die after three years. If the red line is not running through the pupil, the disease can be cured."

邪客第七十一

Chapter 71
Xie Ke
(Retention of the Evil)

黄帝问于伯高曰：夫邪气之客人也，或令人目不瞑，不卧出者〔不卧出者：周学海曰："不卧出者"，疑当作"不汗出者"〕，何气使然？伯高曰：五谷入于胃也，其糟粕、津液、宗气分为三隧。故宗气积于胸中，出于喉咙，以贯心脉，而行呼吸焉。营气者，泌其津液，注之于脉，化以为血，以荣四末内注五脏六府，以应刻数焉。冲气者，出其悍气之慓疾，而先行于四末分肉皮肤之间而不休者也。昼日〔日：《甲乙》卷十二第三并无此字〕行于阳，夜行于阴〔夜行于阴：此后应据《太素》、《甲乙》、《外台》补"其入于阴也"五字〕，常从足少阴之分〔分：《病沅》卷三《虚劳不得眠候》"分"下有"肉"字〕间，行于五藏六府。今厥〔厥：《甲乙》卷十二第三作"邪"〕气客于五藏六府，则卫气独卫其外，行于阳，不得入于藏〔行干阳，不得入于藏：《太素》卷十二《营卫气行》无此八字〕。行于阳则阳气盛，阳气盛则阳跞陷〔陷：《甲乙》卷十二第三并作"满"〕；不得入于阴，阴虚〔阴虚：《太素》卷十二第三"阴"下有"气"字〕，故目不瞑。

Yellow Emperor asked Bogao and said: "When the evil invades the body, one can not sleep with his eyes closed and he has no perspiration, what energy causes it?" Bogao said: "After the five-cereal enters into the stomach, it divides into dross, body fluid and initial energy, which flow to the lower, middle and upper warmers respectively in three routes. The initial energy accumulates in the chest, comes out from the throat, links up the heart and carries out the respiration. The Ying-energy secretes the body fluid and pours into the channels, it turns into blood to nourish the four extremities outside, and pours into the solid and hollow organs inside in the speed of fifty cycles a day and night or one hundred graduations of the clepsydra. The Wei-energy has the disposition of being valiant and swift, it moves along the muscle and the skin unceasingly. In day time, it runs in the Yang portion, in night time, it runs in the Yin portion, it often starts from the muscle of the Foot Shaoyin Channel of Kidney first, then, runs to reach the five solid organs and the six hollow organs. When the evil energy invades the internal organs, the Wei-energy will guard against the exterior of the body solely, when the exterior of the body is guarded, the Yang energy will be overabundant, when the Yang energy is overabundant, the channel energy of Yangqiao Channel will be full, causing the Yang energy fails to enter into the Yin portion. Since the Yin energy is debilitative, the patient will not be able to sleep with his eyes closed."

黄帝曰：善。治之奈何？伯高曰：补其不足，泻其有余，调其虚实，以通其道而去其邪，饮以半夏汤一剂，阴阳已通，其卧立至。黄帝曰：善。此所谓决渎壅塞，经络大通，阴阳和得〔和得：二字误倒，应据《甲乙》乙正〕者也。愿闻其方。伯高曰：其汤方以流水千里以外者八升，扬之万遍，取其清五升煮之，炊以苇薪火〔火：《太素》卷十二《营卫气行》作"大""大沸"自为句〕，沸置秫米一升，治半夏五合，徐炊，令竭为一升半，去其滓，饮汁一小杯，日三稍益，以知为度。故其病新发者，复杯则卧，汗出则已矣。久者，三饮而已也。

Yellow Emperor asked: "How to treat the disease of insomnia?" Bogao said: "Invigorate the Yin which is insufficient and purge the Yang which is having a surplus, adjust the partial asthenia and partial sthenia, in this way, it will cause the passage of the Wei energy to become unimpeded, and the disturbing evil energy removed. At the same time, the patient should take the decoction of pinelliae (tuber), so as the Yin and Yang energies can be dredged and the patient can fall into sleep immediately." Yellow Emperor said: "Good. This therapy is like the dredging of the block of the water course, to cause the channels and collaterals to have a good circulation and the Yin and Yang to become harmonious. I hope to hear about the prescription of pinellia." Bogao said: "In forming the prescription of pinellia, take eight litres of flowing water, stir for ten thousand times, after the precipitation of dust, take five litres of clear water from it and boil it with burning reeds, after the great boiling, put in one litre of husked sorghum, half litre of processed pinelliae and boil slowly, when the decoction water being condensed into one and half litres, remove the dregs of the decoction. Administer the patient with the decoction of a small cup each time and three times a day, the dose may be a little bit larger to attain the curative efficacy. If the disease is in the initial stage, the patient can sleep after the administration, and after perspiration, the disease will be recovered; in the protracted disease, it will be recovered after taking three decoctions."

黄帝问于伯高曰：愿闻人之肢节，以应天地奈何？伯高答曰：天圆地方，人头圆足方以应之。天有日月，人有两〔两：《素问·四季调神大论》王注引《灵枢经》作"眼"〕目。地有九州〔地有九州：《五行大义》卷五第二十三作"天有九星"〕，人有九窍。天有风雨，人有喜怒。天有雷电，人有音声。天有四时，人有四肢。天有五音，人有五藏。天有六律，人有六腑。天有冬夏，人有寒热。天有十日，人有手十指。辰有十二，人有足十指、茎、垂以应之；女子不足二节，以抱人形。天有阴阳，人有夫妻。岁有三百六十五日，人有三百六十节。〔六十：《太素》卷五"十"下有"五"字〕地有高山，人有肩膝。地有深谷，人有腋腘。地有十二经水，人有十二经脉。地有泉脉〔泉脉：《太素》卷五作"云气"〕，人有卫气。地有草蓂，人有毫毛。天有昼夜，人有卧起。天有列星，人有牙齿。地有小山，人有小节。地有山石，人有高骨。地有林木，人有募筋。地有聚邑，人有䐃肉。岁有十二月，人有十二节。地有四〔四：《甲乙》卷五无此字〕时不生草，人有无子。此人与天地相应者也。

Yellow Emperor said to Bogao: "I hope to hear about the correpondance of human extremities and joints with the heaven and earth." Bogao said: "The heaven is round and the earth is square, the head of a man is round and his foot is square, so, heaven and earth correspond with man. In heaven, there are the sun and moon, in man, there are the eyes; in heaven, there are the nine stars, in man, there are the nine orifices; in heaven, there are wind and rain, in man, there are overjoy and anger; in heaven, there are thunder and lightning, in man, there is voice; in heaven, there are the four seasons, in man, there are the four extremities; in heaven, there are the five tones, in man, there are the five solid organs; in heaven, there are the six standards for setting the tone, in man, there are the six hollow organs; in heaven, there are the ten celetial stems (decimal cycles), in man, there are the ten fingers; in heaven, there are the twelve earthen branches (duodecimal cycles) in man, there are ten toes, penis and the testicles which are corresponding to the heaven, in woman, she has no penis and testicles, but she can conceive; in heaven, there are Yin and Yang, in man there are husband and wife; in a year, there are three hundred and sixty five days, in human body, there are three hundred and sixty five acupoints; on earth, there are the high mountains, in human body, there are the shoulders and knees; on earth, there are deep valleys, in human body, there are the armpits and poplitea; on earth, there are twelve large rivers, in human body, there are twelve main channels; on earth, there is cloud, in human body, there is the Wei-energy; on earth, there are grasses overgrown, in human body, there are fine hairs growing; in heaven, there are day and night, in man there are sleep and rise; in heaven, there are the stars, in man, there are the teeth; on earth, there are the small hills, in man, there are the small bone joints; on earth, there are the rocks, in human body, there are the eminent head of bones (like cheeks, shoulders, knees and ankles); on earth, there are woods, in human body, there are the aponeurosis; on earth, there are cities throng with people, in human body, there are the protruding muscles; in a year, there are twelve months, in human body, there are twelve large joints in the four extremities; on earth, sometimes the grass does not grow, in man, one may have no offspring in his whole life. These are the conditions of a man corresponding to the heaven and earth."

黄帝问于岐伯曰：余愿闻持针之数，内针之理，纵舍之意，扞皮开腠理，奈何？脉之屈折，出入之处，焉至而出，焉至而止，焉至而徐，焉至而疾，焉至而入？六腑之输于身者，余愿尽闻。少序〔少序：《太素》卷九《脉行同异》作“其序”〕别离之处，离而入〔入：《太素》卷建筑物《脉行同异》作“行”〕阴，别而入阳，此何道而从行？愿尽〔尽：《太素》卷九《脉行同异》无此字〕闻其方。岐伯曰：帝之所问，针道毕矣。

Yellow Emperor asked Qibo and said: "I hope to know how to manipulate the technique of acupuncture, the principle of inserting the needle, the meaning of the therapies of the deferred pricking, and exempt from pricking, and the therapy of dividing the skin equally to open the striae, besides, I hope to know the places where the channels turn, come in and go out, the starting points and the terminals of the channel energy, the places where it becomes faster and the places where it becomes slower, the places where it enters and the conditions of the pouring of the six hollow organs to the whole body, besides, I hope to hear the flowing sequence of the energy, the places where it branches out from Yang to Yin and from Yin to Yang and the routes they pass. Furthermone, I hope to hear their reasons." Qibo said: "Your questions are comprising all the principles in pricking."

黄帝曰：愿卒闻之。岐伯曰：手太阴之脉，出于大指之端，内屈，循白肉际，至本节之后太渊留以澹，外屈。上于本节下，内屈，与阴诸络会于鱼际，数脉并注，其气滑利，伏行壅骨之下，外屈，出于寸口而行，上至于肘内廉，入于大筋之下，内屈，上行臑阴，入腋下，内屈走肺，此顺行逆数之屈折也。心主之脉。出于中指之端，内屈，循中指内廉以上留于掌中，伏行两骨之间，外屈，出两筋之间，骨肉之际，其气滑利，上二寸〔上二寸：《太素》《脉行同异》作“上行三寸”〕，外屈，出行两筋之间，上至肘内廉，入于小筋之下，留两骨之会，上入于胸中，内络于心脉。

Yellow Emperor said: "I hope to hear them in details." Qibo said: "The energy of the Hand Taiyin Channel starts from the tip of the thumb (Shaoshang point), turns inside along the white flesh to the Taiyuan point behind the basic joint and has pulsation there, then it turns outside, ascends below the basic joint and turns inside again and joins the various Yin collaterals on the thenar eminence, the Hand Taiyin, Hand Shaoyin and the Hand Jueyin channels pour in combination of which the energy current is quite slippery, the energy runs in hiding under the first metacarpal bones of the thenar eminence, then it turns outside and ascends along the Cunkou pulse to reach the inner side of the elbow, then, it enters into the lower part of the large tendon, turns inside, ascends to reach the inner side of the upper arm, then, it enters into the armpit and turns inside to reach the lung. These are the agreeable (vertical) and adverse (Horizontal) running routes of the energy of the Hand Taiyin Channel of Lung. The energy of the Hand Jueyin Channel of pericardium starts from the tip of the middle finger (Zhongchong point), it turns inside, ascends along the inner side of the middle finger to reach the Laogong point, runs in hiding between the basic joints of the middle finger and the forefinger, then, it turns outside, runs above the tendons of the forearm and the side of the palm and the muscle and bone by the wrist and its energy is quite slippery, then, the channel turns outside to ascend to three inches above the wrist, passing the Daling point between the two tendons, ascends to reach the inner side of the elbow, and enters to the lower side of the small tendon and the convergence of the two bones (Quze point), then, it ascends to reach the chest and links the channel of heart."

黄帝曰：手少阴之脉独无腧，何也？岐伯曰：少阴，心脉也。心者，五脏六腑之大主也，精神之所舍也，其藏坚固，邪弗能容也。容之则心伤，心伤则神去，神去则死矣。故诸邪之在于心者，皆在于心之包络，包络者，心主之脉也，故独无腧焉。

Yellow Emperor asked: "Why is it that the Hand Shaoyin Channel has no acupoint solely?" Qibo said: "The Hand Shaoyin Channel is the channel of heart and it is the main dominator of the five solid organs and the six hollow organs, it is the place where the mind stores, as it is firm, the exogenous evil can hardly intrude into it; if the exogenous evil penetrates, the heart will be injured, if the heart is injured, the spirit will be dispersed, if the spirit is dispersed, the patient will die. Therefore, all the exogenous evils retaining on the system of heart are located on the pericardium and the Pericardium Channel is dominated by the heart. Since the pericadium receives the evil for the heart, the Hand Shaoyin Channel of Heart has no acupoint."

黄帝曰：少阴独无腧者，不病乎？岐伯曰：其外经〔经：《甲乙》卷三第二十六“经”下并有“脉”字〕病而藏不病，故独取其经于掌后锐骨之端。其余脉出入屈折，其行之徐疾，皆如少阴心主之脉行也。故本输者，皆因其气之虚实疾徐以取之，是谓因冲而泻，因衰而补，如是者，邪气得去，真气坚固，是谓因天之序。

Yellow Emperor asked: "Since the Hand Shaoyin Channel has no acupoint, would it not contract disease?" Qibo said: "The Heart Channel outside may be ill, but the heart itself will not be ill, when the Heart Channel outside is ill, it can prick the Shenmen point of the Heart Channel on the tip of the sharp bone behind the palm. The turning of all other channels, their coming in and going out, the fast and slow running speed of the channel energy are similar with the Hand Taiyin and the Hand Pericardium Channels. So, the Shenmen point should be pricked according to the conditions of asthenia and sthenia, and the fast and slow speed of the channel energy, that is, purge when it is hyperactive and invigorate when it is debilitative. When one treats in this way, the evil energy can be removed, and the health energy will become firm and substantial. This is the therapy in accordance with the sequence of the four seasons."

黄帝曰：持针纵舍奈何？岐伯曰：必先明知十二经脉之本末，皮肤之寒热，脉之盛衰滑涩。其脉滑而盛者，病日进；虚而细者，久以持；大以涩者，为痛痹，阴阳如一者，病难治。其本末尚热者，病尚在；其热已衰者，其病亦去矣。持其尺，察其肉之坚脆、大小、滑涩、寒温〔温：《甲乙》卷五第七作"热"〕、燥湿。因视目之五色，以知五脏而决死生。视其血脉，察其色，以知其寒热痛痹。

Yellow Emperor asked: "When holding the needle in pricking, there are the deferred therapy and the exemption from pricking therapy. What are they like?" Qibo said: "One must know the starting of the twelve channels, the belongings of the skin to the cold and heat, the overabundant or debilitative, and the smooth and choppy of the pulse condition in advance. If the pulse is abundant and slippery, the disease will become worse day after day, when the pulse condition is asthenic and fine, the disease will be protracted, when the pulse condition is gigantic and choppy, it is the disease of arthralgia aggravated by cold, when the pulse condition appears to be the Yin and Yang are about the same which can hardly be distinguished, the disease can hardly be cured, when the heat is remaining in the four extremities, chest and abdomen, it shows the disease is still existing, if the heat in the chest, abdomen and the four extremities are disappearing, the disease will be recovered. Examine the skin of the anterolateral side of the forearm to observe whether the muscle is firm or crisp, whether the pulse condition is gigantic or small, slippery or choppy, and whether the disease is belonging to the cold, heat, dryness or wetness. Besides, examine the five colours of the eye to know the internal change of the five solid organs, thereby to anticipate the survival or death of the patient, furthermore, examine the green, black, yellow, red and white colour of the skin to determine whether the syndrome is of cold, heat, pain or bi."

黄帝曰：持针纵舍，余未得其意也。岐伯曰：持针之道，欲端以正，安以静，先知虚实，而行疾徐，左手〔手：周本，当注本并作"指"〕执骨，右手循之，无与肉〔肉：藏本作"内"〕果〔果：《甲乙》卷五第七作"裹"〕，泻欲端以正，补必闭肤，辅〔辅：《甲乙》卷五第七作"转"〕针导气，邪〔邪：《甲乙》卷五第七"邪"下有"气不"二字〕得淫泆，真气得居。黄帝曰：扞皮开腠理奈何？岐伯曰：因其分肉，在别其肤，微内而徐端之，适神不散，邪气得去。

Yellow Emperor said: "I do not quite understand the meaning of the deferred pricking therapy and the exemption pricking therapy." Qibo said: "In the manipulation of pricking, one should be upright and calm. He should know the asthenia and sthenia of the disease first, and then, decides the speed of the needle insertion. In the insertion, hold the bone of the patient with the fingers of the left hand, and press the acupoint with the fingers of the right hand to avoid the tangle of the needle by the fibre of the muscle. In pricking, the needle must be kept straight, and the insertion should be right forward; in invigorating, the needle hole on the skin must be sealed up, apply the manipulation of twisting the needle to guide the energy to keep it not to run rashly, and in this way, the healthy energy can be stabilized." Yellow Emperor asked: "How to defend the skin and open the striae?" Qibo said: "It should prick according to the agreeable vein of the muscle and insert the needle lightly when the muscles are being divided, and the pricking must be accurate without deviation. If the acupuncturist concentrates his mind in doing it, the evil can certainly be removed."

黄帝问于岐伯曰：人有八虚，各何以候？岐伯答曰：以候五脏。黄帝曰：候之奈何？岐伯曰：肺心有邪，其气留于两肘；肝有邪，其气流于两腋；脾有邪，其气留于两髀；肾有邪，其气留于两腘。凡此八虚者，皆机关之室，真气之所过，血络之所游，邪气恶血，固不得住留，住留则伤筋〔筋：周本与注本并作“经”〕络，骨节机关不得屈伸，故痀〔痀：胡本熊本周本作“拘”〕挛也。

Yellow Emperor asked Qibo and said: "In human body, there are eight places which are debilitative, how to determine one's disease from them?" Qibo said: "It can determine the diseases in the five organs." Yellow Emperor asked: "How to determine them respectively?" Qibo said: "When there is evil energy in the lung, the energy must be retained in the two elbows; when there is evil energy in the liver, the energy must be retained in the two armpits; when there is evil energy in the spleen, the energy must be retained in two upper halves of the two thighs: when there is evil in the kidney, the energy must be retained in the two poplitea. The two elbows, two armpits, two upper thighs and the two poplitea are the eight locations of asthenia, they are the places where the joints and pivots locate, the healthy energy comes and goes, and the places where the blood and the collaterals converge. In these places, the evil energy and the malicious blood can hardly retain. If it retained, the channel and collaterals would be injured, causing the bone joints fail to stretch and bend to have the syndrome of the contracture of limbs."

通天第七十二

Chapter 72
Tong Tian
(The Different Types of Man)

黄帝问于少师曰：余尝闻人有阴阳，何谓阴人，何谓阳人？少师曰：天地之间，六合之内〔六合之内：《甲乙》卷一第十六无此四字〕，不离于五，人亦应之，非徒一阴一阳而已也，而略言耳，口弗能徧明也。黄帝曰：愿略闻其意，有贤人圣人，心能备而行之乎，少师曰：盖有太阴之人，少阴之人，太阳之人，少阳之人，阴阳和平之人。凡五人者，其态不同，其筋骨气血各不等。

Yellow Emperor asked Shaoshi and said: "I am told that there are different kinds of men belonging to Yin and Yang. What is called the man belongs to Yin and what is called the man belongs to Yang?" Shaoshi said: "Between the heaven and earth, all things can not be divorced from the scope of the five elements, and the human body corresponds to the five elements also, but this is only an approximate speaking, as there are not only the oppositing one Yin and one Yang, and the complicated condition can hardly be expounded by words." Yellow Emperor said: "I hope to hear about the general condition. For the sages and the saints, can they attain the state of keeping the Yin and Yang in complete balance?" Shaoshi said: "Generally speaking, some people belong to Taiyin, some people belong to Shaoyin, some people belong to Taiyang, some people belong to Shaoyang, and some people belong to both mild in Yin and Yang. In a word, in the five types of people, their appearances are different, the strong and weak conditions of their tendons and bones are different, and the overabundant or the debilitative condition of their energy and blood are also different."

黄帝曰：其不等者，可得闻乎？少师曰：太阴之人，贪而不仁，下齐〔齐：《甲乙》卷一第十六作"济"〕湛湛，好内而恶出，心和〔和：《甲乙》卷一第十六作"抑"〕而不发，不务于时，动而后之〔之：《甲乙》卷一第十六作"人"〕，此太阴之人也。

Yellow Emperor asked: "Can you tell me the different conditions?" Shaoshi said: "A man of the Taiyin type is greedy, being not sincere and not generous, avaricious to his subordinates, be fond of taking and have an aversion to giving, he restrains his heart activities to be unexposed, does not care about doing anything good, being time-serving and behaves after others. This is the type of man who belongs to Taiyin like.

少阴之人，小贪而贼心，见人有亡，常若有得，好伤好害，见人有荣，乃反愠怒，心疾〔疾：《甲乙》卷一第十六作"嫉"〕而无恩，此少阴之人也。

"A man of the Shaoyin type keeps on gaining petty advantages and harbours the intention of harming others, he is happy when someone is injured as if he has gained something for paying nothing, he is fond of doing harm to others, angry at the honour of others, jealous and has no sympathy with others. This is the type of man who belongs to Shaoyin like.

太阳之人，居处于于，好言大事，无能而虚说，志发于四野，举措不顾是非，为事如常自用，事虽败而常无悔，此太阳之人也。

"A man of the Taiyang type is usually self-satisfied, he is fond of talking about major events, he is incompetent but often talks big Without the slightest hesitancy. He disregards the right or wrong of his behaviour and considers himself being always in the right, when he fails, he usually does not repent. This is the type of man who belongs to Taiyang like.

少阳之人，諟谛好自贵，有小小官，则高自宜〔宜:《甲乙》卷一第十六作"宣"〕，好为外交而不内附，此少阳之人也。

"A man of the Shaoyang type is usually cautious in dealing with things, he likes to boast his prestige, when he has a lower official post, he thinks he is remarkable and publicizes externally, he likes social communication, but he fails to keep close to the one he should love. This is the type of man who belongs to Shaoyang like.

阴阳和平之人，居处安静，无为惧惧，无为欣欣，婉然从物，或与不争，与时变化，尊则谦谦〔尊则谦谦:《甲乙》卷一第十六作"尊而谦让"〕，谭而不治〔谭而不治:《甲乙》卷一第十六作"卑而不谄"〕，是谓至治。古之善用针艾者，视人五态乃治之，盛者泻之，虚者补之。

"A man of the both mild in Yin and Yang type is calm, he has no accidental fright and excessive joy, he is concordant in submitting to work, if there is some small advantages, he does not bother about striving for it, he accommodates himself to the changes of the situation, when he is in the honourable status, he remains modest, when he is in a lower position, he is not subservient to the higher authorities. The version about the five types of men state above is really a wonderful truth. In ancient times, the physician who is good at acupuncture examines the appearances of the five types of man in advance, then he treats according to the different conditions respectively, purges the patient whose energy is overabundant and invigorates the patient whose energy is debilitative."

黄帝曰：治人之五态奈何？少师曰：太阴之人，多阴而无阳，其阴血浊，其卫气涩，阴阳不和，缓筋而厚皮，不之疾泻，不能移之。少阴之人，多阴少阳，小胃而大肠，六腑不调，其阳明脉小而太阳脉大，必审调之，其血易脱，其气易败也。

Yellow Emperor asked: "How to treat the five different types of men?" Shaoshi said: "To a man of Taiyin who has plenty of Yin without Yang, as his Yin blood is turbid, his Wei-energy is choppy, his Yin and Yang are not harmonious at all, and he has the characteristics of the flaccid tendon and the thick skin, if the rapid purging therapy is not applied to this kind of man, his disease can hardly be removed. To a man of Shaoyin type who has more Yin and little Yang, as his stomach is small and his intestine is large, the functions of his six hollow organs are not harmonious, since the energy of his Foot Yangming Channel is smaller, and the energy of his Hand Taiyang Channel is larger, when treating, one must be very careful, as his blood can easily become exhausted, his energy can easily be injured also.

太阳之人，多阳而少阴〔少阴：《甲乙》卷一第十六作“无阴”〕，必谨调之，无脱其阴，而泻其阳，阳重〔阳重：当注本，张注本并作“阴重”〕脱者易狂，阴阳皆脱者，暴死不知人也。少阳之人，多阳少阴，经小而络大，血在中而气〔气：《甲乙》卷一第十六“气”下有“在”字〕外，实阴而虚阳，独泻其络脉，则强气脱而疾，中气不足，病不起也。

“To the one who belongs to the Taiyang type who has plenty of Yang without Yin, he should be treated cautiously to avoid the exhaustion of Yin, and it is only Yang that can be purged. When Yin is consumed greatly, the patient will become manic due to the overabundance of Yang; if both the Yin and Yang are exhausted, the patient will be unconcious or die suddenly. The man who belongs to Shaoyang type has more Yang and little Yin, his channels are small and his collaterals are large, and his blood is inside and his energy is outside. When treating, it should substantialize the Yin channels and purges the Yang collaterals. But, if one solely purge the Yang collaterals excessively, the Yang energy will be exhausted quickly causing the insufficiency of the middle-warmer energy, and the disease can hardly be cured.

阴阳和平之人，其阴阳之气和，血脉调，谨诊其阴阳，视其邪正，安容仪，审有余不足，盛则泻之，虚则补之，不盛不虚，以经取之。此所以调阴阳，别五态之人者也。

“The man who belongs to the type of both mild in Yin and Yang, his Yin energy and Yang energy are harmonious and his channels are concordant. In treating, one should examine the changes of the Yin and Yang carefully to know the overabundance or debility of the evil energy and the health energy, observe the patient's appearance to determine which side is having a surplus and which side is deficient, when the evil is overabundant, apply purge therapy, when the healthy energy is deficient, apply the invigorating therapy, if the disease is of neither overabundant nor deficient, prick the channel where the disease resides. This is the criterion for adjusting the Yin and Yang and distinguishing the five different types of men.”

黄帝曰：夫五态之人者，相与毋故，卒然新会，未知其行也，何以别之？少师答曰：众人之属，不如〔如：周本，与注本，作“知”〕五态之人者，故五五二十五人，而五态之人不与焉。五态之人，尤不合于众者也。黄帝曰：别五态之人奈何？少师曰：太阴之人，其状黮黮然黑色，念然下意，临临然长大，腘然未偻，此太阴之人也。

Yellow Emperor asked: “For the five types of people, since we are not friends we do not know their daily behavior. when we meet abruptly, We do not know how to distinguish them.” Shaoshi said: “In the various types of men, the characteristics of the five types stated above are not known, so, there are twenty five types of man in Yin and Yang, but the five types of men stated above are excluded, and they are quite different from common people.” Yellow Emperor asked: “How to distinguish the five types of men?” Shaoshi said: “For a man of the Taiyin type, his skin is dark and black, he appears to be solemn, but he is modest in consciousness, his body is tall with his muscle of the neck protruding like a hunchback but actually, he has no rickets. This is the appearance of a man who belongs to the Taiyin type.

少阴之人，其状清然窃然，固以阴贼，立而躁崄，行而似伏，此少阴之人也。

"For a man in Shaoyin type, his appearance is cool and shallow, he likes to injure others with insidiousness especially, he stands impetuosly and slant, and walks like in prostration. This is the appearance of the man who belongs to the Shaoyin type.

太阳之人，其状轩轩储储，反身折腘，此太阳之人也。

"For a man of the Taiyang type, he appears to be relaxed and gay, he is self-satisfied, his chest is sticking out and his abdomen is protruding as if his poplitea are bending. This is the appearance of the man who belongs to the Taiyang type.

少阳之人，其状立则好仰，行则好摇，其两臂〔其两臂:《甲乙》卷一第十六，此三字属上读〕两肘则常出于背〔两肘则常出于臂:《甲乙》卷一第十六作"两臂肘皆出于臂"〕，此少阳之人也。

"For a man of the Shaoyang type, he tosses his head when standing and sways when walking, and he often puts his two arms and two elbows in his back. This is the appearance of the man who belongs to the Shaoyang type.

阴阳和平之人，其状委委然，随随然，颙颙然，愉愉然，䁥䁥然，豆豆然，众人皆曰君子，此阴阳和平之人也。

"For a man of both mild in Yin and Yang type, his appearance is nice, he appears to be obedient, gentle and respectful, he is amiable and pleasant with kind, benign looks, and people call him a gentleman. This is the appearance of the man who belongs to both mild in Yin and Yang type."

官能第七十三

Chapter 73
Guan Neng
(Each According to His Ability)

黄帝问于岐伯曰：余闻九针于夫子，众多矣不可胜数，余推而论之，以为一纪。余司诵之，子听其理，非则语余，请其正道，令可久传，后世无患，得其人乃传，非其人勿言。岐伯稽首再拜曰：请听圣王之道。

Yellow Emperor asked Qibo and said："I have heard a lot of your expositions about the nine kinds of needles in acupuncture of which the times are uncountable, and I have deliberated and studied it for twelve years. Now, let me relate the content over to you, and I hope you can point out the errors in it, so that it may be handed down to the later generations for a long time without doing any harm; I can impart it to the one who has aspiration for acupuncture and keep silent to the one who has no aspiration for it." Qibo bowed time and again and said; "I hope to hear the acupuncture principle from you, the sagacious king."

黄帝曰：用鍼之理，必知形气之所在，左右上下，阴阳表里，血气多少，行之逆顺，出入之合，谋伐有过。知解结，知补虚泻实，上下气门〔气门：《太素》卷十九《知官能》作"之气"〕，明通于四海，审其所在，寒热淋露，以〔以：《太素》卷十九《知官能》《图经》卷三并作"荥"〕输异处，审于调气，明于经隧，左右肢络，尽知其会。寒与热争，能合而调之，虚与实邻，知决而通之，左右不调，把而行之，明于逆顺，乃知可治，阴阳不奇，故知起时，审于本末，察其寒热，得〔得：《图经》卷三引作"知"〕邪所在，万刺不殆，知官九针，刺道毕矣。

Yellow Emperor said: "In applying the principle of acupuncture, one must know the fleshy or emaciate condition of the patien's body and the asthenic or sthenic condition of his energy, the different positions of the internal organs, the relation of the superficies and the interior of Yin and Yang, the plenty or little amount of the blood and energy, the agreeable or adverse flowing direction of the channel energy in the whole body, the convergence of the energies, the locations where it enters into the superficies from the interior and from interior into the superficies, it is only in this way, can the evil energy and blood be eliminated by treating. Besides, one must know the places where the Yin and Yang accumulate, know how to invigorate and purge the asthenic and sthenic energy of the hand and foot channels, comprehend explicitly the functions of the sea of energy, sea of marrow and the sea of water and cereals and know the places of asthenia and sthenia. If the cold and heat are protracted, it is due to the positions of the Xing point and the Shu point are different, so, it should adjust the channel energy carefully and make clear the positions of the channels, collaterals and the collateral-branches scattering on the left and right. If the cold and heat are combating, it must treat according to its synthetic condition; to the disease of which the asthenia and the sthenia are similar, it should make a firm decision of what is right and what is wrong; when the disease is not coordinating in the left side and the right side, it should scrape the acupoint with finger to scatter the energy before pricking. One must understand the agreeable or adverse condition of the disease before treating, and it is only not emphasizing on the Yin nor Yang can one know the relation between the cause of disease and the season. When one observes the change of cold and heat to know the location where the evil energy resides in advance, no accident will occur even in the ten thousand times of pricking. When one knows the principles of the nine kinds of needles and applies accordingly, the principle of acupuncture is supposed to be exhaustive.

明于五输，徐疾所在，屈伸出入，皆有条理，言阴与阳，合于五行，五藏六府，亦有所藏，四时八风，尽有阴阳，各得其位，合于明堂，各处色部，五藏六府，察其所痛，左右上下，知其寒温，何经所在，审皮肤之寒温滑涩，知其所苦，膈有上下，知其气所在。先得其道，稀而疏之，稍深以留，故能徐入之。大热在上，推而下之，从下上者，引而去之，视前痛〔痛：张注本作"病"〕者，常先取之。大寒在外，留而补之，入于中者，从合泻之。针所不为，灸之所宜，上气不足，推而扬之，下气不足，积而从之，阴阳皆虚，火自当之，厥而寒甚，骨廉陷下，寒过于膝，下陵三里，阴络所过，得之留止，寒入于中，推而行之，经陷下者，火则当之，结络坚紧，火所治之。不知所苦，两跅之下，男阴女阳，良工所禁，针论毕矣。

"In acupuncture, the swift and slow pricking to the shu-points of the internal organs, the bending or stretching posture of the patient during pricking and the methods of inserting and pulling the needle are all having certain rules. When one explains the Yin and Yang of the body, it should be in accordance with the five elements. The five solid organs and the six hollow organs are having the functions of storing the spirit and the cereals respectively, and changes of the four seasons and the winds from the eight directions are related with Yin and Yang; on one's face, there are the different positions belonging to the Yin, Yang and the five elements respectively and they combine on the nose; from the different colours displayed on the various part of the face, can the disease of the internal organs be determined. When one examines the location of the patient's pain, and integrates with the colours displayed on the left, right, upper and the lower sides of the face, he will be able to know whether the disease is belonging to the cold or heat and which channel is diseased. In treating, examine the cold, warm, slippery or choppy conditions of the skin of the anterolateral side of the forearm to know what disease is distressing the patient, then, examine the location above and below the diaphragm (lung and stomach) to know where the evil is. One must know the route of the channel first, then, prick the acupoint; the pricking should be few and accurate, prick deeply and retain the needle to cause the health energy to enter slowly. When the patient has high fever in the upper part, prick and cause it to descend, when the evil is developing from below to above, prick and induce it to descend, and then remove it. Besides, note the case histroy of the patient and prick the patient according to the previous condition to treat the cause of the disease. When cold appears on the suface of the body, prick and retain the needle to invigorate so as to produce heat, if the cold-evil has penetrated inside, prick and retain the needle for purging. To the diseases which are not suitable for pricking, apply moxibustion. To the one whose upper warmer energy is insufficient, prick and raise the energy; to the one whose lower-warmer energy is insufficient, prick to accumulate and smooth the energy; to the one whose Yin and Yang are both asthenic, apply moxibustion therapy. When the patient has cold feet and the cold is quite severe, or the muscles by the bone are bogging down, or the extending cold has exceeded the two knees, it should apply moxibusion to the Sanli point; when the cold retains on the location where the Yin collateral passes, and when the cold-evil has penetrated into the internal organs, prick to disperse the energy; when the channel is bogging down, apply the moxibustion therapy; when the collateral is knotty and firm, apply moxibustion also. If the patient is not painful but not numbly , it should prick the Shenmen point of the Yangqiao channel and the Zhaohai point of the Yinqiao Channel, if the Yinqiao Channel is pricked erroneously to a man or the Yangqiao Channel is pricked erroneously to a woman, it is the contraindication for an acupuncturist of higher level. The cardinal principles of acupuncture hereto are expounded completely.

用针之服，必有法则，上视天光，下司八正，以辟奇邪，而观百姓，审于虚实，无犯其邪。是得天之露，遇岁之虚，救而不胜，反受其殃，故曰：必知天忌，乃言针意。法于往古，验于来今，观于窈冥，通于无穷，粗之所不见，良工之所贵，莫知其形，若神髣髴。

"When learning the application of the needle, one must follow a definite rule. One should observe the revolving law of the sun, moon and stars above, and understand the normal condition of the eight solar terms below, so that one can remind people to examine the asthenia and the sthenia, to take precaution against their invasion. When the wind and rain are abnormal in coming or the weather is not in conformity with the season, if the physician can not rescue the patient according to the weather change, it will cause the disease to become dangerous, thus, one must know the seasonal contraindication, then can he understand the acupuncture therapy. Following the examples of the ancient people's learning and verify it with the present situation and examining the invisible things in the body to know the endless changes of the disease are the things that a physician of lower level does not understand and the physician of a higher level appreciates. Since they are invisible without any trace, being subtle as if existing and as if not existing, so, they are hard to be underastood.

邪气之中人也，洒淅动形。正邪之中人也微，先见于色，不知于其身，若有若无，若亡若存，有形无形，莫知其情。是故上工之取气，乃救其萌芽；下工守其已成，因败其形。

"When the evil energy invades the body, the phenomenom of shivering with cold will occur. When one is affected by the cold-evil after perspiration, the disease will appear slightly on the complexion, but the body feels nothing wrong, the patient seems to have disease, yet seems to have no disease, the disease seems to have faded away, yet seems to be remaining, seems to have the morbidity yet seems to have no morbidity, and the actual state of illness can hardly be known.

是故工之用针也，知气之所在，而守其门户，明于调气，补泻所在，徐疾之意，所取之处。泻必用员，切而转之，其气乃行，疾而〔而：《太素》卷十九《知官能》作“入”〕徐出，邪气乃出，伸而迎之，遥〔遥：《太素》卷十九《知官能》并作“摇”〕大其穴，气出乃疾。补必用方，外引其皮，令当其门，左引其枢，右推其肤，微旋而徐推之，必端以正，安以静，坚心无解，欲微以留，气下而疾出之，推其皮，盖其外门，真气乃存。用针之要，无忘其神。

Therefore, in pricking, the physician should know the route of the channel energy and prick the corresponding acupoint. At the same time, he should know the clue of adjusting, under what condition should it be invigorated and under what condition should it be purged, and know whether the swift or slow insertion should be applied. In purging, it should apply the fluent and flexible manipulation, insert the needle to the focus straightly and twist the needle to cause the health energy to operate normally, when one inserts the needle swiftly and pulls it slowly, the evil energy will excrete along with the pulling of the needle, when one extends the needle to receive the coming energy and sways the needle hole before pulling out the needle, the evil energy will come out very quickly. In invigorating, one should prick with a upright and leisure manipulation, knead the skin right on the spot of the acupoint, hold the needle with left hand and insert the needle into the skin with the right hand, twist slightly and insert slowly, when inserting, the body of the needle must be straight, the spirit of the acupuncturist must be calm, resolute without any slackness, when the energy arrives, retain the needle for a moment and pull out the needle swiftly, after the energy has moved away, press the skin on the acupoint and seal the needle hole so that the healthy energy will not excrete. The clue of pricking is one must not forget to recuperate the spirtit."

雷公问于黄帝曰：针论曰：得其人乃传，非其人勿言。何以知其可传？黄帝曰：各得其人，任之其能，故能明其事。雷公曰：愿闻官能奈何？黄帝曰：明目者，可使视色。聪耳者，可使听音。捷疾辞语者，可使传论语。徐而安静，手巧而心审谛者，可使行针艾，理血气而调诸逆顺，察阴阳而兼诸方。缓节柔筋而心和调者，可使导引行气。疾毒言语轻人者，可使唾痈咒病。爪苦手毒，为事善伤者，可使按积抑痹。各得其能，方乃可行，其名乃彰。不得其人，其功不成，其师无名。故曰：得其人乃言，非其人勿传，此之谓也。手毒者，可使试按龟，置龟于器下而按其上，五十日而死矣；手甘者〔手甘：《太素》卷十九《知官能》作“甘手”〕，复生如故也。

Leigong asked Yellow Emperor and said: "It was stated in the《On Acupuncture》: 'You can only impart acupuncture skill to a right person but keeps silent to a wrong person.' But how can one know who is the right person and who is not?" Yellow Emperor said: "When imparting, a proper person of talent must be found, teach him the skill which is competent for him so that he can understand perfectly the task." Leigong said: "I hope to hear how to employ people according to their talents." Yellow Emperor said: "When the one is keen in seeing, he can be induced to examine the colours of the complexion; when the one is keen in hearing, he can be induced to distinguish the voice of the patient; when the one is glib in talking and is gifted with a silver tongue, he can be induced to transmit the speech of others;

when the one is slow and calm in speech, deft in hands and is level-headed, he can be induced to manipulate the acupuncture and moxibustion to dredge the blood and energy, to adjust the agreeable or adverse energies and the abnormal disease, to observe the Yin and Yang changes and apply various treatments; when the one is slow in action, has soft tendons, good nature and agreeable disposition, he can be guided to treat by inducing the energy; when the one is jealous, caustic, despising others when speaking, he can be taught to curse the disease by spit on and incantation; when the one whose finger nails are thick, ruthless in actions and apt to hurt others in doing things, he can be taught to massage the mass and treat the bi-syndrome. In a word, induce one to learn the skill each according to his ability, and it is only in this way, can the various therapies of acupunture be put into practice and one's reputation can widely be made know. If the knowledge is imparted to the wrong person, not only the function of pricking can not be brought into full play, but also the teacher will be discredited. This is what the 'impart to the right person and keep silent to the wrong person' means. As to the method of testing whether the one is having a ruthless hand, it can be distinguished by pressing a turtle: put a turtle under a ware, when the one who is having a ruthless hand presses the ware with his hand, the turtle will die in fifty days, if the one is not having a ruthless hand, the turtle will remain alive in fifty days."

论疾诊尺第七十四

Chapter 74
Lun Ji Zhen Chi
(To Determine the Disease by Inspecting the Skin of the Anterolateral Side of the Forearm)

黄帝问于岐伯曰：余欲无视色持脉，独调〔调：据《太素》卷十五《尺诊》杨注应作“诊”〕其尺，以言其病，从外知内，为之奈何？岐伯曰：审其尺之缓急、小大、滑涩，肉之坚脆，而病形定矣。

Yellow Emperor asked Qibo and said: "I wish to explain the reasons of the disease and know the internal changes from outside without inspecting the complexion and palpating the pulse condition of the patient, but only examine the positions on the skin of the anterolateral side of the forearm, how should I do it?" Qibosaid: "When examining the rapid or slow, large or small, slippery or choppy conditions of the skin of the anterolateral side of the forearm and the firm and crisp conditions of the muscle, the location of the disease can be determined.

视人之目窠〔窠：《太素》卷十五《尺诊》作“果”〕上微痈〔痈：《脉经》卷八第八作“拥”〕，如新卧起伏，其颈脉动，时咳，按其手足上，窅〔窅：《脉经》卷八第八作“陷”〕而不起者，风水肤胀〔肤胀：《脉经》卷八第八无此二字〕也。

"When the eyelides of the patient appear to be slightly swelling as if he has just got up from sleep, his Renying pulse on the neck is pulsating obviously and he coughs now and then, when pressing his hand and foot, and the place being pressed is bogging down deeply and unable to rise up again with the lifting up of the hand, it is the syndrome of edema caused by wind-evil.

尺肤滑〔滑：《太素》卷十五《尺诊》作“温”〕其淖泽者，风也。尺肉〔肉：《脉经》卷四第一作“内”〕弱者，解㑊，安卧脱肉者，寒热，不治，尺肤滑而泽脂者，风也。尺肤涩者，风痹也。尺肤粗如枯鱼之鳞者，水泆饮也。尺肤热甚，脉盛躁者，病温也，其脉盛而滑者，病〔病：《太素》卷十五《尺诊》作“汗”〕且出也。尺肤寒，其〔其：《脉经》卷四第一作“甚”。“寒甚”断句〕脉小〔小：《甲乙》卷四第二上任务“急”〕者，泄、少气。尺肤炬然，先热后寒者，寒热也。尺肤先寒，久大之而热者，亦寒热也。

"When the skin of the anterolateral side of the forearm of the patient is warm, soft, smooth and lustrous, it is the disease of wind. When the muscle of the skin of the anterolateral side of the forearm is crisp and weak, the patient is fatigue, fond of sleeping with emaciation of the muscle, it is the consumptive disease due to cold and heat which can hardly be cured. When the skin of anterolateral side of the forearm is unsmooth without any lubricious feeling, it is the disease of arthralgia due to wind-evil. When the skin of anterolateral side of the forearm is coarse like the fish scale, it is the watery phlegm-retention syndrome. When the skin of anterolateral side of the forearm is very hot, and the pulse condition is gigantic and impetuous, it is the seasonal febrile disease; if the pulse condition is gigantic and slippery, the patient will soon be sweating. When the skin of anterolateral side of the forearm is very cold and the pulse condition is small and fine, it is the disease of diarrhea or the deficiency of energy. When the skin of anterolateral side of the forearm is hot like fire, being hot previously and then becomes cold, it is the disease of cold and heat; when being pressed by hand and it appears to be cold, but becomes hot gradually after enduring pressing, it is also the disease of cold and heat.

肘所独热者，腰以上热；手所独热者，腰以下热。肘前独热者，膺前热；肘后独热者，肩背热。臂中独热者，腰腹热；肘后粗〔粗：《甲乙》卷四第二作“廉”〕以下三四寸热者，肠中有虫〔肠中有虫：按：“虫”疑是“热”之误字〕，掌中热者，腹中热；常中寒者，腹中寒。鱼上〔上：《甲乙》卷四第一作“际”〕白肉有青血脉者，胃中有寒。

"When the skin on the elbow is hot solely, it shows there is heat above the loins; when the hand is hot solely, it shows there is heat below the loins; when the front of the elbow is hot solely, it shows there is heat in the front chest; when the rear of the elbow is hot solely, it shows there is heat in the back; when the inside of the arm is hot solely, it shows the heat is in the loins and the abdomen; when the place three inches under the rear of the elbow is hot, it shows there is heat in the intestine; when the palm is hot, it shows there is heat in the abdomen; when the palm is cold, it shows there is cold in the abdomen; when the green collateral appears on the white flesh of the thenar, it shows there is cold in the stomach.

尺〔尺：《甲乙》卷四第二上“尺”下有“肤”字〕炬然热，人迎大者，当〔当：《脉经》卷四第一作“尝”〕夺血。尺坚大〔坚大：《脉经》卷四第一作“紧人迎”三字〕，脉小甚，少气，悗有加，立死。

"When the skin of anterolateral side of the forearm is so hot to scorch the hand and the Renying pulse is gigantic, it shows the loss of blood of the patient; when the skin of anterolateral side of the forearm is tight and the Renying pulse is small, it shows the patient's energy is deficient, if the complexion appears to be green and white again, the patient will die immediately.

目赤色者病在心，白在肺，青在肝，黄在脾，黑在肾。黄色不可名者，病在胸中。

"When one's eyes are red, the disease is in the Heart Channel, when it is white, the disease is in the lung, when it is green, the disease is in the liver, when it is yellow, the disease is in the spleen, when it is black, the disease is in the kidney, when it is yellow mixing with other colours which can hardly be told, the disease is in the diaphragm.

诊目痛〔痛：《脉经》卷五第四作“病”〕，赤脉从上下者，太阳病；从下上者，阳明病；从外走内者，少阳病。

"When inspecting the disease of the eye, if there is a vertical red channel descending in the eye, it is the disease belonging to the Foot Taiyang Channel; if there is a vertical red channel ascending in the eye, it is the disease belonging to the Yangming Channel; if there is a horizontal red channel running from the outer canthus to the inner canthus, it is the disease belonging to the Shaoyang Channel.

诊寒热，赤脉上下至瞳子，见一脉一岁死，见一脉半一岁半死，见二脉二岁死，见二脉半二岁半死，见三脉三岁死。

"When inspecting the disease of scrofula of cold and heat, and there is a vertical red channel penetrating through the pupil, if the red channel is one of them, the patient will die in a year, if the red channels are one and half of them, the patient will die in one and half years, if the red channels are two of them, the patient will die in two years, if the red channels are two and half of them, the patient will die in two and half years, if the red channels are three of them, the patient will die in three years.

诊龋齿痛，按其阳〔阳："阳"下脱"明"字应据《甲乙》卷十二第六补〕之〔之：《脉经》卷五第四"之"下有"脉"字〕来，有过者独〔独：孙鼎宜曰："独"当作"为"〕热，在左左热，在右右热，在上上热，在下下热。

"When inspecting the dental caries which is painful, press the coming route of the hand and foot Yangming Channels, if the channel is hyperactive, it shows there is heat, when the left side is hyperactive, the heat is on the left, when the right side is hyperactive, the heat is on the right, when the upper part is hyperactive, the heat is in the upper part, when the lower part is hyperactive, the heat is in the lower part.

诊血脉者，多赤多热，多青多痛，多黑为久痹，多赤、多黑、多青皆见者，寒热。

"When inspecting the collaterals, if the red colour is plenty, it shows the patient has plenty of heat, if the green colour is plenty, it shows the patient has plenty of pains, if the black colour is plenty, it shows the patient has protracted bi-syndrome, if the red, black and green colours appear to be plenty simultaneously, it is the disease of cold and heat.

身痛而〔而：《病沅》卷十二并作"面"〕色微黄，齿垢黄，爪甲上黄，黄疸也，安卧，小便黄赤，脉小而涩者，不嗜食。

"When the patient is painful in the body, slightly yellow of the complexion, his tartus is yellow and his nails are yellow, it is the disease of jaundice. When the patient is fond of sleeping, has deep-coloured urine and the small and choppy pulse condition, the patient will have the syndrome of loss of appetite.

人病，其寸口之脉，与人迎之脉小大等及其浮沉等者，病难已也。

"When the patient's Cunkou pulse and the Renying pulse are having the same power in pulsating and their extends of floating and sinking are similar, the disease can hardly be cured.

女子手少阴脉动甚者，妊子。

"When inspecting a woman, if her Hand Shaoyin Channel of Heart is pulsating severely, it shows she is pregnant.

婴儿病，其头毛皆逆上者，必死。耳间青脉起者，掣痛〔痛：《甲乙》卷十二第十一"痛"上有"腹"字〕。大便赤瓣〔赤瓣：《脉经》卷九第九作"赤青瓣"〕，飧泄，脉小〔脉者：

《甲乙》卷十二第一“小”作“大”〕者，手足寒，难已；飧泄，脉少，手足温，泄易已。

“When an infant has disease with his hair standing upward, he will die. If he has green channel being bulge around the ear, it shows he has convulsion of the muscle and the abdominal pain. When the green clottings are seen in the stool, it shows he has indigestion, if his pulse condition is gigantic and he has cold hands and feet, he can hardly be cured, if the patient has indigestion and small pulse condition but his hands and feet are warm, the disease of diarrhea can easily be cured.

四时之变，寒暑之胜，重阴必阳，重阳必阴，故阴主寒，阳主热，故寒甚则热，热甚则寒，故曰：寒生热，热生寒，此阴阳之变也。故曰：冬伤于寒，春生瘅热〔瘅热：《素问·阴阳应象大论》作“温病”〕；春伤于风，夏生后泄肠澼；夏伤于暑，秋生痎疟；秋伤于湿，冬生咳嗽。是谓四时之序也。

“The weather changes of the four seasons are the alternations of cold and heat; when the Yin is overabundant, it will turn into Yang, when the Yang is overabundant, it will turn into Yin; as Yin dominates the cold and Yang dominates the heat, so, when the cold is excessive it will turn into heat when the heat is excessive, it will turn into cold. Thus, the extreme cold can produce heat and the extreme heat can produce cold, and this is the principle of the relative change of Yin and Yang. Therefore, when one is injured by cold in winter, he will have seasonal febrile disease in spring. When one is injured by wind in spring, he will have diarrhea in summer. When one is injured by summer-heat in summer, he will have malaria in autumn. When one is injured by wetness in autumn, he will cough in winter. This is the law of the diseases caused by the weather changes of the four seasons.”

刺节真邪第七十五

Chapter 75
Ci Jie Zhen Xie
(The Criterions of Pricking and the Difference Between Healthy Energy and the Evil Energy)

黄帝向于岐伯曰：余闻刺有五节奈何？岐伯曰：固有五节：一曰振埃，二曰发蒙，三曰去爪〔爪："爪"疑当作"水"〕，四曰彻〔彻：张注本作"撤"〕衣，五日解惑。黄帝曰：夫子言五节，余未知其意。岐伯曰：振埃者，刺外经，去阳病也。发蒙者，刺府输，去府病也。去爪者，刺关节肢〔肢：《太素》卷二十二《五节刺》作"之支"二字〕络也。彻衣者，尽刺诸阳之奇输也。解惑者，尽知调阴阳，补泻有余不足，相倾移也。

Yellow Emperor asked Qibo and said："I am told there are five criterions in pricking, what are they?" Qibo said："No doubt, there are five criterions. They are the Zhen-ai (shake off the dust), Fameng (enlighten the ignorance), Qushui (remove the edema), Cheyi (take off the clothes) and Jiehuo (relieve perplexion)." Yellow Emperor said："I don't understand the meaning of the five criterions you said." Qibo said："The Zhen-ai pricking therapy is to prick the acupoints on the four extremities and the skin to treat the disease of Yang; the Fameng pricking therapy is to prick the shu-points of the six hollow organ to treat the diseases of the six organs; the Qushui pricking therapy is to prick the collateral-branches of the joints; the Cheyi pricking therapy is to prick the large collaterals of the six hollow organs; the Jiehuo pricking therapy is to invigorate the insufficiency and purge the surplus after understanding thoroughly the functions of adjusting the Yin and Yang and pricks flexibly and reversely in extraordinary conditions."

黄帝曰刺节言振埃，夫子乃言刺外经，去阳病，余不知其所谓也，愿卒闻之。岐伯曰：振埃者，阳气大逆，上〔上：《太素》卷二十二《五节刺》无此字〕满于胸中，愤〔愤：《太素》卷二十二《五节刺》作"烦"〕䐜肩息，大气逆上，喘喝坐伏，病恶埃烟，饲不得息，请言振埃，尚疾于振埃。黄帝曰：善。取之何如？岐伯曰：取之天容。黄帝曰：其咳上气，穷诎胸痛者，取之奈何？岐伯曰：取之廉泉。黄帝曰：取之有数乎？岐伯曰：取天容者，无过一里，取廉泉者，血变而止。帝曰：善哉。

Yellow Emperor said："The Zhen-ai pricking therapy you said is to prick the external channels for treating the diseases of Yang, I do not know what you are indicating, I hope you can tell me in details." Qibo said："The Zhen-ai pricking therapy is to treat the severe adverseness of the Yang energy, apply the therapy when the patient has fullness and distention in the chest, shrugging of the shoulders with rapid respiration, when his breath in the chest is reversing up, coughs and perspires rapidly, feels uneasy when sitting or prostrating, has dyspnea like his throat is being choked. This therapy is called Zhen-ai to analogize the curitive efficacy of pricking is as quick as shaking off the dust. "Yellow Emperor said:"Good. But which acupoint should be pricked?" Qibo said: "It should prick the Tianrong point." Yellow Emperor asked:"If the patient has cough and dyspnea caused by the adverse rising of lung energy, obstruction of the breath and pain in the chest, which acupoint should be pricked?" Qibo said: "It should prick the Lianquan point." Yellow Emperor asked: Is there any rule when pricking the two acupoints?" Qibo said: "When pricking the Tianrong point, the insertion must not exceed one inch; when pricking the Lianquan point, the pricking should be ceased when the complexion of the patient has changed." Yellow Emperor said: "Good."

黄帝曰：刺节言发蒙，余不得其意。夫发蒙者，耳无所闻，目无所见。夫子乃言刺腑输，去腑病，何输使然？愿闻其故。岐伯曰：妙乎哉问也！此刺之大〔大：《太素》卷二十三《五节刺》无此字〕约，针之极也，神明之类也，口说书卷，犹不能及也，请言发蒙耳，尚疾于发蒙也。黄帝曰：善。愿卒闻之之。岐伯曰：刺此者，必于日中，刺其听宫，中其眸子，声闻于耳〔耳《甲乙》卷十二第五作"外"〕，此其输也。黄帝曰：善。何谓声闻于耳？岐伯曰：刺邪〔刺邪：《甲乙》卷十二第五作"已刺"〕以手坚按其两鼻窍而〔而：《甲乙》卷十二第五作"令"〕疾偃，其声必应于针也。黄帝曰：善。此所谓弗见为之，而无目视，见而取之，神明相得者也。

Yellow Emperor said: "I don't understand the meaning of the Fameng pricking therapy. The function of the Fameng pricking therapy is to treat the disease of one who can not hear and can not see, but you said it is to prick the shu-points of the six hollow organs for treating the diseases of the six hollow organs, by pricking which shu-point can the result be achieved? I hope to hear the reasons about it." Qibo said: "You have asked a wonderful question! It is the essentials in pricking, and the summit of the skill of acupuncture which belongs to the divinity kind, it can not be expressed even by writing down after oral relating. The name of Fameng is analogizing its treating efficacy being faster than the enlightening of the ignorance." Yellow Emperor said: "Good. I hope you explain it in details." Qibo said: "When treating the disease of which one can not hear by ears and can not see by eyes, the Tinggong point should be pricked at noon, the needling response will affect the pupil straightly and cause the ear to hear sounds. This is the main shu-point for treating the disease." Yellow Emperor said: "Good. But what causes the ear to hear sounds?" Qibo said: "When the needle has inserted, ask the patient to press the two nostrils tightly and lie on his back quickly, then, there must be sounds responding the pricking." Yellow Emperor said: "Good. This is the so-called seeing not what has done, although nothing is seen by the eyes, yet operating the needling like seeing the coming and going of the channel. When the physician has every thing under perfect control like this, he has really attained the extent of divinity."

黄帝曰：刺节言去爪，夫子乃言刺关节肢络，愿卒闻之。岐伯曰：腰脊者，身之大关节也。肢胫〔肢胫：《甲乙》卷九第十一并作"股胻"〕者，人之管〔管：《太素》卷二十二《五节刺》作“所”〕以趋翔也。茎垂者，身中之机，阴精之候，津液之道也。故饮食不节，喜怒不时，津液内溢，乃下留于睾，血〔血：《太素》卷二十二《五节刺》作“水”〕道不通，日大不休，俯仰不便，趋翔不能，此病荣然有水，不上不下，铍石所取，形不可匿，常不得蔽，故命曰去爪。帝曰：善。

Yellow Emperor said: "The Qushui pricking therapy you said is to prick the collateral-branches of the joints, I hope to hear the details." Qibo said: "The loins and the spine are the larger joints of the body; the lower extremities and the shanks are the organs for walking; the penis is the reproductive organ of the body, it can discharge the sperm and it is the exit of the body fluid. When one does not practise temperance in taking food and drink, and has improper overjoy and anger to cause the body fluid to overflow inside, and then flow to the scrotum, as the water course is impeded, the edema of the scrotum will become larger day after day, and the patient will have difficulty in facing up and down and can not walk. This kind of disease is due to the accumulation of the water, obstruction of the upper-warmer energy and the failure of the urine to excrete below. In this case, it can apply the swordshaped needle or the stone needle to remove the water." Yellow Emperor said: "Good."

黄帝曰：刺节言彻衣，夫子乃言尽刺诸阳之奇输，未有常处也，愿卒闻之。岐伯曰：是阳气有余而阴气不足，阴气不足则内热，阳气有余则外热，内热相搏，热于怀炭，外畏绵帛近〔近：《甲乙》作“衣”〕，不可近身，又〔又：《甲乙》卷七第一上作“身热”〕不可近席，腠理闭塞，则汗不出，舌焦唇槁，腊干嗌燥，饮食不让美恶。黄帝曰：善。取之奈何？岐伯曰：取之于其天府、大杼三痏，又刺中膂，以去其热，补足手太阴以去其汗，热去汗稀，疾于彻衣。黄帝曰：善。

Yellow Emperor said: "The Cheyi pricking therapy you said is to prick the side collaterals of the six hollow organs which have no definite positions. I hope to hear the details about it." Qibo said: "It is to treat the disease when the Yang energy is having a surplus and the Yin energy is deficient. When the Yin energy is deficient, the internal heat will produce; when the Yang energy is having a surplus, the external heat will produce, when the two heats are combating each other, the patient will be hot like cherrishing the charcoal. He is afraid of attaching the materials of cotton and silk outside, detests pressing close to the clothes and approaching the matress, he has no sweat due to the obstruction of the striae, he has dry tongue, withered lips, dry muscle, dry throat and overabundant internal heat, he has no appetite and fails to distinguish whether the taste of the food is nice or not." Yellow Emperor said: "Good. But how to treat it by pricking?" Qibo said: "Prick the Tianfu point of the Hand Taiyin Channel and the Dazhu point of Foot Taiyang Channel for three times each, then, prick the Zhonglu point which is the Shu-point of the Foot Taiyang Channel to remove the heat, invigorate the Foot Taiyin Channel of Spleen and the Hand Taiyin Channel of Lung to cause perspiration, when the heat is removed and the sweat is reduced, the disease will be recovered, and the curative efficacy is quicker than taking off the clothes." Yellow Emperor said: "Good."

黄帝曰：刺节言解惑，夫子乃言尽知调〔调：《甲乙》卷十第二下"调"下有"诸"字〕阴阳，补泻有余不足，相倾移也，惑〔惑：《甲乙》卷十第二下无此字〕何以解之？岐伯曰：大风在身，血脉〔血脉：按："血脉"疑当作"血气"〕偏虚，虚者不足，实者有余，轻重不得，倾侧宛伏，不知东西，不知南北，乍上乍下，乍反乍复，颠倒无常，甚于迷惑。黄帝曰：善。取之奈何？岐伯曰：泻其有余，补其不足，阴阳平复，用针若此，疾于解惑。黄帝曰：善：请藏之灵兰之室，不敢妄出也。

Yellow Emperor said: "The Jiehuo pricking therapy you said is to understand thoroughly the functions of Yin and Yang first, then, invigorate that is insufficient and purge that is having a surplus, and interchange the conditions of asthenia and sthenia, but how to know the pathological phenomenon?" Qibo said: "When one contracts the wind severely, his blood and energy will become asthenic, when one is asthenic, his healthy energy must be insufficient, when one is sthenic, his evil energy must be having a surplus, in this way, his extremities will be loss of balance, his body will be slanting and he can not tolerate the oblique of the body and the limbs, he can not make distinction of the orientations. The syndrome is now up and now down, now slight and now severe, and has no regular pattttern in attacking. The patient is abnormal in daily life, and the disease condition is more serious than the loss or partial loss of consciousness." Yellow Emperor said: "Good. But how to treat it by pricking?" Qibo said: "Purge when it is having a surplus and invigorate when it is insufficient, adjust the Yin and Yang to become normal, when applying the pricking therapy like this, the curative efficacy will be faster than relieving the perplexity." Yellow Emperor said: "Good. I will keep the papers of the principle you said in the royal library and not to leak it out rashly."

黄帝曰：余闻刺有五邪，何谓五邪？岐伯曰：病有持痈者，有容〔容：《甲乙》卷五第五无此字〕大者，有狭〔狭：《甲乙》卷五第五无此字〕小者，有热者，有寒者，是谓五邪。黄帝曰：刺五邪奈何？岐伯曰：凡刺五邪之方，不过五章，瘅热消灭，肿聚散亡，寒痹益温，小者益阳，大者必去，请道其方。

Yellow Emperor said: "I am told there is the pricking therapy for treating the five evils, what are the five evils?" Qibo said: "In diseases, some belong to the fat and clumsy type, some belong to the sthenic type, some belong to the asthenic type, some belong to the heat type and some belong to the cold type, and they are called the five evils." Yellow Emperor said: "How to treat them by pricking?" Qibo said: "There are only five articles in treating the five evils: to the disease of heat, the heat-evil should be eliminated; to the disease of swelling and mass, the swelling should be dissipated; to the disease of cold-type arthralgia, it should be warmed; to the debilitating evil, the Yang energy should be reinforced; to the evil of sthenic-type, it should remove the evil-energy. Now, let me explain to you the methods."

凡刺痈邪，无迎陇，易俗移性不得脓，脆〔脆：《甲乙》卷五第二作"越"〕道更行，去〔去：《太素》卷二十二《五邪刺》"去"上有"行"字〕其乡，不安〔不安：《太素》卷二十二《五邪刺》"不安"下有"其"字〕处，所〔所：按"所"疑当作"邪"〕乃散亡。诸阴阳过〔过：《甲乙》卷五第二校语作“遇”〕痈〔痈：《太素》卷二十二《五邪刺》“痈”下有“所”字〕者，取之其输泻之。

“When pricking the mass or carbuncle, one must not prick head on rashly against the flourishing evil, it should treat patiently like diverting the customs or transferring one's disposition, if there is no pus in the mass, one should prick with other therapy and divorce from the definite pricking location, in this way, the evil can be dissipated. It is important to purge by pricking the points on the related Yin and Yang channels which pass the carbuncle.

凡刺大邪日以小，泄夺〔夺：按“夺”字衍〕其有余，乃益虚。剽其通〔通：《太素》卷二十二《五邪刺》作“道”〕，针其邪，肌肉亲，视之毋有反其真。刺诸阳分肉间。

“When treating the pathogentic factor of excess type, which is the sthenic evil the pricking is for reducing it, when purging the surplus, it can cause the hyperactive condition to become normal. When pricking, dredge the evil-energy hastily and hit the location of the evil-energy to cause the muscles to become attaching to each other, cease the pricking when seeing the evil-energy has been removed and the health energy has been recovered. It should be noted that most of the sthenic evils are in the three Yang channels, and the pricking should be on the muscles along the various Yang channels.

凡刺小邪，日以大，补其不足乃无害，视其所在迎之界，远近尽至，其不得外，侵而行之乃自费。刺分肉间。

“When pricking the asthenic evil, it is for substantializing the health energy. When the insufficiency is invigorated, the asthenic evil will not be able to do harm. In invigorating, inspect the location of the asthenia to know its demarcation with the health energy, induce the health energy that is far and near to the sphere of asthenia without exception. If the invigorating is excessive, it will cause injury, so, the pace between the muscles should be pricked.

凡刺热邪，越而苍，出游不归乃无病，为开通〔通：当注本，张注本，并无“通”字〕辟门户，使邪得出病乃已。

“When pricking the heat-evil, it is for causing the heat evil to turn into cold, when the evil is dissipated, the patient will have no heat and he will be recovered. In pricking, enlarge the needle hole to excrete the heat-evil and the disease can be recovered.

凡刺寒邪，日以温，徐往徐来〔徐来：《太素》卷二十二《五邪刺》任务“疾去”〕致其神，门户已闭气不分，虚实得调其气存也。

“When pricking the cold-evil, it is for warming the health energy, the insertion of the needle should be slow, and the pulling out of it should be swift to induce the spirit. When pulling out the needle, the needle hole will close, the energy will not disperse, the sthenia and the asthenia will be adjusted and the health energy will retain inside.”

黄帝曰：官针奈何？岐伯曰：刺痈者用铍针，刺大者用锋针，刺小者用员利针，刺热者用鑱针，刺寒者用毫针也。

Yellow Emperow asked: “In pricking the five evils, what kind of needle should be applied?” Qibo said: “When pricking the carbuncle, apply the sword-shaped needle; when pricking the asthenic evil, apply the ovoid-tip needle; when pricking the sthenic evil, apply the ensiform needle; when pricking the heat-evil, apply the sagital needle; when pricking the cold-evil, apply the filiform needle.

请言解论〔解论：按“论”似应作“结”〕，与天地相应，与四时相副，人参天地，故可为解。下有渐洳，上生苇蒲，此所以知形气之多少也。阴阳者，寒暑也，热则滋雨〔雨：《太素》卷二十二《五邪刺》无此字〕而在上，根荄少汁。人气在外，皮肤缓，腠理开，血气减，汁大泄，皮淖泽。寒则地冻水冰，人气在中，皮肤致，腠理闭，汗不出，血气强，肉坚涩。当是之时，善行水者，不能往冰；善穿地者，不能凿冻；善用针者，亦不能取四厥〔厥：《甲乙》卷七第三作“逆”〕；血脉凝结，坚搏不往来者亦未可即柔。故行水者，必待天温冰释冻解〔冻解：《甲乙》卷七第三“冻解”上有“穿地者必待“五”字〕。而水可行，地可穿也。人脉犹是也，治厥者，必先熨调和其经，掌与腋、肘与脚、项与脊以调之〔之：《甲乙》作“其气”〕，火气〔火气《甲乙》卷七第三作“大道”〕已通，血脉乃行，然后视其病，脉淖泽者刺而平之，坚紧者，破而散之，气下乃止，此所谓以解结者也。

Now, let me tell you the theory of removing the accumulative evil. Since it is acclimatized to heaven and earth and is in accordance with the four seasons, and man coordinates with heaven and earth, so, it can be used to explain what the removing of the accumulative evil means. For instance, when there are water and wetness below, and there are reeds above, when seeing the prosperous or being withered of the reeds, the large or small size of the water area can be estimated. Thus, when seeing the strong or weak of the body from outside, the plenty or few of one's energy and blood can be estimated. As to the changes of Yin and Yang, it can analogize the cold and heat of the four seasons, when the heat is evaporating above, the roots of the grass and wood will be in lack of moisture, when one's energy of the body is fumigated, his skin will be loose, his striae will be open, he will perspire greatly, his blood and energy will be greatly discharged and become debilitative, and his skin will be moist. In the cold weather, when the earth is frozen and the water is iced up, the Yang energy of man will subside inside, his skin will be dense, his striae will be closed, he will have no perspiration, his blood and energy will be strong and his muscle will be firm and choppy. In a cold weather like this, the one who is good at sailing can not sail a boat on the ice; the one who is good at penetrating the earth can not chisel up the frozen stratum, likewise the one who is good at acupuncture can not prick the four extremities of Jueni, if the channel is condensed due to cold in which the blood is stagnant and fails to flow smoothly, it should not be massaged. Thus, for a sailor, he must wait until the weather is warm and the ice is thawed, then can he start the sailing; for the one penetrating the earth, it must wait until the ground has thawed out, then can he chisel the earth. The condition of the channel in human body is similar, when treating the Jueni, it must apply the topical application of heated drugs to adjust the channels first, apply the therapy to the two palms, two armpits, two elbows, the two feet and the joints of the neck, back and spine, when the warm energy has come, the channel will resume its operation; then , one should inspect the condition of the disease, if the pulse is slippery excessively, it shows the Wei energy is floating, prick to cause it to become normal; if the pulse is firm and tight, it shows the evil energy is sthenic, prick to disperse the stagnation, but cease the pricking when the energy of jueni has descended. This is the so called therapy of removing the accumulative evil.

用针之类，在于调气，气积于胃，以通营卫，各行其道。宗气留于海，其下者注于气街，其上者走于息道。故厥在于足，宗气不下，脉中之血，凝而留止，弗之火调，弗能取之。

In the law of pricking, it is mainly the adjusting of the energy. The refined energy of water and cereals accumulated in the stomach can communicate the Ying-energy and the Wei-energy and cause them to circulate over the whole body respectively. The initial energy retains in the sea of energy in the chest, when it descends, it pours into the Qijie point; when it ascends, it goes to the respiratory tract. When one has cold limbs, it is due to the initial energy fails to descend along the channel and the blood in the channel to retain by stagnating, if the topical application of heated drugs in not applied in advance, it is not proper to carry on the pricking.

用针者，必先察其经络之实虚，切而循之，按而弹之，视其应〔应：《太素》卷二十二《五邪刺》作"变"〕动者，乃后取之〔之：此字是衍文〕而下之。六经调者，谓之不病，虽病，谓之自已也。一经上实下虚而不通者，此必有横络盛加于大经，令之不通，视而泻之，此所谓解结也。

When treating with acupuncture, one must inspect the asthenia and sthenia of the channels and the collaterals carefully, palpate the pulse and trace the evil, press and knead the skin and flick the acupoint and inspect the changes first, then, prick the proper acupoints to remove the disease. If the six hand and foot channels are harmonious, it shows there is no disease, even if there is a slight disease, it can be recovered by itself. If a certain channel is impeded with the situation of sthenic in the upper part and asthenic in the lower, the collaterals which are horizontal must have been invaded by the evil, and the evil has transmitted to the channels which is vertical to cause obstruction. When one can perceive the condition and purge, it is the so called applying the therapy of removing the accumulative evil.

上寒下热，先刺其项太阳，久留之，已刺〔刺：《太素》卷二十二《五邪刺》无此字〕则〔则：《甲乙》卷七第三"则"下有"火"字〕熨项与肩胛，令热下合乃止，此所谓推而上之者也。

When one is cold above the loins and hot below the loins, it should prick the acupoints of the Foot Taiyang Channel on the neck, and retain the needle longer, after pricking, apply topical application of heated drugs on the neck and the scapula, cease the pricking when the heat descends to combine with the heat below. This is the so called the therapy of pushing up the heat.

上热下寒，视其虚脉而陷之于经络者取之，气下乃止，此所谓引而下之者也。

When one is hot above the loins and cold below the loins, inspect which deficient pulse is bogging in the channel and collateral, treat by pricking the proper acupoint and cease the pricking after the Yang energy has arrived. This is the so called the pricking therapy of inducing the heat to descend.

大热遍身，狂而妄见、妄闻、妄言、视足阳明及大络取之，虚者补之，血而〔而：《甲乙》卷七第三作“如”〕实者泻之，因其〔其：《太素》卷二十二《五邪刺》作“令”〕偃卧，居其头前，以两手四指挟按颈动脉，久持之，卷而切推，下至缺盆中，而复止〔止：《太素》卷二十二《五邪刺》作“上”〕如前，热去乃止，此所谓推而散之者也。

When one has high fever all over the body, becomes maniac to see and hear things which are not really existing, and he speaks nonsense, prick the proper acupoint after inspecting the Foot Yangming Channel of Stomach and its collaterals, if the channel and collaterals are asthenic, apply the invigorating therapy, if there is the stagnated blood and the syndrome is of sthenic, apply purging therapy. Besides, cause the patient to lie on his back, the physician situates in front of the patient's head, clip and press the patient's Renying pulse on his neck with the two thumbs for a longer time, then, press up and down by bending the fingers, push to cause the heat to reach the supraclavicular fossa, continue the up and down pressing until the heat is removed. This is the so called the therapy of disperse by pushing."

黄帝曰：有一脉生数十病者，或痛、或痈、或热、或寒、或痒、或痹、或不仁，变化无穷，其故何也？岐伯曰：此皆邪气之所生也。黄帝曰：余闻气者，有真气，有正气，有邪气，何谓真气？岐伯曰：真气者，所受于天，与谷气并而充身也。正气者，正风也，从一方来，非实风，又〔非实风，又：《甲乙》卷十第一下无此四字〕非虚风也。邪气者〔邪气者：《甲乙》卷十第一下“邪气者”下有“虚风也”三字〕，虚风之贼伤人也，其中人也深，不能自去。正风者，其中人也浅，合而自去，其气来〔来：《甲乙》卷十第一下《灵枢略》并无此字〕柔弱，不能胜〔胜：《甲乙》卷十第一作“伤”〕真气，故自去。

Yellow Emperor said: "There may be diseases of ten kinds occur in a channel, it can be pain, carbuncle, heat, cold, itching, bi-syndrome or numbness, and the various changes are endless, what is the reason?" Qibo said: "They are all produced from the evil energy." Yellow Emperor said: "I am told that the energies are different. What is the true energy? What is the health energy? What is the evil energy?" Qibo said: "The true energy is the congenital energy man received from heaven, it combines with the energy of water and cereals from the food to nourish the whole body; the health energy which is also called the normal wind is the wind stem from one side in accordance with the weather-change of the four-season which is different from the asthenia-wind against the four-season; the evil energy which is also called the asthenia-wind, it can hurt the body so deeply that it can not dissipate by itself, the normal wind can only hurt the body slightly, and it can be dissipated all by itself. this is because the energy of the normal wind is weak, it can not injure the health energy of the body, so, it can be dissipated all by itself.

虚邪之中人也，洒淅动形，起毫毛而发腠理。其入深，内搏于骨，则为骨痹。搏于筋，则为筋挛。搏于脉中，则为血闭不通，则为痈。搏于肉，与卫气相搏，阳胜者则为热，阴胜者则为寒，寒则真气去，去则虚，虚则寒。搏于皮肤之间〔之间：《甲乙》卷十第一下无此二字〕，其气外发，腠理开，毫毛摇，气往来行，则为痒。留而不去则痹。卫气不行，则为不仁。

When the debilitating evil attack the body, the shivering with cold, standing up of the fine hairs, opening of the striae will appear outside. If the evil penetrates to injure the bone inside, the bone bi-syndrome will occur; when the evil injures the tendon, constriction of the tendon will occur; when the evil injures the channel, the arthralgia due to blood disorder will occur, as the blood circulation is obstructed, it will develope tinto carbuncle; when the evil injures the muscle, it will combine with the Wei-energy, if the Yang-evil is partial overabundant, the heat-syndrome will occur; if the Yin-evil is partial overabundant, the cold syndrome will occur. The cold-evil can force the health energy to depart and cause the Yang-deficiency, when the Yang energy is deficient, the cold energy of Yin will hurt the skin, it will cause the opening of the striae and the fall of the fine hair. When the evil energy comes and goes, it will cause itching, when the evil energy is retaining, it will cause the bi-syndrome, when the Wei-energy fails to flow fluently, it will cause the disease of numbness.

虚邪偏客于身半，其入深，内居〔居：《灵枢略》作“干”〕荣卫，荣卫稍衰，则真气去，邪气独留，发为偏枯。其邪气浅者，脉〔脉：“脉”似应为“为”之误字〕偏痛。

When the debilitating evil hits one side of the body, the evil-energy penetrates inside to invade the Rong-energy and the Wei-energy causing their functions to decline, the health energy will depart and the evil-energy will retain in the body solely, the syndrome of hemiplegia will occur, if the attack of the evil-energy is only slightly, one will have partial pain in the body.

虚〔虚：《甲乙》卷十一九下无此字〕邪之入于身也深，寒与热相搏，久留而内著，寒胜其热，则骨疼肉枯，热胜其寒，则烂肉腐肌为脓，内伤骨，内伤骨为骨蚀。有所疾前筋〔有所疾前筋：楼英曰“疾前”二字衍文，筋当作“结”〕，筋屈不得伸，邪气居其间而不反，发于〔于：周本，张注本并作“为”〕筋溜〔溜：《甲乙》卷十一第九下作“瘤”〕。有所结，气归之，卫气留之，不得反，津液久留，合而为肠溜〔肠溜：“溜”应作“瘤”〕，久者数岁乃成，以手按之柔。已有所结，气归之，津液留之，邪气中之，凝结日以易〔易：按：“易”是“益”之误字〕甚，连以聚居，为昔瘤，以手按之坚。有所结，深中骨，气因于骨，骨与气并，日以益大，则为骨疽〔骨疽：“骨疽”应作“胃瘤”〕。有所结，中于肉，宗气归之，邪留而不去，有热则化而为脓，无热则为肉疽，凡此数气者，其发无常处，而有常名也。

When the debilitating evil penetrates into the body, the cold energy will combat with heat, when the cold-evil retains and resides protractedly, if the cold overcomes the heat, the syndromes of pain in the bone and the withering up of the muscle will occur; if the heat overcomes the cold, it will cause the rotten and suppuration of the muscle, When it penetrates to hit the bone, it will cause corrosion of the bone. When the accumulative evil-energy hits the tendon, the tendon will fail to stretch. When the accumulative evil energy retains protractedly without retreating, the tendinous tumor will occur. If the evil energy is stagnated to obstruct the energy causing the Wei-energy also to become stagnated and fails to circulate normally, the body fluid will retain in the stomach and the intestine for a long time, the intestinal tumor will occur, sometimes, the disease takes a longer time to shape up, it may take several years to take form, and it is soft when being pressed by hand. When the evil energy stagnates inside, the body fluid retains, and the evil energy is attacking the body, the blood and energy will become stagnated day after day, the continued accumulation will cause the fleshy tumor to become is hard when being pressed by hand. When the accumulative evil penetrates into the skeleton, as the bone has injured, the combination of bone -injury and the evil energy will become larger and larger day after day, and finally, the osteoma will occur. When the accumulative evil energy hits the muscle and stagnates there, if the evil energy retains and there is heat inside, the myoma will occur. The several kinds of evil energy stated above have no definite location in the out set, but they are all having the certain name of the disease."

卫气行第七十六

Chapter 76
Wei Qi Xing
(Then Circulation of Wei-energy)

黄帝问于岐伯曰：愿闻卫气之行，出入之合，何如？岐伯曰：岁有十二月，日有十二辰，子午为经，卯酉为纬。天周〔天周：《甲乙》卷一第九作“周天”〕二十八宿，而一面七星，四七二十八星，房昴为纬，虚张为经。是故房至毕为阳，昴至心为阴，阳主昼，阴主夜。故卫气之行，一日一夜五十周于身，昼日行于阳二十五周，夜行于阴二十五周，周于五脏。

Yellow Emperor asked Qibo and sad: " I hope to know the circulation of the Wei-energy and its coming in and going out in the Yin and Yang channels. What are their conditions?" Qibo said: " There are twelve months in a year and there are twelve double-hour in a day. The Zi and Wu are in the south and north respectevely, their connecting line is the vertical longtitude; the Mao and You is in the east and the west respectively, their connecting line is the horizontal latitude. Then celetial bodies go in circulation among the twenty eight stars, and in each orientation, there are seven stars, in the four orientations, there are altogether twenty eight stars. From the Fang star in the east to the Mao star in the west is the latitude, from the Xu star in the north to the Zhang star in the south is the longtitude. Thus, from the Fang star to the Bi star is Yang, from the Mao star to the Xin star is Yin, the Yang dominates the day and the Yin dominates the night, so, the circulations of the Wei-energy in the body are fifty cycles in a day and night. In day time, it circulates in the Yang for twenty five cycles, and in night time, it circulates among the internal organs for twenty five cycles.

是故平旦阴〔阴：《太素》卷十二《卫五十周》“阴”下并有“气”字〕尽，阳气出于目，目张则气上行于头，循项下足太阳，循背下至小指之端。其散者，别于目锐眦，下手太阳，下至手小指之间外侧。其散者，别于目锐眦，下足少阳，注小指次指之间。以上循手少阳之分，侧下至小指之间。别者以上至耳前，合于颔脉，注足阳明，以下行至跗上，入五指之间。其散者，从耳下下手阳明，入大指〔《灵枢约注》卷上《经络第二》“大指”当作“次指”〕之间。入掌中。其至于足也，入足心，出内踝下，行阴分，复合于目，故为一周。

So, by the time of the dawn when the Yin energy is exhausted, the Yang energy will be floating out from the eyes, when the eyes are open, the energy will ascend to the head, then, descends along the neck to reach the Foot Taiyang channel, then descends along the back to reach the Zhiyin point on the tip of the small toe. Its branch branches out from the outer canthus, descends along the Hand Taiyang Channel to reach the Shaoze point on the tip of the outer flank of the small finger. Another branch branches out from the outer canthus, descends along the Foot Shaoyin Channel to reach the Qiaoyin point between the small toe and the fourth toe. From the Foot Shaoyang Channel, it enters into the Hand Shaoyang Channel to reach the Guanzhong point on the tip of the small finger. Another branch ascends to reach the front of the ear, assembles in the mandible pulse, then, pours into the Foot Yangming Channel, descends to the dorsum of foot and reaches the tip of the middle toe. Another branch descends along the Hand Yangming Channel below the ear to reach the Shangyang point on the tip of the fore finger, then its energy enters into the palm. When the Wei-energy reaches the foot, it enters into the centre of the sole, comes out from the inner ankle, ascends to the Yin portion, then, it ascends to converge with other branch on the inner canthus of the eye. This is the circulative cycle of the Wei-energy.

是故日行一舍，人气行〔人气行：《甲乙》卷一第九“行”下并有“于身”二字〕一周与十分身之八；日行二舍，人气行三周于身〔三周于身：《甲乙》卷一第九作“于身三周”〕与十分身之六；日行三舍，人气行于身五周与十分身之四；日行四舍，人气行于身七周与十分身之二；日行五舍，人气行于身九周；日行六舍，人气行于身十周与十分身之八；日行七舍，人气行于身十二周在身与十分身之六；日行十四舍，人气二十五周于身有奇分与十分身之二，阳尽于阴，阴受气矣。其始入于阴，常从足少阴注于肾，肾注于心，心注于肺，肺注于肝，肝注于脾，脾复注于肾为周。是故夜行一舍，人气行于阴脏一周与十分脏之八，亦如阳行之二十五周，而复合于目。阴阳一日一夜，合有奇分十分身之四〔四：黄校本作“二”〕，与十分藏之二，是故人之所以卧起之时有早晏者，奇分不尽故也。

Thus, when the sun travels the distance of one star (From a star to the next star), the Wei-energy will circulate 1 8/10 cycle in the body, when the sun travels the distance of two stars, the Wei-energy will circulate 3 6/10 cycles in the body, when the sun travels the distance of three stars the Wei-energy will circulate 5 4/10 cycles in the body, when the sun travels the distance of four stars, the Wei-energy will circulate 7 2/10 cycles in the body, when the sun travels the distance of five stars, the Wei-energy will circulate 9 cycles in the body, when the sun travels the distance of six stars, the Wei-energy will circulate 10 8/10 cycles in the body, when the sun travels the distance of seven stars, the Wei-energy will circulate 12 6/10 cycles in the body, when the sun travels the distance of fourteen stars, the Wei-energy will circulate 25 2/10 cycles in the body, when the Wei-energy finishes its course of Yang portion in day time, the Yin portion in night time will undertake the energy. When the Wei-energy begins to pour into the Yin portion, commonly it starts from the Foot Shaoyin Channel and pours into the kidney, then, it pours from the kidney to the heart, then it pours from the heat to the lung, then, it pours from the lung to the liver, then, it pours from the liver to the spleen, and then, it pours from the spleen to the kidney again to become one cycle. So, when the sun travels the distance of one star in night time, the Wei-energy circulates 1 8/10 cycles in the Yin viscera of the body, it circulates twenty five cycles in the Yin portion like that in the day time, and finally, they combine on the inner canthus of the eye. In the Yin portion and the Yang portion circulations in a day and night there are the remainder of 2/10 in the body and 2/10 in the Yin viscera. As the early or late of going to sleep and getting up of men are different, so, there are the remainder in calculation."

黄帝曰：卫气之在于身也，上下往来不以〔不以：《甲乙》卷一第九作“无已”〕期〔期：《甲乙》卷一第九作“其”，属下读〕，候气而刺之奈何？伯高曰：分有多少，日〔日：应作“至”〕有长短，春秋冬夏，各有分理，然后常以平旦为纪，以夜尽为始。是故一日一夜，水下百刻，二十五刻者，半日之度也，常如是毋已，日入而止，随日之长短，各以为纪而刺之。谨候其时，病可与期，失时反候者，百病不治〔治：《甲乙》卷一第九作“除”〕。故曰：刺实者，刺其来也；刺虚者，刺其去也。此言气存亡之时，以候虚实而刺之。是故谨候气之所在而刺之，是谓逢时。在〔在：“在”上脱“病”字。应据《太素》补〕于三阳，必候其气在于阳〔阳：《太素》卷十二《卫五邪刺》“阳”下并有“分”字〕而刺之；病在于三阴，必候其气在阴分而刺之。

Yellow Emperor said: “When the Wei-energy is in the human body, it operates unceasingly to go up and down in coming and going, when one wants to wait for the coming of normal sensation during acupuncture treating, what should one do?” Bogao said: “The lengths of the days at Spring Equinox and at Autumn Equinox are different, the lengths of the day at Summer Solstice and at Winter Solstice are also different and the lengths of the day and night in spring, summer, autumn and winter are all having their regular patterns, so, it should take the dawn as the criterion, and take the end of the night as the beginning of the Wei-energy to circulate in the Yang portion. In a day and night, the leaking of water in the clepsydra is one hundred graduations, and twenty five graduations are the number of half the day. It continues to circulatte unceasingly, when the sun sets, it is considered to be the end of the day time. When treating, one must prick according to the various criterions of the length of time from sun-rise to sun-set. If one can wait carefuily the opportunity of the arriving time of the energy and prick, he will be able to predict the date of the disease's recovery; if one misses the opportunity of pricking, or he violates the to weather change of the season, the disease can hardly be removed. Thus, when treating the sthenia-evil, it should purge by pricking the coming energy (sthenic energy); when treating the disease of the deficiency of vital energy, it should invigorate by pricking the leaving energy (asthenic energy). That is to say, when the energy is prosperous or debilitative, prick after inspecting the asthenia and the sthenia. Thus, one must wait for the energy, inspect the location of the energy and prick in time, which is called the meeting of the proper time. When the disease is in the three Yang channels, one must wait until the energy is in the Yang portion, then, start the pricking; when the disease is in the three Yin channels, one must wait until the energy is in the Yin portion, then, start the pricking.

水下一〔一：《太素》卷十二《卫五十周》无此字〕刻，人气在太阳；水下二刻，人气在少阳；水下三刻，人气在阳明；水下四刻，人气在阴分。水下五刻，人气在太阳；水下六刻，人气在少阳；水下七刻，人气在阳明；水下八刻，人气在阴分。水下九刻，人气在太阳；水下十刻，人气在少阳；水下十一刻，人气在阳明；水下十二刻，人气在阴分。水下十三刻，人气在太阳；水下十四刻，人气在少阳；水下十五刻，人气在阳明；水下十六刻，人气在阴分。水下十七刻，人气在太阳；水下十八刻，人气在少阳；水下十九刻，人气在阳明；水下二十刻，人气在阴分。水下二十一刻，人气在太阳；水下二十二刻，人气在少阳；水下二十三刻，人气在阳明；水下二十四刻，人气在阴分。水下二十五刻，人气在太阳，此半日之度也。从房至毕一十四舍，水下五十刻，日行半度〔日行半度：《甲乙》卷一第九作“半日之度也”。此下并有“以昴至心，亦十四舍，水下五十刻，终日之度也“十八字〕，回〔回：作“日”〕行一舍，水下三刻与七分刻之四。大要曰常以日之加于宿上也，人气在太阳。是故日行一舍，人气行三阳行与阴分，常如是无已，天与〔天与：当注本作“与天”〕地同纪，纷纷盼盼，终而复始，一日一夜，水下百刻而尽矣。

When the water level is on the first graduation of the clepsydra, the Wei-energy is in the Hand and Foot Taiyang Channels; when it is on the second graduation, the Wei-energy is in the Hand and Foot Shaoyang Channels; when it is on the third graduation, the Wei-energy is in the Hand and Foot Yangming Channels; when it is on the fourth graduation, the Wei-energy is in the Yin portion. When the water level is on the fifth graduation of the clepsydra, the Wei-energy comes out to the Yang portion to pour into the Hand and Foot Taiyang Channels, when it is on the sixth graduation, the Wei-energy is in the Hand and Foot Shaoyang channels; when it is on the seventh graduation, the Wei-energy is in the Hand and Foot Yangming Channels; when it in on the eighth graduation, the Wei-energy is in the Yin portion. When the water level of the clepsydra is on the ninth graduation, the Wei-energy is in the Hand and Foot Taiyang Channels; when it is on the tenth graduation, the Wei-energy is in the Hand and Foot Shaoyang Channels; when it is on the eleventh graduation, the Wei-energy is in the Hand and Foot Yangming Channels; when it is on the twelfth graduation, the Wei-energy is in the Yin portion. When the water level is on the thirteenth graduation of the clepsydra, the Wei-energy is in the Hand and Foot Taiyang Channels; when it is on the fourteenth graduation, the Wei-energy is in the Hand and Foot Shaoyang Channels; when it in on the fifteenth graduation, the Wei-energy is in the Hand and Foot Yangming Channels; when it is on the sixteenth graduation, the Wei-energy is in the Yin portion. When the water level is on the seventeenth graduation of the clepsydra, the Wei-energy is in the Hand and Foot Taiyang Channels; when it is on the eighteenth graduation, the Wei-energy is in the Hand and Foot Shaoyang Channels; when it is on the nineteenth graduation, the Wei-energy is in the Hand and Foot Yangming Channels; when it is on the twentieth graduation, the Wei-energy is in the Yin portion. When the water level is on the twenty first graduation of the clepsydra, the Wei-energy is in the Hand and Foot Taiyang Channels; when it is on the twenty second graduation, the Wei-energy is in the Hand and Foot Shaoyang Channels; when it is on the twenty third graduation, the Wei-energy is in the Hand and Foot Yangming Channels; when it is on the twenty fourth graduation, the Wei-energy is in the Yin portion. When the water level of the clepsydra is on twenty fifth graduation, the Wei-energy is in the Hand and Foot Taiyang Channels again. These are the graduations for the Wei-energy to circulate in half a day. If a whole day is calculated, the sun travels from the Fang star to the Bi star are fourteen stars, it is about fifty graduations under the water level in the clepsydra, and it is the graduation for the sun to travel in half a day; the sun travels from the Mao star to the Xin star are fourteen stars, and it is also fifty guaduations of the water level in the clepsydra, when they are combined, it is the time period for the sun to travel the entire cycle in a day and night. Whenever the sun travels from a star to the next star, it takes 3 4/7 graduations. It was stated in《Essentials》of the ancient classics: ' When the sun travels the course of one star, the Wei-energy will circulate in the Hand and Foot Taiyang Channels'. Thus, when the sun travels the distance of a star, the Wei-energy will travel through the three Yang channels and the Yin portions. The Wei-energy operates unceasingly in accordance with the law of the change of heaven and earth, it seems confusing but it is orderly, it starts again from the terminal. In a day and night when the graduations of the clepsydra is one hundred, the Wei-energy will complete its circulation of fifty cycles in the human body."

九宫八风第七十七

Chapter 77
Jiu Gong Ba Feng
(The Nine Palaces and the Eight Winds)

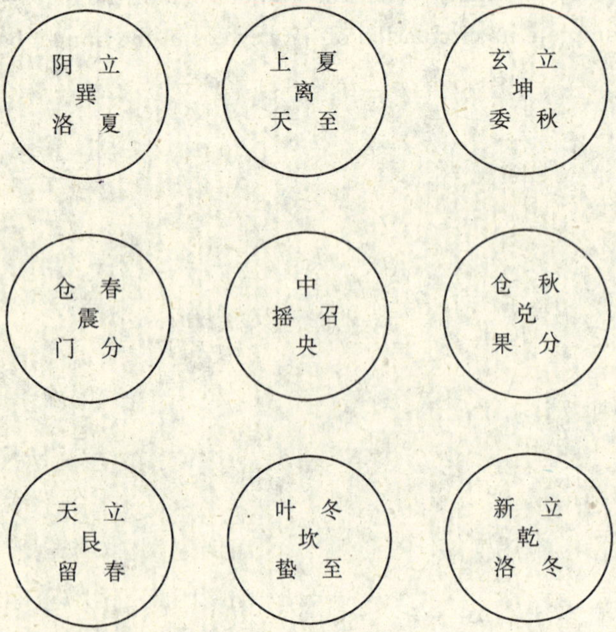

立夏	四	阴洛 东南方	夏至	九	上天 南方	立秋	二	玄委 西南方
春分	三	仓门 东方	招摇	五	中央	秋分	七	仓果 西方
立春	八	天留 东北方	冬至	一	叶蛰 北方	立冬	六	新洛 西北方

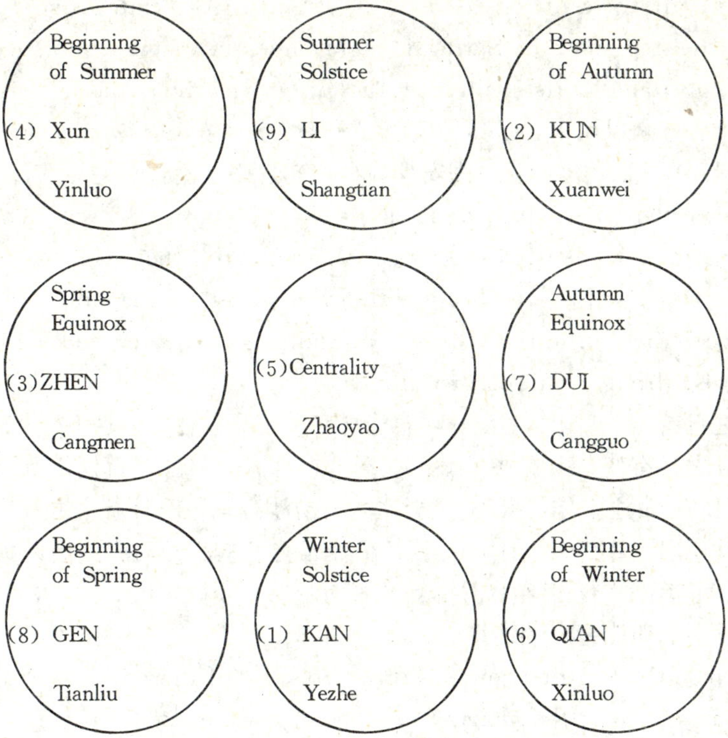

太一常以冬至之日，居叶蛰之宫四十六日，明日居天留四十六日，明日居仓门四十六日，明日居阴洛四十五日，明日居天宫四十六日，明日居玄委四十六日，明日居仓果四十六日，明日居新洛四十五日，明日复居叶蛰之宫，曰冬至矣。

On the day of Winter Solstice, the Polaris usually situates in the Yezhe Palace which is in the right north for forty six days; the next day after the period, it transfers and situates in the Tianliu Palace which is in the northeast for forty six days; the next day after the period, it transfers to the Cangmen palace which is in the right east for forty six days; the next day after the period, it transfers to the Yinluo Palace which is in the southeast for forty five days; on the next day of the period, it transfers to the Shangtian Palace which is in the right south for forty six days; the next day after the period, it transfers to the Xuanwei Palace which is in the southwest for forty six days; the next day after the period, it transfers to the Cang-guo Palace which is in the right west for forty six days; the next day after the period, it transfers to the Xinluo Palace which is in the northwest for forty five days; the next day after the period, it returns to the Yezhe Palace, and it is Winter Solstice again.

太一日游，以冬至之日，居叶蛰之宫，数所在，日从〔从：《图经》卷三《针灸避忌太一之图序》作“徙”〕一处，至九日，复反于一，常如是无已，终而复始。

In the locations where the Polaris situates in the various day; the Polaris begins to situate in the Yezhe Palace which is the Kan position of one in Solstice Winter, it moves to a new palace every day, and on the ninth day, it returns again to the kan position of one (the Winter Solstice is one, the Beginning of Autumn is two, the Spring Equinox is three, the Beginning of Summer is four, the centrality is five, the Beginning of Winter is six, the Autumn Equinox is seven, the Beginning of Spring is eight, and the Summer Solstice is nine). It moves on unceasingly, and starts again from the terminal without end.

太一移日，天必应之以风雨，以其日风雨则吉，岁美〔岁美：《太素》卷二十八《九宫八风》"美"作"矣"、"岁矣"属上读〕民安少病矣，先之则多雨，后之则多汗。

In the day when the Polaris passing from a palace to another palace, there must be the wind and rain appearing. If the wind and rain are harmonious, there will be a good harvest in the year, and the people will live healthily with few diseases. If the wind and rain occur in a few days in advance, the rain in the year will be abundnant; if the wind and rain occur in a few days afterwards, drought will occur in the year.

太一在冬至之日有变，占在君；太一在春分之日有变，占有相；太一在中宫之日有变，占在吏；太一在秋分之日有变，占在将；太一在夏至之日有变，占在百姓。所谓有变者，太一居五宫之日，病〔病：张注本作"疾"〕风折树木，扬沙石。各以其所主占贵贱，因视风所从来而占之。风从其所居之乡来为实风，主生，长养万物。从其冲后来为虚风，伤人者也，主杀主害者〔主杀主害者：《甲乙》卷六第一作"主杀者"〕。谨候虚风而避之，故圣人日避虚邪之道，如避矢石然，邪弗能害，此之谓也。

On the day when the Polaris is in the Winter Solstice, if there is the change of weather, the forecast will come true to the monarch; on the day when the Polaris is in the Spring Equinox, if there is the change of weather, the forecast will come true to the prime minister; on the day when the Polaris is in the Zhao Yao Palace of the centrality (the eighteenth day of every season), if there is the change of weather, the forecast will come true to the officials; on the day when the Polaris is in the Autumnal Equinox, if there is the change of weather, the forecast will come true to the generals; on the day when the Polaris is in the Summer Solstice, if there is the change of weather, the forecast will come true to the common people. The so-called the change of weather is indicating the occurrence of the breaking of the woods and the raising of sands and stones by the tempest on the day when the Polaris situates respectively in the five-palace stated above. One can divine according to the orientation of the Polaris dominating to know the nobility and the humbleness of the patient, and ascertain the consequence of the disease according to the direction of the coming of the wind. When the wind comes from the dominating orientation, it is the sthenia-wind which can nourish all things and it associates with growth. When the wind comes from the opposite dominating direction , it is the asthenia-wind, it can injure people and it associates with killing. One should calculate carefully the occurrence of the asthenia wind and avoid it. It was stated by the sages that one should avoid the asthenia-wind like avoiding the arrows and the hitting stones. In this way, one will not be hurt by the invasion of the exogenious evil.

是故太一入〔入：当注本，张注本并无此字〕徙立于中宫，乃朝八风，以占吉凶也。风从南方来，名曰大弱风，其伤人也，内舍于心，外在于脉，气主热。风从西南方来，名曰谋风，其伤人也，内舍于脾，外在于肌，其气主为弱。风从西方来，名曰刚风，其伤人也，内舍于肺，外在于皮肤，其气主为燥。风从西北方来，名曰折风，其伤人也，内舍于小肠，外在于手太阳脉，脉绝则溢，脉闭则结不通，善暴死。风从北方来，名曰大刚风，其伤人也，内舍于肾，外在于骨与肩背之膂筋〔与肩背之膂筋：《素问・移精变气论》引无“与肩”六字〕，其气主为寒也。风从东北方来，名曰凶风，其伤人也，内舍于大肠，外在于两胁腋骨下及肢节〔外在于两胁胠骨下及肢节：《素问・移精变气论》作“外在于掖胁”〕。风从东方来，名曰婴儿风，其伤人也，内舍于肝，外在于筋纽〔纽：《太素》卷二十八《九宫八风》作纫”〕其气主为身湿。风从东南方来，名曰弱风，其伤人也，内舍于胃，外在肌肉，其气主体重。此八风皆从其虚之乡来，乃能病人。三虚相搏，则为暴病卒死。两实一虚，病则为淋露寒热。犯其雨湿之地，则为痿。故圣人避风。如避矢石焉。其有三虚而偏中于邪风，则为击仆偏枯矣。

Thus, it is only when the Polaris enters into the central palace to face the eight winds, can one calculate the good or evil omen of the disease. Such as, when the wind is from the south, it is the Daruo-wind (great weak wind), its injury to a man is to invade the heart inside and retains in the channel outside, its energy can cause the disease of heat. When the wind is from the southwest, it is the Mouwind (Scheming wind), its injury to a man is to invade the spleen inside and retains in the muscle outside, its energy can cause the disease of debility. When the wind is from the west, it is the Gang-wind (firm wind), its injury to a man is to invade the lung inside and retains in the skin outside, its energy can cause the disease of dryness. When the wind is from the northwest, it is the Zhe-wind (folding wind), its injury to man is to invade the small intestine inside and retains in the Hand Taiyang Channel outside, if the pulse is severed, it is the overflowing of the evil energy, if the pulse is blocked up, it is the stagnation due to obstruction, and the patient can die suddenly. When the wind is from the north, it is the Dagang-wind (great firm wind), its injury to man is to invade the kidney inside and retains in the skeleton outside, its energy can cause the disease of cold. When the wind is from the northeast, it is the Xiong-wind (fierce wind), its injury to man is to invade the large intestine inside and retains in the two armpits and the two hypochondria. When the wind is from the east, it is the Ying-er -wind (infant wind), its injury to a man is to invade the liver inside and retains in the joints of the tendons outside, it can cause the disease of wetness. When the wind is from the southeast, it is the Ruo-wind (weak wind), its injury to a man is to invade the stomach inside and retains in the muscle outside, its energy can cause the disease of increasing the body-weight. In summary, the eight kinds of wind from different directions are stemmed from the debilitative regions and they can cause disease. It should be noted that when a debilitative man encounters the asthenia-year, and again, he is invaded by the asthenia-wind, the three asthenia can cause sudden disease, and the patient can die suddenly. If there are two sthenia and one asthenia, the disease will be of the fatigue mixed with cold and heat kind. If one is hit by wetness in the wet and rainy region, he will contract the flaccidity-syndrome. Thus, a wise man avoids the wind evil like avoiding the arrow and the hitting stones. If one has all the three asthenia, and again is hit by the wind-evil, he will fall on the ground and has hemiplegia.

九针论第七十八

Chapter 78
Jiu Zhen Lun
(On the Nine Kinds of Needle)

黄帝曰：余闻九针于夫子，众多博大矣，余犹不能寤，敢问九针焉生？何因而有名？岐伯曰：九针者，天地之大〔大：《甲乙》卷五第二无此字〕数也，始于一而终于九。故曰：一以法天，二以法地，三以法人，四以法时，五以法音，六以法律，七以法星，八以法风，九以法野。

Yellow Emperor said："I am told that the learning of the nine kinds of needles are abundant, profound and extensive, but I don't understand how the nine kinds of needles are produced, and why do they have different names?" Qibo said："The nine in the needle is a number in heaven and earth, it commences in one and terminals in nine. The first kind of needle is following the example of heaven, the second kind of neeale is following the example of earth, the third kind of needle is following the example of man, the fourth kind of needle is following the example of the four seasons, the fifth kind of needle is following the example of the five tones, the six kind of needle is following the example of the six laws of the music, the seventh kind of needle is following the example of the seven stars, the eighth kind of needle is following the example of the winds from the eight directions, the ninth kind of needle is following the example of the nine divisions of prefecture."

黄帝曰：以针应九之数奈何？岐伯曰：夫圣人之起天地之数也，一而九之，故以立九野，九而九之，九九八十一，以起黄钟数焉，以针应数也。

Yellow Emperor asked："How to analogize the needle with the nine numbers?" Qibo said："The numbers established by the sages are to express the changes of heaven and earth and the Yin and Yang, it takes one to nine as the fundamental numbers, and after this, the nine prefectures are established. Nine times nine is eighty one and the number of Huang Zhong (bell determining the middle note of music) of eighty one fen (8.1 inches) is set up. When one analogizes with the number, there occurs the names of the nine kinds of needle.

一者天也，天者阳也，五脏之应天者肺，肺者五脏六腑之盖也，皮〔皮：《素问·欬论》"皮"下并有"毛"字〕者肺之合也，人之阳也。故为之治〔治：《甲乙》卷五第二"治"下有"鑱"字〕针，必以大其头而锐其末，令无得深入而阳气出。

The first kind of needle is analogizing the heaven and heaven belongs to Yang. In the five solid organs of the human body, the lung corresponds to heaven. The lung is in the highest position, it is the canopy of the five solid organs and the six hollow organs, and the skin and the fine hair which belong to the surface of the body correspond to the lung. In order to treat the disease of the skin and the fine hair, the sagital needle is made, its head is large and its tip is sharp, so that is can not be pricked deeply to excrete the Yang energy.

二者地〔地也:《甲乙》卷五第二“地也”下有“地者土也”四字〕也，人之所以应土者肉也。故为之治〔治:《甲乙》卷五第二“治”下有“员”字〕针，必筩其身而员其末，令无得伤肉分〔肉分:《圣济总录》卷一百九十二“肉”下无“分”字〕，伤则气得竭。

The second kind of needle is analogizing the earth in human body, earth corresponds to the muscle. In order to treat the disease of the muscle, the ovoid-tip needle is made, the body of the needle is straight and its tip is round, so that it can avoid to injure the muscle; if the muscle is hurt, the energy will become debilitative.

三者人也，人之所以成生者血脉也。故为之治〔治:《甲乙》卷五第二“治”下有“鍉”字〕针，必大其身而员其末，令可以按脉勿陷，以至其气，令邪气〔令邪气:《甲乙》卷五第二作“使邪”〕独出。

The third kind of needle is analogizing the man, and the growth of man depends upon the unceasing operation of the channel. In order to treat the disease of the channel, the blunt-tip needle is made, the body of the needle is large and its tip is round so that it can massage the channel and the collateral without bogging down into the muscle, it can induce the health energy to become unimpeded and remove the evil energy from inside individually.

四者时也，时者，四时八风之客于经络之中，为瘤病者也。故为之治针，必筩其身而锋其末，令可以泻热出血，而痼病竭。

The fourth kind of needle is analogizing the four seasons. When one's channel and collateral inside are invaded by the evils from the eight directions of the four seasons, the protracted disease will occur. In order to treat this kind of disease, the ensiform needle is made, the body of the needle is straight and its tip is sharp, which can excrete the heat, let out the blood and purge the chronic disease.

五者音也，音者冬夏之分，分于子午，阴与阳别，寒与热争，两气相搏，合为痈脓〔脓:《甲乙》卷五第二作“肿”〕者也。故为之治〔治:《甲乙》卷五第二“治”下有“铍”字〕针，必令其末如剑锋，可以取大脓。

The fifth kind of needle is analogizing the five tones, the number of five situates in the middle between the numbers of one and nine. Among the nine palaces, one stands for the winter Solstice and Zi, nine stands for the Summer Solstice and Wu, as five is at the centre, it divides the winter and the summer, since the winter and the summer are divided, the Zi and Wu are also divided. It analogizes that there is the difference of Yin and Yang in human body and there is combat between the cold-energy and the heat-energy, when the two energies combine, the disease of carbuncle will occur. In order to treat this kind of disease, the sword-shaped needle is made, its tip resembles the tip of a sword for to pierce the carbuncle and eliminate the pus.

六者律也，律者，调阴阳四时而合十二经脉，虚邪客于经络而为暴痹者也。故为之治〔治:《甲乙》卷五第二“治”下有“员利”二字〕针，必令尖如氂，且员且锐，中身微大，以取暴气。

The sixth kind of needle is analogizing the six laws in music; as the six laws harmonize the high and low notes and the Yin and Yang, it can be used to explain the twelve channels of man. If the Yin and Yang in the human body is not harmonious and the exogenous evil takes chance to invade the channels, the acute bi-syndrome will occur. In order to treat the bi-syndrome of this kind, the horse-tail-shaped needle is made, its tip is round and sharp and is as thin as the hair, but the body of the needle is rather thick, so that it can be used to treat the sudden attack of the bi-syndrome.

七者星也，星者人之七窍，邪之所〔之所：覆刻《太素》卷二十一《九针所象》无此二字〕客于经，而为痛痹，舍于经络者也。故为之治〔治：《甲乙》卷五第二“治”下有“毫”字〕针，令尖如蚊虻喙，静以徐往，微以久留，正气因之，真邪俱往，出针而养者也。

The seventh kind of needle is analogizing the seven stars and the seven stars are like the seven orificies of man. If one's channel is invaded by the exogenous evil to cause the cold-type arthralgia, the evil will retain in the channel. In order to treat this kind of disease, the filiform needle is made, of which the tip of the needle is fine like the proboscis of a mosquito, when treating, insert the needle calmly and slowly and retain the needle for a short time, and it will cause the health energy to become substantial; as the channel energy and the evil energy are both affected by pricking, when the needle is drawn out, press the needle hole for a longer time to avoid the excretion of the energy.

八者风也，风者人之股肱八节也，八正之虚风，八风〔八风：《甲乙》卷五第二无此二字〕伤人，内舍于骨解腰脊节腠理〔理：《甲乙》卷五第二、覆刻《太素》卷二十一并无此字〕之间，为深痹也。故为之治〔治：《甲乙》卷五第二“治”下有“长”字〕针，必长其身〔必长其身：《甲乙》卷五第二作“薄其身”〕，锋其末，可以取深邪远痹。

The eighth kind of needle is analogizing the eight winds, the winds come from the eight different directions are like the eight sections of the arms and the legs in human body. When the debilitative winds from the eight solar terms (the two Equinoxes, the two Solstices and the four Beginnings) injure the body of a man, they penetrate into the seams and the joints between the bones and the spine to become the deep-seated bi-syndrome. In order to treat the disease, the long needle is made, the body of the needle is thin and its tip is sharp so that it can treat the deep-seated evil energy and the protracted bi-syndrome.

九者野也，野者人之节解皮肤之间也，淫邪流溢于身，如风水之状，而溜〔而溜：《甲乙》卷五第二无此字〕不能过于机关大节者也。故为之治〔治：《甲乙》卷五第二“治”下有“大”字〕针，令尖如挺，其锋微员，以取大气之不能过于关节者也。

The ninth kind of needle is analogizing the nine prefectures, the nine prefectures are used to explain the joints and the skins of the whole body. If the evil energy is overabundant to overflow all over the body like the wind and water, it will fail to pass through the joints and become stagnant. In order to treat this kind of disease, the large needle is made, its tip is like the broken bamboo with somewhat round shape, it is for to treat the diseases of the retention of the water energy and the failure of the air to pass the joints."

黄帝曰：针之长短有数乎？岐伯曰：一曰镵针者，取法于巾针〔巾针：《圣济总录》一百九十二并作“布针”〕，去末寸半〔寸半：《甲乙》卷五第二作“半寸”〕，卒锐之，长一寸六分，主热在头身也。二曰圆针，取法于絮针，筩其身而卵其锋，长一寸六分，主治分间气。三曰鍉针，取法于黍粟之锐，长三寸半，主按〔主按：《圣济总录》卷一百九十二作“以接”〕脉取气，令邪出。四曰锋针，取法于絮针，筩其身，锋其末，长一寸六分，主痈热〔痈：《甲乙》卷五第二作“泻”〕出血。五曰铍针，取法于剑锋，广二分半，长四寸，主大痈脓，两热争者也。六曰员利针，取法于氂，针微大其末，反小其身，令可深内也，长一寸六分、主取痈痹者也。七曰毫针，取法于毫毛，长一寸六分，主寒热痛痹在络者也。八曰长针、取法于綦针，长七寸，主取深邪远痹者也。九曰大针，取法于锋针，其锋微员、长四寸，主取大气不出关节者也。针形毕矣，此九针大小长短法也。

Yellow Emperor asked: “Is there any difference in the length of the needles?” Qibo said: “The first kind of needle is called the sagital needle, it is made following the example of the cloth needle (needle for stitching the cloth), it becomes suddenly sharp in the location half inch from the tip, its length is one inch and six fen, and it is mainly for treating the heat-evil in the head and the body. The second kind is called the ovoid-tip needle, it is made following the wadding-needle, the body of the needle is straight and round, its tip is round and sharp like an egg, its length is one inch and six fens and it is mainly for treating the evils between the muscles. The third kind of needle is called the blunt-tip needle, it is made following the example of the glutinous millet which is round and some what sharp, its length is three and half inches and it is mainly for pricking the energy after palpating to excrete the evil. The fourth kind of needle is called the ensiform needle, it is made following the example of the wadding-needle also, the body of the needle is straight and round, its tip is sharp, its length is one inch and six fen and it is mainly for purging the heat and let out the blood. The fifth kind of needle is called the sword shaped needle, it is made following the example of the tip of the sword, it is two and half fen in width, four inches in length, and it is mainly for treating the mass and pus and the combating of the cold and heat. The sixth kind of needle is called the horse-tail-shaped needle, it is made following the example of the yak's hair which is long and stiff, its tip is larger and its body is rather small to enable the needle to penetrate deeply, its length is one inch and six fen, and it is mainly for treating the carbuncle and the bi-syndrome. The seventh kind of needle is called the filiform needle, it is made following the example of the fine hair which is very thin, its length is one inch and six fen and it is mainly for treating the cold and heat, the cold-type arthralgia and the evils in the collaterals. The eighth kind of needle is called the long needle, it is made following the example of the long needle, its length is seven inches and it is mainly for treating the deep-seated evil and the protracted bi-syndrome. The ninth kind of needle is called the large needle, it is made following the example of the ensiform needle, the tip of the needle is some what round, its length is four inches and it is mainly for treating the impediment of the air between the joints. The above-mentioned are the shapes, sizes and the length of the nine kinds of needles.”

黄帝曰：愿闻身形应九野〔九野：《千金翼方》卷二十三《疮痈上》作“九宫”〕奈何？岐伯曰：请言身形之应九野也，左足应立春，其日戊寅己丑。左胁应春分，其日乙卯。左手应立夏，其日戊辰己巳。膺喉首头应夏至，其日丙午。右手应立秋，其日戊申己未。右胁应秋分，其日辛酉。右足应立冬、其日戊戌己亥。腰尻下窍应冬至，其日壬子。六府膈下三藏应中州，其大禁，大禁太一所在之日及诸戊己。凡此九者，善候八正所在之处，所主左右上下身体有痈肿者，欲治之，无以其所直之日溃治之，是谓天忌日也。

Yellow Emperor said: " I hope to hear how the shape of the human body corresponds with the nine palaces in the eight diagrams" Qibo said: " Let me tell you the correspondant condition of the body's shape with the nine palaces. The left foot corresponds with the Beginning of Spring, its duty days are the Wu Yin and the Ji Chou. The left hypochondrium corresponds with the Spring Equinox, its duty day is Yi Mao. The left hand corresponds with the Beginning of Summer, its duty days are the Wu Chen and the Ji Si. The throat and head correspond with the Summer Solstice, its duty day is the Bing Wu. The right hand corresponds with the Beginning of Autumn, its duty days are the Wu Shen and the Ji Wei. The right hypochondrium corresponds with the Autumn Equinox, its duty day is the Xin Chou. The right foot corresponds with the Beginning of winter, its duty days are the Wu Xu and the Ji Hai. The loins, buttock, external genitalis and the anus correspond with the Winter Solstice, its duty day is the Ren Zi. The six hollow organs and the liver, spleen , kidney, which are under the diaphragm correspond with the central palace, the contraindicative prickings are on the days when the Polaris situates and the various days of Wu Ji. From the nine palaces stated above, one can determine the situation of the Polaris and the upper and lower, left and right correspondant parts of the body. To the patient with carbuncle, it must not prick on the duty days, as they are the great contraindication-days.

形乐志苦，病生于脉，治之以灸刺。形苦志乐，病生于筋，治之以熨引，形乐志乐，病生于肉，治之以针石。形苦志苦，病生于咽喝，治之以甘药。形数惊恐，筋脉不通，病生于不仁，治之以按摩醪药。是谓形。

When one is comfortable in the body but is suffering in the spirit, his disease is in the channel, when treating, it should apply the acupuncture. When one is toilsome in the body but is joyful in the spirit, if he has disease, the disease is in the tendon, when treating, it should use the topical application of heated drugs. When one is comfortable in the body and is joyful in the spirit, if he has disease, the disease is in the muscle, when treating, apply the acupuncture and the stone needle. When one is toilsome in the body and is gloomy in the spirit, if he has disease, the disease is in the throat, it should be recuperated with the medicine of sweet taste. When one is frightened repeatedly and his channel and collateral are impeded, if he has disease, it is the numbness of the extremities, when treating, massage and medical wine should be applied. These are the so-called the diseases in the body and spirit.

五藏气〔五藏气：《素问·宣明五气》作“五气所病”〕：心主噫，肺主咳，肝主语，脾主吞，肾主欠。六府气：胆为怒，胃为气逆哕，大肠小肠为泄，膀胱不约为遗溺，下焦溢为水。

"When the energy of the five viscera is maladjusted, different syndromes will occur. In heart, it is mainly the eructation; in lung, it is mainly the cough; in liver, it is mainly the polylogia; in spleen, it is mainly the swallowing; in kidney, it is mainly the yawning; when the energies of the six hollow organs are maladjusted, one will apt to get angry due to the disorder of gallbladder; apt to hiccup due to the disorder of stomach; apt to have diarrhea due to the disorder of the large intestine and the small intestine; when one's bladder is out of control, he will apt to have enuresis; when one's lower warmer is overflowing, he will apt to have edema.

五味〔五味:《素问·宣明五气》"五味"下并有"所入"二字〕:酸入肝,辛入肺,苦入心,甘入脾,咸入肾,淡入胃〔《类说》卷三十七引并无"淡入胃"三字〕,是谓五味。

"When the five tastes of food enter into the stomach, each of them enters into the viscus it prefers. The sour taste enters into the liver first; the acrid taste enters into the lung first; the bitter taste enters into the heart first; the salty taste enters into the kidney first; the sweet taste enters into the spleen first. These are the conditions of the five tastes entering into the viscera respectively.

五并:精气并肝则忧,并心则喜,并肺则悲,并肾则恐,并脾则畏,是谓五精之气并于脏也。

"When the refined energy stored in the kidney produces by the five viscera merges into a viscus, disease will occur. When the refined energy merges into the liver, one will be melancholy; when the refined energy merges into the heart, one will be joyful and becoming laughing; when the refined energy merges into the lung, one will be sorrowful; when the refined energy merges into the kidney, one will be terrified; when the refined energy merges into the spleen, one will apt to get hungry. These are the various syndromes caused by the merging of the refined energy into the five viscera when being debilitative.

五恶:肝恶风,心恶热,肺恶寒,肾恶燥,脾恶湿,此五藏气所恶也。

"The liver detests the wind, the heart detests the heat, the lung detests the cold, the kidney detests the dryness, the spleen detests the wetness. These are the five detestations of the viscera to the various energies.

五液:心主汗,肝主泣,肺主涕,肾主唾,脾主涎,此五液所出也。

"For the five viscera, each of them produces a certain kind of liquid respectively. The heart produces the liquid of sweat; the liver produces the liquid of tear; the lung produces the liquid of the nasal discharge; the kidney produces the liquid of the sputum; the spleen produces the liquid of saliva. These are the conditions of the five liquid productions in various viscera.

五劳〔五劳:《素问·宣明五气》作"五劳所伤"〕:久视伤血,久卧伤气,久坐伤肉,久立伤骨,久行伤筋,此五久劳所病也。

"The five kinds of over-fatigue will cause injuries to different parts of the body. The protracted seeing will injure the blood, the protracted lying will injure the energy, the protracted sitting will injure the muscle, the protracted standing will injure the bone, the protracted walking will injure the tendon. These are the diseases caused by the five kinds of over-fatigue.

五走：酸走筋，辛走气，苦走血〔苦走血，咸走骨：《太素》卷二《调食》杨注为“苦走骨，咸走血”〕，咸走骨，甘走肉，是谓五走也。

“When the five tastes enter into the five viscera, each of them moves to a certain part of the body respectively . The sour taste moves to the tendon; the acrid taste moves to the energy; the bitter taste moves to the bone; the salty taste moves to the blood; the sweet taste moves to the muscle. These are the conditions of the moving of the five tastes.

五裁：病在筋，无食酸；病在气，无食辛；病在骨，无食咸；病在血，无食苦；病在肉，无食甘。口嗜而欲食之，不可多也，必自裁也，命曰五裁。

“When one takes the food of the five tastes, it should practise temperance. When one's disease is in the tendon, he must not take a lot of sour taste; when his disease is in the energy, he must not take a lot of acrid taste; when his disease is in the bone, he must not take a lot of salty taste; when his disease is in the blood, he must not take a lot of bitter taste; when his disease is in the muscle, he must not take a lot of sweet taste. When one takes the five tastes, he must not take excessively, he should control the intake himself, and this is the so-called five self-controls.

五发：阴病发于骨，阳病发于血，以味发于气〔以味：《素问·宣明五气》作“阴病发于肉”〕，阳病发于冬，阴病发于夏。

“In the occurrences of the diseases of the five viscera, they occur in different positions and different seasons. The disease of the kidney occurs in the bone marrow; the disease of heart occurs in the channel; the disease of spleen occurs in the muscle; the Yang disease of liver occurs in the winter; the Yin disease of liver occurs in the summer.

五邪〔五邪：《素问·宣明五气》作“五邪所乱”〕：邪入于阳，则为狂；邪入于阴，则为血痹；邪入于阳，转〔转：《太素》卷二十七《邪传》作“搏”〕则为癫〔癫：素问·宣明五气》作“癫”〕疾；邪入于阴，转则为瘖；阳入之于阴，病静；阴出之于阳，病喜怒。

“When the five viscera are invaded by the evil, diseases will occur: when the evil enters into Yang, the patient will become maniac; when the evil enters into Yin, arthralgia due to blood disorder will occur; when the evil enters into Yang, and Yang combats with the evil, the disease of head will occur; when the evil enters into Yin, and Yin combats with the evil, aphonia will occur; when the evil enters into Yin from Yang, the disease will be calm; when the evil comes out from Yin to Yang, the patient will get angry often.

五藏〔五藏《素问·宣明五气》作“五藏所藏”〕：心藏神，肺藏魄，肝藏魂，脾藏意，肾藏精志也。

“Each of the five viscera stores or controls the mental activities respectively. The heart stores the spirit, the lung stores the inferior spirit, the liver stores the mood (soul), the spleen stores the idea, the Kidney stores the essence and will.

五主〔五主：《素问·宣明五气》作“五藏所主”〕：心主脉，肺主皮，肝主筋，脾主肌，肾主骨。

“Each of the five viscera dominates a certain part of the body, the heart dominates the channel, the lung dominates the skin, the liver dominates the aponeurosis, the spleen dominates the muscle and the kidney dominates the bone marrow.

阳明多血多气，太阳多血少气，少阳多气少血，太阴多血少气，厥阴多血少气，少阴多气少血。故曰刺阳明出血气，刺太阳出血恶气，刺少阳出气恶血，刺太阴出血恶气，刺厥阴出血恶气，刺少阴出气恶血也。

"The Hand and Foot Yangming Channels have plenty of blood and plenty of energy, the Hand and Foot Taiyang Channels have plenty of blood and little energy, the Hand and Foot Shaoyang Channels have plenty of energy and little blood, the Hand and Foot Taiyin Channels have plenty of blood and little energy, the Hand and Foot Jueyin Channels have plenty of blood and little energy, the Hand and Foot Shaoyin Channels have plenty of energy and little blood. Therefore, when pricking the Yangming Channels, both the blood and the energy can be excreted; when pricking the Taiyang Channels, the blood can be let out, but the energy must not be excreted; when pricking the Shaoyang Channels, the energy can be excreted, but the blood must not be let out; when pricking the Taiyin Channels, the blood can be let out, but the energy must not be excreted; when pricking the Jueyin Channels, the blood can be let out, but the energy must not be excreted; when pricking the Shaoyin Channels, the energy can be excreted, but the blood must not be let out.

足阳明太阴为表里，少阳厥阴为表里，太阳少阴为表里，是谓足之阴阳也。手阳明太阴为表里，少阳心主为表里，太阳少阴为表里，是谓手之阴阳也。

"The Foot Yangming Channel of Stomach and the Foot Taiyin Channel of Spleen are the superficies and the interior, the Foot Shaoyang Channel of Gallbladder and the Foot Jueyin Channel of Liver are the superficies and interior, the Foot Taiyang Channel of Bladder and the Foot Shaoyin Channel of Kidney are the superficies and interior; these are the superficies and interior relations between the three foot Yin channels and the three foot Yang channels. The Hand Yangming Channel of Large Intestine and the Hand Taiyin Channel of Lung are the superficies and interior, the Hand Shaoyang Channel of Triple Warmer and the Hand Jueyin Channel of Pericardium are the superficies and the interior, the Hand Taiyang Channel of small Intestine and the Hand Shaoyin Channel of Heart are the superficies and interior, these are the superficies and interior relations between the hand three Yin channels and the hand three Yang Channels.

岁露论第七十九

Chapter 79
Sui Lu Lun
(On the Dew of the Year)

黄帝问于岐伯曰：经言夏日伤暑，秋〔秋：《外治》卷五《疗疟方》"秋"下并有"必"字〕病疟，疟之发以时，其故何也？岐伯对曰：邪〔邪：《素问·疟论》"邪"下并有"气"字〕客于风府，病〔病：《素问·疟论》并无此字〕循膂而下，卫气一日一夜，常大会于风府，其明日日下一节，故其日作晏。此其先客于脊背也，故每至于风府则腠理开，腠理开则邪气入，邪气入则病作，此所以日作尚晏也。卫气之行风府，日下一节，二十一日下至尾底〔底：当注本，张注本并作"骶"〕，二十二日入脊内，注于伏冲〔伏冲：《甲乙》卷七第五作"太冲"〕之脉，其行〔其行：《素问·疟论》"其"下并有"气上"二字〕九日，出于缺盆之中，其气上行〔上行：《素问·疟论》并作"日高"〕，故其病稍益至〔至：按"至"字误，《素问》《甲乙》《病源》作"早"〕。其内搏〔搏：《素问·疟论》并作"薄"〕于五藏，横连募原，其道远，其气深，其行迟，不能日作，故次〔次：《病源》卷十一作"间"〕日乃稸积而作焉。

Yellow Emperor asked Qibo and said: "It was stated in the classics: 'When one is injured by the summer-heat in summer, he will contract malaria in autumn, and the time of its onset is definite. What is the reason?" Qibo answered: "When the evil energy invades the Fengfu point, it moves along the spine and descend day by day; as the Wei-energy converges at the Fengfu point after circulating for a day and night, and on the next day, it moves up for one vertebra, the onset of malaria will be one day later day after day which is due to the evil energy has invaded the spine in advance. Whenever the Wei-energy reaches the Fengfu point, the striae there will open, and from there, the evil energy will invade into the body; when the evil energy invades, the disease will attack the body, and this is the reason that the time of the disease's onset is often later. When the Wei-energy leaves the Fengfu point, it moves down a vertebra every day, on the twenty first day, it reaches the coccyx, on the twenty second day, it enters into the spine and pours into the Taichong Channel, then, it ascends along the channel to reach the supraclavicular fossa (the Tiantu point) on the ninth day, the energy moves higher day after day, so, the time of the disease's onset will be ahead of schedual slightly. If the evil-energy draws near to the five viscera to reach the portion between the diaphragm and the pleura, its distance of travelling is rather long, its location of harbouring of the evil energy is rather deep, and the time of the cycling is rather late and it can not attack every day, so, it attacks every other day after the gathering of the evil energy."

黄帝曰：卫气每至于风府，腠理乃发，发则邪入〔发则邪入：《素问·疟论》"邪入"下并有"入则病作"四字〕焉。其卫气日下一节，则不当风府奈何？岐伯曰：风府无常〔风府无常：《素问·疟论》并作“风无常府”〕，卫气之所应〔应：《素问·疟论》并作“发”〕，必开其腠理，气之所舍节〔舍节：《太素卷二十五“舍”下并无“节”字〕，则其府也〔府也：《甲乙》卷七第五作“病作”〕。

Yellow Emperor said: “The stria opens whenever the Wei-energy reaches the Fengfu point, and when the stria opens, the evil-energy will take chance to invade the body and causes disease. Now, the Wei-energy moves down a vertebra every day, if the cycling of the Wei-energy has not reached precisely the Fengfu point, what will be the condition?” Qibo said: “The place where the evil-energy invades is not definite, but the stria will certainly open when the Wei-energy and the evil energy is in combat, when the evil-energy is retained, disease will attack the body.”

黄帝曰：善。夫风之与疟也，相与同类，而风常在，而疟特以时休何也？岐伯曰：风气留其处，疟气随经络沉以内搏，故卫气应乃作也。帝曰：善。

Yellow Emperor said: “Good. The conditions of the wind-evil and the malarial evil are similar, they all belong to the evil-energy kind, but the disease of wind-evil is lasting, but the attack of the malarial evil stops now and then, what is the reason?” Qibo said: “The disease caused by the wind-evil ususlly retains on the location of the disease, but the malaria is transmitting to the internal organs in turn along with the channel and collateral, when the Wei-energy corresponds with the malarial evil, they will attack. Yellow Emperor said: “Good.”

黄帝问于少师曰：余闻四时八风之中人也，故有寒暑，寒则皮肤急而腠理闭，暑则皮肤缓而腠理开。贼风邪气，因得以入乎？将必须八正虚〔虚：《甲乙》卷六第一作“风”〕邪，乃能伤入乎？少师答曰：不然。贼风邪气之中人也，不得以时。然必因其开也，其入深，其内极病〔其内极病：《甲乙》卷六第一“极病”作“亟而疾”〕，其病人也卒暴；因其闭也，其入浅以留，其病〔病：按“病”下脱“人”之〕也徐以迟〔迟：《太素》卷二十八《三虚三实》作“持”〕。

Yellow Emperor asked Shaoshi and said: “I am told when the human body is injured by the eight kinds of wind from the four seasons is due to the weather difference of cold and heat, when the body is cold, the skin will be tightened and the striae will become dense, when the body is hot, the skin will be loosen and the striae will be open . Whether the injury of the body is due to the heat and cold difference causing the invasion of the thief wind and the evil energy when the striae open, or due to the injury of the debilitative evil of the eight winds?” Shaoshi said: “Neither of them is correct, when the thief wind and the evil-energy injure man, there is no definite time, but when the evil-energy injures man, it can penetrate deeply and fastly and it causes the patient to contract the disease suddenly; when the striae are closed, the evil-energy can only penetrate shallowly and retains on the surface to cause the patient to contract the disease slowly and potractedly.”

黄帝曰：有寒温和适，腠理不开，然有卒病者，其故何也？少师答曰：帝弗知邪人乎？虽〔虽：《甲乙》卷六第一“虽”上有“人”字〕平居，其腠理开闭缓急，其故〔其故：《太素》卷二十八《三虚三实》并作“固”〕常有时也。黄帝曰：可得闻乎？少师曰：人与天地相参也，与日月相应也。故月满则海水西盛，人血气积，肌肉充，以肤致，毛发坚，腠理郄，烟垢著。当是之时，虽遇贼风，其入浅不深。至其月郭空，则海水东盛，人气血虚，其卫气去，形独居，肌肉减，皮肤纵，腠理开，毛发残，膲理薄〔膲理薄：《甲乙》卷六第一无此三字〕，烟垢落。当是之时，遇贼风则其入深，其病人也卒暴。

Yellow Emperor said："Somebody can adapt to the cold and heat properly，his striae do not open，but he can contract disease suddenly，and what is the reason?" Shaoshi said："Don't you know the condition when the evil-energy invades? Although a man can lead a calm life，yet the closing or the openning of the striae and the loose and dense of the skin can be changing in different times." Yellow Emperor said："Can you tell me the condition?" Shaoshi said："Man correlates with heaven and earth，and corresponds with the shifting of the sun and moon；when the moon is full，the water in the west sea will be abundant and one's body will be strong，one's blood and energy will be lucid，his muscle will be substantial，his skin will be dense，his hair will be firm，his striae will be closed，and the surface of his body will be black and thick，if he is invaded by the thief wind by this time，the invasion will be shallow. When the moon is in the wane，the water in the east sea will be abundant，the human body will be weak，one's blood and energy will be debilitative，the Wei-energy will be scattering and the shape of the body will be existing alone，his muscle will be emaciated，his skin will be loose，his striae will be open，his hair will be incomplete and his black and thick healthy outer appearance will be declined，if he encounters the invasion of the thief wind by this time，the invasion will be deep，and the attack of the disease will be quick."

黄帝曰：其有卒然暴死暴病〔暴病：《甲乙》卷六第一无此二字〕者何也？少师答曰：三虚〔三虚：《甲乙》卷六第一"三虚"上并有"得"字〕者，其死暴〔暴：《甲乙》卷六第一无此字〕疾也；得三实者，邪不能伤人也。黄帝曰：愿闻三虚。少师曰：乘年之衰，逢月之空，失时之和，因为贼风所伤，是谓三虚。故论不知三虚，工反为粗。帝曰：愿闻三实。少师曰：逢年之盛，遇月之满，得时之和，虽有贼风邪气，不能危之〔危之：《甲乙》卷六第一作"伤"〕也。黄帝曰：善乎哉论！明乎哉道！请藏之金匮。命曰三实，然此一夫之论也。

Yellow Emperor said："Someone dies all of a sudden，and why is it?" Shaoshi answered："When one encounters the three asthenia，he will not be injured by the evil-energy." Yellow Emperor said："I hope to hear about the three asthenia." Shaoshi said："When one is injured in the asthenia-year of which the year-energy is insufficient，again，the wane of moon is encountered，and the weather of four-season is not harmonious，it is called the three-asthenia encountering. If a physician does not understand the three-asthenia in treating，he is only a physician of lower level." Yellow Emperor said："I hope to hear the condition of three-sthenia." Shaoshi said："It is in the year when the year-energy is having a surplus，again，the day of full moon is encountered and the weather of the four-season is harmonious，although there is the thief wind and the evil energy，yet they can not injure the body." Yellow Emperor said："Your discourse is excellent，and your explanation is also incisive. Please store your statements in the golden cabinet and call it the 'Three-Asthenia'；but your statement above is only indicating the condition of an individual person."

黄帝曰：愿闻岁之所以皆同病者，何因而然？少师曰：此八正之侯也。黄帝曰："侯之奈何？少师曰：侯此者〔侯此者：当注本无此三字〕，常以冬至之日，太一立于叶蛰之宫，其至也，天必应之以风雨者矣。风雨从南方来者，为虚风，贼伤人者也。其以夜半〔半：《太素》卷二十八《八正风候》无此字〕至也，万民皆卧而弗犯也，故其岁民少病。其以昼至者，万民懈惰而皆中于虚风，故万民多病。虚邪入客于骨而不发于外，至其立春，阳气大发，腠理开，因立春之日，风从西方来，万民又皆中于虚风，此两邪相搏，经气结〔结：《太素》卷二十八《八风正候》作"绝"〕代者矣。故诸逢其风而遇其雨者，命曰遇岁露焉。因岁之和，而少贼风者，民少病而少死；岁多贼风邪气，寒温不和，则民多病而死矣。

Yellow Emperor said："I hope to know what energy causes the diseases in the year?" Shaoshi said："It must observe the winds from the eight orientations for determining." Yellow Emperor asked："How to observe them?" Shaoshi answered："One must observe on the day of Winter Solstice when the Polaris situates in the Yezhe Palace, because there must be wind on the day of the Polaris shifting. If the wind is from the south, it is called the debilitative wind which can injure the body. If the wind comes in the night time when most people are sleeping without violating it, few people will contract disease in the year. If the wind comes in day time when many people neglect to defend it, so, many people will contract disease in the year. If the debilitative evil penetrates into the bone in winter and the evil has not excreted to outside, the Yang energy will break out and the striae will open after the Beginning of Spring. When the wind is from the west on the day of the Beginning of Spring, people will be hit by the debilitative wind of the west, the harbouring evil of winter will combat with the recent evil of spring causing the stagnacy of the energy and the disease. Therefore, the wind or rain from a certain orientation is called the dew of the year. When the year-energy is harmonious with few thief wind, few people will contract disease and few people will die; if there are a lot of thief winds and evil energies in the year, the weather is changeful with cold and heat which is not harmonious, many people will contract disease, and many will die."

黄帝曰：虚邪之风，其所伤贵贱何如？侯之奈何？少师答曰：正月朔日太一居天留〔留：《太素》卷二十八《八正风候》作"溜"〕之宫，其日西北风，不雨，人多死矣。正月朔日，平旦北风，春，民多死。正月朔日，平旦北风行，民病多者，十有三也。正月朔日，日中北风，夏，民多死。正月朔日，夕时北风，秋，民多死。终日北风，大病死者十有六。正月朔日，风从南方来，命曰旱乡，从西方来，命曰白骨，将国有殃，人多死亡。正月朔日，风从东方来，发屋，扬沙石，国有大灾也。正月朔日，风从东南方行，春有死亡。正月朔，天和温不风，籴贱，民不病；天寒而风，籴贵，民多病。此所谓侯岁之风，戕伤人者也。二月丑不风，民多心腹病。三月戌不温，民多寒热。四月巳不暑，民多瘅病。十月申不寒，民多暴死。诸所谓风者，皆发屋，折树木，扬沙石，起毫毛，发腠理者也。

Yellow Emperor asked："How to observe the severe or slight injury to man by the debilitative wind?" Shaoshi said："On the first day of the first lunar month, the Polaris moves to the Tianliu Palace, if the wind is from the northwest without rain, many people will die caused by disease; if the wind is from the north in the dawn on the day of the first day of the first lunar month, many people will die in spring of the year due to disease; if the wind is from the north at the noon on the first day of the first lunar month, many people will die in summer of the year; if the wind is from the north in the evening on the first day of the first lunar month, many people will have disease in autumn of the year; if the wind is from the north for the whole day, the diseases will be prevailing, and sixty per cent of the people will die. When the wind is from the south on the first day of the first lunar month, it is called the wind from the dry region; when the wind is from the west, it is called the wind from the region of the dried skeletons, there will be great calamities prevailing in the whole country and many people will die of disease. If the wind is from the east to shake the buildings and carry away the sand and stones, there will be great calamities in the whole country; if the wind in from the southeast on the first day of the first lunar month, and many people will die in spring; if the weather is warm wthout any wind on the first day of the first lunar month, the price of the rice will be moderate and people will be healthy in the year. This is the general condition of observing the winds which injure the human body. When there is no wind on the Chou day of the second lunar month, people will contract the diseases of heart and abdomen mostly; when it is not warm on the Wu day of the third lunar month, people will contract the disease of cold and heat mostly; when it is not hot on the Ji day of the fourth lunar month, people will contract the disease of dan-heat mostly; when it is not cold on the Shen day of the tenth lunar month, people will contract the disease of sudden death mostly. The so-called wind stated above is indicating the wind which can shake the buildings and break the woods, carry away the sands and the stones, it can cause one's hair to stand up and the striae of the body to open, and it is quite different from the ordinary wind."

大惑论第八十

Chapter 80
Da Huo Lun
(On the Big Perplexity)

黄帝问于岐伯曰：余尝上于清泠之台，中阶而顾，匍匐而前则惑。余私异之，窃内怪之，独瞑独视，安心定气，久而不解。独博〔博：《太素》卷二十七《七邪》作“转”〕独眩，披发长跪，俯而视之，后久之不已也。卒然自上〔上：《太素》卷二十七《七邪》并作“止”〕，何气使然？岐伯对曰：五藏六府之精气，皆上注于目而为之精〔精：《千金》卷六上作“睛”〕。精之窠为眼，骨之精为瞳子，筋之精为黑眼，血之精为络，其窠气之精为白眼，肌肉之精为约束，裹撷筋骨血气之精而与脉并为系，上属于脑，后出于项中。故邪中于项，因逢其身之虚，其入深，则随眼系以入于脑，入于脑则脑转，脑转则引目系急，目系急则目眩以转矣。邪〔邪：《太素》卷二十七《七邪》“邪”下有“中”字〕其精〔其精：《太素》卷二十七《七邪》不重此二字〕，其精所中不相比也则〔则：《甲乙》卷十二第四“则”上叠“不相比”三字〕精散，精散则视歧〔视歧：《千金》卷六上并作“故”字〕，视歧见两物。目者，五藏六府之精也，营卫魂魄之所常营也，神气之所生也。故神劳则魂魄散，志意乱。是故瞳子黑眼法于阴，白眼赤脉法于阳也，故阴阳合传而精明也。目者，心使也，心者，神之舍也，故神精乱而不转，卒然见非常处，精神魂魄，散不相得，故曰惑〔惑：周本，日刻本，张注本并作“感”〕也。黄帝曰：余疑其然。余每之东苑，未曾不惑，去之则复，余唯独为东苑劳神议乎？何其异也？岐伯曰：不然也。心有所喜，神有所恶，卒然相感，则精气乱，视误故惑，神移乃复。是故间者为迷，甚者为惑。

Yellow Emperor asked Qibo and said: “I mounted to the Cool Platform before and looked around in the flight of steps, I scrambled forward, and I felt dim in sight, I was amazed secretly, so, I closed my eyes and then opened them to stablize my mind, but the phenomenon could not be eliminated for a long time, and I felt my head was rotative and dazzling. so, I loosened my hair, bowed down my head and overlooked downward for quite a long time, and the dizziness still could not be eliminated, but suddenly, the phenomenon disappeared. What energy makes it so?” Qibo answered: “The refined energies of the five solid organs and the six hollow organs of human body are pouring upward to the eyes to enable one to see. The nest of the refined energy is the eye, the essence of the bone is the pupil, the essence of the tendon is the black of the eye, the essence of blood is in the superficial venules of the two canthus and the two eye sockets, the essence of the breathing air of the body is the white of the eyes, the essence of the muscle is in the eyelid; when the refined energies of the tendon, bone, blood and energy combine with the channel and collateral of the eye, it forms the ocular connectors. The ocular connectors connect the brain above and reach the middle of the neck behind, thus, when the evil energy hits the neck, and the debility of the body is encountered, the evil-energy will penetrate inside, when the evil-energy reaches the brain one will feel the dizziness of the brain and the ocular connectors will be tense due to it. When the ocular connectors are tense, one'e eyes will be dazziling, and the things seen will be like turning. If the evil-energy invades the refined energy of the eye, and the refined energy invaded can not keep harmonious, it will cause the refined energy to disperse, when the refined energy of the eye is dispersed, diplopia will occur, and the thing seen is like two of them. The eye is the place where the refined enregies of the five solid organs and the six hollow organs converge, and it is the place where the Ying-energy, the Wei-energy, the soul and the inferior spirit come and go, thus, the spirit and energy of the eye plays the main role of seeing things. When the spirit and the energy are overfatigue, the soul and the inferior spirit will be rising in the air and one's will will be confused. So, the pupil and the black of the eye belong to the internal organs of Yin, and the red channels of the white of the eye belong to the internal oragns of Yang, when the Yin energies of the bone, tendon, liver and kidney converge with the Yang energies of the blood, energy, heart and lung, the ability of seeing of the eye can be maintained. The eye serves the heart, and the heart is the place where the spirit situates, so, when one's spirit is dispersed and his essence is disorderly without converging, if an extraordinary place is seen, the spirit, the soul and the inferior spirit will become disorderly and disharmonious, as a result, the phenomenon of perplexity of the patient will occur." Yellow Emperor said: "I am sceptical about what you said. Whenever I come to the Cool Platform in the East Yard, I always get confused, but when I left the Cool Platform, I become normal again. Am I consuming my spirit in the East Yard only? Why is it so strange?" Qibo said: "It is not strange at all. When one likes something in the mind, but detests it in the spirit, when the moods of like and dislike mingle all of a sudden, it will cause the spirit to become disorderly, one will be seeing things in double and being perplexed. After the spirit and the consciousness are shifted, one will resume to normal state again. In the conditions stated above, when the case is slight, it is called the perplexity, when the case is severe, it is called the puzzle."

黄帝曰：人之善忘者，何气使然？岐伯曰：上气不足，下气有余，肠胃实而心肺虚，虚则营卫留于下，久之不以时上，故善忘也。

Yellow Emperor asked: "When one is forgetful, what energy causes it?" Qibo said: "It is due to the energies of the internal organs in the upper part is insufficient, and the energies of the internal organs in the lower are having a surplus; that is, the energies of the stomach and intestine are substantial and the energies of the heart and lung are debilitative. When the energies of the heart and lung are deficient, the Ying-energy and the Wei-energy will retain in the intestine and the stomach and fail to spread to the whole body for a long time, when both the energy and the blood are deficient, the disease of forgetfulness will occur."

黄帝曰：人之善饥而不嗜食者，何气使然？岐伯曰：精气并于脾，热气留于胃，胃热则消谷，谷消故善饥。胃气逆上，则胃脘寒，故不嗜食也。

Yellow Emperor asked: "Someone gets hungry often but he is reluctant to eat, what energy causes it?" Qibo said: "The refined energy which is of Yin assembles in the spleen, and the heat which is of Yang retains in the stomach, When the heat in the stomach is vigorous, the digestion will be promoted and one will get hungry often. when the stomach energy is up-reversing, it causes the asthenia-cold of the gastric cavity and one will be reluctant to eat."

黄帝曰：病而不得卧者，何气使然？岐伯曰：卫气不得入于阴，常留于阳。留于阳则阳气满，阳气满则阳跻盛，不得入于阴则阴气虚，故目不瞑矣。

Yellow Emperor asked: "When one can not fall into sleep due to sickness, what energy causes it?" Qibo said: "As the Wei-energy should travels in the Yang portion in day time and travels in the Yin portion in night time, but when it retains in the Yang portion and fails to enter into the Yin portion constantly, it will cause the Yang energy to become prosperous and the pulse energy of Yangqiao to become partial overabundant. As the Wei-energy fails to enter into the Yin portion causing the deficiency of the Yin energy, one will not be able to fall into sleep.:

黄帝曰：病目而〔病目而：当注本"目而"作"而目"〕不得视者，何气使然？岐伯曰：卫气留〔留：《甲乙》卷十二第三作"行"〕于阴，不得行〔行：《甲乙》卷十二第三作"入"〕于阳。留于阴则阴气盛，阴气盛则阴跻满，不得入于阳则阳气虚，故目闭也。

Yellow Emperor asked: "When one shuts his eyes and can see nothing due to sickness, what energy causes it?" Qibo said: "It is due to the Wei-energy travels in the Yin portion only, and fails to enter into the Yang portion. When the Wei-energy travels in the Yin portion, it causes the Yin energy to become prosperous, when the Yin energy is partial overabundant, the pulse energy of the Yinqiao will be full. Since the Wei-energy fails to enter into the Yang portion, the Yang energy will be deficient which will cause one fail to close his eyes and sleep."

黄帝曰：人之多卧者，何气使然？岐伯曰：此人肠胃大而皮肤湿〔湿：《太素》卷二十七《七邪》作"涩"〕，而分肉不解焉。肠胃大则卫气留久，皮肤湿则分肉不解，其行迟。夫卫气者，昼日〔日：《甲乙》卷十二第三无此字〕常行于阳，夜行于阴，故阳气尽则卧，阴气尽则寤。故肠胃大，则卫气行留久；皮肤湿，分肉不解，则行迟。留于阴也久，其气不清〔清：胡本、熊本、周本并作"精"〕，则欲瞑，故多卧矣。其肠胃小，皮肤滑以缓，分肉解利〔分肉解利：按"利"字疑误，《医学纲目》卷十五引"利"作"则"属下读〕，卫气之留于阳也久，故少瞑焉。

Yellow Emperor asked: "When one is fond of lying, what energy causes it?" Qibo said: "The intestine and stomach of this kind of man are thick and large, his skin is coarse and unsmooth and his muscle is not slippery. As his intestine and stomach are thick and large, the retaining period of the Wei-energy will be long; when the skin is coarse and unsmooth, his muscle is not slippery, the operation of the Wei-energy will be slow. Since the Wei-energy travels in the Yang portion in day time and travels in the Yin portion in night time, so, in night time, the Yang energy is deficient and one wants to sleep, and when the Yin energy is deficient at dawn he will awake. When the Wei-energy retains in the Yin portion for a long period, the energy will not be refined, one will like to close his eyes and sleep. If one's intestine and stomach are small, his skin is moist and smooth, his muscle must also be slippery, the Wei-energy will retain in the Yang portion for a long time, and one will be reluctant to lie and sleep."

黄帝曰：其非常经也，卒然多卧者，何气使然？岐伯曰：邪气留于上膲，上膲闭而不通，已食若饮汤，卫气留久〔留久：《太素》卷二十七《七邪》作“歹留”〕于阴而不行，故卒然多卧焉。

Yellow Emperor asked: "If one is not fond of sleep usually but he is suddenly fond of sleep, what energy causes it?" Qibo said: "It is because the evil energy retains in the upper warmer causing the energy of the triple warmer to become impeded, or one eats his fill or drinks water excessively, causing the Wei-energy to retain in the Yin portion and fails to reach the Yang portion, one will like to sleep suddenly."

黄帝曰：善。治此诸邪奈何？岐伯曰：先〔先：《甲乙》卷十二第三“先”下有“视”字〕其藏府，诛其小过，后调其气，盛者泻之，虚者补之，必先明知其形志之苦乐，定乃取之。

Yellow Emperor said: "Good. But how to treat the evil energies?" Qibo said: "One must examine the conditions of the internal organs, eliminate the evil-energy which is slight, then, adjust the Ying-energy and the Wei-energy. When the evil-energy is overabundant, apply the purging therapy, when the health energy is deficient, apply the invigorating therapy. One must know explicitly the joyous or miserable mood of the patient, and after having a mature understanding, treat by pricking the acupoints."

痈疽第八十一

Chapter 81
Yong Ju
(On Carbuncle and Deep-Rooted Carbuncle)

黄帝曰：余闻肠胃受谷，上焦出气，以温分〔分：《灵枢略·六气论》作爪"〕肉，而养骨节，通腠理。中焦出气如露〔露：《甲乙》卷十一第九上作“雾”〕，上〔上：《鬼遗方》卷四无此字〕注谿谷，而渗孙脉，津液和调，变化而赤为血，血和则孙脉先满溢〔溢：《太素》卷二十六《痈疽》作“满”，属下读〕，乃注于络脉，皆盈，乃注于经脉。阴阳已张，因息乃行，行有经〔经：《千金翼方》卷二十三并作“纲”〕纪，周有道理，与天合同，不得休止。切而调之，从虚去实，泻则不足，疾则气减，留则先后。从实去虚，补则有余。血气已调，形气乃持。余已知血气之平与不平，未知痈疽之所从生，成则之时，死生之期，有〔有：《医心方》卷十五“有”上并有“期”字〕远近，何以度之，可得闻乎？

Yellow Emperor said："I am told when the intestine and the stomach receive the cereals, the Wei-energy issues from the upper warmer to moisturize the nails and muscles, and nourish the bone and joints and dredge the striae; the Ying-energy issues from the middle warmer to pour into the groove between the strips of muscles and penetrates into the minute collaterals like mists. When one's body fluid is harmonious, it turns into the red fluid of blood, when the blood is harmonious, it will fill the minute collateral, and when it is being filled, the blood will pour into the collateral branch of the large channel, when it is filled, the blood will pour into the channel, when the Ying-energy and the Wei-energy are fully filled, the blood will spread to the whole body along with the respiration. The circulation of the energy and blood has a certain rule like the revolution of the sun and moon in certain degrees, it operates unceasingly like the universe. To the diseases of asthenia and sthenia, one must treat whole heartedly. Eliminate the sthenia-evil by purging therapy, but if the purging is excessive, it will injure the healthy energy to cause insufficiency. In pricking, the pulling out of the needle should be quick to reduce the evil-energy. If the times of the needle retention in different cases are all the same, the disease can hardly take a turn for the better. Apply the therapy supporting the healthy energy to eliminate the deficiency, but if the invigoration is excessive, it will cause the sthenia to have a surplus and promotes the remainder evil. When the energy and blood are harmonious, the relation between the physical body and the energy will remain normal. Now, I have known the principle of the balance and imbalance of the energy and blood, but I don't know from where the carbuncle and the deep-rooted carbuncle produce, the date of their shaping and dispersing, the date of the patient's recovery, death and the way of inferring the remote or recent date of them. Can you tell me the principle about them?"

岐伯曰：经脉留行不止，与天同度，与地合纪。故天宿失度，日月薄蚀，地经失纪，水道流溢，草萓〔萓：《医心方》卷十五并作"虚"《医心方》旁注："虚死草也"〕不成，五谷不殖，径路不通，民不往来，巷聚邑居，则〔则：《太素》卷二十六《痈疽》并无此字〕别离异处，血气犹然，请言其故。夫血脉营卫，周流不休，上应星宿，下应经数。寒邪〔邪：《病源》卷三十二《痈利候》、《久痈候》均作"寒气"〕客于经络〔经络：《灵枢略》作"经脉"〕之中则血泣，血泣则不通，不通则卫气归之，不得复反，故痈肿。寒气化为热，热胜则腐肉，肉腐则为脓，脓不泻则烂筋，筋烂则伤骨，骨伤则髓消，不当骨空，不得泄泻，血枯空虚，则筋骨肌肉不相荣，经脉败漏，熏于五藏，藏伤故死矣。

Qibo said: "The channel cycles unceasingly like the operation of heaven, and it suits the thoroughfare of the earth, so, if the sun, moon and stars divorce from their common practice, the sun and moon will turn into red and yellow or the eclipses will occur; if the earth divorces from its common pratice, the rivers will be over-flowing, the grasses will not be able to grow and the cereals will not be able to multiply. It is just like when the paths are obstructed and men can not communicate with each other, they are crowded on the street and lane or stay in the suburbs scattering in different places. The condition of the circulation of the blood and energy is similar, and I will tell you the reason about it. The channel energy, the Ying-energy and the Wei-energy are circulating unceasingly, it symbolizes the stars above and symbolizes the tunnel below. If the cold energy invades the channel, the channel will become obstructed and becomes stagnant, the obstruction will cause the accumulation of the Wei-energy and it can hardly operate normally, and thus, the carbuncle is formed. The cold-evil can turn into heat, and when heat is excessing it will corrupt the muscle, and when the muscle is corrupted, it will change into pus, when the pus is not eliminated, it will corrupt the tendon, when the tendon is corrupted, it will injure the bone, when the bone is injured, it will consume the marrow, when the marrow is consumed, the bone will be empty, when the bone is empty, the energy will not be spreading, the blood will suffer heavy losses and the tendon, bone and the muscle will not be able to nourish each other, as a result, the channel will be corrupted, which will affect the internal five solid organs, when five solid organs are injured, the patient will die."

黄帝曰：愿尽闻痈疽之形，与忌曰〔曰：《太素》卷二十六《痈疽》作"日"〕名。岐伯曰：痈发于嗌中，名曰猛疽，猛疽不治，化为脓，脓不泻，塞咽，半日死；其化为脓者，泻则合〔合：《太素》卷二十六《痈疽》作"含"〕豕膏，冷食〔冷食：《外台》卷二十四"冷食"上并有"毋"字〕，三日而已。

Yellow Emperor said: "I hope to hear the forms of the carbuncle and the deep-rooted carbuncle, their contraindication days and their various names."Qibo said: "The deep-rooted carbuncle which is in the pharynx is called the retropharyngeal abscess, if it was not treated hastily, the blood will turn into pus rapidly, if the pus is not removed, it will obstruct the throat, and the patient will die in half a day. If one has suppuration, keep the lard in the mouth to remove the pus, and avoid the cold food, he can be recovered in three days.

发于颈，名曰夭疽，其痈〔痈：《外治》卷二十四并作“状”〕大以赤黑，不急治，则热气下入渊腋，前伤任脉，内熏肝肺〔肺：《鬼遗方》卷四作“脉”〕，熏肝肺〔熏肝肺：《千金翼方》并无此三字〕十余日而死矣。

“When the carbuncle is in the neck, it is called the carbuncle over the mastoid and it is large, red and black, if it is not treated in time, the heat-evil will reach the Yuanye point (three inches under the armpit) to hurt the Ren Channel in front, and will scorch the liver channel inside, the patient will die in ten days.

阳留大发，消脑留项，名日脑烁，其色不乐〔乐：《病源》卷三十二《疽候》作“荣”〕，项〔《甲乙》卷九“项”上有“脑”字〕痛而如刺以针，烦心者死不可治。

“When the Yang-evil is hyperactive to injure the brain and pours into the neck, it is called the Yin-type carbuncle on the nape, it is not red nor swelling, but the head, brain and the neck of the patient are painful like being pricked by needle. If the patient is fretful, it is a fatal disease.

发于肩及臑，名曰疵痈，其状赤黑，急治之〔急治之：《千金翼方》卷二十三作“不急治”〕，此令人汗出至足，不害五藏，痈发四五日逞焫之。

“When the carbuncle is in the shoulder and the upper arm, it is called pyogenic infection of bone and it is red and black. If it is not treated in time, it will cause the patient to perspire down to the feet, but it can not go so far as to injure the five solid organs. It should be treated by moxibustion on the four or five days after the onset.”

发于腋下赤坚者，名曰米〔米：《千金翼方》卷二十三并作“朱”〕疽，治之以砭石，欲细而长，疏〔疏：《太素》卷二十六《痈疽》作“数”〕砭之，涂以豕膏，六日已，勿裹之。其痈坚而不溃者，为马刀挟瘿，急治之。

“When the carbunele is red and firm under the armpit, it is called the red carbuncle. When treating, it should apply the thin and long stone needle to prick for several times, then, smear with ointment and it will recover in six days, and it is not neeessary to bind up the carbuncle. If the carbuncle is hard and does not burst, it is the carbuncle of the sabre kind which should be treated immediately.

发于胸，名曰井疽，其状如大豆，三四日起，不早治，下入腹，不治〔不治：《外台》卷二十四“不治”上有“入腹”二字〕，七〔七：《外台》卷二十四并作“十”〕日死矣。

“When the carbuncle is on the chest, it is called abscess in the 'well'. Its shape is like the soybean, if it is not treated in the first three or four days, the toxic-evil will descend to the abdomen, if it is not treated after reaching the abdomen, the patient will die in ten days.

发于膺，名曰甘疽，色青〔色青：《鬼遗方》卷四无此二字〕，其状如穀实菰𦼮，常苦〔苦：《鬼遗方》卷四无此字〕寒热，急治之，去其寒热〔去其寒热：《甲乙》卷十一第九下“去其寒热”下有“不急治”三字〕，十岁死，死后出脓。

“When the deep-rooted carbuncle is on the two sides of the chest it is called the cellulitis of chest. Its shape is like the paper mulberry fruit and the Mongolian snakegourd. As the patient has the syndrome of cold and heat often, it should be removed immediately, if it is not treated in time, the patient will die in ten days, and the pus will flow out all by itself after the death of the patient.

发于胁，名曰败疵，败疵者女子之病也，灸〔灸：周本作“久”〕之，其病大痈脓，治之，其中乃有生肉大如赤小豆，剉蔆蘸草根各一升，以水一斗六升煮之，竭为取三升，则强饮，厚衣坐于釜上，令汗出至足，

"When the carbuncle is in the hypochondrium, it is called Baizi (the corrupted malady) which is a disease easy for a woman to contract. When it is protracted, it can change into a large carbuncle with pus and a polyp in a size of adzuki bean in the pus. When treating, take a litre of weeping golden bell and grass root each, put them into sixteen litres of water and boil it until the decoction is three litres left, then drink it with difficulty, the patient should sit by a hot pot with thick dresses to have a thorough perspiration to the foot, the disease will be recovered.

发于股胫，名曰股胫疽，其状不甚变，而痈脓搏骨，不急治，三〔三：《甲乙》卷十一第九下并作“四”〕十日死矣。

"When the carbuncle is in the leg, it is called the osteomyelitis of femur and tibia. There is no prominent change in shape, but it is swelling with pus attacking the bone. If it is not treated in time, the patient will die in forty days.

发于尻，名曰锐疽，其状赤坚大，急治之，不〔不：《鬼遗方》卷四“不”下有“速”字〕治，三〔三：《病源》卷三十二作“四”〕十日死矣。

"When the carbuncle is in the buttock, it is called the carbuncle on coccygeal region, it is red, large and firm in shape, and it should be treated immediately, otherwise, the patient will die in forty days.

发于股阴，名曰赤施，不急治，六十〔十：《医心方》卷十五并无此字〕日死，在两股之内，不治，十〔十：《鬼遗方》卷四并作“六”〕日而当死。

"When the carbuncle is in the inner flank of the thigh, it is called the red exerted carbuncle, if it is not treated in time, the patient will die in six days. When the carbuncles are on the both sides of the thigh, the patient will die in six days.

发于膝，名曰疵〔疵：《鬼遗方》卷四作“雌”〕痈，其状大痈，色不变，寒热，如〔如：《鬼遗方》卷四并作“而”〕坚石〔石：《医心方》卷十五并无此字〕，勿石，石〔石：《鬼遗方》卷四作“破”〕之者死，须其柔，乃石之者生。

"When the carbuncle is on the inner flank of the knee, it is called the female carbuncle. It is large and swelling, but the colour of the skin remains unchanged. If the patient has cold and heat, and if the carbuncle is hard, it must not be broken by pricking, if it is broken, the patient will die. If it is kneaded by hand slowly, the patient may survive.

诸痈疽之发于节而相应者，不可治也。发于阳者，百日死；发于阴者，三〔三：鬼遗方》卷四并作四〕十日死。

"When the carbuncle is on the symmetrical position to the above, below, left and right of the joint, it will not be cured, When it is on the position of the Yang Channel, the patient will die in one hundred days; when it is on the position of the Yin Channel, the patient will die in forty days.

发于胫，名曰兔啮，其状赤至骨〔其状赤至骨：《甲乙》卷十一第九下作“其状如赤豆至骨”〕，急治之，不〔不：《甲乙》卷十一第九下“不”下并有“急”字〕治害人也。

“When the carbuncle in on the tibia below the knee, it is like the red bean and it reaches the bone. It should be treated immediately, otherwise, it will injure man.

发于内踝，名曰走缓，其状痈也〔痈也：《太素》卷二十三并无二字〕，色不变，数石其输，而止其寒热，不死。

“When the carbuncle is on the ankle, it is called the retarded movement of the toxicant, and the colour of the muscle remains unchanged. When it is treated with moxibustion frequently, and if the cold and heat are removed, the patient will not die.

发于足上下，名曰四淫，其状大痈，急〔《鬼遗方》卷四“急”上并有“不”字〕治之，百日死。

“When the carbuncle is on the foot, it is called the inflammatory disease of foot. Its appearance is like an ordinary carbuncle, and if it is not treated in time, the patient will die in one hundred days.

发于足傍，名曰厉痈，其状不大，初如小指发，急治之，去其黑者，不消辄益，不治，百日死。

“When the carbuncle is on the side of the foot, it is called carbuncle of the foot, It is not large and it is intiate from the small toe, it should be treated hastily to remove the one which is black. If it is not removed, the diseass will become aggravated and the patient will die in one hundred days.

发于足指，名脱痈，其状赤黑，死不治；不赤黑，不死。不衰，急斩之，不〔不：《甲乙》卷十一第九下“不”下并有“去”字〕则死矣。

“When the carbuncle is on the toe, it is called the gangrene of toe, when it is red and black, it is a fatal disease, if it is not red and black, the patient will not die, but if the disease is not alleviated after treating, cut off the toe and the patient can survive; if it is not being cut off, the patient will die.”

黄帝曰：“夫子言痈疽，何以别之？岐伯曰：营卫〔卫：《甲乙》卷十一第九下作“气”〕稽留于经脉之中，则血泣而不行，不行则卫气从之而不通，壅遏而不得行，故热。大热不止，热胜则肉腐，肉腐则为脓。然不能陷，骨髓不为燋枯，五藏不为伤，故命曰痈。

Yellow Emperor asked:“What is the difference of the carbuncle and the deep-rooted carbuncle you said above?” Qibo said:“When the Ying-energy retains in the channel and collateral for long, the blood will be stagnant and stop flowing, and the Wei-energy will be impeded due to obstruction. In this case, the great heat will produce, When the heat is excessive, it will cause the deterioration of the muscle and will turn it into pus easily, but it will not be able to bog into the marrow, nor to dry the marrow, and thus the five solid organs will not be injured. The disease is called carbuncle.”

黄帝曰：何谓疽？岐伯曰：热气淳〔淳：《鬼遗方》卷一作“浮”〕盛，下陷肌肤，筋髓枯〔枯：《甲乙》卷十一第九作“骨肉”〕，内连五脏，血气〔血气：《太平圣惠方》卷十六《痈疽论》“血气”下有“涸”字〕竭，当其痈〔痈：《太平圣惠方》卷六十一《痈疽论》作

“痈”〕下，筋骨良肉皆无余，故命曰疽。疽者，上之皮夭以坚，上〔上：《甲乙》卷十一第九作“状”〕如牛领之皮。痈者，其皮上薄以泽。此其候也。

Yellow Emperor asked: “What is called the deep-rooted carbuncle?” Qibo said: “When one's heat is overabundant, the toxic-evil bogs into the skin, tendon, marrow, bone and the muscle and then reaches the five solid organs inside to cause the exhaustion of the energy and blood. On the painful positions, all the tendons and muscles are deteriorated and the disease is called the deep-rooted carbuncle. In the deep-rooted carbuncle, the colour of the skin is black and dark, unmoist and firm like the skin under the neck of the cow. In carbuncle, the skin is thin with bright colour. These are the distinguishing methods of the carbuncle and the deep-rooted carbuncle.”

附录

原文校注据本书名：

素问王冰注　　四部丛刊影印明顾氏本
黄帝内经太素　　东洋医学丛书影印本　　简称太素
难经集注　　四部丛刊影印佚存丛书本
伤寒论　　重庆人民出版社排印本
脉经　　四部丛刊影印元广勤书堂刊本
甲乙经　　人民卫生出版社刘衡如校本　　简称甲乙
鬼遗方　　人民卫生出版社影印本
中藏经　　丛书集成本
诸病源候论　　人民卫生出版社影印本　　简称病源
备急千金要方　　人民卫生出版社影印本　　简称千金
千金翼方　　人民卫生出版社影印本
外台秘要　　人民卫生出版社影印本　　简称外台
太平圣惠方　　人民卫生出版社排印本
铜人针灸腧穴图经　　人民卫生出版社影印本　　简称图经
医心方　　人民卫生出版社影印本
校证活人书　　丛书集成本
伤寒补亡论　　梁园豫医双璧本

schleimig-eitrigem Tränenfluß, mitunter auch Nasenausfluß; die Episkleralgefäße sind injiziert, die Konjunktiven stark gerötet, chemotisch verquollen und mit schleimigem bis fibrinösem Exsudat überzogen; ihre als multiple kleine weiße Herde erkennbaren Lymphfollikel sind m. o. w. deutlich geschwollen. Die Hornhaut ist dabei jedoch – im Gegensatz zur infektiösen bovinen Keratokonjunktivitis – nur selten, und zwar im Sinne einer von peripher nach zentral fortschreitenden Trübung beteiligt und ulzeriert nicht. In der zweiten Hälfte der Trächtigkeit befindliche Tiere können verkalben.

■ **Diagnose:** Während der ersten Krankheitswoche läßt sich BHV-1 aus Konjunktivaltupfern anzüchten oder im Bindehautabstrich fluoreszenzimmunologisch nachweisen; außerdem nehmen im Serum BHV-1-spezifische Antikörper deutlich zu.

■ **Behandlung:** Die gegen bakterielle Sekundärkeime gerichtete Therapie der Herpesvirus-bedingten Bindehautentzündung umfaßt Isolierung der Patienten im abgedunkelten Stall sowie 1- bis 2mal täglich vorzunehmender Instillation von kortikosteroidfreier, antibiotischer Augensalbe. Die *Vorbeuge* besteht in der gegen Infektiöse Bovine Rhinotracheitis gerichteten Impfung der Herde (Kap. 5.1.3.1).

11.1.4 Parasitär bedingte Krankheiten der Augen

Abgesehen von dem im folgenden zu schildernden Augenwurmbefall können auch *Demodikose* (Kap. 2.2.4.3), *Stephanofilariose* (Kap. 2.2.4.5), *Besnoitiose* (Kap. 2.2.4.6) und *Sarkozystiose* (Kap. 9.16.1) zu Augenliderkrankung führen. Starker *Fliegenbefall* (Kap. 2.2.4.1) fördert Moraxellen-, Chlamydien-, Mykoplasmen- und Virus-bedingte Keratokonjunktivitis sowie die nachstehend zu besprechende Thelaziose.

11.1.4.1 Augenwurmbefall

■ **Definition:** Als *Thelaziose* wird die von entzündlicher Reaktion begleitete Besiedlung des Konjunktivalsackes und anderer Adnexe des Auges mit Rundwürmern der Gattung Thelazia bezeichnet.

■ **Vorkommen, Ursachen:** Die weltweit verbreiteten, in Bindehautsack, Nickhaut- und Tränendrüsengängen sowie Tränennasenkanal des Rindes parasitierenden Augenwürmer sind *Thelazia gulosa* (s. *alfortensis*), *Th. skrjabini*, *Th. rhodesi* sowie *Th. bubali*. Ihre Differenzierung richtet sich nach der Morphologie der Männchen. Exenterierte Augen von Schlachtrindern erweisen sich zu 15–50% als von Thelazien parasitiert; Befallsstärke und Anteil juveniler Stadien sind in fliegenreichen Sommer- und Herbstmonaten am höchsten. In diesem Zeitraum enthalten 3–6% der bovikolen Musca-autumnalis-Fliegen Thelazienlarven.

■ **Parasitenkreislauf:** Geschlechtsreife Thelazien sind weißlich, 5–20 mm lang und fadenstark (Abb. 11-30); ihre Lebensdauer beträgt einige Monate bis 1 Jahr. Die viviparen Weibchen setzen Larven ab, die – zusammen mit Tränenflüssigkeit oder Nasensekret – von Fliegen (*Musca autumnalis, larvipara, amica, vitripennis, corvina, convexifrons* oder *sorbens*) aufgenommen werden und sich in deren Leibeshöhle binnen 15–30 Tagen zu invasionstüchtigen III. Larven entwickeln. Als solche werden sie über den Rüssel der befallenen Fliege auf die Konjunktiven anderer Rinder übertragen, wo sie sich innerhalb weiterer 3–6 Wochen zur Geschlechtsreife fortentwickeln. Die Überwinterung erfolgt offenbar am Rind, nicht aber im Zwischenwirt (Fliegen).

■ **Pathogenese:** Die krankmachende Wirkung der Augenwürmer ist gering; ihr Maximum erreicht sie vermutlich bei massiver Invasion unreifer Stadien (d. h. in der warmen Jahreszeit) von Th. rhodesi sowie bei jüngeren Rindern. An klinisch unauffälligen Augen sind mitunter über 50 reife Thelazien festzustellen. Bei Schlachttierkontrollen wurden zudem bei thelazienbefallenen Augen nur ~ 5% mehr krankhaft verändert befunden als bei vergleichsweise geprüften parasitenfreien Augen. Etwaiger Juckreiz kann das Krankheitsgeschehen wesentlich verschlimmern. Überstandene Augenwurminvasion hinterläßt keine Immunität gegenüber diesen Parasiten.

■ **Symptome:** Bei Thelaziose mitunter festzustellende Symptome, wie Augen- und Nasenausfluß, Lichtscheu, katarrhalische bis eitrige Bindehautentzün-

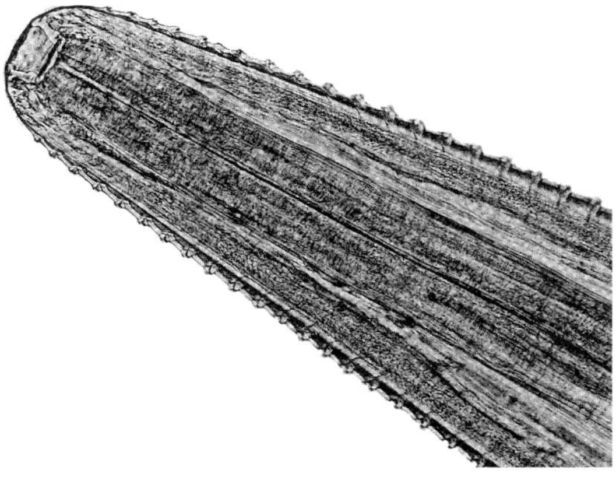

Abbildung 11-30 Vorderende eines *Thelazia-rhodesi*-Männchens (60fache Vergrößerung; Niutta et al., 1992)

dung, lokaler Juckreiz, subkonjunktivale Blutungen, Iridozyklitis, Hornhauttrübung und -geschwür, Lidphlegmone oder -abszeß, ausnahmsweise auch Panophthalmie, lassen sich nicht immer eindeutig auf den Augenwurmbefall zurückführen.

■ **Sektion:** Zur Überprüfung auf etwaige Besiedlung mit Thelazien ist das betreffende Auge samt Bindehautsack und Lidern aus der Orbita herauszulösen, der Konjunktivalsack umzustülpen und unter Ausdrücken von Tränenkarunkel, Tränenpunkten, Tränendrüsenausführungsgängen sowie Rückseite des dritten Augenlids (Nickhautdrüsengänge) auf Parasiten abzusuchen; erforderlichenfalls ist auch der Tränennasenkanal durchzuspülen oder der Länge nach aufzuschneiden. Die Nachsuche sollte gleich nach dem Tod oder der Schlachtung des Wirtsrindes erfolgen, weil die Augenwürmer sonst abwandern können. N. B.: Im unversehrten Augapfel selbst enthaltene Fadenwürmer sind i. d. R. *Setarien* (Kap. 10.4.10).

■ **Diagnose:** Bei Vorstellung augenkranker Rinder ist stets auch an primären oder sekundären Augenwurmbefall zu denken und hierauf zu untersuchen: Einträufeln eines Lokalanästhetikums in den Konjunktivalsack; Hervorziehen und Umklappen des dritten Augenlids mittels Augenpinzette; vorsichtig-wischendes Austasten des Bindehautsackes mit gazeüberzogenem Finger; erforderlichenfalls auch Spülung des Tränennasenganges der betreffenden Seite von seiner innen am lateralen Nasenflügel, auf der medialen Seite der Flügelfalte gelegenen Mündung her mit einem milden Desinfiziens (Abb. 11-31); Überprüfen der Gaze bzw. des Bodensatzes der am medialen Augenwinkel aufgefangenen Spülflüssigkeit. Zur parasitologischen Identifikation vorgesehene Augenwürmer sind in 5%iger Formaldehydlösung oder 70%igem Alkohol einzusenden.

Differentialdiagnostisch sind v. a. infektiöse Keratokonjunktivitis (Kap. 11.1.3), photosensibilitätsbedingte Binde- und Hornhautentzündung (Kap. 2.2.7.3) sowie akzidentelle Augenirritationen in Betracht zu ziehen.

■ **Beurteilung:** Am klinisch unauffälligen Auge festgestellter Thelazienbefall gilt als harmloser Befund. Bei gleichzeitigem Vorliegen krankhafter Veränderungen ist zwar oft nicht erkennbar, ob sie tatsächlich Folge (oder nur Anlaß) des Augenwurmbefalls sind; in solchen Fällen erscheint eine antiparasitäre Behandlung jedoch angebracht, wenn das betreffende Auge nicht bereits panophthalmisch verändert ist (Kap. 11.1.2.11).

■ **Behandlung:** Einträufeln von 3%iger Piperazinadipat-, 1%iger Levamisol- oder 0,1%iger Ivermectinlösung in den Konjunktivalsack, besser aber subkutane Gabe von 0,2 mg Ivermectin/kg LM oder 5 mg Levamisol/kg LM, orale Verabreichung von 15 mg Levamisol/kg LM oder Aufgießen von 0,5 mg Ivermectin oder Doramectin/kg LM auf den Rücken.

■ **Prophylaxe:** Fliegenabwehr (Kap. 2.2.4.1).

11.1.5 Fütterungs-, mangel- und vergiftungsbedingte Krankheiten der Augen

Das *Sehvermögen* ist bei Vergiftung durch *Blei* (Kap. 10.5.12), *Kochsalz* (Kap. 10.5.2), *Sulfide* (Kap. 10.5.14), *Fleckschierling* (Kap. 10.5.32), *Nachtschattengewächse* (Kap. 10.5.28), *Methylimidazol* (Kap. 10.5.26) oder gewisse *Trematodizide* (Kap. 10.5.21) eingeschränkt oder aufgehoben. Bezüglich vergiftungsbedingter *Miosis* und *Mydriasis* wird auf Kapitel 11.1.2.6 ver-

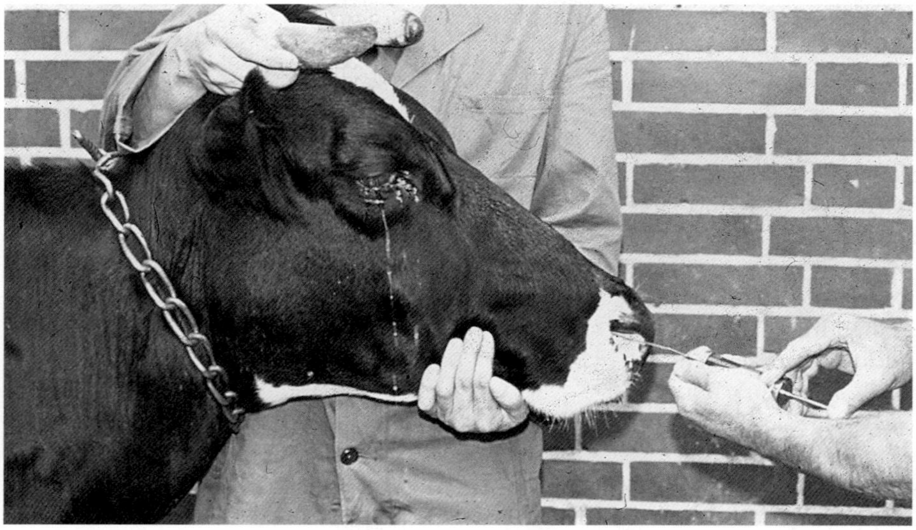

Abbildung 11-31
Spülen des Tränennasenganges

wiesen. Die unter anderem mit Blindheit einhergehende *Vitamin-B_1*-Mangel-bedingte Hirnrindennekrose wird bei den Krankheiten des zentralen Nervensystems besprochen (Kap. 10.5.5). *»Nervöse«* Ketose (Kap. 10.5.7) kann das Sehvermögen ebenfalls beeinträchtigen.

11.1.5.1 Vitamin-A-Mangel

Definition: Ausreichende Versorgung mit Vitamin A oder seinen Vorläufern, den Karotinen, ist Voraussetzung für ständige Regeneration des Sehpurpurs, geregeltes Wachstum der knöchernen Hüllen des ZNS sowie Erhaltung der normalen Epithelstruktur von Haut, Schleimhäuten, Drüsen und Netzhaut (»Epithelschutzvitamin«, »Retinol«). Bei weiblichen Tieren ist Vitamin A auch für die ungestörte intrauterine Entwicklung der Frucht, bei männlichen für die Samenqualität mitverantwortlich. Schwerwiegender Mangel an Vitamin A führt bei Feten zu Augenmißbildungen; bei Kälbern und Jungrindern verursacht anhaltende Hypovitaminose A m.o.w. ausgeprägte Beeinträchtigung des Sehvermögens sowie nervöse Erscheinungen; bei adulten Rindern bedingt unzureichende Vitamin-A-Versorgung verminderte Fruchtbarkeit. Außerdem wird über Vitamin-A-unabhängige fertilitätsfördernde Wirkungen von β-Karotin diskutiert.

Ursachen: Außer in künstlich damit angereicherten Futtermitteln steht Pflanzenfressern Vitamin A nur in Form seiner Provitamine, und zwar vorwiegend als β-Karotin zur Verfügung. Solches ist im Grünfutter einschließlich Rübenblatt sowie in Mohr-, gelben Kohl- und Stoppelrüben (nicht aber in anderen Futter- oder Zuckerrüben) reichlich enthalten. Während des Weideganges reicht das Karotinangebot daher zur Deckung des laufenden Bedarfs sowie zur Ansammlung beträchtlicher, v. a. in Leber und Fett eingelagerter Vorräte an Vitamin A aus (Übersicht 11-1). Unter günstigen Bedingungen gewonnenes gutes Heu enthält zunächst noch ~ 60%, künstlich getrocknetes Grün sogar ≤90% des ursprünglich in ihm vorhandenen Karotins. Frisch gewonnene Silage ist karotinreicher als zuvor angewelktes Silagegut: Unmittelbar nach dem Einsilieren beträgt der Karotingehalt darin noch 80 bzw. 50%. Auf dem Halm verdorrtes sowie verregnetes und ausgebleichtes Heu ist dagegen ausgesprochen karotinarm. Beim Lagern der genannten Futtermittel treten noch weitere, mitunter recht erhebliche Karotinverluste ein. Selbst bei sonst guter, aber Vitamin-A-Zulagen-freier Ernährung muß deshalb gegen Ende der Stallhaltungsperiode auf körpereigene Vitamin-A-Reserven zurückgegriffen werden. Magermilch und Magermilchpulver, Getreideschrote, Kraftfuttermehle sowie die zur Fütterung von Wiederkäuern üblichen Industrieabfälle (Schlempe, Treber, Schnitzel, Rückstände der Ölgewinnung u. ä. m.) sind äußerst arm an Karotin oder praktisch frei davon, wenn es ihnen nicht in Form von Grünmehlen oder als Vitamin A beigemengt wird.

Die Synthese von Vitamin A aus Karotinen erfolgt bei Wiederkäuern nicht nur in der Darmwand, sondern in wesentlichem Umfange auch in der Leber. Bei optimaler Versorgung entwickelt 1 mg β-Karotin so die Wirkung von 400 IE Vitamin A. Unzureichende oder übermäßige Karotinzufuhr bedingen jedoch wesentlich schlechtere Ausnutzungsraten. Karotinresorption und -umwandlung zu Vitamin A können zudem durch folgende Begleitumstände behindert werden, die u. U. zu sekundärem Mangel führen: Lebererkrankungen (Kap. 6.13), hoher Nitratgehalt von Nahrung oder Tränke (Kap. 4.3.5.3), Jodmangel (Kap. 2.3.5.1), unzulängliche oder überreichliche Phosphatzufuhr (Kap. 9.17.5), hohe Umgebungstemperatur (Kap. 10.6.4) oder Vergiftung mit höherchlorierten Naphthalinen (Kap. 12.3.15). Schließlich ist die Verwertbarkeit des im Futter enthaltenen Karotins auch von den in Leber und gelbem Körperfett gespeicherten Vitamin-A-Vorräten abhängig; sie wird bei fortschreitender Erschöpfung dieser Depots immer geringer.

Da Karotine die Plazenta nicht passieren, kann es bei Vitamin A-Mangel des Muttertieres zur Entwicklung amaurotischer und meist auch mit innerem Hydrozephalus behafteter Feten kommen (Kap. 10.1.1.4, 11.1.1.11). Neugeborene Kälber sind bis zum Alter von 6 Wochen auf Zufuhr von Vitamin A angewiesen, da sie bei Geburt nur über geringe Reserven davon verfügen und noch nicht befähigt sind, Karotin auszunutzen. Die vielschichtigen Zusammenhänge von Karotin- und Vitamin-A-Versorgung erschweren die Ermittlung des Bedarfs für Rinder, der zudem von Rasse, Verwendungszweck, Lebensalter, Gesundheitszustand und besonderen Belastungen abhängt.

Zur Vermeidung schwerwiegender Mangelerscheinungen werden 40 IE *Vitamin A* pro kg LM und Tag benötigt. Zur optimalen Versorgung werden für Kälber 100–300 IE, für Jungrinder, gravide und laktierende Tiere 100–160, für Zuchtbullen 80–90 IE Vitamin A pro kg LM und Tag empfohlen. In *β-Karotin* ausgedrückt beträgt der Minimalbedarf zur Verhütung von Nachtblindheit 30 μg, zur Sicherung des normalen Ablaufs der Trächtigkeit 200 μg, und zur Erhaltung der Fruchtbarkeit bei Bullen 50 μg pro kg LM und Tag.

Vorkommen, Verbreitung: Deutliche Hypovitaminose A setzt bei *erwachsenen Rindern* i. d. R. erst nach mehrmonatiger schwerer Mangelversorgung ein, wie sie etwa während der Stallhaltung bei Verabfolgung

Übersicht 11-1 Beurteilung des Vitamin-A- und β-Karotingehalts von Leber, Blutplasma und Milch bei Verdacht auf Mangelversorgung

Probenmaterial	Altersstufe	Vitamin-A-Gehalt normal	knapp	unzureichend
Leber[1] (µg/g FS):	Feten:	0,5–15		
	Kälber			
	bei Geburt:	> 0,6–3,0	0,3–0,6	< 0,3
	nach Kolostrumgabe:	10–50	2–10	< 2
	erwachsene Rinder:	> 50–300	3–50	< 3
Blutplasma[2] (µg/dl):	Feten:	19		
	Kälber			
	bei Geburt:	0,6–8,0		
	nach Kolostrumgabe:	> 12–> 30	7–12	< 7
				< 10
	erwachsene Rinder:	> 25–80	10–25	
Milch[4] (µg/dl):	erwachsene Rinder			
	Winter/Frühjahr:	> 80	50–80	< 50
	Sommer/Herbst:	< 170		
	Kolostralmilch:	150–350		

Probenmaterial	Altersstufe	β-Karotingehalt normal	knapp	unzureichend
Leber[1] (µg/g FS):	Kälber, bei Geburt:	0,25–05		
	erwachsene Rinder:	4–50	0,5–4	< 0,5
Blutplasma[3] (µg/dl):	Kälber			
	bei Geburt:	0,8–6,5		
	nach Kolostrumgabe oder Grünfütterung:	30–> 100	10–30	< 10
	erwachsene Rinder			
	Winter/Frühjahr:	200–500	60–200	< 60
	Sommer/Herbst:	500–1500		
Milch[4] (µg/dl):	erwachsene Rinder			
	Winter/Frühjahr:	≥ 30	20–30	< 20
	Sommer/Herbst:	≤ 370		
	Kolostralmilch[5]:	210–850		

[1] Zur Beurteilung von Versorgung und Bevorratung sind die an Leberbiopsieproben gewonnenen Ergebnisse am zuverlässigsten.
[2] Bei unzureichender Zufuhr von Vitamin A und/oder β-Karotin fällt der Vitamin-A-Spiegel im Blutplasma oft erst nach Verbrauch der Leberreserven und Einsetzen klinischer Mangelsymptome auf pathognostische Werte ab.
[3] Der Karotingehalt des Blutplasmas sinkt während der Trächtigkeit bis zum Puerperium hin innerhalb der normalen Schwankungsbreite ab.
[4] Fütterungsbedingt sind Vitamin-A- und β-Karotingehalt des Milchfetts starken jahreszeitlichen Schwankungen unterworfen.
[5] Die Vitamin-A-Konzentration in der Kolostralmilch ist in hohem Maße von den Leberreserven des Muttertieres, d. h. von seiner Vitamin-A- und/oder β-Karotinversorgung während der Hochträchtigkeit abhängig.

eines aus schlechtem oder überlagertem Heu, Stroh, Spreu, Futterrüben und Getreideschrot bestehenden »Durchhaltefutters« oder bei einseitiger Ernährung mit Maissilage, während des Weideganges dagegen im Verlauf längerer Dürreperioden eintreten kann. Auch Intensivmast auf Grundlage industrieller Futtermittel ohne oder mit nur wenig Grün und Heu führt nach einigen Monaten zu entsprechenden Folgen, wenn die Nahrung nicht durch Vitamin-A-Zulagen ergänzt wird.

Feten sind für Vitamin-A-Mangel besonders anfällig. Gleiches gilt für *Kälber* und *Jungrinder*, deren bei Kolostrumaufnahme angelegte Vitamin-A-Reserven wegen ihres hohen Bedarfs bald aufgebraucht sind, wenn ihre Nahrung (Magermilch, Magermilchpulver, Kälbermehl, Kraftfutter) nicht entsprechende Zusätze enthält. Selbst die Vollmilch suboptimal Karotin- und Vitamin-A-versorgter Muttertiere erweist sich mitunter als unzulänglich. Daher erkranken v. a. ältere Kälber und ≤3 Jahre alte Mastrinder an manifestem Vitamin-A-Mangel; es können aber auch bei adulten Tieren Versorgungsengpässe eintreten, die sich klinisch in unspezifischen Störungen bemerkbar machen.

Pathogenese, Symptome, Verlauf: Intrauteriner Vitamin-A-Mangel kann Abort, Totgeburt und *angeborene Augenmißbildungen*, wie Anophthalmie, Mikrophthalmie oder amaurotische Blindheit, außerdem Hydrozephalus, Verdickung von Hinterhaupts- und Keilbein sowie der Karpalgelenke bedingen.

Erste klinische Anzeichen von 5–12 Monate lang anhaltender postuteriner Hypovitaminose A sind bei 8- bis 20monatigen *Jungrindern* fast immer Beeinträchtigungen des Sehvermögens; dabei pflegen männliche Tiere eher und schwerer zu erkranken als weibliche: Mitglieder betroffener Gruppen zeigen sich zunächst nur im Dunkeln desorientiert (Nachtblindheit), was meist unbemerkt bleibt. Bald darauf setzt völlige Blindheit ein. Nicht selten wird das Leiden aber auch dann noch nicht erkannt, weil sich die Patienten in gewohnter Umgebung unauffällig bewegen. Sonst fallen die meist gut genährten Kranken dadurch auf, daß sie über Unebenheiten stolpern und in unbekanntem Terrain gegen Hindernisse laufen oder sich von den übrigen Tieren absondern. Ihre Augen erscheinen bis auf leichten oder mäßigen Exophthalmus (»Froschaugen« mit vorgewölbter Hornhaut; Abb. 11-32), maximale Erweiterung der auf Lichteinfall nicht reagierenden Pupille, Fehlen des Drohreflexes, blaugrünlich-reflektorischen Schimmer des Tapetum lucidum, unscharf abgesetzten Sehnervenkopf (Stauungspapille), peripapilläre Netzhautblutungen und -narben sowie auffallende Schlängelung der Fundusgefäße unverändert (= Amaurose oder »Schönblindheit«). Im Laufstall fällt auf, daß alle betroffenen Tiere Kopf und Ohren gleichzeitig und gleichsinnig nach Umgebungsgeräuschen ausrichten; entsprechend den Lichtverhältnissen leuchtet ihr Augenhintergrund dabei auf, wenn er dem Betrachter zugewandt wird. Im weiteren Verlauf kann es ausnahmsweise zu xerophthalmiebedingtem Tränenfluß, Bindehautentzündung und Hornhauttrübung kommen. Vor oder nach der Erblindung sind bei anhaltendem Vitamin-A-Mangel zudem Speicheln, Freßunlust, rauhes Haarkleid, schuppige Haut, Durchfall und verminderte Hitzetoleranz, gelegentlich auch zentralnervöse Symptome zu beobachten. Letztere werden, ebenso wie Papillenstauung und Sehstörungen, durch den auf 200–300 (statt 70–120) mm Wassersäule erhöhten Liquordruck verursacht; diese Druckzunahme beruht auf Einengung von Schädelhöhle und Wirbelkanal infolge abnormer Aktivität der Osteoblasten sowie auf Abnahme der Liquorresorption. Hiervon betroffene Patienten zeigen ataktisch-tappenden, schwankenden oder überkötenden Gang, Bewegungsinkoordination, vermehrte Erregbarkeit, Zittern, Zähneknirschen, plötzliches Niederstürzen oder Festliegen in Brustlage und/oder epileptiforme Krämpfe mit Opisthotonus, vorübergehender Bewußtlosigkeit und Laufbewegungen.

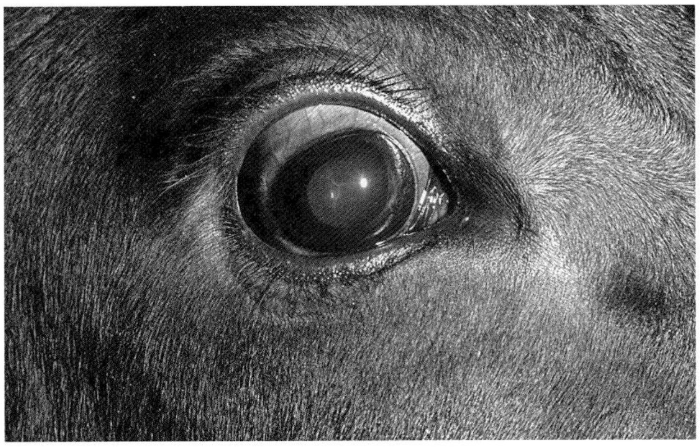

Abbildung 11-32 »Frosch«-Auge eines karotinarm ernährten jungen Mastbullen mit Exophthalmus, Vorwölbung der Hornhaut, ständig weitgestellter Pupille und »Schönblindheit« (Amaurose) infolge Vitamin-A-Mangels

Von Hypovitaminose A betroffene *Kälber* und *Jungrinder* fallen durch struppig-gelichtetes Haarkleid auf und neigen vermehrt zu Infektionen von Haut, Atmungs- und/oder Verdauungsapparat (Husten, Nasenausfluß, Bronchopneumonie, Durchfall). Heute steht zwar fest, daß der kolostral vermittelte Schutz gegenüber solchen Krankheiten in erster Linie auf dem hohen Gehalt der Biestmilch an γ-Globulinen und der durch sie vermittelten passiven Immunität des Kalbes gegenüber den Erregern dieser Leiden beruht; unzureichender Versorgung mit Vitamin A kommt in der Pathogenese derartiger, an den Epithelien von Respirations- oder Digestionstrakt angreifender Infekte aber offenbar ebenfalls Bedeutung zu. Dabei ist des weiteren zu bedenken, daß die Ausnutzung von oral zugeführtem Vitamin A oder β-Karotin bei Enteritis behindert ist.

Mastrinder mit Hypovitaminose A zeigen außer amaurotischer Blindheit z. T. auch schlechtere Futterverwertung sowie bei körperlicher Anstrengung oder Beunruhigung gelegentlich Ohnmachtsanfälle. Mitunter stellen sich bei ihnen zudem ödematöse Anschwellungen am Triel und an den Gliedmaßenenden ein, die bis zum Schulter- und Sprunggelenk reichen können (»Wassermänner«). Hierfür werden Serumeiweißverschiebungen (Hypalbuminämie) verantwortlich gemacht. In der Pathogenese der bei Mastochsen nicht seltenen Harnsteinbildung (Kap. 7.2.4.1) scheint Vitamin-A-Mangel entgegen früherer Annahme keine wichtige Rolle zu spielen.

Bei *erwachsenen Rindern* äußert sich Hypovitaminose A meist in m. o. w. ausgeprägter Störung der Fruchtbarkeit: Dabei wird bei *weiblichen Tieren* weniger die Konzeptionsrate (verzögerter Wiedereintritt der Brunst p. p., embryonaler Fruchttod) als der normale Ablauf der Trächtigkeit gestört, was von Fall zu Fall in Abort, Tot- oder Frühgeburt, blind oder lebensschwach geborenem oder infektionsanfälligem Kalb, Nachgeburtsverhaltung und/oder unbefriedigender Milchleistung zum Ausdruck kommt. Zudem wirkt sich die Verabreichung von Vitamin A in manchen Fällen therapieresistenter »Winter«-Azetonämie offenbar günstig aus. Bei *männlichen Rindern* führt schwerer, vor der Geschlechtsreife einsetzender Vitamin-A-Mangel zu Unfruchtbarkeit infolge irreparabler Schädigung der Keimepithelien (Ausbleiben der Spermiogenese); fällt die Hypovitaminose A dagegen mit der beginnenden Zuchtreife zusammen, so sind die Veränderungen größtenteils reversibel. Bei erwachsenen Bullen beeinträchtigt mäßiger Vitamin-A-Mangel zwar die Samenqualität (→ Verminderung von Volumen, Spermiendichte und -beweglichkeit sowie Haltbarkeit des Ejakulats), doch bleibt ihre Libido meist erhalten. In besonders schweren Fällen kann das Aufsprungvermögen allerdings infolge Verengerung der Zwischenwirbellöcher und hierdurch bedingter Kompression der Spinalnervenwurzeln gestört sein.

Als von der Vitamin-A-Versorgung unabhängige, rein *Karotinmangel-bedingte Fertilitätsstörungen weiblicher Rinder* werden Brunstschwäche, Verzögerung der Ovulation, Entwicklung kleiner karotinarmer Gelbkörper, Rückgang der Progesteronbildung sowie Zunahme von Eierstockszysten, embryonalem Frühtod und Aborten genannt; diese Beobachtungen sind allerdings nicht unumstritten. Gleiches gilt für die Vermutung spezifisch *karotinbedingter Auswirkungen auf die Fruchtbarkeit von Jungbullen.*

Sektion: Konnatale Mikrophthalmie gibt sich durch erbsen- bis walnußgroße, in der Tiefe der Orbita liegende Bulbi zu erkennen; bei angeborener, Vitamin-A-Mangel-bedingter Blindheit ist außer Verengerung des Sehnervenkanals nicht selten innere Hydrozephalie festzustellen. Bei verendeten Saug- und Tränkekälbern zu beobachtende grauweißliche hyperkeratotische Epithelverquellungen in Maul, Rachen, Schlund und Vormägen werden ebenso wie zudem vorliegende pneumonische oder enteritische Veränderungen als Folge unzureichender Vitamin-A-Versorgung angesehen. Bei Jungrindern mit postnataler Vitamin-A-Mangel-Amaurose ist als kennzeichnender makroskopischer Befund eine dorsoventrale Einengung des Canalis opticus mit Ersatz des Sehnervs durch fibröses Gewebe zu ermitteln. *Histologisch* zeigen sich Schwund der Optikusganglienschicht der Netzhaut, Ödem der Sehnervenpapille, Degeneration von Stäbchen und Zapfen des Neuroepithels, Verfettung und WALLERsche Entartung des N. opticus. Die Hypophyse solcher Tiere weist multiple Zysten auf. Als pathognostisches Merkmal gilt die bei Hypovitaminose A schon frühzeitig einsetzende metaplastische Verhornung des Ohrspeicheldrüsengangs.

Diagnose: Bei Häufung konnataler Amaurose oder anderer Augenanomalien unter *Neugeborenen* ist durch Überprüfen des präkolostralen Vitamin-A-Gehalts der Leber festzustellen, ob es sich um Hypovitaminose A handelt; sonst sind erblich und viral bedingte Augendefekte in Betracht zu ziehen (Kap. 11.1.1). Bei *Kälbern und Jungrindern* geben bestandsweise gehäuftes Auftreten von Nachtblindheit oder völliger amaurotischer Blindheit sowie einseitige karotinarme Fütterung meist klare Hinweise auf Hypovitaminose A. Das Blutserum erscheint bei Vitamin-A-Mangel farblos-wasserklar. *Differentialdiagnostisch* ist an Bleivergiftung (Kap. 10.5.12), Milchkälbertetanie (Kap. 10.5.4.4), Listeriose (Kap. 12.2.10), Hirnrindennekrose (Kap. 10.5.5), Meningoenzephalitis (Kap. 10.3.1) sowie exogene und idiopathische Hitzeintoleranz (Kap. 10.6.4, 12.3.4) zu denken. Bei Fruchtbarkeitsstörungen *erwachsener Rinder*, die sich nicht auf Genitalinfektionen oder Primärerkrankungen anderer Organe zurückführen lassen, sollte die Fütterung auf Karotinmangel überprüft werden. Läßt sich der Verdacht einer Unterversorgung dabei nicht abklären, so liefert die vor Umstellung der Ernährung vorzunehmende Untersuchung bioptisch oder bei Schlachtung entnommener Lebergewebeproben auf ihren Vitamin-A-Gehalt Anhaltspunkte (s. Übersicht 11-1).

Beurteilung: Bei Vorliegen Hypovitaminose-A-bedingter zentralnervöser Symptome besteht keine Heilungsaussicht mehr; solche Fälle enden m. o. w. rasch tödlich. Auch bei bereits erblindeten Patienten ist von etwaiger Behandlung keine Wiederherstellung des Sehvermögens zu erwarten; die Patienten erweisen sich zudem meist als unwirtschaftlich oder erliegen interkurrenten enteritischen oder pneumonischen Infektionen. Dagegen lassen sich subklinische Auswirkungen der Hypovitaminose A, wie Nachtblindheit bei Jungtieren oder Fruchtbarkeitsstörungen erwachsener Rinder, durch Gaben von Vitamin A bzw. Steigerung der Karotinzufuhr meist gut beeinflussen. Die Fütterung solcher Tiere sollte jedoch stets auch auf anderweitige Mängel überprüft und erforderlichenfalls entsprechend ergänzt werden.

Behandlung: Die Umstellung der Ernährung auf karotinreiche Pflanzen oder Anreicherung des Futters mit Vitamin A (s. *Prophylaxe*) reicht für sich allein zur raschen Behebung schwerwiegender Mangelerscheinungen nicht aus. Intramuskulär injiziertes wasserdispergierbares Vitamin A ist seiner besseren Ausnutzung wegen therapeutisch wirksamer und wirtschaftlicher als oral verabreichtes oder als i.m. applizierte ölige Emulsionen. Von parenteralen Karotingaben ist kein nennenswerter Effekt zu erwarten. Die i.m. zu injizierende therapeutische Dosis von Vitamin A beträgt mindestens 400 IE pro kg LM (d.h. 20000–40000 IE für Kälber, 50000–200000 IE für Jungrinder, 250000–500000 IE für erwachsene Tiere); bei Kälbern sollte sie eine Woche lang täglich, bei Tieren der übrigen Altersgruppen nach 2 Wochen einmal wiederholt werden.

■ **Prophylaxe:** Besonderer Wert ist auf reichliche Karotinversorgung *tragender Rinder* zu legen. Um die Anlage körpereigener Reserven zu sichern und den Vitamin-A-Gehalt der Kolostralmilch zu steigern, sollte ihre Fütterung etwa 300 mg β-Karotin pro Tier und Tag enthalten. Für laktierende Tiere werden bei Milchleistungen von 10, 20 bzw. 30 l täglich 300, 500 bzw. 700 mg β-Karotin empfohlen. Läßt sich der Bedarf auf diese Weise, d. h. mit Grünfutter, gutem Heu, Luzernemehl oder -pellets, nicht decken, so müssen mit dem Kraftfutter Zulagen von künstlichem Vitamin A (50000–100000 IE pro Tier und Tag) verabreicht werden, das – im Gegensatz zu Karotin – auch den Fetus erreicht. Hierzu sind wegen der Oxidationsempfindlichkeit des Vitamin A stabilisierte Zubereitungen vorzuziehen, die nach 6monatiger Lagerung noch mindestens 50% ihrer ursprünglichen Wirksamkeit aufweisen. Dabei ist zu beachten, daß selbst stabilisiertes Vitamin A in Gegenwart von Mineral- oder Spurenelementsalzen nicht haltbar ist; solche dürfen daher erst kurz vor dem Verfüttern beigemengt werden.

Neugeborene Kälber sollten in den ersten 4–6 h p. p. Kolostralmilch erhalten (Kap. 1.2.3.1, 6.10.19). Nur wenn die Fütterung der tragenden Muttertiere (Winter, Frühjahr) karotinarm war, empfiehlt sich zudem, am 1.–3. Lebenstag je 30000–50000 IE Vitamin A p. o. oder i.m. zu verabreichen. Dabei ist zu bedenken, daß *Überdosierung von Vitamin A* die als *»Hyänenkrankheit«* bezeichnete Fehlentwicklung des Skeletts (Kap. 9.17.7) auslöst.

11.1.6 Haltungs- und sensibilitätsbedingte Krankheiten der Augen

Die Augenlider sind nicht nur bei *Nesselfieber/Urtikaria* (»Nilpferdkopf«, Kap. 2.2.7.1), sondern auch bei *Photosensibilitätsreaktionen* (Kap. 2.2.7.3) am Krankheitsgeschehen beteiligt; sonnenlichtbedingte Auswirkungen auf die Lider zeigen sich v. a. bei Rindern, deren Haut im Augenbereich unpigmentiert ist. Über diese Leiden ist angegebenenorts Näheres nachzulesen. Die Entwicklung von *»Weidekeratitis«* (Kap. 11.1.3.1) und *»Krebsauge«* (Kap. 11.1.7.1) wird offensichtlich durch Exposition gegenüber UV-Strahlen gefördert.

11.1.7 Tumorkrankheiten der Augen

Die Augenlider des Rindes werden nur sehr selten von nichtkarzinomatösen Geschwülsten betroffen, über welche Näheres bei den *Tumoren der Haut* (Kap. 2.2.9) nachzulesen ist (Abb. 11-33, 11-34). *Tumoröse Leukose* (Kap. 3.1.3.1) der retrobulbären Lymphfollikel kann Vorstülpung der Bindehaut, se-

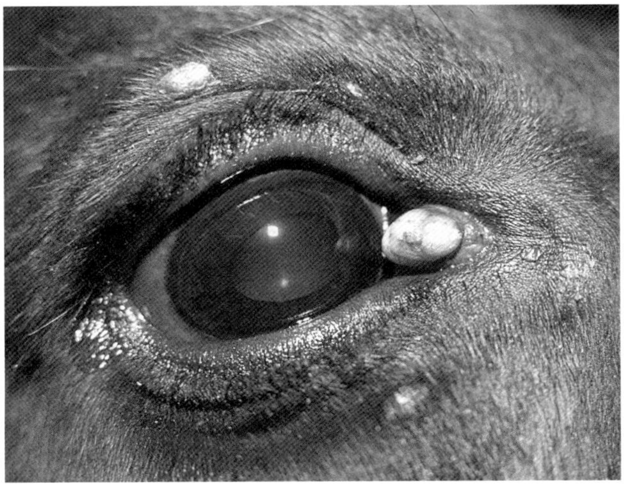

Abbildung 11-33 Der Lidbindehaut im medialen Augenwinkel aufsitzendes fungiformes Papillom (s. auch Kap. 2.2.3.4)

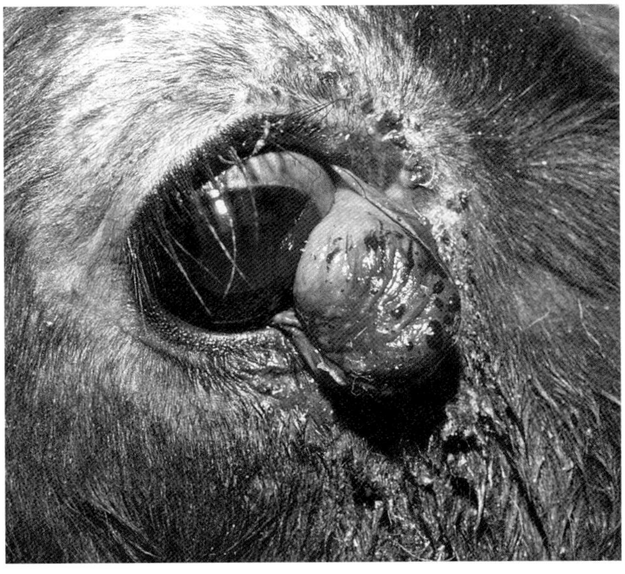

Abbildung 11-34 Von der Konjunktiva des dritten Augenlids ausgehendes Fibrom

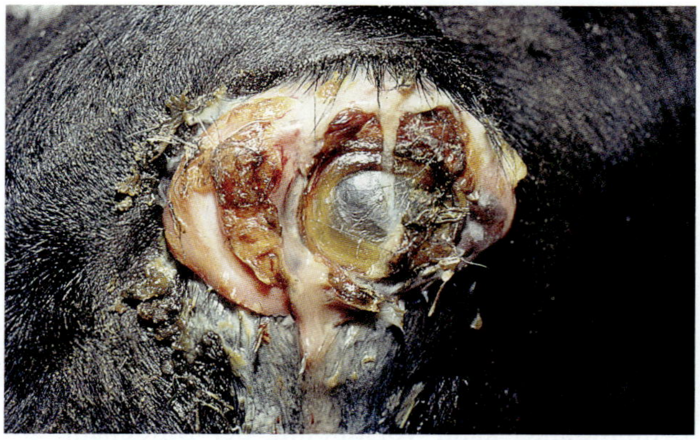

Abbildung 11-35 Panophthalmie infolge tumorösen Vorwucherns der retrobulbären Lymphfollikel und dadurch bedingter Austrocknung der Hornhaut bei enzootischer Erwachsenenleukose (s. auch Kap. 3.1.3.1)

kundären Ex- und Xerophthalmus sowie eitrige Panophthalmie bedingen (Abb. 11-35). Zudem sei auf die beim »Augenkrebs« (Kap. 11.1.7.1) unter *Differentialdiagnose* erwähnten Leiden verwiesen.

11.1.7.1 »Augenkrebs«

■ **Definition:** Maligne Entartung der Epithelien von Augenlid, Konjunktiva und/oder Hornhaut im Sinne eines Plattenepithelkarzinoms mit Neigung, auf benachbarte Organe überzugreifen. *Andere Bezeichnungen:* »Cancer eye«, bovine ocular squamous cell carcinoma.

■ **Vorkommen, Ursachen:** Neben Enzootischer Leukose ist Augenkrebs das häufigste Geschwulstleiden der Boviden. Das weltweit bekannte »Cancer eye« kann bei Schlachtrindern – je nach deren regionaler Exposition – Frequenzen von $\leq$ 0,9% erreichen und zum produktionsmindernden Faktor werden. Es betrifft v. a. intensiv gefütterte adulte Masttiere solcher Rassen, bei denen Augenlider und Hornhaut-Skleraübergang unpigmentiert sind (Herefords, Höhenfleckvieh/Simmentaler, Ayrshires, Charolais), wird aber nach verschleppter augennaher Verletzung auch bei Rindern mit pigmentierten Augenlidern beobachtet. Als weitere karzinogene Faktoren gelten massierte Haltung auf engem Raum, intensive Sonneneinwirkung (vermehrtes Vorkommen in Tropen und Subtropen sowie in Gebirgslagen), Rückgang der vor übermäßiger UV-Bestrahlung schützenden stratosphärischen Ozonschicht (was deutliche Zunahme des Leidens in den letzten Jahrzehnten bedingte) und mechanische Irritation (Staub, Fliegen- oder Augenwurmbefall). Möglicherweise kommt unzureichender Karotinzufuhr (Kap. 11.1.5.1), Keratokonjunktivitis-Erregern (Kap. 11.1.3), Herpes- oder Papillomatose-Viren (Kap. 5.1.3.1, 2.2.3.4) ebenfalls augenkrebsfördernde Wirkung zu. Die Beteiligung eines onkogenen Virus am Krankheitsgeschehen wird zwar vermutet, ist bislang aber nicht erwiesen. In tropischen Gebieten mit vermehrtem Vorkommen von bovinem Augenkrebs wird bei Weiderindern auch Hautkrebs des unpigmentierten Vulvabereichs gehäuft beobachtet.

■ **Pathogenese:** Bei der von der Außenfläche eines Augenlids, der Bindehaut von Ober-, Unter- oder drittem Augenlid, meist aber vom Augapfel, und zwar vom Hornhaut-Sklera-Übergang (lateraler oder medialer Limbus) ausgehenden Entwicklung der bösartigen Geschwülste sind 4 Stadien zu unterscheiden, die innerhalb von ¼ bis 2 Jahren durchlaufen werden:

➤ *Konjunktivale Plaque oder kutanes Akanthom/Keratom:* gutartiger linsengroßer, scharf umschriebener und infolge Epithelverdickung leicht erhöhter perlgrauer Schleimhautbereich mit glatter Oberfläche bzw. hauthornartige Zubildung auf der Lidaußenseite;
➤ *Konjunktivales oder epidermales Papillom:* erbsen- bis gut bohnengroße, an ihrer Oberfläche rauh-zerfranste, flach oder gestielt aufsitzende hyperkeratotische Gewebezubildung (s. Abb. 11-33);
➤ *Nicht-invasives Karzinom:* langsam größer werdende, aber noch abgegrenzte Gewebezubildung mit granulomatöser oder ulzerierender, m. o. w. blutiger Oberfläche;
➤ *Invasives Karzinom:* rasch wachsender, oberflächlich m. o. w. blumenkohlähnlich zerklüfteter, bröcklig-nekrotisierender, mit Blut, Schleim, Fibrin und/oder Eiter bedeckter, breitaufsitzender und in Nachbargewebe einwuchernder Tumor (Abb. 11-36).

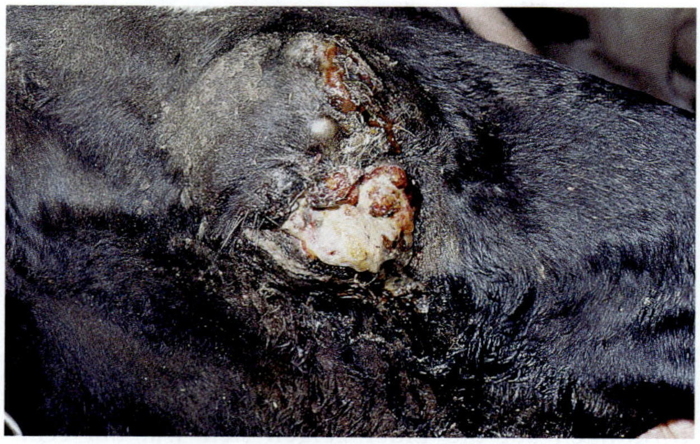

Abbildung 11-36 Durch verschleppte Augen- und Lidverletzung ausgelöstes Plattenepithelkarzinom (»cancer eye«) mit massiver Zerstörung der knöchernen Orbita

Bei der meist ein Auge, seltener beide Augen oder mehrere Lokalisationen eines Auges zugleich betreffenden Entwicklung der o. a. Geschwulststadien kommt es in etwa einem Drittel der Fälle zu spontaner Regression der Plaques oder Papillome; ein Drittel von ihnen kann allerdings später rezidivieren. Das manifeste okuläre Plattenepithelkarzinom befällt bei seiner invasiv-infiltrativen Ausbreitung auch Haut, Tränen- und Speicheldrüsen, regionale Lymphknoten, Schädelknochen und/oder Hirnnerven; lymphogene Metastasen in thorakalen Lymphknoten, Lunge, Pleura, Herz und/oder Nieren treten i. d. R. erst im Endstadium auf. Augenkrebsbedingte immunologische Reaktionen des Rindes waren Gegenstand mehrerer Untersuchungen; Immunprophylaxe und -therapie des Leidens sind aber noch nicht praxisreif.

Symptome: Die mäßig festen, sich immer weniger vom Nachbargewebe absetzenden und größer werdenden knotigen Umfangsvermehrungen bedingen Lidschwellung, zunehmenden Exophthalmus, eingeschränkte Beweglichkeit von Augenlidern und/oder Bulbus, Verschmutzung der Augapfeloberfläche und Expositionskeratitis; später kommt es zu ulzerierender bis perforativer Keratitis, Panophthalmie, übelriechender Exsudation (Abb. 11-36), Fliegen- oder Fliegenmadenbefall, Niedergeschlagenheit, schließlich auch zu Freßunlust sowie Anschwellung regionaler Lymphknoten.

Verlauf: Die Tumoren an Augenlid, Bindehaut oder Hornhaut wachsen zunächst wochen- bis monatelang nur langsam, dann aber rascher. Bei invasivem Einbruch in Nachbargewebe sind außer Blindheit des betroffenen Auges z. T. auch Schlingbeschwerden und/oder gleichseitige nervöse Ausfallserscheinungen (Lähmung des N. mandibularis oder des N. facialis) zu beobachten.

Histologie: Plaques zeigen Hyperplasie der Stachelzellschicht, Papillome dagegen Hyper- und Parakeratose. Die invasiven Tumoren sind typische oder anaplastische Plattenzellkarzinome mit deutlicher mitotischer Aktivität und Bildung von »Keratinperlen«.

Diagnose: Fortgeschrittener Augenkrebs ist aufgrund der geschilderten Veränderungen, insbesondere bei Rindern der o. a. Rassen, meist klar zu erkennen. In fraglichen Fällen sind *differentialdiagnostisch* Fibropapillomatose von Augenlid oder Hornhaut (Kap. 2.2.3.4), keratokonjunktivale Dermoide (Kap. 11.1.1.6), Komplikationen der infektiösen Keratokonjunktivitis (Kap. 11.1.3.1), Orbital- und Lidphlegmone, Leukose der retrobulbären Lymphfollikel (Kap. 3.1.3.1), angeborenes oder erworbenes Augenmelanom, Hornkrebs (Kap. 2.4.4.1), Stirnbeinosteosarkom (Kap. 2.4.4.2) und Siebbeinkarzinom (Kap. 5.1.7.1) in Betracht zu ziehen, was i. d. R. die histologische Untersuchung einer bioptisch entnommenen Gewebeprobe erfordert. Die an PAPANICOLAOU-gefärbten Abstrich- oder Abklatschpräparaten vorzunehmende zytologische Beurteilung auf Gut- oder Bösartigkeit bedarf entsprechender Erfahrung; für »Cancer eye« sprechen Chromatinverdichtung, deutliche Nukleolen, Anisonukleose, bizarre Mitosen, Mehrkernigkeit und Zunahme der Kern-Zytoplasma-Relation.

Beurteilung: Bei nur selten zur Vorstellung gelangenden frischen Fällen kann durch chirurgisches Eingreifen Heilung erzielt werden. Fortgeschrittene Karzinomatose des Auges und/oder seiner Adnexe gilt dagegen, v. a. bei Lymphknoten- oder Knochenbeteiligung, als prognostisch ungünstig; gegebenenfalls muß selbst bei radikalem operativen Vorgehen innerhalb von 4–8 Monaten mit Rezidiven gerechnet werden.

Behandlung: Frühestmögliche Exstirpation des Initialtumors im gesunden Nachbargewebe unter Schonung des Augapfels (z. B. Totalresektion des 3. Augenlids); bei nennenswertem Befall von Lidern und Bindehaut oder Beteiligung des Bulbus dagegen Eviszeration der Orbita (Kap. 11.1.8.6) und sorgfältige Resektion allen erkennbaren Geschwulstgewebes; sachgemäße postoperative Pflege, parenterale Gabe von Vitamin A. In frischen Fällen soll auch die intratumorale Verabreichung von BCG (Bacille CALMETTE-GUÉRIN) oder anderer, m. o. w. spezifischer Eiweißpräparate die Heilung fördern. Aufwendigere Verfahren (Hyperthermie, Kryochirurgie, Einlegen radioaktiver Pellets in das Geschwulstgewebe) sind unter Praxisbedingungen zu kompliziert und ebenfalls rezidivgefährdet.

Prophylaxe: Meiden der unter *Pathogenese* genannten Ursachen; exponierten Weiderindern schattengebende Schutzdächer anbieten. Bei Rinderrassen und -linien, deren Haut im Augenbereich unpigmentiert ist, Zuchtwahl auf Elimination dieses Merkmals ausrichten; die Augen solcher Tiere sollten alle 4 Monate überprüft und etwaige, über 5 mm große Plaques reseziert werden.

11.1.8 Operative Eingriffe im Augenbereich

Vorbereitungen: Zur Entfernung von Fremdkörpern aus dem Konjunktivalsack genügt es meist, diesen durch Einträufeln eines Lokalanästhetikums empfindungslos zu machen (Abb. 11-37). Blutige Eingriffe am Auge sollten jedoch stets am niedergelegten, sedierten und sachgemäß betäubten Patienten vorgenommen werden. Die Anästhesie erfolgt, je nach vorzunehmender Operation, durch rhombenförmige subkutan-subkonjunktivale Infiltration der Augenlider (dünne Kanüle, Abb. 11-38), durch Leitungsanästhesie des R. auriculopalpebralis Ni. facialis (subkutane Infiltration desselben im augenwärtigen Bereich der Ohrbasis mit 5–10 ml Lokalanästhetikum) sowie durch Blockade des am For. orbitorotundum zu erreichenden N. ophthalmicus (Abb. 11-39). Für letztere wird entweder eine leicht gebogene, 8–12 cm lange Kanüle vom medialen Augenwinkel her durch die Haut des Unterlids und nackenwärts der Unterwand der Orbita entlanggleitend bis zum hinteren Augenpol (nicht aber in den Sehnervenkanal) eingestochen, oder eine ebensolange gerade Hohlnadel unmittelbar im Winkel zwischen Proc. temporalis und Proc. frontalis des Jochbeins senkrecht bis zum Grund der Orbita eingeschoben. Hierhin wird dann ein Depot von 10 ml Betäubungsmittel injiziert. Danach wird das Operationsfeld behutsam, aber gründlich gewaschen, rasiert, trockengetupft, desinfiziert und situationsgerecht mit Schlitztuch oder -folie abgedeckt, ohne die Nasenatmung zu behindern.

➤ *Ophthalmo-chirurgische Regeln:* Wenn die Augenbewegungen während der Operation stören (Dermoid- oder Flügelfellresektion), läßt sich der Bulbus mittels zweier durch die sklerale Bindehaut geführter Haltezügel fixieren. Während des Eingriffes ist auf Blutstillung sowie knappe, aber vollständige Entfernung etwa krankhaft veränderten Gewebes besonders zu achten. Als Nahtmaterial ist im allgemeinen feiner resorbierbarer Faden vorzuziehen. Die Nähte sind zwei- oder dreischichtig und möglichst in Form von Einzelknopfheften auszuführen. An den Lidern zu setzende Hefte sollten stets konjunktivafern und neben (nicht auf) der Wunde geknüpft sowie in ihrem der Haut aufliegenden Bereich mit Zell- oder Kunststoffschaum unterpolstert, oder durch ein elastisches Plastikschläuchlein passender Stärke und Länge geführt werden, um Drucknekrosen vorzubeugen.

➤ *Postoperative Versorgung:* Örtliche Antibiose, bedarfsweise auch Einlegen eines Drains; Aufkleben oder Anheften eines Beetverbandes, der vorteilhafterweise noch mit einem über den Stirnschädel zu ziehenden Strumpfnetz fixiert wird; Unterbringen des Patienten in abgedunkeltem Anbindestall (die nicht

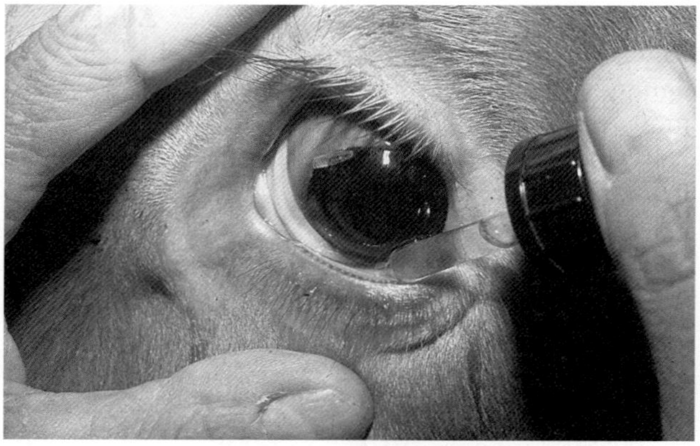

Abbildung 11-37 Örtliche Betäubung für Eingriffe im Lid-, Bulbus- und Orbitalbereich: Einträufeln eines Oberflächenanästhetikums in den Bindehautsack mit Hilfe einer Tropfpipette

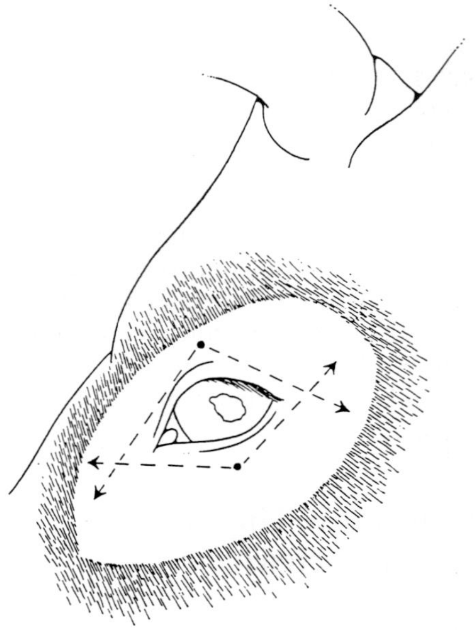

Abbildung 11-38 Subkutane (= subkonjunktivale) Infiltrationsanästhesie parallel zu den Lidrändern

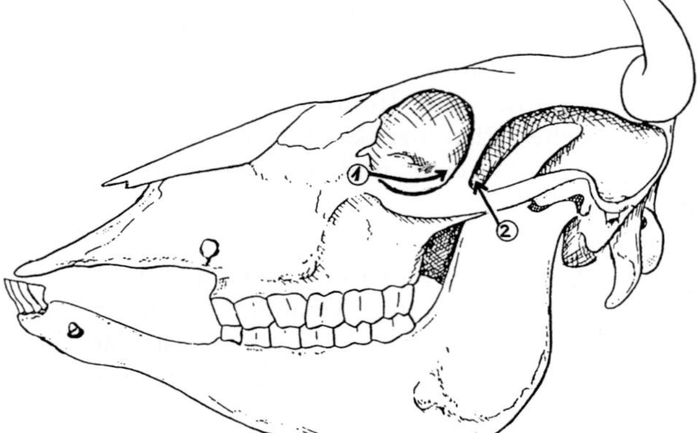

Abbildung 11-39 Leitungsanästhesie des N. ophthalmicus am For. orbitorotundum nach Einstich durch das Unterlid (1) oder im Winkel zwischen Stirn- und Schläfenfortsatz des Jochbeins (2) (nach Pasquini, 1982)

operierte Körperseite zur Wand gerichtet), vorzugsweise in einer Einzelbox; Anlegen eines Vergrittungsgeschirrs, um das den Heilvorgang u. U. in Frage stellende Kratzen der Wunde mit den Hinterklauen zu verhüten; Fliegenbekämpfung (Kap. 2.2.4.1); zunächst täglich, später alle 2–3 Tage vorzunehmende Kontrolle des Heilverlaufs am gut fixierten Kopf: Verbandswechsel, Drainkürzung/-erneuerung, Wundrevision, erneute lokale antibiotische Versorgung; bedarfsweise mehrtägige parenterale Keimhemmung mit Breitbandantibiotika. Bei Anbindehaltung sollte das betreffende Tier nach Ausheilung an das seinem operativ behandelten Auge entsprechende Ende der Standreihe gestellt werden. Wenn die Augenerkrankung auf Hornstoß beruhte, ist Enthornung der Herde (Kap. 2.4.5.2) zu erwägen.

11.1.8.1 Dermoidresektion

Die Hautinsel (Kap. 11.1.1.6; s. Abb. 11-4) wird mittels Pinzette, Arterienklemme oder kleiner Faßzange leicht vorgezogen und, falls sie der Bindehaut entspringt, durch Scherenschlag entfernt, falls sie der Hornhaut aufsitzt, jedoch schichtweise vorsichtig mit dem Skalpell abgetragen, bis alle Haarfollikel beseitigt sind. Der bei Resektion des Dermoids entstandene konjunktivale Defekt wird durch Einzelhefte mit resorbierbarem Faden vernäht und das unverbunden bleibende Auge bis zur Abheilung 2mal täglich mit antibiotischer Augensalbe versorgt. Falls die Kornea angegangen werden mußte, empfiehlt es sich, eine temporäre Bindehautschürze anzulegen.

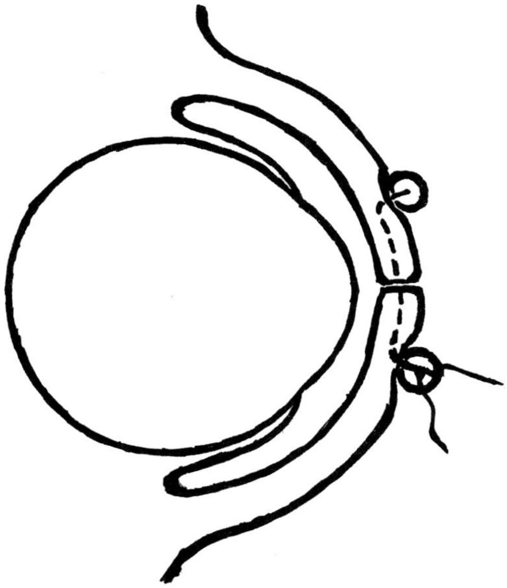

Abbildung 11-40 Temporäre Bindehautschürze (Blepharorrhaphie; schematisch): Nahtführung im Vertikalschnitt durch das Auge

11.1.8.2 Temporäre Bindehautschürze

Das mit Stallhaltung und zweckmäßigerweise mit subkonjunktivaler Injektion eines antibiotischen Depots zu kombinierende 4- bis 8tägige Abdecken des Augapfels mit der Lidbindehaut ist der Heilung schwerwiegender Hornhautreizungen und -defekte dienlich. Hierzu kann man den freien Rand von Unter- und Oberlid durch drei nur die Haut des Lidrandes, nicht aber die Bindehaut durchstechende und den medialen Augenwinkel offen lassende Doppel-U-Hefte miteinander vereinigen (= *Tarso- oder Blepharorrhaphie*; Abb. 11-40, 11-41). Den gleichen Effekt bietet die sogenannte *»Nickhautschürze«*, bei welcher die Konjunktiva des dritten Augenlids sowie der Blinzknorpel mit einem die bulbuswärtige Bindehaut nicht durchstechenden Fadenzügel erfaßt, gegen den lateralen Augenwinkel gezogen und dort verankert werden. Bei beiden Verfahren empfiehlt es sich, die auf der Haut zu liegen kommenden Abschnitte der Hefte elastisch zu unterpolstern oder durch ein Plastik- oder Gummischläuchlein zu führen. Der Zustand der Bindehautschürze ist regelmäßig zu kontrollieren und der Konjunktivalsack täglich mit antibiotischer Augensalbe zu versorgen. Falls sich zeigt, daß die ergriffene Maßnahme den Augapfel irritiert, müssen die Fäden vorzeitig entfernt werden.

11.1.8.3 Blepharoplastik

➤ *Lidverletzungen* lassen sich nur frisch, 6–12 h nach Entstehung, oder erst nach dem Einsetzen sauberer Granulation erfolgreich operativ angehen. Wenn der Patient mit verschlepptem Lidtrauma, d. h. mit phlegmonösen, eiternden oder nekrotisierenden Läsionen, vorgestellt wird, sollte er zunächst 8–14 Tage lang regelmäßig konservativ (Spülungen, Auf-/Einbringen salbenförmiger Antibiotika auf die Wundränder und

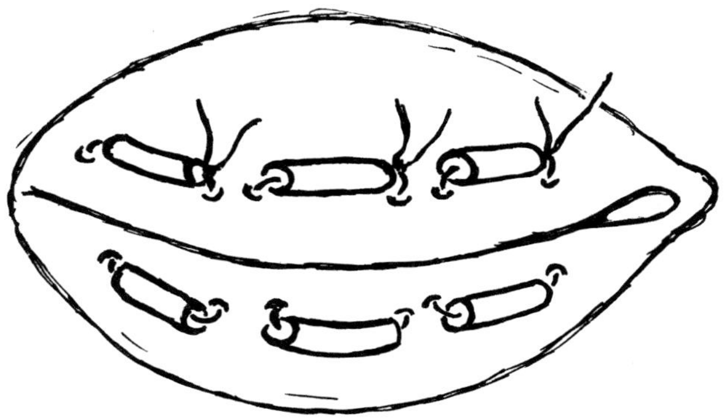

Abbildung 11-41 Blepharorrhaphie-Naht in der Aufsicht: Die drei U-Hefte berühren die Hornhaut nicht; ihre auf der Lidhaut liegenden Abschnitte wurden durch Plastik- oder Gummischläuchlein geführt (→ Polsterung)

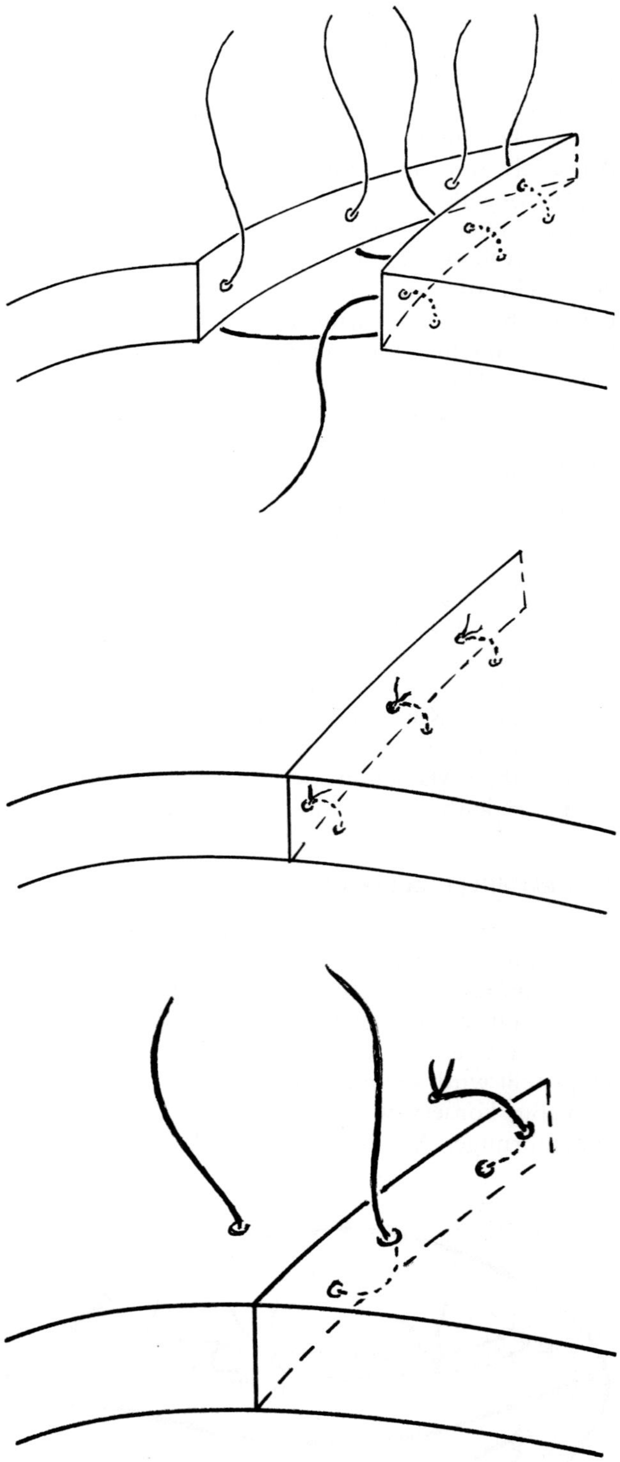

Abbildung 11-42 bis 11-44 Nahtführung bei Lidverletzungen (schematisch; Lidhaut oben, Lidbindehaut unten): Oben: Nach Wundrevision und situationsgerechter Resektion des Defekts werden die konjunktivalen Wundränder durch Einzelhefte miteinander vereinigt; Mitte: Bindehauthefte subkonjunktival verknotet; unten: Setzen der die Lidwundränder vereinigenden Einzelhefte und Verknoten derselben neben dem Wundrandverlauf

in den Bindehautsack) behandelt werden, bis die Demarkation abgeschlossen ist und die Verletzung zu granulieren beginnt. Danach sind die schonend aufgefrischten Wundränder durch situationsgerechte, im Bereich von Lidhaut und -bindehaut zu setzende Einzelknopfhefte (resorbierbarer Faden) miteinander zu vereinigen (Abb. 11-42 bis 11-44).

➤ *Entropium:* Die Korrektur des eingerollten Augenlids erfolgt durch Abpräparieren eines breitenmäßig dem Grad der Einrollung anzupassenden spindelförmigen Hautlappens, ohne die Bindehaut zu durchtrennen; die lidrandwärtige Kurvatur des Lappens ist etwa 5 mm vom Lidrand und parallel zu diesem zu setzen. Diese Resektionswunde wird in subkonjunktival zu legenden Einzelknopfheften vernäht.

11.1.8.4 Exenteration des Bulbus

Dieser Eingriff ist nur bei nicht auf die Adnexe übergreifender schwerwiegender Erkrankung des Augapfels angezeigt. Hierzu wird der Bulbus mittels Hornhaut-Kreuzschnitts eröffnet und sein Inneres mit dem scharfen Löffel ausgeräumt (Abb. 11-45). In der Folge ziehen sich die fibrösen Schichten des Augapfels unter wiederholter örtlicher Antibiose allmählich vernarbend zusammen, doch besteht Gefahr bleibender, u. U. eitriger Konjunktivitis.

11.1.8.5 Enukleation des Augapfels

Bei dieser Operation wird der Bulbus nacheinander aus episkleraler Bindehaut, TENONscher Kapsel und Augenmuskeln herausgeschält (Abb. 11-46). Dann wird er leicht vorgezogen und der Sehnerv mit gebogener Schere durchtrennt. Die anschließend antibiotisch zu versorgende und zu tamponierende Wundhöhle bedarf bis zur völligen Ausgranulierung regelmäßiger Kontrolle und Nachversorgung. Der Eingriff ist komplikationsträchtig (Neigung zu Orbitalphlegmone).

11.1.8.6 Eviszeration der Augenhöhle

Dieses Vorgehen hat im Vergleich zu den beiden vorgenannten Techniken den Vorteil, daß der unheilbar erkrankte Bulbus samt etwa mitbetroffenen Adnexen entfernt und die Lider weitgehend verschlossen werden, was gute Heilungsaussichten bietet (Abb. 11-47 bis 11-55). Zunächst wird die Haut von Ober- und Unterlid 0,5 cm vom Lidrand entfernt und parallel zu diesem gespalten, ohne die Lidbindehaut zu durchtrennen. Von diesem spitzelliptischen Schnitt aus wird ringsherum subkutan/subkonjunktival stumpf bis auf den knöchernen Rand der Orbita vorgegangen. Dann werden die abgetrennten Lidränder mittels Faßzange oder Arterienklemme aneinandergedrückt und leicht vorgezogen. An Ober- und Unterlid sind Haltezügel anzulegen und jeweils situationsgerecht so anzuspannen, daß der Augapfel nun samt Anhangsorganen (TENONsche Kapsel, Tränendrüsen, Muskeln) aus der Orbita freipräpariert werden kann. Nach dem Durchtrennen von N. opticus und A. centralis retinae setzt eine durch Drucktamponade zu beherrschende Blutung ein. Nach Resektion sämtlicher krankhaft veränderter Gewebereste wird die Orbita gut mit antibiotisch getränkter Gaze austamponiert. Schließlich sind die Wundränder beider Augenlider durch lateral beginnende fortlaufende Naht so miteinander zu vernähen, daß der Gazedrain am medialen Augenwinkel etwas aus dem Wundspalt vorsteht. Ein mittels Netzstrumpf fixierter Beetverband schließt den Eingriff ab. Bei den regelmäßig vorzunehmenden Nachkontrollen ist der Drain jeweils stückweise zu entfernen, im Falle starker Wundexsudation oder Geruchsabweichung dagegen zu erneuern. Der aus nicht resorbierbarem Material zu wählende Faden des künstlichen Ankyloblepharons ist nach 2–3 Wochen zu ziehen. Die »entleerte« Augenhöhle füllt sich im Zuge der Heilung mit Granulationsgewebe.

Bei Eviszeration der Orbita von »Augenkrebs«-Patienten (Kap. 11.1.7.1) wird es nicht selten erforderlich, tumorös verändertes Lidgewebe zu entfernen; gegebenenfalls ist ein ordnungsgemäßer Wundverschluß nur nach *V-, H- oder Löffelstiel-Lappenschnitt* und *situationsgerechter Adaptation der abpräparierten Hautränder* möglich (= Verschiebeplastik). Näheres hierzu ist dem ophthalmo-chirurgischen Schrifttum zu entnehmen.

11.2 Krankheiten der Ohren

M. STÖBER/H. SCHOLZ

Im Vergleich zu den Ohrenleiden von Hund und Katze sind diejenigen des Rindes wesentlich seltener; im Hinblick auf Tierschutz und leistungsmindernde Auswirkungen verdienen sie jedoch Beachtung. Im folgenden sollen die *idiopathischen Erkrankungen* der Ohren und ihrer Anhangsorgane besprochen werden,

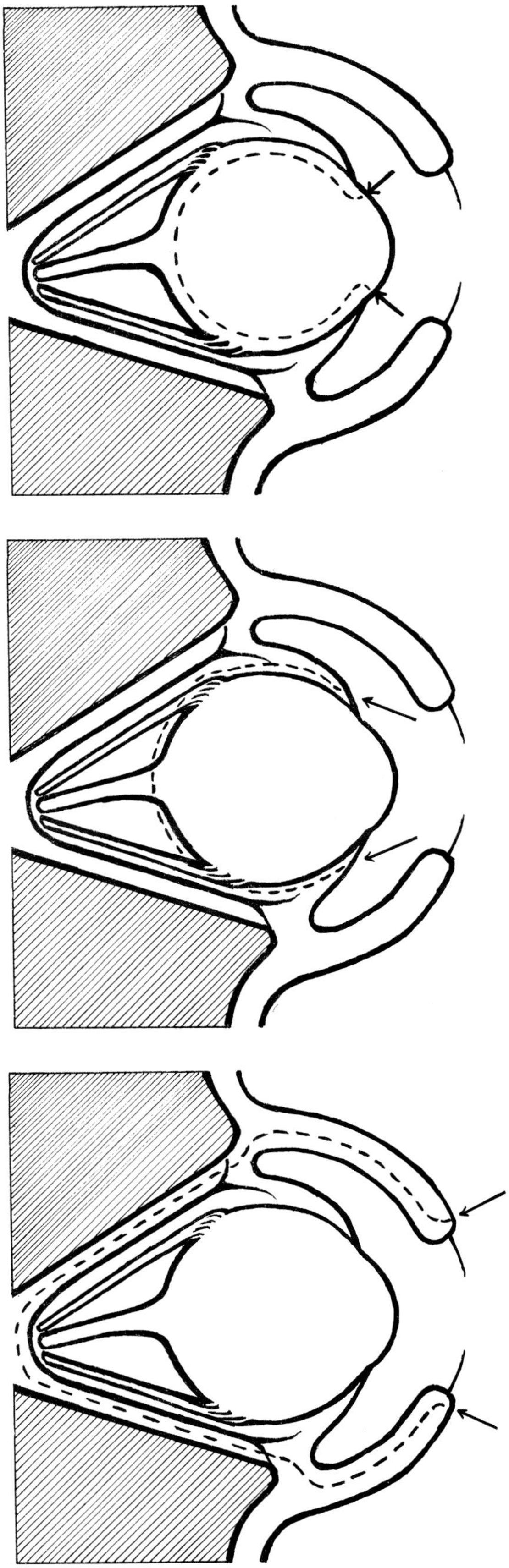

Abbildung 11-45 bis 11-47 Operative Eingriffe am Augapfel (Längsschnitt, schematisch; Orbitalknochen schraffiert mit periorbitalem Periost, tiefer Orbitalfaszie, Bulbus und Adnexen; Schnittführung jeweils an den Pfeilen beginnend und der gestrichelten Linie folgend). Oben: Exenteration des Augapfelinhalts; Mitte: Enukleation des Bulbus ohne dessen Adnexe; unten: Eviszeration der Orbita

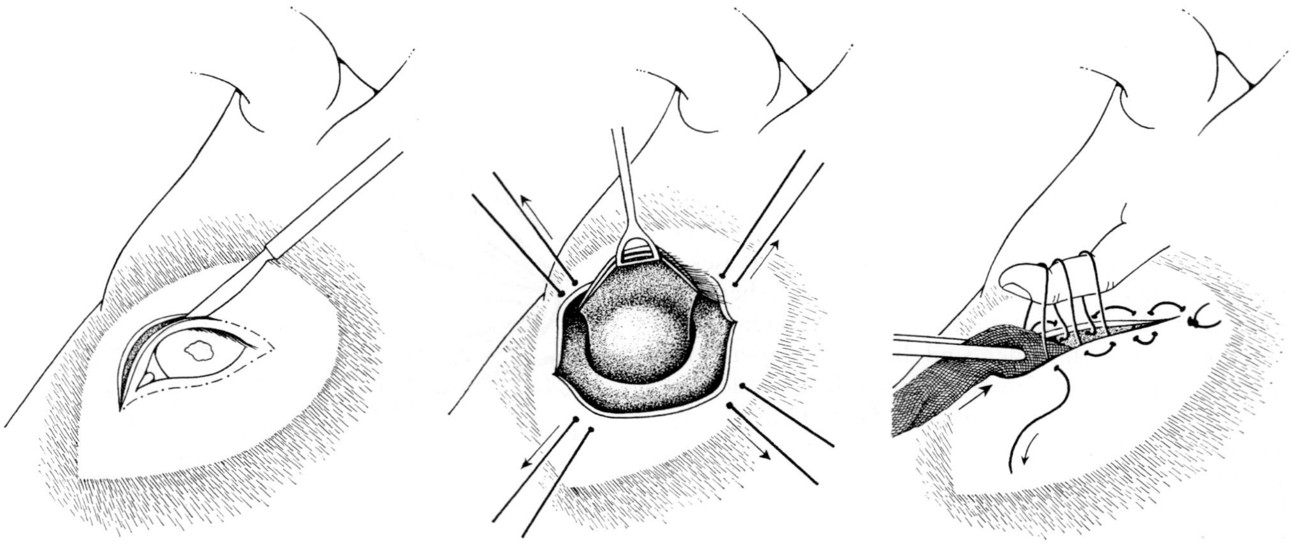

Abbildung 11-48 bis 11-50 Eviszeration der Augenhöhle (Aufsicht). Links: Spalten der Lidhaut parallel zum Lidrand; Mitte: stumpfes subkonjunktival-extrafasziales Freipräparieren des Augapfels samt seiner Adnexe, der hierzu mit einer auf die Lidränder gesetzten Faßzange vorgezogen und dann auf dem Grund der Orbita abgesetzt wird (Operationsfeld mittels Haltezügeln situationsgerecht freigehalten); unten: Vernähen der Lidränder (Ankyloblepharon) und Einlegen eines antibiotisch getränkten Gazedrains in die ausgeräumte Orbita (Drucktamponade)

während ihre *symptomatische Beteiligung* an anderweitigen Krankheiten jeweils beim primär befallenen Organsystem erwähnt wird; entsprechende *differentialdiagnostische Seitenverweise* werden im Rahmen dieses Kapitels gegeben.

11.2.1 Erbliche und andersbedingte Mißbildungen der Ohren

■ **Definition:** Angeborene Anomalien der Ohrmuschel kommen bei Kälbern weit seltener vor als solche der Augen. Sie treten teils ein-, teils beidseitig auf und sind in ausgeprägten Fällen meist mit Fehlentwicklungen von Mittel- und Innenohr verbunden.

■ **Symptome:** Als *Anotie* (Ohrlosigkeit) wird das Fehlen einer oder beider Ohrmuscheln samt Adnexen bezeichnet; beim Polnischen Rotbunt-Rind tritt diese Anomalie zusammen mit erblicher Hornhauttrübung (Kap. 11.1.1.7) auf. *Mikrotie*, d. h. Unterentwicklung einer oder beider Ohrmuscheln (Klein- oder Stummelohrigkeit; Abb. 11-56), kommt teils selbständig, teils zusammen mit unilateral-divergierendem Schielen, bei mandibulo-aurikulärer Dysostose, Akroteriasis (Kap. 9.10.12) oder Ichthyosis congenita (Kap. 2.2.1.3) vor. Angeborene *Ohrrandkerben* (notched ears) wurden bei Ayrshire-, Jersey- und Highland-Kälbern als beidseitig auftretender einfach autosomal-dominanter Erbfehler mit unvollständiger Penetranz beobachtet; sie sind wegen Fehlens narbiger Retraktionen leicht von ansaug- oder verletzungsbedingten Krüppelohren (Kap. 11.2.2.3) zu unterscheiden. Echte *Polyotie*, d. h. das Vorkommen zusätzlicher, knorpelgestützter Ohrmuscheln im Stirn- oder Schläfenbereich (Mehrohrigkeit), darf nicht mit den bei erblicher Lymphgefäßstauung (Kap. 3.1.1.1) im ohrnahen Bereich auftretenden Hautanhängseln verwechselt werden. Als *Otodystopie* wird abnormer, meist weiter halswärts gelegener Ansatz der Ohren am Kopf bezeichnet. *Otozephale Synotie* gibt sich durch ein einzelnes, meist halswärts gelegenes »zusammengewachsenes« Ohr und Fehlen der Unterkiefer, mitunter auch durch Zyklopie (Kap. 11.1.1.3) zu erkennen; solche Kälber sterben vor oder während der Geburt.

■ **Ursachen, Beurteilung:** Die Pathogenese angeborener Ohrdefekte bleibt meist unaufgeklärt; lebensfähige Merkmalsträger sollten nicht zur Zucht benutzt werden.

11.2.2 Unspezifisch bedingte Krankheiten der Ohren

11.2.2.1 Abnorme Ohrhaltung

Fehlhaltung eines oder beider, im übrigen aber gesunder Ohren kann wertvolle Hinweise auf Erkrankungen anderer Organsysteme geben: rückwärts gestellte Ohren bei *Tetanus* (Kap. 10.3.8) und *Weidetetanie*

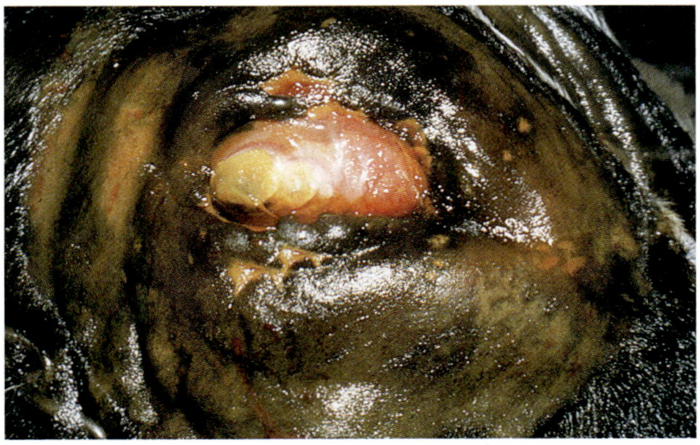

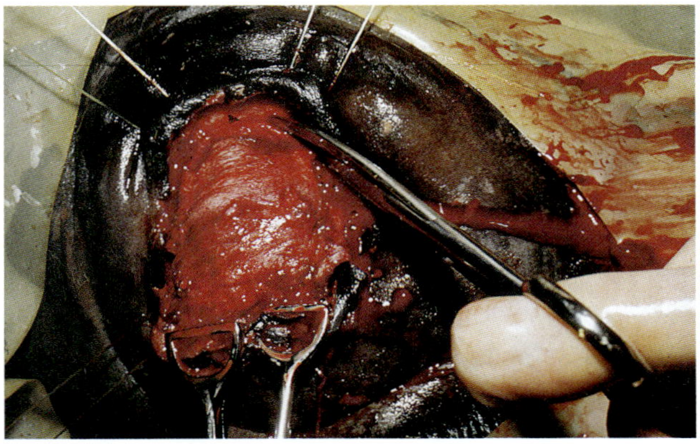

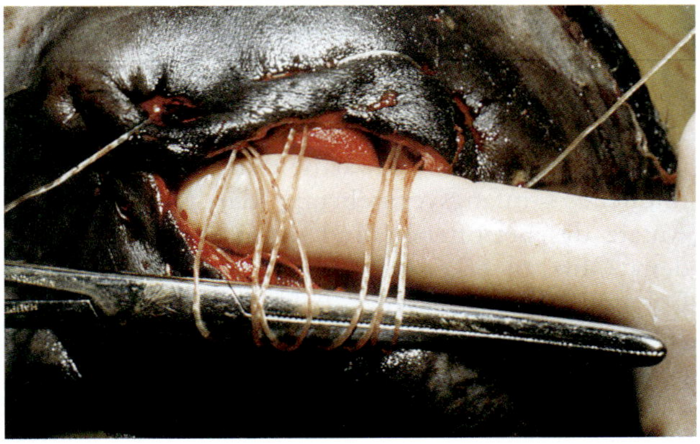

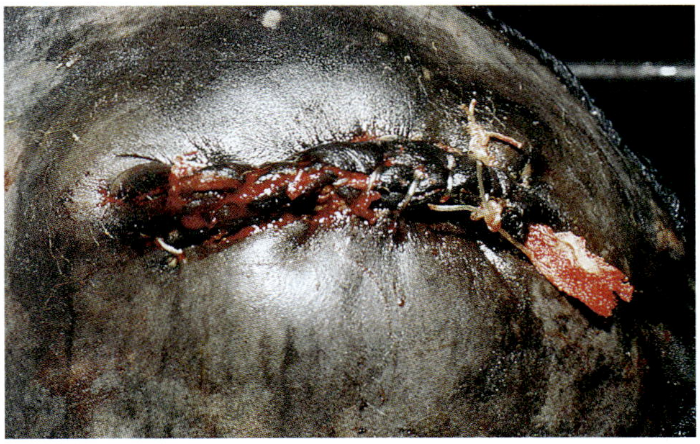

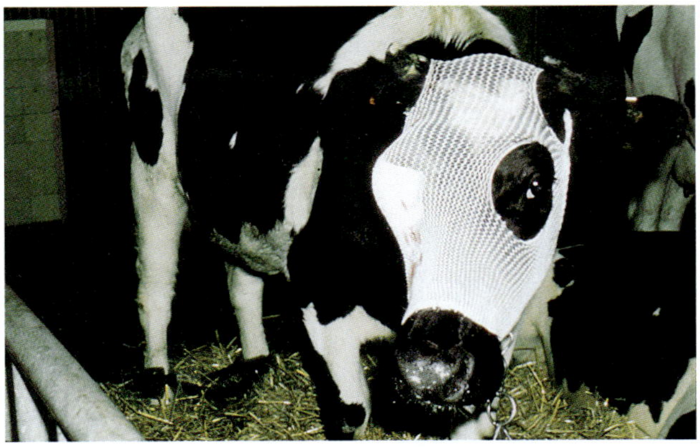

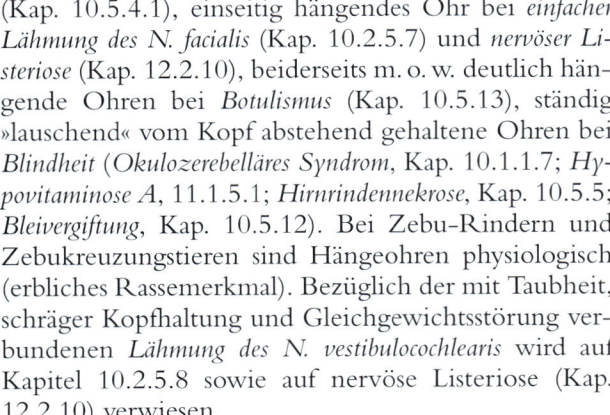

Abbildung 11-51 bis 11-55 Eviszeration der Orbita (am Tier).
Oben links: Operationsfeld anästhesiert, rasiert und desinfiziert;
oben rechts: Herausschälen des Bulbus samt Adnexen (Lidspalte mittels Faßzange verschlossen);
Mitte links: Drucktamponade der ausgeräumten Augenhöhle, Beginn der Lidnaht;
Mitte rechts: Ankyloblepharon beendet, Drainende im medialen Augenwinkel;
unten links: Netzstrumpf-Schutzverband

(Kap. 10.5.4.1), einseitig hängendes Ohr bei *einfacher Lähmung des N. facialis* (Kap. 10.2.5.7) und *nervöser Listeriose* (Kap. 12.2.10), beiderseits m. o. w. deutlich hängende Ohren bei *Botulismus* (Kap. 10.5.13), ständig »lauschend« vom Kopf abstehend gehaltene Ohren bei *Blindheit* (*Okulozerebelläres Syndrom*, Kap. 10.1.1.7; *Hypovitaminose A*, 11.1.5.1; *Hirnrindennekrose*, Kap. 10.5.5; *Bleivergiftung*, Kap. 10.5.12). Bei Zebu-Rindern und Zebukreuzungstieren sind Hängeohren physiologisch (erbliches Rassemerkmal). Bezüglich der mit Taubheit, schräger Kopfhaltung und Gleichgewichtsstörung verbundenen *Lähmung des N. vestibulocochlearis* wird auf Kapitel 10.2.5.8 sowie auf nervöse Listeriose (Kap. 12.2.10) verwiesen.

11.2.2.2 Ohrzittern

Tremor auris ist Begleiterscheinung vieler, mit zentralnervöser Erregung verbundener Krankheiten ohne eigene pathognostische Bedeutung.

11.2.2.3 Verletzungen der Ohrmuschel

Solche Läsionen sind beim Rind vergleichsweise häufig. Sie beruhen von Fall zu Fall auf *Kerbkennzeichnung* (Abb. 11-57), *Ausreißen der Ohrmarke*, *Stacheldrahtriß* oder auf *Bissen wildernder Hunde*. Tierärztliche Hilfe wird i. d. R. nur bei anhaltender Blutung oder langwieriger Eiterung erbeten (Abb. 11-58). Dabei ist

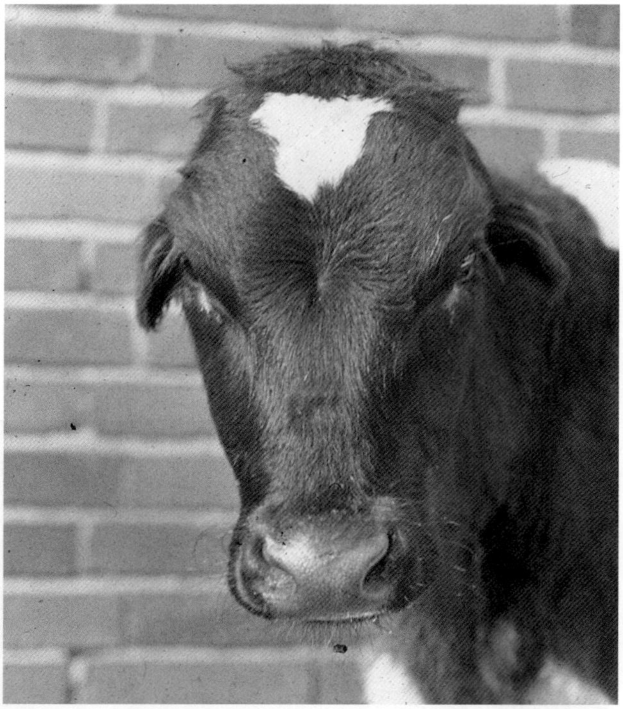

Abbildung 11-56 Beiderseitige Stummelohrigkeit (Mikrotie)

nach den Regeln der Wundversorgung (Kap. 2.2.2.7) vorzugehen sowie darauf zu achten, daß sich kein Exsudat im äußeren Gehörgang ansammelt und sich das Tier nicht mit den Hinterklauen am verletzten Ohr kratzt (Anbindehaltung und Vergrittungsgeschirr). Mit bleibender Deformation der Ohrmuschel muß gerechnet werden (Abb. 11-59).

11.2.2.4 Othämatom

Bei gruppengehaltenen Tränkekälbern werden als Folge gegenseitigen Besaugens gelegentlich Blutergüsse am Ohr beobachtet; bei älteren Tieren kommen Othämatome mitunter als Folge lokalen Juckreizes vor. Das betreffende Ohr weist dabei eine bis zu faustgroße subkutan-fluktuierende Anschwellung auf und hängt gewichtsbedingt herab (Abb. 11-60, 11-61). Zur Behandlung ist die Haut des betreffenden Bereichs mit resorptionsfördernder Salbe zu bestreichen; operatives Ausräumen des Blutergusses ist meist nicht erforderlich. Wichtig ist es jedoch, das Besaugen zu unterbinden (Kap. 10.6.1.2) bzw. eine etwaige, zum Kratzen führende parasitär-, fremdkörper- oder andersbedingte Gehörgangsentzündung (Kap. 11.2.3.2) zu ermitteln und zu beheben. Nach Resorption des Blutergusses bleibt meist ein m. o. w. verschrumpeltes Krüppelohr, mitunter aber ein sklerodermes Ohr (Elefantiasis) zurück.

11.2.3 Infektionsbedingte Krankheiten der Ohren

Die Haut der Ohrmuschel kann von *Aktinobazillose* (Kap. 3.1.3.3), *Fibropapillomatose* (Kap. 2.2.3.4), *Trichophytie* (Kap. 2.1.3.1), *Dermatophilose* (Kap. 2.2.3.6) und *Hautknotenkrankheit* (Kap. 2.2.3.7) betroffen sein; mit *Boviner Leukozyten-Adhäsions-Defizienz* (Kap. 4.3.1.6) behaftete Kälber zeigen mitunter als ersten Hinweis auf diesen Erbfehler überschießende und stark sezernierende Granulation an dem beim Einziehen der Ohrmarke gesetzten Hautdefekt. Über diese Krankheiten ist angegebenenorts Näheres nachzulesen.

11.2.3.1 Ohrbasisphlegmone

Dieses Leiden gibt sich als faust- bis kindskopfgroße, mäßig derbe, vermehrt warme und berührungsempfindliche Umfangsvermehrung der Unterhaut am Ansatz des betroffenen und dabei zudem »hängenden« Ohrs zu erkennen (Abb. 11-62). Eine solche Entzündung ist entweder Folge verschleppter infizierter Verletzungen oder einer versehentlich neben (statt in) die Ohrvene erfolgten Dauertropfinfusion. Das Vorkommnis erfordert Ruhigstellung (Anbindehaltung, Vergrittungsgeschirr), sachgemäße Wundversorgung (Kap. 2.2.2.7) bzw. Auftragen kühlender Salbe/Paste sowie mehrtägige parenterale Antibiose. Bei ausbleibender Behandlung muß mit ständigem Juckreiz, zentraler Verjauchung, Hautnekrose, Verlust des Ohrs und maligner Entartung beteiligter Gewebe gerechnet werden.

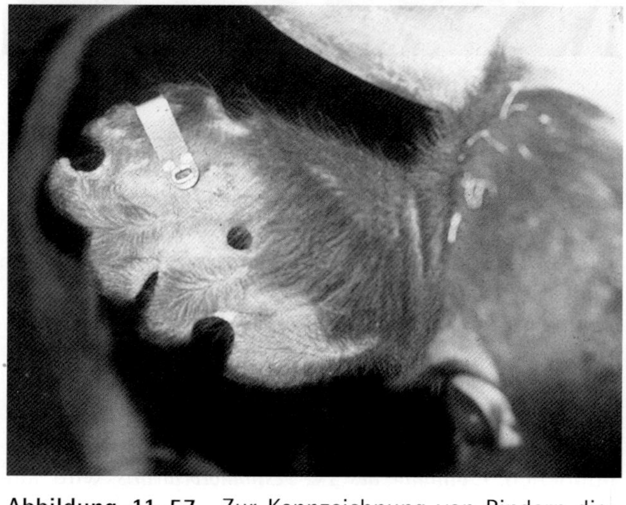

Abbildung 11-57 Zur Kennzeichnung von Rindern dienende Kerbung des Ohrrandes

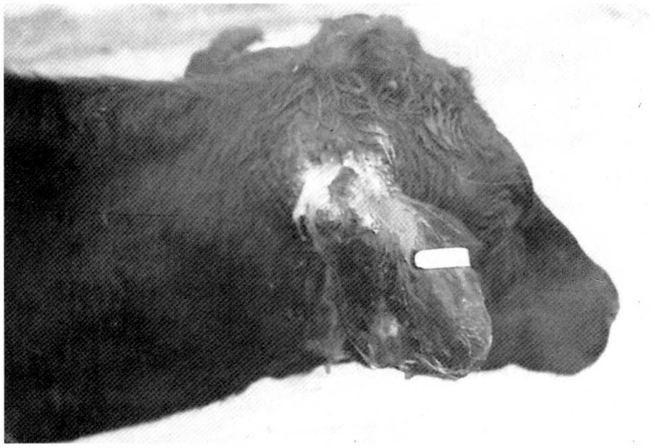

Abbildung 11-58 Ohrmuschelverletzungen: phlegmonös-eiternde Hundebißverletzung an der Ohrbasis

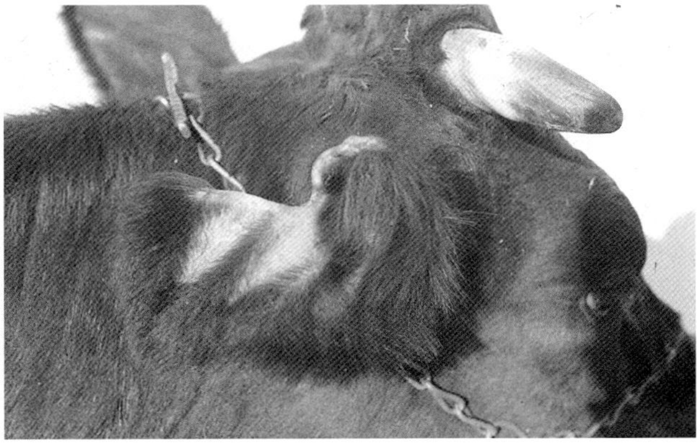

Abbildung 11-59 Vernarbtes »Schlitzohr« infolge Ausreißens der Ohrmarke

11.2.3.2 Entzündung von äußerem Gehörgang, Mittel- oder Innenohr

Definition: Über die Hörtrompete, hämatogen oder von außen her eingeschleppte, mit m. o. w. ausgeprägter Störung von Allgemeinbefinden, Hörvermögen und/oder Gleichgewichtssinn verbundene Infektion des Ohres mit saprophytären und pyogenen Keimen (*Otitis media, interna* bzw. *externa*).

Vorkommen: Bei Tränkekälbern ist das Leiden nicht selten und wird mitunter sogar zum Bestandsproblem. In bestimmten Gruppen erkranken 10–20% der Tiere, und zwar meist innerhalb der ersten 3 Wochen nach Einstellung. Manchmal tritt die bovine Otitis aber erst im Jährlingsalter in Erscheinung. Je nach den Begleitumständen wird sie vereinzelt auch beim erwachsenen Rind beobachtet.

Ursachen, Pathogenese: Im Rahmen septikämisch verlaufender Kälberkrankheiten kann es zur *hämatogenen* Besiedlung des Innenohrs mit pyogenen Keimen kommen, die meist von lokaler Meningitis begleitet

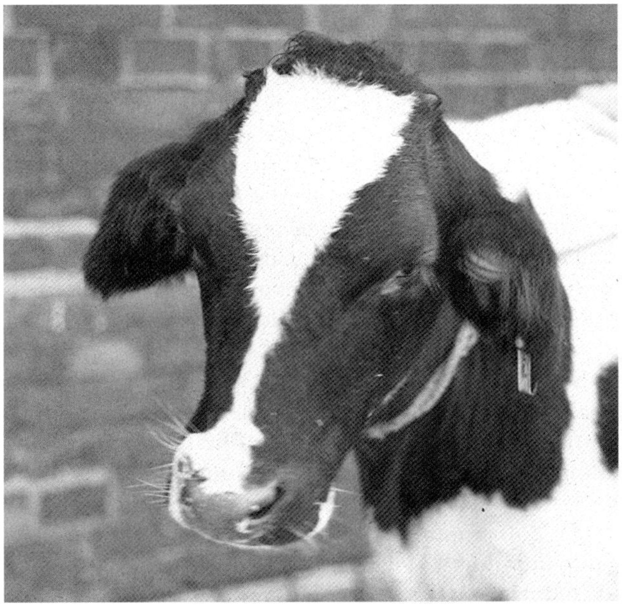

Abbildung 11-60 Beiderseitiges ansaugbedingtes Othämatom bei einem gruppengehaltenen offeneimergetränkten Kalb

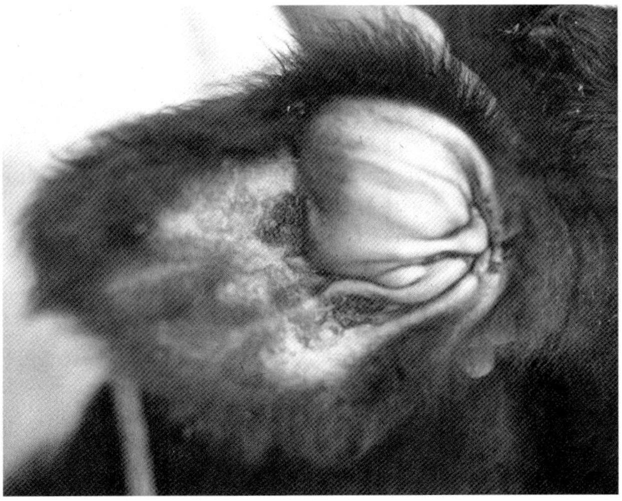

Abbildung 11-61 Ansicht eines der beiden Blutergüsse der Abb. 11-60 von der Ohrinnenseite her

wird. Bei gruppengehaltenen Aufzucht- oder Mastkälbern und -jungbullen erfolgt die Infektion des Ohrs entweder *über die EUSTACHische Röhre*, und zwar in Zusammenhang mit Affektionen der oberen Luftwege, bei Verabreichung der Milch von Kühen mit Mykoplasmen-Mastitis sowie beim Übergang zur Fütterung mit Trockenfutter (Schrot, Schnitzel, Preßlinge) oder aber *über den äußeren Gehörgang*, und zwar infolge gegenseitigen Besaugens der Ohren (Kap. 10.6.1.2). Die Begleitumstände der tubogenen Pathogenese können eine auffallende Häufung von Otitisfällen bedingen. Bei Rindern aller Altersstufen führt mitunter auch Verunreinigung des äußeren Gehörgangs (Zeckenbäder, Staub, Getreidegrannen) oder Parasitenbefall der Ohren (Kap. 11.2.4) sowie damit verbundener Juckreiz zu m. o. w. schwerwiegender Otitis. Bakteriologisch sind von Fall zu Fall *Staphylo-* und *Streptokokken, Mycoplasma bovis, Pseudomonas, A. pyogenes, E. coli, Neisserien, Haemophilus somnus, Pasteurellen, F. necrophorum* und/oder *C. pseudotuberculosis* festzustellen; falls neben Otitis auch bronchopneumonische Veränderungen vorliegen, beruhen beide meist auf den gleichen Erregern.

■ **Symptome, Verlauf** (Abb. 11-63 bis 11-65): Im Falle *otogener* Infektion besteht ein- oder beidseitiger intermittierender oder anhaltender Ohrausfluß, der teils dünnflüssig, grau-bräunlich und muffig, teils zähflüssig-eitrig, gelblichgrün und übelriechend ist; mitunter ist die Ansammlung von Exsudat im äußeren Gehörgang nur durch wiederholtes Zusammenpressen des Ohrs an seiner Basis zu erkennen (»Quatschohr«). Bei Patienten mit *tubogener* Otitis media sind häufig beide Ohren betroffen; zu Otorrhoe nach außen kommt es aber erst nach Durchbruch des Trommelfells.

Das kranke Ohr »hängt« und zeigt kein »Spiel« mehr. Die durch Übergreifen der Entzündung von der Paukenhöhle auf den N. facialis bewirkte Lähmung dieses Nerven gibt sich in gleichseitigem Absinken von Oberlid und Oberlippe zu erkennen. Die örtliche Reizung bedingt zudem Kopfschütteln, mitunter auch Scheuern des Ohrs und/oder Tränenfluß. Bei Beteiligung des Labyrinths wird der Kopf auf der kranken Seite tiefer gehalten als auf der gesunden; bei beidseitiger Innenohrentzündung wird er insgesamt tief getragen. Schwere Otitis interna zieht des weiteren Gleichgewichtsstörungen, wie breitbeiniges Stehen, ataktisch-inkoordinierten Gang, Kreisbewegungen oder plattes Festliegen auf der kranken Seite, nach sich. Das Allgemeinbefinden ist oft deutlich beeinträchtigt: Niedergeschlagenheit, Inappetenz, hohes Fieber, Abmagerung. Zusätzliche, von Fall zu Fall festzustellende Erscheinungen erlauben Rückschlüsse auf den Infektionsweg: Konjunktivitis, Tränen- und Nasenausfluß, Schluckbeschwerden, Husten, Enzootische Bronchopneumonie (= Hinweise auf tubogene Infektion) oder Juckreiz bzw. naßgeleckte, milchverschmutzte oder verschrumpelte Ohren (= Hinweis auf Ektoparasitenbefall, Ohrfremdkörper bzw. Ansaug-Otitis).

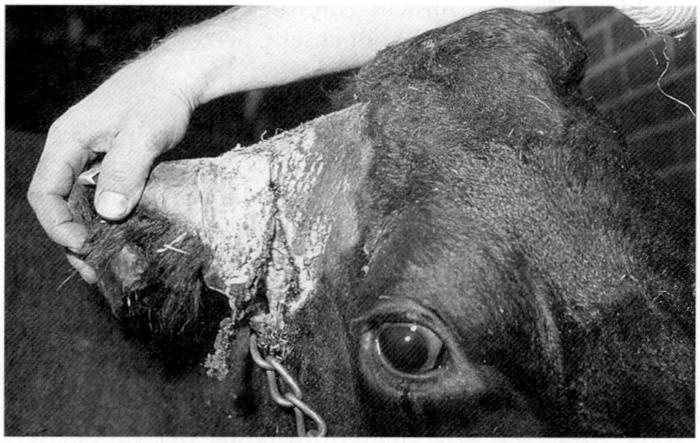

Abbildung 11-62 Gangräneszierende Ohrbasisphlegmone infolge paravenöser Dauertropfinfusion

■ **Sektion:** Bei Beteiligung des Innenohrs zeigen sich nach Aufsägen des Felsenbeins: Zerstörung von Trommelfell und Gehörknöchelchen, Verdickung der Paukenhöhlenwand und Knocheneiterung.

■ **Diagnose:** Allgemeine und örtliche Befunde lenken den Verdacht auf eine Mittel- oder Innenohrerkrankung. Klärung ist durch Untersuchung des äußeren Gehörgangs und endoskopische Überprüfung des Rachens (bei gleichzeitigem Spülen des äußeren Gehörgangs) zu erlangen: Wenn Exsudat oder Spülflüssigkeit am rachenwärtigen Ende der Ohrtrompete austritt (was i. d. R. Schluckbewegungen auslöst) und u. U. auch aus der Nase abläuft, ist das Trommelfell perforiert und das Mittelohr beteiligt. Der jeweiligen Pathogenese (Atemwegserkrankungen, gegenseitiges Besaugen, Fremdkörper oder Parasiten im Ohr) ist möglichst nachzugehen. *Differentialdiagnostisch* sind zu bedenken: Othämatom (Kap. 11.2.2.4), traumatisch ausgelöste Fazialislähmung (Kap. 10.2.5.7), nervöse Listeriose (Kap. 12.2.10), Hirnnervenscheidentumorose (Kap. 10.7.2), Tortikollis (Kap. 9.1.7), enthornungsbedingte zentralnervöse Komplikationen (Kap. 2.4.5.2) und Stirnhöhlenentzündung (Kap. 5.1.2.4).

■ **Beurteilung:** Otitispatienten mit Beeinträchtigung des Gleichgewichtssinnes haben kaum noch Aussichten auf Heilung; solche mit Ohrlähmung und Kopfschiefhaltung bedürfen lokaler und allgemeiner Behandlung; bei bloßer Beteiligung des äußeren Ohrs sind mitunter örtliche Maßnahmen ausreichend. Als Folgeerscheinung kann Fazialislähmung (Kap. 10.2.5.7) zurückbleiben.

■ **Behandlung:** Patient(en) in Einzelbox(en) verbringen. Ohrmuschel und äußeren Gehörgang am gut fixierten Kopf vorsichtig, aber gründlich reinigen (lange Arterienklemme/Zellstoff, elastische Ohrtupfer). Äußeren Gehörgang anschließend mit Hilfe eines dünnen Schlauches spülen (körperwarme physiologische Kochsalz-, 0,75%ige Polyvidon-Jod-, 3%ige Wasserstoffperoxid- oder verdünnte Chlorhexidinlösung) und nach Ablaufenlassen der Flüssigkeit sowie Trockentupfen des Ohres mit einem Breitspektrumantibiotikum (in wäßriger Lösung; bei starker Entzündung oder Juckreiz u. U. mit Glukokortikoidzusatz) versorgen. Diese Maßnahmen sind bis zum Abklingen

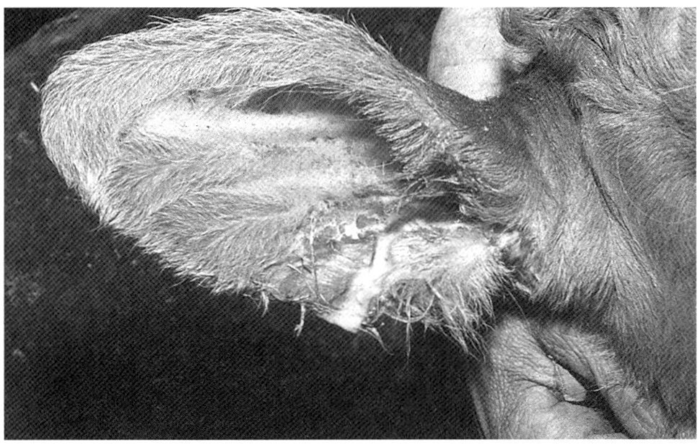

Abbildung 11-63 Otitis: eitriger Ohrausfluß *(Otorrhoe)* und normale Ohrhaltung bei Entzündung des äußeren Gehörgangs

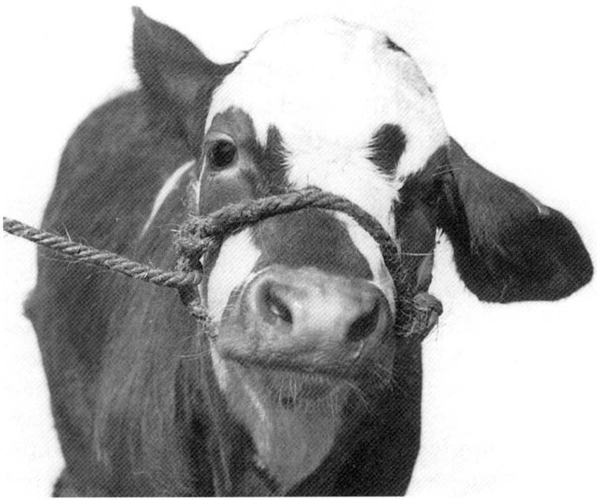

Abbildung 11-64 Hängendes Ohr bei Otitis media

von Ohrausfluß und Allgemeinstörung in 1- bis 2tägigen Abständen fortzusetzen. Zur parenteralen Antibiose wird mehrtägige Verabreichung von Amoxicillin, Kanamycin, Polymyxin, Neomycin, Lincomycin, Spectinomycin, Oxytetracyclin oder Enrofloxacin empfohlen. Das keimeinschleppende Kratzen des Ohres mit den Hinterklauen kann durch Anlegen eines Vergrittungsgeschirrs unterbunden werden.

■ **Prophylaxe:** Verhüten der Ursachen, d. h. etwaiger Infektionen der oberen Luftwege (Kap. 5.2.2, 5.3.3), des gegenseitigen Besaugens (Kap. 10.6.1.2) und des Befalls der Ohren mit Parasiten (s. u.).

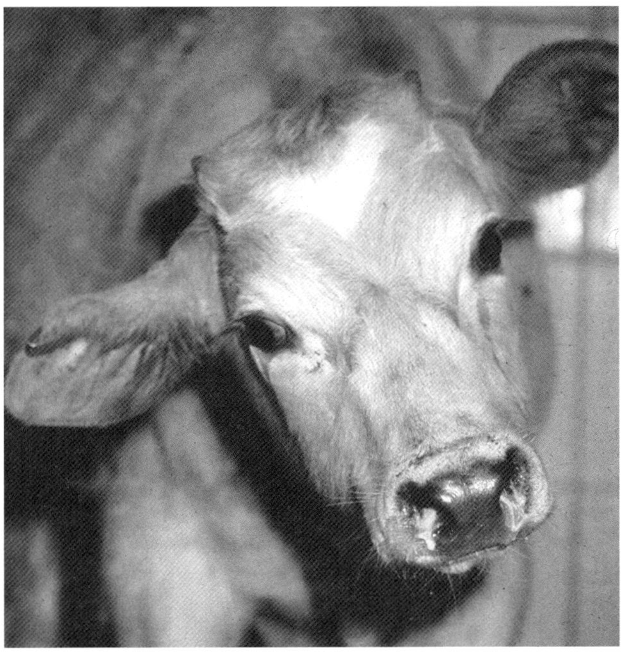

Abbildung 11-65 Kopfschiefhaltung bei rechtsseitiger Mittel- und Innenohrentzündung

11.2.4 Parasitär bedingte Krankheiten der Ohren

Außer bei den im folgenden beschriebenen Parasitosen können die Ohren des Rindes auch bei *Zeckenbefall* (Kap. 2.2.4.4), *Sarkoptes-* oder *Psoroptes-Räude* (Kap. 2.2.4.2) und bei *Besnoitiose* (Kap. 2.2.4.6) der Haut primär betroffen oder beteiligt sein. Näheres hierzu ist angegebenenorts nachzulesen.

11.2.4.1 Ohrmilbenbefall

Raillietia auris kommt bei Rindern (insbesondere Zebus) weltweit und mitunter regional gehäuft als Parasit des äußeren Gehörgangs, gelegentlich auch des Mittelohres vor *(Otocariasis)*. Seine Entwicklung von Ei über Larve, Proto- und Deuteronymphe zur adulten männlichen und weiblichen Milbe dauert nur 4–5 Tage. Der Befall mit den etwa 1 mm großen weißlichen Larven und adulten Milben (Beine und Schild braun; Abb. 11-66) ist klinisch bis auf vermehrte Ohrschmalzbildung meist inapparent und wird deshalb i. d. R. gar nicht erkannt oder bei otoskopischer Betrachtung mit Larven der Ohrzecke (*Otobius megnini*, s. u.) verwechselt. Bei schwerwiegendem, verschlepptem Verlauf kann sich eine eitrig-ulzerative Otitis externa entwickeln, die nach Beschädigung des Trommelfells u. U. zu Otitis media mit Schiefhaltung und/oder Schütteln des Kopfes, Ohr

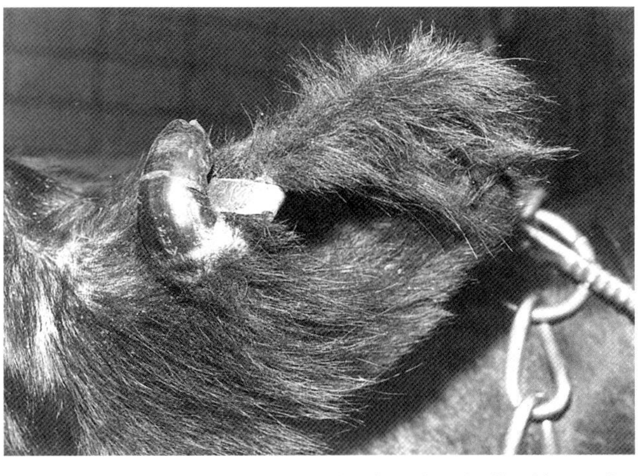

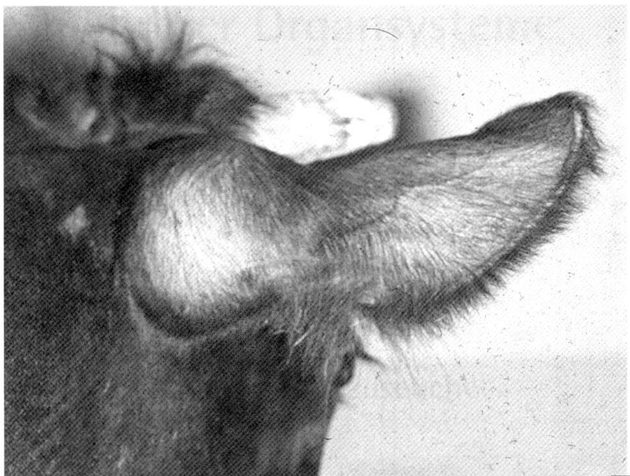

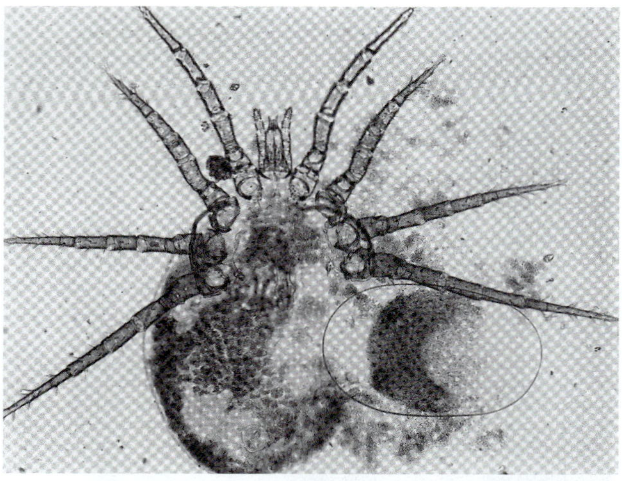

Abbildung 11-66 Ohrmilbenweibchen *(Raillietia auris)* mit Ei (HEFFNER & HEFFNER, 1983)

scheuern, Gehörverlust, ipsilateraler Fazialislähmung und Gleichgewichtsstörungen (Kap. 11.2.3.2) führt. Der Parasit läßt sich intra vitam bzw. postmortal durch mikroskopische Untersuchung von Ohrtupferproben bzw. Ohrspülflüssigkeit nachweisen. Zur Behandlung sind die gleichen Maßnahmen wie beim Ohrwurmbefall zu versuchen.

11.2.4.2 Ohrzeckenbefall

In Afrika und Amerika parasitieren Larven und Nymphen der Lederzecke *Otobius megnini* an den Ohren (sowie unter dem Schwanz) von Rind und Schaf *(Otobiiasis)*. Allgemeingültiges über Zeckenbefall ist bei den Parasitosen der Haut nachzulesen (Kap. 2.2.4.4).

11.2.4.3 Ohrwurmbefall

In Ostafrika wird der äußere Gehörgang von Nutzrindern nicht selten von *Rhabditis bovis*, einem saprophytär-viviparen Nematoden parasitiert *(Otorhabditiasis)*. Innerhalb betroffener Herden können ≤ 70% der Tiere erkrankt sein; die Verlustrate kann ≤ 10% erreichen. Als Ursache für die Zunahme des früher vermutlich nur durch Fliegen sowie Kratzen der Ohren mit verschmutzten Hinterklauen verschleppten Ohrnematodenbefalls gilt das regelmäßige, mit Untertauchen verbundene Baden in sogenannten Zecken-Dips (Kap. 2.2.4.4). Leichte aurikuläre Rhabditiose verläuft klinisch inapparent, doch sind die 1–2 mm langen weißlichen Parasiten dabei in der Tiefe des Ohres mit bloßem Auge erkennbar. Schwerwiegendere Fälle äußern sich in Trägheit und Kopfschütteln *(Otitis externa)*, nach längerem Befall auch in dunkelbraunem Ohrausfluß, verminderter Freßlust (Übergreifen der Entzündung auf Tuba eustachii und Rachen), Abmagerung, Kopfschiefhaltung, gleichseitigem Lidödem, phlegmonöser Anschwellung der Ohrbasis, Hängenlassen oder Absterben der Ohrmuschel, u. U. auch in Festliegen mit tödlichem Ausgang *(Otitis media/interna)*; vielfach besteht zudem sekundärer Schmeißfliegenbefall. Bei der *Zerlegung* erweisen sich äußerer Gehörgang und Mittelohr, mitunter auch Innenohr und angrenzende Hirnbezirke als entzündlich bis nekrotisch verändert und die regionalen Lymphknoten als geschwollen. Die antiparasitäre *Behandlung* durch subkutane Injektion von 0,2 mg Ivermectin/kg LM ist erfolgreich, wenn noch keine zentralnervösen Komplikationen vorliegen. Bezüglich der örtlichen Otitisbehandlung wird auf Kapitel 11.2.3.2 verwiesen. Zur *Vorbeuge* der aurikulären Rhabditiose wird die Zugabe von 2 ppm Nikotin zur Badeflüssigkeit (→ Abtötung der in ihr sonst saprophytisch weiterlebenden Ohrnematoden) sowie Fliegenabwehr empfohlen.

11.2.5 Fütterungs-, vergiftungs- und sensibilisierungsbedingte Krankheiten der Ohren

Bei manchen der auf alimentäre, toxische oder allergene Ursachen zurückzuführenden systemischen Krankheiten der Haut sind auch die Ohren beteiligt, z. B. bei *Ergotismus mumificans* (Kap. 12.3.3), *Jodismus* (Kap. 2.2.5.2), *Vergiftung durch höherchlorierte Naphthaline* (Kap. 12.3.15), *Urtikaria* (Kap. 2.2.7.1), *Photosensibilitätsreaktionen* (Kap. 2.2.7.3) oder *Zitrinin-Toxikose* (Kap. 12.3.8). Patienten mit *Bleivergiftung* (Kap. 10.5.12), *Hirnrindennekrose* (Kap. 10.5.5) oder manifestem *Vitamin-A-Mangel* (Kap. 11.1.5.1) orientieren sich blindheitsbedingt v. a. mit Hilfe des Gehörs, was sich in »radarartigem« Abstehen beider Ohren äußert. An *Botulismus* (Kap. 10.5.13) erkrankte Rinder lassen beide Ohren herabhängen.

11.2.6 Haltungsbedingte Krankheiten der Ohren

Das Auftreten verschmutzter, erodierter, blutergußbehafteter oder narbig verschrumpelnder Ohren bei Kälbern oder Jungrindern ist ein Hinweis auf *gegenseitiges Besaugen* (Kap. 10.6.1.2).

11.2.7 Tumorkrankheiten der Ohren

Die Haut der *Ohrmuschel* kann von den gleichen gut- oder bösartigen Neubildungen betroffen werden wie die übrige Haut des Rindes (Abb. 11-67, 11-68). Unter ihnen sind *Fibropapillome* (Kap. 2.2.3.4) und *Hauthörner* (Kap. 2.2.9) am häufigsten. Am Ohr und im

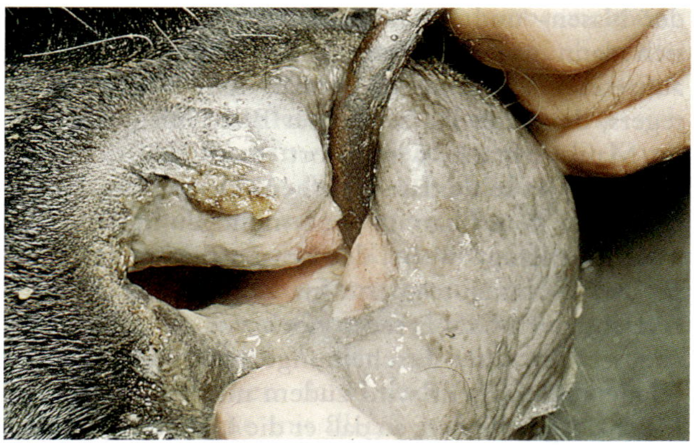

Abbildung 12-1 Maul- und Klauenseuche: Geplatzte Aphthe im Naseneingang

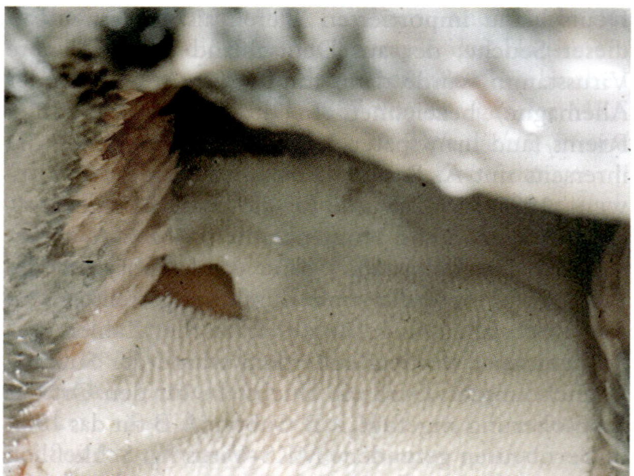

stung geht je nach Schwere der Erkrankung zurück. An den Zitzen können Sekundäraphthen auftreten, die das Melken sehr erschweren und bei Beteiligung des Strichkanals u. U. aszendierende Mastitis auslösen. Entwickeln sich im Zuge der Generalisation auch Blasen im Zwischenklauenspalt, so wird dieser schon zuvor als druckempfindlich befunden. Der anonyme Autor des Werkes »Von der Klauenseuche« schreibt hierzu 1799: *»Nebst gemeinen fieberhaften Zufällen stellt sich unversehens das Hinken ein, die Klauen werden brennendheis, und das Fleisch über ihnen geschwilt; gleichwohl findet sich nichts eingetretenes im Fuß«*; und später: *»Ist die Maulseuche zugleich vorhanden, so ist der Umstand freilich um vieles schlimmer«*. Das Fortschreiten der aphthösen Entzündung auf Kronsaum, Ballen und/oder Afterklauen kann Festliegen, Doppelsohlenbildung oder Verlust des Klauenschuhs (= sekundäres »Ausschuhen«, Kap. 9.14.8) zur Folge haben.

Je nach dem der Erkrankung zugrundeliegenden MKS-Virusstamm kann die Erkrankung, insbesondere bei Jungtieren, auch Myokardschädigung mit plötzlichem Herztod (»bösartige« MKS) oder chronisches, mit starker Abmagerung verbundenes Siechtum bedingen; tragende Tiere können verkalben.

Im Regelfall heilen die aphthösen Epitheldefekte aber rasch aus, weil das Stratum germinativum dieser Stellen intakt bleibt. Von komplikativen Sekundärinfektionen abgesehen, kehren auch Körpertemperatur und Futteraufnahme der Patienten innerhalb weniger Tage zur Norm zurück. Die Milchleistung bleibt in der betreffenden Laktation jedoch, je nach Erkrankungsgrad, um 20–50% niedriger als erwartet.

■ **Sektion:** Gemäß der derzeitigen, gesetzlich verankerten Vorgehensweise dürfte die Zerlegung eines an MKS verendeten oder nach Stellung dieser Diagnose getöteten Rindes nur ausnahmsweise möglich sein. Gegebenenfalls finden sich neben äußerlich erkennbaren und m. o. w. weit entwickelten oder sekundär bakteriell infizierten Aphthen auch solche in der Tiefe von Nasen- und Maulhöhle, mitunter zudem umschriebene verschorfende Veränderungen an den Pansenpfeilern und auf den Psalterblättern. Bei jungen sowie bei stark geschwächten, im Rahmen der MKS plötzlich verendeten Rindern werden v. a. im Myokard, mitunter aber auch/oder statt dessen in der Skelettmuskulatur helle, undurchblutete Streifen sichtbar, die auf Vermehrung des MKS-Virus in den Muskelzellen beruhen; nach längerem Siechtum können hier nekrotisierende, verjauchende oder abszedierende Herde vorliegen.

■ **Diagnose:** Selbst wenn die Diagnose »MKS« aufgrund der klinischen Symptome zweifelsfrei gestellt ist, muß sie – wegen der besonderen Bedeutung dieser Seuche – durch Erregernachweis bestätigt werden. Dieser ist in einem offiziell hierfür benannten nationalen Labor zu führen. Die Entnahme der dazu erforderlichen Proben erfolgt durch den zuständigen Amtstierarzt, nachdem ihm der Verdacht eines MKS-Ausbruchs vom Tierbesitzer oder Tierarzt gemeldet wurde. Dabei werden Blutproben sowie Blasenmaterial entnommen und letzteres in Pufferlösung verbracht; das Untersuchungsgut wird dann samt einschlägigen Formblättern auf raschestem Wege dem national zuständigen Institut* zugesandt. Zum Erregernachweis sowie zur (Sub-)Typenbestimmung können zwar nach wie vor KBR, Gewebekultur und Mäusetest eingesetzt werden; in den meisten Anstalten stützt man sich heute aber auf ELISA und PCR mit Sequenzierung. Reid et al. (1998) wiesen jedoch darauf hin, daß PCR allein hierfür nicht genüge, weil damit nur bestimmte Abschnitte der viralen RNS erfaßt werden. Andererseits gelang Marquardt et al. (1995) der Nachweis von MKS-Virus in Nasentupferproben asymptomatischer Rinder mit RT-PCR innerhalb von 24 h. Niedbalski et al. (1998) konnten damit selbst 14 Tage nach der Infektion noch 10^6–10^8 Virusgenome aus 10^7 Zungenepithelzellen ermitteln.

Probenmaterial erhalten auch das MKS-Weltreferenzzentrum in UK-Pirbright sowie die Laboratorien der Vakzinebanken (s. *Prophylaxe*). Nach Bestätigung der Diagnose wird der MKS-Ausbruch außer den obersten nationalen Veterinärbehörden auch der Europäischen Kommission in Brüssel sowie dem Internationalen Tierseuchenamt in Paris gemeldet.

■ **Differentialdiagnose:** Da MKS in den meisten Ländern Europas seit Jahrzehnten nicht mehr großflächig aufgetreten ist, kennen viele der heute berufstätigen Tierärzte ihr klinisches Bild nicht aus eigener Erfahrung. Somit kommt der kritischen Abgrenzung der MKS von Krankheiten ähnlicher Symptomatologie besondere Bedeutung zu. Das gilt v. a. für einige, mit Nasenausfluß und Speicheln einhergehende virale Infektionskrankheiten, aber auch für bestimmte andere Leiden: Mit *Epithelio-* oder *Keratogenesis imperfecta* (Kap. 2.2.1.5, 2.2.1.6) behaftete neugeborene Kälber weisen zwar MKS-verdächtige Epithelveränderungen an Flotzmaul, Maulschleimhaut und im Klauenbereich auf, sind aber fieberfrei und übertragen ihr Leiden nicht auf Nachbartiere. *Infektiöse Bovine Rhinotracheitis* (Kap. 5.1.3.1) beginnt wie MKS mit Fieber,

* Deutschland: Bundesforschungsanstalt für Viruskrankheiten der Tiere, Paul-Ehrlich-Str. 28, D-72076 Tübingen; Österreich: Bundesanstalt für Virusseuchenbekämpfung bei Haustieren, Emil-Behring-Weg 3, A-1233 Wien; Schweiz: Institut für Viruskrankheiten und Immunprophylaxe, Sensematt-Str. 293, CH-3147 Mittelhäusern.

serösem Nasenausfluß und Milchrückgang; auch können dabei mehrere Tiere zugleich erkranken; selbst bei vermehrtem Speichelfluß sind aber weder im Naseneingang noch im Maul Blasen feststellbar. Beim *Bösartigen Katarrhalfieber* (Kap. 12.2.2) erkranken i. d. R. nur Einzeltiere, und zwar hochfieberhaft an rasch zunehmender diffuser Entzündung aller Kopfschleimhäute einschließlich der Konjunktiven (Lichtscheu, Hornhauttrübung); auf der Euterhaut kann sich ein Exanthem entwickeln, Aphthen treten jedoch nirgends auf. *Stomatitis papulosa* (Kap. 6.1.5) befällt bevorzugt Jungtiere, die mäßig fiebern und speicheln können; an Flotzmaul, Lippen oder Maulschleimhaut sind dabei anstelle von Blasen einzelne bis mehrere kokardenähnliche Papeln festzustellen. Kennzeichnend für *Mucosal Disease* (Kap. 6.10.20) sind Durchfall, Erosionen und Nekrosen der Nasen- und Maulschleimhaut, mitunter auch des Zwischenklauenspalts, sowie die Abwesenheit von Blasen. Die vorwiegend Jungrinder betreffende *Infektion mit dem Bovinen Respiratorischen Synzytialvirus* (Kap. 5.3.3.3) äußert sich in akuter, mit Atemnot und Temperaturanstieg verbundener Erkrankung, bei der sich vor Nase und Maul Schaum ansammeln kann, im Bereich beider aber keine Gewebeveränderungen auftreten. Das bei *Stomatitis vesicularis* (Kap. 6.1.6) zu beobachtende Krankheitsbild ist klinisch nicht von MKS zu unterscheiden; dieses auch Schweine und Pferde befallende Leiden ist in feucht-warmen Regionen Süd- und Mittelamerikas endemisch und kommt auch im Südwesten der USA vor. *Blue tongue* (Kap. 6.1.7) verläuft beim Rind oft subklinisch, manchmal aber mit Speichelfluß und Stomatitis. AUJESZKY*sche Krankheit* (Kap. 10.3.7) bedingt beim Rind zwar hochfieberhafte, mit m. o. w. ausgeprägtem Juckreiz, Belecken sowie Speicheln einhergehende Erkrankung, führt aber nicht zur Blasenbildung und endet schon nach kurzer Zeit tödlich. *Bleivergiftete Rinder* (Kap. 10.5.12) fallen durch roboterähnliches, mit Zähneknirschen verbundenes »Leerkauen« und schaumiges Speicheln auf, zeigen aber ebenfalls keine Blasen im Maul und sind zudem blind.

Beurteilung: Bei sachgemäßer, in MKS-freien Ländern allerdings verbotener palliativer Behandlung und gründlicher, eitrig-nekrotisierende Sekundärinfektionen im Klauenbereich verhütender Pflege heilen MKS-Erkrankungen meist innerhalb weniger Tage aus. Dann sistiert i. d. R. auch die Virusausscheidung. In lymphehaltigen Spalten des Klauenhorns, etwa einer »Doppelsohle«, kann der MKS-Erreger jedoch u. U. 8 Monate lang infektionstüchtig bleiben. MKS-bedingte Todesfälle betreffen vorwiegend Jungtiere sowie großrahmige erwachsene Rinder (Altbullen); sie machen ~ 3% aller Erkrankungen aus und beruhen teils auf viral bedingter Herz- und/oder Skelettmuskelschädigung (»bösartige« MKS), teils auf dem Einbruch sekundärer bakterieller Infekte in Gelenke (→ Festliegen) oder Euter.

Behandlung: Wegen der Gefährlichkeit des Erregers sind gemäß MKS-VO nicht nur Impfungen gegen MKS, sondern auch Heilversuche an MKS-kranken und -verdächtigen Tieren verboten. Zu Forschungszwecken vorgenommene Behandlungen mit Sulfonamiden und/oder Antibiotika führen zwar zur alsbaldigen Genesung der Kranken, können die Virusausscheidung aber nicht beeinflussen (STRAUB, unveröffentlicht).

Prophylaxe: Die vor Einführung der Nichtimpfpolitik in Europa zur MKS-Vorbeuge üblichen, in regelmäßigen Zeitabständen vorgenommenen obligatorischen *Impfungen* stützten sich auf inaktivierte Vakzinen. Das dazu erforderliche MKS-Virus wurde zunächst aus dem Zungenepithel von Versuchsrindern, später aus Gewebekulturen gewonnen. Zur Abtötung des Erregers wurde früher Formalin verwandt; nachdem aber zahlreiche MKS-Ausbrüche auf unzureichend inaktivierte Vakzinen zurückzuführen waren (STROHMAIER & BÖHM, 1984), werden hierfür heute Ethylenimin-Derivate bevorzugt (STROHMAIER & STRAUB, 1995). Als Adjuvans wird anstelle von Aluminiumhydroxid zunehmend Öl benutzt. Synthetische »Peptid«-Impfstoffe befinden sich erst in Erprobung (YOU YONGJIN et al., 1997; ZAMORANO et al., 1998).

Alle bisher eingesetzten MKS-Vakzinen sind mit dem Mangel einer *unzureichenden Dauer des Impfschutzes* behaftet: Er beginnt nach Überzeugung GIRARDS & MACKOWIAKS (1950) schon 6 Monate nach der Vakzination zu schwinden; entsprechende Untersuchungen zeigten, daß der Impfschutz gegen den dem Vakzinevirus homologen Erregerstamm zwar monatelang anhält, gegenüber einem seiner Sequenzanalyse nach nur leicht veränderten Virus jedoch nur wenige Wochen dauert (STRAUB, 1990, 1995) oder ausbleibt. Hieraus ist zu schließen, daß die nach den Regeln der Europäischen Pharmakopöe vorzunehmende Impfstoffprüfung unzulänglich ist; sie sollte auch die verschiedenen Erregertypen sowie Subtypen berücksichtigen und die Testinfektion erst 6 (statt 3) Wochen nach der Vakzination ansetzen.

Bezüglich der bei MKS-Schutzimpfungen mitunter beobachteten *allergischen Sofort- und Spätreaktionen* wird auf Kapitel 2.2.7.1 bzw. 2.2.7.2 verwiesen.

Um im Falle einer Einschleppung von MKS in kürzester Zeit Vakzine für eine *Ringimpfung* verfügbar zu haben, sind in verschiedenen Ländern *Vakzinebanken* eingerichtet worden, in Deutschland z. B. die Bayovac-MKS-Vakzine-Reservebank. Sie ist durch Vertrag mit 14 Bundesländern zur laufenden Produktion, Lagerung und ggf. Lieferung von 10 Millionen Dosen äquivalentem Viruskonzentrat und 1 Millionen Dosen monovalenter MKS-Vakzine verpflichtet. Herstellung und Zulassung dieses Impfstoffs unterliegen strenger nationaler und internationaler Kontrolle.

Bekämpfung: FLÜCKIGER konstatierte schon 1992, daß es unmöglich ist, die MKS allein durch Schutzimpfung zu tilgen. Gemäß TSeuG (Fassung vom 20. 12. 1995) ist MKS anzeigepflichtig; nach dem EU-weiten Verbot der Flächenimpfung wurde wegen der besonderen Gefährdung der Klauentierbestände durch das MKS-Virus eine MKS-VO (Fassung vom 1. 2. 1994; geändert durch VO vom 27. 3. 1995) erlassen und dazu ein Bundesmaßnahmenkatalog erstellt. Hierüber sind die praktizierenden Tierärzte durch Broschüren und Fortbildungsveranstaltungen informiert worden. Gemäß MKS-VO sind Impfungen gegen MKS sowie Heilversuche an seuchenkranken und -verdächtigen Tieren verboten. Die VO führt des weiteren die vor und nach amtlicher Feststellung des Ausbruchs von MKS seitens der zuständigen Behörde zu treffenden Schutzmaßregeln auf: Einschränkung von Personen- und Tierverkehr innerhalb betroffener Bestände, Tötung und unschädliche Beseitigung sämtlicher Klauentiere einschließlich deren Teile und Erzeugnisse, Einrichtung von Sperrbezirk und Beobachtungsgebiet (Radius 3 bzw. 10 km), Desinfektion und Aufhebung der Schutzmaßregeln. Ähnliche Vorkehrungen sind für den Fall des Verdachts eines Ausbruchs von MKS vorgesehen. Je nach Seuchenlage kann von der obersten Landesbehörde im Benehmen mit dem BMELF eine Gebietsimpfung angeordnet werden (s. *Prophylaxe*: Ringimpfung und Vakzinebank); die Impflinge sind durch Ohrmarken mit den Buchstaben I.MKS zu kennzeichnen und dürfen während der folgenden 12 Monate nur zur Schlachtung aus dem Impfbezirk entfernt werden; nach Schlachtung sind Kopf sowie Rachenraumgewebe samt Tonsillen unschädlich zu beseitigen.

Bei den jüngsten MKS-Ausbrüchen im Vereinigten Königreich, in Frankreich und den Niederlanden sind unterschiedliche Bekämpfungsmaßnahmen getroffen worden: In Frankreich und den Niederlanden wurden die Klauentiere der betroffenen und verdächtigen Bestände getötet und unschädlich beseitigt. In den Niederlanden wurde zudem eine Ringimpfung mit einer monovalenten O-Vakzine vorgenommen, die ausreichenden Schutz vermittelte, obwohl Feld- und Impfvirus-Stamm nicht identisch waren (MARQUARDT, 2001b). Das Vereinigte Königreich hielt sich dagegen an das Impfverbot (s. *Behandlung* sowie *Prophylaxe*), obwohl ein Ende des eskalierenden Seuchenzugs nicht abzusehen war.

12.2.2 Bösartiges Katarrhalfieber

M. STÖBER

Definition, Vorkommen, Ursachen: Das Bösartige Katarrhalfieber (BKF) ist eine beim Hausrind und anderen im Stall, auf der Weide, in Wildgehegen oder zoologischen Gärten in m. o. w. engen Kontakt mit erregerausscheidenden Schafen, Ziegen, Gnus, Oryxgazellen oder Säbelantilopen gelangenden Rindern (oder Büffeln, Bantengs, Gaurs, Wisents, Bisons) sowie weiteren Wiederkäuern (Kudu, Okapi, Elch, Rentier und verschiedene Hirscharten) weltweit sporadisch bis bestandsweise gehäuft auftretende Infektionskrankheit. Das Leiden ist durch meist akut und hochfieberhaft-tödlichen Verlauf, erosiv-fibrinoide Veränderungen an den Schleimhäuten des Kopfes und des Magen-Darm-Traktes, Exanthem der Haut sowie Gehirnbeteiligung gekennzeichnet; es wird vom erkrankten Rind nicht weiterübertragen. Pathologisch-anatomisch und -histologisch ist das BKF des Rindes einheitlich; epidemiologisch ist es an vorherigen Kontakt mit selbst gesund erscheinenden *Schafen* (= Schaf-assoziiertes BKF) bzw. mit ebenfalls selbst klinisch unauffälligen, aber erregerverbreitenden *Gnus* (= Gnu-assoziiertes BKF) gebunden; die Ausscheidung des krankmachenden Agens ist offenbar v. a. während der Ablamm- bzw. Kalbesaison der ebengenannten Überträgerspezies massiv. Das seit Ende des 18. Jh. bekannte, Schaf-assoziierte BKF kommt vorwiegend in Europa, Nordamerika, Australien und Asien vor. Gnu-gebundenes BKF ist bislang (abgesehen von Kontakten zwischen zoogehaltenen Rindern und Gnus) nur in Afrika beobachtet worden. Erreger des Gnu-assoziierten BKF ist das *alkelaphine Gamma-Herpes-Virus-1* (AHV_1 = BHV_3); für das Schaf-gebundene BKF wird ein *ovines Gamma-Herpes-Virus-2* (OHV_2) als krankmachender Keim vermutet. Das Rind gilt als Endglied der Infektionskette beider Erreger. *Andere Bezeichnungen des Leidens*: Koryza gangraenosa boum, Malignant Head Catarrh (MHC), Snotziekte, »Kopfkrankheit«.

Bedeutung: Die wirtschaftliche Rolle des *schafgebundenen BKF des Hausrindes* ist – insgesamt gesehen – zwar gering, da es sich auf Betriebe mit gemeinsamer Haltung von Schafen *und* Rindern beschränkt; im einzelnen Bestand können die durch dieses Leiden verursachten Tierverluste jedoch erheblich sein. Seine differentialdiagnostische Abgrenzung von anderen, klinisch ähnlich verlaufenden Krankheiten ist jedoch von praktischer Relevanz. In Ländern mit intensivem Hirsch-»Farming« kann das BKF der Zerviden erhebliche ökonomische Verluste bedingen.

Pathogenese: Das AHV_1 ist unter Gnus weit verbreitet, ohne diese krank zu machen; es wird mit ihren Ausscheidungen (Fruchtwasser [?]; Tränen- und Nasensekret der Neugeborenen) in einer für Rinder infektiösen, nicht-zellgebundenen Form verbreitet und in Aerosolform über die oberen Luftwege aufgenommen. Entsprechendes trifft vermutlich für den vom Schaf übertragenen BKF-Erreger zu, so daß – außer dem unmittelbaren Kontakt mit Schafen – wahrscheinlich auch die bloße Exposition gegenüber ihren vorgenannten Ausscheidungen krankmachend sein kann. Ob und inwieweit Lästlinge oder Ektoparasiten bei der Übertragung der BKF-Erreger eine Rolle spielen, ist bislang ungeklärt. Die Inkubationszeit beim Rind beträgt 3 Wochen bis 6 Monate, was den Nachweis des exponierenden Schaf- oder Gnukontakts mitunter erschwert. BKF-kranke Rinder beherbergen den Erreger in zellgebundener Form und scheiden ihn auch so aus; sie tragen daher nicht zu seiner Weiterverbreitung bei (Ausnahme: Transfusion von Blut BKF-kranker auf -empfängliche Rinder).

Die beim Rind zu beobachtenden BKF-bedingten histologischen Veränderungen lassen vermuten, daß der Keim – als Voraussetzung für das Haften der Infektion – in T-Lymphozyten eindringen muß. Betroffene Rinder sind meist 2–3 (selten mehr) Jahre alt, aber nur ausnahmsweise jünger. Mitunter werden regelrechte BKF-Ausbrüche beobachtet, bei denen ≤50% des beteiligten Rinderbestandes erkranken; die Letalität beträgt > 95%. Überstehen des BKF hinterläßt beim Rind lebenslange Prämunität.

■ **Symptome, Verlauf** (Abb. 12-6 bis 12-10): Traditionsgemäß werden zwar vier Erscheinungsformen des BKF, nämlich *perakute, Kopf-Augen-, Darm-* und *milde Form,* unterschieden; von perakut verlaufenden Fällen abgesehen, ist das Krankheitsbild aber meist komplex, d. h., es umfaßt m. o. w. ausgeprägte Erscheinungen sowohl der »Kopf-Augen«- als der »Darm-Form« und zentralnervöse Symptome sowie ein papulo-krustöses Exanthem der Haut; das weiße Blutbild zeigt anfangs Lymphozytose, später Lymphopenie:

➤ *Perakut verlaufendes BKF* bedingt plötzlich auftretende schwerwiegende Allgemeinstörung mit hohem Fieber, starkem Milchrückgang, Sistieren von Futteraufnahme und Wiederkauen, Niedergeschlagenheit, vielem Liegen, Muskelzittern, Injektion der Episkleralgefäße sowie wäßrigem bis blutigem Durchfall; eine solche Erkrankung führt in 1–3 Tagen zum Tode, ohne daß sich an den äußerlich zugänglichen Schleimhäuten deutliche Veränderungen entwickeln.

➤ Die am häufigsten zu beobachtende, akut verlaufende *Kopf-Augenform des BKF (»malignant head catarrh«, »Kopfkrankheit«)* ist gekennzeichnet durch: plötzlich einsetzendes und meist anhaltendes Fieber (40–42 °C), Zunahme von Herz- und Atemfrequenz, Milchrückgang; Muskelzittern, allgemeine Schwäche, Nachlassen des Appetits und rasche Gewichtsabnahme; generalisierte Lymphknotenschwellung; serös-schleimiger, später kruppös-rötlicher und schließlich eitrig-gelber, auf der zunehmend erodierenden Flotzmaul- und Nasenschleimhaut verkrustender Nasenausfluß (»snotziekte«), der infolge Einengung der Nasengänge schniefende Atmung, u. U. sogar Maulatmung bedingt; Exsudat und Gewebezerfall verleihen der Atemluft abstoßenden Geruch; beim Versuch, Wasser (vermehrter Durst) oder Futter aufzunehmen, können Masseterzittern, zögernd-vorsichtiges Kauen und/oder gequält erscheinender Husten einsetzen; Zahnfleisch, Zungen- und übrige Maulschleimhaut sind deutlich gerötet; im Laufe der Erkrankung entwickeln sie unregelmäßig begrenzte, teilweise fibrinbedeckte feuerrote Epitheldefekte, die bei der stets mit heftiger Abwehr verbundenen Untersuchung des Maules leicht bluten, und ständiges zähflüssig-fadenziehendes Speicheln, Schmatzen sowie üblen Maulgeruch auslösen. Auffallend ist die beide Augen zugleich betreffende Keratokonjunktivitis und Iridozyklitis, welche hochgradige Injektion der Episkleralgefäße, Lidödem, Fibrinansammlung in der vorderen Augenkammer, zentripetal fortschreitende Hornhauttrübung, Lichtscheu und starken Augenausfluß von gleicher Beschaffenheit wie der Nasenausfluß bedingt. Zudem sind fast immer auch katarrhalische Rötung der Scheidenschleimhaut, nervöse Erscheinungen, exanthematöse Hautveränderungen sowie terminaler Durchfall festzustellen, bevor nach 2–7, längstens aber 14 Tagen der Tod eintritt.

➤ Die *nervösen Symptome des BKF* werden durch eine histologisch bei allen Erscheinungsformen des Leidens nachweisbare nichteitrige Vaskulo-Enzephalitis ausgelöst und äußern sich in m. o. w. schwerwiegender Depression mit Aufstützen oder unphysiologischer Haltung des Kopfes, manchmal dagegen in Berührungsempfindlichkeit, tobsuchtartiger Erregung, Aggressivität oder Zwangsbewegungen.

➤ Die *BKF-bedingten Hautveränderungen* bestehen in einem v. a. die dünnhäutigen Bezirke an Hals, Flanke, Unterbauch, Achsel, Schenkelinnenfläche, Perineum, Präputium und Hodensack bzw. Euterspiegel und Zitzen betreffenden, meist erst im Verlauf der Erkrankung und bei näherer Untersuchung erkennbar werdenden Exanthem. Es ist durch multiple stecknadelkopf- bis münzengroße rundliche Papeln gekennzeichnet und kann Juckreiz bedingen. Die Papeln erscheinen im unpigmentierten Bereich zunächst gerötet, später bräunlich und bedingen Induration oberflächlicher Hautschichten. Die Behaarung ist im Bereich der Papeln gesträubt und infolge seröser Hautausschwitzungen verklebt. Außerdem kann es zur Ablösung des Hornsaumes der Klauen und Hör-

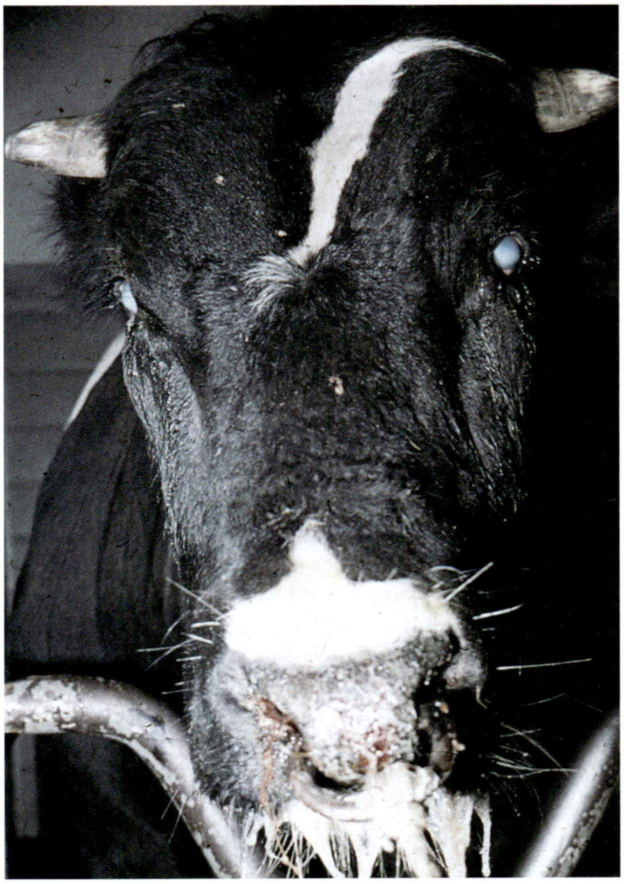

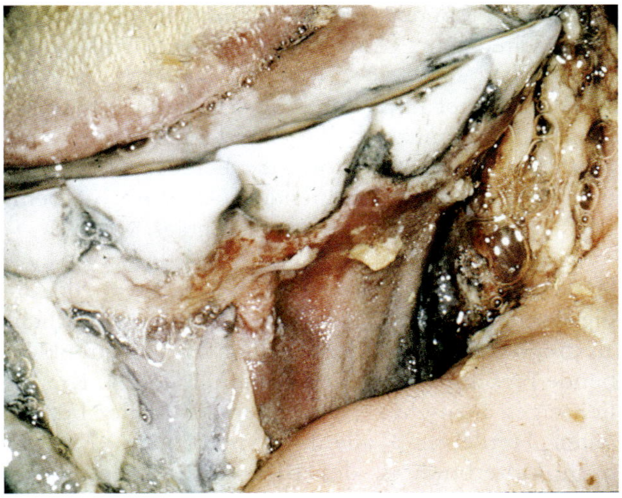

Abbildung 12-6 bis 12-10 Bösartiges Katarrhalfieber: Links oben: schwerwiegende, mit Hornhauttrübung einhergehende beiderseitige Keratokonjunktivitis, Erosionen am Flotzmaul, Nasenausfluß;
rechts oben: Erosionen und pseudomembranöse Auflagerungen am Schneidezahnfleisch;
links Mitte: Erosionen am harten Gaumen;
links unten: papulöses Exanthem an Oberarm und Seitenbrust;
unten rechts: papulöses Exanthem an Perineum und Euterspiegel

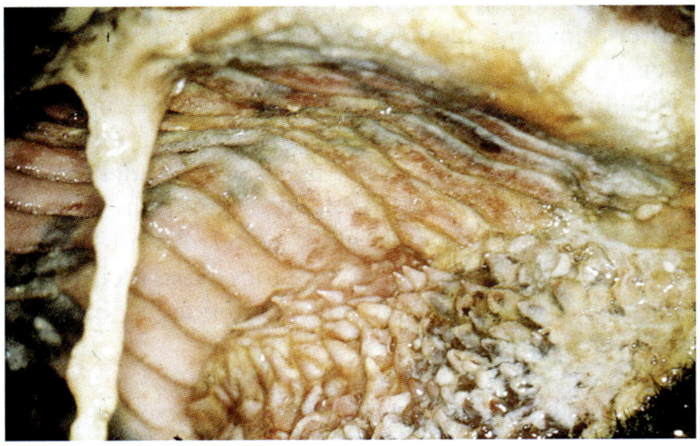

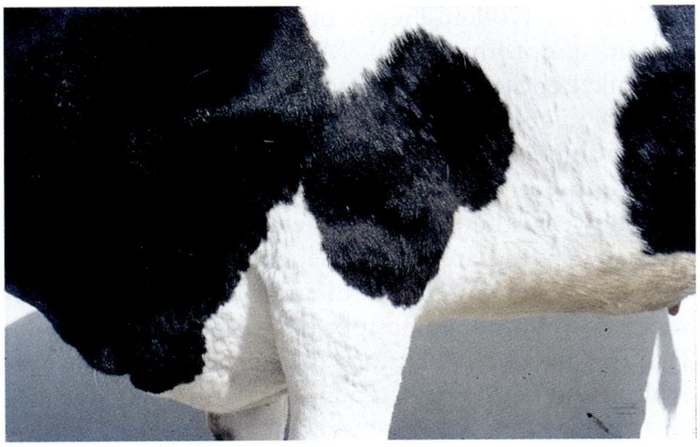

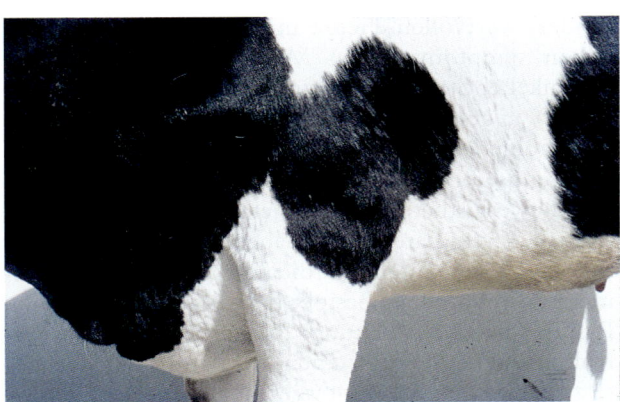

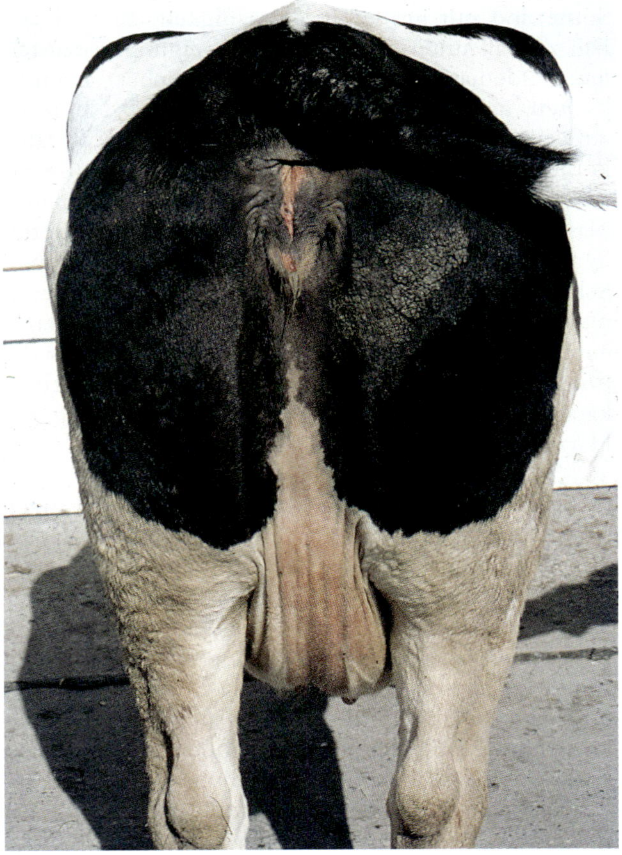

ner, nach besonders langem Krankheitsverlauf auch zu regelrechtem »Ausschuhen« oder »Aushornen« kommen.

➤ Die in erster Linie durch übelriechenden blutigen Durchfall gekennzeichnete, meist aber auch Symptome der Kopf-Augenform des Leidens umfassende und ebenfalls akut verlaufende *»Darmform«* ist beim BKF der Zerviden besonders ausgeprägt.

■ **Beurteilung:** BKF endet beim Rind – unabhängig vom klinischen Bild – fast ausnahmslos tödlich; als prognostisch günstiges Zeichen sind erhaltenbleibende Freßlust sowie das Überstehen des 14. Krankheitstages anzusehen *(»milde Form«)*. In der betroffenen Herde muß allerdings noch ≤ 6 Monate nach Unterbindung des BKF-auslösenden Schaf- bzw. Gnukontaktes mit weiteren Neuerkrankungen gerechnet werden. Das gelegentliche Vorfinden von Antikörpern gegen ein gemeinsames Epitop beider BKF-Viren (mittels kompetitiven Hemmungs-ELISA) bei gesunden Hausrindern sowie großen Wildwiederkäuern weist darauf hin, daß offenbar auch nichtletal verlaufende Infektionen vorkommen.

■ **Zerlegungsbefunde:** Nach perakut tödlichem Verlauf ist das Sektionsbild oft weit »harmloser«, als es die schweren klinischen Erscheinungen vermuten ließen. Sonst sind mit großer Regelmäßigkeit, aber in von Fall zu Fall unterschiedlicher Ausprägung festzustellen: Ödematöse Schwellung sämtlicher Lymphknoten, die z. T. auch Hämorrhagien und Nekrosen aufweisen; hyperplastische Milzschwellung; Keratokonjunktivitis, Iridozyklitis; erosiv-fibrinoide (bis ulzerativ-nekrotisierende) Entzündung von Flotzmaul-, Nasen-, Maul- und Rachenschleimhaut mit Beteiligung der Mukosen von Luftröhre, Bronchen und Schlund; epikardiale Blutungen, Herzmuskeldegeneration; katarrhalische bis hämorrhagische Abomasoenteritis; miliare grauweiße subkapsuläre Herde in der Nierenrinde (= nichteitrige interstitielle Nephritis); katarrhalische bis hämorrhagische Entzündung der Harnblasenschleimhaut.

■ **Histologie:** Die mikroskopischen Veränderungen umfassen lymphoide Infiltration, nicht-eitrige Vaskulitis, v. a. der kleinen Arterien sämtlicher Lokalisationen, sowie Epithelnekrosen; die BKF-bedingte anfängliche T-lymphozytäre Proliferation sämtlicher lymphoider Gewebe und die späteren, von einfachem »Cuffing« mit Infiltration der Adventitia durch Lymphozyten und Lymphoblasten bis zu fibrinoider Nekrose und zu Thrombose reichenden vaskulitischen Prozesse entsprechen einem Autoimmun-Geschehen; dabei spielen zytotoxische T-Lymphozyten eine entscheidende Rolle.

■ **Diagnose:** Die Erkennung des BKF stützt sich auf das kennzeichnende klinische Bild, den voraufgegangenen Schaf- bzw. Gnukontakt, den Zerlegungsbefund (Schleimhautläsionen) sowie die histologische Untersuchung von Gehirn-, Nieren-, Leber- und Lymphknotengewebe (Gefäßveränderungen). Das OHV_2 läßt sich in Blutlymphozyten der an Schaf-assoziiertem BKF erkrankten Rinder (sowie bei klinisch gesunden Schafen) mittels PCR oder CI-ELISA nachweisen. Im Blutserum von Rindern, die Gnu-assoziiertes BKF überstanden haben, sind durch indirekte Immunfluoreszenz, ELISA oder KBR Antikörper gegen AHV_1, in ihrem Blut, Nasen-, Augenausfluß und Urin mittels Gensonde erregerspezifische DNA-Fragmente feststellbar. Klinisch inapparente AHV_1- und OHV_2-Trägertiere lassen sich durch PCR-Prüfung ihrer Blutlymphozyten ermitteln; mit dem gleichen Verfahren läßt sich OHV_2 auch in Gewebeproben nachweisen.

Differentialdiagnostisch und von BKF abzugrenzen: Mucosal Disease (betroffene Tiere meist jünger, keine ausgeprägte Beteiligung von Augen- und Nasenschleimhaut, d. h. kein Schniefen, Erregernachweis; Kap. 6.10.20), Rinderpest (blutiger Durchfall, Erregernachweis; Kap. 12.2.3), Maul- und Klauenseuche sowie Stomatitis vesicularis (bläschenförmige Veränderungen an Maulschleimhaut, Zitzen und im Zwischenklauenpalt, Augen unbeteiligt, Erregernachweis; Kap. 12.2.1, 6.1.6), Blue tongue (ausgeprägte Klauenlahmheit, Augen und Gehirn nicht beteiligt, Miterkrankung kleiner Wiederkäuer, Erregernachweis; Kap. 6.1.7), Infektiöse Bovine Rhinotracheitis (Maulhöhle und übriger Verdauungsapparat meist unbeteiligt, Erregernachweis; Kap. 5.1.3.1), infektiöse Keratokonjunktivitis (nur Augen und Bindehaut erkrankt; Kap. 11.1.3.1), Herpes-Konjunktivitis (i. d. R. nur Bindehaut betroffen; Kap. 11.1.3.4) und Besnoitiose (chronischer Verlauf, anfangs Anasarka, später Sklerodermie der Haut im Kopfbereich, Erregernachweis; Kap. 2.2.4.6).

■ **Behandlung, Prophylaxe:** Therapieversuche kommen wegen geringer Erfolgsaussichten nur bei besonders wertvollen Tieren in Betracht und umfassen neben symptomatischen Maßnahmen (ruhiger abgedunkelter Stall, Schlappfütterung, Tränken aus dem Eimer) regelmäßige Spülungen von Nasen- und Maulhöhle mit milden Desinfizienzien, reichliche intravenöse Flüssigkeitszufuhr und Ausgleich der speichelverlustbedingten metabolischen Azidose (Kap. 4.3.6.2), parenterale Gaben von Breitband-Antibiotika sowie nicht-steroidalen Entzündungshemmern. Die Vorbeuge besteht in strikter Trennung von Rinder- und Schafhaltung; Rinder sollten nicht einmal vorübergehend in einem zuvor mit Schafen besetzt gewesenen Stall untergebracht oder dort geweidet werden, wo kürzlich Schafe gelammt haben. In Wildgehegen und zoologischen Gärten sind BKF-Virus-Überträger- und -Empfängerspezies möglichst weit voneinander entfernt zu halten. Bislang gibt es keine ungefährliche und zugleich wirksame BKF-Vakzine für Rinder.

Bekämpfung: In Deutschland ist Bösartiges Katarrhalfieber gemäß VOmTK zum TSeuG meldepflichtig.

12.2.3 Rinderpest

L. Haas

Definition: Rinderpest ist eine akut bis subakut verlaufende, durch nekrotisierende Entzündung der Schleimhäute, insbesondere derjenigen des Verdauungstrakts, schwere Diarrhoe und Dehydratation charakterisierte virale Infektionskrankheit, die außer Rindern auch andere Paarzeher befällt. Morbidität und Mortalität können bei *epizootischen* Seuchenzügen > 90% betragen, doch kommen auch weniger schwerwiegende *enzootische* Verlaufsformen vor. Als wohl einzige Rinderkrankheit ist Rinderpest im fremdsprachigen Ausland unter ihrem deutschen Namen bekannt; *andere Bezeichnungen*: pestis bovina, cattle plague, peste bovine, veeziekte, plage bovina.

Geschichte: Rinderpest ist eine der gefürchtetsten Seuchen der Boviden, weil sie große Rinder- und Büffelpopulationen nahezu ausrotten kann. In vergangenen Jh. löste sie so immer wieder Hungersnot aus und richtete großen sozioökonomischen und politischen Schaden an (s. Abb. 1-8). Vermutlich asiatischen Ursprungs ist die Rinderpest im Verlauf kriegerischer Ereignisse wiederholt, erstmals wohl im 1. Jh. v. d. Z., nach *Europa* eingeschleppt worden und hat hier mit ihren verlustreichen Seuchenzügen sogar den Verlauf der Geschichte beeinflußt. Unter anderem ist ihr die Gründung der ersten tierärztlichen Bildungsstätten zu verdanken. Zur Bekämpfung der Rinderpest wurden in Österreich und Preußen bereits 1711, also lange vor dem erst 1902 durch Nicolle & Adil Bey erbrachten Nachweis der Virusnatur ihres Erregers, strenge veterinärpolizeiliche Eradikationsmaßnahmen festgelegt (= Vorläufer des heutigen Tierseuchengesetzes); mit ihrer Hilfe ist Deutschland seit 1889 rinderpestfrei geblieben.

Nach *Afrika* wurde die Rinderpest erst gegen Ende des 19. Jh. (Abessinischer Krieg), und zwar durch Importe infizierten Viehs aus Indien eingebracht. Die dadurch ausgelöste verheerende panafrikanische Epizootie breitete sich vom Horn von Afrika bis nach Südafrika aus und vernichtete 80–95% aller Hausrinder, Büffel, Schafe und Ziegen sowie unzählige Wildpaarzeher. Die vorläufig letzte Rinderpestepizootie suchte die Subsahara-Region 1982–1984 heim (Abb. 12-11).

Häufigster *Anlaß für Neu- oder Wiederauftreten der Rinderpest* sind Nachlassen der Impfbemühungen, mangelnde Grenzüberwachung, politische Instabilität sowie militärische Auseinandersetzungen. So wurde die Seuche 1991 als Folge des Golfkrieges aus dem Irak in den anatolischen Teil der Türkei eingeschleppt. Die letzten Ausbrüche von Rinderpest in Europa ereigneten sich 1920 in Belgien sowie 1949 im Zoo von Rom. Ersterer war Mitanlaß zur Gründung des Internationalen Tierseuchenamtes (OIE) in Paris.

Vorkommen, Bedeutung: In einigen ostafrikanischen Gebieten, in Pakistan, Afghanistan und bestimmten Regionen Asiens spielt Rinderpest bei Rindern sowie Büffeln heute noch eine bedeutsame *enzootische* Rolle; Indien gilt derzeit als »provisionally free«. Im Mittleren und Nahen Osten wird das Leiden jedoch wieder vermehrt beobachtet, das zudem in einigen dieser Länder dazu neigt, bodenständig zu werden.

Enzootisch von Rinderpest befallene Gebiete stellen eine fortwährende Gefährdung für benachbarte, rinderpestfreie Regionen dar. Bei derart ausgelösten und dann zur *epizootischen* Ausbreitung neigenden Neuausbrüchen muß mit einer Mortalität von ≤90% und enormen wirtschaftlichen Folgeschäden gerechnet werden. In *enzootisch* befallenen Regionen mit extensiver Viehhaltung ist die Mortalität dagegen mit nur 10–30% wesentlich geringer.

Unter natürlichen Bedingungen umfaßt das *Wirtsspektrum* des Rinderpestvirus praktisch alle Paarzeher. Von den domestizierten Tieren sind insbesondere Rinder (Tauriden, Zebus, Yaks) und Wasserbüffel gefährdet; bei ersteren sind europäische Rassen empfänglicher als Zeburassen. Schafe und Ziegen sowie Schweine asiatischer Rassen können ebenfalls an Rinderpest erkranken; Schweine europäischer Rassen lassen sich zwar infizieren, werden aber nicht krank. Kamele zeigen nur mild verlaufende oder subklinische Infektionen; sie sind deshalb kein bedeutsamer Faktor in der Epidemiologie der Rinderpest. Die Rolle wildlebender Paarzeher im Rinderpestgeschehen Afrikas ist früher überschätzt worden. Heute wird angenommen, daß das Leiden zwar vom Hausrind in die Wildtierfauna getragen wird, dort aber m. o. w. bald wieder erlischt; Wildpaarzeher gelten daher nicht mehr als ständiges Reservoir ihres Erregers. In Asien ist die vom Wild ausgehende Rinderpestgefährdung von Haustieren noch geringer einzuschätzen. Offenbar kann sich das Rinderpestvirus auch in Hunden vermehren, da sie nach Aufnahme infizierten Fleisches serokonvertieren, allerdings ohne Krankheitserscheinungen zu zeigen.

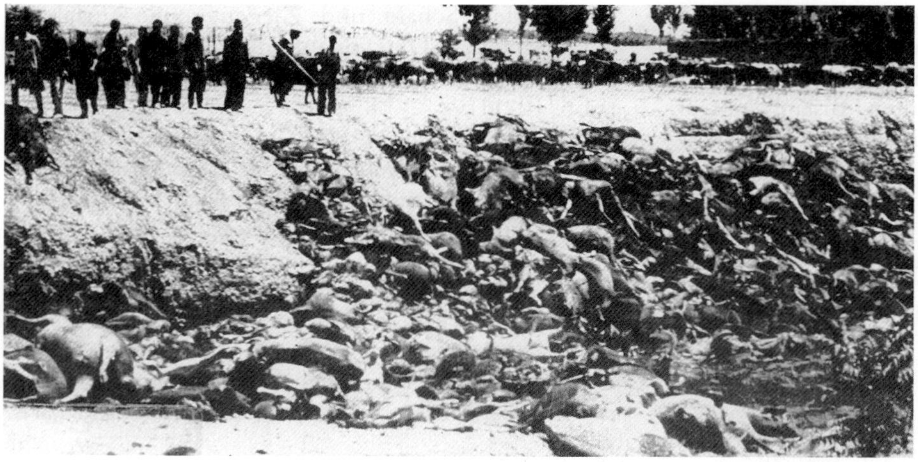

Abbildung 12-11 Rinderpest-Ausbruch in Ostafrika 1982/1984: Einsammeln und Vernichtung angefallener Kadaver (FOOD AND AGRICULTURE ORGANIZATION, 1983; s. auch Abb. 1-8)

■ **Ursachen:** Mit anderen Morbilliviren (Masern, Staupe, Peste-des-petits-Ruminants) gehört das Rinderpestvirus zur Familie der Paramyxoviren. Seine Virionen sind ihrer Struktur wegen durch Austrocknung, Sonnenlicht, UV-Strahlung sowie durch Lipoidlösungsmittel und detergenzhaltige Desinfektionsmittel leicht inaktivierbar; auch außerhalb des pH-Bereichs von 5,0–10,0 verlieren sie ihre Infektiosität rasch. Antigen ist dieser Erreger recht einheitlich, d. h., es gibt keine Serotypen. Molekularbiologisch lassen sich asiatische und afrikanische Isolate des Rinderpestvirus unterscheiden. Letzere bilden zwei, Typ 1- und Typ 2-Viren genannte Linien.

Mit Rinderpestvirus infizierte Paarzeher entwickeln neutralisierende Antikörper gegenüber den in der Virushülle verankerten Glykoproteinen H und F. Hinsichtlich ihrer Virulenz unterscheiden sich die einzelnen Stämme und Isolate des Rinderpestvirus zwar erheblich, doch ist der molekulare Hintergrund dieses Phänomens noch nicht geklärt. Attenuierte Stämme, insbesondere der KABETE-0-Stamm, sind Grundlage der heute gebräuchlichen Lebendimpfstoffe.

■ **Verbreitung:** Die *Übertragung* des Rinderpestvirus erfolgt durch unmittelbaren oder engen mittelbaren Kontakt mit klinisch oder subklinisch erkrankten Paarzehern als oro-nasopharyngeale Infektion mit erregerhaltigen Se- und Exkreten. Infizierte Tiere scheiden den Keim bereits 1–2 Tage vor Einsetzen des Fiebers – also schon in der Inkubationsphase – über Tränenflüssigkeit, Nasensekret, Speichel, Milch, Harn und Kot aus; vor dem Einsetzen klinischer Erscheinungen sind auch Blut und die meisten Organe erregerhaltig. Demgegenüber spielen indirekte Übertragungen des Leidens durch infiziertes Tränkwasser, Dung, unter günstigen klimatischen Bedingungen auch über kontaminierte Weiden, aufgrund der geringen Tenazität des Virus keine bedeutsame Rolle.

■ **Pathogenese:** Nach Befall der Schleimhäute des oberen Respirationstrakts erfolgt die primäre Vermehrung des Erregers in den lymphatischen Einrichtungen des Nasenrachenraums. Dann ist das Virus, eng an mononukleäre Zellen gebunden, im Blut zu finden. Die Virämie geht den klinischen Erscheinungen um 1–2 Tage voraus. Nun vermehrt sich der Keim in den Schleimhäuten des Verdauungs- und Atmungstrakts, in der Lunge sowie sämtlichen lymphoiden Geweben, was mit deutlicher Lymphopenie einhergeht. In dieser Phase wird Rinderpestvirus mit allen Se- und Exkreten, insbesondere mit Augen- und Nasenausfluß sowie den Fäzes, ausgeschieden. Beim Überstehen der Rinderpestvirus-bedingten Infektion setzen Immunisierungsvorgänge ein, die den Erreger eliminieren; daher wurden bisher keine persistierend infizierten Tiere (carriers) beobachtet.

■ **Symptome, Verlauf** (Abb. 12-12 bis 12-14): Das klinische Bild der Rinderpest kann in Abhängigkeit von der Empfänglichkeit des Wirts und der Virulenz des Erregers variieren:

➤ Bei *Epizootien* in zuvor nicht von ihr befallenen Gebieten verläuft Rinderpest als akute fieberhafte Erkrankung hoher Morbidi- und Mortalität. Ihre Inkubationszeit beträgt 3–5 Tage (bei geringer Virulenz ≤2 Wochen). Während der *Prodromalphase* werden Apathie, Anorexie, herabgesetzte Vormagentätigkeit, Zähneknirschen, Milchrückgang sowie gesteigerte Atem- und Herzfrequenz beobachtet. Die Körpertemperatur steigt auf 41–42 °C und bleibt mindestens 4 Tage lang fieberhaft. In der anschließenden *Schleimhautphase* zeigen die Patienten, v. a. an Nasen- und Maulschleimhaut sowie Konjunktiven, katarrhalische Entzündung mit hochgradigem serösen Ausfluß, der rasch mukopurulent werden kann, sowie Lichtscheu. Vom 3.–5. Tag an treten als kennzeichnende Veränderung multiple stecknadelkopfgroße, weißgelbliche epitheliale Nekroseherde auf der Schleimhaut von

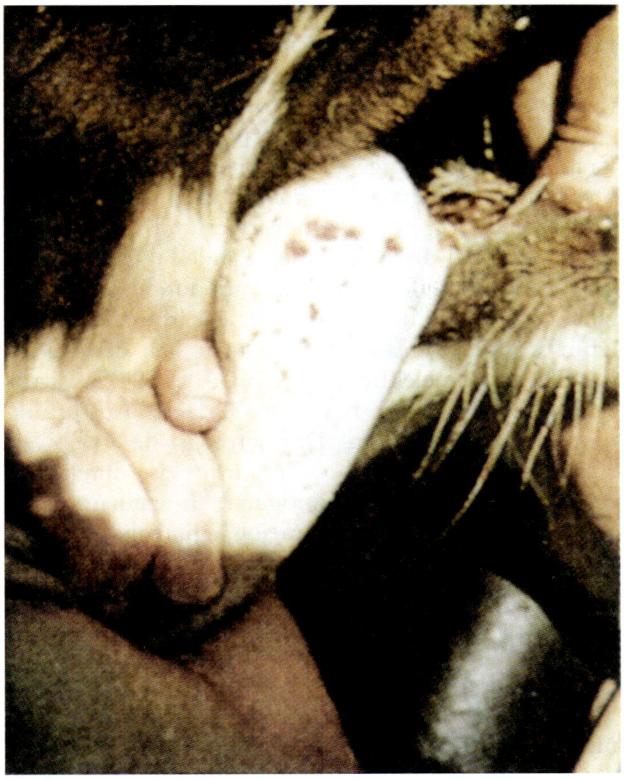

Abbildung 12-12 Rinderpest: Zunge eines ostafrikanischen Rindes mit rinderpestbedingten Erosionen (LIESS & PLOWRIGHT, 1962)

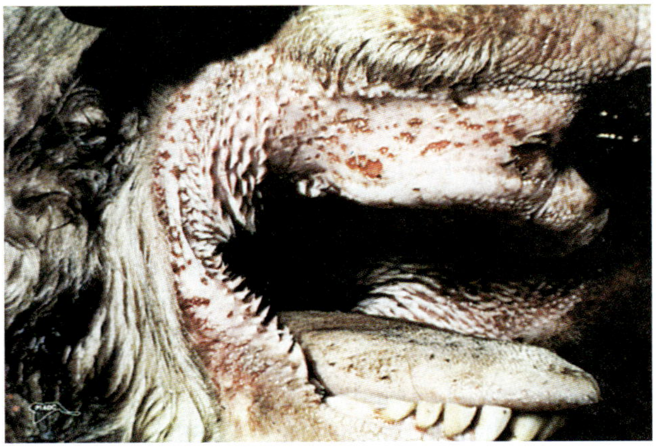

Abbildung 12-13 Rinderpest: Erosiv-nekrotisierende Veränderungen im Bereich der Lippen (CALLIS et al., 1982)

Unterlippe, Maulwinkel, Zahnfleisch, Zungen, Backenpapillen sowie Dentalplatte und Gaumen auf, die dabei sensibel und rauh wird. In den folgenden Tagen nehmen die Mukosaläsionen an Zahl und Größe zu, wobei ihre unregelmäßig-lakunenartigen Ränder konfluieren; schließlich erscheinen die genannten Schleimhäute insgesamt wie »mit Kleie bestreut«. Diese käsig-schmierigen diphtheroiden Beläge sind

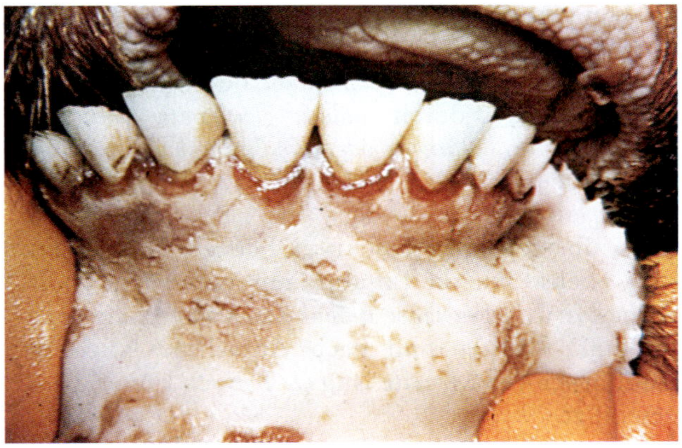

Abbildung 12-14 Rinderpestbedingte Läsionen des Schneidezahnfleischs (CALLIS et al., 1982)

dann leicht abstreifbar und hinterlassen unregelmäßig geformte rote Erosionen. Zugleich setzen Zähneknirschen, profus-schaumiges Speicheln und übler Maulgeruch ein. Die Kranken haben nun vermehrten Durst, und ihr Flotzmaul wird trocken-rissig. Von Fall zu Fall kann sich eine *diarrhöische Phase* anschließen, während der das Fieber meist zurückgeht; sie gilt als prognostisch ungünstiges Zeichen. Solche Patienten zeigen profusen hämorrhagischen Durchfall und Tenesmen; ihr Kot enthält oft Epithelfetzen und fibrinöse Darmausgüsse. Das führt infolge rapider Dehydratation zu erheblichem Gewichtsverlust und körperlicher Schwächung. Schließlich äußern die Kranken bei zunehmender exspiratorischer Dyspnoe kurzes, schmerzhaftes Husten und Stöhnen sowie vermehrte Neigung, sich hinzulegen; unmittelbar vor dem Tode liegen sie mitunter in »Milchfieberhaltung« fest.

Hochgradige Schleimhautschädigungen sowie die virusbedingte Immunsuppression fördern nicht selten die Entwicklung bakterieller oder hämoprotozoärer *Sekundärinfektionen*, als deren Folge eitrige Geschwüre, purulente Bronchopneumonie, Pleuritis oder Peritonitis bzw. Babesiose oder Trypanosomose auftreten, die dann ihrerseits zum tödlichen Verlauf beitragen. Trächtige Patientinnen können *abortieren*.

Die früher häufiger erwähnten *rinderpestbedingten Hautläsionen* werden heute nur noch selten gefunden. Dabei entwickeln sich in dünnhäutigen Bereichen (Euter, Skrotum, Schenkelinnenflächen) oder am gesamten Körper punkt- bis linsengroße Papeln, verkrustende Bläschen und Blutungen, über denen die Haare büschelweise verkleben.

Falls die Diarrhoe ausnahmsweise ausbleibt, können sich mehrwöchige *Rekonvaleszenz* und *Heilung* anschließen.

➤ In *enzootisch rinderpestverseuchten Gebieten* verläuft die Erkrankung beim Einzeltier sowie innerhalb betroffener Herden meist wesentlich milder. Dabei wird das klinische Bild nicht nur von *Pathogenität und Virulenz des jeweiligen Erregers* sowie von der *Resistenzlage der betroffenen Paarzeherpopulation* bestimmt, sondern oft auch noch durch *andere, gleichzeitig vorliegende Leiden* sowie *haltungs- oder ernährungsbedingte Streßfaktoren* beeinflußt (= *subklinische* bzw. *Mischformen der Rinderpest*).

Im übrigen hinterläßt das Überstehen der Infektion, ebenso wie die Impfung mit attenuiertem Rinderpestvirus, *lebenslange Immunität*. Kälber rinderpestimmuner Mütter sind nach Aufnahme kolostraler Antikörper 4–8 Monate lang (z. T. noch länger) passiv geschützt.

■ **Sektion:** Tierkörper abgemagert und dehydratisiert, Körperöffnungen stark verunreinigt. Entsprechend dem klinischen Bild sind v. a. die Schleimhäute des Verdauungstrakts sowie diejenigen von Nase und Scheide betroffen. Sie zeigen m. o. w. diffuse Schwellung und Rötung sowie regionale Erosionen und Nekrosen, die typischerweise mit hämorrhagisch-fibrinösen Auflagerungen bedeckt sind. Sämtliche Lymphknoten sind vergrößert und ödematös. Die Gallenblase kann vergrößert, ihre verdickte Schleimhaut mit Petechien durchsetzt sein. Im Dünndarm sind die PEYERschen Platten nekrotisiert; auch im Ileozäkalbereich sind Ulzerationen zu finden. Im Dickdarm sind die erosiv-geschwürigen Veränderungen der Mukosa i. d. R. wesentlich stärker ausgeprägt; in Zökum, Kolon und Rektum können longitudinal verlaufende hämorrhagische »Zebrastreifen« vorliegen. Etwaiger rinderpestbedingter Abort bedingt Plazentomnekrosen. Von Fall zu Fall sind zudem als Folge der bereits erwähnten Sekundärinfektionen komplikative Veränderungen an weiteren Organen zu finden, die das Sektionsbild u. U. sogar beherrschen.

Histologisch ist der Tropismus des Rinderpestvirus für lymphoide und epitheliale Zellen erkennbar. Hiervon erweisen sich sämtliche lymphatischen Einrichtungen, insbesondere aber Mesenteriallymphknoten und darmassoziiertes lymphatisches Gewebe, als betroffen. Ihre T- und B-Zellbezirke sind v. a. nach Infektion mit virulentem Virus deutlich depletiert. Zudem finden sich nicht selten intrazytoplasmatische und intranukleäre eosinophile Einschlußkörperchen.

■ **Diagnose:** Das durch schwere fieberhafte Allgemeinstörung gekennzeichnete, mit nekrotisch-erosiven Veränderungen der Maulschleimhaut, Durchfall und rascher Ausbreitungstendenz verbundene klinische Bild ist typisch für Rinderpest. Sind jedoch nur einzelne Tiere betroffen, so müssen *differentialdiagnostisch* v. a. Bovine Virusdiarrhoe/Mucosal Disease (Kap. 6.10.20), Bösartiges Katarrhalfieber (Kap. 12.2.2), Maul- und Klauenseuche (Kap. 12.2.1), Infektiöse Bovine Rhinotracheitis (Kap. 5.1.3.1), Stomatitis vesicularis (Kap. 6.1.6), Lungenseuche (Kap. 5.3.3.16), Hämorrhagische Septikämie (Kap. 4.2.3.1), Salmonellose (Kap. 6.10.21) und Paratuberkulose (Kap. 6.10.22) abgegrenzt werden.

Bei etwaigem Ausbruch rinderpestverdächtiger Krankheiten ist zügige *Labordiagnostik* unumgänglich. Der Einsatz der derzeit bekannten Nachweismethoden ist allerdings von ihrer Verfügbarkeit und vom technischen Standard des betroffenen Landes abhängig: Der Nachweis des Rinderpestvirus kann durch Anzucht in Zellkulturen und Immunperoxidase-Färbung erfolgen. Zum Antigennachweis bedient man sich der AGID, der Gegenstromelektrophorese oder des IPOT. Virusnukleinsäure läßt sich bei entsprechender Ausrüstung mittels PCR ermitteln. Der serologische Nachweis rinderpestvirusspezifischer Antikörper ist durch NT oder kompetitiven ELISA möglich. Hierzu kann beim Fehlen einer Kühlkette und unabhängig von der Länge des Einsendungswegs auch an Filterpapier adsorbiertes Blut verwendet werden.

■ **Beurteilung:** Der Verlauf der Erkrankung am Einzeltier und im Bestand hängt weitgehend von der Struktur der betroffenen Herde(n), wie Rasse, Immunitätslage, Konstitution usf. sowie von der Virulenz des beteiligten Erregerstammes ab und ist therapeutisch nicht nennenswert beeinflußbar.

■ **Behandlung, Prophylaxe:** Es gibt keine spezifisch wirksame Therapie der Rinderpest. In Deutschland und anderen europäischen Ländern sind Behandlungsversuche an rinderpestkranken oder -verdächtigen Rindern ebenso wie Impfungen gegen Rinderpest untersagt.

■ **Bekämpfung:** In Deutschland ist Rinderpest gemäß VOaTS anzeigepflichtig. Sollte sie hier erneut auftreten, so würden gemäß § 79 TSeuG bei solcher »Gefahr im Verzuge« sofort die erforderlichen Maßnahmen angeordnet werden. Dabei könnten rechtliche Regelungen als Vorlage dienen, wie sie für andere Tierseuchen, z. B. Maul- und Klauenseuche, detailliert vorgeschrieben sind.

In Afrika basiert die Bekämpfung auf der Impfung mit Zellkultur-Lebendvakzinen. Die damit vorgenommenen international finanzierten Kampagnen (1960er Jahre: Joint Programme 15; 1986: Pan-African Rinderpest Campaign) hatten noch keinen dauerhaften Erfolg. In den 1990er Jahren wurde daher das Global Rinderpest Eradication Program der FAO initiiert, mit dessen Hilfe die Rinderpest bis zum Jahre 2010 weltweit ausgerottet werden soll. Ein Nachteil der ansonsten sehr effizienten Lebendvakzine ist ihre Thermolabilität; sie muß daher bis zur Anwendung am Tier gekühlt bleiben. Deshalb wird versucht, die Haltbarkeit solcher Vakzinen durch Zusätze und schonendes Gefriertrocknen zu verbessern. Außerdem wurden – durch Einschleusen der Gene für die immunogenen H- und F-Proteine des Rinderpestvirus in Vakzinia- oder Kapripoxviren – erfolgversprechende rekombinante Vakzinen entwickelt.

12.2.4 Pararauschbrand, Malignes Ödem

M. Stöber

Definition: Auf nichtkontagiöser *exogener* Infektion perforierender Verletzungen mit bestimmten Clostridien beruhende, unter Entwicklung von Toxinen, Exsudat und Gas zu rasch fortschreitender Schädigung benachbarten Binde- und Muskelgewebes, Bewegungsbehinderung sowie Allgemeinstörungen führende und meist (per-)akut tödlich verlaufende Erkrankung. *Andere Bezeichnungen*: traumatische Gangrän, »Wundrauschbrand«, »Geburtsrauschbrand«, puerperaler Gasbrand, »Kälberrauschbrand«, charbon parasymptomatique, paraboutvuur, blackquarter-like disease. Bei fehlendem oder unklarem Erregernachweis werden Pararauschbrand und Rauschbrand auch unter den Begriffen »bösartige Gasphlegmone« oder »clostridienbedingte Muskelentzündung und -nekrose« zusammengefaßt.

Vorkommen: Das maligne Ödem kommt weltweit ohne besondere örtliche Bindung vor. Beim Rind tritt es sporadisch und ohne Bevorzugung einer bestimmten Altersgruppe auf. Auch Pferd, Schaf oder Schwein werden mitunter, Fleischfresser dagegen nur selten von Pararauschbrand betroffen.

Ursachen, Pathogenese: Als Eintrittspforte für malignes Ödem auslösende Clostridien dienen beim Rind meist tiefere Verletzungen, wie Unfallfolgen, Perforation von Maul- oder Rachenschleimhaut oder des Schlundes, Lazerationen des weichen Geburtswegs oder die Wunden chirurgischer Eingriffe (Enthornung, Kastration, Schwanzamputation o. ä.). Gleiches gilt auch für den bei parenteraler Arzneimittelverabreichung entstehenden Stichkanal, und zwar insbesondere, aber nicht ausschließlich, bei verschmutzter oder nichtdesinfizierter Applikationsstelle, bei Verwendung unsterilen Instrumentariums, nach Gabe verkeimter, örtlich reizender, entzündungshemmender oder gefäßverengender nichtantibiotischer Medikamente, nach intramuskulärer oder subkutaner Applikation großer Arzneimittelvolumina pro Injektionsstelle oder nach paravenöser Einspritzung; solche Begleitumstände können sich bei Reihenmedikation oder -impfung u. U. äußerst schadensträchtig auswirken. Die geschilderten Läsionen bieten miteingebrachten Erregersporen günstige Bedingungen (Anaerobie, absterbendes Gewebe) zur vegetativen Vermehrung und Toxinbildung.

Als offensichtlich krankmachender Keim wird beim Pararauschbrand des Rindes meist *Cl. septicum*, neben ihm aber nicht selten auch *Cl. oedematiens* (s. novyi Typ A), *Cl. perfringens* (s. welchii) Typ A, *Cl. carnis*, *Cl. sordelli*, *Cl. chicamensis*, mitunter auch *Cl. sporogenes* ermittelt. Diese im Erdreich ubiquitär vorkommenden grampositiven Sporenbildner werden von Pflanzenfressern, zu deren Darmflora sie zählen, v. a. während des Weidegangs mit dem Futter aufgenommen und mit ihrem Kot wieder ausgeschieden, d. h. auch verbreitet. Gelegentlich wird sogar *Cl. chauvœi* (Kap. 12.2.5) als Wundkontaminant nachgewiesen. Die genannten Clostridien bilden im betroffenen Gewebe hochwirksame leukozyten-abwehrende, hämolysierende, gewebeabtötende und -auflösende Toxine sowie – mit Ausnahme von Cl. sordelli – Gas.

Symptome: Manche Pararauschbrand-Patienten werden unvermutet tot aufgefunden. Sonst entwickelt sich 1–5 Tage nach der krankmachenden Läsion in deren Umgebung eine subkutan sowie inter- und intramuskulär lokalisierte, anfangs vermehrt warme und druckempfindliche, ödematöse Anschwellung, die im weiteren Verlauf zentral kühler, weicher, unsensibel und m. o. w. deutlich gashaltig wird; ihre Palpation bzw. Perkussion ergibt dann Krepitation bzw. überlauten Klopfschall. Falls die Haut im Bereich der Umfangsvermehrung nicht pigmentiert ist, zeigt sie hier eine dunkle Verfärbung. Das Maligne Ödem breitet sich rasch aus, so daß innerhalb kurzer Zeit eine ganze Körperregion (Zunge/Kehlgang, Kehlgang/Vorbrust, Hals/Schulter, Hinterbacke/Oberschenkel oder Perineum/Euterbereich/Unterbauch) ergriffen sein kann. Das führt zu fortschreitender Einschränkung der Motilität, weshalb sich das kranke Tier immer zögernder fortbewegt und nur schwerfällig niederlegt oder aufsteht (Abb. 12-15). Soweit die regionalen Lymphknoten noch palpierbar sind, erweisen sie sich als geschwollen. Wenn es die Eintrittsstelle der krankmachenden Clostridien erlaubt, entleert sich hier graurötliches übelriechendes und m. o. w. deutlich schaumiges Exsudat. Die Körpertemperatur kann sepsisbedingt bis auf 41 °C ansteigen, fällt dann aber auf normale, im Endstadium sogar auf hypotherme Werte ab. Freßlust, Allgemeinbefinden und Sensorium sind zunehmend beeinträchtigt, der Puls frequent, klein und schwach. In der Mehrzahl der Fälle tritt innerhalb von 2–5 Tagen unter Freßunlust, Versiegen der Milch, zunehmender Benommenheit und allgemeiner Schwäche der Tod ein.

Sektion: Die Zerlegung sollte möglichst innerhalb von 2 h nach dem Verenden erfolgen, weil die postmortale Fäulnis in Kadavern von an Pararauschbrand

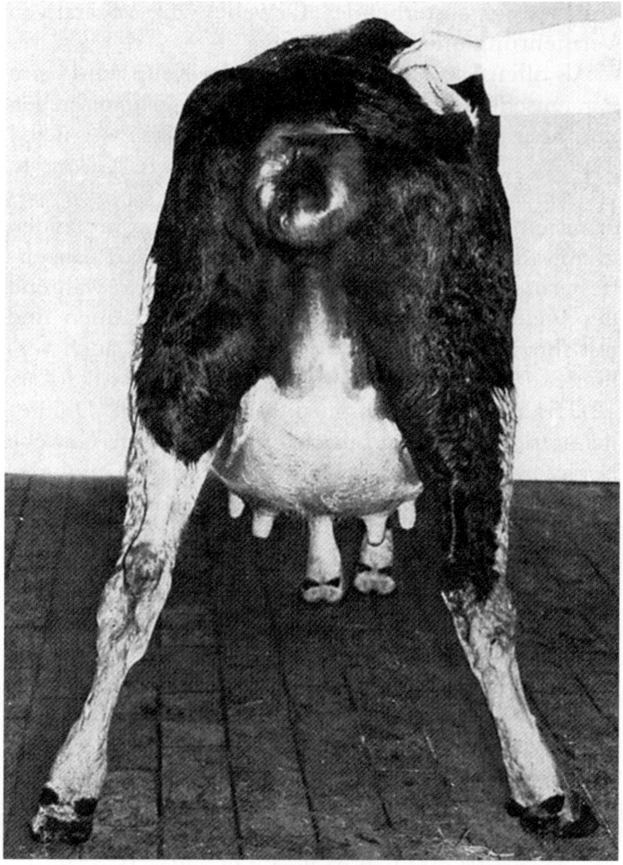

Abbildung 12-15 Malignes Ödem, das sich von der beim Kalben verletzten Scheide und Scham bis zum After sowie auf Euter und Unterbauch ausdehnt

gefallenen Tieren unter gleichzeitiger Tympanie besonders rasch fortschreitet und zum Eindringen von Anaerobiern, z. B. Cl. septicum, aus dem Verdauungstrakt in den Tierkörper beiträgt (→ Verfälschung bakteriologischer Befunde). Entsprechendes gilt für die bei der Sektion erfolgende Entnahme von Proben zum Nachweis der Erreger (Preßsaft oder Tupfpräparat von der Anschnittfläche veränderten Gewebes). Im clostridienbetroffenen Bereich ist das peri- und intermuskuläre Bindegewebe mit reichlich gelblich-rötlichem, sulzigem bis flüssigem Exsudat durchtränkt, das zahlreiche Gasbläschen enthält und aufgrund der sich in ihm entwickelnden flüchtigen Fettsäuren abstoßenden Geruch aufweist. Dieser ist je nach beteiligter Erregerkombination ranzig, süßlich, faulig oder sauer. Benachbartes Muskelgewebe ist dunkelbraun- bis schwarzrot, mitunter dagegen graurot oder fahlgelb, und v. a. im Zentrum des Krankheitsherdes mürbe, aber – im Gegensatz zum Rauschbrand – oft weniger stark verändert als das Bindegewebe. Die Lymphknoten sind geschwollen, die Milz erscheint normal oder durch Gasbläschen aufgetrieben. Zudem bestehen Lungenhyperämie und -ödem. Der Herzmuskel weist brüchige Konsistenz auf. Leber und Nieren enthalten oft postmortal entstandene graugelbe gashaltige Herde; erstere kann sogar schon bald nach dem Tode völlig schwammig-schaumig verändert sein.

■ Diagnose: Die Erkennung des Malignen Ödems stützt sich auf Vorbericht (Hinweise auf exogene Infektion), klinische Erscheinungen (rasch sowie unter deutlicher Beeinträchtigung des Allgemeinbefindens größer werdende Gasphlegmone), Zerlegungsbefunde (Gasödem des Binde- und Gasgangrän des Muskelgewebes) sowie Erregernachweis. Für letzteren eignen sich durch Punktion gewonnenes Exsudat der krankmachenden Anschwellung, bioptisch aus der betreffenden Verletzung entnommenes Gewebe oder von letzterem angefertigte Tupfpräparate, die der Untersuchungsstelle sachgemäß verpackt zuzusenden sind (s. Rauschbrand, Kap. 12.2.5). Der Nachweis stützt sich auf kulturelle Anzüchtung und Differenzierung der beteiligten Keime (DIF, PCR, Morphologie des Sporenstadiums, Toxinanalyse, gaschromatographische Darstellung der von den Clostridien freigesetzten flüchtigen Fettsäuren, Neutralisationsversuch an spezifisch schutzgeimpften Meerschweinchen).

Differentialdiagnostisch sind einfache Ödeme und Phlegmonen (Kap. 2.3.2.1, 2.3.3.1), Abszesse (Kap. 2.3.3.4) und Hämatome (Kap. 2.3.2.3), v. a. aber Rauschbrand (Kap. 12.2.5) und Milzbrand (Kap. 3.2.2.1) zu berücksichtigen.

■ **Beurteilung:** I. d. R. werden von Malignem Ödem betroffene Rinder zu spät vorgestellt, um noch mit Aussicht auf Erfolg behandelt zu werden. Eine Verwertung des Fleisches kommt wegen des septischen Krankheitsgeschehens nicht in Frage.

■ **Behandlung:** Im Hinblick auf die schlechte Prognose sollten Therapieversuche nur in früh zur Vorstellung gelangenden Fällen vorgenommen werden: Einzelaufstallung in eingestreuter Laufboxe; parenterale Gabe von polyvalentem Gasödemserum; 5- bis 8tägige allgemeine Antibiose mit hohen, intravenös und in die Umfangsvermehrung hinein zu verabreichenden Penicillin- oder Tetracyclin-Dosen; Anlegen eines oder mehrerer tiefer vertikaler Hautschnitte im Bereich der Anschwellung und regelmäßig zu wiederholende Spülungen der dabei entstehenden, offen zu haltenden Wundhöhle/n mit 3%igem Wasserstoffperoxid; vorsichtiges Ausräumen abgestorbenen Gewebes. Im Verlauf der Behandlung ist mit erheblicher Abmagerung, nach etwaiger Ausheilung mit bleibender Bewegungsbehinderung und Minderleistung zu rechnen.

■ **Prophylaxe:** Die Vorbeuge des Malignen Ödems besteht in Vermeidung der Ursachen: Einhaltung der erforderlichen Sorgfalt bei parenteraler Arzneimittelverabreichung (Herstellerangaben zur Applikationsweise beachten), geburtshilflichen Maßnahmen und operativen Eingriffen sowie unverzügliche sachgemäße Versorgung perforierender Verletzungen unter gründlicher Resektion veränderten Gewebes. In erfahrungsgemäß von Malignem Ödem bedrohten Beständen kann es ratsam sein, verletzten oder frischoperierten Tieren Gasödemserum zu verabreichen und/oder nachwachsende Jungtiere sowie neueingestellte Rinder generell mit polyvalenter Clostridien-Formolvakzine zu impfen.

■ **Bekämpfung:** Staatlicherseits sind keine Maßnahmen gegen Pararauschbrand vorgesehen.

12.2.5 Rauschbrand, Emphysematöse Gangrän

M. Stöber

■ **Definition:** Nichtkontagiöse und mitunter enzootisch auftretende *endogene* Infektion, d. h. Absiedlung des nach oraler Aufnahme in den Tierkörper gelangten versporten Erregers im Skelett-, Zwerchfell- oder Herzmuskelgewebe, wo er sich – nach anderweitiger Schädigung desselben – unter Toxinbildung und Gasentwicklung vermehrt und eine (per-)akut verlaufende, durch örtliche Anschwellung, Bewegungsstörung sowie Beeinträchtigung des Allgemeinbefindens gekennzeichnete und fast immer tödlich endende Erkrankung auslöst. *Andere Bezeichnungen*: black leg, blackquarter, charbon symptomatique, mal de cuisse, boutvuur. Bei fehlendem oder unklarem Erregernachweis werden Rauschbrand und Pararauschbrand auch unter den Begriffen »bösartige Gasphlegmone« oder »clostridienbedingte Muskelentzündung und -nekrose« zusammengefaßt.

■ **Vorkommen, Ursache:** Im Gegensatz zum Malignen Ödem (Kap. 12.2.4) ist Rauschbrand ein an bestimmte Regionen gebundenes »tellurisches« Leiden, das nur große und kleine Wiederkäuer, und zwar meist (aber nicht ausschließlich) während des Weidegangs befällt. Bei den Gebieten, in denen das äußerst widerstandsfähige sporenbildende und grampositive *Cl. chauvœi* (s. feseri) im Boden angereichert ist, handelt es sich oft um Marschland oder Flußniederungen mit abwechselnder Überflutung und Austrocknung oder um Stellen, an denen früher Rauschbrandkadaver vergraben worden sind. So kann im Umfeld von Erdarbeiten (Grabenaushub o. ä.) bei dort weidenden Rindern völlig überraschend Rauschbrand auftreten. Gleiches gilt für die Verabreichung der von solchen rauschbrandträchtigen Örtlichkeiten stammenden oder dort gelagerten Futtermittel (Heu, mit Erde verunreinigte Silage), was zum Ausbruch von Rauschbrand während der Stallhaltung führen kann.

Von Rauschbrand werden v. a. gut genährte Jung- und Masttiere im Alter zwischen 3 Monaten und 2 (seltener 3) Jahren, und zwar bevorzugt während der warmen Jahreszeit betroffen. In gefährdeten Gegenden gehaltene Rinder immunisieren sich offenbar im Verlauf dieses Zeitraumes aufgrund latenter Exposition aktiv gegen Rauschbrand, während ihre Kälber nach Kolostrumaufnahme zunächst durch maternale Antikörper passiv geschützt sind. Rinder, die aus anderen Gebieten in eine Rauschbrandregion verbracht wurden, erweisen sich dagegen altersunabhängig als rauschbrandanfällig.

Bei näherer Überprüfung von Rauschbrandausbrüchen sind oft, aber nicht immer, Begleitumstände festzustellen, die zu Muskelquetschungen Anlaß gaben (Stoß, Schlag, »Aufreiten«, Rangeleien an Freßplatz oder Tränke, Treiben durch einen Engpaß, Einzwängen im Notstand, Transport o. ä.). Gegebenenfalls kann dann kurz nacheinander bei mehreren derart exponierten Tieren, nicht selten sogar jeweils am gleichen Körperteil, Rauschbrand auftreten.

■ **Bedeutung:** In bestimmten rauschbrandgefährdeten Regionen ist nutzbringende Rinderhaltung nur bei regelmäßiger Rauschbrandschutzimpfung möglich. In Deutschland gelten manche Weidegebiete des nordwestlichen Küstenraumes und bestimmte Täler Oberbayerns als rauschbrandträchtige Territorien.

■ **Pathogenese:** Es ist nicht bekannt, ob Cl. chauvœi im versporten oder vegetativen Stadium oral aufgenommen wird, und auch ungeklärt, auf welchem *endogenen* Wege der Keim dann vom Verdauungskanal aus in den Tierkörper gelangt (zahnwechselbedingte Läsionen der Maulschleimhaut, Fremdkörpertrauma im Vormagenbereich, Darmwandschädigung?). Im Skelett-, Zwerchfells- und/oder Herzmuskel verbleibt er offenbar zunächst in harmloser versporter Form, bis ihm zufällige stumpftraumatische oder hypoxische Schädigungen des Gewebes Gelegenheit zu massiver vegetativer Vermehrung, Toxin- und Gasbildung bieten. Die Toxine hemmen die Abwehrvorgänge des Organismus und bedingen erhöhte Kapillarpermeabilität, Gewebetod sowie -auflösung; zudem sichern sie die zur Proliferation des Erregers erforderliche Anaerobie.

Ausnahmsweise kann Cl. chauvœi auch als *exogen* eindringender Wundkontaminant fungieren (s. Pararauschbrand, Kap. 12.2.4).

■ **Symptome:** Von plötzlichen Todesfällen abgesehen, löst Rauschbrand im Bereich der betroffenen Muskelgruppe eine rasch zunehmende Anschwellung aus, die sich palpatorisch zunächst als vermehrt warm und druckempfindlich, später als unsensibel, kühl und

»brandig«, d.h. puffig-knisternd, erweist. Die Haut über der Umfangsvermehrung wird bald derb und rissig; falls sie in diesem Bereich unpigmentiert ist, erscheint sie dann landkartenartig dunkel verfärbt. Die m.o.w. unförmig werdende Anschwellung wird von Niedergeschlagenheit, Bewegungsunlust, Inappetenz und hoher Herzfrequenz begleitet; die Episkleralgefäße sind injiziert und verwaschen; die Körpertemperatur ist anfangs fieberhaft erhöht, später aber subnormal. Wegen der »Selbstabschottung« des intramuskulären Krankheitsherdes ergibt die Überprüfung des Blutserums auf Kaliumgehalt und CK-Aktivität mitunter normale Werte. Innerhalb von 12–55 h führt Rauschbrand dann unter fortschreitender Toxämie zu Muskelzittern, Atemnot, exspiratorischem Stöhnen, Festliegen, Koma und exzitationslosem Tod.

■ **Sektion:** Die Zerlegung sollte alsbald nach dem Verenden erfolgen, da die postmortale Autolyse in Rauschbrandkadavern rasch fortschreitet, wodurch das Ergebnis bakteriologischer Untersuchungen verfälscht werden kann; außerdem werden dabei die Clostridientoxine zerstört. Bei frisch vorgenommener Sektion sind die veränderten Muskelpartien gut vom gesunden Bereich abgegrenzt. Sie erscheinen peripher auffallend dunkel- bis schwärzlichrot gefärbt und feucht, zentral dagegen infolge Durchsetzung mit Gasbläschen heller und trockener bis mürbe (Abb. 12-16). Schnittflächen und ausgepreßtes schmutzigrot-schaumiges Exsudat riechen nach ranziger Butter. Weitere, von Fall zu Fall vorliegende postmortale Veränderungen sind: betroffene Gliedmaße unförmig angeschwollen und steif gestreckt; Blut rasch geronnen; Vermehrung der oft blut- und fibrinhaltigen Körperflüssigkeiten; Degeneration von Leber und Nieren; fibrinöse bis hämorrhagische Pleuritis; Blutfülle, interstitielles Ödem und Blutungen in der Lunge; Herzmuskel blaß-mürbe; Endokardblutungen; Milz vergrößert mit breiiger Pulpa. Mitunter ergibt die Sektion jedoch keine Skelettmuskelläsionen, sondern lediglich Zwerchfell- oder Herzmuskelveränderungen oder serofibrinöse Perikarditis und Pleuritis. Für die Erregerdarstellung empfiehlt es sich, Tupfpräparate von Muskelgewebeproben anzufertigen, die am Rande des krankhaft veränderten Bereichs entnommen wurden. Miteinzusendendes Muskelgewebe, Preßsaft aus diesem sowie Blut oder Körperhöhlenflüssigkeit sind in lecksicheren Behältern gekühlt zu verschicken.

■ **Diagnose:** Klinisch und postmortal sind Rausch- und Pararauschbrand mitunter nur schwer zu unterscheiden. Für Rauschbrand sprechen das Auftreten bei jüngeren oder zugekauften Rindern im Umfeld einer bekanntermaßen rauschbrandträchtigen Örtlichkeit, das Fehlen krankmachender perforierender

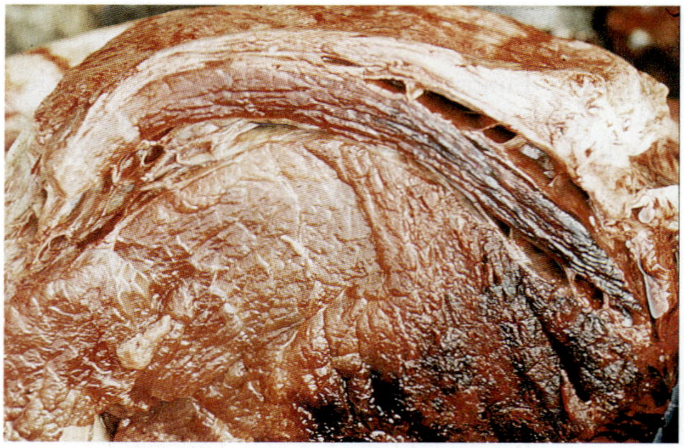

Abbildung 12-16 Rauschbrand: dunkelbraunrote Verfärbung der mit Blutungen und Gasbläschen durchsetzten Skelettmuskulatur eines Rindes

Verletzungen, das Überwiegen gangränöser Muskelveränderungen (im Vergleich zur Ödematisierung desperimuskulären Bindegewebes) und die Ermittlung von Cl. chauvœi in Reinkultur. Für den Erregernachweis eignet sich das am lebenden Tier aus dem Zentrum der Anschwellung gewonnene Aspirat oder der postmortal aus verändertem Muskelgewebe entnommene Preßsaft. Die Keimdifferenzierung erfolgt mittels DIF oder PCR.

Differentialdiagnostisch sind v.a. Pararauschbrand (Kap. 12.2.4), aber auch Milzbrand (Kap. 3.2.2.1), Hämorrhagische Septikämie (Kap. 4.2.3.1), Enterotoxämie (Kap. 6.10.23), Bazilläre Hämoglobinurie (Kap. 4.3.3.2) sowie andersbedingte plötzliche Todesfälle (Weidetetanie, Kap. 10.5.4.1; Blitz- oder Stromschlag, Kap. 10.6.3) zu bedenken.

■ **Beurteilung:** Klinisch manifester Rauschbrand ist prognostisch aussichtslos; zudem besteht dann Schlachtverbot (FlHVO).

■ **Behandlung:** Vor etwaigen Therapieversuchen ist die bei Rauschbrand und Rauschbrandverdacht bestehende Anzeigepflicht zu beachten, da die zuständige Behörde die Tötung der kranken und erkrankungsverdächtigen Tiere anordnen kann. Wiederholte parenterale und intrafokale Gaben von Rauschbrandserum und/oder hoher Dosen von Penicillin oder Tetracyclin haben nur in ganz frischen Fällen einige Aussicht auf Erfolg. Bei behördlicher Zustimmung können die übrigen Tiere des betroffenen Bestandes vorsorglich mit Rauschbrandserum geimpft, d.h. passiv immunisiert werden.

■ **Prophylaxe:** Anfallende Tierkadaver stets ordnungsgemäß über die regional zuständige TKBA entsorgen, d.h. nicht vor Ort vergraben. Erfahrungsgemäß mit Rauschbranderregern verseuchte Örtlichkeiten nicht zum Beweiden oder zur Futtergewinnung nutzen. In solchen Gebieten empfiehlt sich die je nach Gefährdung jährlich zu wiederholende prophylaktische Vakzination der über 3 Monate alten Jungtiere mit polyvalentem Clostridien-Totimpfstoff.

Bekämpfung: Rauschbrand ist gemäß VOaTS zum TSeuG anzeigepflichtig und unterliegt strengen veterinärpolizeilichen Vorschriften (VO zum Schutz gegen den Milzbrand und den Rauschbrand vom 23.5.1991): Die Schlachtung rauschbrandkranker oder -verdächtiger Tiere ist untersagt. Wird Rauschbrand erst nach der Schlachtung bakteriologisch oder serologisch festgestellt, so ist der gesamte Tierkörper als für menschlichen Genuß untauglich zu beurteilen. Zudem kann die zuständige Behörde bei Vorliegen von Rauschbrand oder Rauschbrandverdacht die gleichen Maßregeln wie bei Milzbrand (Kap. 3.2.2.1) anordnen.

12.2.6 Tuberkulose

G. Trautwein

Definition: In ihrer klassischen Form ist die i.d.R. durch *Mycobacterium bovis*, seltener durch *M. avium* oder *M. tuberculosis* bedingte Tuberkulose eine sich meist schleichend entwickelnde Infektionskrankheit zahlreicher Haus- und Wildtierarten und des Menschen. Kennzeichnend für dieses Leiden sind granulomatöse Entzündung mit knötchenförmigen Veränderungen (= »Tuberkel«) an der Eintrittspforte und in regionären Lymphknoten (= Primärkomplex) sowie phasenweiser Verlauf mit Frühgeneralisation (= Miliartuberkulose), chronischer Organtuberkulose und Spätgeneralisation während der Niederbruchsphase. *Andere Bezeichnungen*: Perl- oder Schwindsucht, »Franzosenkrankheit«, Skrofulose, pommelière, consumption, pearl disease, grapes. Hiervon abzugrenzen sind die durch atypische oder opportunistische Mykobakterien hervorgerufenen *Mykobakteriosen*.

Ursache: Haupterreger der Rindertuberkulose ist das außer beim Rind auch beim Menschen sowie verschiedenen Haus-, Zoo- und Wildtierarten vorkommende *Mycobacterium bovis*. Es gehört mit *M. tuberculosis, M. africanum* und *M. microti* zum *M.-tuberculosis-Komplex*. Weitere Mykobakterien, wie diejenigen des *M.-avium-intracellulare-Komplexes, M. kansasii, M. scrofulaceum, M. aquae, M. smegmatis* und *M. fortuitum*, sind für Rinder zwar wenig oder nicht pathogen, spielen bei ihnen aber als Ursache unspezifischer Tuberkulinreaktionen (s. *Diagnose*) eine wichtige Rolle. Tuberkelbakterien sind 1,5–4,0 µm lange, 0,2–0,6 µm dicke, unbewegliche, grampositive, säure- und alkoholfeste, nicht versporende Stäbchen. Bakterioskopisch lassen sie sich am besten mittels Ziehl-Neelsen-Färbung darstellen. Gegen äußere Einflüsse recht widerstandsfähig, überlebt *M. bovis* in Trachealschleim 30–40 Tage, in eingetrocknetem Auswurf ≤100 Tage. In Rinderkot geht der Erreger bei Sonneneinstrahlung in ≤2 Tagen, bei feuchtem Sommerwetter in ≤2 Wochen, im Winter erst in ≤5 Monaten zugrunde. Im Abwasser bleibt er ≤15 Monate lang lebensfähig. In Milch werden Tuberkelbakterien durch Erhitzen auf 65 °C abgetötet. Epidemiologisch bedeutsam ist die Infektionstüchtigkeit von *M. bovis* in Rohmilch und hieraus stammenden Produkten: Sie bleibt in Sauer- und Buttermilch, Joghurt, Kefir und Quark ≤14, in Butter ≤10 Tage, in Weich- und Halbweichkäsen ≤ 300 Tage lang erhalten. In Hartkäsen, deren Reifung 4–5 Monate dauerte, ist *M. bovis* nicht mehr feststellbar. *M. avium* ist noch resistenter als *M. bovis* und kann in der Umwelt ≤ 4 Jahre lang überleben.

Vorkommen, Verbreitung: Die meisten entwickelten Länder sind heute frei von Rindertuberkulose; das gilt in Europa für Dänemark, Deutschland, Finnland, Luxemburg, die Niederlande, Österreich und Schweden. Vorkommendenfalls breitet sie sich in enger Abhängigkeit von bestimmten *Risikofaktoren*, wie Haltungsweise, Besatzdichte, Lebensalter, Tierverkehr und Produktionsrichtung, aus. So ist Tuberkulose bei Milchvieh i.d.R. stärker verbreitet als bei Mastvieh. Stallhaltung und Lebensalter erhöhen Expositionsgrad und Infektionsrate im Gegensatz zur Extensivweide; auch Weidetiere unterliegen jedoch hoher Ansteckungsgefahr, wenn Sammeltränke oder Kraftfuttertrog akzidentell mit *M. bovis* verkeimt sind. Außer bei Haus-, Gehege- und Wildwiederkäuern kommt Tuberkulose in unterschiedlicher Prävalenz bei allen anderen Haus-, Zoo- und Wildtierarten sowie dem Menschen vor; ihrer Übertragbarkeit auf den Menschen wegen stellt bovine Tuberkulose *eine der wichtigsten Zoonosen* dar.

Reinfektionen zuvor als tuberkulosefrei anerkannter Rinderbestände mit *M. bovis* sind zwar selten; die seuchenpolizeilich bedeutsame epidemiologische Aufklärung solcher Vorkommnisse kann aber erhebliche Schwierigkeiten bereiten. Mögliche Quellen erneuter Ansteckung von Rindern sind tuberkulöse Katzen und Wildtiere, verkeimte Weiden oder stehende Gewässer, unkontrollierter Zukauf tuberkulöser Rinder, u.U. auch Betriebsangehörige mit offener, *M.-bovis*-bedingter Lungen- oder Nierentuberkulose. Im Vereinigten Königreich und in Irland wurden nach zunächst unerklärlichen *M.-bovis*-Neuinfektionen von Rindern wilde Dachse *(Meles meles)* als Erregerreservoir ermittelt: Mit ihrem Kot oder Harn können tuberkulöse Dachse ≤ 3,5 Jahre lang *M. bovis* ausscheiden, wonach der Keim im Erdreich ≤ 2 Jahre lang überlebt. Bovine Infektionen kommen dann vermutlich durch Einatmung erregerhaltigen Staubs und/oder orale Aufnahme kontaminierten Futters oder Wassers zustande. In Neuseeland fungieren Fuchskusus *(Trichosurus vulpecula)* als lebende *M.-bovis*-Infektionsquelle für Weidevieh.

■ **Pathogenese:** Rinder infizieren sich direkt oder mittelbar durch Herdengenossen, seltener durch andere Tiere (z. B. Rotwild), die mit ihren Se- oder Exkreten zeitweise oder dauernd *M. bovis* ausscheiden. Die Ansteckung erfolgt meist *aerogen*, so daß der tuberkulöse Primärkomplex erwachsener Rinder in > 90% (bei Kälbern nur in ~ 35%) aller Fälle die Lunge betrifft und Rinder mit »offener« Lungentuberkulose die wichtigste Erregerquelle darstellen. Dabei handelt es sich teils um Tröpfcheninfektionen, teils um Inhalation aufgewirbelter, keimtragender Staubteilchen. Die bei Kälbern überwiegende *alimentär-enterogene* Ansteckung erfolgt über die Tränke (Milch eutertuberkulöser Kühe, ungenügend erhitzte Rück- oder Magermilch aus Molkereien). Uterustuberkulose kann *omphalogene* Infektion des Fetus bedingen (→ Primärkomplex in Leber und periportalen Lymphknoten). Weitere, wesentlich seltenere Übertragungswege von *M. bovis* sind *genitale* bzw. *galaktogene* Infektion infolge Gebärmutter-, Scheiden-, Penis-, Hoden- oder Nebenhodentuberkulose bzw. Eindringen des Erregers aus verkeimter Streu in den Strichkanal. Zustandekommen und Verlauf der tuberkulösen Erkrankung werden von äußeren und inneren *Risikofaktoren* beeinflußt; begünstigend wirken Aufenthalt in überbesetztem, mangelhaft belüftetem Stall, wenig Auslauf in frischer Luft, Ernährungsmängel sowie Schwächung durch andere Leiden.

Die vorwiegend über Bronchalschleim und m. o. w. schubweise erfolgende *Ausscheidung sowie Verbreitung* von *M. bovis* ist am massivsten, wenn die phthisische Lunge Einschmelzungsherde enthalten oder tuberkulöse Geschwüre in Luftröhre und Bronchen vorliegen (= »offene« Tuberkulose). Mit solchem Auswurf abgeschluckte sowie aus tuberkulösen Darmläsionen stammende Erreger werden mit dem Kot ausgeschieden. Bei Nieren- und Gebärmuttertuberkulose ist *M. bovis* in Harn und Genitalsekret enthalten. Die bei vulvovaginaler bzw. Penis-, Hoden- oder Nebenhodentuberkulose mögliche Elimination über Vaginalschleim bzw. Sperma ist vergleichsweise selten. Eutertuberkulose, insbesondere Mastitis caseosa, ist indessen wegen der über die Milch erfolgenden Ausscheidung von *M. bovis* von großer epidemiologischer Bedeutung.

Im infizierten Organismus sind bestimmte *Phasen des tuberkulösen Krankheitsgeschehens* (Übersicht 12-1) zu unterscheiden:

Übersicht 12-1 Phasenverlauf des tuberkulösen Krankheitsgeschehens

Erstinfektionsperiode:	Primärkomplex - Ausheilung (Vernarbung, Verkalkung) - evtl. Reinfektion
	Frühgeneralisation - Miliartuberkulose - protrahierte Generalisation
Postprimäre Prozesse:	chronische Organtuberkulose
- Exazerbation - Superinfektion	} Lunge, Euter, Nieren u. a.
Niederbruchsphase:	Spätgeneralisation - Miliartuberkulose - Pneumonia caseosa - Mastitis caseosa

➤ Im Rahmen der *Erstinfektionsperiode* entwickelt sich an der Ansiedlungsstelle von *M. bovis* eine kennzeichnende granulomatöse Entzündung mit Tuberkelbildung. Gleichsinnige Miterkrankung des/der regionalen Lymphknoten ergibt den *tuberkulösen Primärkomplex*. Bei pulmonalem Primärkomplex findet man z. B. in einem Lungenlappen (und zwar meist im Zwerchfellslappen) einen einzelnen erbsen- bis walnußgroßen tuberkulösen Herd sowie tuberkulöse Veränderungen im zugehörigen tracheobronchalen oder mediastinalen Lymphknoten. Bei günstigem Verlauf kann der Primärkomplex unter Vernarbung und Verkalkung ausheilen.

➤ In anderen Fällen mit schwächerer Abwehr wird der tuberkulöse Prozeß nach längerem Ruhen wieder aktiviert. Dabei gelangen die noch im Primärkomplex vorhandenen Tuberkelbakterien auf dem *Lymph- und Blutwege* in weitere Organe, wo sich dann im Rahmen der *Frühgeneralisation* multiple Tuberkel entwickeln; hierbei erkranken die regionären Lymphknoten stets mit. Erfolgt diese Aussaat rasch und unter massiver Vermehrung der Erreger, so entstehen in den befallenen Organen massenhaft hirsekorngroße tuberkulöse Herdchen *(Miliartuberkulose)*. Bei *schubweise-protrahierter Generalisation* entwickeln sich dagegen gleichenorts nacheinander Herde unterschiedlicher Größe.

➤ Wiederaufflackern der tuberkulösen Erkrankung nach der Erstinfektionsperiode *(Exazerbation)* oder erneute exogene Ansteckung des Patienten *(Superinfektion)* leiten die *postprimären Prozesse* ein. Sie sind durch Fortschreiten des Krankheitsgeschehens entlang anatomisch vorgegebener Wege, wie Bronchen, Luftröhre, Darm oder Milchgänge, gekennzeichnet. Diese *kanalikuläre Ausbreitung* bedingt die charakteristischen Veränderungen der *chronischen* oder *isolierten Organtu-*

berkulose, z. B. azinöse und azinös-nodöse Lungentuberkulose oder lobulär-infiltrierende Eutertuberkulose. Während solcher postprimären Prozesse bleiben die regionären Lymphknoten i. d. R. unverändert.

➤ Unter zusätzlicher Belastung durch Hunger, anderweitige Erkrankung, Transport, Trächtigkeit, Abkalbung oder Hochlaktation können die zellulären Abwehrkräfte des tuberkulosekranken Tierkörpers versagen. Das führt zur *Niederbruchsphase,* in deren Verlauf es zu erneuter lympho-hämatogener Erregeraussaat, d. h. zur *Spätgeneralisation* kommt. Dabei entstehen in den jeweils betroffenen Organen wiederum miliare Tuberkel. Lunge und Euter entwickeln zudem unter rasch fortschreitender, »galoppierender« tuberkulöser Nekrotisation verkäsende Pneumonie bzw. Mastitis.

Symptome, Verlauf: Das klinische Bild der bovinen Tuberkulose ist entsprechend der Mannigfaltigkeit seiner Pathogenese je nach Phase und Lokalisation sowie Erkrankungsgrad vielgestaltig und stets unspezifisch. Das Leiden ist daher nur bei Zuhilfenahme der Tuberkulinprobe und bakteriologischer Untersuchungsverfahren sicher zu diagnostizieren. Wegen seiner langen Inkubationszeit können bis zur offensichtlichen Erkrankung Monate oder Jahre vergehen. Der pulmonale Primäraffekt bleibt klinisch i. d. R. stumm. Symptome setzen meist erst dann ein, wenn es zu Frühgeneralisation, chronischer Organtuberkulose oder Spätgeneralisation (Niederbruchsphase) gekommen ist. Die Generalisation geht mitunter mit Fieber, Freßunlust, Mattigkeit, Anämie und/oder rascher Abmagerung einher; sie kann innerhalb weniger Wochen zum Tode führen. Weitere Erscheinungen weisen von Fall zu Fall auf die Beteiligung bestimmter Organe hin:

➤ *Lungentuberkulose* deutet sich durch matten Husten an, der sich im weiteren Verlauf anfallsweise verstärkt und schleimigen Auswurf bedingt. Die v. a. nach körperlicher Anstrengung oder in schwüler Umgebung beschleunigte und/oder erschwerte Atmung wird dann mitunter von Stöhnen begleitet. Auskultatorisch kann das broncho-bronchuläre Atemgeräusch stellenweise verstärkt oder vermindert sein oder völlig fehlen; in fortgeschrittenen Fällen sind statt dessen knatternde oder pfeifende Rasselgeräusche zu vernehmen; etwaiges »Krugatmen« und übler Geruch des Exspiriums lassen auf offene tuberkulöse Kavernen schließen. Atemhemmung löst meist stoß- bis anfallsweises Husten, u. U. auch Expektoration aus. Perkutorisch sind tuberkulöse Herde nur dann als Dämpfung erfaßbar, wenn sie mindestens Hühnerei- bis Faustgröße erreicht haben und nicht mehr als 3–4 Fingerbreiten weit von der Brustwand entfernt sind. Die tuberkulöse Vergrößerung mediastinaler Lymphknoten kann Kompression des Schlundes mit rezidivierender Tympanie, die Beteiligung der im Brusteingang gelegenen Lymphknoten dagegen Stauung der Drosselvenen bedingen.

➤ *Pleura- und Perikardtuberkulose* führt nur selten zu auskultatorisch deutlich wahrnehmbaren Reibegeräuschen oder zu nennenswerter Einengung der Herztätigkeit (→ Venenstauung).

➤ *Tuberkulose der oberen Luftwege:* Beteiligung der *Nase* äußert sich von Fall zu Fall in schleimig-eitrigem Ausfluß, graugelben Knötchen und Geschwüren auf der Nasenschleimhaut sowie knotig-derber Vergrößerung der Kehlgangslymphknoten. Tuberkulose der *Rachenlymphknoten* bedingt mit der Zeit Pharynxstenose (→ schnarchend-röchelnde atmungssynchrone Geräusche, Schlingbeschwerden). In *Kehlkopf* und/oder *Luftröhre* gelegene tuberkulöse Veränderungen können fauchenden bis pfeifenden Stridor, mitunter auch kräftigen, schmerzhaften Husten bedingen und schließlich sogar die Stimme beeinträchtigen.

➤ *Tuberkulose der Verdauungsorgane:* Bei *Zungen-, Gaumen-* oder *Rachentuberkulose* sind die betroffenen Schleimhäute mit graugelben Knötchen oder Geschwüren bedeckt. Tuberkulose des *Darmes* ist klinisch oft inapparent, kann aber auch Durchfall, Kotverhaltung oder Kolik auslösen. Bei rektaler Exploration solcher Patienten sind die veränderten Gekröslymphknoten u. U. als bis zu kartoffelgroße derbhöckrige Gebilde fühlbar. *Lebertuberkulose* gibt sich klinisch nicht zu erkennen. Tuberkulöse Knötchen des *Bauchfells* (»Perlsucht«) sind bei rektaler Betastung fühlbar.

➤ *Nierentuberkulose* kann zu Proteinurie (→ trüb-übelriechender Harn) und rektal tastbarer knotiger Induration einzelner Renkuli führen. Die Harnleiter solcher Tiere sind mitunter ebenfalls von höckriger Beschaffenheit.

➤ *Tuberkulose des weiblichen Genitales:* Die meist exogen, d. h. deckaktbedingten tuberkulösen Veränderungen von *Vulva* und *Vestibulum vaginae* äußern sich als m. o. w. umfangreiche, fühl- und später auch sichtbare Knoten mit derbem Zentrum, die geschwürig aufbrechen können. Die i. d. R. endogen, d. h. durch lympho-hämatogene Generalisation oder kanalikulär (vom Bauchfell her über die Bursa ovarica deszendierend bzw. von der Vulva her über die Vagina aszendierend) ausgelöste Tuberkulose von *Gebärmutter* und/oder *Eileiter* äußert sich in trübgelblichem Scheidenausfluß, Ausbleiben der Brunst, Umrindern oder Verkalben. Rektal sind dabei unregelmäßige knotig-derbe Veränderungen der Uteruswand und/oder perlschnurartige Indurationen am Ovidukt festzustellen.

➤ *Eutertuberkulose* entwickelt sich meist hämatogen (Generalisation), seltener galaktogen. Bei *miliar-tuberkulöser Mastitis* (Frühgeneralisation) sind innerhalb des Parenchyms, v. a. dem der Hinterviertel, hirsekorn- bis erbsengroße, schmerzlose derbe Knötchen palpierbar. Die Milch ist hierbei allenfalls leicht wäßriggrau verändert; die Euterlymphknoten sind derbgeschwollen. Bei *chronischer, lobulär-infiltrierender Eutertuberkulose* (postprimäre Prozesse) sind größere Drüsenabschnitte oder ganze Viertel induriert, aber weder druckempfindlich noch vermehrt warm. Im weiteren Verlauf wird das Sekret zunehmend wäßrig-graugelb und flockig. *Mastitis caseosa* (Niederbruchsform) tritt dagegen als akute Entzündung auf und bedingt schmerzhafte, vermehrt warme und derbe Vergrößerung ganzer Viertel sowie sulziges Ödem der Unterhaut des Euters. Dabei ist nur wenig wäßrig-gelbliches, flockenhaltiges Sekret zu ermelken; die Euterlymphknoten sind dann deutlich vergrößert und druckempfindlich.

➤ *Tuberkulose des männlichen Genitales* bedingt schmerzlose derbe Knoten in Hoden oder Nebenhoden, die nach außen fisteln können.

➤ *Tuberkulose des zentralen Nervensystems*: Je nach Lokalisation und Umfang der Veränderungen kann eine i. d. R. hämatogen entstandene tuberkulöse Leptomeningitis allgemeine zerebrale Erscheinungen (Kap. 10.2.1), zerebrale Herdsymptome (z. B. das Hirnbasis-Syndrom; Kap. 10.2.3) und/oder spinale Parese oder Paralyse (Kap. 10.2.10) auslösen. Das angegebenenorts nachzulesende klinische Bild pflegt sich dabei allmählich zu verschlimmern.

➤ *Augentuberkulose* ist sehr selten und i. d. R. hämatogen bedingt. Nach Auftreten kleiner gelblicher Knötchen in Iris und Ziliarkörper kommt es zu fortschreitenden intraokulären Trübungen und Adhäsionen, schließlich zur Umwandlung des gesamten Augeninneren in eine käsig-granuläre Masse.

➤ *Tuberkulose der Knochen* betrifft von Fall zu Fall einzelne Rippen, Wirbel- oder Schädelknochen (→ umschriebene derbe Umfangsvermehrung, u. U. Fistelbildung, Beteiligung regionärer Lymphknoten, zerebrale oder spinale Ausfallserscheinungen). *Gelenktuberkulose* befällt meist den rumpfnahen Gliedmaßenbereich und ist wie Knochentuberkulose fast immer hämatogen bedingt; die Veränderungen beginnen dabei zunächst an einer Epiphyse und greifen dann allmählich auf das betreffende Gelenk über (derbe Verdickung, zunehmende Bewegungsstörung, Lymphknotenbeteiligung).

➤ Bei *Tuberkulose von Haut und Unterhaut* entwickeln sich unter Mitbefall regionärer Lymphknoten erbsen- bis walnußgroße, derb-unempfindliche und u. U. auch fistelnde Knoten.

■ **Sektion:** Die Zerlegung tuberkulöser Rinder ergibt typische Veränderungen im Bereich eines oder mehrerer Organe (Abb. 12-17 bis 12-21):

➤ Der *Atmungsapparat*, insbesondere *Lunge* und *Lungenlymphknoten*, erweist sich als am häufigsten betroffen. Der *respiratorische Primärkomplex* besteht meist aus einem einzelnen, am Rand eines Hauptlappens gelegenen Knoten, dessen Schnittfläche gelblichweiß verkäst und m. o. w. verkalkt ist. Die regionären Lymphknoten sind stets ebenfalls tuberkulös verändert. Später kapseln sich solche Lungenherde ab und werden inaktiv. Bei *Frühgeneralisation* finden sich in allen Lungenlappen hirsekorngroße, trübgelbliche Knötchen (= miliare Epitheloidzelltuberkel), bei *protrahierter Generalisation* auch erbsen- bis haselnußgroße Knoten mit verkäsendem bis verkalkendem Zentrum. Beteiligte bronchale und mediastinale Lymphknoten sind vergrößert; ihre Schnittfläche erscheint grautrübe-brüchig sowie durch verbliebene Bindegewebszüge radiär gestreift (= strahlige Verkäsung). Verkäste Lymphknotenbezirke neigen zur baldigen Verkalkung.

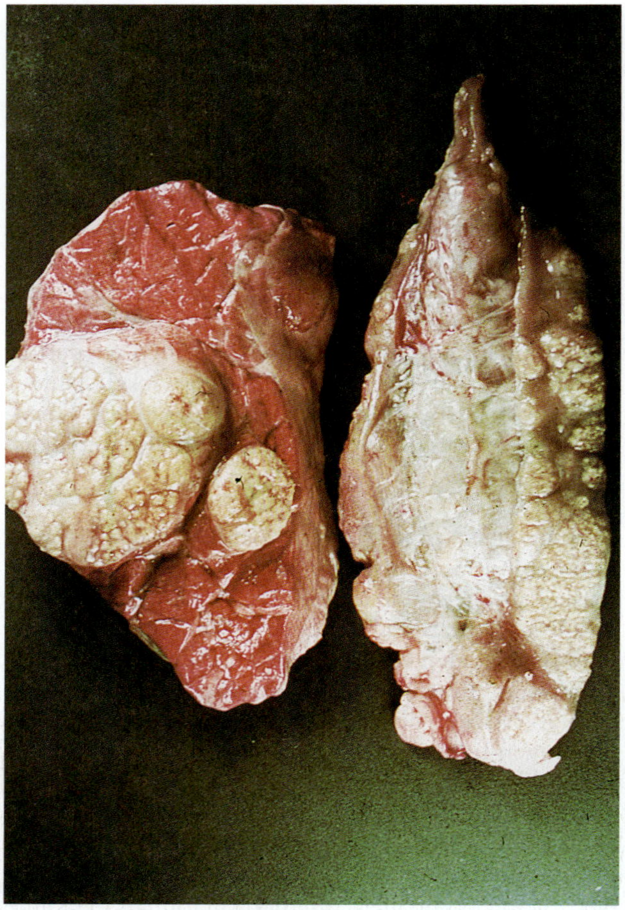

Abbildung 12-17 Bovine Tuberkulose von Lunge (links) und Mediastinallymphknoten (rechts); protrahierte Frühgeneralisation

Im Rahmen *postprimärer Prozesse* entwickelt sich infolge kanalikulärer Ausbreitung die *chronische Lungentuberkulose*. Ihre azinösen Herde besitzen lagebedingt kleeblatt- bis weintraubenartige Gestalt; infolge endobronchaler Ausdehnung vergrößern sie sich zu azinös-nodösen und nodös-lobulären Herden, die

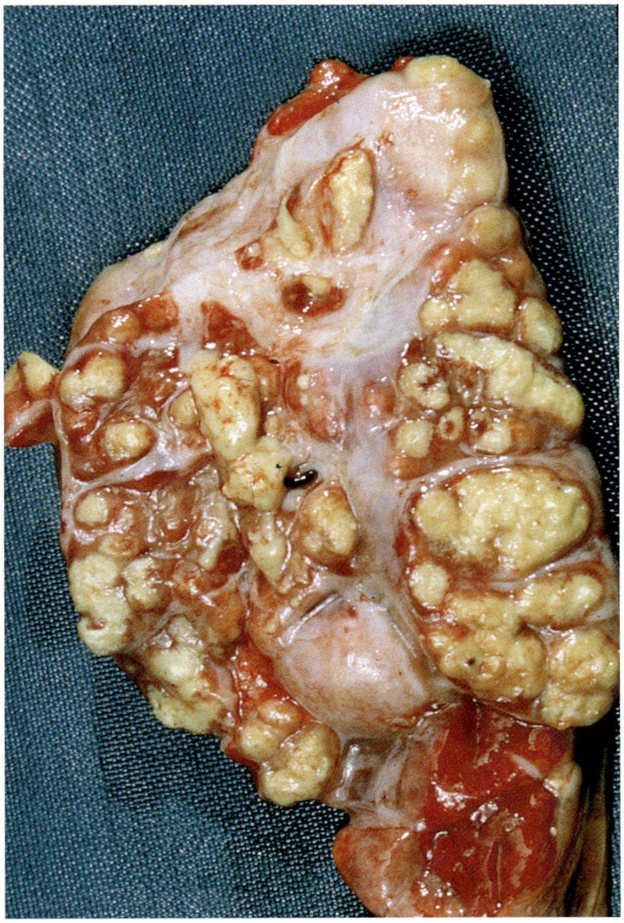

Abbildung 12-18 Chronische azinös-nodöse Lungentuberkulose

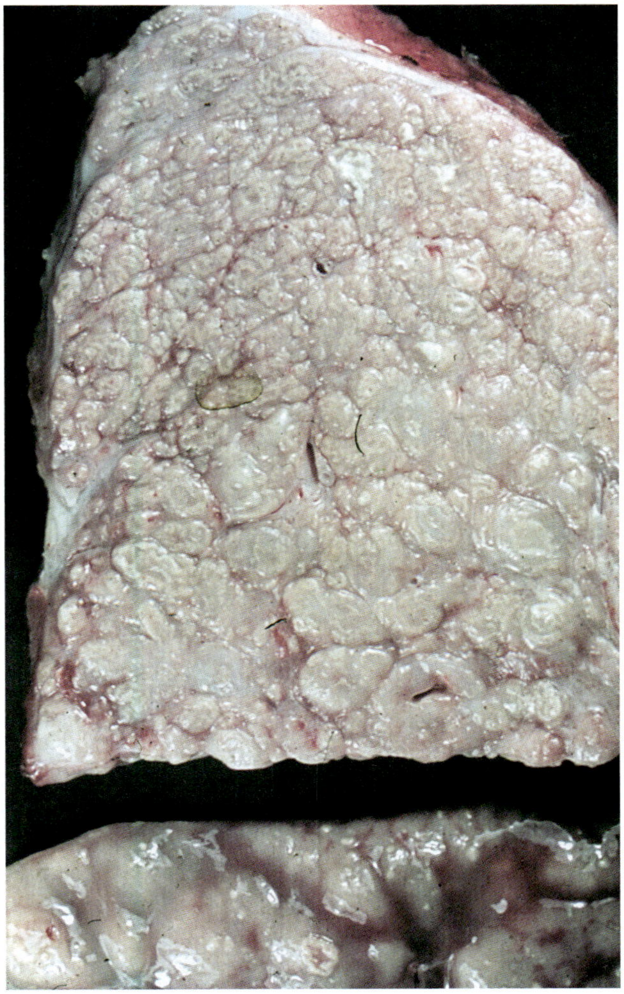

Abbildung 12-19 Lobulär-verkäsende Tuberkulose des Euters, dessen Lymphknoten aus der Frühgeneralisation stammende verkalkte Herde aufweisen

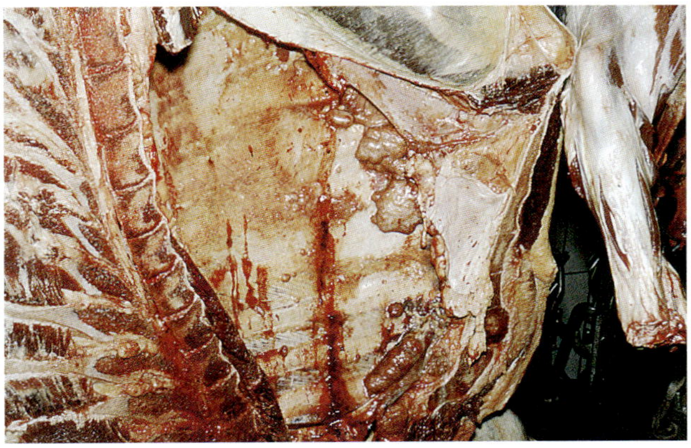

Abbildung 12-20 Tuberkulöse Pleuritis (»Perlsucht«)

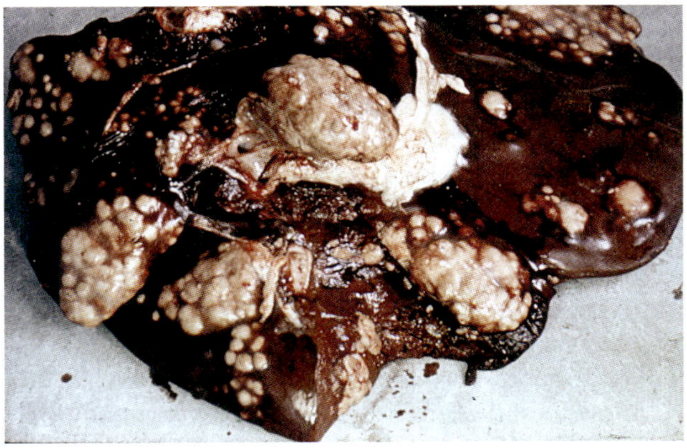

Abbildung 12-21 Chronische Organtuberkulose der Leber mit Beteiligung der Portallymphknoten

schließlich Faustgröße erreichen können. Ältere tuberkulöse Herde grenzen sich bindegewebig vom lufthaltigen Lungengewebe ab. In fortgeschrittenen Fällen entstehen haselnuß- bis faustgroße bronchektatische Kavernen, die eine eiterähnliche gelbliche Masse enthalten. Zudem weist die Schleimhaut von Luftröhre und Bronchen geschwürige Veränderungen auf. In der *Niederbruchsphase* finden sich in der Lunge frische miliare Tuberkel und lobulär-verkäsende pneumonische Herde unterschiedlicher Größe. Ihre Schnittfläche ist trüb-gelblich und mit punktförmigen Blutungen durchsetzt. Die regionären Lymphknoten zeigen frische tuberkulöse Verkäsung. In *Nasenhöhle, Rachen* und *Kehlkopf* zeigt sich Tuberkulose in Form graugelblicher Knötchen und Geschwüre, seltener als polypöse Knoten; die regionären Lymphknoten sind mitbetroffen.

➤ Von den *serösen Häuten* ist v. a. das *Brustfell*, gelegentlich auch das *Bauchfell* tuberkulös verändert und zeigt dann entweder zottig-proliferative oder knotige Serositis (»Perlsucht«); die Flüssigkeit der erkrankten Körperhöhle kann vermehrt sein.

➤ Am *Herzen* findet man chronisch-fibrosierende, von käsigen Herden durchsetzte tuberkulöse Perikarditis (»Panzerherz«).

➤ *Darmtuberkulose* äußert sich in linsen- bis erbsengroßen Knötchen und rundlichen Geschwüren der Schleimhaut; die regionären Lymphknoten sind beteiligt.

➤ *Leber:* miliare Tuberkel (Früh- oder Spätgeneralisation) oder bis zu faustgroße, bindegewebig abgegrenzte tuberkulöse Knoten (protrahierte Generalisation); Miterkrankung der Leberlymphknoten.

➤ *Milz:* miliare Tuberkel (Früh- oder Spätgeneralisation) oder grobe Knoten (protrahierte Generalisation).

➤ *Nieren:* verkäsende und verkalkende Rindenknoten (Frühgeneralisation), tuberkulöse Markherde mit Einbruch in Harnkanälchen (Ausscheidungstuberkulose); trocken-käsige, mit Blutungen durchsetzte Bezirke (Niederbruchsphase); tuberkulöse Pyonephrose; Lymphknotenbeteiligung.

➤ *Harnleiter:* verkäsende Ureteritis.

➤ *Gebärmutter:* miliar-tuberkulöse Endometritis; chronische knotige und diffus-verkäsende Endometritis; verkäsende Plazentitis (→ Abort).

➤ *Eileiter:* miliartuberkulöse Oophoritis oder größere Tuberkel in der Eileiterwand.

➤ *Euter:* miliare bis erbsengroße verkäste und verkalkte Tuberkel (Frühgeneralisation); chronisch lobulär-infiltrierende Eutertuberkulose (postprimäre Prozesse); Mastitis caseosa (Niederbruchsphase).

➤ *Hoden, Nebenhoden:* verkäsende Orchitis und Epididymitis (intratubuläre Ausbreitung).

➤ *Zentrales Nervensystem:* verkäsende Leptomeningitis, bevorzugt im Hirnbasisbereich.

■ **Diagnose:** Die Erkennung der Tuberkulose kann sich auf klinische, bakteriologische, serologische, allergische, molekularbiologische und pathologisch-anatomische Befunde stützen:

➤ *Klinisch* berechtigen außer schleichender Entwicklung des Leidens, allmählichem Rückgang des Nährzustandes und schubweisem Fieber v. a. die Symptome einer chronischen Lungenerkrankung sowie Mitbeteiligung von Körperlymphknoten zum Verdacht auf Tuberkulose. Ähnliches gilt, v. a. in bekanntermaßen tuberkulosebefallenen Beständen, für seltener von ihr betroffene Organe (s. *Symptome*).

➤ Der *bakteriologische Nachweis* von *M. bovis* in Trachealschleim, Milch, Kot, Vaginalausfluß oder Fistelleiter sowie in Punktaten erkrankter Lymphknoten, Gelenke oder Genitalorgane gilt als beweisend für das Vorliegen von Tuberkulose. Bei trotz begründeten Verdachts negativ ausfallendem Befund empfiehlt es sich, die mikrobiologische Untersuchung zu wiederholen. Zum Nachweis des Erregers eignen sich ZIEHL-NEELSEN-Färbung, Fluoreszenzmikroskopie, Kultur auf Spezialnährböden sowie Tierversuch (Meerschweinchen, Kaninchen). Die beiden letztgenannten Verfahren waren zur Differenzierung der klassischen Mykobakterien *(M. bovis, M. avium, M. tuberculosis)*, insbesondere bei Aufklärung von Neuinfektionen oder unspezifischen Tuberkulinreaktionen in zuvor tuberkulosefreien Rinderbeständen, bislang unerläßlich; heute werden sie durch molekularbiologische Methoden (s. u.) ergänzt.

➤ Unter den gegen Mykobakterien gerichteten *Immunreaktionen des Tierkörpers* überwiegt die durch Lymphozyten und Makrophagen vermittelte Immunantwort. Als bewährtes Mittel zur Diagnose der Rindertuberkulose gilt daher seit langem die intrakutane *Tuberkulinprobe* und neuerdings auch der *IFNγT*.

➤➤ *Serologische Methoden* zum Nachweis etwaiger, gegen M. bovis gerichteter Antikörper (KBR, HAT, Hämolyse-Test, Kaolin-Agglutinationstest, IIFT) sind weit weniger empfindlich als die intrakutane Tuberkulinprobe. Bei chronischer Organtuberkulose fallen sie oft negativ aus und eignen sich wegen mangelnder Spezifität auch nicht zur Abklärung fraglicher oder falschpositiver Tuberkulinreaktionen. Entsprechendes gilt für einen kürzlich in Irland bzw. den USA entwickelten ELISA.

➤➤ Die *intrakutane Tuberkulinprobe* ist die wichtigste Methode zum Tuberkulosenachweis am lebenden Tier. Überempfindlichkeit gegenüber Tuberkulin (= aus Tuberkelbakterien gewonnene lösliche Substanzen) beruht auf der vorwiegend zellulär gesteuerten Immunantwort des mykobakteriell infizierten Organismus (= allergische Reaktion verzögerten Typs): Positivenfalls entwickelt sich am Injektionsort infolge Ansammlung von T-Lymphozyten und Makrophagen sowie Ausschüttung von Zytokinen und histaminähnlichen Substanzen innerhalb von 24–48 h eine umschriebene Entzündung mit Schwellung, Rötung, Gewebeinduration und Druckempfindlichkeit, u. U. auch mit Beteiligung des regionären Lymphknotens. Zu der beim Rind anzuwendenden intrakutanen Tuberkulinisierung wird in Deutschland bislang aus *M.-bovis*-Kulturen gewonnenes albumosefreies *Rindertuberkulin* angewandt; internationale Bestrebungen zielen jedoch auf Einsatz des leichter standardisierbaren PPD-Tuberkulins (PPD = purified protein derivative; 0,15 mg PPD entsprechen 5000 TE [Tuberkulin-Einheiten] oder 2000 GE [Gemeinschafts-Einheiten] Tuberkulin). Ein entsprechender, aus *M. avium* gewonnener Extrakt wird als *Geflügeltuberkulin* bezeichnet.

▸▸ Die *einfache intrakutane Tuberkulinprobe* ist gemäß Tuberkulose-VO (1997) wie folgt vorzunehmen: Scheren der Haare im Bereich der handbreit vor der Schulterblattgräte zu wählenden Injektionsstelle; Messen der Hautdicke mit dem Federkutimeter; intrakutane Injektion von 0,1 ml Rindertuberkulin (mindestens 5000 TE oder 2000 GE Tuberkulin) mit der Zylinderampullenspritze; Ablesen und Beurteilen der Reaktion mittels erneuter Hautdickenmessung (Federkutimeter) und Berücksichtigung etwaiger lokaler Veränderungen nach Ablauf von 72–96 h. Dabei gilt eine von örtlicher Druckempfindlichkeit, Exsudation oder Nekrose, von Lymphgefäß- oder -knotenbeteiligung begleitete Zunahme der Hautdicke um ≥ 4,0 mm als positive, ein Hautdickenzuwachs von 2,0–3,9 mm dagegen als zweifelhafte Reaktion (Abb. 12-22). Obwohl die diagnostische Sicherheit der intrakutanen Tuberkulinprobe im positiven wie im negativen Falle ~ 97 % erreicht, ist ihr Ausfall kritisch zu beurteilen. So besteht kein Zusammenhang zwischen der bei einem Patienten ermittelten Reaktionsstärke und dem Umfang seines tuberkulösen Prozesses. Während der ~ 4–6 Wochen p. inf. dauernden *präallergischen Phase* fällt die Tuberkulinprobe noch negativ aus. Dann nimmt die Reaktivität des Organismus deutlich zu und hält, langsam nachlassend, jahrelang an. *Falschnegative Ergebnisse* treten v. a. bei älteren Tieren mit kleinen verkalkten Residuen chronischer Organtuberkulose oder in der Niederbruchsphase auf *(Anergie)*; ähnliches trifft mitunter auch für kurz vor bis 6 Wochen nach dem Kalben stehende Kühe zu *(Immunsuppression)*. Weiterhin können falschnegative Tuberkulinreaktionen auf Desensibilisierung infolge vorangegangener Tuberkulinisierungen, Verabreichung von Kortikosteroiden, Antihistaminika oder nichtsteroidalen Entzündungshemmern oder auf Verwendung unwirksamen Tuberkulins beruhen. *Falschpositive* oder *fragliche Tuberkulinreaktionen* sind bei Rindern zu beobachten, die zuvor durch andere Mykobakterien als *M. bovis* bzw. durch unspezifische Einflüsse (Paratuberkulose, Dermatitis nodosa, knotig-tuberkuloide Entzündung der Zitzen- oder

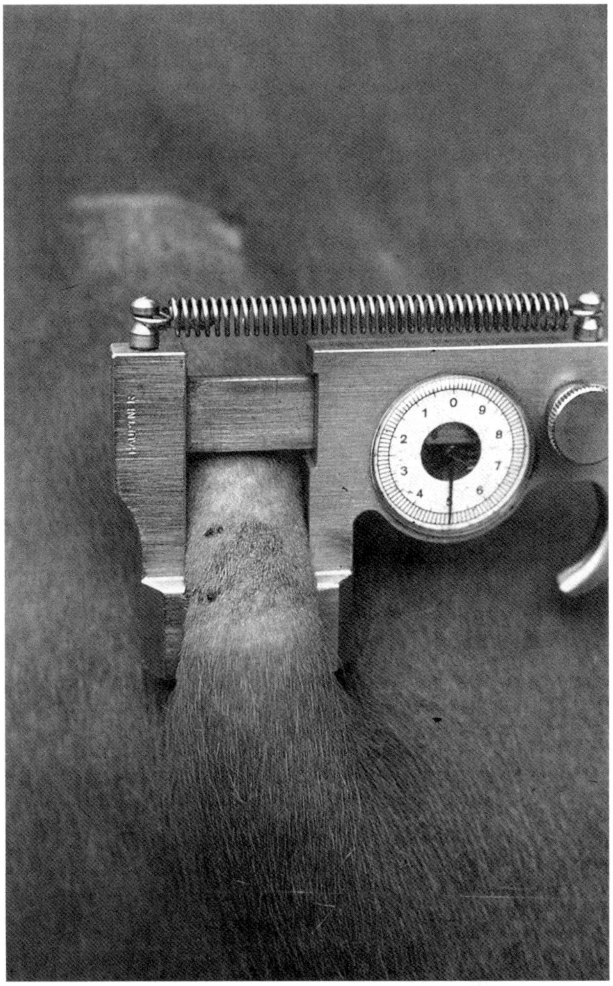

Abbildung 12-22 Deutlich positive intrakutane Tuberkulinprobe (Hautdickenzunahme binnen 3 × 24 h : 15 mm)

Hodensackhaut, Brucellose, Aktinomykose, Dasselbefall, Insektenstiche) sensibilisiert wurden (*parallergischer* bzw. *hetero- oder pseudoallergischer Zustand*). Solche *unspezifischen Reaktionen* haben im Laufe der Tilgung der Rindertuberkulose an Häufigkeit zugenommen. Sie beruhen von Fall zu Fall auf einer der folgenden Ursachen:

Die Infektion des Rindes mit dem vom Menschen stammenden *M. tuberculosis* bedingt mitunter einen unvollständigen Primärkomplex in Form kleiner intralymphonodaler Knötchen und damit einhergehend zeitweilige Empfindlichkeit gegenüber Rindertuberkulin. Eine solche unspezifische Reaktionsweise ist selbst durch Simultantestung mit monovalenten Tuberkulinen nicht sicher abklärbar. Gegebenenfalls ist nach der Infektionsquelle zu fahnden und durch wiederholtes Tuberkulinisieren zu prüfen, ob die Reaktivität innerhalb von 6–9 Monaten verschwindet.

Wichtigster Anlaß *parallergischer Tuberkulinreaktionen* sind Infektionen mit *M. avium*. Hiervon werden v. a. jüngere Rinder betroffen, deren Futter oder Tränke mit dem Kot tuberkulöser Hühner verunreinigt war. Auf solche, i. d. R. selbstlimitierend verlaufenden und keine oder nur geringfügige Organveränderungen hinterlassenden Infektionen entfallen zwei Drittel aller Störungen der Tuberkuloseüberwachung beim Rind. Die Abklärung derartiger Befunde erfolgt durch *simultane Tuberkulinisierung mit bovinem und aviärem Tuberkulin.*

›› Die *simultane Tuberkulinprobe* ist frühestens 6 Wochen nach der hierzu Anlaß gebenden Tuberkulinisierung vorzunehmen. Dabei wird an zwei 12 cm voneinander entfernten Stellen einer Halsseite oder an je einer vor rechter und linker Schulter gelegenen Stelle 0,1 ml *Rinder-* bzw. *Geflügeltuberkulin* intrakutan injiziert und die Reaktion nach Ablauf von 72 h beurteilt. Das Ergebnis gilt als Hinweis auf bovine Tuberkulose, wenn die durch bovines Tuberkulin erzielte Hautdickenzunahme ≥ 4,0 mm größer ist als diejenige der Vergleichsstelle. Entsprechendes gilt auch für den Fall, daß im Bereich der bovinen Tuberkulinprobe klinische Veränderungen (Druckempfindlichkeit, Exsudation oder Lymphgefäßschwellung) auftreten. Die simultane Tuberkulinprobe wird auch zur Abgrenzung der Rindertuberkulose von *Mykobakteriosen* angewandt, die auf Infektion mit atypischen Mykobakterien beruhen (s. *Differentialdiagnose*); sie erbringt hierbei aber nicht immer klare Resultate.

›› Der *Interferon-γ-Test* (IFNγT) ist das derzeit brauchbarste aller immunologischen Verfahren zum Nachweis der Rindertuberkulose, die wegen gewisser Unzulänglichkeiten der intrakutanen Tuberkulinprobe (geringe Spezifität für *M. bovis*, vereinzelt auch falschpositive oder -negative Reaktionen) entwickelt wurden. Hierzu werden zunächst Blutleukozyten des betreffenden Tieres mit bovinem Tuberkulin inkubiert; nach 24 h wird dann das im Zellkulturüberstand freigesetzte IFNγ mittels EIA quantifiziert. In Australien gilt der IFNγT seit 1991 als offiziell anerkannte Methode zur Diagnose der Rindertuberkulose; in Neuseeland, Irland, Kanada und den USA wird er inzwischen ebenfalls zu ihrer Bekämpfung eingesetzt.

›› *Molekularbiologischer Nachweis von M. bovis:* Da die traditionelle Kultivierung und Differenzierung von Mykobakterien auf Spezialnährböden u. U. 2–3 Monate erfordert, sind molekularbiologische Verfahren entwickelt worden, mit denen sich *M. bovis* in Blut, Organen oder Milch innerhalb von 48 h nachweisen läßt: Mit der hochspezifischen und -sensitiven Polymerase-Kettenreaktion (PCR) ist dieser Erreger selbst in geringer Zahl sicher festzustellen und von anderen Mykobakterien zu unterscheiden. Mittels Restriktions-Enzymanalyse (REA) gelingt es sogar, Subtypen innerhalb der Spezies *M. bovis* zu differenzieren. Solche Typisierungen sind von epidemiologischer Bedeutung, etwa zur Aufklärung der Übertragung von boviner Tuberkulose von Rind zu Rind oder von Wildtieren (Rot-, Reh-, Damwild, Dachs) auf Rinder.

➤ Die *postmortal festzustellenden pathologisch-anatomischen Veränderungen* lassen sich im Gegensatz zu den am lebenden Patienten erhobenen klinischen Befunden meist eindeutig einem bestimmten Tuberkulosestadium (s. *Pathogenese*) zuordnen. In Zweifelsfällen ist durch zusätzliche histologische und bakteriologische Untersuchung Klärung zu erzielen.

Differentialdiagnostisch sind bei Tuberkuloseverdacht zu berücksichtigen: Aktinomykose (Kap. 9.1.4), Aktinobazillose (Kap. 3.1.3.3), anderweitige infektiöse Lymphangitiden (Kap. 3.1.3.4, 3.1.3.5), Nocardiose (Kap. 12.2.7), Pneumonomykosen (Kap. 5.3.3.18), Mesotheliose der Serosen (Kap. 5.4.5.2, 6.15.6), Hautknotenkrankheit (Kap. 2.2.3.7), Vulvakarzinom (Kap. 2.2.9) und Mykobakteriosen. Unter letzteren sind Infektionen mit ubiquitär, in Erdboden, Wasser oder Sägemehl, vorkommenden *»atypischen Mykobakterien«* zusammengefaßt, welche die mit bovinem Tuberkulin vorgenommene Intrakutanprobe vorübergehend oder dauerhaft im Sinne einer positiven Reaktion beeinflussen können. Zu diesen Keimen gehören *M. intracellulare, M. fortuitum, M. kansasii, M. scrofulaceum, M. aquae, M. cooki* und *M. smegmatis. M. aquae* gilt als Erreger der tuberkuloiden Entzündung von Zitzen- oder Skrotalhaut (Kap. 2.2.3.5) und der Dermatitis nodosa (Kap. 2.3.3.5); *M. intracellulare* und *M. fortuitum* wurden aus granulomatös veränderten Lymphknoten, *M. fortuitum* und *M. smegmatis* bei Mastitiden isoliert.

■ **Behandlung:** Zwar wäre bei Außerachtlassen der Kostenfrage auch beim tuberkulösen Rind Heilung mit humanmedizinischen Tuberkulostatika erzielbar, doch sind solche Therapieversuche in Deutschland verboten (Tuberkulose-VO, 1997).

■ **Bekämpfung:** Die gemäß VOaTS zum TSeuG anzeigepflichtige Rindertuberkulose ist in Deutschland seit 1962 praktisch getilgt; 1990 wurden bei einem Gesamtbestand von 19,5 Mio. Rindern nur 16 Fälle festgestellt. Die heute in den meisten entwickelten Ländern vollzogene Tilgung der Rindertuberkulose stützt sich auf:

➤ Ermittlung aller mit M. bovis infizierten Rinder durch intrakutane Tuberkulinprobe, die in fraglichen Fällen durch molekularbiologische Methoden ergänzt werden kann (→ Abgrenzung unspezifischer Tuberkulinreaktionen).

➤ Absonderung und Ausmerzung aller auf Tuberkulin positiv reagierenden Rinder, da sie früher oder später zu Keimausscheidern und damit zur Ansteckungsquelle für tuberkulosefreie Artgenossen und andere Tiere werden können.

➤ Tuberkulosefreie Aufzucht der Jungtiere zum sicheren und einfachen Aufbau eines tuberkulosefreien Bestandes.

Nach Tilgung der Rindertuberkulose muß versucht werden, *Neuinfektionen* zu verhindern oder frühestmöglich zu erkennen und ihre Ursache zu klären. Die hierfür erforderlichen Maßnahmen werden in Deutschland durch die *Tuberkulose-VO* (1997) geregelt. Sie sieht die bei Verdacht auf Rindertuberkulose, d. h. bei Feststellung tuberkuloseverdächtiger Symptome oder Veränderungen an einem lebenden, verendeten oder geschlachteten Tier anzuordnende Tuberkulinisierung aller Rinder des betreffenden Bestandes vor. Hierzu sind gemäß Tierimpfstoff-VO zugelassene *Tuberkuline* zu verwenden. Fällt die einfache Tuberkulinprobe fraglich aus, so kann eine vom beamteten Tierarzt mittels Simultantest vorzunehmende Nachuntersuchung angeordnet werden. Nach Ausmerzung der tuberkulösen Rinder eines Bestandes folgt als wichtige Begleitmaßnahme die *Entkeimung des Stalles* (samt Behältern, Gerätschaften, Dung und flüssigen Abgängen) in Form von Zwischen- und Schlußdesinfektion. Hierzu dürfen nur geprüfte Desinfektionsmittel benutzt werden, deren Wirksamkeit derjenigen von 3%iger Formaldehydlösung entspricht: 3- bis 4%ige Karbol- und Kresolschwefelsäure, Präparate mit $\geq$ 4% aktivem Chlor (Chlorkalkmilch, Rohchloramin) oder 2%ige Natronlauge; zur Grobdesinfektion eignen sich Lysovet PA® oder Tegodor 73® 3%ig bei 6stündiger Einwirkung.

In Deutschland, das nach Abschluß der Rindertuberkulose-Sanierung zum Schutzgebiet erklärt wurde, dürfen Rinder gemäß TSeuG (2001) nur mit amtstierärztlicher Bescheinigung über die Tuberkulosefreiheit ihres Herkunftsbestandes zu Nutz- und Zuchtzwecken eingeführt oder von einem Ort zum anderen verkauft werden. Bei laut intrakutaner Tuberkulinprobe oder bakteriologischem Befund festgestellter Tuberkulose ordnet die zuständige Behörde die Tötung des/der betreffenden Rindes/Rinder an; gleiches gilt für den Fall, daß Tuberkulinprobe, bakteriologischer, klinischer und/oder pathologisch-anatomischer Befund den Ausbruch von Tuberkulose befürchten lassen. Der Entschädigung wird der »gemeine Wert« zugrunde gelegt. Rinder aus nicht als tuberkulosefrei anerkannten Beständen dürfen nur zur Schlachtung abgegeben werden. Von tuberkulösen Kühen stammende Milch ist unschädlich zu beseitigen. Gegen Rindertuberkulose gerichtete Schutz- und Heilimpfungen sind verboten. Für die amtliche Wiederanerkennung eines nach Sanierung erneut tuberkuloseinfizierten Bestandes sind negative Ergebnisse von je 2 aufeinanderfolgenden Tuberkulinproben bei allen über 6 Wochen alten Rindern des Bestandes erforderlich; von diesen Tuberkulinisierungen ist die erste frühestens 6 Monate nach Entfernung aller tuberkulosekranken und -verdächtigen Rinder, die zweite nach Ablauf weiterer 6 Monate vorzunehmen.

Die *fleischhygienerechtliche Beurteilung* tuberkulöser Schlachtrinder wird nach dem FlHG und der FlHVO geregelt. Hiernach kann die Schlachterlaubnis versagt werden, wenn die obligatorische Untersuchung des lebenden Schlachttieres Tuberkulose oder Verdacht auf solche ergibt. Wird Tuberkulose erst nach der Schlachtung festgestellt, so ist das betreffende Tier samt Blut als zu menschlichem Genuß untauglich zu beurteilen. Liegen in Lymphknoten herdförmige Veränderungen vor, die durch atypische Mykobakterien verursacht sein können, sind die zugehörigen Organe als untauglich zu beurteilen.

■ **Forensik:** Strafbare Vorfälle können sich ergeben, wenn gegen das inzwischen erlassene Bundesrecht (TSeuG 2001, Tuberkulose-VO 1997) und/oder gegen EU-Recht (Richtlinie 64/432 EWG, 1994) verstoßen wird. In den Jahren der Tuberkulosetilgung hatten bestimmte betrügerische Manipulationen der Tuberkulinreaktion (z. B. Desensibilisierung) beachtliche forensische Bedeutung.

12.2.7 Nocardiose

M. Stöber

Nocardia asteroides, ein aerober, grampositiver, säurefester Erdbodensaprophyt und Mastitis-Erreger des Rindes, löst vom infizierten Euter her gelegentlich (septikämisch?) Abort aus. Auf gleichem Wege oder aerogen dringt er mitunter in die Lunge und deren Lymphknoten ein, was – u. U. gefördert durch Kortikosteroidbehandlung – respiratorische Erscheinungen bedingen kann. Am lebenden Tier sind dann serologisch spezifische AK nachweisbar (KBR, SNT, ELISA); außerdem gibt es einen Intrakutan-Test. Die durch N. asteroides verursachten Gewebeveränderungen sind tuberkuloseähnlich, nämlich verkäsend-eitrig bis verkalkend. Der Erregernachweis bedarf der histologischen Untersuchung (Gram-Färbung: verzweigte Myzelien) oder der Anzüchtung (Sabouraud-Agar). Die Behandlung (Erythromycin, Miconazol) ist nicht sehr erfolgversprechend. Die Vorbeuge besteht in ordnungsgemäßer Melkhygiene sowie keimfreiem Arbeiten beim Einbringen von Medikamenten durch den Strichkanal.

Bezüglich der durch *Nocardia farcinogenes* verursachten Lymphgefäß- und Lymphknotenentzündung wird auf Kapitel 3.1.3.4 verwiesen.

12.2.8 Melioidose

M. Stöber

Die auch als »Pseudorotz« bezeichnete, durch aerogene, orale, perkutane oder intrazisternale Infektion mit *Burkholderia pseudomallei*, einem opportunistischen Saprophyten, hervorgerufene Melioidose ist beim Rind wesentlich seltener als bei Wildnagern, Mensch, kleinen Wiederkäuern, Pferd und Schwein. Sie kommt v. a. in feuchtwarmen Gebieten Südostasiens und Afrikas, und zwar in der Regenzeit vor, weil Überleben und Verbreitung des Erregers in der Umwelt durch solches Klima sowie durch keimstreuende Nagetiere begünstigt werden. Melioidose ist aber auch in Australien sowie Frankreich beim Rind beobachtet worden und verdient zudem als für den Menschen fatale Zoonose Beachtung. Das klinische Bild ist vom Verlauf (septikämisch-akut oder abszedierend-schleichend) und der Lokalisation der Rotz-ähnlichen Eiterungen abhängig: Bei Lungenbeteiligung treten respiratorische, bei Befall von Gehirn und Rückenmark zentralnervöse Ausfallserscheinungen (Lähmungen), nach Septikämie u. U. Abort oder Polyarthritis auf. Gelegentlich fanden sich nach plötzlichem Tod oder anfänglicher Mastitis Abszesse in Milz (mit Ruptur in die Bauchhöhle) oder Leber, die sahnig-weißen Eiter enthielten; solche Abszesse kommen, verbunden mit starker Schwellung regionaler Lymphknoten, auch in der Lunge oder der Unterhaut vor. Zudem wurden Burkholderia-pseudomallei-bedingte Aborte beschrieben. Am lebenden Tier läßt sich der Erreger von Fall zu Fall in Eiter, Nasenschleim oder Durchfallkot nachweisen (Kultur, Agglutination mit Antiserum oder Tierversuch); außerdem ist die Infektion durch Melioidin-Intrakutanprobe feststellbar. Serologisch sind mittels IHA, KBR, ELISA und IFT spezifische AK zu ermitteln. Differentialdiagnostisch ist an Tuberkulose (Kap. 12.2.6), Pneumonomykosen (Kap. 5.3.3.18), Aktinobazillose (Kap. 3.1.3.3), Nocardiose (Kap. 12.2.7) oder Lymphgefäßentzündung (Kap. 3.1.2) zu denken. Eine gezielte Behandlung kommt wegen meist fehlender Diagnose und Gefahr der Übertragung auf den Menschen nicht in Betracht; B. pseudomallei ist in vitro empfindlich gegen Tetracyclin, Kanamycin, Sulfonamide und Trimethoprim-Sulfamethoxazol. Die Vorbeuge besteht in unschädlicher Beseitigung von Streu und Dung, Stall- und Auslaufdesinfektion sowie Tränkewasserhygiene.

12.2.9 Q-Fieber

M. Stöber

Definition, Ursache, Verbreitung: Das auch als *Query-* (= Fragezeichen) oder *Queensland-Fever* sowie als *Coxiellose* bezeichnete Q-Fieber ist eine durch die Rikkettsie *Coxiella burnetii* bedingte, weltweit vorkommende Zoonose von erheblicher Bedeutung für den Menschen: Bei diesem äußert sich das Leiden nach aerogener (windbegünstigte Staub- oder Tröpfchen-), oraler (Rohmilchgenuß) oder perkutaner (geburtshilfebedingter Schmier-) Infektion meist als akut verlaufende grippeähnliche Allgemeinerkrankung mit Fieber, Abgeschlagenheit, Kopf- und Gliederschmerzen, Schlaflosigkeit, »atypischer« Pneumonie, u. U. auch Hepatitis oder Meningoenzephalitis, bei chronischem Verlauf dagegen als Endokarditis oder Osteomyelitis. Bei Angehörigen exponierter Berufsgruppen – wie Tierärzte, Landwirte, Schäfer, Tierpfleger, Schlachter, Gerber, Wolleverarbeiter, Tierpräparatoren, Laborpersonal – sind spezifische AK häufiger und in höheren Titern nachzuweisen als bei der übrigen Bevölkerung. Coxiella burnetii ist in der unbelebten Umwelt (Staub) sehr resistent; der Keim kann sich offenbar nicht nur in der freien Natur (in Zecken, Wildsäugern, Vögeln) zyklisch vermehren und verbreiten sowie von hier aus zur Infektion von Haustieren (kleine Wiederkäuer, Rind u. a.) führen, sondern – unabhängig vom Wildreservoir – auch bei Rind und Schaf zyklisch halten (= Stall- oder Herdeninfektionszyklus). Diese beiden Tierarten sind die Haupterregerquelle für den Menschen, der sich über Fruchtwasser, Nachgeburtsteile, Lochialsekret, Milch oder Zeckenkotstaub anstecken kann, wobei nicht selten plötzlich mehrere bis zahlreiche Personen zugleich erkranken. Serologische Überprüfungen der Seuchenlage zeigen, daß der Anteil positiver Reagenten beim Rind, wohl infolge der in der Tierproduktion eingetretenen Konzentration, im Zunehmen begriffen ist. Das trifft nicht nur für den traditionell endemisch betroffenen süddeutschen Bereich (= Verbreitungsgebiet der erregerübertragenden Zecke *Dermacentor marginatus*), sondern auch für die übrigen Landesteile und andere Länder mit intensiver Rinderhaltung (insbesondere für Bestände mit Fruchtbarkeitsstörungen) zu. Wegen seines zeckengebunden häufigen Vorkommens in Südeuropa wird das Q-Fieber auch *»Balkan-Grippe«* genannt.

Symptome: Beim Rind verläuft die Infektion mit C. burnetii in aller Regel völlig inapparent als latente Besiedlung von Genitale und Euter; gelegentlich, ausnahmsweise aber bestandsweise gehäuft, kommt es zum Abort nach dem 6. Trächtigkeitsmonat. Auch traten in Herden mit großem Anteil hoher spezifischer AK-Titer vorberichtlich häufiger respiratorische Erkrankungen, Aborte, Totgeburten, Nachgeburtsverhaltungen oder Metritiden auf als in Vergleichsbeständen mit unverdächtigem serologischem Befund. Die experimentelle Infektion löst beim Rind Pneumonie aus. Bullen können *C. burnetii* mit dem Sperma ausscheiden, möglicherweise auch übertragen.

Sektion: Am toten Tier sind keine erregerspezifischen Veränderungen festzustellen. Bei histologischer Untersuchung infizierter Nachgeburtsteile läßt sich C. burnetii mittels KÖSTER-, STAMP- oder IPO-Färbung nachweisen.

Diagnose: Meist ergibt sich der Verdacht auf Vorliegen von Q-Fieber beim Haustier aus der plötzlichen grippeähnlichen Erkrankung betreuender Personen. Dabei können von Fall zu Fall aber auch Menschen erkranken, die nicht direkt mit dem Keimausscheider in Berührung gekommen sind, etwa Anwohner einer von Wanderschafen begangenen Straße. Zur Diagnose bedarf es blut- und/oder milchserologischer Untersuchungen (AK-Nachweis mittels HA, KBR, ELISA bzw. Antigen-Nachweis durch IIFT oder PCR). *Differentialdiagnostisch* sind andere Abortursachen in Betracht zu ziehen.

Behandlung, Prophylaxe: Bei feststehender Diagnose sollten etwaige, am Rind vorzunehmende therapeutische Maßnahmen mit dem Amtstierarzt abgesprochen werden; ggf. empfiehlt sich Tetracyclin. Patienten mit Nachgeburtsverhaltung oder Metritis sind gesondert aufzustallen. Zur Prophylaxe wurden verschiedentlich versuchsweise inaktivierte Vakzinen eingesetzt; sie scheinen nichtinfizierte Rinder zu schützen, verursachen z.T. aber erhebliche lokale Impfreaktionen.

Bekämpfung: Q-Fieber ist gemäß VOmTK zum TSeuG meldepflichtig. Je nach vermutetem Ursprung der Erkrankung werden dann Folgeuntersuchungen bei den für menschliche Infektionen in Frage kommenden Tieren vorgenommen. Handelt es sich dabei um Rinder, so werden von Fall zu Fall angeordnet: Bestandssperre, blut- und milchserologische Kontrollen sowie Ausmerzung aller Reagenten, zumindest aber der C.-burnetii-Ausscheider, Pasteurisieren der Milch, unschädliches Beseitigen der Nachgeburten, Stalldesinfektion, u.U. auch Vakzination der serologisch negativ reagierenden Tiere. In endemisch verseuchten Gebieten empfehlen sich Maßnahmen zur Zeckenbekämpfung (Kap. 2.2.4.4).

12.2.10 Listeriose

M. STÖBER

Definition: Eine durch Listeria monocytogenes bedingte, v.a. Haus- und Wildwiederkäuer, aber auch andere Tierarten befallende Infektionskrankheit, die beim Rind meist als *Meningoenzephalitis* mit herdförmig eitriger Enzephalitis des Stammhirns (= zentralnervöse Listeriose), seltener als *Abort, Sepsis, Keratokonjunktivitis* oder *Mastitis* auftritt. *Andere Bezeichnungen* der zentralnervösen Form: Listerellose, Drehkrankheit, circling disease, silage sickness, tournis, maladie de l'ensilage, malattia da insilati, torneo, marcha en circulos, modorra.

Ursachen: Der Erreger, *Listeria monocytogenes* (L. m.) ist ein mikroaerophiles, grampositives, kokkoides bis stäbchenförmiges, bewegliches Bakterium, das in der Umwelt, insbesondere im Erdreich, auf Pflanzen sowie in kothaltigen Verunreinigungen (Abwässer, Gülle, Mist), weit verbreitet und fakultativ pathogen ist; z.B. ist der Keim im Darmtrakt und im Kot gesunder Rinder, v.a. während des Winters, häufig nachzuweisen. Von den 6 bekannten Serotypen (mit 17 Subtypen) werden beim Rind meist L. m. serovar 1/2a oder 4b ermittelt; pathogene L.-m.-Stämme zeigen i.d.R. β-Hämolyse. Außer durch Geophilie zeichnet sich L. m. durch Psychrophilie (Vermehrung bei 3–45 °C), Oligotrophie (Wachstum auch in nährstoffarmem Medium) und Resistenz gegen niedrigen Umwelt-pH ($\geq$ 5,0) sowie Austrocknung aus. Ein ideales Milieu findet L. m. in schlechtvergorenen Randbezirken erdreichverschmutzter Mais-, aber auch in unsauber gewonnener, unsachgemäß gelagerter oder verpilzter Gras-, Roggen-, Hafer- und Leguminosen-, nicht jedoch in Rübenblatt-Silage.

Vorkommen, Verbreitung: Außer bei Haus- und Wildwiederkäuern kommen listerienbedingte Erkrankungen bei Chinchilla, Kaninchen, Schwein, Geflügel, Hund, Katze und Pferd, Kaltblütern sowie beim Menschen vor. Dabei wird der Erreger offensichtlich meist nicht von Tier zu Tier übertragen, sondern jeweils durch individuelle Schmutzinfektion aufgenommen; deshalb ist die in gemäßigten und kalten Klimaten nördlicher und südlicher Breiten, nicht aber in den Tropen heimische Listeriose nicht als Zoonose, sondern als *Sapronose* anzusehen. Beim Rind ist v.a. die *zentralnervöse*, aber auch die *abortauslösende Listeriose* im Zunehmen begriffen; diese beiden, sporadisch bis enzootisch auftretenden Leiden werden heute allerdings auch besser diagnostiziert als früher. Die übrigen Formen boviner Listeriose, nämlich *Septikämien, Keratokonjunktivitiden* und *Mastitiden* sind vergleichsweise selten, wegen der mit ihnen verbundenen Keimstreuung aber bedeutsam.

Die L.-m.-Infektion *prädisponierter Menschen* (Schwangere, Neugeborene sowie ältere, kranke oder immungeschwächte Personen) erfolgt in aller Regel nicht am Listeriose-kranken Tier (Ausnahme: perkutaner Infekt nach Hilfeleistung bei Listerien-Abort), sondern über Lebensmittel (Rotschmiereweichkäse, Schlachtgeflügel, Rohwurst, Hackfleisch, Aufschnitt), die bei ihrer Verarbeitung mit L. m. verkeimt wurden. Pro Million Einwohner ist jährlich mit 3–10

Erkrankungen (Exanthem, Meningoenzephalitis, Abort oder Sepsis) mit saisonaler Häufung von Juni bis September zu rechnen, von denen etwa ein Fünftel tödlich verläuft.

Pathogenese: Bei Rindern tritt Listeriose oft 10 Tage bis 3 Wochen nach Beginn der Verfütterung von Silage aus einem neuangebrochenen oder längere Zeit offenbelassenen Silo auf; dabei erkranken meist nur einzelne, innerhalb der nächsten Wochen aber mitunter mehrere Tiere nacheinander. *Zentralnervöse* und *abortauslösende Listeriose* zeigen in der nördlichen Hemisphäre eine deutliche jahreszeitliche Häufung (März bis Juni); beide pflegen aber nur selten nebeneinander im gleichen Bestand und nur ausnahmsweise am selben Tier aufzutreten. Im Hinblick auf das verbreitete Vorkommen von L. m. in der Umwelt des Rindes sowie in Trägertieren ist anzunehmen, daß beim Zustandekommen boviner Listeriose Hilfsfaktoren eine Rolle spielen, die noch nicht näher geklärt sind (Erregerdichte und/oder Resistenzschwächung infolge massierter, unhygienischer Haltungsweise, Kältebelastung oder fehlerhafter Ernährung):

- *Listerien-Enzephalitis* kann ruminierende Rinder aller Altersstufen (aber bevorzugt solche $\leq$ 3 Jahre, darunter auch tragende Tiere) befallen und innerhalb einiger Wochen $\leq$ 10% des betreffenden Bestandes erfassen. Dabei findet der Erreger offenbar über Schleimhaut- oder Hautläsionen im Bereich des Kopfes (z. B. beim Zahnwechsel) Zugang zu Zweigen des N. trigeminus, um an diesem entlang intraaxonal zum Hirnstamm zu gelangen und dort eine mikroabszedierende Enzephalitis auszulösen (→ vorwiegend unilaterale Schädigung der Kerngebiete einzelner oder mehrerer Hirnnerven).
- *Listerien-bedingte Aborte* machen regional 1–2% aller bovinen Aborte aus; sie betreffen v. a. Färsen im 6.–9. Trächtigkeitsmonat und beruhen vermutlich auf Listerien-Sepsis des Muttertieres; als Erreger ist meist L. m., mitunter aber L. ivanovii zu ermitteln.
- *Listerien-Sepsis* ist entweder auf intrauterine Infektion (Neugeborene), orale Aufnahme (Durchbrechen der Darmschranke: »viszerale« Listeriose) oder Einatmung von L. m. zurückzuführen.
- *Listeriöse Keratokonjunktivitis* kann nicht nur Teilerscheinung sowohl der Listerien-Enzephalitis als der Listerien-Sepsis sein, sondern kommt auch unabhängig hiervon, durch direkten Kontakt von Horn- oder Bindehaut mit verkeimtem Silagegut vor; dabei können Rinder aller Altersstufen und innerhalb einer Stallhaltungsperiode $\leq$ 50% eines Bestandes erkranken.
- Die sehr seltene *Listerien-Mastitis* beruht vermutlich meist auf galaktogener Keimeinschleppung, mitunter aber auf L.-m.-Abort oder L.-m.-Sepsis.

Symptome, Verlauf: Das klinische Bild ist je nach befallenem Organ unterschiedlich:

- Bei *zentralnervöser Listeriose* ist das nach 2- bis 3wöchiger Inkubation einsetzende Krankheitsbild zwar von Fall zu Fall, je nach Lokalisation und Grad der Hirnschädigung, unterschiedlich und m. o. w. stark ausgeprägt; die Ausfallserscheinungen sind – im Gegensatz zu den meisten differentialdiagnostisch abzugrenzenden Leiden – jedoch fast immer einseitig (d. h. unsymmetrisch) und umfassen als »Grundmuster« ziemlich regelmäßig Gegen-die-Wand-Drängen, einseitige Fazialislähmung sowie Im-Kreis-Gehen (Abb. 12-23 bis 12-31).

Anfängliches Fieber oder Unruhe sind beim Einsetzen zentralnervöser Symptome meist abgeklungen; dann ist auch die Anteilnahme an der Umgebung herabgesetzt; weidende Patienten sondern sich von der Herde ab. Die Lähmung des N. facialis äußert sich in Herabhängen des Ohres, »heruntergerutschtem« Ober- und Unterlid (infolge Lähmung des Stirnhautmuskels), Schlaffheit von Ober- und Unterlippe sowie Ausfall der Atembewegungen am Nasenloch der betreffenden Seite. Die Haut dieser Gesichtshälfte erweist sich als hyp- oder anästhetisch (Beteiligung des N. trigeminus). Bei Lähmung des M. orbicularis oculi werden die Augenlider der betroffenen Seite bei Prüfung von Droh- und Palpebralreflex nicht zugekniffen; der Ausfall des Lidschlages bedingt mit der Zeit m. o. w. schwerwiegende Expositionskeratitis. Die Lähmung von Ober- und Unterlippe der kranken Seite gibt sich durch Speichelfluß aus dem betreffenden Maulwinkel zu erkennen; sie ist bei vergleichendem Betasten beider Flotzmaulhälften auch gut zu fühlen und bedingt mit der Zeit Braunfärbung der Schneidezähne dieser Seite. Schädigung des N.-abducens-Kerns bewirkt Einwärtsschielen des Auges der befallenen Seite. Beteiligung des Ramus mandibularis Ni. trigemini äußert sich in Schlaffheit des gleichseitigen M. masseter, Ansammlung eines Futter-»Priems« in der zugehörigen Backentasche, u. U. auch durch Absinken des Unterkiefers dieser Seite (→ »Schiefmaul«). Schädigungen im Kerngebiet des N. vestibulocochlearis geben sich durch Schräghalten des Kopfes (kranke Seite tiefer als gesunde), Hemiparese und -ataxie (Kopf-gegen-die-Wand-Drücken; seitliches Anlehnen mit Schulter oder Hüfte; »drall«-artiges Nach-vorn-und-seitwärts-Drängen; stets in gleicher Richtung entlang der Wand oder Einzäunung erfolgendes, m. o. w. stolperndes Im-Kreis-Gehen), mitunter auch in Nystagmus zu erkennen; das stereotype Wandern im Kreise führt bei Stallhaltung zur Aufschürfung der Haut im Bereich des Jochbogens der wandwärtigen Kopfseite. Mitbetroffensein von N. glossopharyngeus und N. vagus bewirkt m. o. w. ausgeprägte Schlingbeschwerden (Speicheln, Ansammeln von Futter im Rachen, mitunter auch Regurgitieren von Schlund- oder Panseninhalt). Die Beteiligung des N. hypoglossus führt zu Zungenvorfall, diejenige des N. accessorius zur Wendung von Kopf und Hals auf die gesunde Seite hin (Torticollis); in seltenen Fällen besteht Opistho- oder Emprosthotonus. Nach versuchsweiser Korrektur listeriosebedingter Haltungsanomalien kehrt der betreffende Körperteil stets »hartnäckig« wieder in die abnorme Position zurück. Beim Führen eines mit Listerien-Enzephalitis behafteten Rindes ist wegen des oft ungestümen, stets in gleicher Weise nach vorn-seitwärts gerichteten Bewegungsdranges Umsicht geboten, damit keine Helfer umgerannt werden. Die Lähmungen im Kopfbereich bewirken m. o. w. schwerwiegende Behinderung der Futter- und Tränkeaufnahme, bei dauerndem Speichelverlust oft auch fortschreitende Dehydratation (Einsinken der Augäpfel, Verminderung des Hautturgors, Eindickung von Panseninhalt und Kot) sowie metabolische Azidose (→ Steigerung von Atemintensität und -frequenz). Die zunehmenden Bewegungsstörungen führen schließlich unter ständigem »Rotieren« oder wiederholtem seitlichem Umfallen zum Festliegen in einer den individuellen Ausfallserscheinungen entsprechenden, »nicht korrigierbaren« Haltung; in Brustlage festliegende Patienten kriechen dabei zunächst noch weiterhin im Kreis herum, während in platter Seitenlage festliegende Kranke Ruderbewegungen ausführen. Unbehandelt endet klinisch manifeste Listerien-Enzephalitis mit seltenen Ausnahmen innerhalb von 1–2 Wochen tödlich (Atemstillstand).

➤ *Listerien-bedingte Aborte, Tot- und Frühgeburten* treten im Experiment 6–8 Tage nach intravenöser Infektion ein. 10% der spontanen Fälle gehen mit Nachgeburtsverhaltung einher. Bei gegen Ende der Gravidität erfolgendem Listerien-Abort kann das Muttertier fieberhaft erkranken.

➤ Klinisch manifeste *Listerien-Sepsis* betrifft meist neugeborene Kälber $\leq$ 2 Lebenswochen, gelegentlich aber ältere und sogar erwachsene Tiere. Bei ersteren äußert sich das Leiden in allgemeiner, von Fieber begleiteter Schwäche; mitunter besteht zudem Hornhauttrübung, Iritis, Dyspnoe und/oder Opisthotonus; solche Erkrankungen enden meist schon innerhalb von 12 h tödlich. Ältere Patienten zeigen dagegen Diarrhoe mit wäßrigem, übelriechenden Kot; dabei können in rascher Folge mehrere Tiere erkranken und verenden.

➤ *Listeriöse Keratokonjunktivitis* kommt einseitig und mechanisch bedingt bei Listerien-Enzephalitis (s. d.), beidseitig und mit hämatogener Iritis oder Ophthalmie verbunden bei Listerien-Sepsis (s. d.) vor. Außerdem wird ein- oder beidseitige listerienbedingte Keratokonjunktivitis auch als selbständige Erkrankung beobachtet: Sie betrifft v. a. Rinder, die Rundballensilage aus hochangebrachter Fütterungsstelle erhalten oder deren Augen anderweitig mit Grassilage in Kontakt geraten. Diese Binde- und Hornhautentzündung ist gekennzeichnet durch ein- oder beidseitigen Tränenfluß, Photophobie, bläuliche Verfärbung der Kornea und Fältelung der Iris (Iridozyklitis, Kap. 11.1.2.6); später entwickeln sich weiße bis gelbe Flekken auf der Hornhaut; mitunter kommt es zu Hypopyon, Keratokonusbildung oder Panophthalmie.

➤ Die *Listerien-Mastitis* des Rindes verläuft von Fall zu Fall akut oder chronisch und erweist sich oft als therapieresistent; gelegentlich wird L. m. allerdings auch vom klinisch normalen Euter ausgeschieden.

■ **Sektion:** Bei *Listerien-Enzephalitis* ist der makroskopische Zerlegungsbefund, abgesehen von Blutfülle der Hirnhäute und leichter Liquorvermehrung, unauffällig. *Histologisch* finden sich, außer nichteitriger Leptomeningitis bulbaris, Hirnnerven-Neuritis und perivaskulären lympho-monozytären Infiltraten, kennzeichnende Mikroabszesse im Bereich des Hirnstammes, bei denen die Beteiligung von polymorphkernigen Leukozyten allerdings oft weniger ausgeprägt ist als beim listeriosekranken Schaf. N. B.: Unter Tollwutverdacht eingesandte, aber rabiesnegativ befundene Wiederkäuergehirne sollten stets auch auf listeriöse Veränderungen überprüft werden.

➤ Beim *Listerien-Abort* ist der Fetus mäßig bis deutlich autolytisch; seine Leber weist häufig miliare Nekroseherde, die Labmagenschleimhaut kleine Erosionen auf; das Muttertier zeigt Plazentitis und Metritis.

➤ *Listerien-Sepsis* äußert sich in mukofibrinöser bis hämorrhagischer Abomasoenteritis, multiplen miliaren Abszessen innerer Organe, insbesondere der Leber, sowie serofibrinöser Polysynoviitis (und Meningitis), mitunter auch in Ophthalmie.

■ **Diagnose, Differentialdiagnose:** Bei *Listerien-Enzephalitis* lenken klinisches Bild und Überprüfung der verfütterten Silage den Verdacht auf dieses Leiden. Dabei ist zu bedenken, daß nicht jede beim Rind vorkommende Listerieninfektion silagebedingt ist. Die Liquoruntersuchung ergibt positivenfalls mittelgradige Zellvermehrung mit Vorherrschen von Mono- und Lymphozyten sowie leicht erhöhten Glukose- und Eiweißgehalt. L. m. ist jedoch in der Hirnrükkenmarks-Flüssigkeit listeriosekranker Rinder fast nie nachweisbar. Bei versuchsweiser antibiotischer Behandlung eintretende deutliche Besserung der Symptomatik ist als Bestätigung der Diagnose zu werten, die sich intra vitam bislang anderweitig nicht sichern läßt: Serologische Befunde sind ohne diagnostische Aussagekraft. Zur *postmortalen Klärung* ist das Gehirn (Hirnstamm) einzusenden, und zwar die den klinischen Ausfallserscheinungen entsprechende Hälfte zur histologischen Untersuchung (typische, mikroabszedierende Enzephalitis; IF- oder PAP-Färbung des L.-m.-Antigens), die andere Hälfte zum kulturellen

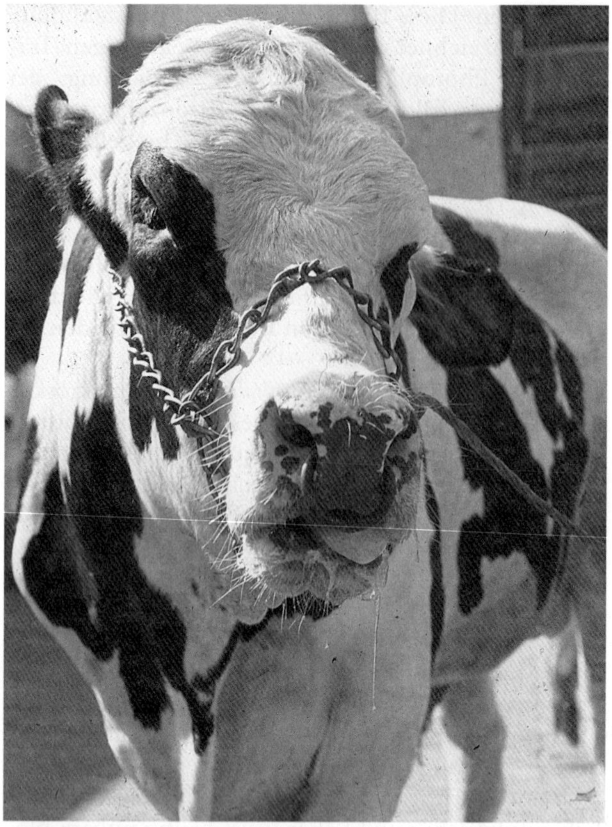

Abbildung 12-23 Nervöse Form der Listeriose: Linksseitige zentrale Fazialisparese (Ptosis von Ohr, Oberlid und Nasenloch/Flotzmaul) mit Beteiligung des linken N. hypoglossus (Zungenvorfall), Dehydratation

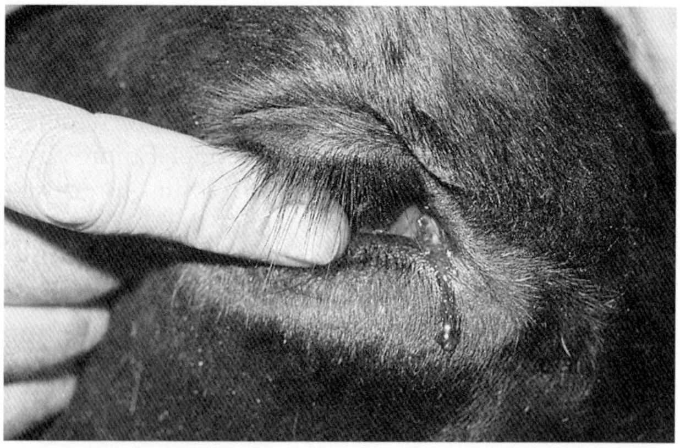

Abbildung 12-24 Nervöse Listeriose: Einseitiger Ausfall des Lidreflexes

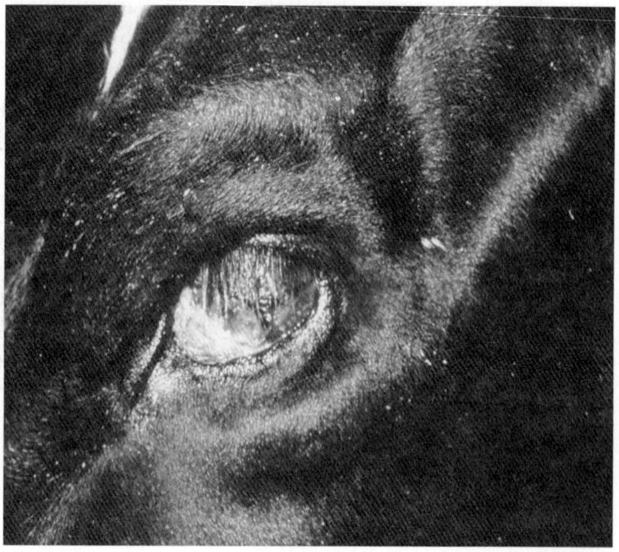

Abbildung 12-25 Nervöse Listeriose: Einseitige Expositionskeratitis

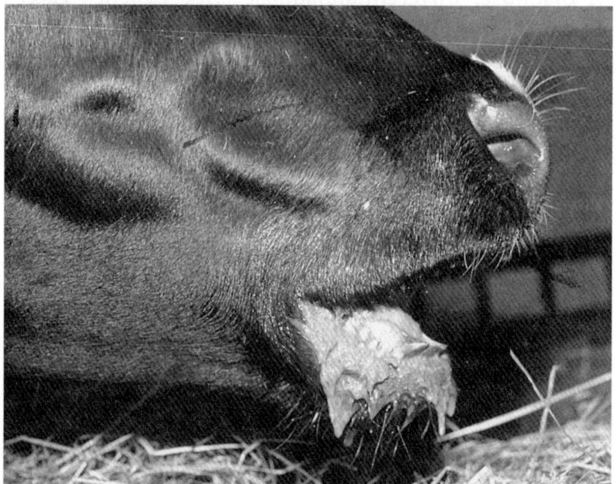

Abbildung 12-26 Nervöse Listeriose: Lähmung der rechten Ober- und Unterlippe (→ Verbleiben und Herausfallen von Futterresten auf der betroffenen Seite)

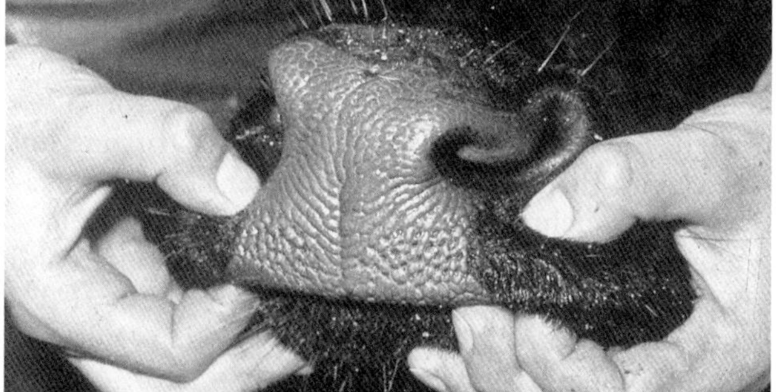

Abbildung 12-27 Nervöse Listeriose: Palpatorischer Vergleich der Konsistenz beider Oberlippenhälften (rechte Seite gelähmt)

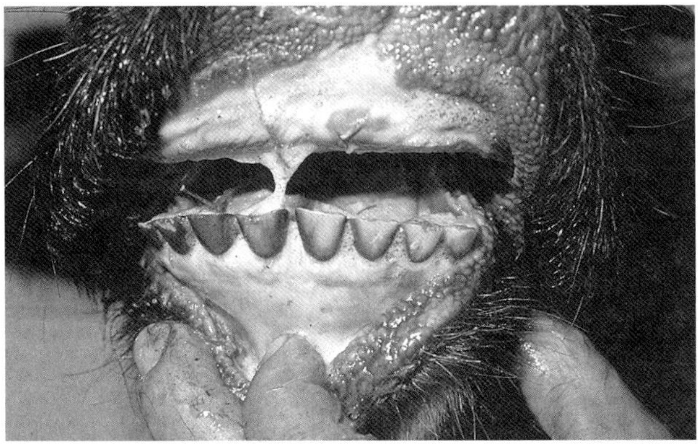

Abbildung 12-28 Nervöse Listeriose: Braunfärbung der Schneidezähne des Tieres von Abb. 12-27 auf der gelähmten Seite

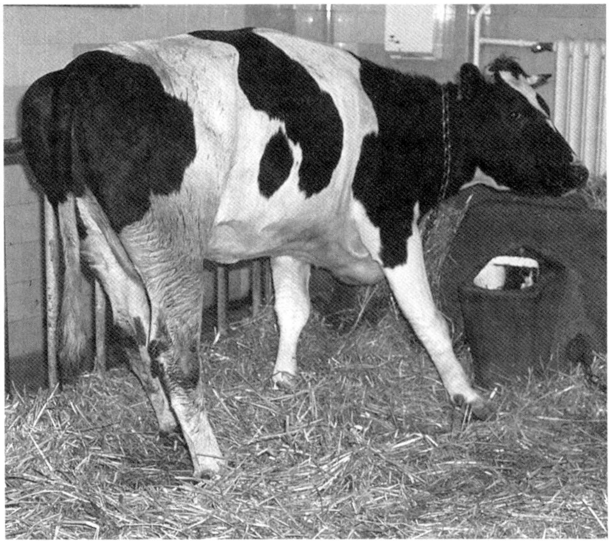

Abbildung 12-29 Nervöse Listeriose: Anlehnbedürfnis infolge Beteiligung des N. vestibulo-cochlearis

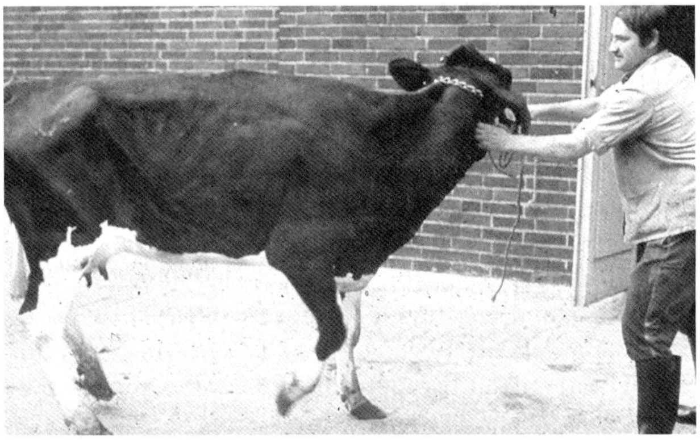

Abbildung 12-30 Nervöse Listeriose: Drängen nach vorn und zur Seite

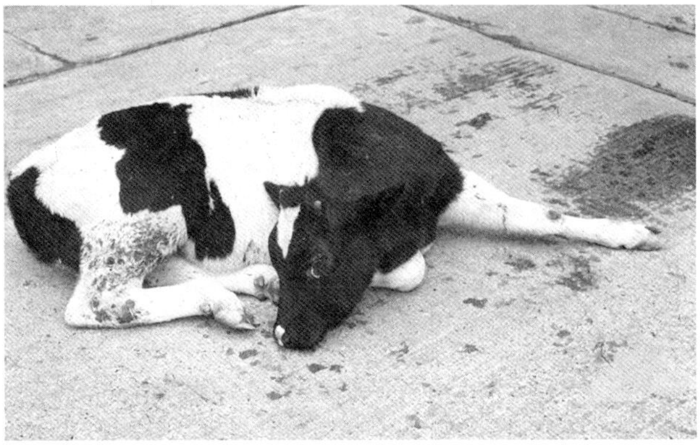

Abbildung 12-31 Nervöse Listeriose: Ständiges gleichsinniges Im-Kreis-Rutschen

Listeriennachweis (Kälteanreicherung); letzterer kann allerdings mehrere Monate benötigen. *Differentialdiagnostisch* sind andersbedingte Lähmungen des N. facialis* (Kap. 10.2.5.7), z. B. bei Otitis media (Kap. 11.2.3.2), außerdem Tollwut (Kap. 10.3.6), Stirnhöhlenentzündung (Kap. 5.1.2.4), Hirnabszeß (Kap. 10.3.2), Hirnbasis-Syndrom (Kap. 10.2.3, 10.3.3), Hirnnervenscheiden-Tumoren (Kap. 10.7.2), Infektiöse septikämisch-thrombosierende Meningoenzephalomyelitis (Kap. 10.3.4), sporadische Meningoenzephalitis (Kap. 10.3.10), nervöse Ketose (Kap. 10.5.7) und Botulismus (Kap. 10.5.13) zu berücksichtigen.

* Nicht jede, aber die meisten einseitigen Fazialislähmungen des Rindes sind listerienbedingt; nicht bei jeder listerienbedingten Meningoenzephalitis, aber doch bei den meisten, kommt es auch zur Fazialislähmung.

➤ Bei *Listerien-Abort* können Hinweise auf im gleichen Bestand bereits vorgekommene L.-m.-bedingte Verkalbungen zur Abgrenzung von andersbedingten Störungen der Trächtigkeit dienlich sein. Zum Erregernachweis eignen sich Fetus (Leber, Labmageninhalt, Lunge, Mekonium), Plazentome/Nachgeburt, Fruchtwasser oder Lochien; dabei ist i. d. R. keine Kälteanreicherung erforderlich.

➤ Bei *Listerien-Sepsis* sind zum Erregernachweis Gewebeproben veränderter Organe (Leber, Lunge, Nieren, Milz), am lebenden Tier Blut einzusenden.

➤ Die verschiedenen Formen *L.-m.-bedingter Keratokonjunktivitis* lassen sich untereinander anhand der Begleitumstände, von andersbedingten Binde- und Hornhautentzündungen (Kap. 11.1.2.5, 11.1.3.1 bis 11.1.3.4) dagegen durch Konjunktivaltupfer (→ Erregerdifferenzierung) unterscheiden.

➤ *Listerien-Mastitis* ist durch Nachweis von L. m. in der Milch zu diagnostizieren.

Beurteilung: Bei rechtzeitiger sachgemäßer, auch etwaige Dehydratation und Azidose berücksichtigender Behandlung ist mehr als die Hälfte aller Fälle von *zentralnervöser boviner Listeriose* heilbar. Allerdings können Lähmungserscheinungen (abnorme Ohr- oder Kopfhaltung u. ä.) mitunter noch einige Zeit oder dauernd bestehen bleiben. Unbehandelt führt L.-m.-Enzephalitis dagegen nach längstens 14 Tagen zum Tode. Bis zu 2 Wochen nach Absetzen der betreffenden Silage können noch weitere Fälle von L.-m.-Enzephalitis auftreten.

➤ *Listerien*-Sepsis verläuft bei Neugeborenen i. d. R. rasch tödlich; bei älteren Patienten soll rechtzeitige Pencillinbehandlung aussichtsreich sein.

➤ L.-m.-Abort und -Metritis bedingen keine dauerhafte Fruchtbarkeitsstörung.

➤ Kühe, die mit ihrer *Milch L. m. ausscheiden*, sind wegen der hiermit für Betreuungspersonal und Verbraucher verbundenen Gefahr auszumerzen.

Behandlung: Fragliche Silage, insbesondere verdorbene oder Randpartien nicht mehr verfüttern.

➤ Patienten mit noch nicht allzuweit fortgeschrittenen *zentralnervösen Erscheinungen* in gut eingestreute Einzellaufbox verbringen; 10 Tage lang je 40000–50000 IE Penicillin (oder Ampicillin)/kg LM oder 5 Tage lang je 5–10 mg Oxytetracyclin/kg LM parenteral verabreichen. Außerdem, je nach Störung der Futter- und Wasseraufnahme des Patienten: intravenöse Zufuhr traubenzuckerhaltiger Elektrolytlösung (nötigenfalls als Dauertropfinfusion); bei mäßigem bzw. starkem Speichelverlust auch Ausgleich der Azidose durch tägliche orale Gabe von 25–50, bzw. 50–100 g Natriumbikarbonat/100 kg LM in 2–4 bzw. 4–8 l Wasser; Pansensaftübertragung. Bei belastungsbedingter Muskelschädigung (Kap. 9.9.7) ist zudem die parenterale Gabe eines Vitamin-E-Selen-Präparates angezeigt.

➤ *»Silagebedingte« Keratokonjunktivitis* spricht nicht immer auf übliche lokale Behandlung (wiederholte Instillation antibiotika- und kortikosteroidhaltiger Augensalbe) an; deshalb sollte die betreffende Silage nicht mehr so hoch vorgelegt werden, daß sie den Tieren auf den Kopf fallen kann; des weiteren empfiehlt sich die Anwendung von Rundballen-Raufen.

Prophylaxe: Silage in Betonhochsilos statt in Betonflach- oder Erdsilos einlagern; Silos vor Einfüllen neuen Silagegutes gründlich reinigen und desinfizieren; beim Beschicken von Silos und beim Abpacken von Plastikfolien-Ballensilage auf Sauberkeit des Silageguts achten (kein Grün von maulwurfbefallenen Flächen ensilieren; kein Erdreich in Fahrsilos einschleppen); Silierungsprozeß durch Zusatzstoffe fördern. Offensichtlich verdorbene (übelriechende oder schimmelige) Silagepartien (pH > 5,0, Aschegehalt > 50 ppm TM) nicht verfüttern. Keine Geflügeleinstreu in Rinderstallungen einbringen. Nach jedem Abort gründliche Stalldesinfektion vornehmen. Über den Nutzen der Listeriose-Schutzimpfung von Rindern liegen keine gesicherten Erkenntnisse vor.

Zur Verhütung *menschlicher Listeriose*: Bei Geburtshilfeleistung am Rind und Schaf stets Schutzkleidung tragen. Der für L.-m.-Infektionen prädisponierte Personenkreis sollte bestimmte Nahrungsmittel (s. *Vorkommen*) meiden oder nur gekocht genießen; Gewinnung und Lagerung dieser Viktualien sollten unter gebotener Hygiene erfolgen. Die Listeriose des Rindes gehört ihrem Wesen nach zu den Krankheiten, bei denen laut FlHVO von 1986 das Blut als für menschlichen Genuß untauglich, Tierkörper und Organe dagegen als bedingt tauglich zu beurteilen sind.

Bekämpfung: Bovine Listeriose ist gemäß VOmTK zum TSeuG meldepflichtig.

12.2.11 Bovines Ephemeral-Fieber

M. Stöber

Definition: Das auch Dreitagekrankheit genannte Bovine Ephemeral-Fieber (BEF) ist eine arthropodenübertragene virusbedingte Krankheit von Rindern und Wasserbüffeln. *Andere Bezeichnungen:* Three day stiff sickness, bovine epizootic fever. Das BEF-Virus kann auch Kaffernbüffel sowie einige Wildwiederkäuerarten befallen, die dabei aber meist nicht erkranken.

Ursachen: Der Erreger des BEF ist ein Rhabdovirus, von dem bislang 4 antigenetisch differenzierbare Stämme bekannt sind.

Vorkommen, Verbreitung, Bedeutung: Das Leiden tritt heute vielerorts in Afrika, Süd- und Südostasien sowie Australien endemisch, stellenweise aber m. o. w. periodisch wiederkehrend und unter rascher Ausbreitung epizootisch auf. Es wird durch blutsaugende Arthropoden übertragen und ist nicht kontagiös. Seine Vektoren können sich offenbar in bestimmten Jahren bzw. Jahresszeiten klimabedingt (feuchtwarmer Sommer/Herbst, anhaltende Regenfälle) stark vermehren oder m. o. w. rasch durch den Wind verbreitet werden, was dann, ebenso wie das Vorhandensein empfänglicher Rinder, die Epidemiologie des BEF bestimmt. Die mit massivem Auftreten des BEF verbundenen wirtschaftlichen Verluste sind erheblich.

Pathogenese: Die Morbidität des BEF kann bei schweren Ausbrüchen ≤ 80% betragen. Bei Milch- und Fleischrindern sowie bei BEF-Epizootien ist sie

i. d. R. höher und der Krankheitsverlauf schwerwiegender als bei Wasserbüffeln bzw. in endemisch betroffenen Regionen; während bei BEF-Epizootien meist alle Altersstufen betroffen werden, erkranken in endemisch verseuchten Gebieten oft nur jüngere, d. h. noch nicht immune Tiere. Die Mortalität überschreitet nur selten 1–2 %. Die 4–5 Tage nach Erkrankungsbeginn eintretende sterile Immunität hält ~ 2 Jahre lang an; erneute Infektion mit dem gleichen Erregertyp bedingt oft nur Zunahme des Antikörperspiegels.

Symptome, Verlauf: Das innerhalb von 2–10 Tagen nach Exposition abrupt einsetzende und meist innerhalb von 3–4 Tagen abklingende Krankheitsbild umfaßt Fieber, Freßunlust, plötzlichen Milchrückgang, Muskelzittern, Tränen-, Nasenaus- und Speichelfluß, Rückgang der Vormagenmotorik, Atembeschwerde, Tachykardie, Lymphknotenschwellung, Niedergeschlagenheit, allgemeine Steifigkeit sowie Lahmheit wechselnder Lokalisation. Manche Patienten liegen sogar zeitweilig fest; ihr Serum kann einen verminderten Kalziumgehalt aufweisen. Während der Fieberphase zeigt das Blut Neutrophilie, Kernlinksverschiebung und Lymphopenie, danach 1–2 Wochen lang anhaltende Zunahme des Fibrinogengehalts.

Sektion: Serofibrinöse Polyserositis sämtlicher Körperhöhlen und ebensolche Polysynoviitis der Gelenke und Sehnenscheiden; ödematös-blutige Durchtränkung aller Lymphknoten; Lungenödem und -emphysem. *Histologisch* sind obliterierende Bronchulitis sowie erhöhte Durchlässigkeit subseröser und subsynovialer Blutgefäße (→ Ödematisierung, Infiltration mit Neutrophilen) kennzeichnend.

Diagnose: Klinisches Bild und Verlauf sowie örtlich gehäuftes Auftreten in bekanntermaßen endemisch befallenem oder an ein solches grenzendem Gebiet lenken den Verdacht auf BEF. Der Nachweis erregerspezifischer Serokonversionen (NT, IFAT, AGID, ELISA) gilt als Bestätigung. Das BEF-Virus ist in den Ergüssen der Körperhöhlen und Gelenke sowie in Lungen-, Milz- und Lymphknotengewebe feststellbar (IFAT).

Differentialdiagnostisch sind bei Erkrankung einzelner Tiere v. a. andersbedingte Lahmheiten (Kap. 9), Hypokalzämische Gebärparese (Kap. 12.3.1) und Fremdkörpererkrankung (Kap. 6.6.2) zu bedenken.

Beurteilung: Nach Überstehen des BEF kehrt die volle Milchleistung in der laufenden Laktation meist nicht mehr zurück. Hochtragende Kühe können abortieren; Kälber von während der Trächtigkeit mit dem BEF-Virus infizierten Kühen weisen keine Mißbildungen auf. Schwere, großrahmige Tiere, insbesondere Bullen, können stark abmagern; bei letzteren erweist sich zudem die Fruchtbarkeit während der auf die BEF-Erkrankung folgenden Monate oft als beeinträchtigt.

Behandlung, Prophylaxe: Ruhigstellung; nichtsteroidale Entzündungshemmer und/oder Metamizol 2–3 Tage lang parenteral, bei Anzeichen von Hypokalzämie (Kap. 12.3.1) auch Kalziumboroglukonat intravenös; zur Verhütung von Sekundärinfektionen wird Tetracyclin empfohlen. In gefährdeten Gebieten werden empfängliche Rinder mit attenuiertem Erreger schutzgeimpft.

12.3 Fütterungs-, stoffwechsel-, mangel- und vergiftungsbedingte Krankheiten mit Beteiligung mehrerer Organsysteme

An den im folgenden zu besprechenden Leiden vorgenannter Ätiologie sind mehrere Organapparate beteiligt. Weitere, alimentär, metabolisch oder defizienzbedingte Rinderkrankheiten, bei denen ebenfalls mehrere Organsysteme zugleich erkranken, werden anderenorts geschildert, weil ihr klinisches Bild sich i. d. R. auf eines von ihnen konzentriert. Das gilt z. B. für *Enzootische Myodystrophie* und *Paralytische Myoglobinurie* (Kap. 9.17.1, 9.17.2), die bei den Krankheiten des Bewegungsapparates besprochen werden, obwohl bei ihnen außer der lokomotorischen auch Atmungs- und Herzmuskulatur m. o. w. stark mitbetroffen sind.

12.3.1 Hypokalzämische Gebärlähmung

J. Martig

Definition: Bei der Hypokalzämischen Gebärlähmung handelt es sich um eine i. d. R. kurz nach dem Kalben auftretende akute Störung des Kalziumstoffwechsels von Milchkühen; sie führt zum Festliegen und in schweren Fällen zum Koma. *Andere Bezeichnungen:* Gebärparese, puerperales Festliegen, Milchfieber, Kalbefieber, Gebärkoma, parturient hypocalcemia, parturient paresis, milk fever, kalfziekte, melkziekte, fièvre vitulaire, paraplégie puérpérale, colasso puerperale.

Vorkommen, Bedeutung: Das Leiden tritt weltweit in Betrieben mit intensiver Milchviehhaltung auf. Die durchschnittliche Inzidenz dürfte 5–10 % aller adulten Milchkühe betragen. Hochleistungskühe sind anfälliger als solche mit geringer Milchproduktion.

Weit deutlicher als die Leistungsdisposition ist die mit zunehmendem Alter verbundene erhöhte Anfälligkeit. So erkranken Primipare praktisch nie an Hypokalzämischer Gebärlähmung, während das Gebärpareserisiko für Kühe bis zu einem Alter von 6 Jahren linear zunimmt. Typischerweise tritt das Leiden 1–2 Tage nach dem Abkalben auf. Da die Störung ätiologisch mit dem Einsetzen der Milchsynthese in Zusammenhang steht (s. u.), kann das durch Kalziummangel bedingte Festliegen auch schon vor, während oder unmittelbar nach dem Partus auftreten. In Ausnahmefällen tritt Hypokalzämische Gebärlähmung auch erst 3–7 Tage nach dem Kalbedatum oder noch später auf.

■ **Ätiologie, Pathogenese:** Die dem Leiden zugrundeliegende Hypokalzämie hat ihre Ursache in der zum Kalbetermin einsetzenden Laktation und der damit verbundenenen Steigerung des Kalziumbedarfs. Der rasch verfügbare Anteil des im Körper der Kuh vorhandenen Kalziums beträgt lediglich ungefähr 0,3%, nämlich 15–20 g. Der Großteil ist im Skelett gelagert. Der Pool des rasch verfügbaren Kalziums wird mit dem aus dem Darm aufgenommenen und dem aus dem Knochen resorbierten Kalzium ergänzt (wobei ein Teil davon auch wieder im Skelett eingelagert wird); ein gewisser Anteil (~ 8 g pro Tag) wird über die Nieren und mit dem Kot ausgeschieden. Aus dem Pool des frei verfügbaren Kalziums wird während der Trächtigkeit das für die Skelettbildung des Feten benötigte, während der Laktation das in der Milch enthaltene Kalzium zur Verfügung gestellt. Ein Liter Milch enthält etwa 1,25 g Kalzium; der Gehalt im Kolostrum ist mit 1,8–2,5 g/l sogar noch höher. Während des Trockenstehens beträgt der Bedarf an Kalzium für den Aufbau des fetalen Skeletts 4–5 g pro Tag. Mit dem Beginn der Milchproduktion nimmt somit der Bedarf an rasch verfügbarem Kalzium innerhalb von 1–2 Tagen um ein Mehrfaches zu. Dadurch sinkt zu diesem Zeitpunkt bei allen Kühen der Gehalt an frei verfügbarem Kalzium im Körper ab, was sich in einer Hypokalzämie äußert, die aber im Normalfall den Wert von 1,9 mmol/l im Serum nicht wesentlich unterschreitet. Bei Kühen, welche an Gebärparese erkranken, sinkt dieser Wert unter 1,5 mmol/l. Der Grund hierfür liegt in ungenügender, v. a. zu langsamer Adaptation des Stoffwechsels an die rasch gestiegenen Bedürfnisse.

Die Kalziumhomöostase wird durch das in der Nebenschilddrüse gebildete Parathormon (PTH), den Vitamin-D_3-Metaboliten 1,25-Dihydroxycholekalziferol (1,25$[OH]_2D_3$) und das von den C-Zellen der Schilddrüse abgesonderte Thyreokalzitonin (TC) gewährleistet. Vitamin D wird von der Kuh aus 7-Dehydrocholesterol in der Haut synthetisiert oder teilweise aus dem Futter resorbiert und in der Leber zu 25-Hydroxycholekalziferol hydrolysiert. In dieser Form zirkuliert Vitamin D in einer Konzentration von 20–50 ng/ml Plasma. In der Niere wird es zu 1,25-Dihydroxycholekalziferol, die stoffwechselaktive Form des Vitamins D_3, umgewandelt. Dieser Hydroxylierungsschritt wird hauptsächlich durch PTH reguliert. Das 1,25-Dihydroxycholekalziferol fördert die Resorption von Kalzium aus dem Darm und, gemeinsam mit PTH, diejenige aus dem Knochen. Parathormon vermindert zudem die Rückresorption von Phosphor in der Niere und führt somit zu einer vermehrten Ausscheidung von Phosphor und dadurch zum Absinken seines Gehalts im Plasma. Die renale Ausscheidung von Kalzium wird dagegen durch PTH und 1,25-Dihydroxycholekalziferol gedrosselt. Die Thyreokalzitoninsekretion wird bei abnormer Zunahme des Ca-Plasmaspiegels stimuliert. Thyreokalzitonin fördert den Einbau von Kalzium im Knochen.

Mit dem Einsetzen der Laktation weisen alle Kühe eine negative Kalziumbilanz und somit eine Hypokalzämie auf. Die dadurch bedingte vermehrte Ausschüttung von Parathormon führt zum Anstieg des 1,25-Dihydroxycholekalziferols. Mit einer Latenzzeit von 24 h verbessert sich dann die aktive Kalziumresorption aus dem Darm. Bis die Resorption von Kalzium aus dem Knochen wirksam wird, dauert es 48 oder mehr Stunden. Warum es bei gewissen Kühen nach dem Abkalben zu einem Absinken des Kalziumgehalts im Plasma auf pathologische, zum Festliegen führende Werte kommt, ist bislang, trotz intensiver Forschung auf diesem Gebiet, nur teilweise geklärt. Heute ist unbestritten, daß auch bei Kühen, welche zum Festliegen kommen, die Parathormonausschüttung normal erfolgt. Bei den meisten Kühen steigt unmittelbar danach auch der Spiegel des 1,25-Dihydroxycholekalziferols an. Kühe, welche an Hypokalzämie erkranken, unterscheiden sich von den anderen dadurch, daß ihre Endorgane (Darm und Knochen) ungenügend oder verspätet auf diese hormonellen Stimuli reagieren. Das als Hormon wirkende 1,25$(OH)_2$-Vitamin D_3 bindet an spezifischen Rezeptoren, sogenannten Vitamin-D_3-Rezeptoren (VDR), in den Zellen der Endorgane. Ein Grund für die Entstehung des Festliegens liegt in der mit zunehmendem Alter abnehmenden Anzahl solcher Rezeptoren. Ein weiterer Grund für die refraktäre Reaktion auf hormonelle Stimuli liegt darin, daß bei reichlichem Angebot von Kalzium im Futter am Ende des Trockenstehens die Kuh ihren Bedarf fast ausschließlich mit dem passiv resorbierten Kalzium zu decken vermag. Die an die Wirkung der Stoffwechselhormone gebundene aktive Resorption wird nicht beansprucht, weil die Sekretion von Parathormon wegen des hohen Gehalts von Kalzium im Plasma und somit auch die Bildung von 1,25$(OH)_2$-Vitamin D_3 unterdrückt wird. Dadurch nimmt auch die Zahl der VDR ab. Bei vergleichenden Untersuchungen über den Gehalt von Knochenmarkern bei gesunden und festliegenden Kühen wurde festgestellt, daß auch bei der festliegenden Kuh der Knochenstoffwechsel aktiviert wird. Daraus läßt sich ableiten, daß der Resorptionsstörung aus dem Darm vermutlich größere ätiologische Bedeutung zukommt als der gestörten Mobilisation aus dem Knochen. Es konnte auch gezeigt werden, daß im Zustand von metabolischer Alkalose sowohl die Nieren als auch die Knochen auf den Stimulus des bei Hypokalzämie in normalen Mengen ausgeschütteten Parathormons nicht oder erst mit zeitlicher Verzögerung reagieren. Eine Überproduktion von Thyreokalzitonin wird heute nicht mehr als Ursache des hypokalzämischen Festliegens in Betracht gezogen.

Aus dem bisher Gesagten geht hervor, daß das Alter der Kuh und die Fütterung während der Trockenzeit für die Entstehung der Hypokalzämischen Gebärparese von großer ursächlicher Bedeutung sind und daß auch die Höhe der Milchleistung, insbesondere zu Beginn der Laktation, eine gewisse Rolle spielt. Zwar wurde für verschiedene Rinderrassen eine unterschiedlich hohe Anfälligkeit für Hypokalzämische Gebärparese beschrieben; die errechnete Heritabilität dieses Leidens wird jedoch allgemein als gering eingestuft. Die Erkenntnisse über die Pathogenese der Hypokalzämischen Gebärparese sind wegweisend für die Empfehlungen zu Therapie und Prophylaxe (s. d.).

Nicht eindeutig geklärt ist der Zusammenhang zwischen der Hypokalzämie und der zum Festliegen führenden schlaffen Muskellähmung. Kalziumionen spielen sowohl bei der Erregungsausbreitung am Nerven und an der Muskelzelle als auch für die Übertragung der Erregung an der motorischen Endplatte sowie für die Muskelkontraktion selbst eine wichtige Rolle. Bei der Untersuchung von Muskelbiopsien von Kühen mit hypokalzämischem Festliegen ergaben sich Hinweise, daß der intrazelluläre Gehalt an Kalium dabei erniedrigt, derjenige von Natrium erhöht wird. Falls diese Beobachtung mit einer exakten Meßmethode bestätigt werden könnte, würde dies bedeuten, daß durch Erniedrigung der extrazellulären Kalziumkonzentration die Durchlässigkeit der Muskelzellmembran für Natrium und Kalium erhöht wird. Die dadurch bedingte Verminderung des Membranpotentials würde zuerst zu einer Übererregbarkeit der Zelle und bei weiterem Absinken zu einem Nichtmehransprechen auf Reize und somit zur schlaffen Lähmung führen. Ebenfalls viel diskutiert wird die Hypothese, wonach die Übertragung des Reizes an der motorischen Endplatte nicht zustande kommt, weil das für die Ausschüttung von Azetylcholin essentielle Kalzium fehlt. Neuere experimentelle Untersuchungen oder klinische Studien zu dieser Frage sind in der Literatur nicht zu finden. Ebensowenig ist die genaue Pathogenese des gestörten Sensoriums und des im fortgeschrittenen Stadium auftretenden Komas bekannt. Neben einer Beeinträchtigung der Herzfunktion und Blutdruckabfall kommt auch ein direkter Einfluß des Kalziummangels auf das zentrale Nervensystem in Frage.

Symptome, Verlauf: Klinisch unterscheidet man drei Stadien, wobei das erste von kurzer Dauer sein kann und nicht selten übersehen wird; das dritte tritt nur bei hochgradiger Hypokalzämie auf und ist deshalb nicht in jedem Fall zu beobachten: Zu Beginn sind die klinischen Erscheinungen nicht sehr auffällig. Solche Kühe zeigen eine leicht verkrampfte Körperhaltung. Manchmal drängen sie nach vorne, entlasten abwechslungsweise die Gliedmaßen und weisen fibrilläre Muskelzuckungen, vorzugsweise in der Schultergegend, auf. Wiederkauen und Pansenmotorik sind vermindert. Bei Patientinnen mit Retentio placentae stellt man mitunter einen stark verminderten Tonus der Gebärmutterwand und nur geringe Haftung der Nachgeburt fest; solche Befunde ergeben deutliche Hinweise auf das Vorliegen einer Hypokalzämie, auch wenn noch keine äußerlichen klinischen Symptome wahrnehmbar sind. Zu Beginn des zweiten Stadiums ist das Stehvermögen meist noch erhalten. Die Kranken weisen jedoch bereits einen schläfrigen Gesichtsausdruck auf, sind in ihrem Verhalten träge, stehen ungern und ungelenk auf und sperren sich trotz Nachhandschwäche gegen das Abliegen. Später liegen sie mit schlaffer Lähmung der Muskulatur in Sternallage fest und machen auch nach Anrufen und Antreiben keine Versuche aufzustehen (puerperales Festliegen, Gebärparese, Gebärlähmung). Die Somnolenz nimmt zu, der Kopf wird auf der Krippe oder auf der Seitenbrust aufgestützt (Abb. 12-32, 12-33). Bei der klinischen Untersuchung stellt man normale oder leicht erniedrigte Körpertemperatur und eine normale oder leicht erhöhte Herzschlagfrequenz fest. Der Herzschlag ist, bei meist noch normalem Herzrhythmus, oft pochend. Die Pansentätigkeit ist deutlich vermindert. Meist wird weder Kot noch Harn abgesetzt. Die Hautsensibilität im Bereich von Kreuz und Nachhand ist nicht selten schon in dieser Phase herabgesetzt. Im dritten Stadium (Milchfieber, Kalbefieber, Gebärkoma) nimmt die allgemeine Paralyse noch zu. Solche Tiere liegen schnarchend oder röchelnd (Lähmung des Gaumensegels) mit m. o. w. stark aufgetriebenem Abdomen (beeinträchtigter Ruktus) in Seitenlage und reagieren nicht mehr auf äußere Reize. Ihre Körperoberfläche ist nicht nur an den Akren, sondern meist auch am Rumpf kühl; auch die Rektaltemperatur ist erniedrigt. Die Herzschlagfrequenz ist erhöht, manchmal in Verbindung mit Arrhythmie und Stauung der Jugularvenen. Die Atmung ist oberflächlich und sehr oft unregelmäßig. Lid- und Kornealreflex sowie die Hautsensibilität sind stark herabgesetzt.

Laborbefunde: Neben der Hypokalzämie ist bei festliegenden Kühen i. d. R. ein deutlich erniedrigter Serumgehalt an anorganisch gebundenem Phosphor und eine leichtgradige Hypermagnesiämie feststellbar. Bei Verfütterung von rasch gewachsenem Grünfutter kann Hypokalzämische Gebärlähmung allerdings auch mit deutlicher Hypomagnesiämie einhergehen. Der normale Bereich des Kalziums im Serum liegt zwischen 2,1 und 2,7 mmol/l. Unmittelbar nach dem Kalben fällt aus den eingangs erwähnten Gründen die Kalziumkonzentration im Serum auf subnormale Werte ab. Es besteht keine sehr enge Korrelation zwischen dem Grad der Hypokalzämie und dem Symptom des Festliegens: Die meisten Kühe mit Serum-Ca-Konzentrationen von 1,25 mmol/l und darunter liegen fest. Das Stehvermögen kann aber schon bei einem Serum-Ca-Gehalt von 1,75 mmol/l verlorengehen. Im Stadium III mißt man manchmal Konzentrationen von 0,5 mmol/l. Bei den hier aufgeführten Werten handelt es sich um das gesamte im Serum gemessene, d. h. das freie und das an Protein und andere organische Komplexe gebundene Kalzium. Für die Funktion der Muskel- und Nervenzellen ist nur das freie, ionisierte Kalzium von Bedeutung. Zwischen der Konzentration des freien Kalziums und den klinischen Erscheinungen sind denn auch die Beziehungen etwas deutlicher. Die Bestimmung des ionisierten Kalziums ist jedoch an spezielle Apparaturen gebunden, weshalb für die Routinediagnostik i. d. R. das Gesamtkalzium im Serum gemessen wird. Es besteht eine enge und gut gesicherte, lineare Korrelation zwischen Gesamtkalzium und freiem Kalzium. Da aber das Verhältnis zwischen freiem und gesamtem Kalzium neben anderen Faktoren v. a. auch durch den Proteingehalt und den pH des Serums bestimmt wird, leuchtet es ein, daß in einzelnen Fällen die klinischen Erscheinungen schlecht mit dem gemessenen Gehalt des totalen Kalziums übereinstimmen. Die leichtgradige Hypermagnesiämie und die Hypophosphatämie sind durch den sich infolge der Hypokalzämie einstellenden Hyperparathyreoidismus zu erklären, der eine verminderte Ausscheidung von Magnesium und eine vermehrte Elimination von Phosphat über die Niere bewirkt. Nach Behandlung mittels Kalziuminfusion steigt deshalb der Phosphatgehalt im Serum wieder auf normale Werte an, ohne daß Phosphor substituiert wird. Die bei der Hypokalzämischen Gebärlähmung i. d. R. nachweisbare Hyperglykämie läßt sich dadurch erklären, daß durch die Hypokalzämie die Ausschüttung von Insulin gehemmt wird; zudem besteht, z. T. wegen Hyperkortisolämie, auch eine Insulinresistenz. Aus dem gleichen Grund und wegen der Aktivierung des sympathischen Nervensystems wird auch vermehrt Depotfett mobilisiert; als Komplikation der Hypokalzämie kann deshalb eine Leberverfettung (Kap. 6.13.3, 6.13.14) entstehen.

Je nach Ausmaß der durch das Festliegen entstandenen Muskelschäden und somit auch nach der Dauer des Festliegens kommt es zu leicht- bis mittelgradigen Aktivitätserhöhungen bestimmter Enzyme, nämlich der für Muskulatur spezifischen Kreatinkinase (CK) und der auch im Muskel reichlich vorhandenen Aspartat-Amino-Transferase (AST). Bei durch Muskeltraumen bedingtem Festliegen dagegen sind die Aktivitäten dieser Enzyme in viel größerem Maße erhöht, so daß sich mit der Bestimmung der Aktivität muskelspezifischer Enzyme die beiden ursächlich unterschiedlichen Formen des Festliegens unterscheiden lassen. Bei hämatologischer Untersuchung sind keine spezifischen Veränderungen zu erwarten: Das vorangegangene Abkalben und die Erkrankung selbst wirken als Streß und führen zu Neutrophilie, Lympho- und Eosinopenie. Die Beeinträchtigung der Wasseraufnahme hat nicht selten Hämokonzentration zur Folge.

Komplikationen: Die in Zusammenhang mit der Hypokalzämischen Gebärlähmung eintretende Unbeholfenheit beim Niederlegen und Aufstehen kann Verletzungen infolge Ausrutschens oder Sturzes zur Folge haben: Quetschungen und offene Verletzungen der Zitzen, Exkoriationen am Fesselkopf der Hinterbeine, Zerrung oder Zerreißung von Muskeln (Mm. adductores, M. gastrocnemius), Gelenkluxation (Hüfte, Knie) oder Frakturen (Hüfthöcker, Beckenring, Oberschenkel). Umgekehrt läßt das Vorliegen solcher Läsionen bei Kühen nach komplikationslos verlaufenem Abkalben auf vorangegangene und möglicherweise übersehene Gebärparese schließen. Diagnose, Prognose und Therapie dieser Komplikationen werden bei den Krankheiten des Bewegungsapparates besprochen. Bei länger auf harter Unterlage festliegenden Kühen können zudem Druckschädigungen eintreten, die sich als Hautnekrosen (»Liegestellen« an Fesselkopf, seitlich an Tarsus, Knie oder Trochanter femoris), Phlegmonen, als druckischämiebedingte Degeneration und Nekrose der Gliedmaßenmuskulatur (kompartementale Quetschung) oder als Nervenlähmung (N. radialis, fibularis, tibialis) äußern. Eine weitere Gefahr stellt die auf Regurgitation von Panseninhalt oder erzwungener oraler Verabreichung von Medikamenten an eine komatöse Patientin beruhende Aspirationspneumonie dar, die i. d. R. tödlich endet.

Sektion: Bei der Zerlegung von infolge Gebärparese verendeten oder notgeschlachteten Kühen sind keine kennzeichnenden Veränderungen festzustellen. Nach unkompliziertem Verlauf erscheinen lediglich die Unterhautvenen stark blutgefüllt und die Gebärmutter schlecht zurückgebildet, aber ohne abnormen Inhalt. Nach längerdauernder Erkrankung können die Lunge ödem- und emphysemhaltig, Leber und Herzmuskel degeneriert sein. Die oben erwähnten Komplikationen führen zu deutlichen pathologisch-anatomischen Veränderungen: von interstitiellem Emphysem begleitete Bronchopneumonie infolge Verschluckens, subkutane und intramuskuläre Blutungen, fibrilläre Muskelzerreißung, Myonekrosen, Gelenkverletzungen oder Knochenfraktur; in forensischen Fällen kann der Bestimmung des Alters solcher Läsionen Bedeutung zukommen. Bei Zerlegung von Kühen, welche klinisch typische Erscheinungen von Nervenlähmungen zeigten, läßt sich leider die Lokalisation der Nervenschädigung nur in den seltensten Fällen feststellen.

■ **Diagnose:** Anhand der klinischen Befunde, des zeitlichen Auftretens der Erkrankung nach dem Abkalben, dem aus dem Vorbericht bekannten Geburtsverlauf und dem Alter des Tieres läßt sich die klinische Diagnose mit hoher Wahrscheinlichkeit stellen. Das in vielen Fällen gute Ansprechen auf die Infusionstherapie mit Kalzium dient nachträglich als Bestätigung der Diagnose. Da aber diese Therapie, v. a. bei nicht durch Hypokalzämie bedingtem Festliegen, mit erheblichen Risiken verbunden ist, muß in jedem Fall eine gründliche klinische Untersuchung durchgeführt werden (s. *Differentialdiagnose*). Auf eine Bestimmung des Gehalts an Kalzium und anderen Elektrolyten im Serum kann man i. d. R. verzichten. Eine Untersuchung im Labor fällt außer Betracht, weil bis zum Vorliegen des Resultats zu viel Zeit verlorenginge. Für ausgewählte Fälle, insbesondere bei Krankheitsbildern, bei denen die Kalziuminfusion als besonders riskant eingestuft wird und auch bei Nichtansprechen oder Rezidiven nach mehrmaligen Kalziumgaben, steht ein im Stall durchführbarer, semiquantitativer Schnelltest zur Bestimmung der Kalziumkonzentration im Vollblut zur Verfügung (Calcium-Test-Graeub®). Dabei macht man sich zunutze, daß Kalziumionen auch für die Blutgerinnung essentiell sind.

■ **Differentialdiagnose:** Viele andere Ursachen können im frühen Puerperium zum Festliegen führen. Zudem ist zu berücksichtigen, daß gleichzeitig bestehende andere Leiden das klinische Bild wesentlich beeinflussen können. Grundsätzlich muß die Hypokalzämische Gebärlähmung gegenüber anderen metabolischen Störungen, wie Hypomagnesiämie (Kap. 10.5.4), primäre Hypophosphatämie (Kap. 9.17.4) und Lipomobilisationssyndrom (Kap. 6.13.14), abgegrenzt werden. Neben Hypokalzämie können aber traumatische Beschädigungen des Beckengürtels und der Hintergliedmaßen infolge Schwergeburt Ursache für puerperales Festliegen sein. In Frage kommen Luxation des Kreuz-Darmbeingelenks (Kap. 9.4.1), des Hüftgelenks (Kap. 9.4.12), Frakturen an Becken (Kap. 9.4.2) oder Femur (Kap. 9.5.1), Zerrungen des Gastroknemiusmuskels (Kap. 9.5.6) oder der Adduktoren (Kap. 9.5.5) sowie zentrale und periphere Nervenlähmungen (Kap. 10.2.10, 9.5.8 bis 9.5.12). Wie bereits erwähnt, können solche Traumen auch erst als Komplikationen einer Hypokalzämie entstehen. Des weiteren kann eine schwergeburtsbedingte Erschöpfung oder ein Schockzustand infolge großen Blutverlusts (Kap. 4.3.2.1), einer Quetschung oder Ruptur des Dünndarms (Kap. 6.10.10) oder der ableitenden Harnwege (Kap. 7.2.2.4, 7.2.2.5) Ursache des Festliegens sein. Auch Beschädigungen des weichen Geburtswegs, Retentio placentae und verzögerte Involution der Gebärmutter können wegen der damit verbundenen Entzündungen, schweren Infektionen und Schmerzen zum Festliegen führen, besonders, wenn sich daraus, meist endotoxinbedingt, ein Schock entwickelt. Des weiteren sollte man darauf achten, ob eine Toxämie allenfalls durch eine – zu diesem Zeitpunkt nicht selten auftretende – akute Mastitis (»Mastitis paralytica«) bedingt ist. Bei Fütterung von jungem, rasch gewachsenem Gras geht die puerperale Gebärlähmung häufig mit Hypomagnesiämie einher. Das klinische Bild entspricht dabei weitgehend dem oben beschriebenen, wobei allerdings zeitweilig tetanische Erscheinungen und Übererregbarkeit beobachtet werden können. Die durch Phosphormangel bedingte puerperale Hämoglobinurie (Kap. 4.3.5.5) kommt äußerst selten vor und tritt meist erst 1–4 Wochen nach der Kalbung auf. Auch Störungen des Energiestoffwechsels, wie Ketose und Lipomobilisationssyndrom (Kap. 6.13.14), welche bei starker Ausprägung mit Festliegen einhergehen können, treten i. d. R. nicht unmittelbar nach dem Partus auf.

Gegenüber zum Festliegen führenden Verletzungen, welche als direkte Folgen des Abkalbens auftreten, läßt sich die Hypokalzämische Gebärlähmung meist bereits anhand der Beschreibung des Geburtsverlaufs und des zeitlichen Auftretens abgrenzen. Bei Festliegen infolge Schwergeburt stehen die Kühe i. d. R. schon unmittelbar nach dem Kalben nicht mehr auf. Außer beim Vorliegen von sehr schmerzhaften Zuständen sind zudem bei traumatisch bedingtem Festliegen Appetit und Sensorium der Tiere wenig beeinträchtigt. Es gilt allerdings zu bedenken, daß das hypokalzämische Festliegen schon während oder vor dem Partus auftreten kann, und daß andererseits eine Hypokalzämie, z. B. bei Aufstehversuchen, Ursache für zum Festliegen führende Traumata sein kann.

Bei allen puerperalen Erkrankungen mit durch bakterielle Toxämie bedingtem Festliegen kann zwar das Sensorium ebenfalls erheblich gestört sein; solche Zustände gehen aber mit Fieber einher. Schwerere

Schockzustände infolge Toxämie oder großen Blutverlusten lassen sich jedoch von der komatösen Form der Hypokalzämie klinisch nicht in jedem Fall eindeutig unterscheiden.

■ **Prognose:** Unkomplizierte Fälle von Hypokalzämischer Gebärparese sprechen i. d. R. auf die Infusionsbehandlung gut an. Die Patienten erheben sich dann innerhalb einer halben bis 12 h nach ihrer Behandlung. Allerdings ist die Häufigkeit von Rezidiven mit 25–30% relativ hoch. Untersuchungen an Kühen, welche nach einer Kalziuminfusion erneut festlagen, haben ergeben, daß bei solchen Tieren die Hydroxylierung von $25(OH_2)D_3$ in der Niere trotz hohen PTH-Spiegels nur mit einer Verzögerung von 24–48 h wirksam wurde. Wie bereits erwähnt, wird hierfür eine metabolische Alkalose verantwortlich gemacht. Im Durchschnitt ist damit zu rechen, daß 5–10% der erkrankten Kühe auf die Behandlung nicht ansprechen oder wegen meist traumatisch bedingter und weiter vorn beschriebener Sekundärleiden sterben oder getötet werden müssen.

Vereinzelt trifft man festliegende Kühe an, bei denen nach mehrmaliger Behandlung mit Kalziuminfusionen der Kalziumgehalt im Serum auf normale Werte ansteigt, jedoch eine Hypophosphatämie persistiert. Solche Fälle lassen sich mit Infusionen von organischen Phosphorlösungen erfolgreich behandeln. Ein besonderes Problem stellen Kühe dar, welche sich trotz Normalisierung des Kalzium- und Phosphorgehalts im Serum nach mehrtägigem Festliegen nicht mehr erheben können. Nach Korrektur der Hypokalzämie verbessert sich ihr Allgemeinzustand zwar vorübergehend; nach einigen Tagen verschlechtern sich Appetit und Allgemeinbefinden aber erneut. Außer einer leicht- bis mittelgradigen Aktivitätserhöhung von leber- und muskelspezifischen Enzymen, welche jedoch das Festliegen nicht erklären, findet man bei der klinisch chemischen Untersuchung des Serums keine signifikanten Veränderungen. Im angelsächsischen Schrifttum wird dieses prognostisch ungünstige Leiden als »downer cow syndrome« bezeichnet. Bei der Sektion solcher Tiere ist in den meisten Fällen die Ursache des Festliegens nicht feststellbar (s. auch hypokaliämiebedingtes Festliegen, Kap. 9.17.3).

■ **Behandlung:** Neben der ätiotropen Therapie, welche die Wiederherstellung des normalen Kalziumhaushalts zum Ziel hat, kommt den unterstützenden Pflege- und Kontrollmaßnahmen zur Verhütung von Komplikationen große Bedeutung zu:

➤ *Ätiotrope Maßnahmen*: Für die Infusionstherapie kommen Kalziumlösungen, vorzugsweise in Form organischer Verbindungen, wie z. B. Kalziumboroglukonat in 20- bis 35%iger Lösung zur Anwendung. Die Richtdosis beträgt 15–20 mg Kalzium/kg LM, was bei Kühen von durchschnittlichem Körpergewicht mit 500 ml einer 20%igen Kalziumglukonatlösung erreicht wird. Dies entspricht einer Dosis von 9 g Kalzium pro Kuh. Höhere Dosierungen bewirken keinen besseren therapeutischen Effekt und sind wegen des erhöhten Risikos toxischer Nebenwirkungen nicht empfehlenswert. Auch bei normaler Dosierung ist das Risiko von Störwirkungen am Herzen nicht vollständig auszuschließen. Zur Vermeidung von kurzfristig sehr hohen Serumkonzentrationen soll eine Infusionszeit von 6 min nicht unterschritten werden. Damit die Infusion beim Erreichen toxischer Konzentrationen sofort abgebrochen werden kann, muß die Herztätigkeit während der Infusion mit dem Phonendoskop überwacht werden. Normalerweise bewirkt die Kalziuminfusion als Folge einer Hemmung der Reizleitung im Herzen und eines erhöhten Vagotonus Bradykardie. Im weiteren Verlauf der Infusion nimmt die Herzschlagfolge dann wieder zu; als Zeichen einer Überdosierung ist zu werten, wenn ihre Frequenz dabei über Normalwerte hinaus ansteigt. Das gleiche gilt für im weiteren Verlauf der Infusion auftretende Herzrhythmusstörungen in Form von Extrasystolen.

Auch nach der Infusion hält die massive Hyperkalzämie an; perakute Störwirkungen können noch 30 min nach der Infusion auftreten. Es besteht keine Möglichkeit, solche Störwirkungen mit herzwirksamen Medikamenten zu behandeln oder zu verhindern. Bei Infusion von Kalziumchloridlösungen liegt das Kalzium in vollständig ionisierter Form vor; Störwirkungen am Herzen sind deshalb rascher zu erwarten als nach Infusion von Lösungen, in welchen das Kalzium an einen organischen Komplex gebunden ist. Unabhängig von der in der Infusionslösung enthaltenen Kalziumverbindung stellt sich nach relativ kurzer Zeit im Serum ein Gleichgewicht zwischen ionisiertem und gebundenem Kalzium ein; die beiden Behandlungsarten unterscheiden sich somit bezüglich des Risikos von Störwirkungen nicht grundsätzlich voneinander. Bei langsamer Infusion von Kalziumchloridlösungen ist die Behandlung dagegen besser steuerbar. Während der Infusion von Lösungen, welche komplex gebundenes Kalzium enthalten, werden weniger leicht schädlich wirkende Konzentrationen von Kalziumionen erreicht; die Gefahr, daß Störwirkungen noch nach Beendigung der Infusion auftreten, ist jedoch größer.

Kalziumlösungen wirken stark gewebereizend, Kalziumchlorid enthaltende Lösungen ausgeprägter als solche mit organischen Kalziumverbindungen. In jedem Fall ist aber eine einwandfreie Infusionstechnik zu befolgen. Um Abwehrbewegungen vorzubeugen, sollen auch komatöse Tiere vor der Infusion gut fixiert werden, da sie schon unter der Behandlung erwachen können. Sobald der Verdacht besteht, daß die

Infusion nicht mehr streng intravenös erfolgt, muß sie sofort abgebrochen und nach Punktion einer anderen Vene fortgeführt werden. Wegen der besseren lokalen Verträglichkeit können gewisse organische Kalziumlösungen auch subkutan, in Depots bis zu 80 ml injiziert werden. Die alleinige subkutane Verabreichung von Kalzium reicht aber zur wirksamen Erhöhung des Kalziumspiegels im Blut nicht aus; hingegen kann der Rest der Infusionslösung allenfalls subkutan appliziert werden, wenn die Infusion wegen auftretender Rhythmusstörungen abgebrochen werden muß.

Die Kalziuminfusion bewirkt bei somnolenten oder komatösen Tieren i. d. R. eine rasche Verbesserung des Bewußtseins, teilweise wegen der kardiogen bedingten Blutdrucksteigerung, aber auch wegen des erhöhten Vagotonus, der zudem am sich vermehrenden Speichelfluß zu erkennen ist. Aus dem gleichen Grund, aber auch als Folge der direkten Wirkung des Kalziums auf die glatte Muskulatur, setzen die behandelten Tiere Kot und Harn ab. Manchmal ist außerdem Muskelzittern zu beobachten. Vorher in Seitenlage verharrende Tiere lassen sich i. d. R. kurz nach der Infusion leicht in Sternallage verbringen. Behandelte Tiere weisen wieder einen normalen Muskeltonus auf und machen nicht selten schon kurz nach der Behandlung Aufstehversuche (Abb. 12-34). Wegen der oben erwähnten Gefahr von selbst noch nach Abschluß der Infusion einsetzenden perakuten Störwirkungen am Herzen sollte man die Kühe nicht unmittelbar nach der Behandlung zum Aufstehen antreiben. Hingegen ist es sinnvoll, sie umzulagern, da durch das lange Liegen auf einer Seite zusätzlich zur metabolisch bedingten Lähmung auch noch (reversible) Nerven- und Muskelschäden vorliegen können. Aus dem gleichen Grund verhalten sich die Tiere bei ihren ersten Aufstehversuchen nicht selten ungeschickt. Um ein Vergrätschen (Zerrung der Adduktorenmuskeln) zu vermeiden, müssen den festliegenden Tieren die Gliedmaßen oberhalb des Fesselkopfes mit einem Abstand von 30 cm gefesselt werden.

Eine Alternative zur Therapie mittels Kalziuminfusion stellt die *Euterinsufflation* dar (Abb. 12-35). Die Beliebtheit dieser schon vor Einführung der Infusionsbehandlung praktizierten Methode zur Behandlung des hypokalzämiebedingten Festliegens hat in den letzten Jahrzehnten wieder zugenommen, seit ihr Einfluß auf den Gehalt des Kalziums im Serum nachgewiesen werden konnte. Nach gründlicher Desinfektion der Zitzenkuppe führt man einen sterilen Melkkatheter in eine der Zitzen ein und pumpt mit einem zuvor sterilisierten Gebläse, welchem ein Filter zwischengeschaltet ist, Luft in das betreffende Euterviertel, bis eine deutliche Vergrößerung desselben sichtbar wird. Nacheinander werden so alle vier Euterviertel insuffliert. An Stelle des Handgebläses kann auch Druckluft aus einer Flasche mit Reduzierventil eingebracht werden. Zur Verhinderung von Austritt der eingepumpten Luft aus der Zitzenzisterne kann diese durch Anbringen eines zirkulären Heftpflasters verschlossen werden. Zwei Stunden danach muß dieses jedoch wieder entfernt werden, damit keine Zirkulationsstörungen in der Zitzenwand auftreten. Da eine schon bestehende Mastitis durch die Luftinsufflation verschlimmert werden könnte, darf die Behandlung nur an gesunden Eutervierteln vorgenommen werden. Vor der Insufflation muß das Sekret jedes einzelnen Viertels beurteilt werden, was wegen der großen normalen Variabilität der grobsinnlichen Beschaffenheit des Kolostrums und seiner Reaktion im SCHALM-Test nicht immer einfach ist. Der Vorteil der Euterinsufflation gegenüber der Kalziuminfusion liegt darin, daß der Kalziumspiegel im Serum innerhalb von 4 h und nachhaltig auf den Normalwert ansteigt. Weil mit dieser Methode die Entstehung einer vorübergehenden massiven Hyperkalzämie vermieden werden kann, wird die Funktion der Nebenschilddrüse nicht beeinträchtigt; aus diesem Grund kommt es nach Euterinsufflation viel seltener zu Rezidiven als nach der Infusionsbehandlung. Da für jede Insufflation ein sterilisiertes Gerät zur Verfügung stehen muß, wird sich die Anwendung dieser Methode auf Einzelfälle beschränken. Auch die Befürchtung von unsachgemäßer Nachahmung dieser Behandlungsmethode durch Laien schreckt Tierärztinnen und Tierärzte etwas von der Anwendung der Euterinsufflation ab. Für Behandlung von Kühen, welche nach ein- oder mehrmaliger Infusionstherapie erneut festliegen, aber auch für solche, bei denen eine Infusionsbehandlung wegen Störwirkungen am Herzen zu riskant erscheint, ist die Euterinsufflation nach wie vor sehr empfehlenswert.

Falls neben der Hypokalzämie keine anderen Leiden vorliegen, erübrigt sich in dieser Phase jede zusätzliche parenterale Behandlung. Hingegen ist es sinnvoll, die Kuh ergänzend peroral mit Kalziumchlorid in Form von Gel oder dickflüssiger Suspension zu versorgen, sobald dies ohne Verschluckgefahr möglich ist. Damit unterstützt man die Kuh bei der Selbstregulation ihres Kalziumstoffwechsels nach Abklingen der Wirkung der Infusionsbehandlung. Die normalerweise bei der Hypokalzämischen Gebärparese zu beobachtende Hypophosphatämie ist Folge der Stimulierung der Parathyreoidea und verschwindet nach der Kalziuminfusion spontan. Eine zusätzliche Behandlung mit phosphathaltigen Lösungen erübrigt sich deshalb. Wie schon weiter vorn erwähnt, kann bei Verfütterung von rasch gewachsenem Grünfutter gleichzeitig mit der puerperalen Hypokalzämie eine Hypomagnesiämie vorliegen. Die Infusion einer Lösung, welche therapeutische Dosen von Kalzium und Magnesium enthält, ist deshalb unter solchen Bedingungen einer reinen Kalziumlösung vorzuziehen.

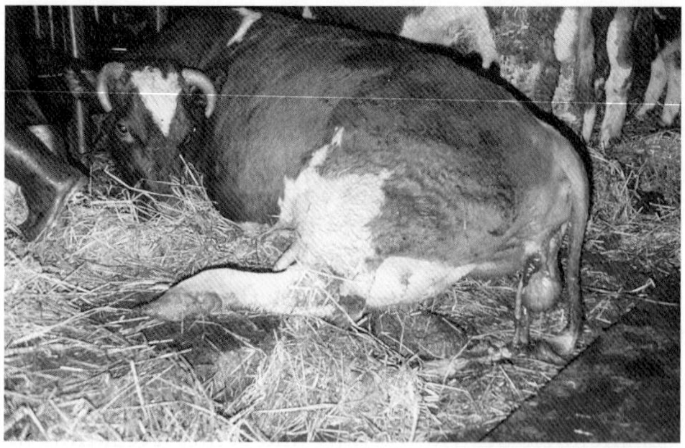

Abbildung 12-32 Hypokalzämische Gebärparese (im Stall): Apathie, Brustseitenlage, autauskultatorische Haltung, Kopf aufgestützt

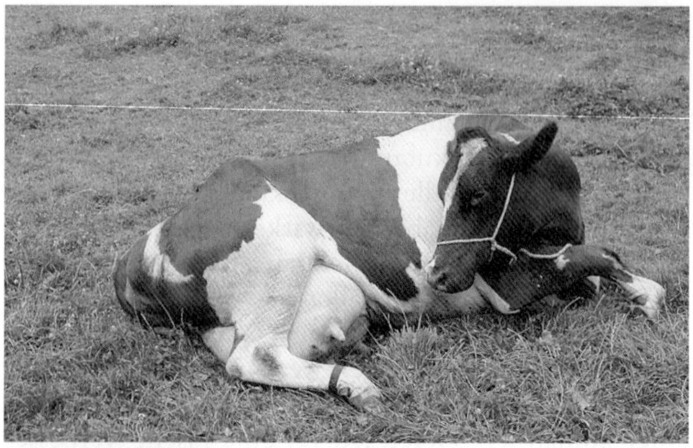

Abbildung 12-33 Hypokalzämische Gebärparese (auf der Weide): Anteilnahme an der Umgebung erloschen, keine Fliegenabwehr, »Milchfieberhaltung«

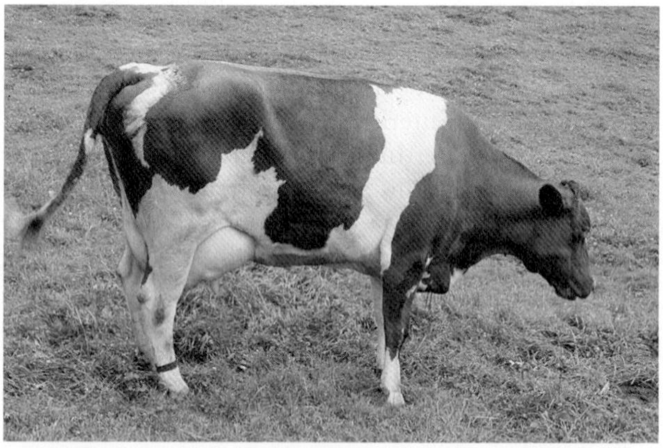

Abbildung 12-34 Hypokalzämische Gebärparese: Nach i.v. Kalziumsalzinfusion ist das Tier von Abb. 12-33 aufgestanden

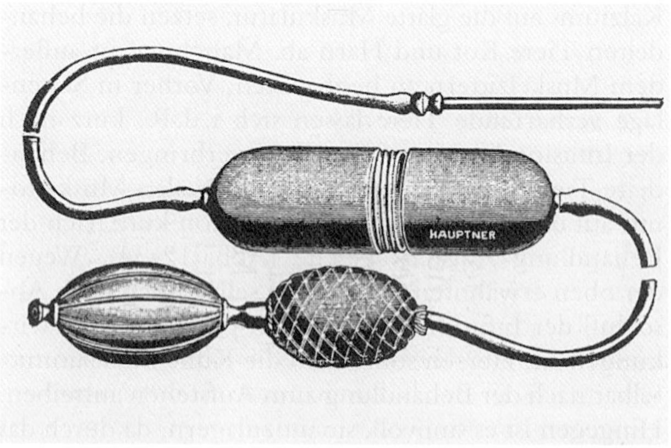

Abbildung 12-35 Filterpumpe nach EVERS zur Luftinsufflation des Euters

➤ *Unterstützende Pflege- und Kontrollmaßnahmen:* Der Betreuung der festliegenden Kuh kommt für den Erfolg der Therapie entscheidende Bedeutung zu. Bereits erwähnt wurde das Umlagern, welches innerhalb 24 h mindestens viermal vorgenommen werden muß. Wichtig ist dabei, daß die Kuh auf trockenem Strohbett liegt. Darunter bedarf es einer rutschfesten Unterlage, welche ihr das Aufstehen erleichtert; auch ist darauf zu achten, daß sie im Kopfbereich genügend Bewegungsfreiheit zum Aufstehen hat. Wie erwähnt, sollen die Hintergliedmaßen bei Aufstehversuchen oberhalb der Fesselgelenke in einem Abstand von ungefähr 30 cm gefesselt werden. Ob man dazu spezielle Gurte oder einfache Seilschlingen verwendet, ist unwesentlich, solange darauf geachtet wird, daß keine Hautverletzungen durch Friktionsbewegungen entstehen können (s. Kap. 9.9.7).

Bei Kühen, welche trotz mehrerer Behandlungen liegenbleiben, sollten andere Ursachen für das Festliegen erwogen werden. Vorausgesetzt, daß anhand einer Bestimmung des Kalziumgehalts im Serum zu diesem Zeitpunkt eine schwere Hypokalzämie ausgeschlossen werden kann oder anhand der klinischen Befunde als wenig wahrscheinlich erscheint, empfiehlt es sich, solche Tiere mit mechanischen Mitteln behutsam aufzuziehen. Diese Maßnahme dient v. a. auch diagnostischen Zwecken und erlaubt es, eine besser fundierte Prognose zu stellen, als dies bei der Beurteilung am liegenden Tier möglich ist. Das Aufziehen mittels Hüftklammer und Flaschenzug bedingt jedoch gewisse Verletzungsgefahren (subkutane Blutungen, Muskelabrisse). Besser eignet sich der »Kuhlift«, ein Gerüst mit Winden, welches über der Patientin zusammengesetzt wird; mit unter Brust und Abdomen durchgezogenen Gurten wird die Kuh vorsichtig in eine stehende Position verbracht. Noch schonender, aber wesentlich aufwendiger, ist das Heben der Kuh mittels faltbarer Wanne oder in einem Tank, die bzw. den man dann mit Wasser auffüllt (Kap. 9.9.7). Welche Methode auch immer zur Anwendung kommt: Falls die Patientin keine Anstrengungen macht aufzustehen, sollte der Versuch abgebrochen werden.

Der festliegenden Kuh soll gut strukturiertes, den Appetit anregendes, die Vormagentätigkeit stimulierendes, gehaltvolles Futter angeboten werden; auch ist zu bedenken, daß sie oft das Becken der Selbsttränke nicht erreichen kann, weshalb ihr mehrmals täglich Wasser aus dem Eimer angeboten werden muß.

■ **Prophylaxe:** Bei den vorbeugenden Maßnahmen ist zwischen den für das Einzeltier bestimmten medikamentösen Behandlungen und der Anpassung der Fütterung der trockenstehenden Kühe zu unterscheiden. Letztere wirkt erst nach einer längeren Latenz, hat aber den Vorteil, daß sie sich für alle gefährdeten Kühe positiv auswirkt; sie ist deshalb v. a. bei gehäuftem Auftreten von Hypokalzämischer Gebärlähmung in einem Bestand in Erwägung zu ziehen:

➤ *Medikamentöse Methoden:* Verabreichung von 10×10^6 IE Vitamin D_3 durch intramuskuläre Injektion 2–5 Tage vor dem erwarteten Kalbetermin. Durch diese Behandlung kann die Resorption von Kalzium aus dem Darm und aus dem Knochen wirksam erhöht werden. Die Wirkung kommt jedoch nicht zustande, wenn das Tier schon vor oder erst nach Erreichen der wirksamen Gewebespiegel abkalbt. Bekanntlich ist die genaue Vorhersage des Gebärtermins aber nicht immer möglich. Von einer Wiederholung der Behandlung, z. B. wenn die Kuh später als erwartet abkalbt, muß abgeraten werden, da dann Gefahr besteht, daß die Kuh infolge Hypervitaminose D_3 an Kalzinose (Kap. 4.2.5.1) erkrankt. 25-Hydroxy-Vitamin-D_3 oder auch Dihydroxy-Verbindungen des Kalziferols haben sich für die Verhinderung der Hypokalzämischen Gebärlähmung als noch wirksamer erwiesen als hohe Dosen von Vitamin D_3, besonders weil auch die Zeitspanne der Wirkung ausgedehnt werden kann. Teilweise wurde aber auch beobachtet, daß bei auf diese Weise behandelten Kühen das Festliegen erst eine Woche nach dem Partus auftritt. In Deutschland, Österreich und der Schweiz sind solche Metaboliten des Vitamins D_3 für das Rind z. Zt. nicht registriert.

Eine weitere medikamentöse Vorbeuge besteht in der peroralen Verabreichung von 4 Einzelgaben Kalziumchlorid oder -propionat (als Gel, dickflüssige Emulsion oder Bolus), die jeweils ~ 50 g Kalzium enthalten. Die erste Dosis wird dem Tier am Tag vor dem erwarteten Abkalben, die zweite zum Zeitpunkt des Partus, die nächsten beiden ein und zwei Tage danach eingegeben. Mit dieser Behandlung kann der Plasmagehalt des Kalziums in der kritischen Phase erhöht und die Häufigkeit des hypokalzämischem Festliegens bei gefährdeten Tieren signifikant vermindert werden. Die Darreichungsform als Gel oder dickflüssige Emulsion wird gewählt, um dem Verschlucken bei der Eingabe an bereits hypokalzämische Tiere vorzubeugen.

➤ *Anpassung der Fütterung:* Die Empfehlungen zur Hypokalzämie-Prophylaxe durch Änderung der Ration in den letzten Wochen a. p. haben zum Ziel, die Kuh auf den Beginn der Laktation so vorzubereiten, daß die Kalziumhomöostase optimal funktioniert. Wie bereits erwähnt, sprechen die Endorgane der Kühe, welche an Festliegen erkranken, ungenügend auf die an sich funktionierenden Mechanismen zur Hebung des Kalziumspiegels an. Bei knapper Kalziumversorgung in der Trockenzeit wird die aktive Resorption aus dem Darm und die Freisetzung von Kalzium aus dem Knochen gefördert. Damit ein solcher Effekt zum Tragen käme, dürften den Kühen nicht mehr als 20 g Kalzium pro Tier und Tag angeboten werden. Mit den üblicherweise zur Verfügung stehenden Futtermitteln ist es jedoch nicht möglich, den Kalziumgehalt der in der Trockenzeit verabreichten Ration so tief zu halten, daß der Gebärparese damit wirksam vorgebeugt werden kann.

Größere Bedeutung kommt der Regulierung des Kationen:Anionen-Verhältnisses der in der Trockenzeit verabreichten Ration zu (s. Kap. 4.3.6.2). Es sollte auf < 0 meq/kg TM reduziert werden. Am besten kann die Inzidenz von Milchfieber mit Rationen vermindert werden, deren Kationen:Anionen-Verhältnis zwischen –100 und –200 meq/kg TM liegt. Mit solchen Rationen bewirkt man eine leichtgradige metabolische Azidose. Bei alkalotischer Stoffwechsellage, die bei Fütterung von Rationen mit Kationenüberschuß vorliegt, sind die Nieren für die Hydroxylierung des 25-Hydroxycholekalziferols gegenüber dem Parathormon refraktär, wodurch die aktive Resorption von Kalzium aus dem Darm und dem Knochen beeinträchtigt wird. Es konnte auch gezeigt werden, daß den starken Kationen Natrium und Kalium größere Bedeutung zukommt als dem Kalzium. Das Kationen:Anionen-Verhältnis kann durch Zugabe von Chloriden, Sulfaten und Phosphaten erniedrigt werden. Die künstliche Ansäuerung der Ration ist nur begrenzt möglich, weil ihre Akzeptanz bei Zugabe von > 300 meq Anionen pro kg TM Futter vermindert wird. Eine Verminderung der Futteraufnahme in dieser kritischen Phase vor dem Abkalben muß jedoch unbedingt vermieden werden, weil sonst das Risiko von Leberverfettung und Ketose zunehmen würde. Voraussetzung für die Verhütung von Hypokalzämischer Gebärlähmung über die Fütterung ist demnach, daß der Gehalt der Ration an Kalium, Natrium, Kalzium, Magnesium, Phosphor, Chlor und Schwefel bestimmt wird. Der Gehalt des Rauhfutters an Kalium variiert stark, je nach botanischer Zusammensetzung und Düngung. Hoher Kationenüberschuß kommt fast immer durch einen zu hohen

Kaliumgehalt der Ration zustande. Da die Zugabe von Anionen zum Futter nur in begrenztem Maß möglich ist, muß bei einem Kationenüberschuß im Futter von > 200 meq/kg TM der Anteil an Kalium in der Ration durch Änderung ihrer Zusammensetzung reduziert werden. Eine weitere Reduktion läßt sich durch Weglassen von allfällig der Ration beigefügtem Kochsalz und Kalziumsalzen erzielen. Die täglich aufgenommene Menge Kalzium sollte 140 g nicht übersteigen. Obschon Phosphat zur Ansäuerung der Ration beiträgt, sollte die Kuh nicht mehr als 60 g anorganisch gebundenen Phosphor pro Tag aufnehmen, weil sonst die Bildung von 1,25-Dihydroxycholekalziferol beeinträchtigt wird. Falls die Reduktion der starken Kationen zur Senkung des Kationen:Anionen-Verhältnisses nicht ausreicht, kann die Ration mit Magnesium- oder Kalziumsulfat bis zu einem Schwefelgehalt von 0,45 % TM oder mit Ammoniumchlorid angesäuert werden.

➤ Eine weiterhin mögliche vorbeugende Maßnahme besteht darin, gefährdete Kühe in den ersten Tagen nach dem Abkalben *nicht vollständig auszumelken*. Hierzu entzieht man ihnen vorerst nur gerade so viel Kolostrum, wie für die Sättigung des Kalbes benötigt wird. Später entzieht man nur die Hälfte der produzierten Milch. Dadurch vermindert man ein übermäßiges Absinken des Kalziumgehalts im Plasma. Mit dieser Maßnahme allein läßt sich jedoch die Hypokalzämische Gebärlähmung meist nicht verhindern. Zudem nimmt das Mastitisrisiko zu, wenn Restmilch im Euter zurückbleibt.

12.3.2 Solaninvergiftung

M. Stöber

■ **Definition, Ursachen, Pathogenese:** Kraut, Blüten, Früchte, grüne Schalen sowie Keimtriebe der Kartoffel enthalten 0,2–1,0% FM des giftigen Glykoalkaloids *Solanin*; in reifen Kartoffelknollen beträgt sein Gehalt dagegen nur 0,002–0,01 % FM. Beim Erhitzen zerfällt Solanin in Zucker, *Solanidin* und *Solanein*; letztere gehen in das Kochwasser über, das deshalb als Tränke ungeeignet ist. Meist bedarf es größerer Mengen solaninhaltiger Abschnitte der Kartoffelpflanze (z. B. einmalige Aufnahme von ~ 5–15 kg oberirdischer Teile), um Intoxikationen beim Rind auszulösen. Solche akut verlaufenden Vergiftungen ereignen sich v. a. dann, wenn aus Unkenntnis oder Futtermangel grüne, keimende oder faulende Kartoffeln oder Kartoffelkraut verabreicht werden oder solches Kraut eingestreut wird. Bezüglich der auf langfristiger Aufnahme von reifen Überschußkartoffeln oder Abfällen kartoffelverarbeitender Betriebe beruhenden »Schlempemauke« wird auf Kapitel 2.2.5.1 verwiesen.

■ **Symptome, Verlauf:** Die Patienten erscheinen, mitunter erst nach kurzfristiger Erregung, freßunlustig und apathisch; ihre Milchleistung geht rasch zurück. Außerdem zeigen sie Speicheln, z. T. Nasenausfluß, entzündliche Rötung/Erosionen der Maulschleimhaut (ausnahmsweise auch Schmatzen) sowie rasch zunehmende Schwäche mit Zittern, Taumeln oder breitbeinigem Stehen, Tympanie und profusem, wäßrig-übelriechendem Durchfall (gelegentlich erst nach vorheriger Verstopfung). Herz- und Atemfrequenz nehmen deutlich zu. Nach kurzer Zeit liegen die Kranken unter ausgeprägter Benommenheit fest. Schwer betroffene Tiere verenden innerhalb von 1–3 Tagen, manchmal sogar schon im nervösen Stadium des Leidens, d. h. vor Einsetzen der Diarrhoe, infolge zentraler Lähmung von Kreislauf und Atmung.

■ **Diagnose:** Klinisches Bild und Fütterungsanamnese lenken den Verdacht auf Solaninvergiftung. *Differentialdiagnostisch* sind andere, mit allgemeiner Lähmung oder Durchfall verbundene Leiden, bei Beteiligung der Maulschleimhaut auch Maul- und Klauenseuche (Kap. 12.2.1) in Betracht zu ziehen.

■ **Behandlung:** Ernährung umstellen; salinische Abführmittel sowie Adsorbenzien p. o., erforderlichenfalls auch Analeptika parenteral.

■ **Prophylaxe:** Keine solaninhaltigen Bestandteile der Kartoffelpflanze verfüttern sowie Zugang zu solchen verhindern.

N. B.: Schwarzer Nachtschatten (*Solanum nigrum*, mitunter auf Rieselfeldern gehäuft auftretend), Bittersüß *(S. dulcamara)* sowie weitere Solanum-Arten enthalten ebenfalls Solanin und außerdem mydriatisch wirkende Tropanalkaloide (Kap. 10.5.28); auch in Tomatenpflanzen *(Lycopersicon esculentum)* befinden sich solaninartige Toxine. Das durch diese Pflanzen ausgelöste Vergiftungsbild ähnelt dem der akuten Kartoffelkrautintoxikation; dabei ist der starre Blick der Patienten (Pupillenerweiterung) auffällig; mitunter treten zudem auch Krämpfe und/oder Kehlkopfödem auf. Zur Verhütung solcher Unfälle sind die genannten Solanazeen zu meiden oder vor Nutzung der betreffenden Grünfläche restlos zu beseitigen.

12.3.3 Mutterkornvergiftung

E. Renner

■ **Definition:** Mutterkornvergiftung oder *Ergotismus* beruht auf Verzehr von Ähren, Körnern, Schrot/Kraftfutter, Silage oder Abfällen verschiedener Getreide, wie Roggen, Weizen, Hafer, Gerste, Hirse, oder bestimmter Gräser, wie australisches oder Wimmera-Weidelgras *(Lolium rigidum)*, deutsches Weidelgras (*Lolium perenne* = englisches Raygras), Knaulgras *(Dactylis glomerata)*, Honiggras *(Holcus lanatus)*, oder wilder Gräser, die mit Sklerotien von Claviceps spp. (*Cl. purpurea*, *Cl. africana* o. a.) befallen sind; ein solcher Befall kann durch voraufgegangene Überschwemmung begünstigt werden. Diese Mykotoxikose verläuft teils akut, als zentralnervöse Erkrankung *(Ergotismus nervosus)*, teils chronisch, als mumifizierende Nekrose der Haut der Körperendigungen *(E. cutaneus s. mumificans)* oder als idiopathische Hitzeintoleranz *(Hyperthermiesyndrom)*; mitunter führt sie auch zum Abort.

Vorkommen: Die genannten Erscheinungsformen der Mutterkornvergiftung sind weltweit verbreitet. Sie treten unter Witterungsbedingungen (feuchtwarme Vegetationsperiode) vermehrt auf, welche den Mutterkornbefall der erwähnten Substratpflanzen begünstigen; dabei werden u. U. auch gleicherweise exponierte Schweine mitbetroffen.

Ursachen: Die Sklerotien von *Cl. purpurea* sind braunschwarze, hörnchenartige derbe Gebilde von 1–3 cm Länge (Abb. 12-36). Sie enthalten mehrere Alkaloide *(Ergometrin, Ergonovin, Ergotamin, Ergotoxin)*, deren relative Konzentrationen vermutlich von Fall zu Fall schwanken und die Variabilität des Krankheitsbildes bestimmen.

Pathogenese: Mutterkornalkaloide bewirken zunehmende Verdickung von Tunica media und intima peripherer Arteriolen. Die dadurch bedingte Einengung des Lumens dieser Blutgefäße löst dann, je nach den Begleitumständen (Stärke des Sklerotienbefalls, Verfügbarkeit unverpilzten Futters, Lebensalter, Umwelttemperatur, etwaige Trächtigkeit), eines oder mehrere der o. a. Krankheitsbilder aus. Oral aufgenommene Ergotalkaloide werden über die Milch ausgeschieden, was bei damit getränkten Kälbern zu nervösen und/oder mumifizierenden Erscheinungen führen kann, ohne daß die betreffenden Mütter selbst erkranken. Bei erwachsenen Rindern sind dagegen 10 Tagesgaben von je 100 g Mutterkorn erforderlich, um Ergotismus hervorzurufen. Unter Feldbedingungen setzen die ersten Symptome frühestens 3 Tage, meist aber erst 2–3 Wochen nach Beginn der Verabreichung mykotoxinhaltiger Futtermittel ein.

Symptome: Die verschiedenen Erscheinungsformen der Mutterkornvergiftung können innerhalb eines Bestandes oder beim Einzeltier zugleich, nacheinander oder unabhängig voneinander auftreten, doch ist der *Verlauf* meist wie folgt: Im Anfangsstadium, das durch fieberhaft erhöhte Körpertemperatur (40,5–41,6 °C) und herabgesetzte Pansentätigkeit gekennzeichnet ist, stehen *nervöse Symptome* im Vordergrund, nämlich Freßunlust, Speicheln, Zittern, Muskelzucken, ataktischer Gang, Taumeln/Gleichgewichtsstörungen, Vorhandschwäche, Niederstürzen, Hochspringen, gegenseitiges Angreifen, später Bewegungsunlust. Herz- und Atemtätigkeit sind beschleunigt, die Schleimhäute blaß. Falls das mykotoxinhaltige Futter in dieser Phase abgesetzt wird, genesen die Kranken innerhalb von ~ 3 Wochen.

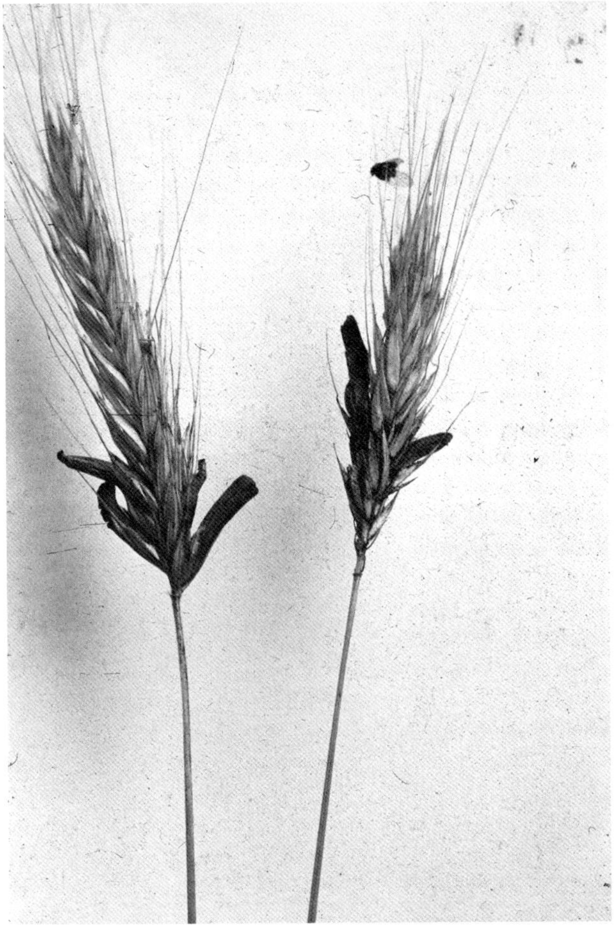

Abbildung 12-36 Mutterkornbefallener Roggen (Merkel, 1968; natürliche Größe)

Die weitere Entwicklung des Leidens ist schleichend und durch *allmähliches Absterben der Extremitätenenden* gekennzeichnet (Abb. 12-37 bis 12-39). Dabei kommt es v. a. distal an den Hintergliedmaßen, ein- oder beidseitig, gelegentlich zudem auch an den Vorderbeinen, zu umschriebenen und vom gesunden proximalen Bereich scharf abgesetzten nichtentzündlichen Anschwellungen, die zunächst deutlich schmerzhaft sind. Die hier mit verkrusteten Haaren bedeckte Haut geht nach zeitweiliger Exsudation in trockene Nekrose über und löst sich schließlich ab. In leichteren Fällen beschränken sich die auffallend kühl erscheinenden Hautveränderungen auf den Bereich

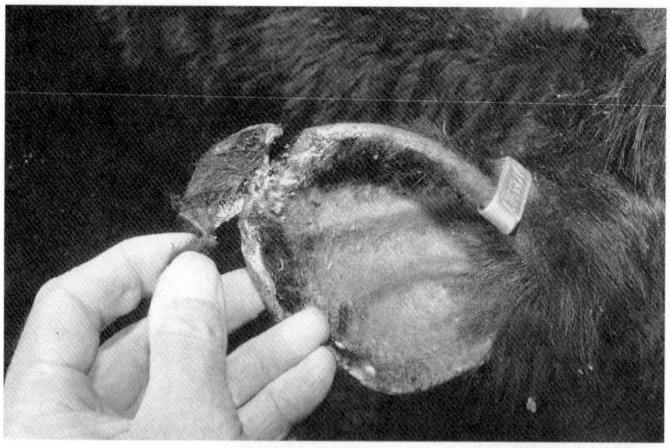

Abbildung 12-37 Ergotismus cutaneus: Mumifikation und beginnende Ablösung des Ohrendes

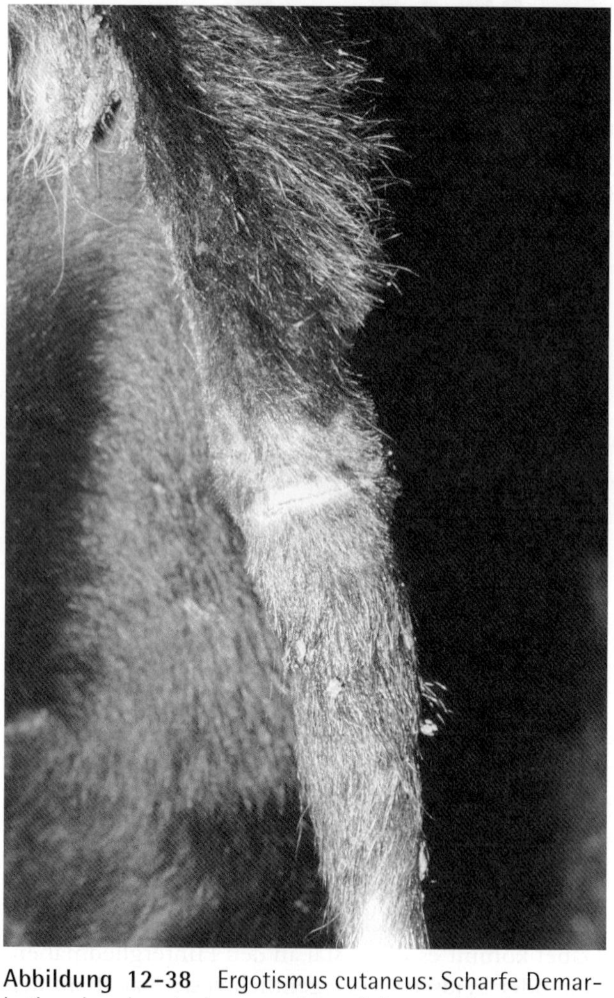

Abbildung 12-38 Ergotismus cutaneus: Scharfe Demarkation des abgestorbenen unteren Schwanzdrittels

zwischen Afterklauen und Klauen. Bei schwerer Mutterkornvergiftung liegt die später schnittlinienartig klaffende Demarkationsgrenze weiter proximal, in Höhe von Fesselgelenk, Röhrbeinmitte oder Sprunggelenk. Dann sind i. d. R. auch tiefergelegene Weichgewebe und der Knochen abgestorben sowie eitrig

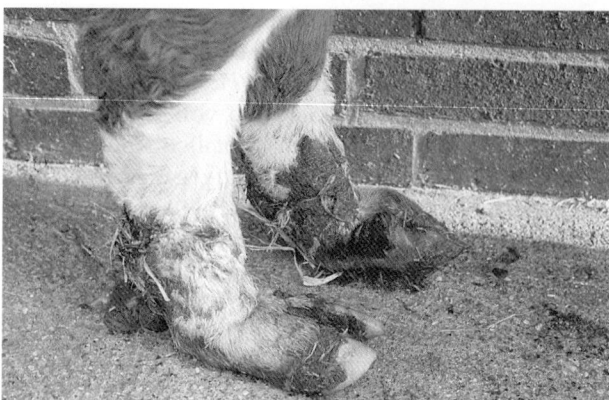

Abbildung 12-39 Ergotismus cutaneus: Fortgeschrittene Abstoßung der Zehen beider Hinterbeine

infiziert, weshalb solche Patienten entweder »ausschuhen« oder die betroffenen Klauen samt Klauenbein verlieren, wenn nicht sogar das gesamte Gliedmaßenende ab Fessel- oder Sprunggelenk schließlich abfällt; der verbleibende Extremitätenstumpf zeigt keine nennenswerte Blutungsneigung. Fortgeschrittene Läsionen sind offenbar ziemlich unempfindlich, da die Patienten trotz der Veränderungen weiterhin laufen. Meist ergreift die Mumifikation auch das Schwanzende, seltener zudem die Ohrspitzen und/oder das Flotzmaul; manche Tiere verlieren nur die Schwanzquaste, andere die Hälfte des Schwanzes oder mehr. Bezüglich der Erscheinungen der ergotbedingten *idiopathischen Hitzeintoleranz* wird auf diesbezügliche Ausführungen bei der Festukose (Kap. 12.3.4) verwiesen. Mutterkornbedingte *Aborte* sollen beim Rind zwar vorkommen, scheinen jedoch ziemlich selten zu sein.

■ **Sektion:** Zerlegungs- und histologische Befunde ergeben bei mumifizierendem, nicht aber bei nervösem Ergotismus die erwähnten Haut- und Gefäßveränderungen im Bereich der Akren.

■ **Diagnose:** Die Mutterkornalkaloide lassen sich im Futter mittels HPLC oder ELISA feststellen. *Differentialdiagnostisch* sind Tollwut (Kap. 10.3.6), Neuromykotoxikosen (Kap. 10.5.41), Rohrschwingelgrasvergiftung (Kap. 12.3.4), traumatisch bedingte Schwanzspitzennekrose (Kap. 9.4.5), Bleivergiftung (Kap. 10.5.12), nervöse Listeriose (Kap. 12.2.10), Herpesenzephalitis (Kap. 10.3.5) sowie exogener Hitzestreß (Kap. 10.6.4) zu berücksichtigen; möglicherweise kann bei jungen Kälbern auch schwere Salmonellose (Kap. 6.10.21) zum Absterben der Hinterbeinenden führen.

■ **Beurteilung:** Mit nekrotisierenden Gliedmaßenenden behaftete Tiere sind aus Gründen des Tierschutzes umgehend zu töten. Wirksame *Behandlungsmaßnahmen* sind nicht bekannt. Die *Vorbeuge* des Ergotismus besteht im Überprüfen verdächtiger Futterpflanzen und -mittel sowie im Vermeiden derjenigen, die mit *Claviceps* spp. befallen sind.

12.3.4 Rohrschwingelgrasvergiftung

E. Renner

Definition: Die auf Verzehr von endophytisch mit *Neotyphodium* (s. *Acremonium*) *coenophialum* befallenem Rohrschwingelgras oder -heu (= *Festuca arundinacea*; Abb. 12-40) beruhende *Festukose* des Rindes umfaßt *mehrere Krankheitsbilder*: Rohrschwingellahmheit (»fescue foot«, »pie de festuca«), idiopathische Hitzeintoleranz (»Sommer«- oder Dysthermie-Syndrom), Fettgewebsnekrose (Liponekrose), mangelhafte Zelluloseverwertung und Störungen der Trächtigkeit.

Vorkommen: Die verschiedenen Formen der Festukose sind v. a. in Ländern gemäßigter Klimazonen bekannt, in denen Rohrschwingel als Weidegras genutzt wird (Australien, Neuseeland, USA, Argentinien, Chile, Uruguay). Solches Gras wird weltweit, insbesondere auf alkalischen Böden, angepflanzt und bietet ein zwar zellulosereich-grobes, aber gutes Futter. Ähnliche Vergiftungen werden gelegentlich auch beim Pferd, wegen des hohen Wuchses der Rohrschwingelweiden aber fast nie bei kleinen Wiederkäuern beobachtet.

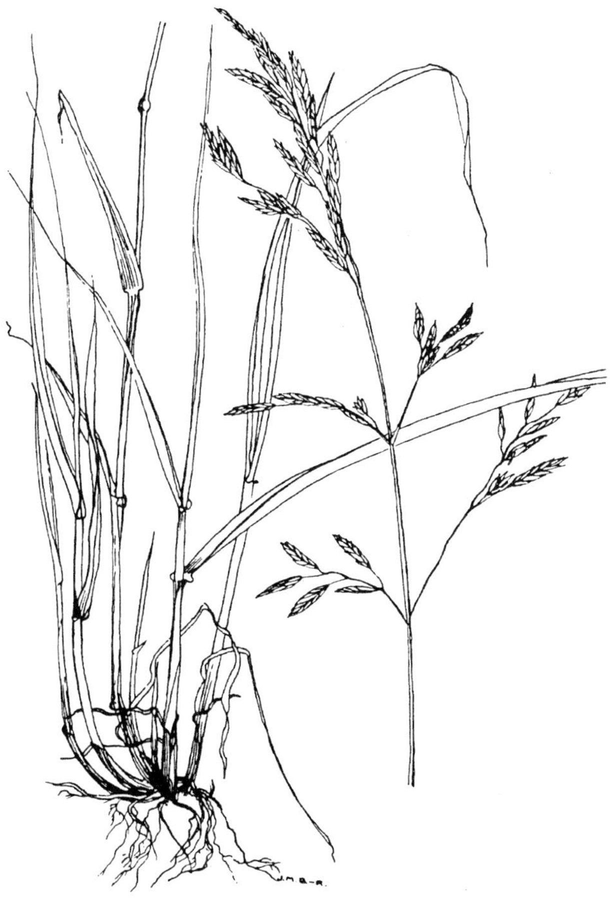

Abbildung 12-40 Rohrschwingelgras (*Festuca arundinacea*; Walton, 1983; natürliche Größe 60–180 cm)

Ursachen: Rohrschwingel kann von einem endophytischen Pilz, *Neotyphodium* (s. *Acremonium*) *coenophialum*, der asexuellen Form von *Epicloe typhina*, befallen sein. Er bildet verschiedene Alkaloide, nämlich Ergonovin, α-Ergokryptin, Ergovalin und N-Azetyllolin, deren Wirkungsweise derjenigen des Mutterkorns (Kap. 12.3.3) ähnelt. In vitro fördern oder hemmen diese Gifte – je nach Konzentration – das Wachstum glatter Gefäßmuskelzellen. Innerhalb befallener Weiden breitet sich der Pilz über Bestockung und Samen aus. Da von ihm parasitierte Pflanzen weniger gern gefressen werden als gesunde, produzieren sie mehr (und zwar pilzbefallene) vegetative Triebe und Samen als jene. Das bedingt, daß eine zunächst ungiftige Rohrschwingelweide innerhalb von 5–7 Jahren toxisch werden kann. Zudem breitet sich Rohrschwingel auf befallenen Grünflächen mattenartig invasiv aus, wodurch andere Gräser sowie Leguminosen regelrecht verdrängt und Mischweiden allmählich in reine Rohrschwingelweiden verwandelt werden. Auch italienisches Ray- oder Weidelgras (*Lolium multiflorum*) kann von *N.* (*A.*) *coenophialum* befallen werden und zur Vergiftung von Weiderindern (in Form des Dysthermie-Syndroms) beitragen. Die Pilztoxine sind gegenüber Heuwerbung und -lagerung resistent; deshalb kann Festukose auch während der Stallhaltung auftreten.

Pathogenese: Die genannten Alkaloide bewirken zunehmende Verdickung von Tunica media und intima der Arteriolen; die damit verbundene Einengung des Lumens dieser Blutgefäße löst je nach den Begleitumständen (Stärke des Pilzbefalls, Verfügbarkeit pilzfreien Futters, Lebensalter, Umwelttemperatur, Trächtigkeit) eines oder mehrere der erwähnten Krankheitsbilder aus. Dabei treten die verschiedenen Syndrome oft unabhängig voneinander, mitunter aber gleichzeitig oder nacheinander auf, was für zeitweilige Verschiebungen im »Angebot« der einzelnen Pilzgifte spricht. (Nach Stickstoffdüngung solcher Weiden nimmt z. B. die Konzentration an Ergovalin, nach Gaben von Geflügelmist das Krankheitsbild der Fettgewebsnekrose zu.)

Symptome, Verlauf: Das klinische Bild der Festukose ist je nach dem dabei im Vordergrund stehenden Syndrom verschieden:

➤ *Rohrschwingellahmheit* tritt v. a. bei niedriger Umwelttemperatur, und zwar bevorzugt bei Rindern mit pigmentloser oder -armer Haut, auf. Entsprechend dem Expositionsgrad des Einzeltieres zeigen sich distal an beiden Hinterbeinen schon 1–2 Wochen oder aber erst Monate nach Aufnahme toxischen Rohrschwingels Rötung und Haarausfall, mitunter auch ödematöse Kronsaumschwellung; später stirbt die dabei kühler und lederartig werdende Zehenhaut ab (Abb. 12-41) und wird unterhalb einer scharfen, meist proximal des Fesselgelenks rings um das Bein verlaufenden Demarkationslinie mumifiziert abgestoßen; die zugehörigen Klauen »schuhen aus«. Hierdurch bloßgelegte Weichgewebe entwickeln kräftige Granulation. Die Erkrankung bedingt zunehmende, zu Abmagerung/Kachexie, Festliegen und Tod führende Lahmheit. Manche Patienten, insbesondere solche, bei denen nur ein Hinterbein betroffen ist, fußen jedoch auf dem verbleibenden, ziemlich unempfindlichen Gliedmaßenstumpf.

➤ *Idiopathische Hitzeintoleranz** ist v. a. im Sommer, bei hoher Umgebungstemperatur, zu beobachten und betrifft insbesondere dunkler oder schwarz pigmentierte taurine Rinder. Gleichermaßen exponierte Zeburinder sowie deren Kreuzungsprodukte (Brangus, Bradford u. a.) zeigen keine oder nur leichte klinische Erscheinungen, da sie pro kg LM über wesentlich mehr Hautoberfläche, d. h. bessere Wärmeregulationsfähigkeit verfügen als erstere. Die Kranken leiden unter übernormaler Körpertemperatur, weshalb sie ständig Schatten aufsuchen oder in Oberflächengewässern stehen; Tränkeverbrauch, Speichelfluß und Harnabsatz sind vermehrt; Serum-Prolaktinspiegel und Milchleistung sind erniedrigt. Zudem magern die Patienten ab, und ihr Haarkleid bleibt trotz der warmen Jahreszeit lang und struppig (»summer slump«). Herz- und Atemfrequenz sind – je nach Lufttemperatur und -feuchtigkeit – beschleunigt, d. h. höher als bei gesunden Vergleichstieren.

➤ *Fettgewebsnekrose:* Bei gut genährten Rindern bedingt die mit dem Verbringen auf toxische Rohrschwingelweide verbundene allgemeine Verengerung arterieller Gefäße mangelhafte Durchblutung der abdominalen Fettdepots, was (viel)herdförmige aseptische Liponekrose auslöst. Das absterbende Fett ist nicht mobilisierbar; es verwandelt sich vielmehr in erbsen- bis faustgroße derbe Knoten, welche – je nach Umfang und Lokalisation – die Labmagen-Darm- oder Harnpassage behindern, d. h. zu Kolik und sogar zum Tod führen können; zudem geht Fettgewebsnekrose (Kap. 6.15.5) meist mit deutlicher Abmagerung einher.

➤ *Unzulängliche Zelluloseverwertung:* Lolin hemmt den Abbau der Zellulose durch die Mikroorganismen im Pansen. Die schlechte Ausnutzung dieses Nährstoffs

* Gleichartige Erscheinungen treten auch bei leichterer Mutterkornvergiftung (Kap. 12.3.3) auf.

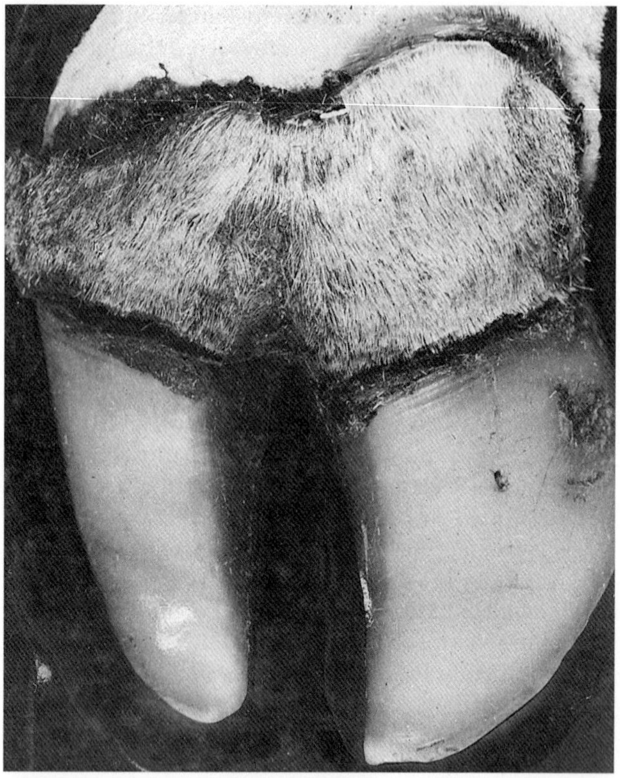

Abbildung 12-41 »Rohrschwingellahmheit« *(Festukose)*: Hinterbeinende einer Färse nach 70tägiger Verfütterung von Rohrschwingelgras: trockene Gangrän und beginnende Demarkation des abgestorbenen Gewebes (Jensen et al., 1956)

betrifft v. a. Jungtiere (Verzögerung des Wachstums oder Abmagerung, struppiges Haarkleid) und Kühe (unterernährungsbedingte Fruchtbarkeitsstörungen).

➤ *Embryonaltod, Aborte, Frühgeburten:* An Festukose erkrankte weibliche Rinder weisen niedrige Prolaktin-Blutspiegel sowie abnorme Konzentrationen anderer Sexualhormone auf, was Zyklusstörungen bedingt. Werden in der zweiten Hälfte der Trächtigkeit befindliche Kühe auf toxische Rohrschwingelweide verbracht, so bewirkt die dadurch ausgelöste mangelhafte Durchblutung von Gelbkörper und Eihäuten verminderte Progesteronbildung sowie fetalen Streß (→ vermehrte Kortisolausschüttung). So kommt es zu vorzeitiger Ausstoßung des lebenden Fetus ohne Retention der Eihäute; das betreffende Kalb kann – entsprechend der von ihm bis dahin durchlaufenen intrauterinen Entwicklung – u. U. überleben.

➤ *Verlängerte Tragezeit:* Dieses Syndrom tritt v. a. bei Pferden, mitunter aber auch bei Rindern auf, die frühtragend auf nicht allzu giftige Rohrschwingelweide getrieben werden. Bei ihnen bewirkt die generalisierte Verengerung von Arteriolen eine pergamentartige Induration der Eihäute, deren Blutgefäße dabei deutlich verdickt sind. Die hiermit verbundene mangelhafte Blutversorgung des Fetus äußert sich in Verzögerung des Geburtstermines (bei Stuten um bis zu 30 Tage).

■ **Sektion:** Der Zerlegungsbefund ergibt kennzeichnende Veränderungen an Akren (Mumifikation und Demarkation der Zehenhaut, »Ausschuhen«), intraabdominalem Fett (gut abgesetzte grauweiße derbe Liponekroseknoten mit »seifiger« Schnittfläche) und/oder indurierte Eihäute sowie Abmagerung. *Histologisch* erweisen sich Tunica media und intima sämtlicher Arteriolen, insbesondere aber derjenigen der Unterhaut der Akren und jener der Eihäute als deutlich verdickt; ihr Lumen ist bis auf ein Zehntel der Norm verringert. Im Bereich der Hautnekrosen sind zudem die Vasa vasorum thrombosiert.

■ **Diagnose:** Die Erkennung des Leidens stützt sich auf klinische Erscheinungen, Vorbericht und Begleitumstände (Fütterung), Sektions- sowie histologische Befunde. *Neotyphodium* (s. *Acremonium*) *coenophialum* ist in den Markzellen der Bestockungssprosse sowie in den Samen mikroskopisch und mittels ELISA nachweisbar. Im Harn von auf endophytbefallenem Rohrschwingelgras weidenden Rindern lassen sich mittels ELISA Ergotalkaloide feststellen.

■ **Differentialdiagnose:** Zur Abgrenung der *Rohrschwingellahmheit* ist v. a. an Ergotismus (Kap. 12.3.3) sowie akzidentelle Abschnürung des Gliedmaßenendes (Kap. 9.7) zu denken; Mutterkornvergiftung wird häufig, Festukose dagegen nur selten von Mumifikation der Haut weiterer Akren (Schwanzspitze, Ohrrand) begleitet. *Festukose-bedingte Fettgewebsnekrose* ist von andersbedingten intraabdominalen Zubildungen (Kap. 6.15.6) und kolikauslösenden Leiden (Kap. 6.10.1) sowie von idiopathischer Fettgewebsnekrose zu unterscheiden. *Idiopathische Hitzeintoleranz* hat zwar Ähnlichkeit mit exogener Hyperthermie (Hitzschlag), doch fehlen bei letzterer die histologischen Blutgefäßveränderungen der Festukose. *Rohrschwingelgrasbedingte Trächtigkeitsstörungen* lassen sich durch mikrobiologische und serologische Untersuchungen (Eihäute, Fetus, Labmageninhalt bzw. Blut) sowie histologische Kontrollen (arterielle Blutgefäße von Akren und Eihäuten) von solchen infektiöser Ursache (Brucellose, Campylobakteriose, Leptospirose, Bovine Virusdiarrhoe, Infektiöse Bovine Rhinotracheitis u. a.) unterscheiden.

■ **Beurteilung:** Die Prognose ausgeprägter Festukosefälle ist schlecht, weil die Verengerungen der Arteriolen irreversibel sind. Mit Zehennekrosen behaftete Patienten kommen meist bald zum Festliegen und verenden in Kachexie.

■ **Behandlung:** Therapieversuche sind daher bei deutlicher Erkrankung i. d. R. erfolglos; in leichteren Fällen läßt sich durch sofortige Futterumstellung allmähliche Besserung erzielen.

■ **Prophylaxe:** Schwach mit *N.* (A.) *coenophialum* befallene Rohrschwingelweiden nicht »alt« werden lassen. Toxische F.-arundinacea-Weiden meiden oder zur Heuwerbung nutzen und das Heu vor dem Verfüttern ammonisieren; weniger sicher ist das Zufüttern von gutem Heu und/oder Kraftfutter während des Weidegangs auf befallenen Flächen. Am wirksamsten ist das Umbrechen mit anschließender Neuansaat eines A.-coenophialum-freien Rohrschwingel-Kultivars.

12.3.5 Aflatoxikose

M. Stöber

■ **Definition, Vorkommen:** Bei diesem, auch *»Erdnußvergiftung«* genannten Leiden handelt es sich um eine auf oraler Aufnahme der von *Aspergillus spp.* produzierten *Aflatoxine* beruhende Hepatomykotoxikose, deren klinisches Bild – je nach Verlauf – von nervösen und/oder digestiven Symptomen beherrscht wird. Aflatoxikose kommt weltweit, v. a. bei Geflügel und Schwein, aber auch bei Kälbern und Jungrindern, nach fortgesetzter Verabreichung Aspergillus-befallenen Futters zudem bei erwachsenen Rindern vor. Ein Teil der früher als »mouldy corn poisoning« bezeichneten Erkrankungen ist gemäß heutiger Kenntnis der Aflatoxikose zuzurechnen. Möglicherweise spielt aflatoxinhaltige Fütterung auch eine Rolle bei der Entstehung des Siebbeinkarzinoms (Kap. 5.1.7.1).

■ **Ursachen, Pathogenese:** Unter feuchtwarmen Witterungs- oder Lagerungsbedingungen können mit Erdnüssen, Sojabohnen, Sonnenblumen, Baumwolle, Mais, Reis oder anderem Getreide bestandene Kulturen, die von ihnen geernteten Früchte oder die hieraus gewonnenen Produkte (Schrot, Mehl, Extraktionskuchen) von *Aspergillus flavus* und *A. parasiticus* befallen werden. Die von diesen Pilzen gebildeten *Aflatoxine* verbinden sich mit Nukleinsäuren und Nukleoproteinen, wodurch sie muta-, terato- und karzinogene sowie immunsuppressorische Wirkung erlangen. Die für Kälber bzw. erwachsene Rinder verträgliche Aflatoxinkonzentration des Futters liegt unter 100 bzw. 300 ppb, d. h., jüngere Tiere sind wesentlich aflatoxinempfindlicher als ältere. Aflatoxinexponierte und dabei selbst u. U. gar nicht erkrankende Kühe können das Pilzgift offenbar schon transplazentar auf ihre Feten, sonst über die Kolostralmilch an ihre Kälber weitergeben, was bei letzteren bereits in der ersten Lebenswoche zu klinisch manifester Intoxikation führt.

■ **Symptome, Verlauf:** *Perakut* bis *akut* einsetzende Fälle äußern sich schon wenige Tage nach Beginn der aflatoxinhaltigen Fütterung. Bei schwerer Erkrankung kommt es entweder zu plötzlichem Tod oder starker tetanoider Erregbarkeit, blindem Anrennen gegen Hindernisse, Muskelzucken, Inkoordination, Überköten, Kreisbewegungen und Festliegen unter Krämpfen; je nach Lebensdauer der Patienten werden an ihnen zudem auch die bei weniger stark betroffenen Bestandsgenossen auftretenden Symptome beobachtet: Kolik, blaß-zyanotische oder ikterische Schleimhäute, Tenesmen, Mastdarmvorfall, schleimig-blutiger Durchfall, Dehydratation, Zähneknirschen, Klauenrehe, Festliegen sowie Tod infolge Kreislaufversagens innerhalb weniger Tage. Im letzten Drittel der Trächtigkeit schwer aflatoxinvergiftete Kühe verkalben und verenden nach mehrtägigem, z. T. von Kopftremor begleitetem Festliegen (→ Nachweis von Aflatoxin im Lebergewebe des Feten). Im Blutserum von Aflatoxikose-Patienten sind die Gehalte an direktem und indirektem Bilirubin sowie die Aktivitäten von AST und γGT erhöht, die Blutgerinnungszeit ist verkürzt; bei Kälbern ist der Serumgehalt an Immunoglobulinen verringert. Im fortgeschrittenen Stadium besteht Bilirubinurie.

Das *subakute bis chronische Krankheitsbild* wird nach mehrwöchiger bis monatelanger Giftaufnahme beobachtet: Niedergeschlagenheit; unbefriedigende Freßlust und körperliche Entwicklung; Abmagerung; verminderte Milchleistung; rauhes Haarkleid; Nasenausfluß und -bluten, Husten, erhöhte Atemfrequenz; verminderte Pansenmotorik; subkutane Ödeme (Kehlgang, Triel, Unterbauch) und Aszites (Zunahme des Bauchumfangs). Die Resistenz gegenüber Infektionen ist deutlich verringert (→ Neigung zu Durchfall, Sepsis, Mastitis und Metritis); außerdem kann bei weiblichen Rindern die Fruchtbarkeit, bei Bullen die Spermaqualität beeinträchtigt sein. Manche Patienten sind zudem photosensibilisiert. Auch solche Fälle enden oft früher oder später tödlich oder durch Notschlachtung.

■ **Sektion:** In akuten Fällen Schwellung und Induration der gelbbraunen Leber, Ödem der Gallenblase, wäßrige Beschaffenheit der Galle sowie oft, aber nicht immer, ausgeprägter Ikterus; mitunter auch subkutane, subepi- und perikardiale, tracheale, renale und vesikale Petechien. In chronischen Fällen: subkutane Ödeme, Leberzirrhose, Aszites, Hydrothorax, Labmagenwand- und Mesenterialödem. *Histologisch* finden sich Proliferation und Fibrose der kleinen Gallengänge, zentrolobuläre Leberzellvakuolisierung und -nekrose, auffallend große, karyomegale Hepatozyten und Pseudolobulation der Leber; nach chronischem Verlauf besteht ausgeprägte diffuse periportale Fibrose der Leber mit Venenokklusion (Abb. 12-42) sowie mäßige Nephrose. Das Gehirn kann die bei hepatogener Enzephalopathie (Kap. 10.5.8) beschriebenen Veränderungen aufweisen.

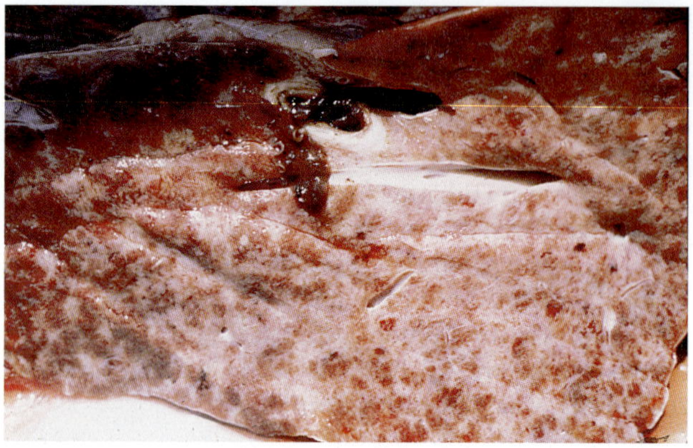

Abbildung 12-42 Hochgradige aflatoxikosebedingte Leberzirrhose (Kap. 12.3.5; Pedugsorn et al., 1979)

■ **Diagnose:** Die Erkennung des Leidens stützt sich auf klinisches Bild, Fütterungskontrolle und Aflatoxinnachweis (im Futter, Harn, Milch, Leber oder Niere: ELISA, HPLC, Fluorometrie). *Differentialdiagnostisch* sind Kreuzkrautvergiftung (Kap. 12.3.6), andere Mykotoxikosen (Kap. 10.5.4.1) und Kokzidiose (Kap. 6.11.5) zu berücksichtigen.

■ **Beurteilung:** Wirksame Behandlungsmaßnahmen sind unbekannt. Toxinhaltige Futtermittel sind umgehend abzusetzen und möglichst zu vernichten. Deutlich erkrankte Patienten bleiben meist unrentabel; bei ikterischen Tieren ist kein Schlachterlös zu erwarten.

■ **Prophylaxe:** Sachgemäße Werbung und Lagerung der eingangs genannten zugekauften oder selbstgeernteten Futtermittel. Importfutter erst nach Überprüfen seines Aflatoxingehalts verabreichen; die hierfür gültigen Höchstgehalte sind in Anl. 5/FMG 1975 festgelegt. Für menschlichen Genuß bestimmte Milch soll nicht mehr als 30 ppb Aflatoxin M_1/kg enthalten (UN-Vereinbarung). Experimentell läßt sich die Ausscheidung von Aflatoxin mit der Milch durch Zufügen von hydriertem Natrium-Kalzium-Aluminium-Silikat zum toxinhaltigen Futter vermindern.

12.3.6 Kreuzkrautvergiftung

M. Stöber

■ **Definition:** Auf längerem Beweiden von mit Kreuzkrautarten oder anderen Pyrrolizidin-haltigen und daher hepatotoxischen Pflanzen bestandenen Weiden oder Verfüttern des von solchen Flächen gewonnenen Heus (oder ebensolcher Silage) beruhende Vergiftung, die durch digestive und mitunter auch zentralnervöse Symptome gekennzeichnet ist. *Andere Bezeichnungen:*

Seneziose, Greiskraut-Toxikose, Pyrrolizidin-Alkaloidose, ragwort poisoning, »straining« oder »walking disease«, dike svinblom-toksikose, »enfermedad de los hinchazones«, enzootische Leberzirrhose.

Verbreitung: Das Leiden ist an *hepatotoxische Senecio- und andere Pflanzenarten* gebunden. Weltweit gibt es über 1200 Kreuzkrautarten, von denen diejenigen der Paucifolii-Gruppe als besonders giftig gelten. In manchen Regionen spielen sie, v. a. auf extensiv genutzten bergigen oder sumpfigen Weiden, und zwar im Frühjahr (nach Regenfällen), nach Herbizidbesprühung und/oder bei Futterknappheit, eine erhebliche wirtschaftliche Rolle.

Ursache: Verzehr von Pyrrolizidin-bildenden Pflanzen, insbesondere der kraut- bis strauchartigen Kreuzkrautarten (*Senecio* spp.; Abb. 12-43), aber auch von *Amsinckia, Crotalaria, Cynoglossum* (Kap. 12.3.7), *Echium, Heliotropum* und *Trichodesma* spp., auf der Weide oder im Stall (u. U. als Streu). Von ihnen werden über 30 verschiedene, ihrer kumulativen Wirkung nach aber ziemlich einheitliche Pyrrolizidinalkaloide gebildet. Als letal toxische Dosis wird eine in weniger als 3 Wochen gefressene Menge von Kreuzkrautgrün angegeben, die 2–8% der LM entspricht; die Aufnahme von 2–20 mg Pyrrolizidinalkaloiden/kg LM und Tag führt zur chronischen Erkrankung.

Pathogenese: Reifes Kreuzkraut wird von Rindern i. d. R. gemieden, wenn ihnen genügend anderes Grün zur Verfügung steht; dagegen wird die toxinreiche junge Pflanze (Knospen- und Vorblütestadium) gern, in Heu oder Silage enthaltenes Kreuzkraut aber zwangsläufig gefressen. Rinder sind Pyrrolizidinen gegenüber weit empfindlicher als kleine Wiederkäuer. Junge sowie hochlaktierende Tiere sind dabei i. d. R. gefährdeter als andere. In der Leber werden die Pyrrolizidine enzymatisch in giftigere Pyrrolabkömmlinge umgewandelt (Bioaktivation), die mit Nukleinsäuren sowie Nukleoproteinen reagieren und bei Ratten karzinogen wirken; Pyrrolizidinmetaboliten passieren die Plazenta und gehen auch in die Milch über, sind aber offenbar unschädlich. Pyrrolizidine hemmen die Leberzellteilung und bedingen Megalozytose; die dadurch ausgelöste Proliferation der Endothelien von zentrolobulären und Lebervenen sowie perivenöse Fibrose führen zu m. o. w. vollständiger Verlegung dieser Gefäße. Zudem entwickelt sich allgemeine Leberzirrhose und Hyperplasie der Gallengänge. Diese Veränderungen beeinträchtigen die Perfusion der Leber und steigern den Blutdruck im Pfortaderbereich.

Symptome: Bei *akuter Vergiftung* setzen vereinzelte bis gehäufte, v. a. Kälber sowie Jungrinder betreffende Erkrankungen schon innerhalb von 1–7 Tagen nach Aufnahme größerer Pyrrolizidinalkaloid-Mengen ein und enden innerhalb von Stunden bis weniger Tage tödlich. Bei *chronischer Intoxikation* kommt es als Folge mehrwöchiger bis monatelanger Ingestion geringerer Mengen von Kreuzkraut (oder anderer der o. a. Pflanzenarten) zu schleichender, einige Wochen bis zu ½ Jahr dauernder Erkrankung, deren Symptombild sich beim Versagen der Funktionstüchtigkeit von Leber und Kreislauf plötzlich verschlimmert; dabei können neben m. o. w. schwerwiegenden digestiven Störungen auch solche einer hepatogenen Enzephalopathie (Kap. 10.5.8) auftreten, die i. d. R. den Tod ankündigt. Die Morbidität beträgt je nach Intensität der Exposition ≤ 20%, die Letalität um 100%. Mitunter kommt es erst einige Zeit nach Abtrieb von kreuzkrautbestandener Weide zu Erkrankungen, was die Diagnose entsprechend erschwert.

Von unerwarteten Todesfällen abgesehen, zeigen die Patienten meist mehrere folgender Symptome: stark nachlassende Milchleistung; Absondern von der Herde; Niedergeschlagenheit; Freßunlust; mitunter vermehrter Durst; ungepflegt-struppiges Haarkleid; herabgesetzte oder fehlende Pansenmotorik; bis zur Kachexie fortschreitende Abmagerung; Fressen von

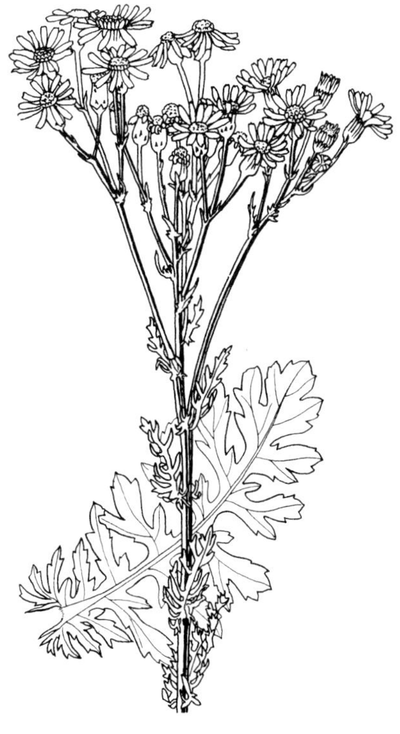

Abbildung 12-43 Jakobskreuzkraut (*Senecio jacobaea*; WEIHE, V., 1972; natürliche Höhe 30–100 cm)

Rinde und Holz; Kot dunkelfarben, durchfällig, oft auch bluthaltig und übelriechend; Koliken oder quälende Tenesmen mit Mastdarmvorfall; Harn bräunlich; in schweren Fällen Ikterus; mitunter auch Photosensibilisierung; subkutanes Senkungsödem an Kehlgang, Triel und Unterbauch; birnenförmige Zunahme des Bauchumfangs. Im fortgeschrittenen Stadium sind Blutleukozytenzahl, Serumaktivitäten von SDH, AST, CK und AP sowie der Gehalt des Serums an Bilirubin, Gallensäuren und Harnstoff erhöht, derjenige an Gesamteiweiß, Albumin, Fibrinogen, Cholesterin, anorganischem Phosphor und Kalzium erniedrigt. Etwaige zentralnervöse Symptome bestehen von Fall zu Fall in Zähneknirschen, ziellosem Umherwandern, Unruhe, tetanoid erhöhter Erregbarkeit, Muskelzittern, Kreisbewegungen, Aufbrüllen, blindem Anrennen gegen Hindernisse oder Angriffslust, Ataxie und Inkoordination, paretischem Nachziehen der Hinterbeine, Taumeln oder Niederstürzen.

Von seneziosekranken Kühen geborene Kälber erwiesen sich als gesund und zeigten keine histologisch nachweisbaren Leberveränderungen; ihre Mütter verendeten dagegen bald nach dem Kalben. An seneziosekranken Kühen saugende Kälber erkrankten ebenfalls nicht. Deshalb wird angenommen, daß solche Milch nicht menschenpathogen ist.

■ **Sektion:** Von akuten Fällen abgesehen, weist der Tierkörper hochgradige Abmagerung, sturzbedingte subkutane Hämorrhagien, Unterhautödem, seröse Fettatrophie und deutliche Vermehrung der Körperhöhlenflüssigkeiten, nicht selten auch Ikterus auf. Die Bauchorgane zeigen mitunter subseröse Petechien; Gekröse, Labmagen und periproktales Bindegewebe sind ödematisiert. Die Leber ist in akuten Fällen leicht bis deutlich vergrößert, stumpfrandig, dunkelrot bis orangebraun gefärbt, von mürber Konsistenz und auffallend blutreich; ihre Schnittfläche weist Muskatnußzeichnung auf. In chronischen Fällen erscheint die Leber gelbbraun, derb und ihre Oberfläche von Knoten durchsetzt. Die Gallenblase ist vergrößert und prall gefüllt, ihre mitunter blutunterlaufene Wand ebenso wie Labmagen, großes Netz und Darmgekröse ödematisiert. Kennzeichnende *histologische Veränderungen* der Leber bestehen bei akuten Fällen in Gallengangshyperplasie, zentrolobulärer hepatozellulärer Nekrose (mit Hämorrhagien) und Megalozytose, periportaler Fibrose sowie Proliferation des Venenendothels (→ Venenokklusion). Nach chronischem Verlauf wird das mikroskopische Bild von schwerer Leberfibrose und -zirrhose beherrscht. Bei Beteiligung des Gehirns zeigt dieses spongiöse Degeneration der weißen Substanz (s. hepatogene Enzephalopathie, Kap. 10.5.8).

■ **Diagnose:** Klinisches Bild und Umwelt-/Futterkontrolle bieten wertvolle Hinweise; Aszites, Lebervergrößerung, Portalvenenstauung und inhomogene Lebergewebsdichte sind ultrasonographisch darstellbar. Durch mikroskopische Untersuchung von Leberbioptaten lassen sich kennzeichnende histologische Veränderungen feststellen. Der Pyrrolizidin-Nachweis in Futter-, Blut- oder Leberproben erfolgt dünnschichtchromatographisch oder mittels HPLC und Massenspektroskopie. *Differentialdiagnostisch* ist v. a. an Aflatoxikose (Kap. 12.3.5), Magendarmwurmbefall (Kap. 6.11.2) und Paratuberkulose (Kap. 6.10.22), aber auch an Tollwut (Kap. 10.3.6), Weidetetanie (Kap. 10.5.4.1), Vergiftung durch Blei oder Hundszunge (Kap. 10.5.12, 12.3.7) sowie Neuromykotoxikosen (Kap. 10.5.41) zu denken.

■ **Beurteilung:** Pyrrolizidingeschädigte Tiere verfallen chronischem Siechtum, wenn sie nicht schon zuvor verenden. Auch bei zunächst nur durch Leberbiopsie als »latent« betroffen befundenen Herdengenossen ist früher oder später mit manifester Erkrankung zu rechnen.

■ **Behandlung:** Sofortige Umstellung auf pyrrolizidinfreie Fütterung; Ausmerzen der erkrankten und leberbioptisch »latent« betroffenen Tiere, da es keine wirksame Medikation gibt.

■ **Prophylaxe:** Aufnahme von *Senecio* spp. und anderen pyrrolizidinhaltigen Pflanzen vermeiden. Die Zufütterung von Mineralstoffen und Vitaminen hat keine protektive Wirkung. Das von befallenen Flächen gewonnene Heu bleibt selbst nach langer Lagerung noch giftig; beim Silieren nimmt der Toxingehalt nur allmählich und nur bis zu einem gewissen Grenzwert ab. Auf Nutzflächen sollten die eingangs genannten Giftpflanzen ausgerottet werden.

12.3.7 Vergiftung durch Hundszunge

M. Stöber

■ **Definition, Vorkommen, Ursachen, Pathogenese:** Intoxikationen durch Hundszunge (*Cynoglossum officinale;* Abb. 12-44) ereignen sich v. a. infolge Verabreichens von stark mit solcher durchsetztem Grünfutter (Esparsette) oder Heu. Von weidenden Rindern wird die durch ihren Gehalt an Pyrrolizidinalkaloiden (≤ 2% TM *Heliotridine*, insbesondere *Heliosupin* und *Ethinatin*) kumulativ giftige Pflanze wegen ihres abstoßenden mäuseartigen Geruchs i. d. R. gemieden. Ihr Verbreitungsgebiet umfaßt Europa und Nordamerika. Bei Kälbern führt einmalige Aufnahme von 60 mg Hundszungenalkaloiden/kg LM innerhalb von

48 h zum Tode; fortgesetzte niedrigere Dosen bedingen chronisches Siechtum.

■ **Symptome, Verlauf:** Anfangs Unruhe, später Niedergeschlagenheit, Freßunlust, übelriechender Durchfall (z. T. blutig), Tenesmen, Taumeln, Ikterus und Verenden nach m. o. w. lang anhaltender Erkrankung; Hypoglykämie, Hypoproteinämie, Serumaktivitäten von AST und γ-GT sowie Serumgehalt an Gallenfarbstoff und -säuren erhöht.

■ **Sektion:** Die Zerlegung ergibt je nach Dauer des Leidens m. o. w. ausgeprägte Abmagerung/Kachexie, Trielödem, Leberschwellung und multiple subseröse sowie submuköse Blutungen der Bauchorgane. *Histologisch* sind in akuten Fällen diffuse Leberzellnekrose mit Anisokaryose, Aniso- und Megalozytose der Hepatozyten und Karyomegalie der Gallengangsepithelien festzustellen.

■ **Diagnose:** Die Erkennung dieser Vergiftung ergibt sich aus klinischem Bild, Umweltkontrolle und Sektionsbefund. *Differentialdiagnostisch* sind Kreuzkrautvergiftung (Kap. 12.3.6) und Aflatoxikose (Kap. 12.3.5) in Betracht zu ziehen.

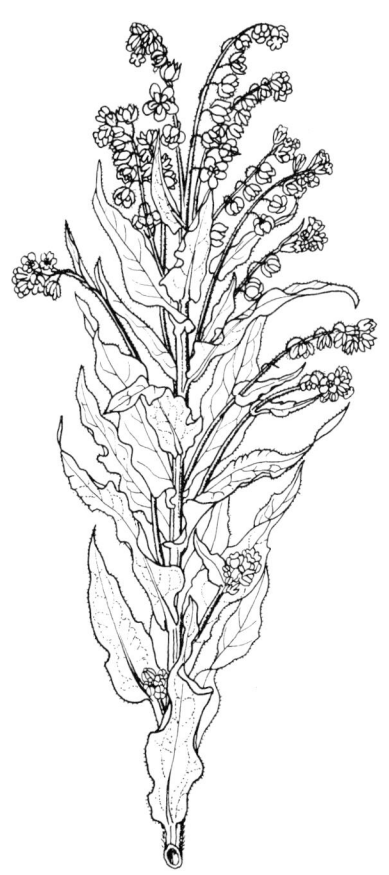

Abbildung 12-44 Hundszunge (*Cynoglossum officinale*; WEIHE, V., 1972; natürliche Höhe 30–80 cm)

■ **Beurteilung:** Nach Diagnosestellung sind auch die weniger schwer erkrankten Tiere als dauerhaft unrentabel und ihre Behandlung als wirkungslos anzusehen.

12.3.8 Pruritus-Pyrexie-Hämorrhagie-Syndrom

M. STÖBER

Das zunächst als *DUIB-Vergiftung* bezeichnete Leiden ist verschiedentlich in Kuhherden beobachtet worden, in denen bestimmte, im allgemeinen gutverträgliche Silierungsverfahren (Zusatz von ICI-Sylade oder Di-Ureido-Iso-Butan) angewandt wurden. Heute wird angenommen, daß das *Pruritus-Pyrexie-Hämorrhagie(= PPH)-Syndrom* eine *Zitrinin-bedingte Mykotoxikose* ist, die meist von besonders gut erscheinender Silage ausgeht. Ihr klinisches Bild umfaßt: Milchrückgang; papulo-erythematöse, später exsudative Hautentzündung mit starkem, bis zum Wundlecken oder -scheuern gehendem Juckreiz sowie m. o. w. großflächigen Haarverlusten an Kopf, Hals, Rücken, Schwanzansatz, Perineum und Euter, mitunter auch im proximalen Bereich der Gliedmaßen, die distal ödematös anschwellen können; deutliche Berührungsempfindlichkeit; nachlassende Freßlust, Verweigern des Kraftfutters; Hyperämie des Flotzmauls, Nasenausfluß, Tränen (Lichtscheu), Husten, Atembeschwerde; fieberhaft erhöhte Körpertemperatur ($\leq$ 41,5 °C); nicht selten auch Durchfall, Abort und/oder Metritis. Die Hautveränderungen werden schließlich hyperkeratotisch (»Elefantenhaut« mit zerklüfteten grauen Krusten). Im fortgeschrittenen Stadium zeigen sich zudem Blutungen an den sichtbaren Schleimhäuten und Blutaustritt aus den Körperöffnungen. Laborbefunde: mäßige Anämie, Neutrophilie und Hyperglobulinämie. Betroffene Tiere sterben innerhalb von 1–8 Wochen oder magern stark ab und werden unwirtschaftlich (Morbidität ~ 10%, Letalität $\leq$ 90%). Bei der Zerlegung sind oft, aber nicht immer, multiple Petechien an inneren Organen, hellgelbe Färbung der Nieren sowie Lungenemphysem festzustellen; histologisch findet man interstitielle Nephritis, nekrotisierende Kardiomyopathie, nichteitrige Enzephalitis sowie multiple herdförmige Entzündungen mit Lymphozyteninfiltration und Riesenzellvorkommen in vielen Organen. Differentialdiagnostisch sind Räude (Kap. 2.2.4.2), Besnoitiose (Kap. 2.2.4.6), Pentachlorphenol- und Chlornaphthalinvergiftung (Kap. 12.3.14, 12.3.15), AUJESZKYsche Krankheit (Kap. 10.3.7), »Schlempemauke« (Kap. 2.2.5.1), Dermatitis solaris (Kap. 2.2.7.3) sowie hämorrhagische Diathesen (Kap. 4.3.5.10) in Betracht zu ziehen.

12.3.9 Selenvergiftung

M. Stöber

Definition: Durch Verzehr von Pflanzen mit übermäßigem Gehalt an organisch oder anorganisch gebundenem Selen, oder durch Überdosierung dieses Spurenelements bedingte Intoxikation *(Selenose)*, die je nach Giftmenge und -aufnahmeweise *akut* (mit zentralnervösen und respiratorischen Erscheinungen) oder *chronisch* (= »alkali disease« mit Auswirkungen auf Gelenke, Leber, Herz, Klauen und Hörner) verläuft. Das Krankheitsbild der früher ebenfalls als chronische Selenvergiftung angesehenen *»blind staggers«* weidender Wiederkäuer ist nach heutiger Kenntnis offenbar weniger Selen- als Pflanzenalkaloid-bedingt.

Vorkommen, Ursachen: Die Viehhaltung bestimmter Gebiete (im mittleren Westen der USA sowie in Kanada, Mexiko, Kolumbien, Irland, Israel, Rußland, Indien, Australien und Südafrika) ist durch bodenständige Selenose stark beeinträchtigt. Für das Zustandekommen solcher Erkrankungen ist die Aufnahme Se-haltiger Pflanzen entscheidend:

- *Primäre »Selensammler«-* (oder *»-indikator«-*) *Pflanzen* gedeihen nur auf Se-reichen Böden, aus denen sie bis zu 10000 ppm TM Se aufnehmen und in toxisch wirkende, wasserlöslich organisch gebundene Form überführen (*Astragalus, Stanleya, Oonopsis* und *Xylorrhizia* spp.). Wegen ihres Se-bedingten knoblauchartigen Geruchs und Geschmacks werden sie von Weidetieren gemieden, solange genügend anderes Futter vorhanden ist. Anderenfalls verursachen sie akute Selenose.
- *Sekundäre »Selensammler«-* (oder *»-umwandler«*)-*Pflanzen* sind dagegen befähigt, sich auf einem mit abgestorbenen primären »Selensammler«-Pflanzen versetzten Boden bis zu einigen Hundert ppm TM mit Selen (vorwiegend in Form von Selenaten) anzureichern (*Aster, Atriplex, Castilleja, Comandra, Grayia, Grindelia, Gutierrezia, Macharenthera* und *Sideranthus* spp.). Nach Ingestion entsprechender Mengen führen sie ebenfalls zu akuter Selenvergiftung.
- Auf Se-reichen Böden können schließlich auch bestimmte *Getreidearten* (Mais, Weizen, Roggen, Hafer) und *Gräser* Gehalte von 10–30 ppm TM an proteingebundenem, relativ wenig wasserlöslichem Selen erreichen; ihre Verfütterung löst chronische Selenose (»alkali disease«) aus.
- Nach Aufklärung der Bedeutung von Selen als Spurenelement wird es allein oder in Kombination mit Vitamin E als *Medikament* zur Vorbeuge der Weißmuskelkrankheit (Kap. 9.17.1) und anderer, auf Selen- und/oder Tokopherolmangel zurückgeführter Leiden (Kap. 9.17.2) viel eingesetzt. Dabei sind infolge unsachgemäßer Zubereitung oder Anwendung verschiedentlich Überdosierungen mit erheblichen Verlusten durch akute Selenose vorgekommen. Entsprechendes gilt für fehlerhafte Zusammensetzung von *Mineralstoffmischungen*.

Pathogenese: *Akute Selenvergiftung* wird oft schon durch einmalige Aufnahme größerer Mengen stark selenhaltiger Pflanzen (~ 2–10 mg Se/kg LM) oder aber durch versehentliche parenterale Gabe von $\geq$ 1 mg Se/kg LM ausgelöst. Bei täglicher Ingestion von $\geq$ 0,15 mg Se/kg LM kommt es dagegen zu *chronischer Selenose*. Das Vergiftungsgeschehen wird durch Trockenheit und Futterknappheit gefördert (→ vermehrter Verzehr von dürrebedingt besonders Se-reich gewordenen Pflanzen), während reichliche Zufütterung von Eiweiß den Intoxikationsprozeß bremst. Im Organismus behindert Se vermutlich aminosäurehaltige Enzyme.

Symptome: Patienten mit *akuter Selenose* fallen durch Niedergeschlagenheit, abnorme Stellung oder Haltung und unsicheren Gang auf. Zudem zeigen sie Speicheln, dunklen wäßrigen Durchfall, erhöhte Körpertemperatur, frequent-schwachen Puls, blasse Schleimhäute und erschwerte, von Stöhnen begleitete Atmung, knoblauchähnlichen Geruch der Atemluft, rötlichen Schaum vor der Nase, Zähneknirschen, Koliken, Tympanie, häufigeren Harnabsatz, weite Pupillen und Zyanose. Innerhalb weniger Stunden bis einiger Tage kommen sie zu apathisch-schlaffem Festliegen, Bewußtlosigkeit und zum Tod durch Versagen der Atmung.

Chronische Selenose (»alkali disease«) ist durch schleichenden Verlauf mit Haarausfall an der Schwanzquaste, Bewegungsunlust und wechselnde Lahmheit, Rissigwerden des Saumbandes der Hörner und der Klauenkrone, Entwicklung zirkulärer Klauenhornspalte und überlanger »Schnabelschuhklauen«, »chronisches Ausschuhen«, Freßunlust, mikrozytäre hypochrome Anämie, Abmagerung, Schwäche, mangelhafte Fruchtbarkeit und vereinzelte Aborte gekennzeichnet.

Verlauf: *Akute Selenose* verläuft meist tödlich; ausgeprägte *chronische Selenose* bedingt i. d. R. Unwirtschaftlichkeit.

Sektion: Bei *akuter Selenose* findet man Leberdegeneration, schlaffmürben Herzmuskel, Vermehrung von Herzbeutel- und Brusthöhlenflüssigkeit, Blutfülle und Ödem der Lunge, fokale Nekrosen in Herzmuskel, Leber und Nieren, multiple Blutungen sowie katarrhalische bis hämorrhagische Enteritis; histologisch zeigen sich perivaskuläre Ödeme in Gehirn, Kleinhirn und verlängertem Mark. An *»alkali disease«* eingegangene Rinder sind abgemagert und weisen, außer den erwähnten Veränderungen an Hörnern und Klauen, Erosionen an den Gelenkknorpeln großer Röhrenknochen, Leberzirrhose und Herzatrophie auf.

Diagnose: Klinisches Bild und Kenntnis der örtlichen Selenosegefahr lenken den Verdacht auf Selenvergiftung. Zur Klärung sind bei akuter Erkrankung Serum-, Leber- und Futterproben, in chronischen Fällen Haar-, Horn-, Blut- und Futterproben auf ihren Se-Gehalt zu untersuchen (s. Übersicht 9-11). *Differentialdiagnostisch* ist akute Selenose von Blausäurevergiftung (Kap. 5.3.5.10), Weideemphysem (Kap. 5.3.5.8) und Arsenvergiftung (Kap. 6.12.10), chronische Selenose dagegen von traumatisch und toxisch bedingter Klauenrehe (Kap. 9.14.8), Osteomalazie (Kap. 9.17.5), mumifizierendem Ergotismus (Kap. 12.3.3) und Rohrschwingellahmheit (Kap. 12.3.4) abzugrenzen.

Behandlung: Wirksame therapeutische Verfahren sind nicht bekannt; Dimerkaptopropanol ist kontraindiziert. Die weitere Verfütterung des selenhaltigen Futters an noch nicht erkrankte Herdenmitglieder ist zu unterbinden. Die *Vorbeuge* besteht im Meiden selenhaltiger Böden sowie der mit Indikator- oder Sammlerpflanzen bestandenen Weiden. Betroffene Futtermittel vernichten oder mit einwandfreiem Futter verschneiden. Bei oraler und parenteraler Selenmangelprophylaxe (Kap. 9.17.1, 9.17.2) sind die für das gewählte selenhaltige Präparat gültige Gebrauchsanweisung und Dosierung einzuhalten.

12.3.10 Manganmangel

M. Stöber

Definition, Vorkommen, Ursachen: Störungen der Mn-Versorgung spielen beim Rind eine ätiopathogenetisch erst teilweise geklärte Rolle. Experimentell lassen sich bei Wiederkäuern Ausfallserscheinungen nur unter extremen Mangelbedingungen (Mn-Gehalt des Futters < 10 ppm TM) auslösen. Vergleichbare Krankheitsbilder werden in den Niederlanden, in Belgien, Frankreich, Deutschland, der Slowakei, Norwegen, dem Vereinigten Königreich, Irland, Kanada, den USA und Südafrika gelegentlich auch in Rinderherden beobachtet, die auf Mn-armen alkalischen, stark gekalkten oder ausgewaschenen Heide-, Moor- oder Lehmböden weiden oder ausschließlich mit betriebseigenem Futter ernährt werden; dabei ist der Mn-Gehalt der Ration aber keineswegs immer knapp, sondern liegt u. U. zwischen 40 und 80 ppm TM. Ähnliche Auswirkungen kann auch die Verfütterung von Maissilage oder Apfelpülpe haben. Solche v. a. bei Fleisch-, mitunter aber auch bei Milchrindern bestandsweise gehäuft auftretenden Syndrome lassen sich zudem durch orale Mn-Gaben beheben. Deshalb wird vermutet, daß sie entweder auf sekundärem Mn-Mangel beruhen oder Folgen einer durch weitere Faktoren komplizierten Mn-Defizienz sind. Die Verwertbarkeit von oral aufgenommenem Mn wird nämlich nicht nur von hohem Ca-, P- oder Fe- (möglicherweise auch Sr-)Gehalt des Futters, sondern auch durch weites Ca:P-Verhältnis der Ration beeinträchtigt; außerdem ist Mn aus Silage offenbar schlechter verwertbar als solches aus Heu gleicher Herkunft. Vom Verdauungskanal her wird Mn nur in geringem Umfang resorbiert und großenteils über Galle und Kot wieder ausgeschieden, so daß der Blutplasma-Mn-Spiegel auf 0,1–0,2 µmol/l gehalten wird. Die tägliche Mn-Retention beträgt beim erwachsenen Rind nur ~ 150 mg. Speicherorgane sind Leber (normaler Mn-Gehalt > 10 ppm TM), Pankreas, Nieren, Knochen und Haare. Wie andere Spurenelemente ist Mn in einigen Enzymen enthalten oder für deren Aktivierung verantwortlich. So ist ausreichende Mn-Versorgung Voraussetzung für normales Knochenwachstum (Bildung der Knochenmatrix, Synthese saurer Mukopolysaccharide); außerdem ist Mn mitverantwortlich für Entwicklung und Funktionstüchtigkeit der weiblichen und männlichen Geschlechtsorgane.

Symptome: Folgende, meist m. o. w. bestandsweise gehäuft, bei unverändert bleibender Fütterung zudem alljährlich erneut auftretende Krankheitsbilder werden als mögliche Folgen primär oder sekundär unzureichender Mn-Versorgung angesehen; ihre Pathogenese ist jedoch vermutlich nicht einheitlich: Bei *geschlechtsreifen Tieren* werden stille oder ausbleibende Brunst bzw. verminderte Spermaqualität, außerdem bräunliche Verfärbung der Spitzen schwarzpigmentierter Haare beschrieben; in schweren Fällen treten bei ihnen vermehrt lebensschwach geborene Kälber, Frühgeburten oder Aborte auf; außerdem wird das Geschlechtsverhältnis der neugeborenen Kälber u. U. zugunsten der männlichen verschoben. *Jungtiere* zeigen außer Entwicklungshemmung und rauh-trockenem, entfärbtem Haarkleid z. T. auch verzögerte Geschlechtsreife und/oder Zungenspielen; die Aktivität ihrer alkalischen Serumphosphatase ist vermindert. *Neugeborene Kälber* extrem Mn-arm sowie silagereich ernährter Mütter sind klein, lebensschwach und weisen m. o. w. starke Verkrümmungen der auffallend kurzen Beine (z. T. auch Einwärtsdrehung vom verdickten Karpus und/oder Tarsus an abwärts) auf; die Bewegungsfähigkeit proximaler Gliedmaßengelenke kann eingeschränkt sein; diejenige distaler Gelenke ist vielfach abnorm vermehrt. Manche Kälber sind infolge Nachhandparese unfähig zu stehen, zeigen kuppelartige Auftreibung der Stirn und/oder Verkürzung von Unter- oder Oberkiefer. Vermutungen, daß angeborene Spinalstenose (Kap. 10.1.2.6) oder Steilstellung und Spastische Parese der Hinterbeine (Kap. 9.8.3) auf Mn-Mangel beruhen, sind bislang noch nicht erwiesen.

■ **Sektion:** Die Zerlegung ergibt nur bei den mißgebildeten *Kälbern* krankhafte Befunde: Nichtproportionierter chondrodystrophischer Zwergwuchs mit verdickten Gliedmaßengelenken und Verkürzung der langen Röhrenknochen, die u. U. schon bei der halben bis einem Drittel der sonst hierfür erforderlichen Belastung brechen; der Höhendurchmesser des Wirbelkanals kann eingeengt und die Schädelhöhle verkürzt sein.

■ **Histologische Befunde:** In den metaphysären Wachstumsscheiben der langen Röhrenknochen und Wirbel sind die Chondrozytenreihen unregelmäßiger angeordnet und kürzer, die Zahl voll hypertrophierter Chondrozyten geringer als bei gesunden Vergleichstieren; im hyalinen Knorpel solcher Kälber ist der Mukopolysaccharidgehalt vermindert. In mit Stenose des Wirbelkanals einhergehenden Fällen ist vorzeitiger herdförmiger Schluß der metaphysären Wachstumsplatten festzustellen.

■ **Diagnose:** Klinisches Bild sowie Überprüfung der Fütterung lenken den Verdacht auf Mn-Mangel. Aus Futteranalysen sind allerdings oft keine brauchbaren Rückschlüsse zu ziehen, weil dabei auch der hemmende Einfluß anderer Nahrungsbestandteile berücksichtigt werden müßte (s. *Pathogenese*). Organproben Mn-normal und Mn-arm gefütterter Rinder unterscheiden sich in ihrem Mn-Gehalt nur geringfügig voneinander. Auch der Mn-Gehalt der pigmentierten Haare gestattet nach heutiger Ansicht keinen sicheren Rückschluß auf die Mn-Versorgung während der voraufgegangenen Fütterungsperiode (Gelfert & Staufenbiel, 1998).

Differentialdiagnostisch kommen bei *Kälbern* mit verkrümmten und/oder abnorm beweglichen Gliedmaßen erblich veranlagter dysproportionierter chondrodystrophischer Zwergwuchs (Kap. 9.10.7.2), angeborene übermäßige Beweglichkeit der Gelenke (Kap. 9.10.13), Neuromyodysplastische Arthrogrypose (Kap. 9.10.4), Akabane-Disease (Kap. 9.10.8), »Crooked Calf Disease« (Kap. 9.10.5), Osteogenesis imperfecta (Kap. 9.10.10) und Osteopetrose (Kap. 9.10.11) in Betracht. Bei *Jungtieren* ist an Rachitis (Kap. 9.17.4), chronische Bleivergiftung (Kap. 10.5.12) und Kupfermangel (Kap. 12.3.11), bei *erwachsenen Rindern* zunächst an andersbedingte Fruchtbarkeitsstörungen zu denken. Ansprechen des Krankheitsbildes auf Mn-Zulagen spricht für Vorliegen einer Mn-Unterversorgung.

■ **Prophylaxe:** Zur Vermeidung von Mangelerscheinungen gilt ein Mn-Gehalt der Gesamtration von 40 ppm TM als ausreichend. Das kann erforderlichenfalls durch Kraftfutterzulagen erzielt werden. Auf bestimmten Weiden soll die Fruchtbarkeit allerdings selbst bei einem Mn-Gehalt des Grases von 80 ppm TM nicht befriedigend sein.

■ **Behandlung:** Reversible Mn-Mangelerscheinungen lassen sich durch Zulagen von Mn-Sulfat beheben (*Kälber* 0,5–1,0 g, *Jungrinder* und *erwachsene Tiere* 2–4 g/Tag p. o.); das Anbieten einer mit 6 g Mn/kg angereicherten Mineralsalzmischung ist ebenfalls wirksam. Dagegen hat sich das Düngen Mn-armer Weiden mit Mn-haltigem Kunstdünger nicht bewährt.

➤ *Manganvergiftung:* Bis zu 3monatige Aufnahme extremer Mn-Mengen (> 800–5000 ppm TM der Ration) bedingt bei Kälbern lediglich Verminderung von Freßlust und LM-Zunahme, u. U. auch Reduktion des Hb-Gehalts im Blut; dabei werden Zellulose-, Eisen-, Kobalt- und Zinkverwertung beeinträchtigt sowie der Mn-Gehalt des Blutplasmas auf > 20 µmol/l und derjenige der Leber auf 10–1800 ppm angehoben. Ähnliche, aber mit Ikterus und Cholangiohepatitis verbundene Symptome wurden in Südafrika bei Kälbern beobachtet, die zuvor beim Beweiden Fe-armer/Mn-reicher Böden auffallende Geophagie gezeigt hatten. Bei Kühen soll ein Mn-Gehalt des Futters von ≥ 80 ppm sekundären Zn-Mangel (Kap. 2.2.5.4) auslösen.

12.3.11 Kupfermangel

Ch. Laiblin/M. Stöber

■ **Definition, Ursachen:** Bei der vorwiegend während des Weideganges, im Falle alleiniger Verabreichung betriebseigenen Futters jedoch auch während der Stallhaltung auftretenden unzureichenden Versorgung mit Kupfer ist zwischen *primärer* (= einfacher) und *sekundärer* (d. h. durch andere Faktoren [mit]bedingter) *Hypokuprose* zu unterscheiden (Übersicht 12-2). Erstere wird durch absolut unzulängliches Cu-Angebot in Grünfutter, Silage und Heu ausgelöst, welche von Böden mit niedrigem Cu-Gehalt oder geringer Cu-Verfügbarkeit stammen. Letztere ist dagegen auf die Cu-antagonistische Wirkung von in der Nahrung oder Tränke enthaltenem Molybdän (Kap. 12.3.12), Schwefel (Kap. 10.5.14) und/oder Eisen zurückzuführen. Auch weitere alimentäre Faktoren (Gehalt des Futters an Zink, Kadmium, Blei oder Kalziumkarbonat) oder anderweitige Erkrankungen können die Verwertung des mit der Nahrung aufgenommenen Cu behindern. Gefahr für das Auftreten sekundärer

Hypokuprose besteht v.a. dann, wenn die Ration eine Cu:Molybdän-Relation von ≤ 2–3 oder > 3 g Schwefel/kg TM aufweist. Massive Aufnahme von Eisen (> 350 mg Fe/kg FTM) infolge Mitfressens von Erde bedingt ebenfalls eine Zunahme des Cu-Bedarfs.

Pathogenese: Cu aus frischem Grünfutter ist i.d.R. schlechter verfügbar als solches aus Heu und faserarmem Futter, wie Getreide und Brassikazeen. Am schlechtesten verfügbar ist das in Silage enthaltene Cu. Die Fähigkeit zur Verwertung des Nahrungs-Cu ist beim Rind weniger stark erblich verankert als beim Schaf; immerhin zeigen Angus-Rinder eine höhere Fähigkeit zur Cu-Absorption als Charolais- oder Simmentaler Vieh. Bei Wiederkäuern ist ausreichende Cu-Versorgung Voraussetzung für den normalen Ablauf wichtiger, enzymgesteuerter Lebensvorgänge: Einbau von Eisen in das Hämoglobin, Färbung und Verhornung der Haare, Myelinisierung der Nervenscheiden, Osteoblastentätigkeit im Skelett sowie Funktion des Elastin- und Kollagenstoffwechsels mit Auswirkungen auf quergestreifte Muskulatur, Gefäßwände und Darmepithel. Die bei Cu-Mangel zu erwartenden Ausfallserscheinungen umfassen daher Blutarmut, Pigment- und Strukturverlust des Haarkleids, Ataxie, abnorme Knochenentwicklung, Atrophie und Fibrose von Herz- und Skelettmuskulatur, Gefäßrupturen sowie Diarrhoe. Aus Neuseeland wird über das Auftreten einer offensichtlich mit Hypokuprose in Zusammenhang stehenden puerperalen Hämoglobinurie (Kap. 4.3.5.5) berichtet. Schließlich soll Cu-Mangel auch die Entwicklung der auf übermäßiger Schwefelaufnahme beruhenden Hirnrindennekrose (Kap. 10.5.5, 10.5.14) fördern. Der früher als unmittelbare Folge des Cu-Mangels angesehene »Weide«-Durchfall ist nach heutigem Wissen Auswirkung eines relativen oder absoluten Molybdänüberschusses (Kap. 12.3.12). Dabei behindern die in den Vormägen entstehenden Tri- und Tetra-Thiomolybdenate infolge Bildung von Cu-Komplexen die intestinale Absorption von Cu, während ins Blut gelangte und an Serumalbumin gebundene Di- und Tri-Thiomolybdate den intermediären Cu-Stoffwechsel, insbesondere einige Cu-haltige Enzyme (Übersicht 12-3) hemmen. Entsprechend dem Cu-, Mo-, S- und Fe-Gehalt der Nahrung führt dieses Zusammenwirken mit der Zeit zur Entleerung des Cu-Vorrats der Leber und erst später zu klinischer Hypokuprose.

Vorkommen: Der in vielen Ländern ökonomisch bedeutsame Cu-Mangel ist i.d.R. an ausgesprochen Cu-arme Böden (ausgewaschener diluvialer Sand,

Übersicht 12-2 Beurteilung des Kupfer- und Molybdängehalts im Futter bei Verdacht auf primären oder sekundären Kupfermangel⁺

Hypokuprose	unwahrscheinlich	möglich	sicher
Primärer Kupfermangel (bei normalem Mo-Gehalt der Nahrung von < 2–5 ppm):	> 10 ppm Cu	5–10 ppm Cu	< 3–5 ppm Cu
*Sekundärer Kupfermangel** (bei knappem bis normalem Cu-Gehalt der Nahrung von 5–25 ppm):	< 2–5 ppm Mo	5–10 ppm Mo**	> 10 ppm Mo***

⁺ Das Cu:Mo-Mengenverhältnis der Ration sollte ≥ 2 betragen. * Der Cu-antagonistische Effekt des Molybdäns wirkt sich v.a. bei einem Sulfatschwefelgehalt des Futters von > 0,3 % TM aus. ** Bei knapper Kupferversorgung ist dieser Molybdängehalt der Nahrung bereits gefährlich. *** Solche Molybdänkonzentrationen sind nur bei überreichlichem Kupferangebot unschädlich.

Übersicht 12-3 Wirkungsweise und Wirkungsort kupferabhängiger Enzyme

Enzym	Wirkungsweise	Wirkungsort
Zytochrom-c-Oxidase:	Zellatmungsenzym	Mitochondrien
Dopamin-β-Hydroxylase:	Biosynthese und Abbau der Katecholamine	Nebennieren, Nervensystem
Lysiloxidase:	Elastin-Kollagen-Vernetzung (Desaminierung von Lysin und Hydroxylysin)	Bindegewebe (Knochen, Muskel, Gefäßsystem, Lunge)
Superoxid-Dismutase:	antioxidativ (Dismutation von Superoxid-Anionen)	Zytosol aller sauerstoffverbrauchenden Zellen
Zäruloplasmin:	Kupferbindung, Oxidation von Fe^{II} zu Fe^{III}	Blut/Plasma, retikuloendotheliales System, Leber
Tyrosinase:	Pigmentation, Keratinisierung	Haut, Haare

alkalischer Schlicklehm, Flächen mit hohem Grundwasserpegel oder Überschwemmungsland) gebunden. Gleichartige Krankheitsbilder treten aber auch in Gebieten auf, in denen Cu im Erdreich (Torf, Sumpf, Moor) zwar in ausreichender Menge vorhanden, dort aber komplex gebunden und deshalb nicht in genügendem Umfang für die Vegetation verfügbar ist; solche Böden sind oft molybdänreich. Betroffen werden weidende Rinder der Fleischrassen, insbesondere die bei Fuß gehenden Kälber, da der Cu-Gehalt der Milch ihren Bedarf schon bei ausreichender Cu-Versorgung der Mütter nicht voll deckt. Mit Mähgras gefüttertes Milchvieh kann ebenfalls erkranken. Das Leiden häuft sich meist im Frühjahr und Sommer, wenn der Cu-Gehalt des Grases am niedrigsten ist.

Örtlich sind folgende Cu-Mangelsyndrome bekannt: »falling disease« oder »sudden death« (Australien) und »enzootische Kälberataxie« (Neuseeland) als *primäre Hypokuprosen,* »peat scours« und »reclaim disease« (Irland, Neuseeland, Kalifornien, Kanada) sowie »pine« der Kälber (Schottland) als *sekundäre Cu-Mangelsyndrome.* Bei der im Nordseeküstenbereich beobachteten »Lecksucht«, der »coast disease« (Australien) und der »salt sickness« (Florida) handelt es sich dagegen um *kombinierten Mangel an Cu und Kobalt* (Kap. 4.3.5.2). Die im Vereinigten Königreich vorkommende »Teart«-Krankheit ist eine bei normalem Cu-Gehalt der Nahrung auftretende *Molybdänose* (Kap. 12.3.12). Die Anfälligkeit des Rindes gegenüber unzureichender Cu-Versorgung nimmt vom Kälber- zum Erwachsenenalter ab, da der Cu-Bedarf während des Wachstums besonders hoch ist. Gefährdet sind aber auch trächtige Tiere, weil die Cu-Versorgung des Fetus Vorrang vor derjenigen des Muttertieres hat; so kann der Leber-Cu-Gehalt des Feten das Zehnfache desjenigen der betreffenden Kuh erreichen. Als Folge der auf Cu-Mangelstandorten und auf Mo-belasteten Böden üblichen Schutzmaßnahmen (s. *Prophylaxe*) ist klinisch manifester Cu-Mangel beim Rind heute im Abnehmen begriffen.

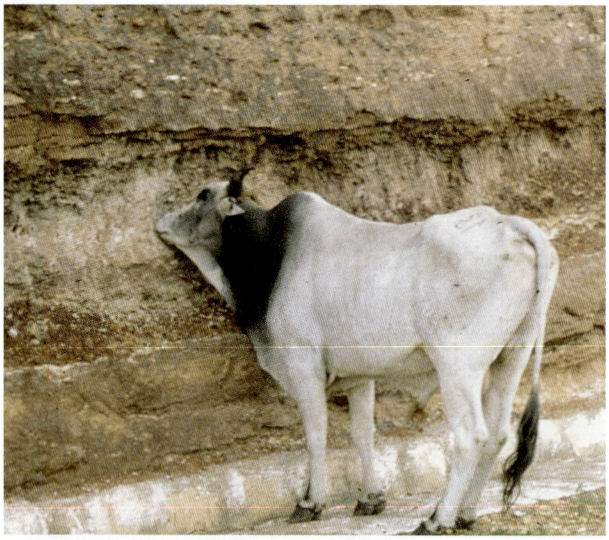

Abbildung 12-45 Kupfermangel: Infolge mangelhafter Kupferversorgung erdefressende Kuh (Brasilien; Tokarnia, 1986)

Symptome, Verlauf: An *primärer Hypokuprose* leidende Wiederkäuer haben wechselnde bis mangelhafte Freßlust; nicht selten sind auch Lecksuchtsymptome (Kap. 10.6.1.1), insbesondere Erdefressen, zu beobachten (Abb. 12-45). Hypokuprotische Kälber und Jungrinder zeigen z. T. steif-stelzenden Gang mit steiler Fesselung und/oder Auftreibungen der distalen metatarsalen und -karpalen Epiphysenfugen (»Blockgelenke«, »gehäuft auftretende Epiphysitis«). Zudem können Lahmheiten oder Frakturen im Extremitätenbereich und/oder vorübergehende Ataxie der Nachhand mit plötzlichem Niederstürzen oder Verharren in hundesitziger Stellung beobachtet werden. In schweren Fällen kommt es zu Apathie und bis zur Kachexie fortschreitender Entkräftung. Erwachsene Patienten entwickeln bei anhaltendem Cu-Mangel eine m. o. w. ausgeprägte hypochrome makrozytäre Anämie. Bei Kranken aller Altersstufen setzt daneben, v. a. im Herbst, gelegentlich Durchfall ein; er ist aber i. d. R. nicht so schwerwiegend und anhaltend wie bei Molybdänose (Kap. 12.3.12) oder sekundärem Cu-Mangel.

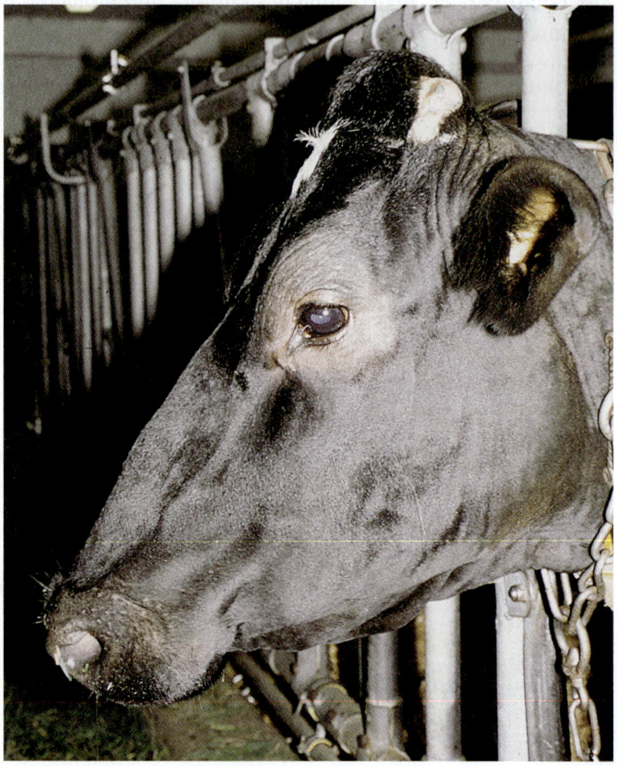

Abbildung 12-46 Ausbleichung des Haarkleids bei sekundärer Hypokuprose

Patienten mit *Mo-bedingtem sekundärem Kupfermangel* bleiben im Entwicklungs- und Nährzustand zurück; Kälber und Jungrinder kümmern; erwachsene Tiere magern ab. Kühe weisen zudem eine bezüglich Menge und Fettgehalt unbefriedigende Milchleistung auf. Die Fruchtbarkeit von Mo-bedingt hypokuprotischen weiblichen und männlichen Rindern kann beeinträchtigt sein, wofür offenbar mehr der Mo-Überschuß als der sekundäre Cu-Mangel entscheidend ist. Auffallend ist mitunter die brillenartig rings um Augen und Flotzmaul einsetzende und später auch auf Backen, Hals, Rücken, Seitenbrust sowie Vorderbeine übergreifende Ausbleichung der Haarfarbe (schwarz → braun- oder mausgrau; rot → fahlgelb: symmetrische Hypochromotrichie; Abb. 12-46). Dabei wird das Haarkleid zudem stumpf-rauh und sein sommerlicher Wechsel verzögert; mitunter besteht auch Juckreiz der Haut (Belecken). Sekundärer Cu-Mangel wird, im Gegensatz zur primären Hypokuprose, oft nicht von Anämie begleitet. Bei Kälbern und Jungrindern schwächt die Abnahme der B-Lymphozytenpopulation die zellvermittelte Infektabwehr.

Die *örtlich unter eigenen Namen bekannten Kupfermangelkrankheiten* zeichnen sich durch folgende Symptome aus:

➤ *»Falling disease«* ist das Endstadium schwerer primärer Hypokuprose und wird v. a. bei laktierenden sowie hochtragenden Kühen, seltener auch bei Bullen, aber nie bei unter 12 Monate alten Rindern beobachtet. Betroffene Tiere werfen aus scheinbar ungestörter Gesundheit heraus, vielfach kurz vor, während oder nach dem Melken oder Treiben, plötzlich den Kopf auf, brüllen laut und stürzen nieder, um sofort oder nach nur wenige Minuten dauernden Laufbewegungen der Gliedmaßen oder Aufstehversuchen und erneutem Brüllen zu verenden (»sudden death«). Ausnahmsweise kann der geschilderte Zustand ≤ 24 h lang anhalten. Solche Patienten senken, nachdem sie wieder auf die Beine gelangt sind, periodisch wiederkehrend den Kopf und drehen sich infolge Inkoordination der Nachhand um die Achse ihrer Vordergliedmaßen; der Tod tritt meist während eines solchen Anfalls ein.

➤ *»Enzootische Kälberataxie«* ähnelt der ebenfalls auf primärem Cu-Mangel beruhenden enzootischen Ataxie der Lämmer, ist aber wesentlich seltener. Nach körperlicher Anstrengung (Treiben) werden die Bewegungen der Hinterhand plötzlich inkoordiniert, so daß die Patienten umfallen oder in hundesitziger Stellung verharren; nach einiger Ruhezeit ist ihr Gang dann wieder normal.

➤ *»Peat scours«* (= Torfdurchfall), eine sekundäre Hypokuprose, gibt sich durch 8–10 Tage nach Weideauftrieb einsetzenden gelblich-grünen bis schwärzlichen, oft auch übelriechenden wäßrig-blasenhaltigen Durchfall zu erkennen; dabei erfolgt der Kotabsatz ohne Drängen und i. d. R. auch ohne Anheben des Schwanzes. In der Folge magern die Kranken dann trotz guter Freßlust unter zunehmender Entkräftung rasch ab.

➤ *»Pine«* (= Dahinsiechen) ist eine weitere Form sekundären Kupfermangels: Betroffene Kälber kümmern, ohne anämisch zu werden, und zeigen, besonders auf der Nachhand, steifstelzenden bis lahmenden Gang; die Gliedmaßenepiphysen sind druckempfindlich. Das Haarkleid erscheint gebleicht; zudem besteht zeitweilig Durchfall. Schwere Erkrankung führt innerhalb von 4–5 Monaten zu Kachexie und Tod.

■ **Sektion:** Bei der Zerlegung von an Cu-Mangel verendeten Rindern sind, abgesehen von der Hypochromotrichie und je nach Schwerpunkt der Erkrankung, bestimmte kennzeichnende Befunde, mitunter aber keine Abweichungen von der Norm zu erheben:

➤ *»Falling disease«:* Venöse Blutfülle, Bauchhöhlenflüssigkeit gelegentlich vermehrt, Leber und Milz relativ groß, Kongestion von Labmagen und Darm, Herz meist groß, schlaff und blaß, Myokard dünnwandig und mit helleren Streifen durchsetzt; *histologisch:* Atrophie, Degeneration und progressive Fibrose des Herzmuskels, Glomerulonephritis sowie Hämosiderose in Leber, Milz und Nieren.

➤ *»Enzootische Kälberataxie«:* In ausgeprägten Fällen Hirnödem und Mikrokavitation mit *histologisch* erkennbarem Myelinschwund und vakuolärer Neuronendegeneration.

➤ Das *Skelett* Cu-arm aufgezogener Kälber zeigt Verbreiterung der metatarsalen und -karpalen Epiphysenfugenknorpel mit Verdickung des distalen Diaphysenendes; solche Fugenknorpel weisen *histologisch* neben aktiven Osteoblasten Zungen unverkalkten Knochens mit verzögerter oder gestörter Primärkalzifikation auf.

■ **Diagnose:** Da die geschilderten klinischen Erscheinungen und Zerlegungsbefunde für eine sichere Erkennung des Cu-Mangels sowie seine Einstufung als primäre oder sekundäre Hypokuprose oft nicht ausreichen, sind möglichst auch Cu- und Mo-Bestimmungen an Futter- und Blutproben vorzunehmen (Übersicht 12-2, 12-4, 12-5). Für letztere sind mindestens 10 % der Herdenmitglieder, und zwar bevorzugt tragende Kalbinnen, bei Mutterkuhhaltung auch kälberführende Kühe sowie deren weidende Nachzucht heranzuziehen. Einzeltieruntersuchungen sind nicht sinnvoll, da ihre Resultate großen individuel-len Schwankungen unterliegen. Auf Cu zu untersuchende Blutproben sind mit Heparin (nicht mit Ca-EDTA oder Oxalat) zu versetzen; ihr Plasma sollte möglichst schon vor dem Versand abzentrifu-

Übersicht 12-4 Beurteilung des Kupfergehalts von Körperflüssigkeiten und Gewebeproben bei Verdacht auf Kupfermangel

Probenmaterial	normaler Kupfergehalt	primäre Hypokuprose*	sekundäre Hypokuprose*
Blutplasma**			
(mg/l):	0,8–1,2	< 0,2	< 0,7
(µmol/l):	12–20	< 3	< 9
Leber***			
(ppm TM):	> 30–350	1,5	5–20
(µmol/kg TM):	> 0,5–5,5	0,02–0,08	0,08–0,3
Milch+ (mg/l):	0,05–0,20	0,01–0,02	–
Haar++ (ppm TM):	6,6–10,4	1,8–3,4	5,5

* Bezüglich dieser Definitionen siehe Übersicht 12-2. ** Bei Entnahme der Blutproben sind Cu-Verunreinigungen (über Kanüle oder Gefäß) zu vermeiden; auch ist zu berücksichtigen, daß der Blut-Cu-Spiegel trotz knappen Cu-Gehalts der Leber noch oder wieder im Normalbereich liegen kann und erst nach völliger Erschöpfung der Cu-Reserven der Leber deutlich absinkt; zudem kann der Blut-Cu-Gehalt bei anderweitiger Erkrankung (Parasitosen, Leberleiden, Unterernährung) vermindert sein, ohne daß echte Hypokuprose vorliegt. *** Der Cu-Gehalt der Leber sollte v. a. während der Trächtigkeit mindestens 30 ppm TS betragen, um die Cu-Versorgung des Fetus zu sichern und die Anlage fetaler Cu-Reserven zu ermöglichen; neugeborene Kälber weisen (auf Kosten ihrer Mütter) einen relativ hohen Leber-Cu-Gehalt (> 300 ppm) auf. + Rindermilch ist als alleinige Cu-Quelle für Kälber auf Dauer unzureichend; Kälber nehmen mit der Milch ihrer Mütter auch Molybdän auf, wenn deren Futter Mo-reich ist. ++ Der Cu-Gehalt des Haares eignet sich zur Ermittlung langfristig bestehender Cu-Mangelzustände; unpigmentiertes Haar enthält 1–2 ppm Cu weniger als pigmentiertes. N. B.: Die Aktivität des *Plasma-Zäruloplasmins* und diejenige der *erythrozytären Kupferoxid-Dismutase* betragen beim Rind normalerweise > 40 U/l bzw. ~ 400 U/g Hb; bei ausgeprägtem Cu-Mangel sinken sie auf < 5 U/l bzw. < 250 U/g Hb ab.

giert werden. Bei Beurteilung der Resultate ist zu bedenken, daß Hypokuprämie oft nicht gleichbedeutend mit unzureichender Cu-Versorgung oder klinischer Hypokuprose ist, weil der Cu-Gehalt des Blutes von anderen Krankheiten beeinflußt sein kann.

Zuverlässige Auskunft über den Cu-Status ergibt der Cu-Gehalt der Leber. Da hierfür Gewebemengen von ~ 5 g erforderlich sind, werden solche Proben meist an Schlachttieren entnommen. Ein Leber-Cu-Gehalt von < 30 mg/kg TM weist auf hochgradige Hypokuprose hin. N. B.: Die Cu-Speicherung in der Leber des Feten bedingt es, daß die Leber-Cu-Werte von Kühen während des letzten Drittels der Trächtigkeit und des ersten Monats der Laktation immer unter dem Herdendurchschnitt liegen. Diagnostische Hinweise ergeben sich auch aus der verminderten Aktivität kupferhaltiger Enzyme (erythrozytäre Superoxid-Dismutase [Vollblut], Zäruloplasmin [Plasma]; Übersicht 12-4).

Differentialdiagnostisch sind im Hinblick auf Cu-mangelbedingte *Diarrhoe* v. a. Molybdänose (Kap. 12.3.12), Magendarmwurmbefall (Kap. 6.11.2), Kokzidiose (Kap. 6.11.5) und infektiös bedingte Enteritiden, bezüglich der *Entfärbung des Haarkleids* dagegen Kobalt- und Zinkmangel (Kap. 4.3.5.2, 2.2.5.4), bei *Skelettbeteiligung* jedoch Rachitis (Kap. 9.17.4) sowie chronische Bleivergiftung (Kap. 10.5.12), bei *zentralnervöser Bewegungsstörung* aber erblich bedingte Ataxien der Nachhand (Kap. 10.1.3) und bei *Herzmuskelschädigung* (»falling disease«) hereditäre Kardiomyopathie (Kap. 4.1.1.7) zu berücksichtigen.

Beurteilung: Abgesehen von Patienten mit fortgeschrittener Schädigung des Herzmuskel-, Nerven- oder Knochengewebes ist die Behandlung diagnostisch gesicherter *primärer* Hypokuprose aussichtsreich; bei *sekundärem Cu-Mangel* sind die durch Cu-Zulagen zu erzielenden Resultate vom Ausmaß der Mo- und S-Zufuhr abhängig. Vor unbegründeter oder zu reichlicher therapeutischer oder prophylaktischer Gabe von Cu-Salzen ist wegen der Gefahr einer Intoxikation zu warnen; letztere äußert sich bei akuter oraler Cu-Vergiftung als Gastroenteritis (Kap. 6.12.8), bei kumulativ-»chronischer« oraler Cu-Überdosierung als hämolytische Anämie, nach übermäßiger parenteraler Cu-Gabe dagegen als hepatogene Enzephalopathie (Kap. 10.5.8).

Behandlung: Der Cu-Bedarf ist als gedeckt anzusehen, wenn die Gesamtration für Kälber 4 mg Cu/kg TM, diejenige für Kühe 10 mg Cu/kg TM, aber keine Cu-antagonistisch wirksamen Mo-, S- oder Fe-Mengen enthält. Bei *primärem Cu-Mangel* sind therapeutisch über einige Wochen hinweg orale Gaben von täglich 1 g Cu-Sulfat/Jungrind bzw. 2 g Cu-Sulfat/erwachsenes Tier, oder solche von wöchentlich 2 bzw. 4 g Cu-Sulfat pro Jungrind bzw. erwachsenes Tier angezeigt. Ähnlich wirksam sind Salzlecksteine, die entsprechend dem Grad des vorliegenden Cu-Mangels 1–5% Cu-Sulfat enthalten. Technisch schwieriger ist die Dosierung einer Cu-Zulage (2–3 mg/l)* über das Tränkewasser. Bei der Behand-

* 1 g Cu ist in 3,93 g $CuSO_4 \cdot 5\, H_2O$ enthalten.

lung von *sekundärem Kupfermangel* sind futtereigene Inhaltsstoffe zu berücksichtigen, welche die Verfügbarkeit des aufgenommenen Cu behindern.

Prophylaxe: Milchaustauscher für Kälber sollten 6 ppm TM Cu enthalten. Zur Depotprophylaxe der Hypokuprose sind verschiedene p. o. einzugebende, im Netzmagen kontinuierlich Cu (z. T. auch Kobalt oder Selen) freisetzende Cu-Oxid-Nadeln und Cu-in-Glas-Boli geeignet. Einige subkutan zu injizierende Cu-Komplex-Präparationen (Cu-Ca-Versenat, Cu-DEA-Oxychinolinsulfonat, Cu-Glyzinat) werden in angelsächsischen Ländern erfolgreich angewandt, sind in Deutschland aber z. Zt. nicht zugelassen. In Cu-Mangel-Gebieten wird diese Art der Cu-Bevorratung bei erwachsenen Rindern im 6./7. Monat der Trächtigkeit sowie nach dem Kalben, bei Kälbern nach dem Absetzen und nach weiteren 6 Monaten angewandt, falls die Fütterung nur aus Weidegang oder anderem betriebseigenem Pflanzengut besteht. Die Schutzwirkung der oralen oder subkutanen Depots hält ~ 6 Monate lang vor.

Bei Vorliegen von Cu-Antagonismen (hoher S- oder Mo-Gehalt des Futters) müssen anorganische Cu-Verbindungen u. U. in Dosen angeboten werden, die das Doppelte des normalen Bedarfs erreichen. Komplexresistente organische Verbindungen, wie Cu-Methionat und Cu-Lysin, werden dagegen kaum antagonistisch beeinflußt. Der Cu-Gehalt von Cu-Mangelböden kann durch Aufbringen Cu-haltigen Kunstdüngers (oder von Schweinegülle) aufgebessert werden; vor dem Beweiden solcher Flächen oder dem Ernten dort heranwachsender Pflanzen müssen jedoch ausgiebige Regenfälle abgewartet werden, um Cu-Vergiftungen (Kap. 4.3.5.9) zu verhüten. Enthält das Tränkwasser (Bohrbrunnen) zuviel Sulfatschwefel, so läßt es sich durch Filtern entschwefeln.

12.3.12 Molybdänvergiftung

Ch. Laiblin/M. Stöber

Definition: Durch übermäßige orale Aufnahme von Molybdän ausgelöster *sekundärer Kupfermangel*, dessen Krankheitsbild sich von demjenigen der primären Hypokuprose (Kap. 12.3.11) meist durch stärker ausgeprägten, anhaltenden Durchfall sowie das Ausbleiben von schwerer Anämie unterscheidet. *Andere Bezeichnungen:* Molybdänose, peat scours, teart, malmagliar.

Vorkommen, Ursachen: Das v. a. Kälber und Jungrinder, mitunter zudem auch Kühe betreffende Leiden wird bei Weidegang auf natürlicherweise Mo-reichen und teilweise auch Cu-armen Böden beobachtet (Moor-, Porphyr-, Granit- und Schieferstandorte, Abfluß-, Sicker- sowie Überschwemmungsgebiete größerer Flüsse und Seen mit hohem Grundwasserspiegel im Vereinigten Königreich, in Irland, den USA, Kanada, Australien und Neuseeland). Das von solchen Grünflächen gewonnene Heu ist weniger gefährlich, weil Mo beim Trocknen des Grases in schlechtlösliche Verbindungen überführt wird. Des weiteren kommt Molybdänose in der Umgebung von Berg- und Legierungswerken, Porzellan- und Farbenfabriken sowie Ölraffinerien vor, die Mo-haltigen Rauch ausstoßen oder Mo-kontaminiertes Abwasser bzw. Öl in die Umwelt entlassen. Entsprechendes gilt für übermäßiges Ausbringen von Mo-haltigem Kunstdünger, Verunreinigungen mit Mo-Sulfid enthaltendem Motorenöl, versehentliches Einmischen von Na-Molybdat in die Ration oder Verwendung Mo-haltiger Flugasche bei weidenahem Straßenbau.

Pathogenese: Wiederkäuer, insbesondere Rinder, sind gegenüber Mo wesentlich empfindlicher als andere Nutztiere. In ihren Vormägen bilden sich aus Molybdaten und den bei der Reduktion S-haltiger Substanzen anfallenden Sulfiden unter mikrobiellem Einfluß Thiomolybdate. Diese behindern durch Komplexbildung die intestinale Resorption von Cu und den intermediären Cu-Stoffwechsel. Gegebenenfalls sinkt der Cu-Gehalt des Lebergewebes von normaliter > 100 ppm auf < 30 ppm FS ab, während sein Mo-Gehalt zunimmt. Somit wird bodenständige Molybdänose durch das Zusammentreffen von hohem Mo-Gehalt des Erdreichs oder von Mo-Verschmutzung der Grünflächen mit knapper Cu-Zufuhr (< 10 ppm FTM) und/oder übermäßiger Aufnahme von Sulfatschwefel (> 3 g/kg FTM) bedingt.

Symptome, Verlauf: Bei weiblichen Rindern wird die Fruchtbarkeit schon im subklinischen Vorstadium der Molybdänose beeinträchtigt (→ verspätete Geschlechtsreife, Stillbrunst, Umrindern); bei männlichen Tieren sind Libido und Spermatogenese vermindert. In manifesten Fällen kommt es zudem 1–2 Wochen nach Weideauftrieb zu anhaltender, durch gasblasenhaltigen flüssigen Kot gekennzeichneter Diarrhoe. Der Durchfall bedingt Wachstumsverzögerung und Abmagerung, bei Kühen auch Milchrückgang; bei Kälbern sind humorale und zellgebundene Immunantwort reduziert. Anhaltende Mo-Exposition führt schließlich zur Entfärbung des rauh und matt werdenden Haarkleids infolge sekundären Cu-Mangels (Kap. 12.3.11) sowie zu gelenkschmerzbedingter Lahmheit; Jungtiere zeigen dabei Auftreibungen der distalen Epiphysenfugen an Metakarpus und Metatarsus (»Blockgelenke«). Nur bei schwerer, industriell bedingter Molybdänose kommt es infolge Knochenmarkschädigung auch zu hypoplastischer Anämie, die Festliegen und tödlichen Ausgang nach sich ziehen kann.

Sektion: Bis auf m. o. w. ausgeprägte Abmagerung, mitunter auch Anämie, sind die Zerlegungsbefunde nach *chronischem* Krankheitsverlauf wenig aussagekräftig. Makro- und mikroskopisch finden sich keine Hinweise auf Darmentzündung. Jungtiere zeigen *histologisch* mitunter Osteoporose sowie unverkalkte »Zungen« innerhalb der obenerwähnten Epiphysenfugen. In *akut* tödlich verlaufenen Fällen sind periazinäre bis diffuse Lebernekrosen und tubuläre Nierennekrosen festzustellen.

Diagnose: Klinisches Bild sowie das an Gebiete mit bekanntermaßen hohem Mo-Gehalt des Bodens oder an die Nachbarschaft zu Mo-ausstoßenden Anlagen gebundene Auftreten des Leidens gestatten die Vermutung eines Mo-bedingten sekundären Cu-Mangels. Günstige Auswirkungen oraler Cu-Zulagen (1–2 g Cu-Sulfat pro Jungrind bzw. Kuh und Tag oder 3 bzw. 5 g Cu-Sulfat pro Woche) werden zwar als Bestätigung für das Vorliegen von Hypokuprose angesehen; ein Beweis für gefährlich hohe Mo- sowie normale oder unzulägliche Cu-Zufuhr ist jedoch nur über Futteranalysen zu erlangen (Übersicht 12-2 und 12-5; s. auch Kupfermangel, Kap. 12.3.11); in fraglichen Fällen ist sinnvollerweise auch der Schwefelgehalt von Nahrung und Tränke (Kap. 10.5.14) zu berücksichtigen.

Differentialdiagnostisch sind primärer Cu-Mangel (Kap. 12.3.11), Magendarmwurmbefall (Kap. 6.11.2), Paratuberkulose (Kap. 6.10.22), Rachitis (Kap. 9.17.4) und chronische Bleivergiftung (Kap. 10.5.12) in Betracht zu ziehen.

Beurteilung: Bei Unterbindung der Mo-Aufnahme und/oder Steigerung der Cu-Zufuhr ist mit rascher Behebung des Durchfalls und allmählichem Verschwinden der übrigen Erscheinungen zu rechnen.

Behandlung, Prophylaxe: Auf Weiden mit einem *natürlichen* Mo-Gehalt von ≤ 5 bzw. > 5 ppm TM kann versucht werden, das Krankheitsbild durch Anbieten von Salzlecksteinen bzw. von Granulat mit einem Cu-Sulfatgehalt von 1 bzw. von 2% zu verhindern; bedarfsgerechte Cu-Mengen werden dabei allerdings i. d. R. nicht aufgenommen. Eine gute Lösung ist die gleichzeitige Einmischung anorganischer und organischer Cu-Verbindungen (Cu-Methionat, Cu-Lysin, Cu-haltige Hefen) in das Mineralfutter, um Mo zu binden und dem Organismus komplexresistentes Cu anzubieten. Das Zumischen von 2–3 mg Cu als Cu-Sulfat pro Liter Tränkewasser ist zwar möglich, auf der Weide aber technisch schwierig. Ein weiterer Weg besteht in der bei Weideauftrieb vorzunehmenden subkutanen Verabreichung von 400 mg Cu in Form einer lokal verträglichen organischen Verbindung (Kap. 12.3.11). Auf *industriell Mo-verunreinigten* Weiden sind diese Maßnahmen oft nicht ausreichend; ggf. muß solcher Boden melioriert oder seine Nutzung aufgegeben werden.

Übersicht 12-5 Beurteilung des Molybdängehalts in Blut-, Kot-, Leber-, Futter-, Boden- und Tränkewasserproben

Molybdänose:	unwahrscheinlich	möglich*	sicher
Blut (mg/l):	0,05	0,1	0,2–1,0
Dünndarmkot (mg/kg FM):	< 2		> 20
Leber (mg/kg FM):	< 2	2–5	> 5
Haar (mg/kg FM):	< 0,3	0,3–1	> 1
Weidegras (ppm)**/***:	< 1	1–3	1–10° > 10°°
Boden (ppm):			> 10–100 > 10–250°°°
Tränkewasser (ppm):			10–> 50⁺

* Die in dieser Spalte angegebenen Mo-Werte sprechen für Molybdänose, wenn die Cu-Versorgung (Kap. 12.3.11) der betreffenden Tiere knapp und/oder der Sulfatgehalt des Futters (Kap. 10.5.14) hoch ist. ** Der Cu:Mo-Quotient des Futters sollte normaliter 6:1 betragen; eine Relation von 2–3:1 ist bedingt verträglich, eine solche von < 2:1 toxisch. *** Leguminosen enthalten etwa zehnmal soviel Mo wie Gräser; der Mo-Gehalt des Grünfutters ist während der Vegetationsperiode höher als in der kalten Jahreszeit; ° falls Cu-Gehalt des Grases < 5 ppm beträgt; °° unabhängig vom Kupfergehalt des Grases; °°° bei industriell bedingter Molybdänose zu findende Werte; ⁺ bei normaler Cu- und S-Zufuhr.

12.3.13 Äthylenglykolvergiftung

M. Stöber

Ursachen, Pathogenese: Das zu verschiedenen technischen Zwecken, insbesondere als Frostschutzmittel eingesetzte Äthylenglykol (*Äthylenalkohol* oder *»Glykol«*), eine süßlich schmeckende farblos-visköse Flüssigkeit, kann bei unachtsamem Umgang Rindern zugänglich und von ihnen aufgenommen werden. Die toxische Dosis beträgt 2 ml/kg LM für Kälber und 5–10 ml/kg LM für erwachsene Tiere. Das innerhalb von 3 Tagen einsetzende Krankheitsbild beruht auf Umwandlung des Giftes in Oxalsäure (→ Oxalatnephrose).

Symptome: Tachypnoe, Niedergeschlagenheit, schwankender Gang, Nachhandparese, in schweren Fällen zudem Nasenbluten, Oligurie, Hämoglobinurie, Festliegen und Tod. Im Blut finden sich Urämie, Hypokalzämie, Neutrophilie, bei tödlichem Verlauf auch Azidose, Hyperosmolalität des Plasmas und hämolytische Anämie. Das Harnsediment enthält Oxalatkristalle.

■ **Sektionsbefunde:** Hämorrhagische Abomasoenteritis, perirenales Ödem, Nieren auffallend dunkelgefärbt, Oxalatablagerungen in den Geweben, v. a. in Nieren und Gehirn.

■ **Diagnose:** Die Erkennung des Leidens stützt sich auf Vorbericht, Umweltkontrolle und Symptome; die *Prognose* klinisch ausgeprägter Fälle ist schlecht.

■ **Behandlung:** Über die bei Kleintieren intravenös angewandten Gegenmittel (Äthylalkohol und/oder 4-Methylpyrazol) bestehen am Rind noch keine Erfahrungen; die intravenöse Verabreichung von Natriumbikarbonat (Kap. 4.3.6.2) erscheint angezeigt.

12.3.14 Pentachlorphenolvergiftung

M. Stöber

■ **Definition, Ursachen, Pathogenese:** Das früher als Fungi-, Herbi- und Molluskizid eingesetzte geruchlose *Pentachlorphenol* (PCP, »Penta«) wird heute noch als Konservierungsmittel für im Freien stehende Holzkonstruktionen verwendet. Technisches Pentachlorphenol enthält i. d. R. geringe Mengen an wesentlich toxischeren *polychlorierten Benzo-Dioxinen* (PCBD), *Benzo-Furanen* (PCBF) und *Biphenylen* (PCB). Es wirkt schleimhautreizend und wird nicht nur nach oraler Aufnahme, sondern auch perkutan sowie bei Einatmung resorbiert, wonach es Stoffwechselsteigerung durch Freisetzung zellulärer Phosphorylierungsvorgänge bewirkt. Reines PCP ist um vieles verträglicher als technisches PCP, dessen für Rinder akut giftige bis letale Dosis ~ 150–200 mg/kg LM einmal p. o., und dessen chronisch toxische Dosis 20–30 mg/kg LM täglich langfristig p. o. beträgt. Außerdem gleichen die Erscheinungen der chronischen Exposition gegenüber technischem PCP denen der Vergiftung durch die o. a. Verunreinigungen. Deshalb wird heute angenommen, daß PCP-Intoxikationen v. a. auf letztere zurückzuführen sind. In den Vormägen hemmt PCP den mikrobiellen Zelluloseabbau. Es wird vorwiegend renal, aber – ebenso wie die genannten Verunreinigungen – auch mit der Milch ausgeschieden.

■ **Vorkommen:** Mit technischem PCP behandeltes Holz sowie von solchem stammende Hobel- und Sägespäne führen zur direkten oralen und/oder perkutanen Intoxikation der mit ihnen in Kontakt geratenden Tiere. Bei wärmebedingtem Verdampfen (heiße Jahreszeit) können die o. a. Gifte auch in die Atemluft sowie in nahebei gelagerte Futtermittel (Heu, Silage) gelangen, deren Verzehr dann ebenfalls toxisch wirkt.

■ **Symptome:** Bei *akuter* Vergiftung zeigen sich Speicheln, Nasenausfluß, Tränen, Rötung der Kopfschleimhäute, Zunahme von Atem- und Pulsfrequenz, Schwitzen, hypertherme Körpertemperatur, Hyperglykämie, Glukosurie, Schwanken, Kollaps, schlaffe Lähmung (keine Krämpfe), Dyspnoe mit asphyktischem Zittern, Tod und rasch eintretende Totenstarre. Die *chronische* Intoxikation äußert sich in schlechter Futterverwertung, Rückgang von Vormagenmotorik und Milchleistung, Abmagerung, Muskelschwäche, Proteinurie und zunehmender depressiver Anämie; gelegentlich werden ihr auch mangelhafte Fruchtbarkeit, Aborte und vermehrte Neigung zu Infekten zugeschrieben.

■ **Sektion:** Vergrößerung von Lunge, Leber und Nieren, verkleinerter Thymus, Labmagenentzündung, Verdickung der Harnblasenwand. *Histologie:* Interstitielle Nephritis, Zystitis, Hyperplasie der Gallengänge und der Gallenblasenschleimhaut, Hyperkeratose der Meibomschen Lidranddrüsen.

■ **Diagnose:** Die Erkennung stützt sich auf klinisches Bild, Umweltkontrolle und PCP- oder PCBD-Nachweis in konserviertem Holz, Futtermitteln, Blut (> 2mg PCP/100 ml) oder Lebergewebe (> 4 mg PCP/100 g FS). *Differentialdiagnostisch* ist an Vergiftung durch polychlorierte Naphthaline (Kap. 12.3.15), Teer oder PCB (Kap. 3.1.5.1) zu denken.

■ **Beurteilung:** Nach Ermittlung und Abstellen der Ursache ist bei akuter Exposition mit baldiger Elimination des Gifts aus dem Tierkörper, nach chronischer Exposition mit längerem Siechtum und Unwirtschaftlichkeit zu rechnen. Fleisch und Milch manifest erkrankter Tiere sind nicht zum Verzehr geeignet. N. B.: PCP-behandeltes Holz gefährdet auch den in solchen Räumen lebenden Menschen.

■ **Behandlung:** Die Therapie ist rein symptomatisch, da kein spezifisches Antidot bekannt ist: Salinische Abführmittel p. o.; Abwaschen etwaiger, auf der Haut befindlicher Giftspuren; bei Hyperthermie auch Abkühlung durch Übergießen mit kaltem Wasser. *Prophylaxe:* Im Wohn-, Tierhaltungs- und Vorratsbereich keine PCP-haltigen Holzschutzmittel anwenden.

12.3.15 Vergiftung durch höherchlorierte Naphthaline

M. Stöber

Definition, Ursachen, Pathogenese: Die früher als Holzschutzmittel, Zusatz zu Schmier-, Dichtungs- und Lösungsmitteln sowie Isolierstoffen (Dachpappe), Wachsen u. ä. mannigfaltig eingesetzten *polychlorierten Naphthaline* waren in Nordamerika und Europa zwischen 1940 und 1955 Ursache gehäuft auftretender und zunächst völlig unerklärlicher Rindererkrankungen *(»X-Disease«)*. Die empfindlichen Verluste ließen sich erst nach langwierig-umfangreichen Untersuchungen auf das Vorkommen von Penta-, Hexa- und Heptachlornaphthalinen in Umwelt (konserviertes Holz, vorbehandeltes Öl) oder Futter (Übergang von Schmierstoffen aus Bearbeitungsmaschinen in die Nahrung) zurückführen. Dabei wurde das Gift teils oral, teils perkutan, seltener pulmonal (aerogene industrielle Emission) aufgenommen. Die Giftigkeit der Chlornaphthaline nimmt mit ihrem Chlorierungsgrad zu. Die Ingestion von 5 mg Hexachlornaphthalin/kg LM und Tag führt beim Kalb innerhalb weniger Tage zu schwerwiegender Intoxikation. Perkutane Giftaufnahme bewirkt v. a. Hautveränderungen und nur schwach ausgeprägte Allgemeinerscheinungen. Nach Resorption behindern polychlorierte Naphthaline die Umwandlung von β-Karotin in Vitamin A, was Veränderungen an Haut und Schleimhäuten bedingt. Das Gift geht auch in die Milch über. Jungtiere sind chlornaphthalinempfindlicher als erwachsene Rinder, weshalb erstere oft akut, letztere meist chronisch erkranken (→ *»bösartige Magen-Darmentzündung«* bzw. *Hyperkeratose*). Da polychlorierte Naphthaline heute praktisch kaum noch angewandt werden, sind solche Vergiftungen selten geworden; infolge Einwirkung unerkannter oder »vergessener« Altlasten (imprägnierte Holzkonstruktionen, Hobelspaneinstreu, Gummimatten, Ölabfälle, Bindegarnwachs) kommt es jedoch gelegentlich noch zu Bestandserkrankungen, die ihrer versteckten Entstehungsweise und schleichenden Entwicklung wegen meist nur schwer aufzuklären sind. N. B.: Höherchlorierte Naphthaline können mit *polychlorierten Biphenylen* (PCB, Kap. 3.1.5.1), aber auch mit *polychlorierten Benzo-Dioxinen* und *Benzo-Furanen* (PCBD, BCBF) verunreinigt sein.

Symptome: Bei *akutem Verlauf* zeigen die Patienten schon wenige Tage nach Beginn von Giftaufnahme oder -kontakt Tränen- und Nasenausfluß, Speicheln, zunehmende Apathie, wechselnde oder abnehmende Freßlust, Durchfall, Polyurie sowie Abmagerung. Bei laktierenden Rindern geht die Milchleistung zurück oder versiegt. An Naseneingang, Flotzmaul, Lippen, Dentalplatte, Gaumen und/oder Zunge entwickeln sich in vielen Fällen erbsen- bis walnußgroße papulös-proliferative Schleimhautwucherungen oder Geschwüre, auf den Wangen Hauterosionen und Ulzera. Vergiftete Tiere neigen in vermehrtem Maße zu Sekundärinfektionen (Nekrobazillose, Abszesse, Bronchopneumonien). Kälber und Jungrinder verenden vielfach schon innerhalb von 1–2 Wochen, vor dem Auftreten von Hautveränderungen.

Chronische Chlornaphthalinvergiftung ist durch eine neben vorgenannten, aber weniger stark ausgeprägten Symptomen einsetzende räudeähnliche Hyperkeratose der Haut gekennzeichnet, die etwa 3–5 Wochen nach Beginn des Giftkontakts, meist an Hals, Widerrist und Schulter, beginnt und sich allmählich auf Backen, Innenfläche der Hinterschenkel, Perineum und Euter oder Hodensack ausdehnt (Abb. 12-47). Die Gliedmaßen bleiben i. d. R. verschont. In den genannten Bereichen wird die sich zunehmend verdikkende Haut unelastisch-derb und weist schließlich eine waschbrettähnliche, von trockenen Schuppen und Borken bedeckte und von zahlreichen senkrecht verlaufenden Rissen durchzogene Fältelung auf. Diese nichtentzündlichen und nichtjuckenden Veränderungen werden von m. o. w. ausgeprägtem Haarausfall begleitet. Mitunter zeigen Hörner und/oder Klauen abnormes Wachstum oder lösen sich ab. Bei tragenden Rindern kommt es zu verminderter Fertilität, Aborten, Geburt toter oder lebensschwacher Kälber sowie zu Nachgeburtsverhaltung, später auch zu Euterentzündungen. Außerdem enthält die Milch hyperkeratosekranker Kühe mitunter genügend Chlornaphthaline, um damit getränkte Kälber zu vergiften. Bei Bullen kann die Fruchtbarkeit infolge Schädigung der Epithelien ihrer akzessorischen Geschlechtsdrüsen ebenfalls beeinträchtigt sein (→ Rückgang von Libido sowie Menge und Spermiengehalt des Ejakulats).

Sowohl bei *akut* als bei *chronisch* Kranken ist der Blutplasmaspiegel an Vitamin A deutlich erniedrigt (5–15 µg/100 ml).

Sektion: Außer Abmagerung und m. o. w. generalisierter Hyperkeratose der Haut finden sich von Fall zu Fall: papulös-proliferative Stomatitis; ulzerative Ösophagitis; kleine weiße Flecken auf der Leberschnittfläche; Vergrößerung und Wandverdickung der Gallenblase; kleines derbes Pankreas; große Nieren mit blaß-feuchter, grauweiß-strahlig gestreifter Rinde; Ödem, Blutungen und/oder Geschwüre der Labmagenschleimhaut. Kennzeichnende *histologische Veränderungen* sind: orthokeratotische Hyperkeratose der Haut mit fingerartig gefächertem Papillarkörper; Umwandlung der Haarfollikel in keratinhaltige Zysten; schuppige Metaplasie der Meibomschen Lidranddrüsen und der Speicheldrüsengänge; periportale Leberfibrose, papilläre Wucherungen und mukoide Reten-

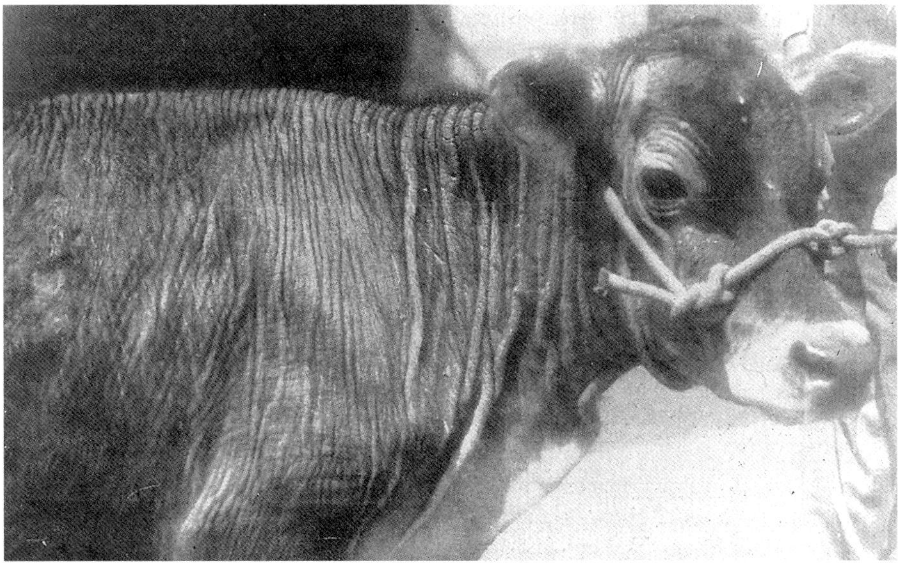

Abbildung 12-47 Hochgradige Hyperkeratose der Haut nach Aufnahme polychlorierter Naphthaline (KRÁL & SCHWARTZMAN, 1964)

tionszysten in der Wand von Hauptgallengängen und Gallenblase; Erweiterung der Nierentubuli, des Nebenhodenkanals, der GARTNERschen Gänge sowie der Krypten der LIEBERKÜHNschen Dickdarmdrüsen.

Diagnose: Klinisches Bild, Verlauf und Umweltkontrolle lenken den Verdacht auf Hyperkeratose infolge Intoxikation mit polychlorierten Naphthalinen. Zur Bestätigung dienen Vitamin-A-Gehalt des Plasmas, histologischer Befund von Gewebeproben (Haut, Lidrand, Leber, akzessorische Geschlechtsdrüsen) und Nachweis polychlorierter Naphthaline in Umgebung oder Futter.

Differentialdiagnostisch sind gegenüber *akuter Chlornaphthalinvergiftung* v. a. Mucosal Disease (Kap. 6.10.20), Bösartiges Katarrhalfieber (Kap. 12.2.2), Stomatitis papulosa (Kap. 6.1.5), in tropischen Gebieten auch Rinderpest (Kap. 12.2.3) zu bedenken. Zur Abgrenzung der *chlornaphthalinbedingten Hyperkeratose* sind Pentachlorphenoltoxikose (Kap. 12.3.14), Räude (Kap. 2.2.4.2), Dermatophilose (Kap. 2.2.3.6), Photosensibilitätsreaktionen (Kap. 2.2.7.3) und Thalliumvergiftung (Kap. 2.1.5.2) in Betracht zu ziehen.

Beurteilung: *Akut* erkrankte Kälber und Jungrinder sind meist verloren. Auch schwer *chronisch* betroffene Tiere bleiben in Entwicklung und Leistung oft unbefriedigend. Bei den übrigen Patienten ist nach Unterbinden der Giftaufnahme und wiederholten parenteralen oder oralen Gaben von Vitamin A und E allmähliche Besserung sowie Rückkehr der Fruchtbarkeit zu erwarten. Bei Fortbestehen der Chlornaphthalinexposition erweist sich jedoch jedwede Behandlung als unwirksam.

Prophylaxe: Etwa noch vorhandene Giftreste (altkonserviertes Holz, Schmiermittelreste, Motorenschrott u. ä.) ordnungsgemäß entsorgen. N. B.: Beim Menschen lösen höherchlorierte Naphthaline Chlorakne aus.

12.3.16 Insektenstiche

M. STÖBER

Definition, Vorkommen, Ursachen: Über Insektenplage (*Dipterenbefall*, Kap. 2.2.4.1), Fliegenmaden- und Dasselbefall (*Myiasis*, Kap. 2.3.4.4; *Hypodermose*, Kap. 2.3.4.1), die i. d. R. nicht mit toxischen Auswirkungen einhergehen, wird bei den Krankheiten der Haut Näheres berichtet. Befall mit Kriebelmücken (*Simuliotoxikose*, Kap. 4.1.5.4) wird seiner Auswirkungen auf den Kreislauf wegen bei dessen Leiden abgehandelt. Unfälle durch *Bienen-, Hummel-, Wespen-* oder *Hornissenstiche* sind beim Rind wesentlich seltener als beim Pferd, welches diese Insekten durch seine Schweißabsonderung und sofortige heftige Abwehr eher auf sich zieht. Das in der Giftdrüse des stachelbewehrten Hinterleibendes aller Akuleaten enthaltene toxische Sekret besitzt neurotoxische, hämolysierende, hämorrhagiebedingende und krampfauslösende Komponenten. Schwerwiegende Intoxikationen treten i. d. R. nur dann auf, wenn ein (Jung-)Rind von einer großen Zahl der genannten Insekten zugleich gestochen wird (Umstoßen eines Bienenkorbs, Zertreten von Nestern, Schwarmanflug). Mitunter können aber schon einzelne Stiche gefährlich werden, z. B. nach Aufnahme solcher Insekten mit dem Futter (hochgradige Behinderung von Atmung und Nahrungsaufnahme infolge Anschwellens von Rachen und Kehlkopfschleimhaut) bzw. beim Anstechen eines Blut- oder Lymphgefäßes (Schockwirkung). Für den Menschen gelten 50–100 Bienenstiche als lebensgefährlich; bei anaphylaktisch veranlagten Personen kann u. U. schon ein einziger Akuleatenstich zum Tode führen.

■ **Symptome:** Während sowie unmittelbar nach dem Insektenüberfall ist der Patient unruhig (Umherrennen, Auf- und Niedergehen, Schlagen mit Beinen und Schwanz, Kopfschleudern), um schon kurze Zeit danach teilnahmslos zu werden. An Rumpf und Gliedmaßen entwickeln sich nun rasch haselnuß- bis handtellergroße, z. T. konfluierende quaddelartige schmerzhafte Umfangsvermehrungen von Haut und Unterhaut, in deren Zentrum bei Bienen- und Hummelstichen noch der Stachel des Insekts samt Giftdrüse erkennbar ist. An Kopf (Lippen, Flotzmaul, Augenlider), Vorhaut, Hodensack, Euter und Perinealbereich können diese entzündlichen Ödeme erhebliches Ausmaß erreichen. Die Herztätigkeit ist beschleunigt-pochend, der Puls klein und hart. Die Schleimhäute erscheinen gerötet, mitunter zyanotisch. Die Atmung kann dyspnoisch, die Körpertemperatur erhöht sein. In bedrohlichen Fällen folgen Zittern, häufigerer Absatz von rötlichem, hämoglobinhaltigem Harn, Schwäche und Festliegen, u. U. auch Krämpfe.

■ **Sektion:** Unterhaut sulzig-blutig durchtränkt, allgemeine Blutfülle der Organe und Neigung zu subserösen Petechien.

■ **Diagnose:** Differentialdiagnostisch sind Urtikaria (Kap. 2.2.7.1), Phlegmonen (Kap. 2.3.3.1, 2.3.3.2, 7.2.2.5, 12.2.4) zu bedenken.

■ **Beurteilung:** Bei ausbleibender Behandlung kann innerhalb weniger Stunden bis 2 Tagen durch schockartigen Kollaps oder Versagen der Atmung der Tod eintreten. Weniger schwer geschädigte Tiere erholen sich langsam wieder; an den Stichstellen können sich in der Folge Nekrosen oder Abszesse entwickeln.

■ **Behandlung:** Betroffene Tiere aus dem Gefahrenbereich entfernen. Steckengebliebene Stacheln mittels Pinzette herausziehen, ohne den Giftapparat zu berühren, oder samt diesem abschneiden. Veränderte Hautpartien während der ersten auf den Unfall folgenden Stunden wiederholt mit kaltem Wasser, verdünntem Essig, essigsaurer Tonerde oder Salmiak begießen, abwaschen oder betupfen. Schwellungen danach mit kortikosteroidhaltiger Salbe bestreichen. In schweren Fällen sind zudem parenterale Gaben von Kalziumboroglukonatlösung, peripher wirksamen Kreislaufmitteln, Antihistaminika oder nichtsteroidalen Entzündungshemmern angezeigt; erforderlichenfalls ist ein Tracheotubus (Kap. 5.2.2.4) einzusetzen.

12.3.17 Spinnenbisse und Skorpionstiche

M. Stöber

Spinnenbiß- oder skorpionstichbedingte Unfälle beschränken sich auf die tropischen und subtropischen Verbreitungsgebiete dieser Gifttiere (Abb. 12-48, 12-49). In Mitteleuropa spielen sie bei Nutzieren praktisch keine Rolle. Die einzelnen Raubspinnen- und Skorpionarten produzieren toxische Sekrete, die teils örtliche, teils schwerwiegende allgemeine Wirkung entfalten. Das äußert sich von Fall zu Fall in entzündlicher bis nekrotisierender Reaktion im Bereich der Biß- oder Stichstelle, oder aber in Hämolyse, Schädigung von Herz und Gefäßen, Berührungsempfindlichkeit und/oder nervösen Störungen. Die Behandlung umfaßt Schockbekämpfung (Kap. 4.2.2.1), lokale Entzündungshemmung (kühlende Umschläge) sowie Verabreichung spezifischer oder polyvalenter Immunseren.

In Spanien und Südafrika, insbesondere aber in Rußland und Chile, sind infolge Bisses von *Latrodectus*-Spinnen (»Schwarze Witwe«) erhebliche Verluste unter Rindern vorgekommen (Tränen, Schwitzen, Speicheln, Mydriasis → Myosis, Tachy- → Bradykardie, Atembeschwerde, Muskelstarre, Krämpfe).

12.3.18 Giftschlangenbiß

M. Stöber

■ **Definition, Ursachen, Pathogenese:** Weltweit sind etwa 400 Giftschlangenarten bekannt. Sie gehören zu den Familien der Nattern (*Elapidae*: Kobras, Schmuckottern, Mambas, Korallenschlangen, Tigerottern), Ottern (*Viperidae*: Bauch-, Erd-, Sand-, Kröten- und Hornvipern, echte Ottern sowie Puffottern), Loch- oder Grubenottern (*Crotalidae*: Dreiecksköpfe, Lanzenottern, Klapperschlangen, Buschmeister) oder Seeschlangen (*Hydrophiidae*). In Deutschland kommt nur der Kreuzotter (*Vipera berus*) praktische Bedeutung zu. Im außerdeutschen Europa finden sich zudem noch: Sandviper (*Vipera ammodytes*), Aspisviper (*V. aspis*), Stülpnasenotter (*V. latasi*), Levanteviper (*V. lebetina*), Wiesenotter (*V. ursini*) und Bergotter (*V. xanthina*). Schlangengifte werden ihrer toxischen Hauptwirkung nach gruppenweise zusammengefaßt: *Viperidengift* bewirkt v. a. Blutgerinnungsstörungen. *Bothropsgift* (Ottern, Lanzenottern, Buschmeister, zentral- und nordamerikanische Klapperschlangen)

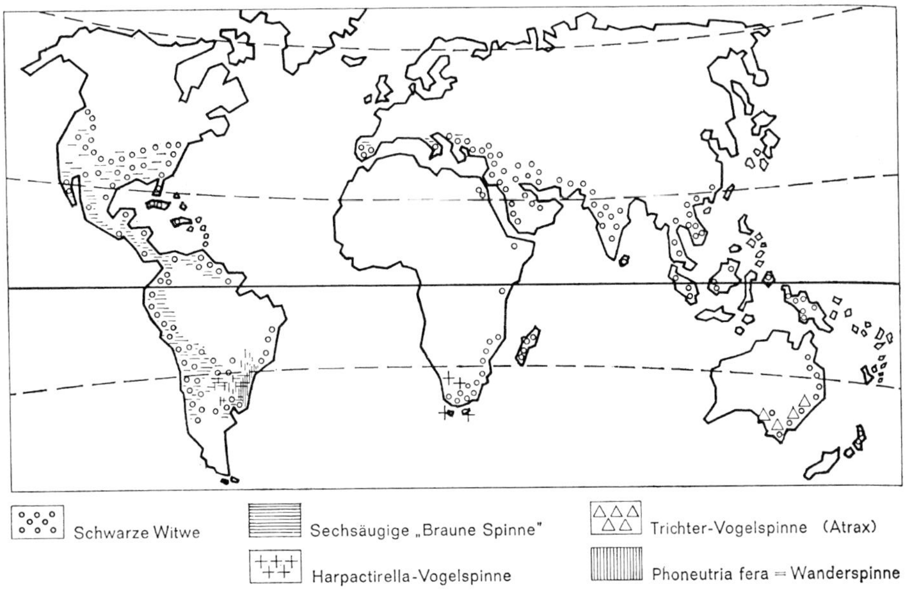

Abbildung 12-48 Verbreitungsgebiete der wichtigsten giftigen Spinnenarten (BÜCHERL, 1966)

bedingt örtliche Nekrose im Bißstellenbereich und Ungerinnbarkeit des Blutes, z. T. auch nervöse Symptome. *Crotalusgift* (südamerikanische Klapperschlangen) besitzt neurotoxische und hämolysierende Eigenschaften. *Elapidengift* verursacht fast ausschließlich nervöse Symptome (Unruhe, Zähneknirschen, Speicheln, unwillkürlicher Harnabgang, Ataxie, Krämpfe, Lähmungen, Tod durch Atemlähmung). *Hydrophiidengift* hat myotoxische Wirkung (reflexlose Bewegungsunfähigkeit, Myoglobinurie). Schadensfälle bei weidenden Haustieren sind in tropischen und subtropischen Regionen wesentlich häufiger als in gemäßigten Klimazonen. Die meisten Giftschlangen beißen nur zu, wenn sie von grasenden Tieren beunruhigt werden.

Symptome: Die punktförmigen »Fangmarken« finden sich i. d. R. am »suchenden« und dabei schlangenstörenden Flotzmaul, an Kopf, Halsunterseite, Unterbauch oder Euter, aber nur selten an den Gliedmaßen. *Bothropsgift* löst örtlich starken Schmerz und rasch zunehmendes entzündliches Ödem (»Nilpferdkopf«) aus, das in Nekrose und verjauchende Gangrän übergeht sowie mit Lymphknotenschwellung verbunden ist, was Atemnot bedingen kann. Nach anfänglicher Unruhe zeigen sich zunehmende Apathie, schwankender Gang oder Festliegen, Anorexie, Fieber, Tachykardie, Poly- und Dyspnoe, z. T. auch Abort; in schweren Fällen kommt es zu Blutungen aus natürlichen Körperöffnungen (einschließlich Hämaturie) und zum Tod durch Kreislaufversagen. Die Folgen von *Crotalusgiftbissen* sind örtliche Ekchymose (→ Nekrose), allgemeine Schmerzempfindlichkeit, motorische Störungen, Lähmung der Augenmuskeln, verminderter Lidreflex, Speicheln, Durst sowie Hämoglobinurie; der Tod beruht auf Nierenschädigung (Protein- und Glykosurie, Verminderung des spezifischen Harngewichts) und Blutungen im ZNS. *Elapidenbisse* führen zu Empfindungslosigkeit rings um die ödematös anschwellende Bißstelle, Beeinträchtigung der Sehkraft, z. T. auch zu Angriffslust, Tortikollis, Ptosis des Oberlids, allgemeiner Schwäche und fortschreitender Lähmung; der Tod tritt durch Ersticken ein.

Diagnose: In Gewebeproben (Bißstelle), Harn oder Blut befindliches Schlangengift ist mittels spezifischer, aber kostspieliger ELISA identifizierbar. *Differentialdiagnostisch* sind v. a. gut- und bösartige Gasödeme (Kap. 2.3.3.2, 12.2.4), allergische Reaktionen (Kap. 1.2.3.1, 2.2.7.1) sowie anderweitige ödematöse und phlegmonöse Anschwellungen von Haut und Unterhaut zu bedenken.

Beurteilung: Kreuzotternbisse verlaufen bei erwachsenen Rindern meist nicht tödlich, doch entwickeln sich im Bißbereich oft umfangreiche Gewebseinschmelzungen. Kälber sind ihrer dünnen Haut und geringeren Körpermasse wegen mehr gefährdet. Nach Bissen durch andere Giftschlangen sind die Heilungsaussichten vielfach weniger günstig, insbesondere, wenn bis zur Antiserumgabe mehr als 4–6 h verstreichen; zudem neigen verschleppte Schlangenbisse zu schwerwiegender Sekundärinfektion (→ Gasphlegmone).

Behandlung: Ruhigstellung des Patienten. Wenn irgend möglich, ist die Schlangenart zu ermitteln, von welcher der Biß ausging, damit spezifisches Antiserum angewandt werden kann. Falls sich der Biß an einer Gliedmaße befindet, ist proximal davon sofort

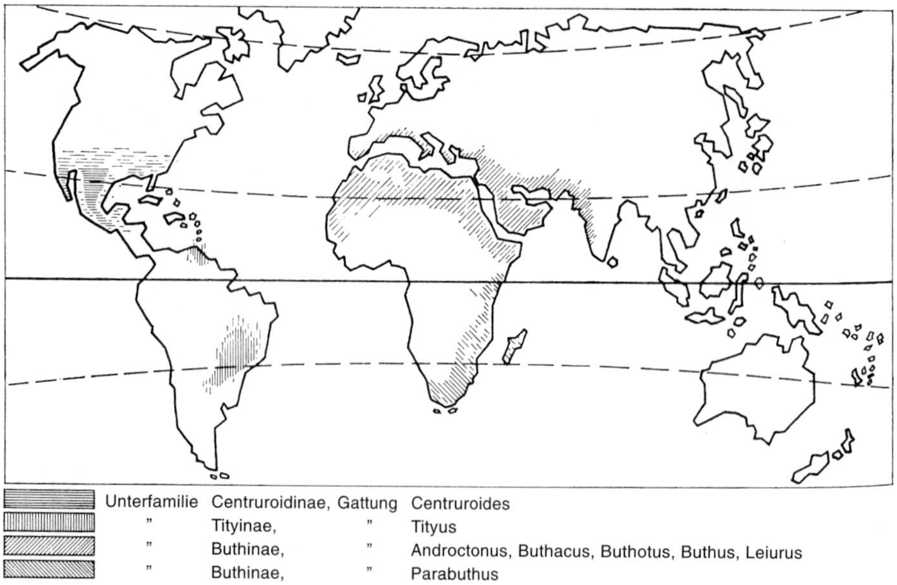

Abbildung 12-49
Verbreitungsgebiete der wichtigsten Skorpiongattungen (Bücherl, 1966)

eine elastische Ligatur anzulegen und erst nach Abschluß der örtlichen Versorgung wieder abzunehmen. Sie besteht in Resektion eines kreisförmigen Stücks Haut samt Unterhaut von etwa 7 cm Durchmesser; wenn dieser Eingriff innerhalb der ersten 2 h erfolgt, werden damit ~ 90% des Gifts entfernt. Die Wunde ist offen zu lassen und antibiotisch zu versorgen. Ausbrennen und Ätzen sind kontraindiziert. Weniger aussichtsreich und zudem komplizierter ist das alsbaldige kräftige Aussaugen der zuvor inzidierten Bißwunde mit Hilfe einer Milchpumpe oder mit dem Mund; im letztgenannten Falle ist der Bißstelle zum Schutz des Behandelnden eine Plastik- oder Gummifolie aufzulegen. Bei verspäteter Hilfeleistung ist die Umgebung der Bißstelle zu rasieren, gründlich zu desinfizieren und zwischen den Fangmarken ein bis in die Unterhaut reichender Schnitt anzulegen; außerdem ist der Patient örtlich und allgemein antibiotisch zu versorgen. Bei erfahrungsgemäß mit Lebensgefahr verbundenen Schlangenbissen sollte binnen 12 h das gegen das Gift der betreffenden Schlangenart wirksame Immunserum, anderenfalls das ortsübliche polyvalente Schlangengiftserum herbeigeschafft und die Gesamtdosis von 50–100 ml zu je einem Drittel als Infiltration des Bißbereichs, intramuskulär bzw. langsam intravenös (= Pferdeserum!) injiziert werden; auch Kälbern und Jungtieren ist die volle Dosis zu verabreichen. Etwaiger biß- oder serumbedingter Schock ist durch intravenöse Infusion von physiologischer Kochsalz-, Traubenzucker- oder Kalziumboroglukonatlösung, bei Bothropsbiß auch mit Blutübertragung (Kap. 4.3.2.1) anzugehen. Von Glukokortikoiden ist nur Schockabwehr und leichte Verminderung der lokalen Gewebsreaktion, andererseits aber Förderung von Sekundärinfektionen zu erwarten. Die Gefahr letzterer erfordert mehrtägige parenterale Breitspektrum-Antibiose, u. U. auch Gabe von Gasödem- und Tetanusserum (Kap. 12.2.4, 10.3.8). Der Patient sollte bis zur Besserung unter Beobachtung bleiben; im allgemeinen ist die unmittelbare Todesgefahr nach 3 Tagen überwunden.

■ **Prophylaxe:** In gefährdeten Gebieten tätige Tierärzte sollten wissen, wo (Krankenhaus, Apotheke, Vergiftungszentrale) im Bedarfsfall das gegen die örtlich vorkommenden Giftschlangenarten wirksame Immunserum verfügbar ist.

12.3.19 Vergiftung durch Blattwespenlarven

M. Stöber

Bei weidenden Schafen bzw. Rindern sind verschiedentlich schwerwiegende bis tödliche Erkrankungen infolge Aufnahme von Sägefliegenlarven (Dänemark: *Lophyrotoma interrupta*; Australien: *Arge pullata*; Uruguay: *Perreya flavipes*) aufgetreten. Das in ihnen enthaltene Peptidgift *Lophyrotomin* bedingt akute Lebernekrose mit hepatogener Enzephalopathie (Kap. 10.5.8). Klinisch zeigen sich bei akutem Verlauf Zittern, Atemnot, Aggressivität, Festliegen, Krämpfe, Stupor und plötzlicher Tod, in subakuten Fällen herabgesetzte Erregbarkeit, Ikterus, Photosensibilisierung und Durchfall. Die Sektion ergibt Lebernekrosen, Blutungen im Labmagendarmkanal und Nephrose, bei länger überlebenden Tieren auch Vermehrung der Körperhöhlenflüssigkeiten. Die symptomatische Behandlung manifest kranker Patienten ist wenig aussichtsreich; Erfahrungen mit spezifischem Anatoxin oder Toxoid liegen noch nicht vor. Zur Vorbeuge wird empfohlen, die Substratpflanzen der Sägefliegenlarven auszurotten oder das Vieh bei Einsetzen des Larvenbefalls auf ungefährdete Weiden umzutreiben.

12.4 Sensibilitätsreaktionen mit Beteiligung des Gesamtorganismus

M. Stöber

Da die *allergisch-anaphylaktische Allgemeinreaktion* des Rindes i. d. R. mit auffälligen Hautveränderungen im Sinne der Urtikaria einhergeht, wird sie bei den Krankheiten der Haut (Kap. 2.2.7.1) besprochen. Näheres über die *Pathogenese von Immunreaktionen* ist in Kapitel 1.2.3.1 nachzulesen.

12.5 Strahlenkrankheit

W. Giese/M. Stöber

Unter obigem Begriff werden die auf extremer Röntgen-*Bestrahlung* und die auf Einwirkung *radioaktiver Strahlen* zurückzuführenden Gesundheitsschädigungen zusammengefaßt. Die auf *Sensibilisierung gegenüber Sonnenstrahlen* des sichtbaren oder ultravioletten Spektralbereichs beruhenden und nur die Haut betreffenden Photosensibilitätsreaktionen werden andernorts besprochen (Kap. 2.2.7.3).

12.5.1 Schädigung durch Röntgen-Strahlen

Definition, Ursachen, Vorkommen: Medizinische Röntgen-Strahlen sind elektromagnetische Strahlen mit Wellenlängen von 0,01–0,1 nm oder Frequenzen von 3×10^{18} bis 3×10^{19} Hz (= weiche bzw. harte Röntgen-Strahlen). Ihr Spektrum liegt somit zwischen dem des UV-Lichts (Kap. 2.2.7.3) und demjenigen der Gamma-Strahlung (Kap. 12.5.2). Ebenso wie letztere gehören Röntgen-Strahlen, deren Quantenenergie $1{,}25 \times 10^4$ bis $1{,}25 \times 10^5$ eV beträgt, zu den ionisierenden Strahlen. In der Buiatrik spielt übermäßige Exposition von Patienten gegenüber diesen Strahlen keine nennenswerte Rolle, da diagnostische Röntgen-Durchleuchtungen und -Aufnahmen, insbesondere aber massive therapeutische Röntgen-Bestrahlungen am Rind nur selten vorgenommen werden.

Symptome: Bei experimenteller Verabreichung stark überhöhter Röntgen-Strahlendosen an Kälber und Rinder sind, je nach deren Exposition, lokale Reaktionen unterschiedlichen Schweregrades (Epilation, Erythem, Dermatitis, Nekrose/Gangrän) ausgelöst worden. Röntgen-Bestrahlung des Hodensacks mit > 1,0 Sv führt bei geschlechtsreifen Bullen zu vorübergehender Azoospermie; Ganzkörper-Röntgen-Exposition gleicher und höherer Größenordnung bedingt m. o. w. schwerwiegende, u. U. tödlich verlaufende Strahlenkrankheit (Hemmung von Lympho-, Myelo-, Thrombo- und Erythropoese, hämorrhagische Diathese, fibrinöse Pleuropneumonie und Perikarditis, Leberzellnekrose, Myokarddegeneration, akute Tubulonephrose, katarrhalische bis diphtheroide Enteritis und sekundäre Unterernährung).

N. B.: Zum Schutze des *Tierarztes* sowie des ihm assistierenden *Personals* sind bei Röntgen-Arbeiten stets die hierfür üblichen Vorschriften (Beantragen der Genehmigung der Anlage, Fachkundenachweis) und Vorsichtsmaßregeln (Überwachung der Sicherheit der Röntgen-Apparatur, Fixation und Sedation des Patienten, Tragen von Bleischürze und -handschuhen, Stativhalterung der Kassetten, regelmäßige Überprüfung der bei dieser Tätigkeit zu tragenden Dosimeter) einzuhalten (s. Röntgen-VO vom 8. 1. 1987 samt Änderungs-VO vom 19. 12. 1990); die in der Röntgen-VO angegebenen Körperteil- und Personendosen sollten nicht überschritten werden.

12.5.2 Schädigung durch radioaktive Strahlung

Definition, Ursachen: Kernwaffendetonationen und Reaktorunfälle (Oak Ridge 1952, Windscale 1957, Tschernobyl 1986) haben wiederholt zu weltweiter Zunahme des Radionuklid-Niederschlags (»Fallout«) geführt. Die damit zusammenhängende Gefährdung verdient daher auch tierärztliche Beachtung. Diagnostischer und experimenteller Einsatz von Tracer-Isotopen sowie Radiotherapie von Tumoren spielen dagegen in der buiatrischen Praxis keine wesentliche Rolle. Je nach Herkunft der Strahlung ist zwischen natürlicher und künstlicher Radioaktivität zu unterscheiden. Erstere geht von den seit jeher vorhandenen radioaktiven Elementen (in Form von Alpha-, Beta- oder Gamma-Strahlen), letztere von den durch Kernspaltung erzeugten Radionukliden (und zwar als Beta- oder Gamma-Strahlung) aus:

- *Alpha-Strahlung* besteht aus beim Kernzerfall ausgestoßenen Heliumkernen (= Alpha-Teilchen); diese Korpuskularstrahlung besitzt hohe Energie (2–8 MeV) und starke Ionisierungs-, aber nur geringe Durchdringungsfähigkeit (in Körpergeweben: 0,07 mm). Daher wird Alpha-Strahlung für Lebewesen erst nach oraler oder pulmonaler Aufnahme (= Inkorporation) radioaktiver Isotope gefährlich, die solche Teilchen aussenden (= Alpha-Strahler), z. B. ^{239}Plutonium (→ Schädigung von Leber und Knochenmark).

➤ *Beta(β^-)-Strahlen* sind ebenfalls korpuskulärer Natur (Beta-Teilchen = Elektronen). Ihre Energie beträgt je nach Herkunftsisotop maximal 3,15 MeV, ihre Ionisationsfähigkeit ist wesentlich geringer als diejenige der Alpha-Strahlung; ihre Durchdringungsfähigkeit beläuft sich auf ~ 3 mm/MeV. Wichtigste Beta(β^-)-Strahler sind ^{131}Jod, ^{89}Strontium und ^{90}Strontium sowie ^{134}Zäsium und ^{137}Zäsium, die sich nach Inkorporation in Schilddrüse (^{131}J), Knochen (^{89}Sr und ^{90}Sr) und Weichgeweben (^{134}Cs und ^{137}Cs) anreichern.

➤ *Gamma-Strahlen* sind den RÖNTGEN-Strahlen ähnelnde elektromagnetische Quantenstrahlen von großer Härte (Wellenlänge 0,1–10^{-4} nm, Frequenz 3×10^{18} bis 3×10^{21} Hz, Quantenenergie ≤ 2,2 MeV) und besonders starker Durchdringungskraft. Sie bewirken nur schwache direkte Ionisierung. Intensive Ganzkörper-Gamma-Bestrahlung löst m. o. w. schwerwiegende Strahlenkrankheit aus. Zu den wichtigsten Gamma-Strahlern gehören ^{131}J sowie ^{134}Cs und ^{137}Cs, die sich postinkorporativ in Schilddrüse bzw. in Muskulatur und inneren Organen anreichern.

➤ *Neutronen*, die bei Kernspaltung und -fusion frei werden, können ebenfalls Atome ihrer Umgebung sekundär aktivieren.

Vorkommen, Pathogenese: Im lebenden Organismus besteht die Schadwirkung radioaktiver Strahlen in der Anregung von Elektronen sowie der Ionisation von Atomen innerhalb ihres Moleküls. Nutztiere können in folgenden Situationen durch radioaktive Strahlung gefährdet sein:

➤ *Aufenthalt im Wirkungsbereich einer Kernwaffendetonation:* Dabei sind Schädigungen durch die extreme *Überdruck-* und anschließende *Unterdruckwelle* (→ direkte Auswirkungen und Verletzungen durch Gebäudetrümmer) sowie die *Hitzestrahlung* (→ Verbrennungen, Verkohlungen) mindestens ebenso schwerwiegend wie die Folgen der ~ 10–15 s dauernden durchdringenden *Initialstrahlung* (= Gamma-Strahlen und Neutronen) samt denen der unmittelbar danach vom radioaktiven Niederschlag ausgelösten *Residualstrahlung* (= Beta- und Gamma-Strahlung der Spaltprodukte von ^{235}Uran und ^{239}Plutonium).

➤ *Aufenthalt im Wirkungsbereich des lokalen »Fallout«:* Das Gebiet, in dem die schwereren Partikel des noch »jungen« und daher stark radioaktiven Niederschlags zu Boden sinken, erstreckt sich – je nach Größenordnung der Kernwaffenexplosion bzw. des Reaktorunfalls und vorherrschender Windrichtung – bis zu mehrere hundert km vom Zentrum des nuklearen Ereignisses. Die innerhalb dieses Bereichs im Freien befindlichen Lebewesen sind v. a. durch *äußere Einwirkung* von Gamma-Strahlen (→ Strahlenkrankheit), u. U. auch von Beta-Strahlen (→ Hautveränderungen) gefährdet. Wenn sie radioaktiven Staub einatmen oder solchen über Futter und Tränke aufnehmen, kommen noch Inkorporationsschäden durch *innere Strahlenwirkung* hinzu; so betrug die auf ^{131}Jod zurückzuführende mittlere Radioaktivität der Schilddrüsen von in der Umgebung von Tschernobyl 1986 geschlachteten, teils mit Hypo-, teils mit Hyperthyreoidismus behafteten Rindern 19,95 MBq/kg. Die Resorption radioaktiver Substanzen durch Hautverletzungen spielt dagegen nur eine untergeordnete Rolle.

➤ *Aufenthalt im Wirkungsbereich des weltweiten »Fallout«:* Die bei atomaren Explosionen und Reaktorzwischenfällen in Tropo- und Stratosphäre aufsteigenden radioaktiven Partikel gelangen erst nach längerer Verteilung allmählich wieder auf den Erdboden. Unter den in solchem Niederschlag enthaltenen Radionukliden sind aufgrund ihrer Konzentration, Halbwertszeit* und biologischen Wirksamkeit v. a. ^{89}Sr und ^{90}Sr (Beta-Strahler) sowie ^{134}Cs und ^{137}Cs (Beta- und Gamma-Strahler), aber auch ^{131}J (Beta- und Gamma-Strahler) von Bedeutung. Sie reichern sich nach Inkorporation zunächst in bestimmten »kritischen« Organen an (Strontium: Skelett; Zäsium: Muskelfleisch, Leber, Nieren → je nach Strahlungsintensität und Dauer Schädigung hämopoetischer Organe; Jod: Schilddrüse → je nach Strahlungsintensität und Dauer Adenome bis Zerstörung). Nach 14tägiger Anreicherung werden sie auch in gewissem Umfang mit der Milch ausgeschieden, und zwar Jod zu 0,8–1,0% sowie Strontium zu 0,1% der täglich weiterhin aufgenommenen Menge pro l Milch, bei Zäsium dagegen 10% der täglich aufgenommenen Menge im Gesamtgemelk. Den genannten radioaktiven Kontaminationen von Luft, Wasser, Boden und Vegetation sind weidende Nutz- und Wildwiederkäuer aufgrund ihrer Lebensweise besonders ausgesetzt.

Symptome, Verlauf: Gewebe mit hoher Vermehrungsrate (Knochenmark, Stratum germinativum von Haut und Schleimhäuten, Keimzellen, Embryonen und Feten) gelten als besonders strahlenempfindlich;

* *Physikalische Halbwertszeit* = Zeitraum, innerhalb dessen die Hälfte der ursprünglich vorhandenen radioaktiven Atomkerne zerfallen ist (^{131}J: 8 Tage; ^{89}Sr: 51 Tage; ^{90}Sr: 28 Jahre; ^{137}Cs: 30 Jahre). *Biologische Halbwertszeit* = Zeitraum, innerhalb dessen die halbe Menge eines inkorporierten radioaktiven Elements auf natürlichem Wege (Kot, Harn, Milch) ausgeschieden wird. Aus der Kombination von physikalischer und biologischer Halbwertszeit ergibt sich die *effektive Halbwertszeit*.

Organparenchyme, Muskel- und Nervenzellen sind vergleichsweise widerstandsfähig. Die Folgen übermäßiger Einwirkung radioaktiver Strahlung äußern sich, je nach Expositionsweise, -intensität und -dauer, als *Strahlenkrankheit* (Ganzkörperirradiation mit Gamma-Strahlen), als *Hautverbrennungen* (residuale Beta[β^-]-Strahlung) oder als *Inkorporationsschäden* (nach Aufnahme radioaktiven Staubes):

➤ *Strahlenkrankheit* wird durch Ganzkörperbestrahlung mit durchdringenden Gamma-Strahlen ausgelöst, wenn dabei kurzfristig Dosen von 1,0–1,3 Sv überschritten werden; die nach Bestrahlung mit ≥ 0,25 Sv/h bei der Hälfte der exponierten Tiere zum Tode führende Gamma-Strahlendosis beträgt 5,0–7,0 Sv, die sicher tödliche Dosis 7,0–11,0 Sv. Kälber und ältere Tiere sind meist strahlenempfindlicher als Jungrinder. Die Erkrankung läuft phasenweise ab:

Während der ersten 3 Tage sind die Patienten scheu bis erregt und zeigen Muskelzittern sowie um 0,5–1,5 °C erhöhte Körpertemperatur *(Prodromalphase)*. Während der folgenden 7–10 Tage erscheint ihr Allgemeinbefinden dann bis auf vereinzelte Diarrhoe ungestört *(Latenzphase)*. Erst 2–3 Wochen nach der Strahlenexposition setzen ausgeprägte Symptome ein *(Hauptreaktionsphase)*: Milchrückgang, Bewegungsunlust, Niedergeschlagenheit und allgemeine Schwäche, Einknicken der Nachhand sowie zunehmende Freßunlust bei vermehrtem Durst; Haarausfall; Hornhauttrübung; schleimig-blutiger Durchfall (*gastrointestinales Strahlensyndrom:* führt bei voller Ausprägung binnen weniger Tage zum Tode). Überlebende Tiere zeigen dann Anschwellen der Beine, Blutungen an Schleimhäuten und inneren Organen; frequent-oberflächliche, später auch keuchende Atmung, z. T. verbunden mit schleimigem bis blutigem Nasenausfluß, Kehlkopfödem oder pneumoniebedingten Nebengeräuschen; Keto- und Proteinurie; in den letzten Tagen vor dem Tod auch septikämiebedingtes Fieber (≤ 43,3 °C) und völliges Verweigern des Futters. Als prognostisch ungünstig sind schwerwiegende Blutbildveränderungen (Granulo-, Lympho- und Thrombozytopenie infolge Knochenmarkschädigung) sowie Blutungsneigung und starke Anämie zu werten (= *hämatopoetisches Strahlensyndrom:* endet bei schwerem Verlauf innerhalb von 30–60 Tagen tödlich). Überlebende Tiere sind zunächst m. o. w. stark abgemagert, erholen sich aber meist gut, wenn sie die ersten 6 Wochen nach der Strahlenexposition überstanden haben *(Restitutionsphase)*; an ihren Augen kann Linsentrübung auftreten. Bei Jungtieren kommt es zur Störung der Skelettentwicklung im Bereich der Epiphysenfugen der langen Röhrenknochen. Gamma-Bestrahlungen tragender Rinder mit 2–4 Sv (0,2–0,4 Sv/h) führen zu Fruchtresorption, Entwicklungsstörungen an den Gliedmaßen ihrer Feten oder Abort; von derart exponierten Müttern geborene Bullenkälber zeigen später ein um 50% verringertes Hodengewicht und eine ebensostark reduzierte Spermienzahl im Ejakulat, während sich die von ihnen stammenden weiblichen Kälber zu 90% als fruchtbar erweisen.

Noch höhere Irradiationsdosen (> 20 Sv) bedingen rascheren, anfangs mit Apathie, später mit Erregung verbundenen und stets tödlichen Verlauf der Erkrankung (*zentralnervöses Strahlensyndrom* → Tod innerhalb von 3 Tagen).

➤ *Beta-Verbrennungen der Haut* sind meist auf lokalen »Fallout« (d. h. im Haarkleid haftende Beta-Partikel) zurückzuführen. Solche Verbrennungen werden nur selten, und zwar bei Tieren beobachtet, die einer letalen Gamma-Ganzkörperbestrahlung entgangen sind. Im Gegensatz zu thermischen Hautverbrennungen treten Beta-Schäden erst einige Zeit nach der Exposition auf. Sie ähneln den durch RÖNTGEN-Strahlen verursachten kutanen Veränderungen (Kap. 12.5.1) und den Photosensibilitätsreaktionen (Kap. 2.2.7.3), doch sind dabei pigmentierte und unpigmentierte Hautbezirke des Rückenbereichs gleichermaßen betroffen: fleckenweiser Haarausfall, Grauwerden ursprünglich pigmentierter Hautstellen und ihrer Behaarung, Abschilferung oberflächlicher Gewebeschichten, Verlust der Hautdrüsen, Akanthose, Hyperkeratose und Entwicklung dicker verhornender Platten, z. T. auch karzinomatöse Entartung des Epithels.

➤ *Weltweiter »Fallout«* betrifft über kontaminierte Luft, Futter und Erdreich v. a. weidende Wiederkäuer. Die dabei nach massiver pulmonaler und/oder oraler Aufnahme radioaktiver Partikel möglicherweise eintretenden *Inkorporationsschäden* sind von Art und Menge der Kontaminationen sowie von deren bevorzugtem Speicherorgan abhängig. Messungen, die nach dem Unfall des Tschernobyl-Reaktors an Weiderindern im Vereinigten Königreich vorgenommen wurden, ergaben für ^{137}Zäsium und ^{134}Zäsium Kontaminationen in der Größenordnung von 4000 bzw. 2000 Bq/kg Muskelfleisch, für ^{131}Jod solche von 2 MBq/kg Schilddrüse; die sich hieraus ableitende Strahlenbelastung betrug für Zäsium etwa 1/1000, für Jod 1/10000 der beim Rind zur Auslösung klinischer Erscheinungen erforderlichen Dosis. In Deutschland wurden im Mai 1986 50–150 Bq ^{131}J/kg Rindfleisch und ≤ 300 Bq ^{137}Cs/l Milch gemessen. Inkorporierte radioaktive Substanzen können aber schon in Dosen, welche Nutztiere noch nicht schädigen, den Verbraucher der von ihnen stammenden Lebensmittel gefährden. Zur Ermittlung der beim Transfer von »Fallout« über Boden → Pflanze → Tier → Mensch, d. h. innerhalb der Nahrungskette, erfolgenden Anreicherung der o. a. Radionuklide sind Rechenmodelle entwickelt worden, mit denen sich diese Gefährdung abschätzen läßt.

Beurteilung, Behandlung: Im nuklearen Katastrophenfall steht auch für den Tierarzt die erste Hilfe bei betroffenen Menschen im Vordergrund der zu ergreifenden Maßnahmen; erst dann kann er sich der Betreuung von Tierbeständen widmen. Dabei gilt es, unter Hinzuziehung von Fachleuten den Grad und die Art der radioaktiven Kontamination radiometrisch zu ermitteln, um dann zu entscheiden, welche Tiere aus Gründen des Tierschutzes oder wegen Gefährdung des Menschen unschädlich zu vernichten, welche zur Sicherung der Ernährung unter entsprechenden Vorsichtsmaßnahmen zu schlachten und welche aufgestallt weiterhin zu nutzen sind. Eine Behandlung strahlenkranker Rinder dürfte wegen des damit verbundenen Aufwands und geringer Erfolgsaussichten nur in Sonderfällen in Betracht kommen. Die durch mäßige Ganzkörper-Gamma-Bestrahlung ausgelösten Folgen lassen sich in gewissem Umfang durch parenterale Verabreichung von Antibiotika und nichtsteroidalen Entzündungshemmern, Flüssigkeitszufuhr (Kap. 4.3.6.1) sowie Blutübertragung (Kap. 4.3.2.1) mildern. Unter den Nachkommen strahlengeschädigter Nutztiere ist mit vermehrtem Auftreten von Mißbildungen zu rechnen.

Vor dem Betreten kontaminierten Geländes ist mittels Radiometer zu prüfen, ob die damit für den Betreffenden verbundene Strahlenexposition vertretbar ist. Rinder können bei einer Wochenbelastung von $\leq$ 0,25 Sv noch gefahrlos auf die Weide gebracht und gewartet werden. Des weiteren muß versucht werden, den Grad der radioaktiven Kontamination von Futtermitteln und Tränke zu bestimmen, um über ihre Verwendbarkeit entscheiden zu können; u. U. muß das Beweiden kontaminierter Flächen untersagt, d. h. Stallhaltung angeordnet und unbedenkliches Futter aus weniger schwer »Fallout«-betroffenen Gebieten herangeschafft werden; des weiteren ist das Verbringen exponierten Viehs in unbelastete Gegenden in Betracht zu ziehen, wo vor etwaiger Schlachtung die Elimination inkorporierter Radionuklide abgewartet werden kann. Für Verbraucher der von radioaktiv exponierten Rindern stammenden Lebensmittel sind v. a. ihre äußere Kontamination und ihr Gehalt an inkorporierten radioaktiven Substanzen von Bedeutung; erstere kann durch Entfernen der äußeren Schicht des betreffenden Lebensmittels beseitigt werden, letzterer sinkt bei Elementen mit kurzer physikalischer Halbwertszeit während der Lagerung nennenswert ab. Durch Zufüttern selektiver Radioisotop-Inhibitoren (Natriumjodid, Kalziumkarbonat bzw. Ammonium-Eisen-Hexazyanoferrat) läßt sich der Radio-Jod-, Radio-Strontium- bzw. Radio-Zäsium-Gehalt von Milch und Fleisch »Fallout«-exponierter Rinder erheblich reduzieren (= Dekorporation). Nähere Einzelheiten zu den im Falle nuklearer Ereignisse zu ergreifenden Überwachungs- und Vorsorgemaßnahmen sind dem Strahlenschutzvorsorge-Gesetz vom 19. 12. 1986 zu entnehmen.

Prophylaxe: Verzicht auf Erprobung und Einsatz nuklearer Waffen; ordnungsgemäße Betreibung, Überwachung und Entsorgung von Atomreaktoren. Bei drohender Gefahr Aufstallung der Rinderbestände und Abdecken der im Freien lagernden Futtervorräte (Plastikplanen). Wildwiederkäuer haben sich als wertvolle Radionuklid-Indikatoren erwiesen.

12.6 Tumorkrankheiten mit Beteiligung mehrerer Organsysteme

M. Stöber

Viele Tumorosen sind zwar plurilokalisiert, doch werden sie im Rahmen dieses Buches bei denjenigen Organsystemen abgehandelt, von deren Geweben sie auszugehen pflegen. So werden die *lymphatischen Leukosen* beim Lymphapparat (Kap. 3.1.3.1, 3.1.6), die *von Knochenmarksabkömmlingen ausgehenden Leukosen* beim Kreislauf (Kap. 4.4.4) besprochen. Die *Mesotheliose* wird bei den Krankheiten der Atmungs- und der Verdauungsorgane (Kap. 5.4.5.2, 6.15.6) abgehandelt, die *bovine Nervenscheidentumorose* bei den Leiden des Nervensystems (Kap. 10.7.1).

Literatur unter http://www.medizinverlage.de/detailseiten/9783830441694.html

Sachwortverzeichnis

Seitenangaben in **Fettdruck** verweisen auf Abbildungen bzw. Tabellen.

C

G

I

J

K

N

O

Q

R